NCLEX-RN® Review

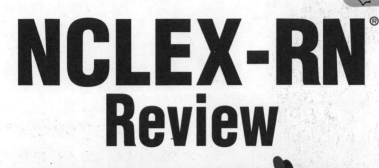

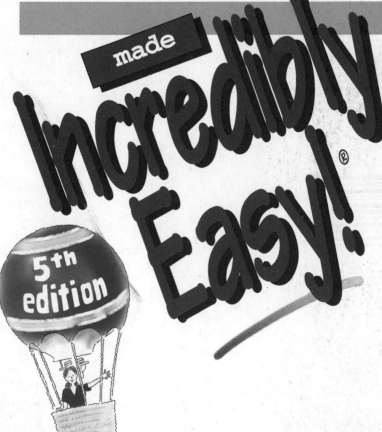

made Incredibly Easy!®

5th edition

NCLEX-RN® Review

made Incredibly Easy!®

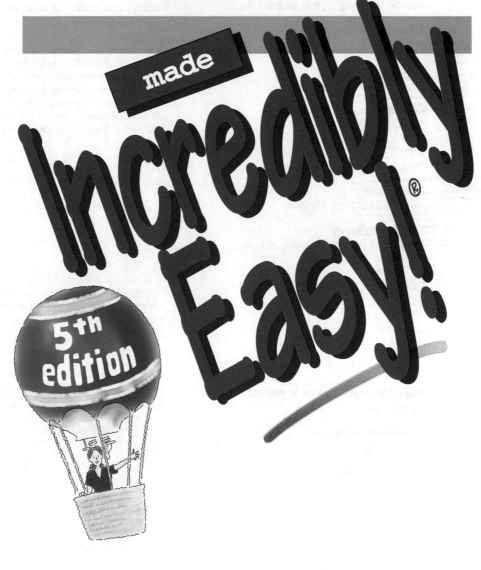

5th edition

Wolters Kluwer Health | Lippincott Williams & Wilkins

Philadelphia • Baltimore • New York • London
Buenos Aires • Hong Kong • Sydney • Tokyo

Staff

Publisher
Chris Burghardt

Clinical Director
Joan M. Robinson, RN, MSN

Clinical Project Manager
Beverly Ann Tscheschlog, RN, MS

Clinical Editor
Jennifer Meyering, RN, BSN, MS, CCRN

Acquisitions Editor
Bill Lamsback

Product Director
David Moreau

Product Manager
Rosanne Hallowell

Editors
Tracy S. Diehl, Jaime Stockslager Buss

Copy Editors
Jerry Altobelli, Tricia Mulvihill

Editorial Assistants
Karen J. Kirk, Jeri O'Shea, Linda K. Ruhf

Art Director
Elaine Kasmer

Designer
Lynn Foulk

Illustrator
Bot Roda

Project Manager, Electronic Products
John Macalino

Manufacturing Manager
Beth J. Welsh

Production Services
SPi Technologies

Printed in China.

RNREVIE5E010710

Library of Congress Cataloging-in-Publication Data

NCLEX-RN review made incredibly easy! — 5th ed.
    p. ; cm.
  Includes bibliographical references and index.
  ISBN 978-1-60831-341-9 (alk. paper)
  1. Nursing—Examinations, questions, etc. 2. National Council Licensure Examination for Registered Nurses—Study guides. I. Lippincott Williams & Wilkins.
  [DNLM: 1. Nursing Care—Examination Questions.
2. Nursing—Examination Questions. WY 18.2 N3366 2011]
  RT55.N74 2011
  610.73076—dc22   2010006909

Contents

Contributors and consultants

Betty Abraham-Settles, RN, MSN
Nursing Instructor
University of South Carolina, Aiken

Judith Alexander, RN, DNS
Associate Professor
Armstrong Atlantic State University
Savannah, Ga.

Bernadette Amicucci, RN, MS, CNE
Nursing Instructor
Cochran School of Nursing
Yonkers, N.Y.

Alicia H. Anderson, RN, MSN
Faculty II
Mercy School of Nursing
Charlotte, N.C.

Melody C. Antoon, RN, MSN
Instructor
Lamar State College
Orange, Tex.

Dometrives Armstrong, RN, MSN, FNP, PHN
Assistant Professor
San Diego City College

Peggy D. Baikie, RN, DNP, PNP-BC, NNP-BC
Program Manager/Nurse Practitioner
Denver Health – Family Crisis Center

Bridget Bailey, RN, MSN
Associate Professor
Iowa Lakes Community College
Emmetsburg

Kathleen C. Banks, MSN, CNS
Assistant Professor
Kent State University, East Liverpool
(Ohio) Campus

Carol A. Blakeman, ARNP, MSN
Professor
Central Florida Community College
Ocala

Kimberly R. Blount, MSN, CRNP, CS
Assistant Professor
Villa Maria School of Nursing
Gannon University
Erie, Pa.

Wendy Bowles, RN, MSN, CPNP
Assistant Professor
Kettering (Ohio) College of Medical Arts

Cheryl L. Brady, RN, MSN
Assistant Professor of Nursing
Kent State University
Salem, Ohio

Noreen R. Brady, PhD, APRN-BC, LPCC
Assistant Professor
Director, Hirsh Institute for Evidence-
Based Nursing Practice
Frances Payne Bolton School of Nursing
Case Western Reserve University
Cleveland

Tamara Bussan, RN, MSN, CCM
Assistant Professor of Nursing
University of Dubuque (Iowa)

Stephanie C. Butkus, RN, MSN, CPNP, CLC
Assistant Professor, Division of Nursing
Kettering (Ohio) College of Medical Arts

Anita L. Carroll, RN, EdD, MSN
Instructor – Nursing
West Texas A&M University
Department of Nursing
Canyon

Joseph T. Catalano, RN, PhD
Professor and Chairman
Department of Nursing
East Central University
Ada, Okla.

Marsha L. Conroy, RN, MSN, APN
Nurse Educator
Chamberlain College of Nursing
Columbus, Ohio
Indiana Wesleyan University
Marion

Kim Cooper, RN, MSN
Nursing Department Chair
Ivy Tech Community College
Terre Haute, Ind.

Linda Carman Copel, PhD, RN, PMHCNS, BC,
CNE, NCC, FAPA
Professor
Villanova (Pa.) University

Lillian Craig, RN, MSN, FNP-C
Family Nurse Practitioner
Amarillo (Tex.) City Cares Clinic
Adjunct Faculty
Oklahoma Panhandle State University
Goodwell

Cheryl DeGraw, RN, MSN, CRNP, CNE
Instructor
Florence-Darlington Technical College
Florence, S.C.

Diane Glasser, MSN, RNC
Faculty – Instructor/Clinical
Instructor
Lebanon (Pa.) County Career and
Technology Center
Staff RN – Neonatal Intensive
Care Unit
The Reading (Pa.) Hospital & Medical
Center

Joyce J. Hamlin, MSN, BC
Research Coordinator
Contract Dental Evaluations
Langhorne, Pa.

Michelle Helderman, RN, MSN
Nursing Instructor
Ivy Tech Community College
Terre Haute, Ind.

Mary A. Helming, PhD, APRN, FNP-BC, AHN-BC
Associate Professor of Nursing and
Family Nurse Practitioner Track
Coordinator
Quinnipiac University Department of
Nursing
Hamden, Conn.

Kathy J. Keister, PhD, RN, CNE
Assistant Professor
Director, BEACON Accelerated BSN
Program
Wright State University College
of Nursing and Health
Dayton, Ohio

Linda Ann Kucher, RN, MSN, CMSRN
Nursing Instructor
St. Joseph School of Nursing
North Providence, R.I.

Allyn L. Kulk, RN, MS
First Year Nursing Instructor
St. John's Riverside Hospital
Cochran School of Nursing
Yonkers, N.Y.

Ronnette C. Langhorne, RN, MS
Assistant Professor
Thomas Nelson Community College
Hampton, Va.

Melissa Langone, PhD, ARNP, CNS
Assistant Professor
Pasco-Hernando Community College
New Port Richey, Fla.

Bernadette Madara, APRN, EDD, BC
Professor-Nursing
Southern Connecticut State University
New Haven

Megan McClintock, RN, MS
Clinical Simulation Lab Coordinator
Redlands Community College
El Reno, Okla.

Carole McCue, RN, MS, CNE
Instructor
Cochran School of Nursing
Yonkers, N.Y.

Joyce Pompey, APRN, DNP, MSN, RN,C
Assistant Professor
University of South Carolina, Aiken School
    of Nursing

Dana Reeves, RN, MSN
Assistant Professor
University of Arkansas-Fort Smith

Roseann Regan, PhD, APRN, BC
Assistant Professor, Adult Health Nursing
    and Behavioral Health Nursing
Gwynedd Mercy College
Gwynedd Valley, Pa.
Thomas Jefferson University
Philadelphia

Kendra S. Seiler, RN, MSN
Nursing Instructor
Rio Hondo College
Whittier, Calif.

Barbara Shaw, MSN, APN
Nurse Practitioner, Clinical Instructor
University of Illinois at Chicago

Allison J. Terry, PhD, RN, MSN
Director, Center for Nursing
Alabama Board of Nursing
Montgomery

Peggy Thweatt, RN, MSN
Nursing Faculty
Medical Careers Institute
Newport News, Va.

Kathleen Tusaie, PhD, APRN, BC
Associate Professor
The University of Akron (Ohio)

Elizabeth A. Waldron, MS, RN, BC
Nurse Administrator
New York University Langone Medical
    Center

Julie A. Will, RN, MSN
Dean, School of Health Sciences
Ivy Tech Community College of Indiana,
    Wabash Valley Region
Terre Haute

Cheryl Zauderer, PhD, CNM, NPP
Instructor
New York Institute of Technology
Westbury

Polly Gerber Zimmermann, RN, MS, MBA,
CEN, FAEN
Associate Professor
Harry S. Truman College
Chicago

Advisory board

Foreword

Congratulations, new graduate! You're almost there! There's only one hurdle left—passing the National Council Licensure Examination for Registered Nurses (NCLEX-RN®). It may seem like a daunting task ahead but if you study hard and prepare yourself for the examination, you can tackle this challenge with success and begin your exciting career as a nurse!

NCLEX-RN Review Made Incredibly Easy, Fifth Edition, is designed to help you review and prepare. This book is the capstone of the *Incredibly Easy* book series. The same user-friendly format and humorous approach you have come to know and love in the *Incredibly Easy* book series is followed in this book as well. It's informative, easy to understand, and provides a light-hearted approach, which helps keep you interested and motivated—all the ingredients for a great study aid for NCLEX-RN preparation!

The text is divided into six parts and 37 chapters. Part I provides an overview of the specifics of the NCLEX-RN examination (including alternate-format questions!) and outlines a plan for NCLEX-RN preparation. Parts II, III, IV, and V address content in the nursing specialty areas: Care of the adult, psychiatric care, maternal-neonatal care, and care of the child. Part VI features two chapters that focus on professional issues. The content is presented in an easy-to-read, concise fashion, and features the *Incredibly Easy* characters who offer encouragement and humor along the way! Other features, such as *Memory joggers*, provide hints and tips to remember key facts.

In addition, you'll find these valuable features in each chapter:
* **Brush up on key concepts** provides an overview of anatomy and physiology appropriate for the client's developmental level.
* **Cheat sheet** serves as a quick overview of the chapter, summarizing each disorder, including key signs and symptoms, test results, treatments, and interventions. It can be used to review and reinforce what you've studied.
* **Keep abreast of diagnostic tests** describes the most common tests used to diagnose disorders and their associated nursing actions to help you ensure client safety—a key component of the NCLEX-RN.
* **Polish up on client care** details nursing care for each disorder, using a nursing process approach. The content outlines provide a quick synopsis of pathophysiology, etiology, diagnostics, medical treatment, priority nursing diagnoses, and nursing management, including client teaching.
* **Pump up on practice questions** allows the reader to practice traditional and alternate-format NCLEX-style test questions related to the content. The answers include the rationale for the correct and incorrect responses, helping to reinforce learning. Each test question is classified according to the *NCLEX Client needs* categories and the cognitive level of the question according to Bloom's taxonomy.

The accompanying Web site is a fantastic resource for NCLEX-RN examination practice. It contains more than 3,250 practice test questions, which you can take in "review" or "test" mode. In addition, you can select the number of questions to include in a practice test—75, 150, 256, all questions, or a random quantity designated by the tester. You can also access an online calculator to assist in answering questions requiring mathematical calculations.

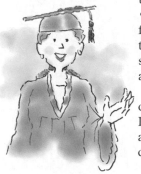

Congratulations! You're well on your way to becoming a licensed registered nurse!

As a faculty member in an accelerated nursing program, I am always searching for resources to facilitate student learning and development of test-taking skills. *NCLEX-RN Review Made Incredibly Easy*, Fifth Edition, addresses both areas. Not only will new nursing graduates preparing for NCLEX-RN examination benefit from this invaluable resource, but students currently enrolled in a nursing program may find it helpful as well. Using this book in conjunction with their regular nursing textbooks can help them prepare for course examinations throughout the nursing curriculum.

All your hard work is about to pay off. This book can help you succeed on the NCLEX-RN examination and realize your goal of becoming a registered nurse. Good luck and best wishes for a long and happy nursing career!

Kathy J. Keister, PhD, RN, CNE
Assistant Professor
Director, BEACON Accelerated BSN Program
Wright State University College of Nursing and Health
Dayton, Ohio

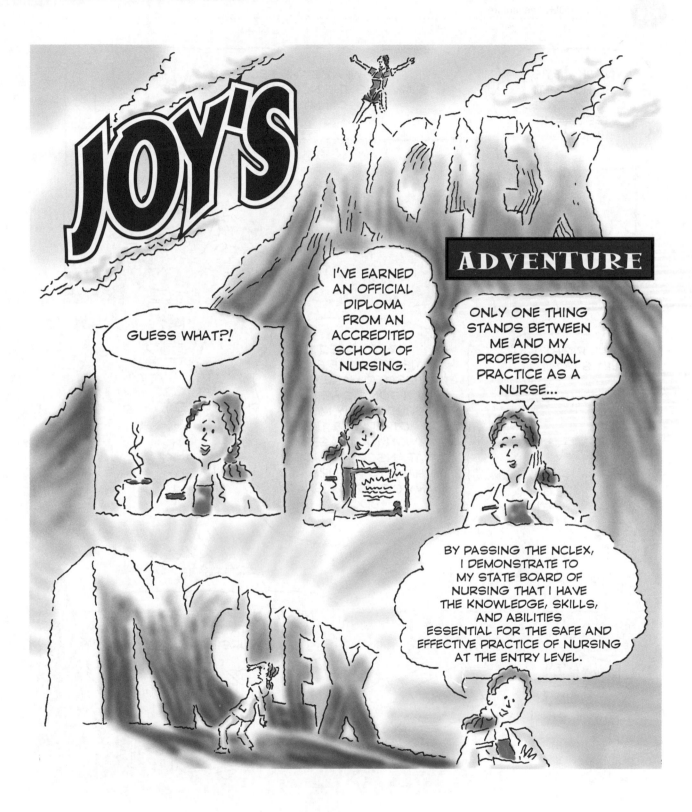

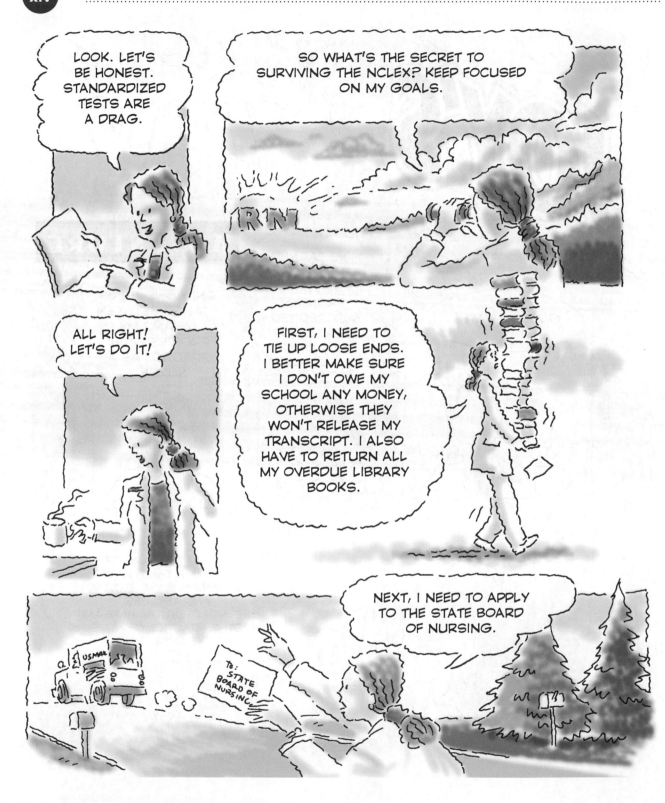

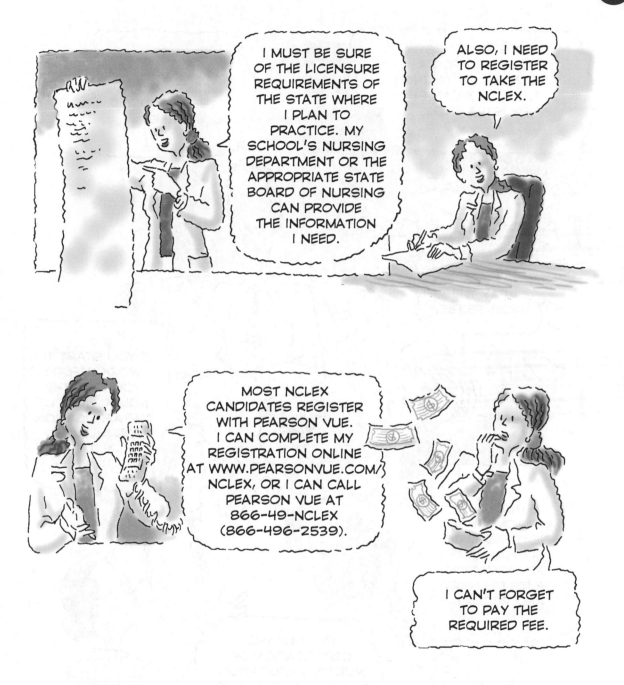

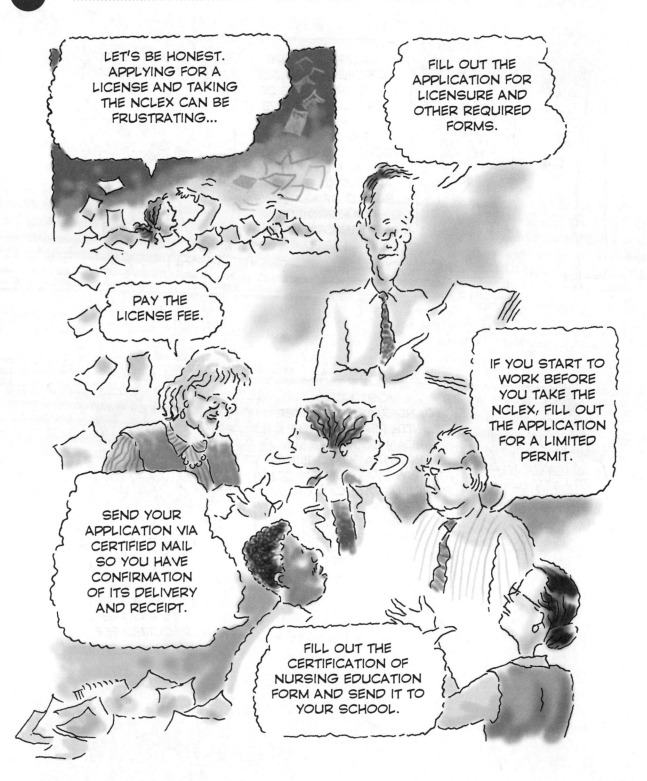

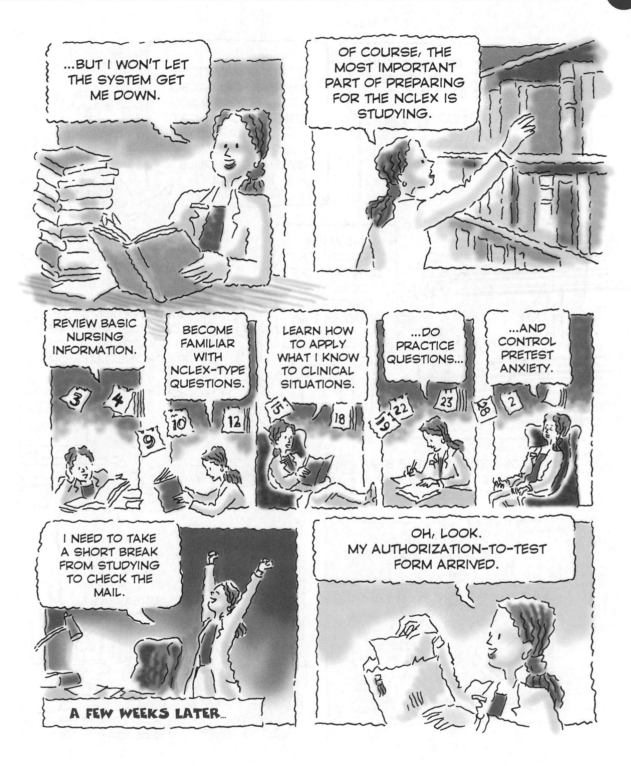

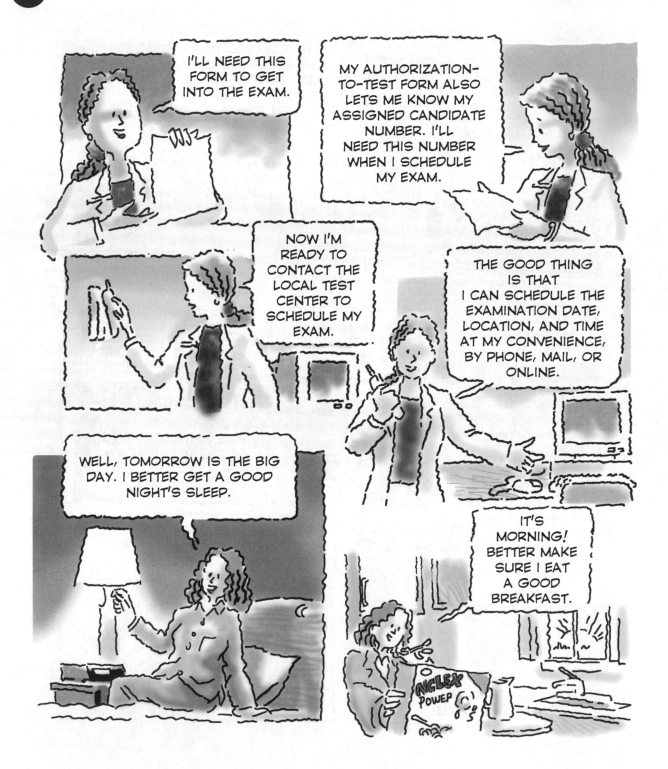

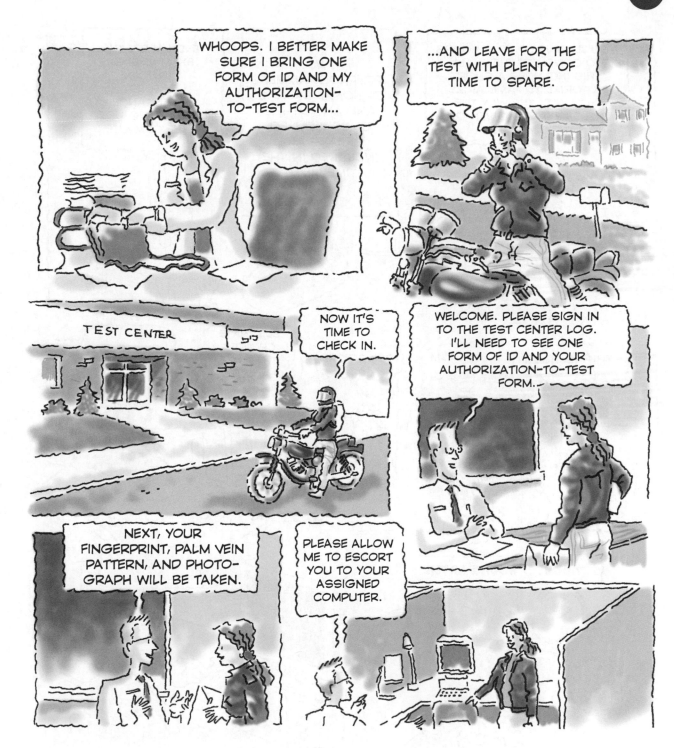

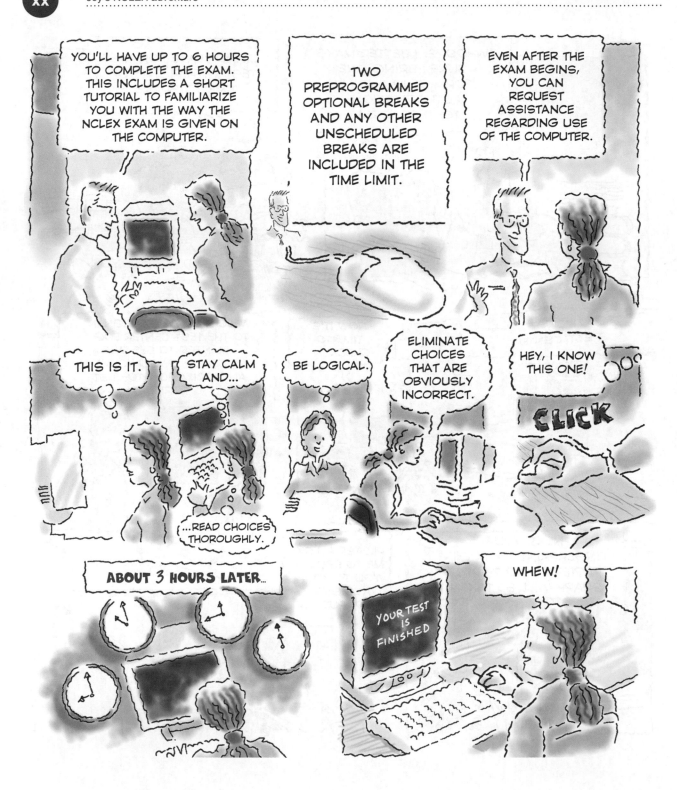

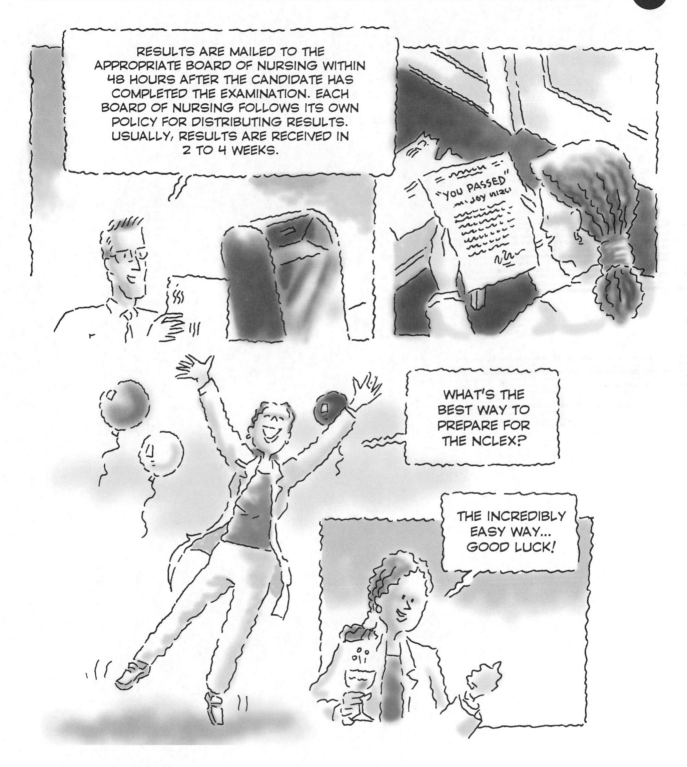

Part I   Getting ready

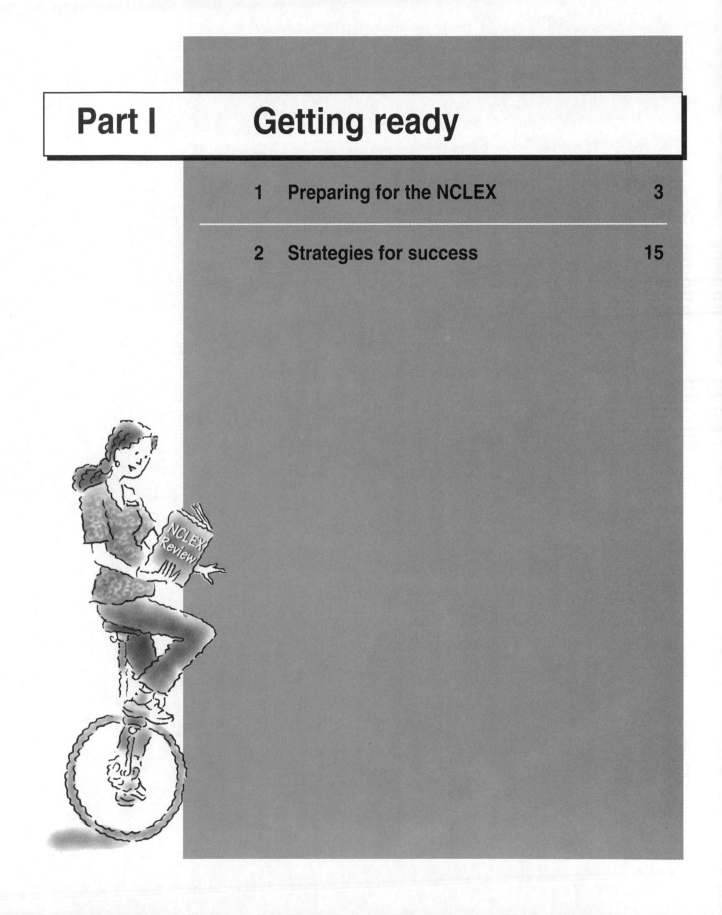

1 Preparing for the NCLEX®

NCLEX basics

Passing the National Council Licensure Examination (NCLEX®) is an important landmark in your career as a nurse. The first step on your way to passing the NCLEX is to understand what it is and how it's administered.

NCLEX structure

The *NCLEX* is a test written by nurses who, like most of your nursing instructors, have an advanced degree and clinical expertise in a particular area. Only one small difference distinguishes nurses who write NCLEX questions: They're trained to write questions in a style particular to the NCLEX.

If you've completed an accredited nursing program, you've already taken numerous tests written by nurses with backgrounds and experiences similar to those of the nurses who write for the NCLEX. The test-taking experience you've already gained will help you pass the NCLEX. So your NCLEX review should be just that — a review. (For eligibility and immigration requirements for nurses from outside of the United States, see *Guidelines for international nurses,* page 4.)

What's the point of it all?
The NCLEX is designed for one purpose: namely, to determine whether it's appropriate for you to receive a license to practice as a nurse. By passing the NCLEX, you demonstrate that you possess the minimum level of knowledge necessary to practice nursing safely.

Mix 'em up
In nursing school, you probably took courses that were separated into such subjects as pharmacology, nursing leadership, health assessment, adult health, pediatric, maternal-neonatal, and psychiatric nursing. In contrast, the NCLEX is integrated, meaning that different subjects are mixed together.

As you answer NCLEX questions, you may encounter clients in any stage of life, from neonatal to geriatric. These clients — clients, in NCLEX lingo — may be of any background, may be completely well or extremely ill, and may have any disorder.

Client needs, front and center
The NCLEX draws questions from four categories of client needs that were developed by the *National Council of State Boards of Nursing* (NCSBN), the organization that sponsors and manages the NCLEX. *Client needs categories* ensure that a wide variety of topics appear on every NCLEX examination.

The NCSBN developed client needs categories after conducting a practice analysis of new nurses. All aspects of nursing care observed in the study were broken down into four main categories, some of which were broken down further into subcategories. (See *Client needs categories*, page 5.)

The whole kit and caboodle
The categories and subcategories are used to develop the *NCLEX test plan,* the content guidelines for the distribution of test questions. Question-writers and the people who put the NCLEX together use the test plan and client needs categories to make sure that a full spectrum of nursing activities is covered in the examination. Client needs categories appear in most NCLEX review and question-and-answer books, including this one. As a test-taker, you don't have to concern yourself with client needs categories. You'll see those categories for each question and answer in this book, but they'll be invisible on the actual NCLEX.

Guidelines for international nurses

To become eligible to work as a registered nurse in the United States, you'll need to complete several steps. In addition to passing the NCLEX® examination, you may need to obtain a certificate and credentials evaluation from the Commission on Graduates of Foreign Nursing Schools (CGFNS®) and acquire a visa. Requirements vary from state to state, so it's important that you first contact the Board of Nursing in the state where you want to practice nursing.

CGFNS CERTIFICATION PROGRAM

Most states require that you obtain CGFNS certification. This certification requires:
• review and authentication of your credentials, including your nursing education, registration, and licensure
• passing score on the CGFNS Qualifying Examination of nursing knowledge
• passing score on an English language proficiency test.

To be eligible to take the CGFNS Qualifying Examination, you must complete a minimum number of classroom and clinical practice hours in medical-surgical nursing, maternal-infant nursing, pediatric nursing, and psychiatric and mental health nursing from a government-approved nursing school. You must also be registered as a first-level nurse in your country of education and currently hold a license as a registered nurse in some jurisdiction.

The CGFNS Qualifying Examination is a paper and pencil test that includes 260 multiple-choice questions and is administered under controlled testing conditions. Because the test is designed to predict your likelihood of successfully passing the NCLEX-RN examination, it's based on the NCLEX-RN test plan.

You may select from three English proficiency examinations—Test of English as a Foreign Language (TOEFL®), Test of English for International Communication (TOEIC®), or International English Language Testing System (IELTS). Each test has different passing scores, and the scores are valid for up to 2 years.

CGFNS CREDENTIALS EVALUATION SERVICE

This evaluation is a comprehensive report that analyzes and compares your education and licensure with U.S. standards. It's prepared by CGFNS for a state board of nursing, an immigration office, employer, or university. To use this service you must complete an application, submit appropriate documentation, and pay a fee.

More information about the CGFNS certification program and credentials evaluation service is available at *www.cgfns.org*.

VISA REQUIRED

You can't legally immigrate to work in the United States without an occupational visa (temporary or permanent) from the United States Citizenship and Immigration Services (USCIS). The visa process is separate from the CGFNS certification process, although some of the same steps are involved. Some visas require prior CGFNS certification and a *VisaScreen*™ Certificate from the International Commission on Healthc are Professions (ICHP). The VisaScreen program involves:
• credentials review of your nursing education and current registration or licensure
• successful completion of either the CGFNS certification program or the NCLEX-RN to provide proof of nursing knowledge
• passing score on an approved English language proficiency examination.

After you successfully complete all parts of the *VisaScreen* program, you'll receive a certificate to present to the USCIS. The visa granting process can take up to one year.

You can obtain more detailed information about visa applications at *www.uscis.gov*.

Testing by computer

Like many standardized tests today, the NCLEX is administered by computer. That means you won't be filling in empty circles, sharpening pencils, or erasing frantically. It also means that you must become familiar with computer tests, if you aren't already. Fortunately, the skills required to take the NCLEX on a computer are simple enough to

Client needs categories

Each question on the NCLEX is assigned a category based on client needs. This chart lists client needs categories and subcategories and the percentages of each type of question that appears on an NCLEX examination.

Category	Subcategories	Percentage of NCLEX questions
Safe and effective care environment	• Management of care • Safety and infection control	16% to 22% 8% to 14%
Health promotion and maintenance		6% to 12%
Psychosocial integrity		6% to 12%
Physiological integrity	• Basic care and comfort • Pharmacological and parenteral therapies • Reduction of risk potential • Physiological adaptation	6% to 12% 13% to 19% 10% to 16% 11% to 17%

allow you to focus on the questions, not the keyboard.

Q&A

When you take the test, depending on the question format, you'll be presented with a question and four or more possible answers, a blank space in which to enter your answer, a figure on which you'll identify the correct area by clicking the mouse on it, a series of charts or exhibits you'll use to select the correct response, items you must rearrange in priority order by dragging and dropping them in place, an audio recording to listen to in order to select the correct response, or a question and four graphic options.

Feeling smart? Think hard!

The NCLEX is a *computer-adaptive test*, meaning that the computer reacts to the answers you give, supplying more difficult questions if you answer correctly, and slightly easier questions if you answer incorrectly. Each test is thus uniquely adapted to the individual test-taker.

A matter of time

You have a great deal of flexibility with the amount of time you can spend on individual

questions. The examination lasts a maximum of 6 hours, however, so don't waste time. If you fail to answer a set number of questions within 6 hours, the computer will determine that you lack minimum competency.

Most students have plenty of time to complete the test, so take as long as you need to get the question right without wasting time. But remember to keep moving at a decent pace to help you maintain concentration.

Difficult items = Good news

If you find as you progress through the test that the questions seem to be increasingly difficult, it's a good sign. The more questions you answer correctly, the more difficult the questions become.

Some students, though, knowing that questions get progressively harder, focus on the degree of difficulty of subsequent questions to try to figure out if they're answering questions correctly. Avoid the temptation to do this, as this may get you off track.

Free at last!

The computer test finishes when one of the following events occurs:
• You demonstrate minimum competency, according to the computer program, which

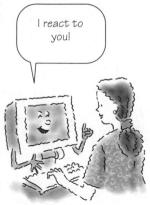

I react to you!

does so with 95% certainty that your ability exceeds the passing standard.
- You demonstrate a lack of minimum competency, according to the computer program.
- You've answered the maximum number of questions (265 total questions).
- You've used the maximum time allowed (6 hours).

Unlocking the NCLEX mystery

In April 2004, the NCSBN added alternate-format items to the examination. However, most of the questions on the NCLEX are four-option, multiple-choice items with only one correct answer. Certain strategies can help you understand and answer any type of NCLEX question.

Alternate formats

The first type of alternate-format item is the *multiple-response question*. Unlike a traditional multiple-choice question, each multiple-response question has one or more correct answers for every question, and it may contain more than four possible answer options. You'll recognize this type of question because it will ask you to select *all* answers that apply — not just the best answer (as may be requested in the more traditional multiple-choice questions).

All or nothing
Keep in mind that, for each multiple-response question, you must select at least one answer and you must select all correct answers for the item to be counted as correct. On the NCLEX, there is no partial credit in the scoring of these items.

Don't go blank!
The second type of alternate-format item is the *fill-in-the-blank* question. These questions require you to provide the answer yourself, rather than select it from a list of options. You will perform a calculation and then type your answer (a number, without any words, units of measurements, commas, or spaces) in the blank space provided after the question. Rules for rounding are included in the question stem if appropriate. A calculator button is provided so you can do your calculations electronically.

Mouse marks the spot!
The third type of alternate-format item is a question that asks you to identify an area on an illustration or graphic. For these *"hot spot" questions*, the computerized exam will ask you to place your cursor and click over the correct area on an illustration. Try to be as precise as possible when marking the location. As with the fill-in-the-blanks, the identification questions on the computerized exam may require extremely precise answers in order for them to be considered correct.

Click, choose, and prioritize
The fourth alternate-format item type is the *chart/exhibit* format. For this question type, you'll be given a problem and then a series of small screens with additional information you'll need to answer the question. By clicking on the tabs on screen, you can access each chart or exhibit item. After viewing the chart or exhibit, you select your answer from four multiple-choice options.

Drag n' drop
The fifth alternate-format item type involves prioritizing actions or placing a series of statements in correct order using a *drag-and-drop* (ordered response) technique. To move an answer option from the list of unordered options into the correct sequence, click on it using the mouse. While still holding down the mouse button, drag the option to the ordered response part of the screen. Release the mouse button to "drop" the option into place. Repeat this process until you've moved all of the available options into the correct order.

Now hear this!
The sixth alternate-format item type is the *audio item* format. You'll be given a set of headphones and you'll be asked to listen to an

The harder it gets, the better I'm doing.

audio clip and select the correct answer from four options. You'll need to select the correct answer on the computer screen as you would with the traditional multiple-choice questions.

Picture perfect
The final alternate-format item type is the *graphic option* question. This varies from the exhibit format type because in the graphic option, your answer choices will be graphics such as ECG strips. You'll have to select the appropriate graphic to answer the question presented.

The standard's still the standard
The NCSBN hasn't yet established a percentage of alternate-format items to be administered to each candidate. In fact, your exam may contain only one alternate-format item. So relax; the standard, four-option, multiple-choice format questions constitute the bulk of the test. (See *Sample NCLEX questions*, pages 8 to 10.)

Understanding the question

NCLEX questions are commonly long. As a result, it's easy to become overloaded with information. To focus on the question and avoid becoming overwhelmed, apply proven strategies for answering NCLEX questions, including:
• determining what the question is asking
• determining relevant facts about the client
• rephrasing the question in your mind
• choosing the best option or options before entering your answer.

DETERMINE WHAT THE QUESTION IS ASKING
Read the question twice. If the answer isn't apparent, rephrase the question in simpler, more personal terms. Breaking down the question into easier, less intimidating terms may help you to focus more accurately on the correct answer.

Give it a try
For example, a question might be, "A 74-year-old client with a history of heart failure is admitted to the coronary care unit with pulmonary edema. He's intubated and placed on a mechanical ventilator. Which parameters should the nurse monitor closely to assess the client's response to a bolus dose of furosemide (Lasix) I.V.?"

The options for this question — numbered from 1 to 4 — might include:
1. Daily weight
2. 24-hour intake and output
3. Serum sodium levels
4. Hourly urine output

Hocus, focus on the question
Read the question again, ignoring all details except what's being asked. Focus on the last line of the question. It asks you to select the appropriate assessment for monitoring a client who received a bolus of furosemide I.V.

DETERMINE WHAT FACTS ABOUT THE CLIENT ARE RELEVANT
Next, sort out the relevant client information. Start by asking whether any of the information provided about the client isn't relevant. For instance, do you need to know that the client has been admitted to the coronary care unit? Probably not; his reaction to I.V. furosemide won't be affected by his location in the hospital.

Determine what you do know about the client. In the example, you know that:
• he just received an I.V. bolus of furosemide, a crucial fact
• he has pulmonary edema, the most fundamental aspect of the client's underlying condition
• he's intubated and placed on a mechanical ventilator, suggesting that his pulmonary edema is serious
• he's 74 years old and has a history of heart failure, a fact that may or may not be relevant.

REPHRASE THE QUESTION
After you've determined relevant information about the client and the question being asked, consider rephrasing the question to make it more clear. Eliminate jargon and put the question in simpler, more personal terms. Here's how you might rephrase the question in the example: "My client has pulmonary edema. He requires intubation and

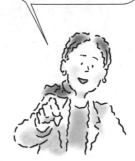

Focusing on what the question is really asking can help you choose the correct answer.

(Text continues on page 10.)

Sample NCLEX questions

Sometimes, getting used to the format is as important as knowing the material. Try your hand at these sample questions and you'll have a leg up when you take the real test!

Sample four-option, multiple-choice question

A client's arterial blood gas (ABG) results are as follows: pH, 7.16; $Paco_2$, 80 mm Hg; Pao_2, 46 mm Hg; HCO_3^-, 24 mEq/L; Sao_2, 81%. These ABG results represent which condition?

1. Metabolic acidosis
2. Metabolic alkalosis
3. Respiratory acidosis
4. Respiratory alkalosis

Correct answer: 3

Sample multiple-response question

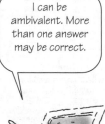
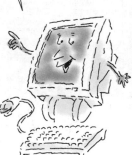

I can be ambivalent. More than one answer may be correct.

A nurse is caring for a 45-year-old married woman who has undergone hemicolectomy for colon cancer. The woman has two children. Which concepts about families should the nurse keep in mind when providing care for this client?

Select all that apply:
1. Illness in one family member can affect all members.
2. Family roles don't change because of illness.
3. A family member may have more than one role at a time in the family.
4. Children typically aren't affected by adult illness.
5. The effects of an illness on a family depend on the stage of the family's life cycle.
6. Changes in sleeping and eating patterns may be signs of stress in a family.

Correct answer: 1, 3, 5, 6

Sample fill-in-the-blank calculation question

An infant who weighs 8 kg is to receive ampicillin 25 mg/kg I.V. every 6 hours. How many milligrams should the nurse administer per dose? Record your answer using a whole number.

_____ milligrams

Correct answer: 200

Sample hot spot question

A client has a history of aortic stenosis. Identify the area where the nurse should place the stethoscope to best hear the murmur.

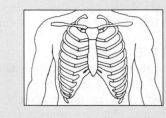

Correct answer:

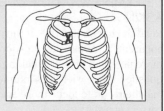

Sample NCLEX questions *(continued)*

Sample exhibit question

A 3-year old child is being treated for severe status asthmaticus. After reviewing the progress notes (shown below), the nurse should determine that this client is being treated for which condition?

Progress notes	
9/1/10 0600	Pt. was acutely restless, diaphoretic, and with dyspnea at 0530. Dr. T. Smith notified of findings at 0545 and ordered ABG analysis. ABG drawn from R radial artery. Stat results as follows: pH 7.28, $Paco_2$ 55 mm Hg, HCO_3- 26 mEg/L. Dr. Smith with pt. now. ———————— J. Collins, RN.

1. Metabolic acidosis
2. Respiratory alkalosis
3. Respiratory acidosis
4. Metabolic alkalosis

Correct answer: 3

Sample drag-and-drop (ordered response) question

When teaching an antepartal client about the passage of the fetus through the birth canal during labor, the nurse describes the cardinal mechanisms of labor. Place these events in the sequence in which they occur. Use all options:

1. Flexion	
2. External rotation	
3. Descent	
4. Expulsion	
5. Internal rotation	
6. Extension	

Correct answer:

3. Descent
1. Flexion
5. Internal rotation
6. Extension
2. External rotation
4. Expulsion

(continued)

Sample NCLEX questions *(continued)*

Sample audio item question

Listen to the audio clip. What sound do you hear in the bases of this client with heart failure?

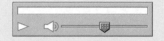

1. Crackles
2. Rhonchi
3. Wheezes
4. Pleural friction rub

Correct answer: 1

Sample graphic option question

Which electrocardiogram strip should the nurse document as sinus tachycardia?

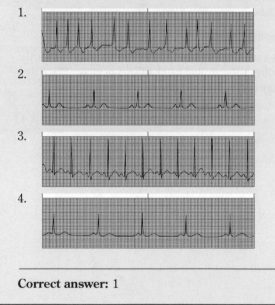

Correct answer: 1

mechanical ventilation. He's 74 years old and has a history of heart failure. He received an I.V. bolus of furosemide. What assessment parameter should I monitor?"

CHOOSE THE BEST OPTION

Armed with all the information you now have, it's time to select an option. You know that the client received an I.V. bolus of furosemide, a diuretic. You know that monitoring fluid intake and output is a key nursing intervention for a client taking a diuretic, a fact that eliminates options 1 and 3 (daily weight and serum sodium levels), narrowing the answer down to option 2 or 4 (24-hour intake and output or hourly urine output).

Can I use a lifeline?

You also know that the drug was administered by I.V. bolus, suggesting a rapid effect. (In fact, furosemide administered by I.V. bolus takes effect almost immediately.)

Monitoring the client's 24-hour intake and output would be appropriate for assessing the effects of repeated doses of furosemide. Hourly urine output, however, is most appropriate in this situation because it monitors the immediate effect of this rapid-acting drug.

Key strategies

Regardless of the type of question, four key strategies will help you determine the correct answer for each question. These strategies are:
- considering the nursing process
- referring to Maslow's hierarchy of needs
- reviewing client safety
- reflecting on principles of therapeutic communication.

Nursing process

One of the ways to answer a question is to apply the nursing process. Steps in the nursing process include:
- assessment
- diagnosis
- planning
- implementation
- evaluation.

First things first
The nursing process may provide insights that help you analyze a question. According to the nursing process, assessment comes before analysis, which comes before planning, which comes before implementation, which comes before evaluation.

You're halfway to the correct answer when you encounter a four-option, multiple-choice question that asks you to assess the situation and then provides two assessment options and two implementation options. You can immediately eliminate the implementation options, which then gives you, at worst, a 50-50 chance of selecting the correct answer. Use the following sample question to apply the nursing process:

A client returns from an endoscopic procedure during which he was sedated.

Before offering the client food, which action should the nurse take?
1. Assess the client's respiratory status.
2. Check the client's gag reflex.
3. Place the client in a side-lying position.
4. Have the client drink a few sips of water.

Assess before intervening
According to the nursing process, the nurse must assess a client before performing an intervention. Does the question indicate that the client has been properly assessed? No, it doesn't. Therefore, you can eliminate options 3 and 4 because they're both interventions.

That leaves options 1 and 2, both of which are assessments. Your nursing knowledge should tell you the correct answer — in this case, option 2. The sedation required for an endoscopic procedure may impair the client's gag reflex, so you would assess the gag reflex before giving food to the client to reduce the risk of aspiration and airway obstruction.

Final elimination
Why not select option 1, assessing the client's respiratory status? You might select this option but the question is specifically asking about offering the client food, an action that wouldn't be taken if the client's respiratory status was at all compromised. In this case, you're making a judgment based on the phrase, "Before offering the client food." If the question was trying to test your knowledge of respiratory depression following an endoscopic procedure, it probably wouldn't mention a function — such as giving food to a client — that clearly occurs only after the client's respiratory status has been stabilized.

Maslow's hierarchy

Knowledge of Maslow's hierarchy of needs can be a vital tool for establishing priorities on the NCLEX. Maslow's theory states that physiologic needs are the most basic human needs of all. Only after physiologic needs have been met can safety concerns be addressed. Only after

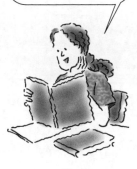

Say it 1,000 times: Studying for the exam is fun... studying for the exam is fun...

safety concerns are met can concerns involving love and belonging be addressed, and so forth. Apply the principles of Maslow's hierarchy of needs to the following sample question:

A client complains of severe pain 2 days after surgery. Which action should the nurse perform first?
1. Offer reassurance to the client that he will feel less pain tomorrow.
2. Allow the client time to verbalize his feelings.
3. Check the client's vital signs.
4. Administer an analgesic.

Phys before psych
In this example, two of the options — 3 and 4 — address physiologic needs. Options 1 and 2 address psychosocial concerns. According to Maslow, physiologic needs must be met before psychosocial needs, so you can eliminate options 1 and 2.

Final elimination
Now, use your nursing knowledge to choose the best answer from the two remaining options. In this case, option 3 is correct because the client's vital signs should be checked before administering an analgesic (assessment before intervention). When prioritizing according to Maslow's hierarchy, remember your ABCs — airway, breathing, circulation — to help you further prioritize. Check for a patent airway before addressing breathing. Check breathing before checking the health of the cardiovascular system.

One caveat...
Just because an option appears on the NCLEX doesn't mean it's a viable choice for the client referred to in the question. Always examine your choice in light of your knowledge and experience. Ask yourself, "Does this choice make sense for this client?" Allow yourself to eliminate choices — even ones that might normally take priority — if they don't make sense for a particular client's situation.

Client safety

As you might expect, client safety takes high priority on the NCLEX. You'll encounter

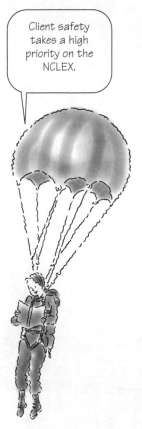

Client safety takes a high priority on the NCLEX.

many questions that can be answered by asking yourself, "Which answer will best ensure the safety of this client?" Use client safety criteria for situations involving laboratory values, drug administration, activities of daily living, or nursing care procedures.

Client first, equipment second
You may encounter a question in which some options address the client and others address the equipment. When in doubt, select an option relating to the client; never place equipment before a client.

For example, suppose a question asks what the nurse should do first when entering a client's room where an infusion pump alarm is sounding. If two options deal with the infusion pump, one with the infusion tubing, and another with the client's catheter insertion site, select the one relating to the client's catheter insertion site. Always check the client first; the equipment can wait.

Therapeutic communication

Some NCLEX questions focus on the nurse's ability to communicate effectively with the client. Therapeutic communication incorporates verbal or nonverbal responses and involves:
• listening to the client
• understanding the client's needs
• promoting clarification and insight about the client's condition.

Room for improvement
Like other NCLEX questions, those dealing with therapeutic communication commonly require choosing the best response. First, eliminate options that indicate the use of poor therapeutic communication techniques, such as those in which the nurse:
• tells the client what to do without regard to the client's feelings or desires (the "do this" response)
• asks a question that can be answered "yes" or "no," or with another one-syllable response
• seeks reasons for the client's behavior
• implies disapproval of the client's behavior
• offers false reassurances

- attempts to interpret the client's behavior rather than allow the client to verbalize his own feelings
- offers a response that focuses on the nurse, not the client.

Ah, that's better!
When answering NCLEX questions, look for responses that:
- allow the client time to think and reflect
- encourage the client to talk
- encourage the client to describe a particular experience
- reflect that the nurse has listened to the client, such as through paraphrasing the client's response.

Avoiding pitfalls

Even the most knowledgeable students can get tripped up on certain NCLEX questions. (See *A tricky question*, page 14.) Students commonly cite three areas that can be difficult for unwary test-takers:

☞ knowing the difference between the NCLEX and the "real world"

☞ delegating care

☞ knowing laboratory values.

NCLEX versus the real world

Some students who take the NCLEX have extensive practical experience in health care. For example, many test-takers have worked as licensed practical nurses or nursing assistants. In one of those capacities, test-takers might have been exposed to less than optimum clinical practice and may carry those experiences over to the NCLEX.

However, the NCLEX is a textbook examination — not a test of clinical skills. Take the NCLEX with the understanding that what happens in the real world may differ from what the NCLEX and your nursing school say should happen.

Don't take shortcuts
If you've had practical experience in health care, you may know a quicker way to perform a procedure or tricks to get by when you don't have the right equipment. Situations such as staff shortages may force you to improvise. On the NCLEX, such scenarios can lead to trouble. Always check your practical experiences against textbook nursing care, taking care to select the response that follows the textbook.

Delegating care

On the NCLEX, you may encounter questions that assess your ability to delegate care. Delegating care involves coordinating the efforts of other health care workers to provide effective care for your client. On the NCLEX, you may be asked to assign duties to:
- licensed practical nurses or licensed vocational nurses
- direct-care workers, such as certified nursing assistants and personal care aides
- other support staff, such as nutrition assistants and housekeepers.

In addition, you'll be asked to decide when to notify a physician, a social worker, or another hospital staff member. In each case, you'll have to decide when, where, and how to delegate.

Shoulds and shouldn'ts
As a general rule, it's okay to delegate actions that involve stable clients or standard, unchanging procedures. Bathing, feeding, dressing, and transferring clients are examples of procedures that can be delegated.

Be careful not to delegate complicated or complex activities. In addition, don't delegate activities that involve assessment, evaluation, or your own nursing judgment. On the NCLEX and in the real world, these duties fall squarely on your shoulders. Make sure that you take primary responsibility for assessing and evaluating the client and for making decisions about the client's care. Never hand off those responsibilities to someone with less training.

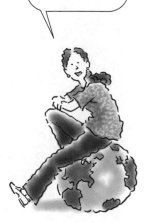

Remember, this is an exam, not the real world.

Normal laboratory values

- Blood urea nitrogen: 8 to 25 mg/dl
- Creatinine: 0.6 to 1.5 mg/dl
- Sodium: 135 to 145 mmol/L
- Potassium: 3.5 to 5.5 mEq/L
- Chloride: 97 to 110 mmol/L
- Glucose (fasting plasma): 70 to 110 mg/dl
- Hemoglobin

    Male: 13.8 to 17.2 g/dl

    Female: 12.1 to 15.1 g/dl
- Hematocrit

    Male: 40.7% to 50.3%

    Female: 36.1% to 44.3%

Advice from the experts

A tricky question

The NCLEX occasionally asks a particular kind of question called the "further teaching" question, which involves client-teaching situations. These questions can be tricky. You'll have to choose the response that suggests the client has *not* learned the correct information. Here's an example:

37. A client undergoes a total hip replacement. Which statement by the client indicates he requires further teaching?
1. "I'll need to keep several pillows between my legs at night."
2. "I'll need to remember not to cross my legs. It's such a bad habit."
3. "The occupational therapist is showing me how to use a 'sock puller' to help me get dressed."
4. "I don't know if I'll be able to get off that low toilet seat at home by myself."

The option you should choose here is 4 because it indicates that the client has a poor understanding of the precautions required after a total hip replacement and that he needs further teaching. Remember: If you see the phrase further teaching or further instruction, you're looking for a wrong answer by the client.

Calling in reinforcements

Deciding when to notify a physician, a social worker, or another hospital staff member is an important element of nursing care. On the NCLEX, however, choices that involve notifying the physician are usually incorrect. Remember that the NCLEX wants to see you, the nurse, at work.

If you're sure the correct answer is to notify the physician, though, make sure the client's safety has been addressed before notifying a physician or another staff member. On the NCLEX, the client's safety has a higher priority than notifying other health care providers.

Knowing laboratory values

Some NCLEX questions supply laboratory results without indicating normal levels. As a result, answering questions involving laboratory values requires you to have the normal range of the most common laboratory values memorized to make an informed decision (See *Normal laboratory values.*)

2 Strategies for success

Study preparations

If you're like most people preparing to take the NCLEX®, you're probably feeling nervous, anxious, or concerned. Keep in mind that most test takers pass the first time around.

Passing the test won't happen by accident, though; you'll need to prepare carefully and efficiently. To help jump-start your preparations:

- determine your strengths and weaknesses
- create a study schedule
- set realistic goals
- find an effective study space
- think positively
- start studying sooner rather than later.

Strengths and weaknesses

Most students recognize that, even at the end of their nursing studies, they know more about some topics than others. Because the NCLEX covers a broad range of material, you should make some decisions about how intensively you'll review each topic.

Make a list
Base those decisions on a list. Divide a sheet of paper in half vertically. On one side, list topics you think you know well. On the other side, list topics you feel less secure about. Pay no attention if one side is longer than the other. When you're done studying, you'll feel strong in every area.

Where the list comes from
To make sure your list reflects a comprehensive view of all the areas you studied in school, look at the contents page in the front of this book. For each topic listed, place it in the "know well" column or "needs review"

column. Separating content areas this way shows immediately which topics need less study time and which need more time.

Scheduling study time

Study when you're most alert. Most people can identify a period of the day when they feel most alert. If you feel most alert and energized in the morning, for example, set aside sections of time in the morning for topics that need a lot of review. Then you can use the evening to study topics for which you just need some refreshing. The opposite is true as well; if you're more alert in the evening, study difficult topics at that time.

What you'll do, when
Set up a basic schedule for studying. Using a calendar or organizer, determine how much time remains before you'll take the NCLEX. (See *2 to 3 months before the NCLEX,* page 16.) Fill in the remaining days with specific times and topics to be studied. For example, you might schedule the respiratory system on a Tuesday morning and the GI system that afternoon. Remember to schedule difficult topics during your most alert times.

Keep in mind that you shouldn't fill each day with studying. Be realistic and set aside time for normal activities. Try to create ample study time before the NCLEX and then stick to the schedule. Allow some extra time in the schedule in case you get behind or come across a topic that requires extra review.

Set goals you can meet
Part of creating a schedule means setting goals you can accomplish. You no doubt studied a great deal in nursing school, and by now you have a sense of your own capabilities. Ask yourself, "How much can I cover in a day?" Set that amount of time aside and

To-do list

2 to 3 months before the NCLEX

With 2 to 3 months remaining before you plan to take the examination, take these steps:
• Establish a study schedule. Set aside ample time to study but also leave time for social activities, exercise, family or personal responsibilities, and other matters.
• Become knowledgeable about the NCLEX-RN, its content, the types of questions it asks, and the testing format.
• Begin studying your notes, texts, and other study materials.
• Answer some NCLEX practice questions to help you diagnose strengths and weaknesses as well as to become familiar with NCLEX-style questions.

then stay on task. You'll feel better about yourself — and your chances of passing the NCLEX — when you meet your goals regularly.

Study space

Find a space conducive to effective learning and then study there. Whatever you do, don't study with a television on in the room. Instead, find a quiet, inviting study space that:
• is located in a quiet, convenient place, away from normal traffic patterns
• contains a solid chair that encourages good posture (Avoid studying in bed; you'll be more likely to fall asleep and not accomplish your goals.)
• uses comfortable, soft lighting with which you can see clearly without eye strain
• has a temperature between 65° and 70° F
• contains flowers or green plants, familiar photos or paintings, and easy access to soft, instrumental background music.

Accentuate the positive
Consider taping positive messages around your study space. Make signs with words of encouragement, such as, "You can do it!" "Keep studying!" and "Remember the goal!" These upbeat messages can help keep you going when your attention begins to waver.

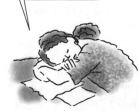

Approach your studying with enthusiasm, sincerity, and determination.

Maintaining concentration

When you're faced with reviewing the amount of information covered by the NCLEX, it's easy to become distracted and lose your concentration. When you lose concentration, you make less effective use of valuable study time. To stay focused, keep these tips in mind:
• Alternate the order of the subjects you study during the day to add variety to your study. Try alternating between topics you find most interesting and those you find least interesting.
• Approach your studying with enthusiasm, sincerity, and determination.
• Once you've decided to study, begin immediately. Don't let anything interfere with your thought processes once you've begun.
• Concentrate on accomplishing one task at a time, to the exclusion of everything else.
• Don't try to do two things at once, such as studying and watching television or conversing with friends.
• Work continuously without interruption for a while, but don't study for such a long period that the whole experience becomes grueling or boring.
• Allow time for periodic breaks to give yourself a change of pace. Use these breaks to ease your transition into studying a new topic.

- When studying in the evening, wind down from your studies slowly. Don't progress directly from studying to sleeping.

Taking care of yourself

Never neglect your physical and mental well-being in favor of longer study hours. Maintaining physical and mental health are critical for success in taking the NCLEX. (See *4 to 6 weeks before the NCLEX*.)

A few simple rules

You can increase your likelihood of passing the test by following these simple health rules:
- Get plenty of rest. You can't think deeply or concentrate for long periods when you're tired.
- Eat nutritious meals. Maintaining your energy level is impossible when you're undernourished.
- Exercise regularly. Regular exercise, preferably 30 minutes daily, helps you work harder and think more clearly. As a result, you'll study more efficiently and increase the likelihood of success on the all-important NCLEX.

Memory powers, activate!

If you're having trouble concentrating but would rather push through than take a break, try making your studying more active by reading out loud. Active studying can renew your powers of concentration. By reading review material out loud to yourself, you're engaging your ears as well as your eyes — and making your studying a more active process. Hearing the material out loud also fosters memory and subsequent recall.

You can also rewrite in your own words a few of the more difficult concepts you're reviewing. Explaining these concepts in writing forces you to think through the material and can jump-start your memory.

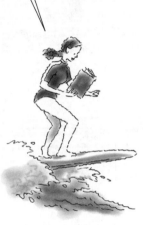

Kowabonga! Regular exercise helps you work harder and think more clearly.

Study schedule

When you were creating your schedule, you might have asked yourself, "How long should I study? One hour at a stretch? Two hours? Three?" To make the best use of your study time, you'll need to answer those questions.

Optimum study time

Consider studying in 20- to 30-minute intervals with a short break in-between. You remember the material you study at the beginning and end of a session best and tend to remember less material studied in the middle of the session. The total length of time in each study session depends on you and the amount of material you need to cover.

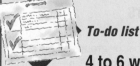

To-do list

4 to 6 weeks before the NCLEX

With 4 to 6 weeks remaining before you plan to take the examination, take these steps:
- Focus on your areas of weakness. That way, you'll have time to review these areas again before the test date.
- Find a study partner or form a study group.
- Take a practice test to gauge your skill level early.
- Take time to eat, sleep, exercise, and socialize to avoid burnout.

To-do list

1 week before the NCLEX

With 1 week remaining before the NCLEX examination, take these steps:
• Take a review test to measure your progress.
• Record key ideas and principles on note cards or audiotapes.
• Rest, eat well, and avoid thinking about the examination during nonstudy times.
• Treat yourself to one special event. You've been working hard, and you deserve it!

To thine own self be true

So what's the answer? It doesn't matter as long as you determine what's best for you. At the beginning of your NCLEX study schedule, try study periods of varying lengths. Pay close attention to those that seem more successful.

Remember that you're a trained nurse who is competent at assessment. Think of yourself as a client, and assess your own progress. Then implement the strategy that works best for you.

Finding time to study

So does that mean that short sections of time are useless? Not at all. We all have spaces in our day that might otherwise be dead time. (See *1 week before the NCLEX.*) These are perfect times to review for the NCLEX but not to cover new material because, by the time you get deep into new material, your time will be over. Always keep some flash cards or a small notebook handy for situations when you have a few extra minutes.

You'll be amazed how many short sessions you can find in a day and how much reviewing you can do in 5 minutes. The following occasions offer short stretches of time you can use for studying:
• eating breakfast
• waiting for, or riding on, a train or bus

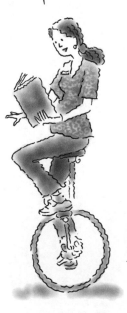

Studying getting dull? Get creative and liven it up.

• waiting in line at the bank, post office, bookstore, or other places
• using exercise equipment, such as a treadmill.

Creative studying

Even when you study in a perfect study space and concentrate better than ever, studying for the NCLEX can get a little, well, dull. Even people with terrific study habits occasionally feel bored or sluggish. That's why it's important to have some creative tricks in your study bag to liven up your studying during those down times.

Creative studying doesn't have to be hard work. It involves making efforts to alter your study habits a bit. Some techniques that might help include studying with a partner or group and creating flash cards or other audiovisual study tools.

Study partners

Studying with a partner or group of students (3 or 4 students at most) can be an excellent way to energize your studying. Working with a partner allows you to test each other on the material you've reviewed. Your partner can give you encouragement and motivation. Perhaps most important, working with a partner can provide a welcome break from solitary studying.

What to look for in a partner

Exercise some care when choosing a study partner or assembling a study group. A partner who doesn't fit your needs won't help you make the most of your study time. Look for a partner who:

• possesses similar goals to yours. For example, someone taking the NCLEX at approximately the same date who feels the same sense of urgency as you do might make an excellent partner.

• possesses about the same level of knowledge as you. Tutoring someone can sometimes help you learn, but partnering should be give-and-take so both partners can gain knowledge.

• can study without excess chatting or interruptions. Socializing is an important part of creative study but, remember, you still have to pass the NCLEX — so stay serious!

Audiovisual tools

Using flash cards and other audiovisual tools fosters retention and makes learning and reviewing fun.

Flash Gordon? No, it's Flash Card!

Flash cards can provide you with an excellent study tool. The process of writing material on a flash card will help you remember it. In addition, flash cards are small and easily portable, perfect for those 5-minute slivers of time that show up during the day.

Creating a flash card should be fun. Use magic markers, highlighters, and other colorful tools to make them visually stimulating. The more effort you put into creating your flash cards, the better you'll remember the material contained on the cards.

Other visual tools

Flowcharts, drawings, diagrams, and other image-oriented study aids can also help you learn material more effectively. Substituting images for text can be a great way to give your eyes a break and recharge your brain. Remember to use vivid colors to make your creations visually engaging.

Hear's the thing

If you learn more effectively when you hear information rather than see it, consider recording key ideas using a handheld tape recorder. Recording information helps promote memory because you say the information aloud when taping and then listen to it when playing it back. Like flash cards, tapes are portable and perfect for those short study periods during the day. (See *The day before the NCLEX*.)

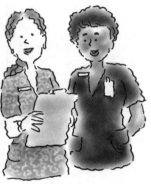

It wasn't easy finding a partner who has the same study habits I do.

To-do list

The day before the NCLEX

With 1 day before the NCLEX examination, take these steps:
• Drive to the test site, review traffic patterns, and find out where to park. If your route to the test site occurs during heavy traffic or if you're expecting bad weather, set aside extra time to ensure prompt arrival.
• Do something relaxing during the day.
• Avoid concentrating on the test.
• Eat well and avoid dwelling on the NCLEX during nonstudy periods.
• Call a supportive friend or relative for some last-minute words of encouragement.
• Get plenty of rest the night before and allow plenty of time in the morning.

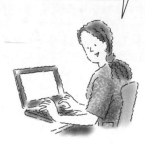

Practice questions provide an excellent means of marking your progress.

Practice questions

Practice questions should be an important part of your NCLEX study strategy. Practice questions can improve your studying by helping you review material and familiarizing yourself with the exact style of questions you'll encounter on the NCLEX.

Practice at the beginning
Consider working through some practice questions as soon as you begin studying for the NCLEX. For example, you might try a few of the questions that appear at the end of each chapter in this book.

If you do well, you probably know the material contained in that chapter fairly well and can spend less time reviewing that particular topic. If you have trouble with the questions, spend extra study time on that topic.

I'm getting there
Practice questions can also provide an excellent means of marking your progress. Don't worry if you have trouble answering the first few practice questions you take; you'll need time to adjust to the way the questions are asked. Eventually you'll become accustomed

to the question format and begin to focus more on the questions themselves.

If you make practice questions a regular part of your study regimen, you'll be able to notice areas in which you're improving. You can then adjust your study time accordingly.

Practice makes perfect
As you near the examination date, you should increase the number of NCLEX practice questions you answer at one sitting. This will enable you to approximate the experience of taking the actual NCLEX examination. Using the Web site associated with this book, you can create practice tests of any number of questions. Note that 75 questions is the minimum number of questions you'll be asked on the actual NCLEX examination. By gradually tackling larger practice tests, you'll increase your confidence, build test-taking endurance, and strengthen the concentration skills that enable you to succeed on the NCLEX. (See *The day of the NCLEX*.)

Part II   Care of the adult

3 Cardiovascular system

Brush up on key concepts

The heart, arteries, and veins make up the cardiovascular system. These structures:
- transport life-supporting oxygen and nutrients to cells
- help remove metabolic waste products
- carry hormones from one part of the body to another.

At the center of the system, the heart propels blood through the body by continuous rhythmic contractions.

At any time, you can review the major points of this chapter by consulting the *Cheat sheet* on pages 24 to 32.

2 atria & 2 ventricles
The heart is a muscular organ composed of two **atria** and two **ventricles.**

A sac
The heart is surrounded by a **pericardial sac** that consists of two layers: the **visceral** (inner) layer and the **parietal** (outer) layer.

3 layers
The heart wall has three layers:
- **epicardium** (visceral pericardium), the outer layer
- **myocardium,** the thick, muscular middle layer
- **endocardium,** the inner layer.

4 valves
There are four heart valves. The **tricuspid valve** (in the right side of the heart) and **mitral valve** (in the left side of the heart) lie between the atria and ventricles; because of their location, they're also called *atrioventricular (AV) valves.* These valves prevent backflow of blood into the atria when the ventricles contract. The **pulmonic semilunar valve** lies between the right ventricle and the pulmonary artery. The **aortic semilunar valve** lies between the left ventricle and the aorta. These valves prevent backflow of blood into the ventricles during diastole.

Pumping it in
The heart itself is nourished by blood from two main arteries, the **left coronary artery** and the **right coronary artery**. As it branches off the aorta, the left coronary artery branches into the left anterior descending (LAD) artery and the circumflex artery. The LAD artery then supplies blood to the anterior wall of the left ventricle, the anterior ventricular septum, and the apex of the left ventricle, while the circumflex artery supplies blood to the left atrium, the lateral and posterior portions of the left ventricle.

The right coronary artery (RCA) fills the groove between the atria and ventricles and gives rise to the acute marginal artery, which becomes the posterior descending artery. The RCA supplies blood to the sinoatrial (SA) and AV nodes, the septum, the right atrium, and the right ventricle. The posterior descending artery supplies the posterior and inferior wall of the left ventricle and the posterior portion of the right ventricle.

Pumping it through (and out)
Blood circulates through the heart following this pathway:
- from the inferior and superior venae cavae to the right atrium
- through the tricuspid valve to the right ventricle
- through the pulmonic valve to the pulmonary artery, to the lungs where blood is oxygenated, through the pulmonary veins to the left atrium
- through the mitral valve to the left ventricle

(Text continues on page 32.)

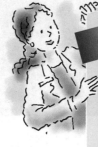

Cardiovascular refresher

ABDOMINAL AORTIC ANEURYSM

Key signs and symptoms
• Commonly asymptomatic

Key test results
• Chest X-ray shows aneurysm.

Key treatments
• Abdominal aortic aneurysm resection

Key interventions
• Assess cardiovascular status, and monitor and record vital signs.
• Monitor intake and output and laboratory studies.
• Observe the client for signs of hypovolemic shock from aneurysm rupture, such as anxiety, restlessness, severe back pain, decreased pulse pressure, increased thready pulse, and pale, cool, moist, clammy skin.

ANGINA

Key signs and symptoms
• Pain that may be substernal, crushing, or compressing; may radiate to the arms, jaw, or back; and usually lasts 3 to 5 minutes; usually occurs after exertion, emotional excitement, or exposure to cold but can also develop when the client is at rest; in women, may manifest as atypical symptoms of pain, such as indigestion, back pain, and less severe complaints of substernal pain

Key test results
• Electrocardiogram (ECG) shows ST-segment depression and T-wave inversion during anginal pain.

Key treatments
• Percutaneous transluminal coronary angioplasty or coronary artery stent placement

Key interventions
• Assess for chest pain and evaluate its characteristics.
• Administer medications, as prescribed. Hold nitrates and notify physician for systolic blood pressure less than 90 mm Hg. Hold beta-adrenergic blocker and notify physician for heart rate less than 60 beats/minute.
• Obtain 12-lead ECG during an acute attack.

ARRHYTHMIAS

Key signs and symptoms
Atrial fibrillation
• Commonly asymptomatic
• Irregular pulse with no pattern to the irregularity
Asystole
• Unresponsive
• Apnea
• Cyanosis
• No palpable blood pressure
• Pulselessness
Ventricular fibrillation
• Unresponsive
• Apnea
• No palpable blood pressure
• Pulselessness
Ventricular tachycardia
• Diaphoresis
• Hypotension
• Weak or absent pulse
• Dizziness

Key test results
Atrial fibrillation
• ECG shows irregular atrial rhythm, atrial rate possibly greater than 400 beats/minute, irregular ventricular rhythm, QRS complexes of uniform configuration and duration, indiscernible PR interval, and no P waves (fibrillation waves).
Asystole
• ECG shows no atrial or ventricular rate or rhythm and no discernible P waves, QRS complexes, or T waves.
Ventricular fibrillation
• ECG shows rapid and chaotic ventricular rhythm, wide and irregular or absent QRS complexes, and no visible P waves.
Ventricular tachycardia
• ECG shows ventricular rate of 140 to 220 beats/minute, wide and bizarre QRS complexes, and no discernible P waves. Ventricular tachycardia may start or stop suddenly.

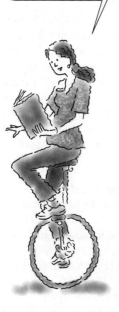

Want a quick overview of this chapter? Check out the Cheat sheet.

Cardiovascular refresher (continued)

ARRHYTHMIAS (CONTINUED)
Key treatments
Atrial fibrillation
• Antiarrhythmics (if client is stable): amiodarone (Cordarone), digoxin (Lanoxin), diltiazem (Cardizem), procainamide, verapamil (Calan)
• Synchronized cardioversion (if client is unstable)
Asystole
• Cardiopulmonary resuscitation (CPR)
• Advanced cardiac life support (ACLS) protocol for endotracheal intubation and possible transcutaneous pacing
• Antiarrhythmics: atropine, epinephrine per ACLS protocol
Ventricular fibrillation
• CPR
• Defibrillation
• ACLS protocol for endotracheal intubation
• Antiarrhythmics: amiodarone (Cordarone), epinephrine, lidocaine (Xylocaine), magnesium sulfate, procainamide, vasopressin per ACLS protocol
Ventricular tachycardia
• CPR, if pulseless
• Defibrillation
• Antiarrhythmics: amiodarone (Cordarone), epinephrine, lidocaine (Xylocaine), magnesium sulfate, procainamide
• ACLS protocol for endotracheal intubation, if pulseless

Key interventions
• If the client's pulse is abnormally rapid, slow, or irregular, watch for signs of hypoperfusion, such as hypotension and altered mental status.
• When life-threatening arrhythmias develop, rapidly assess the level of consciousness, respirations, and pulse.
• Initiate CPR, if indicated.
• If trained, perform defibrillation early for ventricular tachycardia and ventricular fibrillation.
• Administer medications as needed, and prepare for medical procedures (for example, cardioversion) if indicated.
• Provide adequate oxygen and reduce the heart's workload, while carefully maintaining metabolic, neurologic, respiratory, and hemodynamic status. Follow ACLS protocol for endotracheal intubation.

CARDIAC TAMPONADE
Key signs and symptoms
• Muffled heart sounds on auscultation
• Narrow pulse pressure
• Jugular vein distention
• Pulsus paradoxus (an abnormal inspiratory drop in systemic blood pressure greater than 15 mm Hg)
• Restlessness
• Upright, leaning forward posture

Key test results
• Chest X-ray shows slightly widened mediastinum and cardiomegaly.
• Echocardiography records pericardial effusion with signs of right ventricular and atrial compression.
• ECG may reveal changes produced by acute pericarditis. This test rarely reveals tamponade but is useful to rule out other cardiac disorders.

Key treatments
• Surgery: pericardiocentesis (needle aspiration of the pericardial cavity) or surgical creation of an opening to drain fluid, thoracotomy
• Adrenergic agent: epinephrine
• Inotropic agent: dopamine

Key interventions
If the client needs pericardiocentesis
• Keep a pericardial aspiration needle attached to a 50-ml syringe by a three-way stopcock, an ECG machine, and an emergency cart with a defibrillator at the bedside. Make sure the equipment is turned on and ready for immediate use.
• Position the client at a 45- to 60-degree angle. Connect the precordial ECG lead to the hub of the aspiration needle with an alligator clamp and connecting wire. When the needle touches the myocardium during fluid aspiration, an ST-segment elevation or premature ventricular contractions appear.
• Monitor blood pressure and central venous pressure (CVP) during and after pericardiocentesis to monitor for complications such as hypotension, which may indicate cardiac chamber puncture.
• Watch for complications of pericardiocentesis, such as ventricular fibrillation, vasovagal response, or coronary artery or cardiac chamber puncture.
If the client needs a thoracotomy
• Explain the procedure to the client. Tell him what to expect postoperatively (chest tubes and chest tube drainage system, administration of oxygen). Teach him how to turn, deep-breathe, and cough.
• Maintain the chest tube drainage system and be alert for complications, such as hemorrhage and arrhythmias.

(continued)

Cardiovascular refresher (continued)

CARDIOGENIC SHOCK
Key signs and symptoms
- Cold, clammy skin
- Hypotension (systolic pressure below 90 mm Hg)
- Narrow pulse pressure
- Oliguria (urine output of less than 30 ml/hour)
- Tachycardia or other arrhythmias

Key test results
- ECG shows myocardial infarction (MI) (enlarged Q wave, elevated ST segment).

Key treatments
- Intra-aortic balloon pump
- Adrenergic agent: epinephrine
- Cardiac glycoside: digoxin (Lanoxin)
- Cardiac inotropes: dopamine, dobutamine, inamrinone (Amrinone), milrinone
- Diuretics: furosemide (Lasix), bumetanide (Bumex), metolazone (Zaroxolyn)
- Vasodilators: nitroprusside (Nitropress), nitroglycerin
- Vasopressor: norepinephrine (Levophed)

Key interventions
- Assess cardiovascular status, including hemodynamic variables, vital signs, heart sounds, capillary refill, skin temperature, and peripheral pulses.
- Assess respiratory status, including breath sounds and arterial blood gas levels.
- Administer I.V. fluids, oxygen, and medications, as prescribed.

CARDIOMYOPATHY
Key signs and symptoms
- Murmur, third (S_3) and fourth (S_4) heart sounds

Key test results
- ECG shows left ventricular hypertrophy and nonspecific changes.

Key treatments
- Dual-chamber pacing (for hypertrophic cardiomyopathy)
- Beta-adrenergic blockers: propranolol (Inderal), nadolol (Corgard), metoprolol (Lopressor) for hypertrophic cardiomyopathy
- Calcium channel blockers: verapamil (Calan), diltiazem (Cardizem) for hypertrophic cardiomyopathy
- Diuretics: furosemide (Lasix), bumetanide (Bumex), metolazone (Zaroxolyn) for dilated cardiomyopathy
- Inotropic agents: dobutamine, milrinone, digoxin (Lanoxin) for dilated cardiomyopathy
- Oral anticoagulant: warfarin (Coumadin) for dilated and hypertrophic cardiomyopathy

Key interventions
- Monitor ECG.
- Assess cardiovascular status, vital signs, and hemodynamic variables.
- Administer oxygen and medications, as prescribed.

CORONARY ARTERY DISEASE
Key signs and symptoms
- Angina (chest pain) that may be substernal, crushing, or compressing; may radiate to the arms, jaw, or back; usually lasts 3 to 5 minutes; and usually occurs after exertion, emotional excitement, or exposure to cold but can also develop when the client is at rest

Key test results
- Blood chemistry tests show increased cholesterol (decreased high-density lipoproteins, increased low-density lipoproteins).
- ECG or Holter monitoring shows ST-segment depression and T-wave inversion during an anginal episode.

Key treatments
- Activity changes, including weight loss, if necessary
- Dietary changes, including establishing a low-sodium, low-cholesterol, low-fat diet with increased dietary fiber (low-calorie only if appropriate)
- Antilipemic agents: cholestyramine (Questran), lovastatin (Mevacor), simvastatin (Zocor), nicotinic acid (Niacor), gemfibrozil (Lopid), colestipol (Colestid)
- Low-dose aspirin therapy

Key interventions
- Obtain ECG during anginal episodes.
- Assess cardiovascular status, including vital signs and hemodynamic variables.
- Administer nitroglycerin for anginal episodes.
- Administer oxygen therapy during anginal episodes.
- Monitor intake and output.
- Monitor laboratory studies.

ENDOCARDITIS
Key signs and symptoms
- Chills
- Fatigue
- Loud, regurgitant murmur

Key test results
- Echocardiography may identify valvular damage.
- ECG may show atrial fibrillation and other arrhythmias that accompany valvular disease.
- Three or more blood cultures in a 24- to 48-hour period identify the causative organism in up to 90% of clients.

Cardiovascular refresher (continued)

ENDOCARDITIS (CONTINUED)
Key treatments
- Maintaining sufficient fluid intake
- Antibiotics: based on infecting organism
- Aspirin

Key interventions
- Watch for signs of embolization (hematuria, pleuritic chest pain, left upper quadrant pain, and paresis), a common occurrence during the first 3 months of treatment.
- Monitor the client's renal status (blood urea nitrogen [BUN] levels, serum creatinine, creatinine clearance, and urine output).
- Observe for signs of heart failure, such as dyspnea, tachypnea, tachycardia, crackles, jugular vein distention, edema, and weight gain.
- Make sure a susceptible client understands the need for prophylactic antibiotics before, during, and after dental work, childbirth, and genitourinary, GI, or gynecologic procedures.

HEART FAILURE
Key signs and symptoms
Left-sided failure
- Crackles
- Dyspnea
- Gallop rhythm: S_3, S_4
Right-sided failure
- Dependent edema
- Jugular vein distention
- Weight gain

Key test results
Left-sided failure
- B-type natriuretic peptide (BNP) levels are elevated.
- Chest X-ray shows increased pulmonary congestion and left ventricular hypertrophy.
- Arterial blood gas (ABG) levels indicate hypoxemia and hypercapnia.
Right-sided failure
- BNP levels are elevated.
- Chest X-ray reveals pulmonary congestion, cardiomegaly, and pleural effusions.
- ABG levels indicate hypoxemia and hypercapnia.

Key treatments
- Human BNP: nesiritide (Natrecor)
- Angiotensin-converting enzyme (ACE) inhibitors: captopril (Capoten), enalapril (Vasotec), lisinopril (Prinivil)
- Diuretics: furosemide (Lasix), bumetanide (Bumex), metolazone (Zaroxolyn)
- Cardiac glycoside: digoxin (Lanoxin)
- Inotropic agents: dopamine, dobutamine, inamrinone (Amrinone), milrinone
- Nitrates: isosorbide (Isordil), nitroglycerin
- Vasodilator: nitroprusside (Nitropress)

Key interventions
- Assess cardiovascular status, including vital signs and hemodynamic variables.
- Assess respiratory status and oxygenation.
- Keep the client in semi-Fowler's position.
- Administer oxygen.
- Weigh the client daily.

HYPERTENSION
Key signs and symptoms
- Asymptomatic
- Headache
- Vision disturbances, including blindness

Key test results
- Blood pressure measurements result in sustained readings higher than 140/90 mm Hg.

Key treatments
- Activity changes: regular exercise to reduce weight
- Dietary changes: establishing a low-sodium diet and limiting alcohol intake
- ACE inhibitors: captopril (Capoten), enalapril (Vasotec), lisinopril (Prinivil)
- Antihypertensives: methyldopa, hydralazine, prazosin (Minipress), doxazosin (Cardura)
- Diuretics: furosemide (Lasix), spironolactone (Aldactone), hydrochlorothiazide (Microzide), bumetanide (Bumex)

Key interventions
- Take an average of two or more blood pressure readings rather than relying on a single, possibly abnormal reading.

HYPOVOLEMIC SHOCK
Key signs and symptoms
- Cold, pale, clammy skin
- Decreased sensorium
- Hypotension with narrowing pulse pressure
- Reduced urine output (less than 25 ml/hour)
- Tachycardia

(continued)

...ular refresher (continued)

HYPOV...MIC SHOCK (CONTINUED)

Key test results
• Blood tests show elevated potassium, serum lactate, and BUN levels; increased urine specific gravity (greater than 1.020) and urine osmolality; decreased blood pH; decreased partial pressure of arterial oxygen; increased partial pressure of arterial carbon dioxide; and possible decreased hemoglobin and hematocrit (if the client is bleeding).
• ABG analysis reveals metabolic acidosis.

Key treatments
• Blood and fluid replacement
• Control of bleeding

Key interventions
• Record blood pressure, pulse rate, peripheral pulses, respiratory rate, and pulse oximetry every 15 minutes and monitor the ECG continuously. A systolic blood pressure lower than 80 mm Hg usually results in inadequate coronary artery blood flow, cardiac ischemia, arrhythmias, and further complications of low cardiac output. When blood pressure drops below 80 mm Hg, increase the oxygen flow rate and notify the physician immediately.
• Insert large-bore (14G) I.V. catheters and infuse normal saline, lactated Ringer's solution, and appropriate blood products as indicated.
• Insert an indwelling urinary catheter to measure hourly urine output. If output is less than 30 ml/hour in adults, increase the fluid infusion rate but watch for signs of fluid overload such as an increase in pulmonary artery wedge pressure (PAWP). Notify the physician if urine output doesn't improve. An osmotic diuretic such as mannitol (Osmitrol) may be ordered.
• Monitor hemodynamic parameters (CVP, pulmonary artery pressure [PAP], and PAWP).
• During therapy, assess skin color and temperature and note any changes. Cold, clammy skin may be a sign of continuing peripheral vascular constriction, indicating progressive shock.

MYOCARDIAL INFARCTION

Key signs and symptoms
• Crushing substernal chest pain that may radiate to the jaw, back, and arms; lasts longer than anginal pain; is unrelieved by rest or nitroglycerin; may not be present (in asymptomatic or silent MI); in women, possible atypical symptoms of pain or fatigue

Key test results
• ECG shows an enlarged Q wave, an elevated or a depressed ST segment, and T-wave inversion.

Key treatments
• Anticoagulants: aspirin, dalteparin (Fragmin), enoxaparin (Lovenox), heparin I.V. after thrombolytic therapy
• Thrombolytic therapy: alteplase (Activase), streptokinase (Streptase), reteplase (Retavase); should be given within 6 hours of onset of symptoms but most effective when started within 3 hours
• Oxygen therapy
• Nitrate: nitroglycerin I.V.
• Analgesic: morphine I.V.

Key interventions
• Assess cardiovascular and respiratory status.
• Obtain an ECG reading during acute pain.
• Administer medications.

MYOCARDITIS

Key signs and symptoms
• Arrhythmias (S_3 and S_4 gallops, faint S_1)
• Dyspnea
• Fatigue
• Fever

Key test results
• ECG typically shows diffuse ST-segment and T-wave abnormalities (as in pericarditis), conduction defects (prolonged PR interval), and other supraventricular arrhythmias.
• Endomyocardial biopsy confirms the diagnosis, but a negative biopsy doesn't exclude the diagnosis. A repeat biopsy may be needed.

Key treatments
• Bed rest
• Antiarrhythmics: amiodarone (Cordarone), procainamide
• Antibiotics: according to sensitivity of infecting organism
• Cardiac glycoside: digoxin (Lanoxin) to increase myocardial contractility
• Diuretic: furosemide (Lasix)

Key interventions
• Assess cardiovascular status frequently to monitor for signs of heart failure, such as dyspnea, hypotension, and tachycardia. Check for changes in cardiac rhythm or conduction.
• Stress the importance of bed rest. Assist with bathing as necessary; provide a bedside commode. Reassure the client that activity limitations are temporary.

Cardiovascular refresher *(continued)*

PERICARDITIS
Key signs and symptoms
Acute pericarditis
• Pericardial friction rub (grating sound heard as the heart moves)
• Sharp and usually sudden pain that usually starts over the sternum and radiates to the neck, shoulders, back, and arms (unlike the pain of MI, pericardial pain is commonly pleuritic, increasing with deep inspiration and decreasing when the client sits up and leans forward, pulling the heart away from the diaphragmatic pleurae of the lungs)
Chronic pericarditis
• Pericardial friction rub
• Symptoms similar to those of chronic right-sided heart failure (fluid retention, ascites, hepatomegaly)

Key test results
• Echocardiography confirms the diagnosis when it shows an echo-free space between the ventricular wall and the pericardium (in cases of pleural effusion).
• ECG shows the following changes in acute pericarditis: elevation of ST segments in the standard limb leads and most precordial leads without significant changes in QRS morphology that occur with MI, atrial ectopic rhythms such as atrial fibrillation, and diminished QRS voltage in pericardial effusion.

Key treatments
• Bed rest
• Surgery: pericardiocentesis (in cases of cardiac tamponade), partial pericardectomy (for recurrent pericarditis), total pericardectomy (for constrictive pericarditis)
• Antibiotics: according to sensitivity of infecting organism

Key interventions
• Provide complete bed rest.
• Assess pain in relation to respiration and body position.
• Place the client in an upright position.
• Provide analgesics and oxygen, and reassure the client with acute pericarditis that his condition is temporary and treatable.

PERIPHERAL ARTERY DISEASE
Key signs and symptoms
Femoral, popliteal, or innominate arteries
• Mottling of the extremity
• Pallor
• Paralysis and paresthesia in the affected arm or leg
• Pulselessness distal to the occlusion
• Sudden and localized pain in the affected arm or leg (most common symptom)
• Temperature change that occurs distal to the occlusion

Internal and external carotid arteries
• Transient ischemic attacks (TIAs), which produce transient monocular blindness, dysarthria, hemiparesis, possible aphasia, confusion, decreased mentation, headache
Subclavian artery
• Subclavian steel syndrome (characterized by the backflow of blood from the brain through the vertebral artery on the same side as the occlusion into the subclavian artery distal to the occlusion; clinical effects of vertebrobasilar occlusion and exercise-induced arm claudication)
Vertebral and basilar arteries
• TIAs, which produce binocular vision disturbances, vertigo, dysarthria, and falling down without loss of consciousness

Key test results
• Arteriography demonstrates the type (thrombus or embolus), location, and degree of obstruction and collateral circulation.
• Doppler ultrasonography shows decreased blood flow distal to the occlusion.

Key treatments
• Surgery (for acute arterial occlusion): atherectomy, balloon angioplasty, bypass graft, embolectomy, laser angioplasty, patch grafting, stent placement, thromboendarterectomy, or amputation
• Thrombolytic agents: alteplase (Activase), streptokinase (Streptase)

Key interventions
Preoperatively (during an acute episode)
• Assess the client's circulatory status by checking for the most distal pulses and by inspecting his skin color and temperature.
• Provide pain relief as needed.
• Administer I.V. heparin, as needed, using an infusion pump.
• Watch for signs of fluid and electrolyte imbalance, and monitor intake and output for signs of renal failure (urine output less than 30 ml/hour).
Postoperatively
• Monitor the client's vital signs. Continuously assess his circulatory function by inspecting skin color and temperature and by checking for distal pulses. In charting, compare earlier assessments and observations. Watch closely for signs of hemorrhage (tachycardia, hypotension), and check dressings for excessive bleeding.
• In carotid, innominate, vertebral, or subclavian artery occlusion, assess neurologic status frequently for changes in level of consciousness or muscle strength and pupil size.
• In mesenteric artery occlusion, connect a nasogastric tube to low intermittent suction. Monitor intake and output. (Low urine output may indicate damage to renal arteries during surgery.) Assess abdominal status.

(continued)

Cardiovascular refresher *(continued)*

PERIPHERAL ARTERY DISEASE *(CONTINUED)*

• In saddle block occlusion, check distal pulses for adequate circulation. Watch for signs of renal failure and mesenteric artery occlusion (severe abdominal pain) and cardiac arrhythmias, which may precipitate embolus formation.
• In iliac artery occlusion, monitor urine output for signs of renal failure from decreased perfusion to the kidneys as a result of surgery. Provide meticulous catheter care.
• In both femoral and popliteal artery occlusions, monitor peripheral pulses. Assist with early ambulation, but discourage prolonged sitting.

RAYNAUD'S DISEASE

Key signs and symptoms
• Numbness and tingling that are relieved by warmth
• Typically, blanching of the skin on the fingers, which then becomes cyanotic before changing to red (after exposure to cold or stress)

Key test results
• Arteriography reveals vasospasm.

Key treatments
• Activity changes: avoidance of cold
• Smoking cessation (if appropriate)
• Surgery (used in fewer than one-quarter of clients): sympathectomy
• Calcium channel blockers: diltiazem (Cardizem), nifedipine (Procardia)

Key interventions
• Warn against exposure to the cold. Tell the client to wear mittens or gloves in cold weather or when handling cold items or defrosting the freezer.

RHEUMATIC FEVER AND RHEUMATIC HEART DISEASE

Key signs and symptoms
• Carditis
• Temperature of 100.4° F (38° C) or greater
• Migratory joint pain or polyarthritis

Key test results
• Blood tests show elevated white blood cell count and erythrocyte sedimentation rate and slight anemia during inflammation.
• Cardiac enzyme levels may be increased in severe carditis.
• C-reactive protein is positive (especially during the acute phase).

Key treatments
• Bed rest (in severe cases)
• Surgery: corrective valvular surgery (in cases of persistent heart failure)

• Antibiotics: erythromycin (Erythrocin), penicillin (Pfizerpen)
• Nonsteroidal anti-inflammatory drugs: aspirin, indomethacin (Indocin)

Key interventions
• Before giving penicillin, ask the client if he's ever had a hypersensitivity reaction to it. Even if the client has never had a reaction to penicillin, warn that such a reaction is possible.
• Instruct the client to watch for and report early signs of heart failure, such as dyspnea and a hacking, nonproductive cough.
• Warn the client to watch for and immediately report signs of recurrent streptococcal infection — sudden sore throat, diffuse throat redness and oropharyngeal exudate, swollen and tender cervical lymph glands, pain on swallowing, a temperature of 101° to 104° F (38.3° to 40° C), headache, and nausea. Urge the client to stay away from people with respiratory tract infections.

THORACIC AORTIC ANEURYSM

Key signs and symptoms
Ascending aneurysm
• Pain (described as severe, boring, and ripping and extending to the neck, shoulders, lower back, or abdomen)
• Unequal intensities of the right carotid and left radial pulses
Descending aneurysm
• Pain (described as sharp and tearing, usually starting suddenly between the shoulder blades and possibly radiating to the chest)
Transverse aneurysm
• Dyspnea
• Pain (described as sharp and tearing and radiating to the shoulders)

Key test results
• Aortography, the definitive test, shows the lumen of the aneurysm, its size and location, and the false lumen in a dissecting aneurysm.
• Chest X-ray shows widening of the aorta.
• Computed tomography scan confirms and locates the aneurysm and may be used to monitor its progression.

Key treatments
• Surgery: resection of aneurysm with a Dacron or Teflon graft replacement, possible replacement of aortic valve
• Analgesic: morphine
• Antihypertensives: nitroprusside (Nitropress), labetalol (Trandate)
• Negative inotropic: propranolol (Inderal)

Key interventions
• Monitor the client's blood pressure, PAWP, and CVP. Also evaluate pain, breathing, and carotid, radial, and femoral pulses.

Cardiovascular refresher (continued)

THORACIC AORTIC ANEURYSM (CONTINUED)

- Review laboratory test results, which must include a complete blood count, differential, electrolytes, typing and crossmatching for whole blood, ABG studies, and urinalysis.
- Insert an indwelling urinary catheter and monitor intake and output.
- Carefully monitor nitroprusside I.V. infusion rate; use a separate I.V. line for infusion. Adjust the dose by slowly increasing the infusion rate. Meanwhile, check blood pressure every 5 minutes until it stabilizes.
- With suspected bleeding from an aneurysm, prepare to give a blood transfusion.

After repair of thoracic aneurysm

- Evaluate the client's level of consciousness. Monitor vital signs, PAP, PAWP, CVP, pulse rate, urine output, and pain.
- Check respiratory function. Carefully observe and record the type and amount of chest tube drainage, and frequently assess heart and breath sounds.
- Monitor I.V. therapy to prevent fluid excess, which may occur with rapid fluid replacement.
- Give medications as appropriate to help improve the client's condition.

THROMBOPHLEBITIS

Key signs and symptoms

Deep vein thrombophlebitis

- Cramping calf pain (may be painless)
- Edema
- Tenderness to touch

Superficial vein thrombophlebitis

- Redness along the vein
- Warmth and tenderness along the vein

Key test results

- Photoplethysmography shows venous-filling defects.
- Ultrasound reveals decreased blood flow.

Key treatments

- Activity changes: maintaining bed rest and elevating the affected extremity
- Anticoagulants: warfarin (Coumadin), heparin, enoxaparin (Lovenox)
- Anti-inflammatory agents: aspirin, dalteparin (Fragmin)
- Fibrinolytic agent: streptokinase (Streptase)

Key interventions

- Assess pulmonary status.
- Maintain bed rest, and elevate the affected extremity.
- Perform neurovascular checks.
- Monitor laboratory values.
- Apply warm, moist compresses to improve circulation.

VALVULAR HEART DISEASE

Key signs and symptoms

Aortic insufficiency

- Angina
- Cough
- Dyspnea
- Fatigue
- Palpitations

Mitral insufficiency

- Angina
- Dyspnea
- Fatigue
- Orthopnea
- Peripheral edema

Mitral stenosis

- Dyspnea on exertion
- Fatigue
- Orthopnea
- Palpitations
- Peripheral edema
- Weakness

Mitral valve prolapse

- Possibly asymptomatic
- Palpitations

Tricuspid insufficiency

- Dyspnea
- Fatigue

Key test results

Aortic insufficiency

- Echocardiography shows left ventricular enlargement.
- X-ray shows left ventricular enlargement and pulmonary vein congestion.

Mitral insufficiency

- Cardiac catheterization shows mitral insufficiency and elevated atrial pressure and PAWP.

Mitral stenosis

- Cardiac catheterization shows diastolic pressure gradient across valve and elevated left atrial and PAWP.
- Echocardiography shows thickened mitral valve leaflets.
- ECG shows left atrial hypertrophy.
- X-ray shows left atrial and ventricular enlargement.

Mitral valve prolapse

- ECG shows prolapse of the mitral valve into the left atrium.

Tricuspid insufficiency

- Echocardiography shows systolic prolapse of the tricuspid valve.
- ECG shows right atrial or right ventricular hypertrophy.
- X-ray shows right atrial dilation and right ventricular enlargement.

(continued)

Cardiovascular refresher (continued)

VALVULAR HEART DISEASE (CONTINUED)
Key treatments
• Surgery: open-heart surgery using cardiopulmonary bypass for valve replacement (in severe cases)
• Anticoagulant: warfarin (Coumadin) to prevent thrombus formation around diseased or replaced valves

Key interventions
• Watch closely for signs of heart failure or pulmonary edema and for adverse effects of drug therapy.

• Place the client in an upright position.
• Maintain bed rest and provide assistance with bathing.
• If the client undergoes surgery, watch for hypotension, arrhythmias, and thrombus formation. Monitor vital signs, ABG levels, intake and output, daily weight, blood chemistries, chest X-rays, and pulmonary artery catheter readings.

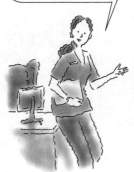

Cardiac output is the total amount of blood ejected from a ventricle per minute.

• through the aortic valve to the aorta and throughout the body.

The body electric
The system that conducts electrical impulses and coordinates the heart's contractions consists of the SA node, internodal tracts, AV node, bundle of His, right and left bundle branches, and Purkinje fibers.

A normal electrical impulse is initiated at the **SA node,** the heart's intrinsic pacemaker, which results in the following chain of events:
• atrial depolarization
• atrial contraction
• impulse transmission to the AV node
• impulse transmission to the bundle of His, bundle branches, and Purkinje fibers
• ventricular depolarization
• ventricular contraction
• ventricular repolarization.

How's it working?
Cardiac function can be assessed by measuring the following parameters:
• **Stroke volume (SV)** is the amount of blood ejected from a ventricle with each beat (normally, 70 ml).
• **Cardiac output (CO)** is the total amount of blood ejected from a ventricle per minute. Cardiac output equals stroke volume multiplied by heart rate (HR) (CO = SV × HR).
• **Ejection fraction** is the percent of left ventricular end-diastolic volume ejected during systole (normally, 60% to 70%).

A system of canals
Blood flows throughout the body via arteries and veins as well as through smaller

vessels such as arterioles, capillaries, and venules:
• **Arteries** are three-layered vessels (intima, media, adventitia) that carry oxygenated blood from the heart to the tissues.
• **Arterioles** are small-resistance vessels that feed into capillaries.
• **Capillaries** join arterioles to venules (larger, lower-pressured vessels than arterioles), where nutrients and wastes are exchanged.
• **Venules** join capillaries to veins.
• **Veins** are large-capacity, low-pressure vessels that return unoxygenated blood to the heart.

Think of these vessels as a series of large and small canals forming an interlocking system of blood flow.

Keep abreast of diagnostic tests

Here are the most important tests used to diagnose cardiovascular disorders, along with common nursing interventions associated with each test.

Graphing the heart's electrical activity
Electrocardiography is a noninvasive test that gives a graphic representation of the heart's electrical activity.

Nursing actions
• Determine the client's ability to lie still for several minutes.

Memory jogger

To remember how blood flows from the heart, think **Arteries away** and **veto**, for **veins to.**

Arteries away — arteries carry oxygenated blood **away** from the heart to the tissues. **Veto** — veins, by contrast, carry blood **to** the heart.

- Reassure the client that electrical shock won't occur.
- Apply the electrodes to clean, dry skin.
- Interpret the electrocardiogram (ECG) for changes, such as life-threatening arrhythmias or ischemia.

24-hour record of the heart

Ambulatory ECG, also known as Holter monitoring, is a noninvasive test that records the heart's electrical activity and cardiac events over a 24-hour period.

Nursing actions
- Explain the purpose of Holter monitoring.
- Instruct the client to keep an activity diary.
- Advise the client not to bathe or shower, operate machinery, or use a microwave oven or an electric shaver while wearing the monitor.

View through a catheter

Cardiac catheterization and arteriography (also called angiography) involve an injection of radiopaque dye through a catheter, after which a fluoroscope is used to examine the coronary arteries and intracardiac structures. The procedure is also used to monitor major intracardiac pressures, oxygenation, and cardiac output.

Nursing actions
Before the procedure
- Withhold the client's food and fluids after midnight.
- Administer daily medications as ordered by the physician.
- Discuss any anxiety the client may have about the procedure.
- Assess and record baseline vital signs and peripheral pulses.
- Make sure that written, informed consent has been obtained.
- Inform the client about possible nausea, chest pain, flushing of the face, or a sudden urge to urinate from the injection of radiopaque dye.
- Note the client's allergies to seafood, iodine, or radiopaque dyes.
After the procedure
- Monitor vital signs, peripheral pulses, and the injection site for bleeding.

- Maintain a pressure dressing and bed rest as ordered after the procedure.
- Encourage fluids unless contraindicated.
- Monitor for complaints of chest pain, and report any complaints immediately.
- If bleeding occurs at the site, apply manual pressure until the bleeding stops.

Echoing heart structures

Echocardiography is a noninvasive examination of the heart that uses echoes from sound waves to visualize intracardiac structures and monitor the direction of blood flow.

Nursing actions
- Determine the client's ability to lie still for 30 to 60 minutes.
- Explain the procedure to the client.

Jog and monitor

An **exercise ECG,** also known as a *stress test,* is a noninvasive test that studies the heart's electrical activity and monitors for ischemic events during levels of increasing exercise.

Nursing actions
- Explain the procedure to the client.
- Withhold food and fluids for 2 to 4 hours before the test.
- Instruct the client to wear loose-fitting clothing and supportive shoes.
- Perform a cardiopulmonary assessment.
- Tell the client to report chest discomfort, shortness of breath, fatigue, leg cramps, or dizziness immediately if it occurs during the test.

No fallout here

Nuclear cardiology examines the heart using radioisotopes. After I.V. injection of the isotopes, a monitor is used to read images of myocardial perfusion and contractility.

Nursing actions
Before the procedure
- Explain the procedure.
- Make sure that written, informed consent has been obtained.
- Determine the client's ability to lie still during the procedure.
After the procedure
- Examine the injection site for bleeding.

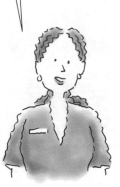

Cardiac catheterization is an invasive procedure. Be aware of the complications that may occur.

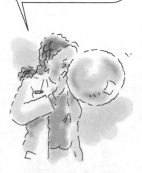

Hemodynamic monitoring uses a balloon-tipped catheter to measure cardiac output.

A complete picture of arterial blood supply

Digital subtraction angiography is an invasive procedure involving fluoroscopy with an image intensifier. This test allows complete visualization of the arterial blood supply to a specific area.

Nursing actions
Before the procedure
- Determine the client's ability to lie still during the test.
- Make sure that written, informed consent has been obtained.

After the procedure
- Monitor the client's vital signs.
- Check the insertion site for bleeding.
- Instruct the client to drink at least 1 qt (1 L) of fluid after the procedure.

Balloon and blood flow

Hemodynamic monitoring, also known as *single procedure monitoring* or *continuous monitoring,* uses a balloon-tipped, flow-directed pulmonary artery catheter to measure intracardiac pressures and cardiac output.

Nursing actions
Before the procedure
- Explain the procedure to the client.
- Make sure that written, informed consent has been obtained.

After the procedure
- Check the insertion site for signs of infection.
- Assess for such complications as arrhythmias, hemorrhage, clot formation, air embolus, and spontaneous wedging of the catheter balloon.
- Monitor the pressure tracings and record readings.

One for the photo album

A **chest X-ray** supplies a radiographic picture that determines the size and position of the heart. It can also detect the presence of fluid in the lungs and other abnormalities such as pneumothorax.

Nursing actions
- Determine the client's ability to hold his breath.

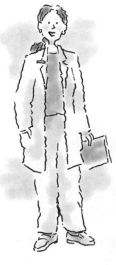

ABGs assess acid-base status.

- Ensure that the client removes all jewelry before the X-ray is taken.

Blood to the lab, part 1

Blood chemistry tests use blood samples to measure blood urea nitrogen (BUN), creatinine, sodium, potassium, bicarbonate, glucose, magnesium, calcium, phosphorus, cholesterol, triglycerides, creatine kinase (CK), CK isoenzymes, aspartate aminotransferase (AST), cardiac troponin levels, myoglobin, lactate dehydrogenase (LD), and LD isoenzymes.

Nursing actions
- Note any drugs the client is taking that may alter test results.
- Restrict the client's exercise before the blood sample is drawn.
- Withhold I.M. injections or note the time of the injection on the laboratory slip (after CK levels).
- Withhold food and fluids, as ordered.
- Assess the venipuncture site for bleeding.

Blood to the lab, part 2

Hematologic studies use blood samples to analyze and measure red blood cell and white blood cell (WBC) counts, erythrocyte sedimentation rate (ESR), prothrombin time, International Normalized Ratio, partial thromboplastin time, platelet count, hemoglobin (Hb) level, and hematocrit (Hct).

Nursing actions
- Note any drugs that might alter test results before the procedure.
- Assess the venipuncture site for bleeding after the procedure.

ABCs of ABGs

An **arterial blood gas (ABG) analysis** assesses arterial blood for tissue oxygenation, ventilation, and acid-base status.

Nursing actions
Before the procedure
- Document the client's temperature.
- Note whether the client is receiving supplemental oxygen and the amount or mechanical ventilation along with the ventilator settings.

After the procedure
- Apply continuous pressure to the puncture site for at least 5 minutes, then apply a pressure dressing for at least 30 minutes.
- Periodically check the site for bleeding.

Hear that sound? It's blood flow
A **Doppler ultrasound** transforms echoes from sound waves into audible sounds, allowing examination of blood flow in peripheral circulation.

Nursing actions
- Determine the client's ability to lie still.
- Explain the procedure.

Visualize the veins
In a **venogram,** a dye is injected to allow visualization of the veins. This picture is then used to diagnose deep vein thrombosis or incompetent valves.

Nursing actions
Before the procedure
- Withhold food and fluids after midnight.
- Assess and record the client's baseline vital signs and peripheral pulses.
- Make sure that written, informed consent has been obtained.
- Note the client's allergies to seafood, iodine, or radiopaque dyes.
- Inform the client about possible flushing of the face or throat irritation from the injection of the dye.
After the procedure
- Check the injection site for bleeding, infection, and hematoma.
- Encourage fluids unless contraindicated.

Oxygen in arterial blood
Pulse oximetry uses infrared light to measure arterial oxygen saturation in the blood. This test helps assess a client's pulmonary status.

To distinguish it from oxygen saturation obtained by ABGs, oxygen saturation obtained by pulse oximetry is abbreviated SpO_2.

Nursing actions
- Protect the sensor from bright light.
- Don't place the sensor on an extremity that has impeded blood flow.

- Attach the monitoring sensor to a fingertip, ear lobe, bridge of the nose, or toe.
- If a fingertip is used, remove artificial nails, nail tips, and nail polish because they may interfere with light transmission.

Polish up on client care

Major cardiovascular disorders include abdominal aortic aneurysm, angina, arrhythmias, cardiac tamponade, cardiogenic shock, cardiomyopathy, coronary artery disease (CAD), endocarditis, heart failure, hypertension, hypovolemic shock, myocardial infarction (MI), myocarditis, pericarditis, peripheral artery disease, Raynaud's disease, rheumatic fever and rheumatic heart disease, thoracic aortic aneurysm, thrombophlebitis, and valvular heart disease.

For all these disorders, the goal of nursing management is to decrease cardiac workload and increase myocardial blood supply. These steps increase oxygenation to the tissues and reduce overall damage to the heart.

Abdominal aortic aneurysm

An abdominal aortic aneurysm results from damage to the medial layer of the abdominal portion of the aorta. Aneurysm commonly results from atherosclerosis, which over time causes a weakening in the medial layer of the artery. Continued weakening from the force of blood flow results in outpouching of the artery and formation of the aneurysm. The aneurysm may then cause a rupture, leading to hemorrhage, hypovolemic shock, and possibly death.

There are four types of abdominal aneurysms:

dissecting (the vessel wall ruptures, and a blood clot is retained in an outpouching of tissue)

false (pulsating hematoma results from trauma)

fusiform (bilateral outpouching)

saccular (unilateral outpouching).

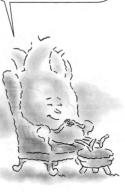

For all cardiac disorders, the goal of nursing care is to decrease cardiac workload and increase myocardial blood supply.

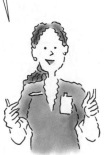

Look for signs of shock when caring for clients with abdominal aortic aneurysm.

CAUSES
- Atherosclerosis
- Congenital defect
- Hypertension
- Infection
- Marfan syndrome
- Syphilis
- Trauma

ASSESSMENT FINDINGS
- Abdominal mass to the left of the midline
- Abdominal pulsations
- Bruits over the site of the aneurysm
- Commonly asymptomatic
- Diminished femoral pulses
- Lower abdominal pain
- Lower back pain
- Systolic blood pressure in the legs that's lower than that in the arms

DIAGNOSTIC TEST RESULTS
- Abdominal computed tomography scan shows aneurysm.
- Abdominal ultrasound shows aneurysm.
- Arteriography shows aneurysm.
- Chest X-ray shows aneurysm.
- ECG differentiates aneurysm from MI.

NURSING DIAGNOSES
- Acute pain
- Anxiety
- Ineffective tissue perfusion: Peripheral
- Risk for deficient fluid volume

TREATMENT
- Abdominal aortic aneurysm resection
- Bed rest

Drug therapy
- Analgesic: oxycodone (OxyContin)
- Antihypertensives: prazosin (Minipress), nitroprusside (Nitropress), nitroglycerin
- Beta-adrenergic blocker: propranolol (Inderal), metoprolol (Lopressor)

INTERVENTIONS AND RATIONALES
- Assess cardiovascular status and monitor and record vital signs. *Tachycardia, dyspnea or hypotension may indicate fluid volume deficit caused by rupture of aneurysm.*
- Monitor intake and output and laboratory studies. *Low urine output and high specific gravity indicate hypovolemia.*

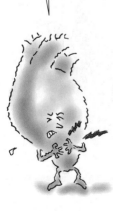

Angina isn't hard to understand. If I don't get enough oxygen, it hurts.

- Observe the client for signs of hypovolemic shock from aneurysm rupture, such as anxiety, restlessness, severe back pain, decreased pulse pressure, increased thready pulse, and pale, cool, moist, clammy skin, *to detect early signs of compromise.*
- Gently palpate the abdomen for distention. *Increasing distention may signify impending rupture.*
- Check peripheral circulation: pulses, temperature, color, and complaints of abnormal sensations *to detect poor arterial blood flow.*
- Assess pain *to detect enlarging aneurysm or rupture.*
- Administer medications, as prescribed, *to reduce hypertension and control pain.*
- Encourage the client to express feelings such as a fear of dying *to reduce anxiety.*
- Maintain a quiet environment *to control blood pressure and reduce risk of rupture.*

Teaching topics
- Explanation of the disorder and treatment plan
- Medications and possible adverse effects
- Signs and symptoms of decreased peripheral circulation, such as change in skin color or temperature, complaints of numbness or tingling, and absent pulses
- Activity limitations, including alternating rest periods with activity, and adhering to prescribed exercise and diet regimen

Angina

Angina is chest pain caused by inadequate myocardial oxygen supply. It's usually caused by narrowing of the coronary arteries, which results from plaque accumulation in the intimal lining.

Angina is generally categorized as one of three main forms: stable, unstable (an acute coronary syndrome), or Prinzmetal's (variant).
- In stable angina, symptoms are consistent and pain is relieved by rest.
- In unstable angina, pain is marked by increasing severity, duration, and frequency. Pain from unstable angina responds slowly to nitroglycerin and isn't relieved by rest.
- In Prinzmetal's angina, pain is unpredictable and may occur at rest.

CAUSES
- Activity or disease that increases metabolic demands
- Aortic stenosis
- Atherosclerosis
- Pulmonary stenosis
- Small-vessel disease (associated with rheumatoid arthritis, radiation injury, or lupus erythematosus)
- Thromboembolism
- Vasospasm

ASSESSMENT FINDINGS
- Anxiety
- Diaphoresis
- Dyspnea
- Epigastric distress
- Palpitations
- Pain that may be substernal, crushing, or compressing; may radiate to the arms, jaw, or back; usually lasts 3 to 5 minutes; usually occurs after exertion, emotional excitement, or exposure to cold but can also develop when the client is at rest; in women, may manifest as atypical symptoms of pain, such as indigestion, back pain, and less severe complaints of substernal pain
- Tachycardia

DIAGNOSTIC TEST RESULTS
- Blood chemistry shows increased cholesterol levels.
- Cardiac enzymes are within normal limits.
- Coronary arteriography shows plaque accumulation.
- ECG shows ST-segment depression and T-wave inversion during anginal pain.
- Holter monitoring reveals ST-segment depression and T-wave inversion.
- Stress test results include abnormal ECG findings and chest pain.

NURSING DIAGNOSES
- Acute pain
- Anxiety
- Decreased cardiac output
- Ineffective tissue perfusion: Cardiopulmonary

TREATMENT
- Diet: low fat, low sodium, and low cholesterol (low calorie if necessary)
- Coronary artery bypass grafting
- Oxygen therapy (typically 2 to 4 L)
- Percutaneous transluminal coronary angioplasty (PTCA), stent placement
- Semi-Fowler's position

Drug therapy
- Anticoagulants: heparin, aspirin
- Beta-adrenergic blockers: propranolol (Inderal), nadolol (Corgard), atenolol (Tenormin), metoprolol (Lopressor)
- Calcium channel blockers: verapamil (Calan), diltiazem (Cardizem), nifedipine (Procardia), nicardipine (Cardene)
- Low-dose aspirin therapy
- Nitrates: nitroglycerin, isosorbide dinitrate (Isordil), topical nitroglycerin, transdermal nitroglycerin (Transderm-Nitro)

INTERVENTIONS AND RATIONALES
- Assess cardiovascular status, hemodynamic variables, and vital signs *to detect evidence of cardiac compromise and response to treatment.*
- Administer oxygen *to increase oxygenation supply.*
- Assess for chest pain and evaluate its characteristics. *Assessment allows for care plan modification as necessary.*
- Administer medications, as prescribed, *to increase oxygenation and to reduce cardiac workload.* Hold nitrates and notify physician for systolic blood pressure less than 90 mm Hg. Hold beta-adrenergic blocker and notify the physician for heart rate less than 60 beats/ minute *to prevent complications that can occur as a result of therapy.*
- Advise the client to rest if pain begins *to reduce cardiac workload.*
- Obtain 12-lead ECG during an acute attack *to assess for ischemic changes.*
- Keep the client in semi-Fowler's position *to promote chest expansion and ventilation.*
- Monitor and record intake and output *to monitor fluid status.*
- Maintain the client's prescribed diet (low-fat, low-sodium, and low-cholesterol; low-calorie, if necessary) *to reduce risk of CAD.*
- Encourage weight reduction, if necessary, *to reduce risk of CAD.*
- Encourage the client to express anxiety, fears, or concerns *because anxiety can increase oxygen demands.*

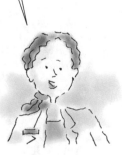

Anginal pain can be difficult to identify. It's usually shorter in duration than pain from MI.

Teaching topics
• Explanation of the disorder and treatment options
• Medications and possible adverse effects
• Taking sublingual nitroglycerin for acute attacks and prophylactically to prevent anginal episodes
• Reducing risk factors through diet, exercise, weight loss, cholesterol reduction, smoking cessation, and stress reduction
• Avoiding activities or situations that cause angina, such as exertion, heavy meals, emotional upsets, and exposure to cold
• Seeking medical attention if pain lasts longer than 20 minutes
• Differentiating between symptoms of angina and symptoms of MI
• Contacting the American Heart Association

Arrhythmias

In cardiac arrhythmias, abnormal electrical conduction or automaticity changes heart rate and rhythm. Arrhythmias vary in severity, from mild and asymptomatic ones that require no treatment (such as sinus arrhythmia, in which heart rate increases and decreases with respirations) to catastrophic ventricular fibrillation (VF), which necessitates immediate resuscitation.

Arrhythmias are generally classified according to their origin (atrial or ventricular). Their effect on cardiac output and blood pressure, partially influenced by the site of origin, determines their clinical significance. The most common arrhythmias include atrial fibrillation, asystole, VF, and ventricular tachycardia (VT).

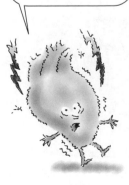

What a shock! A change in electrical conduction breaks my rhythm.

CAUSES
• Congenital
• Degeneration of conductive tissue
• Drug toxicity
• Heart disease
• MI
• Myocardial ischemia

ASSESSMENT FINDINGS
Atrial fibrillation
• Commonly asymptomatic
• Palpitations
• Complaints of feeling faint
• Irregular pulse with no pattern to the irregularity

Asystole
• Unresponsive
• Apnea
• Cyanosis
• No palpable blood pressure
• Pulselessness

Ventricular fibrillation
• Unresponsive
• Apnea
• No palpable blood pressure
• Pulselessness

Ventricular tachycardia
• Chest pain
• Diaphoresis
• Hypotension
• Weak or absent pulse
• Dizziness
• Possible loss of consciousness

DIAGNOSTIC TEST RESULTS
Atrial fibrillation
• ECG shows irregular atrial rhythm, atrial rate possibly greater than 400 beats/minute, irregular ventricular rhythm, QRS complexes of uniform configuration and duration, indiscernible PR interval, and no P waves (fibrillation waves).

Asystole   = Flatline
• ECG shows no atrial or ventricular rate or rhythm and no discernible P waves, QRS complexes, or T waves.

Ventricular fibrillation
• ECG shows rapid and chaotic ventricular rhythm, wide and irregular or absent QRS complexes, and no visible P waves.

Ventricular tachycardia
• ECG shows ventricular rate of 140 to 220 beats/minute, wide and bizarre QRS complexes, and no discernible P waves. VT may start or stop suddenly.

NURSING DIAGNOSES
- Ineffective tissue perfusion: Cardiopulmonary
- Decreased cardiac output
- Impaired gas exchange

TREATMENT
Atrial fibrillation
- Antiarrhythmics (if client is stable): amiodarone (Cordarone), digoxin (Lanoxin), diltiazem (Cardizem), procainamide, verapamil (Calan)
- Permanent pacemaker
- Radiofrequency catheter ablation
- Synchronized cardioversion (if client is unstable)

Asystole
- Cardiopulmonary resuscitation (CPR)
- Advanced cardiac life support (ACLS) protocol for endotracheal intubation and possible transcutaneous pacing
- Antiarrhythmics: atropine, epinephrine per ACLS protocol
- Buffering agent: sodium bicarbonate

Ventricular fibrillation
- CPR
- Defibrillation
- ACLS protocol for endotracheal intubation
- Antiarrhythmics: amiodarone (Cordarone), epinephrine, lidocaine (Xylocaine), magnesium sulfate, procainamide, vasopressin per ACLS protocol
- Implantable cardiac defibrillator
- Buffering agent: sodium bicarbonate

Ventricular tachycardia
- CPR, if pulseless
- Defibrillation
- Antiarrhythmics: amiodarone (Cordarone), epinephrine, lidocaine (Xylocaine), magnesium sulfate, procainamide
- ACLS protocol for endotracheal intubation, if pulseless
- Implantable cardioverter-defibrillator

INTERVENTIONS AND RATIONALES
- Assess an unmonitored client for rhythm disturbances *to promptly identify and treat life-threatening arrhythmias.*

- If the client's pulse is abnormally rapid, slow, or irregular, watch for signs of hypoperfusion, such as hypotension and altered mental status, *to prevent such complications as cerebral anoxia.*
- Document any arrhythmias in a monitored client *to create a record of their occurrence.* Assess for possible causes and effects *so proper treatment can be instituted.*
- When life-threatening arrhythmias develop, rapidly assess level of consciousness, respirations, and pulse *to avoid or treat crisis.*
- Initiate CPR, if indicated, *to maintain cerebral perfusion until other ACLS measures are successful.*
- Evaluate the client for altered cardiac output resulting from arrhythmias. *Decreased cardiac output may cause inadequate perfusion of major organs, leading to irreversible damage.*
- If trained, perform defibrillation early for VT and VF. *Studies show that early defibrillation intervention improves the client's chance of survival.*
- Administer medications as needed, and prepare for medical procedures (for example, cardioversion) if indicated *to ensure prompt treatment of life-threatening arrhythmias.*
- Monitor for predisposing factors — such as fluid and electrolyte imbalance — and signs of drug toxicity, especially with digoxin. Drug toxicity may require withholding the next dose. *Alleviating predisposing factors decreases the risk of arrhythmias.*
- Provide adequate oxygen and reduce the heart's workload, while carefully maintaining metabolic, neurologic, respiratory, and hemodynamic status, *to prevent arrhythmias in a cardiac client.* Follow ACLS protocol for endotracheal intubation.
- Be prepared to assist with temporary pacemaker insertion or transcutaneous pacing, if necessary, *to treat arrythmia.*
- Restrict the client's activity after temporary or permanent pacemaker insertion. Monitor the pulse rate regularly, and watch for signs of decreased cardiac output. *These measures avert permanent pacemaker malfunction.*
- If the client has a permanent pacemaker, warn him about environmental hazards as indicated by the pacemaker manufacturer *to avoid pacemaker malfunction.*

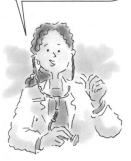

Fluid and electrolyte imbalances can increase the risk of arrhythmias.

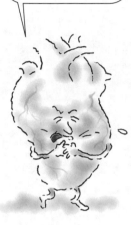

You think the NCLEX creates pressure? In cardiac tamponade, excess fluid puts so much pressure on me, I may need emergency treatment.

Teaching topics

- Explanation of the disorder and treatment options
- Medications and possible adverse effects
- Reporting light-headedness or syncope
- Coming in for regular checkups
- Environmental hazards for clients with permanent pacemakers
- Follow-up permanent pacemaker function tests

Cardiac tamponade

In cardiac tamponade, a rapid rise in intrapericardial pressure impairs diastolic filling of the heart. The rise in pressure usually results from blood or fluid accumulation in the pericardial sac.

If fluid accumulates rapidly, this condition is commonly fatal and necessitates emergency lifesaving measures. Slow accumulation and rise in pressure, as in pericardial effusion associated with cancer, may not produce immediate symptoms because the fibrous wall of the pericardial sac can gradually stretch to accommodate as much as 1 to 2 L of fluid.

CAUSES

- Dressler's syndrome
- Effusion (in cancer, bacterial infections, tuberculosis and, rarely, acute rheumatic fever)
- Hemorrhage from nontraumatic causes (such as rupture of the heart or great vessels or anticoagulant therapy in a client with pericarditis)
- Hemorrhage from trauma (such as gunshot or stab wounds of the chest and perforation by a catheter during cardiac or central venous catheterization or after cardiac surgery)
- MI
- Uremia

ASSESSMENT FINDINGS

- Anxiety
- Diaphoresis
- Dyspnea
- Hepatomegaly
- Increased venous pressure
- Muffled heart sounds on auscultation

- Narrow pulse pressure
- Jugular vein distention
- Pallor or cyanosis
- Pulsus paradoxus (an abnormal inspiratory drop in systemic blood pressure greater than 15 mm Hg)
- Reduced arterial blood pressure
- Restlessness
- Tachycardia
- Upright, leaning forward posture

DIAGNOSTIC TEST RESULTS

- Chest X-ray shows slightly widened mediastinum and cardiomegaly.
- Echocardiography records pericardial effusion with signs of right ventricular and atrial compression.
- ECG may reveal changes produced by acute pericarditis. This test rarely reveals tamponade but is useful to rule out other cardiac disorders.
- Pulmonary artery catheterization detects increased right atrial pressure, right ventricular diastolic pressure, and central venous pressure (CVP).

NURSING DIAGNOSES

- Ineffective tissue perfusion: Cardiopulmonary
- Anxiety
- Decreased cardiac output

TREATMENT

- Surgery: pericardiocentesis (needle aspiration of the pericardial cavity), surgical creation of an opening to drain fluid, or thoracotomy

Drug therapy

- Adrenergic agent: epinephrine
- Heparin antagonist: protamine sulfate in heparin-induced cardiac tamponade
- Inotropic agent: dopamine
- Vitamin K in warfarin-induced cardiac tamponade

INTERVENTIONS AND RATIONALES
If the client needs pericardiocentesis

- Explain the procedure to the client *to alleviate anxiety.*
- Keep a pericardial aspiration needle attached to a 50-ml syringe by a three-way stopcock, an ECG machine, and an

emergency cart with a defibrillator at the bedside. Make sure the equipment is turned on and ready for immediate use *to avoid treatment delay.*
• Position the client at a 45- to 60-degree angle. Connect the precordial ECG lead to the hub of the aspiration needle with an alligator clamp and connecting wire. When the needle touches the myocardium during fluid aspiration, an ST-segment elevation or premature ventricular contractions will be seen. *Monitoring the client's ECG ensures accuracy of the procedure and helps prevent complications.*
• Monitor blood pressure and CVP during and after pericardiocentesis *to monitor for complications such as hypotension, which may indicate cardiac chamber puncture.*
• Infuse I.V. solutions *to maintain blood pressure.* Watch for a decrease in CVP and a concomitant rise in blood pressure, *which indicate relief of cardiac compression.*
• Watch for complications of pericardiocentesis, such as VF, vasovagal response, and coronary artery or cardiac chamber puncture, *to prevent or rapidly treat crisis.*
• Closely monitor ECG changes, blood pressure, pulse rate, level of consciousness, and urine output *to detect signs of decreased cardiac output.*

If the client needs a thoracotomy
• Explain the procedure to the client. Tell him what to expect postoperatively (chest tubes, chest tube drainage system, administration of oxygen). Teach him how to turn, deep-breathe, and cough *to prevent postoperative complications and relieve the client's anxiety.*
• Give antibiotics *to prevent or treat infection* and protamine sulfate or vitamin K as needed *to prevent hemorrhage.*
• Postoperatively, monitor critical parameters, such as vital signs and ABG levels, and assess heart and breath sounds *to detect early signs of complications such as reaccumulation of fluid.*
• Give pain medication as needed *to alleviate pain and promote comfort.*
• Maintain the chest tube drainage system and be alert for complications, such as hemorrhage and arrhythmias, *to prevent further decompensation.*

Teaching topics
• Explanation of the disorder and treatment plan
• Medications and possible adverse effects
• Alerting the nurse if condition worsens

Cardiogenic shock

Cardiogenic shock occurs when the heart fails to pump adequately, thereby reducing cardiac output and compromising tissue perfusion.
    Here's how cardiogenic shock progresses:
• Decreased stroke volume results in increased left ventricular volume.
• Blood pooling in the left ventricle backs up into the lungs, causing pulmonary edema.
• To compensate for a falling cardiac output, heart rate and contractility increase.
• These compensating mechanisms increase the demand for myocardial oxygen.
• An imbalance between oxygen supply and demand results, increasing myocardial ischemia and further compromising the heart's pumping action.

CAUSES
• Advanced heart block
• Cardiomyopathy
• Heart failure
• MI
• Myocarditis
• Papillary muscle rupture

ASSESSMENT FINDINGS
• Anxiety, restlessness, disorientation, and confusion
• Cold, clammy skin
• Crackles in lungs
• Hypotension (systolic pressure below 90 mm Hg)
• Narrow pulse pressure
• Jugular vein distention
• Oliguria (urine output of less than 30 ml/hour)
• Third (S_3) and fourth (S_4) heart sounds
• Tachycardia or other arrhythmias
• Tachypnea, hypoxia
• Weak, thready pulse

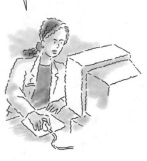

A post-MI client exhibits cold, clammy skin; hypotension; oliguria; and tachycardia. Hmmmm. Probably adds up to cardiogenic shock.

DIAGNOSTIC TEST RESULTS
- ABG levels show respiratory alkalosis initially. As shock progresses, metabolic acidosis develops.
- Blood chemistry tests show increased BUN, creatinine, and cardiac troponin levels.
- ECG shows MI (enlarged Q wave, elevated ST segment).
- Hemodynamic monitoring reveals decreased stroke volume and decreased cardiac output; it also shows increased pulmonary artery pressure (PAP), increased pulmonary artery wedge pressure (PAWP), increased CVP, and increased systemic vascular resistance.

NURSING DIAGNOSES
- Decreased cardiac output
- Ineffective tissue perfusion: Cardiopulmonary
- Ineffective tissue perfusion: Renal
- Anxiety

TREATMENT
- Intra-aortic balloon pump (IABP) (see *IABP action*)
- Oxygen therapy: intubation and mechanical ventilation, if necessary
- Activity changes, including maintaining bed rest and implementing passive range-of-motion and isometric exercises
- Continuous renal replacement therapy
- Dietary changes, including withholding food and oral fluids

Drug therapy
- Adrenergic agent: epinephrine
- Cardiac glycoside: digoxin (Lanoxin)
- Cardiac inotropes: dopamine, dobutamine, inamrinone (Amrinone), milrinone
- Diuretics: furosemide (Lasix), bumetanide (Bumex), metolazone (Zaroxolyn)
- Vasodilators: nitroprusside (Nitropress), nitroglycerin
- Vasopressor: norepinephrine (Levophed)

INTERVENTIONS AND RATIONALES
- Assess cardiovascular status, including hemodynamic variables, vital signs, heart sounds, capillary refill, skin temperature, and peripheral pulses *to monitor the effects of drug therapy and detect cardiac decompensation.*
- Assess respiratory status, including breath sounds and ABGs. *Tachypnea, crackles, and hypoxemia may indicate pulmonary edema.*
- Monitor level of consciousness *to detect cerebral hypoxia caused by reduced cardiac output.*
- Monitor fluid balance, including intake and output, *to monitor kidney function and detect fluid overload leading to pulmonary edema.*
- Administer I.V. fluids, oxygen, and medications, as prescribed, *to maximize cardiac, pulmonary, and renal function.*
- Monitor laboratory studies *to detect evidence of MI, evaluate renal function, and assess oxygen-carrying capacity of the blood.*
- Withhold food and fluids, as directed, *to reduce risk of aspiration with a reduced level of consciousness.*
- Provide suctioning *to aid in the removal of secretions and reduce risk of aspiration.*
- Encourage the client to express feelings such as a fear of dying *to reduce his anxiety.*

Teaching topics
- Explanation of the disorder and treatment plan
- Medications and possible adverse effects
- Recognizing early signs and symptoms of fluid overload
- Maintaining activity limitations, including alternating rest periods with activity

---

IABP action

With an intra-aortic balloon pump (IABP), an inflatable balloon is inserted through the femoral artery into the descending aorta. The balloon inflates during diastole, when the aortic valve is closed, to increase coronary artery perfusion. It also deflates during systole, when the aortic valve opens, to reduce resistance to ejection (afterload) and to reduce cardiac workload.

- Maintaining a low-fat, low-sodium diet
- Monitoring daily weight and notifying the physician of a weight gain greater than 3 lb (1.4 kg)

Cardiomyopathy

In cardiomyopathy, the myocardium (middle muscular layer) around the left ventricle becomes flabby, altering cardiac function and resulting in decreased cardiac output. Increased heart rate and increased muscle mass compensate in early stages; however, in later stages, heart failure develops.

The three types of cardiomyopathy are:
- dilated (congestive), the most common form, in which dilated heart chambers contract poorly, causing blood to pool and reducing cardiac output
- hypertrophic (obstructive), in which a hypertrophied left ventricle is unable to relax and fill properly
- restrictive (obliterative), a rare form, characterized by stiff ventricles resistant to ventricular filling.

CAUSES
Dilated cardiomyopathy
- Chronic alcoholism
- Infection
- Metabolic and immunologic disorders
- Pregnancy and postpartum disorders

Hypertrophic cardiomyopathy
- Congenital
- Hypertension

Restrictive cardiomyopathy
- Amyloidosis
- Cancer and other infiltrative diseases

ASSESSMENT FINDINGS
- Cough
- Crackles on lung auscultation
- Dependent pitting edema
- Dyspnea, paroxysmal nocturnal dyspnea
- Enlarged liver
- Fatigue
- Jugular vein distention
- Murmur, S_3 and S_4 heart sounds

DIAGNOSTIC TEST RESULTS
- Cardiac catheterization excludes the diagnosis of coronary artery disease.
- Chest X-ray shows cardiomegaly and pulmonary congestion.
- ECG shows left ventricular hypertrophy and nonspecific changes.
- Echocardiogram shows decreased myocardial function.

NURSING DIAGNOSES
- Decreased cardiac output
- Impaired gas exchange
- Activity intolerance

TREATMENT
- Dietary changes: establishing a low-sodium diet with vitamin supplements
- Dual-chamber pacing (for hypertrophic cardiomyopathy)
- Surgery (when medication fails): heart transplantation or cardiomyoplasty (for dilated cardiomyopathy); ventricular myotomy (for hypertrophic cardiomyopathy)

Drug therapy
- Beta-adrenergic blockers: propranolol (Inderal), nadolol (Corgard), metoprolol (Lopressor) for hypertrophic cardiomyopathy
- Calcium channel blockers: verapamil (Calan) and diltiazem (Cardizem) for hypertrophic cardiomyopathy
- Diuretics: furosemide (Lasix), bumetanide (Bumex), metolazone (Zaroxolyn) for dilated cardiomyopathy
- Inotropic agents: dobutamine, milrinone, digoxin (Lanoxin) for dilated cardiomyopathy
- Oral anticoagulant: warfarin (Coumadin) for dilated and hypertrophic cardiomyopathy

INTERVENTIONS AND RATIONALES
- Monitor ECG *to detect arrhythmias and ischemia.*
- Assess cardiovascular status, vital signs, and hemodynamic variables *to detect heart failure.*
- Monitor respiratory status *to detect evidence of heart failure, such as dyspnea and crackles.*
- Administer oxygen and medications, as prescribed, *to improve oxygenation and cardiac output.*

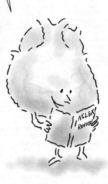

In dilated cardiomyopathy, the muscles around my left ventricle become flabby.

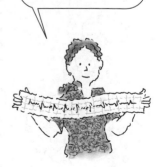

When treating cardiomyopathy, monitor ECGs to detect arrhythmias and ischemia.

- Monitor and record intake and output *to detect fluid volume overload.*
- Keep the client in semi-Fowler's position *to enhance gas exchange.*
- Maintain bed rest *to reduce oxygen demands on the heart.*
- Monitor laboratory results *to detect abnormalities, such as hypokalemia, from the use of diuretics.*
- Maintain the client's prescribed diet. *A low-sodium diet reduces fluid retention.*

Teaching topics
- Explanation of the disorder and treatment plan
- Medications and possible adverse effects
- Early signs and symptoms of heart failure
- Monitoring pulses and blood pressure
- Measuring weight daily and reporting increases over 3 lb (1.4 kg)
- Exercises to increase cardiac output, such as raising arms
- Avoiding straining during bowel movements
- Refraining from smoking and drinking alcohol
- Contacting the American Heart Association

Coronary artery disease

CAD results from the buildup of atherosclerotic plaque in the arteries of the heart. This causes a narrowing of the arterial lumen, reducing blood flow to the myocardium.

CAUSES
- Aging
- Arteriosclerosis
- Atherosclerosis
- Depletion of estrogen after menopause
- Diabetes
- Genetics
- High-fat, high-cholesterol diet
- Hyperlipidemia
- Hypertension
- Obesity
- Sedentary lifestyle
- Smoking
- Stress

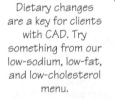

Dietary changes are a key for clients with CAD. Try something from our low-sodium, low-fat, and low-cholesterol menu.

ASSESSMENT FINDINGS
- Angina (chest pain) that may be substernal, crushing, or compressing; may radiate to the arms, jaw, or back; usually lasts 3 to 5 minutes; usually occurs after exertion, emotional excitement, or exposure to cold but can also develop when the client is at rest

DIAGNOSTIC TEST RESULTS
- Blood chemistry tests show increased cholesterol levels (decreased high-density lipoproteins, increased low-density lipoproteins).
- Coronary arteriography shows plaque formation.
- ECG or Holter monitoring shows ST-segment depression and T-wave inversion during anginal episode.
- Stress test reveals ST-segment changes, multiple premature ventricular contractions, and chest pain.

NURSING DIAGNOSES
- Activity intolerance
- Impaired gas exchange
- Acute pain

TREATMENT
- Activity changes, including weight loss, if necessary
- Atherectomy
- Coronary artery bypass surgery
- Coronary artery stent placement
- Dietary changes, including establishing a low-sodium, low-cholesterol, and low-fat diet with increased dietary fiber (low-calorie only if appropriate)
- PTCA

Drug therapy
- Analgesic: morphine I.V.
- Anticoagulants: heparin, dalteparin (Fragmin), enoxaparin (Lovenox)
- Antilipemic agents: cholestyramine (Questran), lovastatin (Mevacor), simvastatin (Zocor), nicotinic acid (Niacor), gemfibrozil (Lopid), colestipol (Colestid)
- Beta-adrenergic blockers: metoprolol (Lopressor), propranolol (Inderal), nadolol (Corgard)

- Calcium channel blockers: nifedipine (Procardia), verapamil (Calan), diltiazem (Cardizem)
- Low-dose aspirin therapy
- Nitrates: nitroglycerin, isosorbide dinitrate (Isordil)

INTERVENTIONS AND RATIONALES

- Obtain an ECG during anginal episodes *to detect evidence of ischemia.*
- Assess cardiovascular status, vital signs, and hemodynamic variables *to detect evidence of compromise.*
- Administer sublingual nitroglycerin and oxygen for anginal episodes *to provide pain relief.*
- Monitor intake and output *to detect changes in fluid status.*
- Monitor laboratory studies. *Evaluate cardiac enzymes to rule out MI. Obtain lipid panel to determine need for diet changes and lipid-lowering drugs.*
- Encourage the client to express anxiety, fears, or concerns *to help him cope with his illness.*

Teaching topics

- Explanation of the disorder and treatment plan
- Medications and possible adverse effects
- Limiting activity, alcohol intake, and dietary fat
- Smoking cessation, if appropriate
- Taking nitroglycerin for chest pain
- Contacting the American Heart Association

Endocarditis

Endocarditis is an infection of the endocardium, heart valves, or a cardiac prosthesis resulting from bacterial or fungal invasion. This invasion produces vegetative growths on the heart valves, the endocardial lining of a heart chamber, or the endothelium of a blood vessel that may embolize to the spleen, kidneys, central nervous system, and lungs. This disorder may also be called infective endocarditis and bacterial endocarditis.

In endocarditis, fibrin and platelets aggregate on the valve tissue and engulf circulating bacteria or fungi that flourish and produce friable verrucous vegetations. Such vegetations may cover the valve surfaces, causing ulceration and necrosis; they may also extend to the chordae tendineae, leading to their rupture and subsequent valvular insufficiency.

Untreated endocarditis is usually fatal, but with proper treatment, about 70% of clients recover. The prognosis is worst when endocarditis causes severe valvular damage, leading to insufficiency and heart failure, or when it involves a prosthetic valve.

CAUSES

- Enterococci
- I.V. drug abuse
- Mitral valve prolapse
- Prosthetic heart valve
- Rheumatic heart disease
- Streptococci (especially *Streptococcus viridans*)
- Staphylococci (especially *Staphylococcus aureus*)

CONTRIBUTING FACTORS

- Coarctation of the aorta
- Degenerative heart disease
- Marfan syndrome
- Pulmonary stenosis
- Subaortic and valvular aortic stenosis
- Tetralogy of Fallot
- Ventricular septal defects

ASSESSMENT FINDINGS

- Anorexia
- Arthralgia
- Chills
- Fatigue
- Intermittent, recurring fever
- Loud, regurgitant murmur
- Malaise
- Night sweats
- Signs of cerebral, pulmonary, renal, or splenic infarction
- Valvular insufficiency
- Weakness
- Weight loss

DIAGNOSTIC TEST RESULTS

- Blood test results may include normal or elevated WBC count, abnormal histiocytes

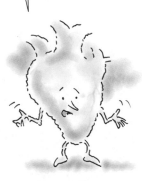

I never promised you a rose garden. Vegetative growths on my valves lead to endocarditis.

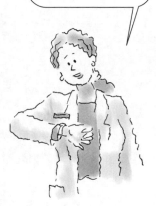

(macrophages), elevated ESR, normocytic normochromic anemia (in 70% to 90% of endocarditis cases), and positive serum rheumatoid factor (in about one-half of all clients with endocarditis after the disease is present for 3 to 6 weeks).
• Echocardiography may identify valvular damage.
• ECG may show AF and other arrhythmias that accompany valvular disease.
• Three or more blood cultures in a 24- to 48-hour period identify the causative organism in up to 90% of clients.

NURSING DIAGNOSES
• Activity intolerance
• Decreased cardiac output
• Risk for injury

TREATMENT
• Bed rest
• Maintaining sufficient fluid intake
• Surgery (in cases of severe valvular damage) to replace defective valve

Drug therapy
• Antibiotics: based on infective organism
• Aspirin

INTERVENTIONS AND RATIONALES
• Before giving antibiotics, obtain a client history of allergies *to prevent anaphylaxis.*
• Observe for signs of infiltration and inflammation, possible complications of long-term I.V. drug administration, at the venipuncture site. Rotate venous access sites *to reduce the risk of these complications.*
• Watch for signs of embolization (hematuria, pleuritic chest pain, left upper quadrant pain, and paresis), a common occurrence during the first 3 months of treatment. *These signs may indicate impending peripheral vascular occlusion or splenic, renal, cerebral, or pulmonary infarction.*
• Monitor the client's renal status (BUN levels, serum creatinine, creatinine clearance, and urine output) *to check for signs of renal emboli or evidence of drug toxicity.*
• Observe for signs of heart failure, such as dyspnea, tachypnea, tachycardia, crackles, jugular vein distention, edema, and weight gain. *Detecting heart failure early ensures*

prompt intervention and treatment and decreases the risk of heart failure progressing to pulmonary edema.
• Provide reassurance by teaching the client and his family about this disease and the need for prolonged treatment. Tell them to watch closely for fever, anorexia, and other signs of relapse about 2 weeks after treatment stops. Suggest quiet diversionary activities to prevent excessive physical exertion. *Having the client and his family involved in care gives them a feeling of control and promotes compliance with long-term therapy.*
• Make sure a susceptible client understands the need for prophylactic antibiotics before, during, and after dental work, childbirth, and genitourinary, GI, or gynecologic procedures *to prevent further episodes of endocarditis.*

Teaching topics
• Explanation of the disorder and treatment plan
• Medications and possible adverse effects
• Recognizing symptoms of endocarditis; notifying the physician immediately if symptoms occur
• Need for prophylactic antibiotics before, during, and after dental work, childbirth, and genitourinary, GI, or gynecologic procedures

Heart failure

Heart failure occurs when the heart can't pump enough blood to meet the body's metabolic needs.

Heart failure can occur as left-sided failure or right-sided failure. Left-sided heart failure causes mostly pulmonary symptoms, such as shortness of breath, dyspnea on exertion, and a moist cough.

Right-sided heart failure causes systemic symptoms, such as peripheral edema and swelling, jugular vein distention, and hepatomegaly.

CAUSES
• Atherosclerosis
• Cardiac conduction defects (in left-sided failure)

- Chronic obstructive pulmonary disease (in right-sided failure)
- Fluid overload
- Hypertension (in left-sided failure)
- Left-sided heart failure (in right-sided failure)
- MI
- Pulmonary hypertension (in right-sided failure)
- Valvular insufficiency
- Valvular stenosis

ASSESSMENT FINDINGS
Left-sided failure
- Anxiety
- Arrhythmias
- Cough
- Crackles
- Dyspnea
- Fatigue
- Gallop rhythm: S_3 and S_4
- Orthopnea
- Paroxysmal nocturnal dyspnea
- Tachycardia
- Tachypnea

Right-sided failure
- Anorexia
- Ascites
- Dependent edema
- Fatigue
- Gallop rhythm: S_3 and S_4
- Hepatomegaly
- Jugular vein distention
- Nausea
- Signs of left-sided heart failure
- Tachycardia
- Weight gain

DIAGNOSTIC TEST RESULTS
Left-sided failure
- B-type natriuretic peptide (BNP) levels are elevated.
- ABG levels indicate hypoxemia and hypercapnia.
- Blood chemistry tests reveal decreased potassium and sodium levels and increased BUN and creatinine levels.
- Chest X-ray shows increased pulmonary congestion and left ventricular hypertrophy.
- ECG shows left ventricular hypertrophy.

- Echocardiography shows increased size of cardiac chambers and decreased wall motion.
- Hemodynamic monitoring reveals increased PAP and PAWP and decreased cardiac output.

Right-sided failure
- BNP levels are elevated.
- Blood chemistry tests show decreased sodium and potassium levels and increased BUN and creatinine levels.
- Chest X-ray reveals pulmonary congestion, cardiomegaly, and pleural effusions.
- ABG levels indicate hypoxemia and hypercapnia.
- ECG shows left and right ventricular hypertrophy.
- Echocardiogram shows increased size of chambers and decrease in wall motion.
- Hemodynamic monitoring shows increased CVP and right ventricular pressure and decreased cardiac output.

NURSING DIAGNOSES
- Decreased cardiac output
- Excess fluid volume
- Impaired gas exchange

TREATMENT
- Oxygen therapy, possibly requiring intubation and mechanical ventilation
- Establishing a low-sodium diet and limiting fluids
- IABP
- Left ventricular assist device (for left-sided failure)
- Paracentesis (for right-sided failure)
- Thoracentesis (for right-sided failure)

Drug therapy
- Human BNP: nesiritide (Natrecor)
- Angiotensin-converting enzyme (ACE) inhibitors: captopril (Capoten), enalapril (Vasotec), lisinopril (Prinivil)
- Diuretics: furosemide (Lasix), bumetanide (Bumex), metolazone (Zaroxolyn)
- Analgesic: morphine I.V.
- Cardiac glycoside: digoxin (Lanoxin)
- Inotropic agents: dopamine, dobutamine, inamrinone (Amrinone), milrinone

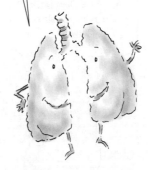

Left-sided heart failure causes pulmonary symptoms.

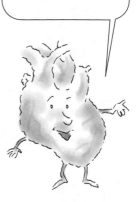

Right-sided heart failure causes systemic symptoms.

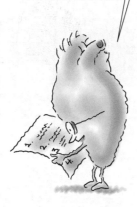

Understanding risk factors for hypertension is important. After all, some of these risk factors can be modified, eliminating the need for drug therapy.

- Nitrates: isosorbide (Isordil), nitroglycerin
- Vasodilator: nitroprusside (Nitropress)

INTERVENTIONS AND RATIONALES

- Assess cardiovascular status, vital signs, and hemodynamic variables *to detect signs of reduced cardiac output.*
- Assess respiratory status and oxygenation *to detect increasing fluid in the lungs and respiratory failure.*
- Keep the client in semi-Fowler's position *to increase chest expansion and improve ventilation.*
- Administer medications, as prescribed, *to enhance cardiac performance and reduce excess fluids.*
- Administer oxygen *to enhance arterial oxygenation.*
- Measure and record intake and output. *Intake greater than output may indicate fluid retention.*
- Monitor laboratory studies *to detect electrolyte imbalances, renal failure, and impaired cardiac circulation.*
- Provide suctioning, if necessary, and assist with turning, coughing, and deep breathing *to prevent pulmonary complications.*
- Restrict oral fluids *because excess fluids can worsen heart failure.*
- Weigh the client daily. *A weight gain of 1 to 2 lb (0.5 to 1 kg) per day indicates fluid gain.*
- Measure and record the client's abdominal girth. *An increase in abdominal girth suggests worsening fluid retention and right-sided heart failure.*
- Maintain the client's prescribed diet (low sodium) *to reduce fluid accumulation.*
- Encourage the client to express feelings, such as a fear of dying, *to reduce anxiety.*

Teaching topics

- Explanation of the disorder and treatment plan
- Medications and possible adverse effects
- Limiting sodium intake and supplementing diet with foods high in potassium
- Recognizing signs and symptoms of fluid overload
- Elevating legs when seated
- Contacting the American Heart Association

Hypertension

Persistent elevation of systolic or diastolic blood pressure (systolic pressure higher than 140 mm Hg, diastolic pressure higher than 90 mm Hg) indicates hypertension. Hypertension results from a narrowing of the arterioles, which increases peripheral resistance, necessitating increased force to circulate blood through the body.

There are two major types of hypertension. Essential hypertension, the most common, has no known cause, though many factors play a role in its development. Secondary hypertension is caused by renal disease or other systemic diseases.

Mild to very severe

Hypertension is classified according to three stages:

prehypertension: systolic 120 to 139 mm Hg or diastolic 80 to 89 mm Hg

stage 1: systolic 140 to 159 mm Hg or diastolic 90 to 99 mm Hg

stage 2: systolic 160 mm Hg or higher or diastolic 100 mm Hg or higher

CAUSES

- Cushing's disease
- No known cause (essential hypertension)
- Hormonal contraceptive use
- Pheochromocytoma
- Pregnancy
- Primary hyperaldosteronism
- Renovascular disease
- Thyroid, pituitary, or parathyroid disease
- Use of drugs, such as cocaine

CONTRIBUTING FACTORS (ESSENTIAL HYPERTENSION)

- Aging
- Atherosclerosis
- Diet (sodium and caffeine)
- Family history
- Obesity
- Race (more common in blacks)
- Sex (more common in males over age 40)
- Smoking
- Stress

ASSESSMENT FINDINGS
- Asymptomatic
- Cerebral ischemia
- Dizziness
- Elevated blood pressure
- Headache
- Heart failure
- Left ventricular hypertrophy
- Papilledema
- Renal failure
- Vision disturbances, including blindness

DIAGNOSTIC TEST RESULTS
- Blood chemistry tests show elevated sodium, BUN, creatinine, and cholesterol levels.
- Blood pressure measurements result in sustained readings higher than 140/90 mm Hg.
- Chest X-ray reveals cardiomegaly.
- ECG shows left ventricular hypertrophy.
- Ophthalmoscopic examination shows retinal changes, such as severe arteriolar narrowing, papilledema, and hemorrhage.
- Urinalysis shows proteinuria, RBCs, and WBCs.

NURSING DIAGNOSES
- Excess fluid volume
- Deficient knowledge (disease process and treatment plan)
- Imbalanced nutrition: More than body requirements

TREATMENT
- Activity changes: regular exercise to reduce weight, if appropriate (see *Treating hypertension: Step-by-step*)
- Dietary changes: establishing a low-sodium diet and limiting alcohol intake (see *Dash into dietary changes,* page 50)

Drug therapy
- ACE inhibitors: captopril (Capoten), enalapril (Vasotec), lisinopril (Prinivil)
- Antihypertensives: methyldopa, hydralazine, prazosin (Minipress), doxazosin (Cardura)
- Beta-adrenergic blockers: propranolol (Inderal), metoprolol (Lopressor), carteolol (Cartrol), penbutolol (Levatol)
- Calcium channel blockers: nifedipine (Procardia), verapamil (Calan), diltiazem (Cardizem), nicardipine (Cardene)
- Diuretics: furosemide (Lasix), spironolactone (Aldactone), hydrochlorothiazide (Microzide), bumetanide (Bumex)
- Vasodilator: nitroprusside (Nitropress)

INTERVENTIONS AND RATIONALES
- Assess cardiovascular status, including vital signs *to detect cardiac compromise.*

Treating hypertension: Step-by-step

The National Institutes of Health recommend a stepped-care approach for treating primary hypertension.

STEP 1
The first step involves lifestyle modifications, including weight reduction, moderation of alcohol intake, reduction of sodium intake, and smoking cessation.

STEP 2
If the client fails to achieve the desired blood pressure, continue lifestyle modifications and begin drug therapy. Preferred drugs include thiazide-type diuretics, angiotensin-converting enzyme (ACE) inhibitors, or beta-adrenergic blockers. If these drugs aren't effective or acceptable, angiotensin receptor blockers or calcium channel blockers may be used.

STEP 3
If desired blood pressure still isn't achieved, drug dosage is increased, another drug is substituted for the first drug, or a drug from a different class is added.

STEP 4
If the client fails to achieve the desired blood pressure or make significant progress, add a second or third agent or a diuretic (if one isn't already prescribed). Second or third agents may include vasodilators, alpha$_1$-antagonists, peripherally acting adrenergic neuron antagonists, ACE inhibitors, and calcium channel blockers.

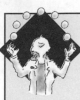

Management moments

Dash into dietary changes

Studies indicate that using the National Institutes of Health Dash into Dietary Changes (DASH) combination diet lowers blood pressure and may also help prevent it. The diet is low in cholesterol; high in dietary fiber, potassium, calcium, and magnesium; and moderately high in protein. If you educate your client about this diet, he may be able to control his blood pressure without the use of medication.

Here's an example of a DASH plan based on a 2,000-calorie diet. Depending on caloric needs, the number of servings in a food group may vary.

Food group	Daily servings	Serving sizes
Grains	7 to 8	1 slice bread 1/2 cup celery 1/2 cup cooked rice, pasta, or cereal
Vegetables	4 to 5	1 cup raw leafy vegetable 1/2 cup cooked vegetable 6 oz vegetable juice
Fruit	4 to 5	6 oz fruit juice 1 medium fruit 1/4 cup dried fruit 1/4 cup fresh, frozen, or canned fruit
Low-fat or nonfat dairy products	2 to 3	8 oz milk 1 cup yogurt 1 1/2 oz cheese
Meat, poultry, and fish	2 or less	3 oz cooked meat, poultry, or fish
Nuts, seeds, and legumes	4 to 5 per week	1 1/2 oz or 1/3 cup nuts 1/2 oz or 2 tablespoons seeds 1/2 cup cooked legumes

• Take an average of two or more blood pressure readings rather than relying on one single abnormal reading *to establish hypertension*.
• Administer medications as prescribed *to lower blood pressure*.
• Assess blood pressure reading in the lying, sitting, and standing positions *to monitor for orthostatic hypotension* (observe for pallor, diaphoresis, or vertigo).
• Assess neurologic status and observe *for changes that may indicate an alteration in cerebral perfusion* (stroke or hemorrhage).
• Monitor and record intake and output and daily weight *to detect fluid volume overload*.

• Maintain the client's prescribed diet *because a high-sodium, high-cholesterol diet may contribute to hypertension*.
• Encourage the client to express feelings about daily stress *to reduce anxiety*.
• Maintain a quiet environment *to reduce stress*.

Teaching topics
• Explanation of the disorder and treatment plan
• Medications and possible adverse effects
• Taking blood pressure daily and recognizing when to notify the physician

- Beginning a smoking cessation program, if appropriate
- Reducing alcohol intake to moderate levels
- Following a low-cholesterol, low-sodium diet
- Following a program of regular exercise
- Losing weight, if appropriate
- Contacting the American Heart Association

Hypovolemic shock

In hypovolemic shock, reduced intravascular blood volume causes circulatory dysfunction and inadequate tissue perfusion. Without sufficient blood or fluid replacement, hypovolemic shock syndrome may lead to irreversible cerebral and renal damage, cardiac arrest and, ultimately, death.

Hypovolemic shock requires early recognition of signs and symptoms and prompt, aggressive treatment to improve the prognosis.

CAUSES
- Acute blood loss (approximately one-fifth of total volume)
- Acute pancreatitis
- Dehydration from excessive perspiration
- Diabetes insipidus
- Diuresis
- Inadequate fluid intake
- Intestinal obstruction
- Peritonitis
- Severe diarrhea or protracted vomiting

ASSESSMENT FINDINGS
- Cold, pale, clammy skin
- Decreased sensorium
- Hypotension with narrowing pulse pressure
- Rapid, shallow respirations
- Reduced urine output (less than 25 ml/hour)
- Tachycardia

DIAGNOSTIC TEST RESULTS
- Blood tests show elevated potassium, serum lactate, and BUN levels; increased urine specific gravity (greater than 1.020) and urine osmolality; decreased blood pH; decreased partial pressure of arterial oxygen, increased partial pressure of arterial carbon dioxide; and possible decreased Hb and HCT (if the client is bleeding).
- Gastroscopy, aspiration of gastric contents through a nasogastric tube, and X-rays identify internal bleeding sites.
- ABG analysis reveals metabolic acidosis.

NURSING DIAGNOSES
- Ineffective tissue perfusion: Cardiopulmonary, renal, cerebral, GI
- Decreased cardiac output
- Deficient fluid volume

TREATMENT
- Blood and fluid replacement
- Control of bleeding

INTERVENTIONS AND RATIONALES
Management of hypovolemic shock necessitates prompt, aggressive supportive measures and careful assessment and monitoring of vital signs. Follow these priorities:
- Check for a patent airway and adequate circulation. If blood pressure and heart rate are absent, start CPR *to prevent irreversible organ damage and death*.
- Record blood pressure, pulse rate, peripheral pulses, respiratory rate, and pulse oximetry every 15 minutes and monitor the ECG continuously. A systolic blood pressure lower than 80 mm Hg usually results in inadequate coronary artery blood flow, cardiac ischemia, arrhythmias, and further complications of low cardiac output. When blood pressure drops below 80 mm Hg, increase the oxygen flow rate and notify the physician immediately. *A progressive drop in blood pressure accompanied by a thready pulse generally signals inadequate cardiac output from reduced intravascular volume.*
- Insert large-bore (14G) I.V. catheters and infuse normal saline or lactated Ringer's solution and appropriate blood products, as indicated, *to correct fluid volume deficit*.
- Insert an indwelling urinary catheter to measure hourly urine output. If output is less than 30 ml/hour in adults, increase the fluid infusion rate but watch for signs of fluid overload, such as an increase in PAWP. Notify the physician if urine output doesn't improve. An osmotic diuretic such as mannitol (Osmitrol)

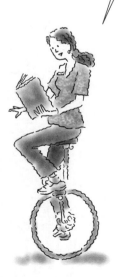

I better back up and study assessment findings again. Early recognition of signs and symptoms of hypovolemic shock are necessary to prevent irreversible damage.

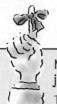

Memory jogger

To remember the signs and symptoms of MI, think DANCE PAD:

Dyspnea

Anxiety

Nausea and vomiting

Crushing substernal chest pain

Elevated temperature

Pallor

Arrhythmias

Diaphoresis

may be ordered *to increase renal blood flow and urine output.*

• Monitor hemodynamic parameters (CVP, PAP, and PAWP) *to determine how much fluid to give.*

• Draw an arterial blood sample to measure ABG values. Administer oxygen and adjust the oxygen flow rate to a higher or lower level as ABG measurements indicate *to ensure adequate oxygenation of tissues.*

• Draw venous blood for complete blood count and electrolytes, type and crossmatch, and coagulation studies *to guide the treatment regimen.*

• During therapy, assess skin color and temperature and note any changes. Cold, clammy skin may be a sign of continuing peripheral vascular constriction, indicating progressive shock.

• Explain all procedures and their purpose. Throughout these emergency measures, provide emotional support to the client and his family *to help them cope with the overwhelming situation.*

Teaching topics

• Explanation of the disorder and treatment plan

• Medications and possible adverse effects

• Cause of hypovolemia and treatment options

Myocardial infarction

In MI (an acute coronary syndrome), reduced blood flow in one of the coronary arteries leads to myocardial ischemia, injury, and necrosis.

In transmural MI, tissue damage extends through all myocardial layers. In subendocardial MI, usually only the innermost layer is damaged.

CAUSES

• Narrowed or occluded coronary vessels

• Anoxia or hypoxia

• Hypovolemia

CONTRIBUTING FACTORS

• Aging

• Decreased serum high-density lipoprotein levels

• Diabetes mellitus

• Elevated serum triglyceride, low-density lipoprotein, and cholesterol levels

• Excessive intake of saturated fats, carbohydrates, or salt

• Hypertension

• Obesity

• Positive family history of CAD

• Postmenopause

• Sedentary lifestyle

• Smoking

• Stress

• Use of amphetamines or cocaine

ASSESSMENT FINDINGS

• Anxiety

• Arrhythmias

• Crushing substernal chest pain that may radiate to the jaw, back, and arms; lasts longer than anginal pain; is unrelieved by rest or nitroglycerin; may not be present (in asymptomatic or silent MI); in women, possible atypical symptoms of pain and fatigue

• Diaphoresis

• Dyspnea

• Elevated temperature

• Nausea and vomiting

• Pallor

DIAGNOSTIC TEST RESULTS

• ECG shows an enlarged Q wave, an elevated or depressed ST segment, and T-wave inversion.

• Blood chemistry studies show increased CK, AST, and lipids; positive CK-MB fraction; and increased troponin T.

• Blood studies show increased WBC count.

NURSING DIAGNOSES

• Decreased cardiac output

• Ineffective tissue perfusion: Cardiopulmonary

• Anxiety

TREATMENT

• Bed rest with bedside commode

• Coronary artery bypass graft

• IABP

• Left ventricular assist device

• Low-calorie, low-cholesterol, low-fat diet

• Monitoring vital signs, urine output, ECG, and hemodynamic status

- Ongoing laboratory studies: ABG levels, CK with isoenzymes, electrolyte levels, cardiac troponins
- Oxygen therapy
- PTCA or coronary artery stent placement
- Pulmonary artery catheterization (to detect left- or right-sided heart failure)

Drug therapy
- Analgesic: morphine I.V.
- ACE inhibitors: captopril (Capoten), enalapril (Vasotec)
- Antiarrhythmics: amiodarone (Cordarone), lidocaine (Xylocaine), procainamide
- Anticoagulants: aspirin, dalteparin (Fragmin), enoxaparin (Lovenox), heparin I.V. after thrombolytic therapy
- Antihypertensive: hydralazine
- Beta-adrenergic blockers: propranolol (Inderal), nadolol (Corgard), metoprolol (Lopressor); beta-adrenergic blockers contraindicated if client also has hypotension, asthma, or chronic obstructive pulmonary disease
- Calcium channel blockers: nifedipine (Procardia), verapamil (Calan), diltiazem (Cardizem)
- I.V. atropine or pacemaker for symptomatic bradycardia or heart block
- Nitrate: nitroglycerin I.V.
- Thrombolytic therapy: alteplase (Activase), streptokinase (Streptase), reteplase (Retavase); should be given within 6 hours of onset of symptoms but most effective when started within 3 hours

INTERVENTIONS AND RATIONALES
- Monitor ECG *to detect ischemia, injury, new or extended infarction, arrhythmias, conduction defects.* (See *Close monitoring for complications,* page 54.)
- Assess cardiovascular and respiratory status *to watch for signs of heart failure, such as an S_3 or S_4 gallop, crackles, cough, tachypnea, and edema.*
- Administer oxygen, as ordered, *to improve oxygen supply to heart muscle.*
- Obtain an ECG reading during acute pain *to detect myocardial ischemia, injury, or infarction.*
- Monitor and record vital signs and hemodynamic variables *to monitor response to therapy and detect complications.*

- Monitor and record intake and output *to assess renal perfusion and possible fluid retention.*
- Follow laboratory values *to detect myocardial damage, electrolyte abnormalities, drug levels, renal function, and coagulation.*
- Maintain bed rest *to reduce oxygen demands on the heart.*
- Maintain the client's prescribed diet *to reduce fluid retention and cholesterol levels.*
- Provide postoperative care, if necessary, *to avoid postoperative complications and help the client achieve a full recovery.*
- Provide emotional support to allay the client's anxiety *because anxiety increases oxygen demand.*
- Administer medications, as ordered, *to improve cardiac function.*

Teaching topics
- Explanation of the disorder and treatment plan
- Medications and possible adverse effects
- Undergoing cardiac rehabilitation
- Maintaining a low-cholesterol, low-fat, low-sodium diet
- Modifying risk factors
- Stopping smoking, if appropriate
- Differentiating between the pain of angina and MI
- Contacting the American Heart Association

Myocarditis

Myocarditis is focal or diffuse inflammation of the cardiac muscle (myocardium). It may be acute or chronic and can occur at any age. Frequently, myocarditis fails to produce specific cardiovascular symptoms or ECG abnormalities, and recovery is usually spontaneous, without residual defects. Occasionally, myocarditis is complicated by heart failure; rarely, it may lead to cardiomyopathy.

CAUSES
- Bacterial infections: diphtheria, tuberculosis, typhoid fever, tetanus, and staphylococcal, pneumococcal, and gonococcal infections
- Chemical poisons such as chronic alcoholism

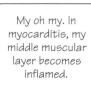

Thrombolytic therapy is most effective when started within 3 hours of onset of MI symptoms.

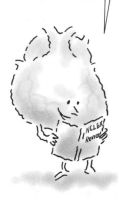

My oh my. In myocarditis, my middle muscular layer becomes inflamed.

Management moments

Close monitoring for complications

After a myocardial infarction (MI), the nurse must closely monitor the client for complications. Early recognition and treatment of these complications can improve the client's outcome.

Complication	What to look for
Arrhythmias	• Premature ventricular contractions on electro-cardiogram • Ventricular tachycardia • Ventricular fibrillation • In inferior wall MI, bradycardia, junctional rhythms, or atrioventricular blocks • In anterior wall MI, tachycardia or atrioventricular blocks
Heart failure	• Shortness of breath • Dyspnea on exertion • Crackles on auscultation of the lungs • Jugular vein distention
Cardiogenic shock	• Hypotension • Tachycardia • Third and fourth heart sounds • Decreased level of consciousness • Decreased urine output • Jugular vein distention • Cool, pale skin
Papillary muscle rupture	• Jugular vein distention • Dyspnea • Holosystolic murmur on auscultation
Pericarditis	• Chest pain that's relieved by sitting up • Friction rub on auscultation

• Helminthic infections such as trichinosis
• Hypersensitive immune reactions, such as acute rheumatic fever and postcardiotomy syndrome
• Parasitic infections, especially South American trypanosomiasis (Chagas' disease) in infants and immunosuppressed adults; also, toxoplasmosis
• Radiation therapy: large doses of radiation to the chest for treatment of lung or breast cancer
• Viral infections (most common cause in the United States and western Europe): coxsackievirus A and B strains and,

possibly, poliomyelitis, influenza, rubeola, rubella, and adenoviruses and echoviruses

ASSESSMENT FINDINGS
• Arrhythmias (S_3 and S_4 gallops, faint S_1)
• Cardiomyopathy
• Chronic valvulitis (when myocarditis results from rheumatic fever)
• Dyspnea
• Fatigue
• Fever

- Mild, continuous pressure or soreness in the chest (unlike the recurring, stress-related pain of angina pectoris)
- Palpitations
- Thromboembolism

DIAGNOSTIC TEST RESULTS

- Blood tests show elevated cardiac enzyme levels (CK, the CK-MB isoenzyme, and AST), increased WBC count and ESR, and elevated antibody titers (such as antistreptolysin-O titer in rheumatic fever).
- ECG typically shows diffuse ST-segment and T-wave abnormalities (as in pericarditis), conduction defects (prolonged PR interval), and other supraventricular arrhythmias.
- Endomyocardial biopsy confirms the diagnosis, but a negative biopsy doesn't exclude the diagnosis. A repeat biopsy may be needed.
- Stool and throat cultures may identify the causative bacteria.

NURSING DIAGNOSES

- Activity intolerance
- Decreased cardiac output
- Hyperthermia

TREATMENT

- Bed rest
- Diet: sodium restriction

Drug therapy

- Antiarrhythmics: amiodarone (Cordarone), procainamide
- Antibiotics: according to sensitivity of infecting organism
- Anticoagulants: warfarin (Coumadin), heparin, dalteparin (Fragmin), enoxaparin (Lovenox)
- Cardiac glycoside: digoxin (Lanoxin) to increase myocardial contractility
- Diuretic: furosemide (Lasix)

INTERVENTIONS AND RATIONALES

- Assess cardiovascular status frequently to monitor for signs of heart failure, such as dyspnea, hypotension, and tachycardia. Check for changes in cardiac rhythm or conduction. *Rhythm disturbances may indicate early cardiac decompensation.*
- Observe for signs of digoxin toxicity (anorexia, nausea, vomiting, blurred vision,

cardiac arrhythmias) and for complicating factors that may potentiate toxicity, such as electrolyte imbalances or hypoxia, *to prevent further complications.*
- Stress the importance of bed rest *to decrease oxygen demands on the heart.* Assist with bathing as necessary; provide a bedside commode, *which puts less stress on the heart than using a bedpan.* Reassure the client that activity limitations are temporary.
- Offer diversional activities that are physically undemanding *to decrease anxiety.*

Teaching topics

- Explanation of the disorder and treatment plan
- Medications and possible adverse effects
- Restricting activities for as long as the physician prescribes
- If taking digoxin at home, checking pulse for 1 full minute before taking the dose and withholding the dose and notifying the physician if pulse rate falls below the predetermined rate (usually 60 beats/minute)
- Resuming normal activities slowly, when appropriate, and avoiding competitive sports

Pericarditis

Pericarditis is an inflammation of the pericardium, the fibroserous sac that envelops, supports, and protects the heart. It occurs in both acute and chronic forms. Acute pericarditis can be fibrinous or effusive, with purulent, serous, or hemorrhagic exudate; chronic constrictive pericarditis is characterized by dense fibrous pericardial thickening. The prognosis depends on the underlying cause but is generally good in acute pericarditis, unless constriction occurs.

CAUSES

- Bacterial, fungal, or viral infection (infectious pericarditis)
- High-dose radiation to the chest
- Hypersensitivity or autoimmune disease, such as acute rheumatic fever (most common cause of pericarditis in children), systemic lupus erythematosus, and rheumatoid arthritis
- Idiopathic factors (most common in acute pericarditis)

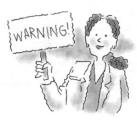

Administer cardiac glycosides carefully. Some clients with myocarditis show a paradoxical sensitivity to even small doses of these drugs.

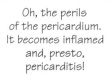

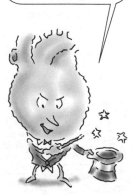

Oh, the perils of the pericardium. It becomes inflamed and, presto, pericarditis!

- Neoplasms (primary or metastasis from lungs, breasts, or other organs)
- Postcardiac injury, such as MI (which later causes an autoimmune reaction [Dressler's syndrome] in the pericardium), trauma, or surgery that leaves the pericardium intact but causes blood to leak into the pericardial cavity
- Uremia

ASSESSMENT FINDINGS
Acute pericarditis
- Pericardial friction rub (grating sound heard as the heart moves)
- Sharp and usually sudden pain that usually starts over the sternum and radiates to the neck, shoulders, back, and arms (Unlike the pain of MI, pericardial pain is commonly pleuritic, increasing with deep inspiration and decreasing when the client sits up and leans forward, pulling the heart away from the diaphragmatic pleurae of the lungs.)
- Symptoms of cardiac tamponade (pallor, clammy skin, hypotension, pulsus paradoxus, neck vein distention)
- Symptoms of heart failure (dyspnea, orthopnea, tachycardia, ill-defined substernal chest pain, feeling of fullness in the chest)

Chronic pericarditis
- Gradual increase in systemic venous pressure
- Pericardial friction rub
- Symptoms similar to those of chronic right-sided heart failure (fluid retention, ascites, hepatomegaly)

DIAGNOSTIC TEST RESULTS
- Blood tests reflect inflammation and may show normal or elevated WBC count, especially in infectious pericarditis; elevated ESR; and slightly elevated cardiac enzyme levels with associated myocarditis.
- Culture of pericardial fluid obtained by open surgical drainage or cardiocentesis sometimes identifies a causative organism in bacterial or fungal pericarditis.
- Echocardiography confirms the diagnosis when it shows an echo-free space between the ventricular wall and the pericardium (in cases of pleural effusion).
- ECG shows the following changes in acute pericarditis: elevation of ST segments in the

standard limb leads and most precordial leads without significant changes in QRS morphology that occur with MI, atrial ectopic rhythms such as AF, and diminished QRS voltage in pericardial effusion.

NURSING DIAGNOSES
- Decreased cardiac output
- Deficient diversional activity
- Acute pain

TREATMENT
- Bed rest
- Surgery: pericardiocentesis (in cases of cardiac tamponade), partial pericardectomy (for recurrent pericarditis), total pericardectomy (for constrictive pericarditis)

Drug therapy
- Antibiotics: according to sensitivity of infecting organism
- Corticosteroid: methylprednisolone (Solu-Medrol)
- Nonsteroidal anti-inflammatory drugs (NSAIDs): aspirin, indomethacin (Indocin)

INTERVENTIONS AND RATIONALES
- Provide complete bed rest *to decrease oxygen demands on the heart.*
- Assess pain in relation to respiration and body position *to distinguish pericardial pain from myocardial ischemic pain.*
- Place the client in an upright position *to relieve dyspnea and chest pain.*
- Provide analgesics and oxygen, and reassure the client with acute pericarditis that his condition is temporary and treatable *to promote client comfort and allay anxiety.*
- Monitor the client for signs of cardiac compression or cardiac tamponade, possible complications of pericardial effusion. Signs include decreased blood pressure, increased CVP, and pulsus paradoxus. Keep a pericardiocentesis set handy whenever pericardial effusion is suspected *because cardiac tamponade requires immediate treatment.*
- Explain tests and treatments to the client. If surgery is necessary, he should learn deep breathing and coughing exercises beforehand *to alleviate fear and anxiety and promote compliance with the postoperative treatment regimen.* Postoperative care is similar to that given after cardiothoracic surgery.

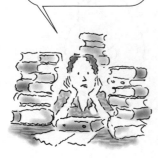

Face it. Cardiovascular care is a huge topic. Feeling overwhelmed by information? Take a break to clear your head.

Teaching topics
- Explanation of the disorder and treatment plan
- Medications and possible adverse effects
- Explanation of all tests and treatments
- Coughing and deep breathing exercises
- Slow resumption of daily activities and scheduled rest periods in daily routine

Peripheral artery disease

In peripheral artery disease, the obstruction or narrowing of the lumen of the aorta and its major branches causes an interruption of blood flow, usually to the legs and feet. Peripheral artery disease may affect the carotid, vertebral, innominate, subclavian, mesenteric, and celiac arteries. Occlusions may be acute or chronic and commonly cause severe ischemia, skin ulceration, and gangrene.

Peripheral artery disease is more common in males than in females. The prognosis depends on the location of the occlusion, the development of collateral circulation to counteract reduced blood flow and, in acute disease, the time elapsed between the occlusion and its removal.

CAUSES
- Atherosclerosis
- Emboli formation
- Thrombosis
- Trauma or fracture

CONTRIBUTING FACTORS
- Age
- Diabetes
- Family history of vascular disorders, MI, or stroke
- Hyperlipidemia
- Hypertension
- Smoking

ASSESSMENT FINDINGS
Assessment findings depend on the site of the occlusion.

Femoral, popliteal, or innominate arteries
- Mottling of the extremity
- Pallor
- Paralysis and paresthesia in the affected arm or leg
- Pulselessness distal to the occlusion
- Sudden and localized pain in the affected arm or leg (most common symptom)
- Temperature change that occurs distal to the occlusion

Internal and external carotid arteries
- Absent or decreased pulsation with an auscultatory bruit over affected vessels
- Stroke
- Transient ischemic attacks (TIAs), which produce transient monocular blindness, dysarthria, hemiparesis, possible aphasia, confusion, decreased mentation, headache

Subclavian artery
- Subclavian steel syndrome (characterized by the backflow of blood from the brain through the vertebral artery on the same side as the occlusion into the subclavian artery distal to the occlusion; clinical effects of vertebrobasilar occlusion and exercise-induced arm claudication)

Vertebral and basilar arteries
- TIAs, which produce binocular vision disturbances, vertigo, dysarthria, and falling down without loss of consciousness

DIAGNOSTIC TEST RESULTS
- Arteriography demonstrates the type (thrombus or embolus), location, and degree of obstruction and collateral circulation.
- Doppler ultrasonography shows decreased blood flow distal to the occlusion.
- EEG and a computed tomography scan may be necessary to rule out brain lesions.
- Ophthalmodynamometry helps determine the degree of obstruction in the internal carotid artery by comparing ophthalmic artery pressure to brachial artery pressure on the affected side. A more than 20% difference between pressures suggests insufficiency.

NURSING DIAGNOSES
- Ineffective tissue perfusion (type depends on the location of the occlusion)
- Fear
- Risk for injury

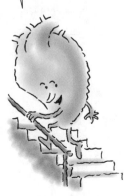

Tickle my toes. Everyone depends on me. If my aorta is obstructed, even the feet feel it.

TREATMENT
- Light exercise such as walking
- Surgery (for acute occlusion): atherectomy, balloon angioplasty, bypass graft, embolectomy, laser angioplasty, patch grafting, stent placement, thromboendarterectomy, or amputation

Drug therapy
- Anticoagulants: heparin, dalteparin (Fragmin), enoxaparin (Lovenox), warfarin (Coumadin)
- Antiplatelets: aspirin, pentoxifylline (Trental)
- Thrombolytic agents: alteplase (Activase), streptokinase (Streptase)

INTERVENTIONS AND RATIONALES
- Advise the client to stop smoking and to follow the prescribed medical regimen *to modify risk factors and promote compliance.*

Preoperatively (during an acute episode)
- Assess the client's circulatory status by checking for the most distal pulses and by inspecting his skin color and temperature. *Decreased tissue perfusion causes mottling; skin also becomes cooler and skin texture changes.*
- Provide pain relief as needed *to help decrease ischemic pain.*
- Administer I.V. heparin as needed *to prevent thrombi.* Use an infusion pump *to ensure the proper flow rate.*
- Reposition the foot frequently *to prevent pressure on any one area.* Strictly avoid elevating or applying heat to the affected leg. *Directly heating extremities causes increased tissue metabolism; if arteries don't dilate normally, tissue perfusion decreases and ischemia may occur.*
- Watch for signs of fluid and electrolyte imbalance, and monitor intake and output for signs of renal failure (urine output less than 30 ml/hour). *Electrolyte imbalances and renal failure are complications that may occur as a result of arterial occlusion and tissue damage.*
- If the client has a carotid, innominate, vertebral, or subclavian artery occlusion, monitor him for signs of stroke, such as numbness in an arm or leg and intermittent blindness, to *detect early signs of decreased cerebral perfusion.*

Postoperatively
- Monitor the client's vital signs. Continuously assess his circulatory function by inspecting skin color and temperature and by checking for distal pulses. In charting, compare earlier assessments and observations. Watch closely for signs of hemorrhage (tachycardia, hypotension) and check dressings for excessive bleeding *to prevent or detect postoperative complications.*
- In carotid, innominate, vertebral, or subclavian artery occlusion, assess neurologic status frequently for changes in level of consciousness or muscle strength and pupil size *to ensure prompt treatment of deteriorating neurologic status.*
- In mesenteric artery occlusion, connect a nasogastric tube to low intermittent suction. Monitor intake and output. (Low urine output may indicate damage to renal arteries during surgery.) Assess abdominal status. *Increasing abdominal distention and tenderness may indicate extension of bowel ischemia with resulting gangrene, necessitating further excision, or peritonitis.*
- In saddle block occlusion, check distal pulses for adequate circulation. Watch for signs of renal failure and mesenteric artery occlusion (severe abdominal pain) and cardiac arrhythmias, which may precipitate embolus formation, *to ensure prompt recognition and treatment of complications.*
- In iliac artery occlusion, monitor urine output for signs of renal failure from decreased perfusion to the kidneys as a result of surgery. Provide meticulous catheter care *to prevent complications.*
- In both femoral and popliteal artery occlusions, monitor peripheral pulses. Assist with early ambulation, but discourage prolonged sitting *to encourage circulation to the extremities.*
- After amputation, check the client's stump carefully for drainage and record its color and amount and the time *to detect hemorrhage.* Elevate the stump, and administer adequate analgesic medication *to treat edema and pain.* Because phantom limb pain is common, explain this phenomenon to the client *to reduce the client's anxiety.*
- When preparing the client for discharge, instruct him to watch for signs of recurrence (pain, pallor, numbness, paralysis, absence of pulse) that can result from graft occlusion or

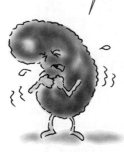

Renal failure may occur as a result of arterial occlusion and tissue damage.

occlusion at another site. Warn him against wearing constrictive clothing. *These measures enable the client to join actively in his care, and allow him to make more informed decisions about his health status.*

Teaching topics
- Explanation of the disorder and treatment options
- Medications and possible adverse effects
- Performing proper foot care
- Recognizing signs of arterial occlusion
- Modifying risk factors

Raynaud's disease

Raynaud's disease is characterized by episodic vasospasm in the small peripheral arteries and arterioles, precipitated by exposure to cold or stress. This condition occurs bilaterally and usually affects the hands or, less often, the feet.

Raynaud's disease is most prevalent in women, particularly between puberty and age 40. A benign condition, it requires no specific treatment and has no serious sequelae.

Raynaud's phenomenon, however, a condition often associated with several connective tissue disorders — such as scleroderma, systemic lupus erythematosus, and polymyositis — has a progressive course, leading to ischemia, gangrene, and amputation. Differentiating the two disorders is difficult because some clients who experience mild symptoms of Raynaud's disease for several years may later develop overt connective tissue disease — most commonly scleroderma.

CAUSES
- Unknown (most probable theory involves an antigen antibody immune response)

ASSESSMENT FINDINGS
- Numbness and tingling that are relieved by warmth
- Sclerodactyly, ulcerations, or chronic paronychia (in longstanding disease)
- Typically, blanching of skin on the fingers, which then becomes cyanotic before changing to red (after exposure to cold or stress)

DIAGNOSTIC TEST RESULTS
- Arteriography reveals vasospasm.
- Plethysmography reveals intermittent vessel occlusion.

NURSING DIAGNOSES
- Ineffective tissue perfusion: Peripheral
- Risk for injury
- Risk for peripheral neurovascular dysfunction
- Acute pain
- Chronic pain

TREATMENT
- Activity changes: avoidance of cold
- Smoking cessation (if appropriate)
- Surgery (used in fewer than one-quarter of clients): sympathectomy

Drug therapy
- Calcium channel blockers: diltiazem (Cardizem), nifedipine (Procardia)
- Vasodilator: phenoxybenzamine (Dibenzyline)

INTERVENTIONS AND RATIONALES
- Warn against exposure to the cold. Tell the client to wear mittens or gloves in cold weather and when handling cold items or defrosting the freezer *to prevent vasospasm, which causes onset of symptoms.*
- Advise the client to avoid stressful situations and to stop smoking *to prevent exacerbation of symptoms.*
- Instruct the client to inspect the skin frequently and to seek immediate care for signs of skin breakdown or infection *to prevent complications.*
- Teach the client about drugs, their use, and their adverse effects *to prevent further complications.*
- Provide psychological support and reassurance *to allay the client's fear of amputation and disfigurement.*

Teaching topics
- Modifying risk factors, including smoking cessation, if appropriate
- Preventive measures such as avoiding cold and stress

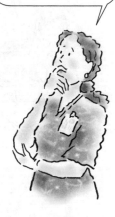

Hmmm... Vasodilators are typically used only in severe cases of Raynaud's disease because the adverse effects of these drugs may be more bothersome than the disease itself.

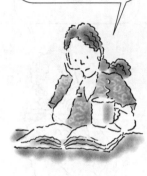

Fever vs. disease. Rheumatic fever follows a group A beta-hemolytic streptococcal infection. Rheumatic heart disease refers to the cardiac manifestations of rheumatic fever.

Rheumatic fever and rheumatic heart disease

Commonly recurrent, acute rheumatic fever is a systemic inflammatory disease of childhood that follows a group A beta-hemolytic streptococcal infection. Rheumatic heart disease refers to the cardiac manifestations of rheumatic fever and includes pancarditis (myocarditis, pericarditis, and endocarditis) during the early acute phase and chronic valvular disease later.

Long-term antibiotic therapy can minimize recurrence of rheumatic fever, reducing the risk of permanent cardiac damage and eventual valvular deformity. However, severe pancarditis occasionally produces fatal heart failure during the acute phase. Of the clients who survive this complication, about 20% die within 10 years.

This disease strikes most often during cool, damp weather in the winter and early spring. In the United States, it's most common in the northern states.

CAUSES
- Hypersensitivity reaction to a group A beta-hemolytic streptococcal infection

ASSESSMENT FINDINGS
- Carditis
- Temperature of 100.4° F (38° C) or greater
- Migratory joint pain or polyarthritis
- Skin lesions such as erythema marginatum (in only 5% of clients)
- Transient chorea (can develop up to 6 months after the original streptococcal infection)

DIAGNOSTIC TEST RESULTS
- Blood tests show elevated WBC count and ESR as well as slight anemia during inflammation.
- Cardiac catheterization evaluates valvular damage and left ventricular function in severe cardiac dysfunction.
- Cardiac enzyme levels may be increased in severe carditis.
- Chest X-rays show normal heart size (except with myocarditis, heart failure, or pericardial effusion).
- C-reactive protein is positive (especially during the acute phase).
- Echocardiography helps evaluate valvular damage, chamber size, and ventricular function.
- ECG shows prolonged PR interval in 20% of clients.

NURSING DIAGNOSES
- Activity intolerance
- Decreased cardiac output
- Risk for infection

TREATMENT
- Bed rest (in severe cases)
- Surgery: corrective valvular surgery (in cases of persistent heart failure)

Drug therapy
- Antibiotics: erythromycin (Erythrocin), penicillin (Pfizerpen)
- NSAIDs: aspirin, indomethacin (Indocin)

INTERVENTIONS AND RATIONALES
- Before giving penicillin, ask the client if he's ever had a hypersensitivity reaction to it. Even if the client has never had a reaction to penicillin, warn that such a reaction is possible *to adequately inform the client about possible treatment complications.*
- Tell the client to stop taking the drug and to immediately report the development of a rash, fever, chills, or other signs of allergy at any time during penicillin therapy *to prevent anaphylaxis.*
- Instruct the client to watch for and report early signs of heart failure, such as dyspnea and a hacking, nonproductive cough, *to prevent further cardiac decompensation.*
- Stress the need for bed rest during the acute phase and suggest appropriate, physically undemanding diversions. *These measures decrease oxygen demands of the heart.*
- After the acute phase, encourage family and friends to spend as much time as possible with the client *to minimize boredom.*
- If the client has severe carditis, help him prepare for permanent changes in his lifestyle *to promote positive coping strategies.*
- Warn the client to watch for and immediately report signs of recurrent streptococcal infection — sudden sore throat, diffuse throat

redness and oropharyngeal exudate, swollen and tender cervical lymph glands, pain on swallowing, a temperature of 101° to 104° F (38.3° to 40° C), headache, and nausea *to prevent complications associated with delayed treatment such as heart valve damage.* Urge the client to avoid people with respiratory tract infections *to prevent reinfection.*
• Make sure the client understands the need to comply with prolonged antibiotic therapy and follow-up care and the need for additional antibiotics during dental surgery *to prevent reinfection.*
• Arrange for a visiting nurse to oversee home care if necessary *to promote compliance.*

Teaching topics
• Explanation of the disorder and treatment plan
• Medications and possible adverse effects
• Watching for and reporting signs of heart failure
• Starting normal activities slowly
• Taking prophylactic antibiotics during dental surgery
• Performing good dental hygiene to prevent gingival infection

Thoracic aortic aneurysm

Thoracic aortic aneurysm is characterized by an abnormal widening of the ascending, transverse, or descending part of the aorta. Aneurysm of the ascending aorta is most common and most commonly fatal.

The aneurysm may be *dissecting,* a hemorrhagic separation in the aortic wall, usually within the medial layer; *saccular,* an outpouching of the arterial wall, with a narrow neck; or *fusiform,* a spindle-shaped enlargement encompassing the entire aortic circumference.

Some aneurysms progress to serious and, eventually, lethal complications such as rupture of an untreated thoracic dissecting aneurysm into the pericardium, with resulting tamponade.

CAUSES
• Atherosclerosis
• Congenital disorders such as coarctation of the aorta

• Fungal infection (infected aneurysm) of the aortic arch and descending segments
• Hypertension
• Syphilis, usually of the ascending aorta (uncommon because of antibiotics)
• Trauma, usually of the descending thoracic aorta, from an accident that shears the aorta transversely (acceleration-deceleration injuries)

ASSESSMENT FINDINGS
Ascending aneurysm
• Bradycardia
• Pain (described as severe, boring, and ripping and extending to the neck, shoulders, lower back, or abdomen)
• Pericardial friction rub caused by a hemopericardium
• Unequal intensities of the right carotid and left radial pulses

Descending aneurysm
• Pain (described as sharp and tearing, usually starting suddenly between the shoulder blades and possibly radiating to the chest)

Transverse aneurysm
• Dry cough
• Dysphagia
• Dyspnea
• Hoarseness
• Pain (described as sharp and tearing and radiating to the shoulders)

DIAGNOSTIC TEST RESULTS
• Aortography, the definitive test, shows the lumen of the aneurysm, its size and location, and the false lumen in a dissecting aneurysm.
• Blood tests may show low Hb levels because of blood loss from a leaking aneurysm.
• Chest X-ray shows widening of the aorta.
• Computed tomography scan confirms and locates the aneurysm and can be used to monitor its progression.
• Echocardiography may help identify a dissecting aneurysm of the aortic root.
• ECG helps distinguish a thoracic aneurysm from MI.
• Transesophageal echocardiography is used to measure the aneurysm in the ascending and descending aorta.

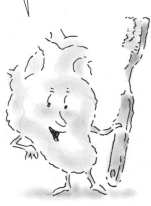
For clients with rheumatic fever, good dental hygiene is necessary to prevent gingival infection.

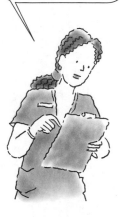
Pain is the key assessment finding with thoracic aortic aneurysm, but the kind of pain depends on the type of aneurysm.

NURSING DIAGNOSES
- Decreased cardiac output
- Ineffective breathing pattern
- Acute pain

TREATMENT
- Surgery: resection of aneurysm with a Dacron or Teflon graft replacement, possible replacement of aortic valve

Drug therapy
- Analgesic: morphine
- Antihypertensives: nitroprusside (Nitropress), labetalol (Trandate)
- Negative inotropic: propranolol (Inderal)

INTERVENTIONS AND RATIONALES
- Monitor the client's blood pressure, PAWP, and CVP *to detect fluid volume deficit.* Also evaluate pain, breathing, and carotid, radial, and femoral pulses *to detect early signs of aneurysm rupture.*
- Review laboratory test results, which must include a complete blood count, differential, electrolytes, typing and crossmatching for whole blood, ABG studies, and urinalysis, *to note Hb levels and ensure that the client can tolerate surgery.*
- Insert an indwelling urinary catheter and monitor intake and output *to evaluate fluid status.*
- Carefully monitor nitroprusside I.V. infusion rate; use a separate I.V. line for infusion. Adjust the dose by slowly increasing the infusion rate. Meanwhile, check blood pressure every 5 minutes until it stabilizes *to note the effectiveness of treatment and prevent hypotension from large dose nitroprusside.*
- With suspected bleeding from an aneurysm, prepare to give a blood transfusion *to adequately replace deficient fluid volume.*
- Explain diagnostic tests. If surgery is scheduled, explain the procedure and expected postoperative care (I.V. lines, endotracheal and drainage tubes, cardiac monitoring, ventilation) *to alleviate the client's anxiety.*

After repair of thoracic aneurysm
- Evaluate the client's level of consciousness. Monitor vital signs, PAP, PAWP, CVP, pulse rate, urine output, and pain *to guide treatment regimen and evaluate its effectiveness.*
- Check respiratory function. Carefully observe and record the type and amount of chest tube drainage and frequently assess heart and breath sounds *to detect early signs of compromise.*
- Monitor I.V. therapy *to prevent fluid excess, which may occur with rapid fluid replacement.*
- Give medications as appropriate *to help improve the client's condition.*
- Watch for signs of infection, especially fever, and excessive wound drainage *to initiate treatment promptly and prevent complications such as sepsis.*
- Assist with range-of-motion exercises of the legs *to prevent thromboembolism due to venostasis during prolonged bed rest.*
- After stabilization of vital signs and respiration, encourage and assist the client in turning, coughing, and deep breathing. If necessary, provide intermittent positive pressure breathing *to promote lung expansion.*
- Help the client walk as soon as he's able *to prevent complications of immobility, such as pneumonia and thromboembolism formation.*
- Before discharge, ensure adherence to antihypertensive therapy by explaining the need for such drugs and the expected adverse effects. Teach the client how to monitor his blood pressure *to prevent complications associated with ineffective blood pressure management such as stroke.*
- Throughout hospitalization, offer the client and family psychological support *to relieve anxiety and feelings of helplessness.*

Teaching topics
- Explanation of the disorder and treatment plan
- Medications and possible adverse effects
- Monitoring blood pressure and reducing hypertension
- Modifying risk factors, including smoking cessation

Thrombophlebitis

Thrombophlebitis is marked by inflammation of the venous wall and thrombus formation. It may affect deep veins or superficial veins.

The thrombus may occlude a vein or detach and embolize to the lungs.

CAUSES
- Hypercoagulability (from cancer, blood dyscrasias, hormonal contraceptives)
- Injury to the venous wall (from I.V. injections, fractures, antibiotics)
- Venous stasis (from varicose veins, pregnancy, heart failure, prolonged bed rest)

ASSESSMENT FINDINGS
Deep vein thrombophlebitis
- Cramping calf pain (may be painless)
- Edema
- Tenderness to touch

Superficial vein thrombophlebitis
- Redness along the vein
- Warmth and tenderness along the vein

DIAGNOSTIC TEST RESULTS
- Hematology reveals increased WBC count.
- Photoplethysmography shows venous-filling defects.
- Ultrasound reveals decreased blood flow.
- Venography shows venous-filling defects.

NURSING DIAGNOSES
- Acute pain
- Activity intolerance
- Ineffective tissue perfusion: Peripheral

TREATMENT
- Activity changes: maintaining bed rest and elevating the affected extremity
- Antiembolism stockings
- Embolectomy and insertion of a vena cava umbrella or filter
- Warm, moist compresses

Drug therapy
- Anticoagulants: warfarin (Coumadin), heparin, enoxaparin (Lovenox)
- Anti-inflammatory agents: aspirin, dalteparin (Fragmin)
- Fibrinolytic agents: streptokinase (Streptase)

INTERVENTIONS AND RATIONALES
- Assess pulmonary status. *Crackles, dyspnea, tachypnea, hemoptysis, and chest pain suggest pulmonary embolism.*

- Assess cardiovascular status. *Tachycardia and chest pain may indicate pulmonary embolism.*
- Assess for bleeding *resulting from anticoagulant therapy.*
- Monitor and record vital signs, such as hypotension, tachycardia, tachypnea, and restlessness. Observe for bruising, epistaxis, blood in stool, bleeding gums, and painful joints. *Tachypnea and tachycardia may suggest pulmonary embolism or hemorrhage.*
- Perform neurovascular checks *to detect nerve or vascular damage.*
- Monitor laboratory values. *Partial thromboplastin time in a client receiving heparin and prothrombin time in a client receiving warfarin should be $1\frac{1}{2}$ to 2 times the control. International normalized ratio should be 2 to 3 for the client receiving warfarin. A falling Hb level and hematocrit indicate blood loss.*
- Maintain bed rest and elevate the affected extremity *to promote venous return and reduce swelling.*
- Administer medications, as prescribed, *to control or dissolve blood clots.*
- Apply warm, moist compresses *to improve circulation to the affected area and relieve pain and inflammation.*
- Measure and record the circumference of thighs and calves. Compare the measurements *to assess for worsening inflammation in the affected leg.*

Teaching topics
- Explanation of the disorder and treatment plan
- Medications and possible adverse effects
- Recognizing signs and symptoms of bleeding and clot formation
- Avoiding prolonged sitting or standing, constrictive clothing, and crossing the legs when seated
- Avoiding hormonal contraceptives

Valvular heart disease

In valvular heart disease, three types of mechanical disruption can occur: stenosis, or narrowing, of the valve opening; incomplete closure of the valve; or prolapse of the valve. These conditions can result from such

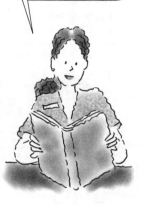

A clot is typically caused by venous stasis, endothelial damage, and hypercoagulability. This is called Virchow's triad.

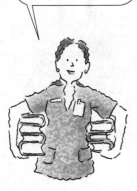

Three types of mechanical disruption can affect heart valves: stenosis, or narrowing, of the valve opening; incomplete closure of the valve; and prolapse of the valve.

disorders as endocarditis (most common), congenital defects, and inflammation, and they can lead to heart failure.

Valvular heart disease occurs in several forms. The most common include:

• aortic insufficiency, in which blood flows back into the left ventricle during diastole, causing fluid overload in the ventricle, which dilates and hypertrophies (The excess volume causes fluid overload in the left atrium and, finally, the pulmonary system. Left ventricular failure and pulmonary edema eventually result.)

• mitral insufficiency, in which blood from the left ventricle flows back into the left atrium during systole, causing the atrium to enlarge to accommodate the backflow (As a result, the left ventricle also dilates to accommodate the increased volume of blood from the atrium and to compensate for diminishing cardiac output.)

• mitral stenosis, in which narrowing of the valve by valvular abnormalities, fibrosis, or calcification obstructs blood flow from the left atrium to the left ventricle (Consequently, left atrial volume and pressure rise and the chamber dilates.)

• mitral valve prolapse (MVP), in which one or both valve leaflets protrude into the left atrium (MVP syndrome is the term used when the anatomic prolapse is accompanied by assessment findings unrelated to the valvular abnormality.)

• tricuspid insufficiency, in which blood flows back into the right atrium during systole, decreasing blood flow to the lungs and left side of the heart. (Cardiac output also lessens. Fluid overload in the right side of the heart can eventually lead to right-sided heart failure.)

CAUSES
Aortic insufficiency
• Endocarditis
• Hypertension
• Idiopathic origin
• Rheumatic fever
• Syphilis

Mitral insufficiency
• Hypertrophic cardiomyopathy
• Left ventricular failure

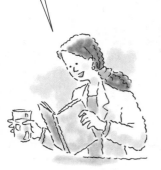

Don't lose your motivation in the middle of your exam preparation. It's important to keep a positive attitude for the long haul.

• Mitral valve prolapse
• Rheumatic fever

Mitral stenosis
• Rheumatic fever

Mitral valve prolapse
• MI involving papillary muscles
• Unknown

Tricuspid insufficiency
• Endocarditis
• Rheumatic fever
• Right-sided heart failure
• Trauma

ASSESSMENT FINDINGS
Aortic insufficiency
• Angina
• Cough
• Dyspnea
• Fatigue
• Palpitations
• Pulmonary vein congestion
• Rapidly rising and collapsing pulses

Mitral insufficiency
• Angina
• Dyspnea
• Fatigue
• Orthopnea
• Peripheral edema

Mitral stenosis
• Dyspnea on exertion
• Fatigue
• Orthopnea
• Palpitations
• Peripheral edema
• Weakness

Mitral valve prolapse
• Chest pain
• Fatigue
• Headache
• Palpitations
• Possibly asymptomatic

Tricuspid insufficiency
• Dyspnea
• Fatigue
• Peripheral edema

DIAGNOSTIC TEST RESULTS

Aortic insufficiency
• Cardiac catheterization shows reduction in arterial diastolic pressures.
• Echocardiography shows left ventricular enlargement.
• ECG shows sinus tachycardia and left ventricular hypertrophy.
• X-ray shows left ventricular enlargement and pulmonary vein congestion.

Mitral insufficiency
• Cardiac catheterization shows mitral insufficiency and elevated atrial pressure and PAWP.
• Echocardiography shows abnormal valve leaflet motion.
• ECG may show left atrial and ventricular hypertrophy.
• X-ray shows left atrial and ventricular enlargement.

Mitral stenosis
• Cardiac catheterization shows diastolic pressure gradient across the valve and elevated left atrial and pulmonary artery wedge pressures.
• Echocardiography shows thickened mitral valve leaflets.
• ECG shows left atrial hypertrophy.
• X-ray shows left atrial and ventricular enlargement.

Mitral valve prolapse
• Color-flow Doppler studies show mitral insufficiency.
• ECG shows prolapse of the mitral valve into the left atrium.

Tricuspid insufficiency
• Echocardiography shows systolic prolapse of the tricuspid valve.
• ECG shows right atrial or right ventricular hypertrophy.
• X-ray shows right atrial dilation and right ventricular enlargement.

NURSING DIAGNOSES
• Activity intolerance
• Anxiety
• Decreased cardiac output

TREATMENT
• Diet: sodium restrictions (in cases of heart failure)
• Surgery: open-heart surgery using cardiopulmonary bypass for valve replacement (in severe cases)

Drug therapy
• Anticoagulant: warfarin (Coumadin) to prevent thrombus formation around diseased or replaced valves

INTERVENTIONS AND RATIONALES
• Watch closely for signs of heart failure or pulmonary edema and for adverse effects of drug therapy *to prevent cardiac decompensation.*
• Place the client in an upright position *to relieve dyspnea.*
• Maintain bed rest and provide assistance with bathing, if necessary, *to decrease oxygen demands on the heart.*
• If the client undergoes surgery, watch for hypotension, arrhythmias, and thrombus formation. Monitor vital signs, ABG levels, intake, output, daily weight, blood chemistries, chest X-rays, and pulmonary artery catheter readings *to detect early signs of postoperative complications and ensure early intervention and treatment.*
• Allow the client to verbalize concerns over being unable to meet life demands because of activity restrictions *to reduce anxiety.*

Teaching topics
• Explanation of the disorder and treatment plan
• Medications and possible adverse effects
• Following diet restrictions and medication schedule
• Need for consistent follow-up care
• Incorporating rest into the daily routine

The heart of the matter is you're almost through with this chapter. Just quiz yourself with the practice questions on the next few pages before moving on.

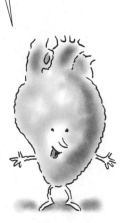

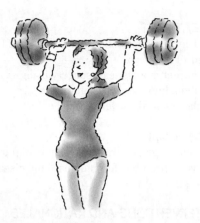

Pump up on practice questions

1. A cardiologist prescribes digoxin (Lanoxin) 125 mcg by mouth every morning for a client diagnosed with heart failure. The pharmacy dispenses tablets that contain 0.25 mg each. How many tablets should the nurse administer in each dose? Record your answer using one decimal place.

_____ tablet(s)

Answer: 0.5. The nurse should begin by converting 125 mcg to milligrams.

$$\frac{125 \text{ mcg}}{1,000} = 0.125 \text{ mg}$$

The following formula is used to calculate drug dosages:

$$\frac{\text{Dose on hand}}{\text{Quantity on hand}} = \frac{\text{Dose desired}}{X}$$

The nurse should use the following equations:

$$\frac{0.25 \text{ mg}}{1 \text{ tablet}} = \frac{0.125 \text{ mg}}{X}$$
$$0.25(X) = 0.125$$
$$X = 0.5 \text{ tablet}$$

➡ NCLEX keys
Client needs category: Physiological integrity
Client needs subcategory: Pharmacological and parenteral therapies
Cognitive level: Application

2. A client is prescribed diltiazem (Cardizem) to manage his hypertension. The nurse should tell the client the diltiazem will:
1. lower his blood pressure only.
2. lower his heart rate and blood pressure.
3. lower his blood pressure and increase his urine output.
4. lower his heart rate and blood pressure and increase his urine output.

Answer: 2. Diltiazem, a calcium channel blocker, will reduce both the heart rate and blood pressure. It doesn't directly affect urine output.

➡ NCLEX keys
Client needs category: Physiological integrity
Client needs subcategory: Pharmacological and parenteral therapies
Cognitive level: Comprehension

3. A client reports substernal chest pain. Test results show electrocardiographic changes and an elevated cardiac troponin level. What should be the focus of nursing care?
1. Improving myocardial oxygenation and reducing cardiac workload
2. Confirming a suspected diagnosis and preventing complications
3. Reducing anxiety and relieving pain
4. Eliminating stressors and providing a nondemanding environment

Answer: 1. The client is exhibiting clinical signs and symptoms of a myocardial infarction (MI); therefore, nursing care should focus on improving myocardial oxygenation and reducing cardiac workload. Confirming the diagnosis of MI and preventing complications, reducing anxiety and relieving pain, and providing a nondemanding environment are secondary to improving myocardial oxygenation and reducing workload. Stressors can't be eliminated, only reduced.

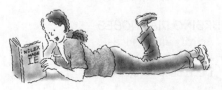

➡ NCLEX keys
Client needs category: Physiological integrity
Client needs subcategory: Reduction of risk
potential
Cognitive level: Analysis

4. A client with a myocardial infarction and
cardiogenic shock is placed on an intra-aortic
balloon pump (IAPB). If the device is functioning properly, the balloon inflates when
the:
1. tricuspid valve is closed.
2. pulmonic valve is open.
3. aortic valve is closed.
4. mitral valve is closed.
Answer: 3. An IAPB inflates during diastole
when the tricuspid and mitral valves are open
and the aortic and pulmonic valves are closed.

➡ NCLEX keys
Client needs category: Physiological integrity
Client needs subcategory: Physiological
adaptation
Cognitive level: Comprehension

5. A client with unstable angina receives
routine applications of nitroglycerin ointment.
The nurse should delay the next dose if the
client has:
1. atrial fibrillation.
2. a systolic blood pressure below
90 mm Hg.
3. a headache.
4. skin redness at the current site.
Answer: 2. Nitroglycerin is a vasodilator and
can lower arterial blood pressure. As a rule,

when the client's systolic blood pressure is
below 90 mm Hg, the nurse should delay the
dose and notify the physician. Nitroglycerin
isn't contraindicated in a client with atrial
fibrillation. Headache, a common occurrence with nitroglycerin isn't a cause for
withholding a dose. Application sites should
be changed with each dose, especially if skin
irritation occurs.

➡ NCLEX keys
Client needs category: Physiological integrity
Client needs subcategory: Pharmacological
and parenteral therapies
Cognitive level: Application

6. A client experiences acute myocardial
ischemia. The nurse administers oxygen and
sublingual nitroglycerin. When assessing an
electrocardiogram (ECG) for evidence that
blood flow to the myocardium has improved,
the nurse should focus on the:
1. widening of the QRS complex.
2. frequency of ectopic beats.
3. return of the ST segment to baseline.
4. presence of a significant Q wave.
Answer: 3. During episodes of myocardial
ischemia, an ECG may show ST-segment
elevation or depression. With successful
treatment, the ST segment should return to
baseline. Widening QRS complex, presence
of a Q wave, and frequent ectopic beats aren't
directly indicative of myocardial ischemia.

➡ NCLEX keys
Client needs category: Physiological integrity
Client needs subcategory: Pharmacological
and parenteral therapies
Cognitive level: Application

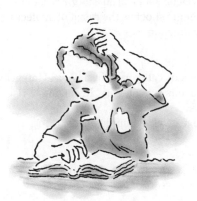

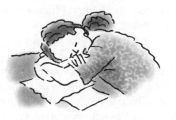

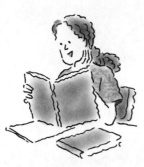

7. Following a left anterior myocardial infarction, a client undergoes insertion of a pulmonary artery catheter. Which finding most strongly suggests left-sided heart failure?
1. A drop in central venous pressure
2. An increase in the cardiac index
3. A rise in pulmonary artery diastolic pressure
4. A decline in mean pulmonary artery pressure

Answer: 3. A rise in pulmonary artery diastolic pressure suggests left-sided heart failure. Central venous pressure would rise in heart failure. The cardiac index would decline in heart failure. The mean pulmonary artery pressure would increase in heart failure.

➡ *NCLEX keys*

Client needs category: Physiological integrity
Client needs subcategory: Physiological adaptation
Cognitive level: Application

8. A client with dilated cardiomyopathy, pulmonary edema, and severe dyspnea is placed on dobutamine. Which assessment finding indicates that the drug is effective?
1. Increased activity tolerance
2. Absence of arrhythmias
3. Negative Homans' sign
4. Blood pressure of 160/90 mm Hg

Answer: 1. Dobutamine should improve the client's symptoms and the client should experience an increased tolerance for activity. The absence of arrhythmias doesn't indicate effectiveness of dobutamine. A negative Homans' sign indicates absence of blood clots, which isn't a therapeutic effect of dobutamine.

➡ *NCLEX keys*

Client needs category: Physiological integrity
Client needs subcategory: Pharmacological and parenteral therapies
Cognitive level: Analysis

9. A nurse administers warfarin (Coumadin) to a client with deep vein thrombophlebitis. Which laboratory value indicates that the client has a therapeutic level of warfarin?

1. Partial thromboplastin time (PTT) $1^{1}/_{2}$ to 2 times the control
2. Prothrombin time (PT) $1^{1}/_{2}$ to 2 times the control
3. International Normalized Ratio (INR) of 3 to 4
4. Hematocrit (HCT) of 32%

Answer: 2. Warfarin is at a therapeutic level when the PT is $1^{1}/_{2}$ to 2 times the control. Values greater than this increase the risk of bleeding and hemorrhage; lower values increase the risk of blood clot formation. Heparin, not warfarin, prolongs PTT. The INR may also be used to determine whether warfarin is at a therapeutic level; however, an INR of 2 to 3, not 3 to 4, is considered therapeutic. HCT doesn't provide information on the effectiveness of warfarin. However, a falling HCT in a client taking warfarin may be a sign of hemorrhage.

➡ *NCLEX keys*

Client needs category: Physiological integrity
Client needs subcategory: Pharmacological and parenteral therapies
Cognitive level: Application

10. A client comes to the emergency department with a dissecting aortic aneurysm. The client is at greatest risk for:
1. septic shock.
2. anaphylactic shock.
3. cardiogenic shock.
4. hypovolemic shock.

Answer: 4. A dissecting aortic aneurysm is a precursor to aortic rupture, which leads to hemorrhage and hypovolemic shock. Septic shock occurs with overwhelming infection. Anaphylactic shock is an allergic response. Cardiogenic shock is the result of ineffective cardiac function.

➡ *NCLEX keys*

Client needs category: Physiological integrity
Client needs subcategory: Reduction of risk potential
Cognitive level: Comprehension

Congrats! You finished the chapter. My advice: Take a break to exercise your body and give your mind a rest.

4 Respiratory system

Brush up on key concepts

The major function of the respiratory system is gas exchange, which includes the transfer of oxygen and carbon dioxide between the atmosphere and the blood. During gas exchange, air is taken into the body through inhalation and travels through respiratory passages to the lungs. In the lungs, oxygen (O_2) takes the place of carbon dioxide (CO_2) in the blood, and the CO_2 is then expelled from the body through exhalation.

The respiratory system is divided into two sections: the upper respiratory tract and the lower respiratory tract. At any time, you can review the major points of this chapter by consulting the *Cheat sheet* on pages 70 to 77.

Upper respiratory tract

Enter here
The **nose** and **mouth** allow air flow into and out of the body. They also humidify inhaled air, which reduces irritation of the mucous membranes. Within the nose, the **nares** (nostrils) contain olfactory receptor sites, providing for the body's sense of smell.

Keep out!
The **paranasal sinuses** are air-filled, cilia-lined cavities within the nose. Their function is to trap particles of foreign matter that might interfere with the workings of the respiratory system.

Going down
The **pharynx** serves as a passageway to the digestive and respiratory tracts. The pharynx maintains air pressure in the middle ear and also contains a mucosal lining. This lining continues the process of humidifying and warming inhaled air in addition to trapping foreign particles.

If you can read this aloud, thank your larynx
The **larynx,** known as the voice box, connects the upper and lower airways. It contains vocal cords that produce sounds. The larynx also initiates the cough reflex, which is part of the respiratory system's defense mechanisms.

C-shaped connector
The **trachea** contains C-shaped cartilaginous rings composed of smooth muscle. It connects the larynx to the bronchi.

Lower respiratory tract

Branching into bronchi
The trachea branches into the right and left **bronchi,** the large air passages that lead to the right and left lungs. The right main bronchus is slightly larger and more vertical than the left.

As they pass into the lungs, the bronchi form smaller branches called **bronchioles,** which themselves branch into terminal bronchioles, alveolar ducts, and alveoli.

Gas exchange center
Alveoli are clustered microscopic sacs enveloped by capillaries. Gas exchange occurs over the millions of alveoli in the lungs as gases diffuse across the alveolar-capillary membrane. The alveoli also contain a coating of surfactant, which reduces surface tension and keeps them from collapsing.

(Text continues on page 77.)

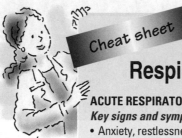

Cheat sheet

Respiratory refresher

ACUTE RESPIRATORY DISTRESS SYNDROME

Key signs and symptoms
- Anxiety, restlessness
- Crackles, rhonchi, decreased breath sounds
- Dyspnea, tachypnea

Key test results
- Arterial blood gas (ABG) levels show respiratory acidosis, metabolic acidosis, hypoxemia that doesn't respond to increased fraction of oxygen.
- Chest X-ray shows bilateral infiltrates (in early stages) and lung fields with a ground-glass appearance and, with irreversible hypoxemia, massive consolidation of both lung fields (in later stages).

Key treatments
- Oxygen (O_2) therapy: intubation and mechanical ventilation using positive end-expiratory pressure (PEEP) or pressure-controlled inverse ratio ventilation
- Antibiotics: according to infectious organism
- Bronchodilator: Albuterol (Ventolin HFA)
- Neuromuscular blocking agents: pancuronium, vecuronium
- Steroids: hydrocortisone (Solu-Cortef), methyl-prednisolone (Solu-Medrol)

Key interventions
- Assess respiratory, cardiovascular, and neurologic status.
- Maintain bed rest, with prone positioning if possible.
- Provide chest physiotherapy.

ACUTE RESPIRATORY FAILURE

Key signs and symptoms
- Decreased respiratory excursion, accessory muscle use, retractions
- Difficulty breathing, shortness of breath, dyspnea, tachypnea, orthopnea
- Fatigue

Key test results
- ABG levels show hypoxemia, acidosis, alkalosis, and hypercapnia.

Key treatments
- O_2 therapy, intubation, and mechanical ventilation (possibly with PEEP)
- Anesthetic: propofol (Diprivan)
- Antianxiety agent: lorazepam (Ativan)
- Bronchodilators: terbutaline, aminophylline, theophylline (Theochron); via nebulizer: albuterol (Proventil-HFA), ipratropium (Atrovent)
- Steroids: hydrocortisone (Solu-Cortef), methyl-prednisolone (Solu-Medrol)

Key interventions
- Assess respiratory status.
- Administer O_2.
- Provide suctioning; assist with turning, coughing, and deep breathing; perform chest physiotherapy and postural drainage.
- Maintain bed rest.

ASBESTOSIS

Key signs and symptoms
- Dry crackles at lung bases
- Dry cough
- Dyspnea on exertion (usually first symptom)
- Pleuritic chest pain

Key test results
- Chest X-rays show fine, irregular, and linear diffuse infiltrates; extensive fibrosis results in a "honeycomb" or "ground-glass" appearance. X-rays may also show pleural thickening and pleural calcification, with bilateral obliteration of costophrenic angles and, in later stages, an enlarged heart with a classic "shaggy" heart border.

Key treatments
- Chest physiotherapy
- Fluid intake: at least 3 qt (3 L)/day unless contraindicated
- O_2 therapy or mechanical ventilator (in advanced cases)

> Because the major function of the respiratory system is gas exchange, focus on keeping airways clear and facilitating breathing.

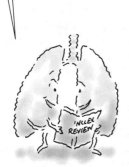

Respiratory refresher *(continued)*

ASBESTOSIS *(CONTINUED)*
• Antibiotics: according to susceptibility of infecting organism (for treatment of respiratory tract infections)
• Mucolytic inhalation therapy: acetylcysteine

Key interventions
• Perform chest physiotherapy techniques, such as controlled coughing and segmental bronchial drainage, with chest percussion and vibration.
• Administer O_2 by cannula or mask (1 to 2 L/minute), or by mechanical ventilation if arterial oxygen can't be maintained above 40 mm Hg.

ASPHYXIA
Key signs and symptoms
• Agitation
• Altered respiratory rate (apnea, bradypnea, occasional tachypnea)
• Anxiety
• Central and peripheral cyanosis (cherry-red mucous membranes in late-stage carbon monoxide poisoning)
• Confusion leading to coma
• Decreased breath sounds
• Dyspnea

Key test results
• ABG measurement indicates decreased partial pressure of arterial oxygen (Pao_2) < 60 mm Hg and increased partial pressure of arterial CO_2 ($Paco_2$) > 50 mm Hg.
• Pulse oximetry reveals decreased hemoglobin saturation with oxygen.

Key treatments
• Bronchoscopy (for extraction of a foreign body)
• O_2 therapy, which may include endotracheal intubation and mechanical ventilation
• Opioid antagonist: naloxone (for opioid overdose)

Key interventions
• Assess cardiac and respiratory status.
• Position the client upright, if his condition tolerates.
• Suction carefully, as needed, and encourage deep breathing.

ASTHMA
Key signs and symptoms
• Lack of symptoms between attacks (usually)
• Wheezing, primarily on expiration but also sometimes on inspiration

Key test results
• Pulmonary function tests (PFTs) during attacks show decreased forced expiratory volumes that improve with therapy and increased residual volume and total lung capacity.

Key treatments
• Fluids to 3 qt (3 L)/day unless contraindicated
• Beta-adrenergic drugs: epinephrine, salmeterol (Serevent)
• Bronchodilators: terbutaline, aminophylline, theophylline (Theochron); via nebulizer: albuterol (Proventil-HFA), ipratropium (Atrovent)
• Mast cell stabilizer: cromolyn (Intal)
• Antileukotrienes: zafirlukast (Accolate), montelukast (Singulair)

Key interventions
• Administer low-flow humidified O_2.
• Assess respiratory status.
• Keep the client in high Fowler's position.

ATELECTASIS
Key signs and symptoms
• Diminished or bronchial breath sounds
• Dyspnea
In severe cases
• Anxiety
• Cyanosis
• Diaphoresis
• Severe dyspnea
• Substernal or intercostal retraction
• Tachycardia

Key test results
• Chest X-ray shows characteristic horizontal lines in the lower lung zones and, with segmental or lobar collapse, characteristic dense shadows associated with hyperinflation of neighboring lung zones (in widespread atelectasis).

Key treatments
• Bronchoscopy
• Chest physiotherapy
• Bronchodilator: albuterol (Proventil-HFA)
• Mucolytic inhalation therapy: acetylcysteine

Key interventions
• Encourage postoperative and other high-risk clients to cough and deep breathe every 1 to 2 hours.
• Teach the splinting technique.
• Encourage ambulation.
• Administer adequate analgesics.

(continued)

Respiratory refresher (continued)

ATELECTASIS (CONTINUED)
- Teach the client how to use an incentive spirometer and encourage him to use it every 1 to 2 hours, while awake.
- Humidify inspired air and encourage adequate fluid intake. Perform postural drainage and chest percussion.
- Assess breath sounds and ventilatory status frequently and be alert for any changes.

BRONCHIECTASIS
Key signs and symptoms
- Chronic cough that produces copious, foul-smelling, mucopurulent secretions, possibly totaling several cupfuls daily
- Coarse crackles during inspiration over involved lobes or segments, rhonchi, wheezing
- Exertional dyspnea
- Anorexia

Key test results
- Chest X-rays show peribronchial thickening, areas of atelectasis, and scattered cystic changes.
- Sputum culture and Gram stain identify predominant organisms.

Key treatments
- Bronchoscopy (to mobilize secretions)
- Chest physiotherapy and incentive spirometry
- O_2 therapy
- Antibiotics: according to sensitivity of causative organism
- Bronchodilator: albuterol (Proventil-HFA)

Key interventions
- Assess respiratory status.
- Provide supportive care and help the client adjust to the permanent changes in lifestyle that irreversible lung damage necessitates.
- Perform chest physiotherapy, including postural drainage and chest percussion designed for involved lobes, several times per day. Encourage use of incentive spirometer every 1 to 2 hours while the client is awake.

CHRONIC BRONCHITIS
Key signs and symptoms
- Dyspnea
- Increased sputum production
- Productive cough

Key test results
- Chest X-ray shows hyperinflation and increased bronchovascular markings.

- PFTs may reveal increased residual volume, decreased vital capacity and forced expiratory volumes, and normal static compliance and diffusion capacity.

Key treatments
- Fluid intake up to 3 qt (3 L)/day, if not contraindicated
- Endotracheal intubation and mechanical ventilation if respiratory status deteriorates
- Antibiotics: according to sensitivity of infective organism
- Bronchodilators: terbutaline, aminophylline, theophylline (Theochron); via nebulizer: albuterol (Proventil-HFA), ipratropium (Atrovent)
- Influenza and Pneumovax vaccines
- Steroids: hydrocortisone (Solu-Cortef), methylprednisolone (Solu-Medrol)
- Steroids (via nebulizer): beclomethasone (Beconase AQ), triamcinolone (Azmacort)

Key interventions
- Administer low-flow O_2.
- Assess respiratory status, ABG levels, and pulse oximetry.
- Assist with diaphragmatic and pursed-lip breathing.
- Monitor and record the color, amount, and consistency of sputum.
- Provide chest physiotherapy, postural drainage, incentive spirometry, and suction.

COR PULMONALE
Key signs and symptoms
- Dyspnea on exertion
- Edema
- Fatigue
- Orthopnea
- Tachypnea
- Weakness

Key test results
- ABG analysis shows decreased PaO_2 (< 70 mm Hg).
- Chest X-ray shows large central pulmonary arteries and suggests right ventricular enlargement by rightward enlargement of cardiac silhouette on an anterior chest film.
- Pulmonary artery pressure measurements show increased right ventricular and pulmonary artery pressures as a result of increased pulmonary vascular resistance.

Key treatments
- O_2 therapy as necessary by mask or cannula in concentrations ranging from 24% to 40%, depending on PaO_2 and, in acute cases, endotracheal intubation and mechanical ventilation

Respiratory refresher *(continued)*

COR PULMONALE *(CONTINUED)*
- Cardiac glycoside: digoxin (Lanoxin)
- Diuretic: furosemide (Lasix)
- Vasodilators: diazoxide, hydralazine, nitroprusside (Nitropress), prostaglandins (in primary pulmonary hypertension)
- Calcium channel blocker: diltiazem (Cardizem)
- Angiotensin-converting enzyme inhibitor: captopril (Capoten)

Key interventions
- Limit the client's fluid intake to 1 to 2 qt (1 to 2 L)/day, and provide a low-sodium diet.
- Reposition the client every 2 hours.
- Provide meticulous respiratory care, including O_2 therapy and, for clients with chronic obstructive pulmonary disease, pursed-lip breathing exercises.
- Monitor ABG levels and watch for signs of respiratory failure such as a change in pulse rate; deep, labored respirations; and increased fatigue produced by exertion.

EMPHYSEMA
Key signs and symptoms
- Barrel chest
- Dyspnea
- Pursed-lip breathing

Key test results
- Chest X-ray in advanced disease reveals a flattened diaphragm, reduced vascular markings in the lung periphery, enlarged anteroposterior chest diameter, and a vertical heart.
- PFTs show increased residual volume, total lung capacity, and compliance as well as decreased vital capacity, diffusing capacity, and expiratory volumes.

Key treatments
- Chest physiotherapy, postural drainage, and incentive spirometry
- Fluid intake up to 3 qt (3 L)/day, if not contraindicated
- O_2 therapy at 2 to 3 L/minute; transtracheal therapy for home O_2 therapy
- Antibiotics: according to sensitivity of infective organism
- Bronchodilators: terbutaline, aminophylline, theophylline (Theochron); via nebulizer: albuterol (Proventil-HFA), ipratropium (Atrovent)
- Influenza and Pneumovax vaccines
- Steroids: hydrocortisone (Solu-Cortef), methylprednisolone (Solu-Medrol)
- Steroids (via nebulizer): beclomethasone (Beconase AQ), triamcinolone (Azmacort)

Key interventions
- Assess respiratory status, ABG levels, and pulse oximetry.
- Assist with diaphragmatic and pursed-lip breathing.
- Monitor and record the color, amount, and consistency of sputum.
- Provide chest physiotherapy, postural drainage, and suction.

IDIOPATHIC PULMONARY FIBROSIS
Key signs and symptoms
- Dyspnea
- Dry, hacking, paroxysmal cough
- Rapid, shallow breathing

In late cases
- Cyanosis
- Profound hypoxemia
- Pulmonary hypertension

Key test results
- Lung biopsy findings vary based on the stage of the disease. In general, the alveolar walls are swollen with chronic inflammatory infiltrates. In the late disease stages, the alveolar walls are destroyed and are replaced by honeycombing cysts.

Key treatments
- Lung transplant: in younger, otherwise healthy clients
- O_2 therapy
- Corticosteroids and cytotoxic drugs: to suppress inflammation, but are usually unsuccessful

Key interventions
- Assess respiratory status.
- Monitor oxygen levels and administer O_2 as needed.
- Encourage activity to the extent that the client is able.
- Provide emotional support.

LUNG CANCER
Key signs and symptoms
- Cough, hemoptysis
- Weight loss, anorexia

Key test results
- Chest X-ray shows a lesion or mass.

Key treatments
- Resection of the affected lobe (lobectomy) or lung (pneumonectomy)
- Radiation therapy

(continued)

Respiratory refresher (continued)

LUNG CANCER (CONTINUED)
• Antineoplastics: cyclophosphamide, doxorubicin (Doxil), cisplatin (Platinol), vincristine

Key interventions
• Assess the client's pain level and administer analgesics, as prescribed.
• Provide suctioning and assist with turning, coughing, and deep breathing.
• Track laboratory values, and monitor for bleeding, infection, and electrolyte imbalance due to effects of chemotherapy.

PLEURAL EFFUSION AND EMPYEMA
Key signs and symptoms
• Decreased breath sounds
• Dyspnea
• Fever
• Pleuritic chest pain

Key test results
• Chest X-ray shows radiopaque fluid in dependent regions.
• Thoracentesis shows lactate dehydrogenase (LD) levels less than 200 international units and protein levels less than 3 g/dl (in transudative effusions); ratio of protein in pleural fluid to serum greater than or equal to 0.5, LD in pleural fluid greater than or equal to 200 international units, and ratio of LD in pleural fluid to LD in serum greater than 0.6 (in exudative effusions); and acute inflammatory white blood cells and microorganisms (in empyema).

Key treatments
• Thoracentesis (to remove fluid) with chest tube insertion if necessary
• Thoracotomy if thoracentesis isn't effective
• Antibiotics for empyema: according to sensitivity of causative organism

Key interventions
• Administer O_2.
• Administer antibiotics.
• Provide meticulous chest tube care, and use sterile technique for changing dressings around the tube insertion site.
• Ensure chest tube patency by watching for bubbles in the underwater seal chamber.
• Record the amount, color, and consistency of chest tube drainage.

PLEURISY
Key signs and symptoms
• Pleural friction rub (a coarse, creaky sound heard during late inspiration and early expiration)
• Sharp, stabbing pain that increases with respiration

Key test results
• Although diagnosis generally rests on the client's history and the nurse's respiratory assessment, diagnostic tests help rule out other causes and pinpoint the underlying disorder.

Key treatments
• Bed rest
• Analgesic: acetaminophen with oxycodone (Percocet)
• Anti-inflammatories: indomethacin (Indocin), ibuprofen (Motrin)

Key interventions
• Stress the importance of bed rest and plan your care to allow the client as much uninterrupted rest as possible.
• Administer antitussives and pain medication as necessary.
• Encourage the client to cough and deep breathe. Teach him to apply firm pressure at the pain site during coughing exercises.

PNEUMOCYSTIS PNEUMONIA
Key signs and symptoms
• Generalized fatigue
• Low-grade, intermittent fever
• Nonproductive cough
• Shortness of breath
• Weight loss

Key test results
• Chest X-ray may show slowly progressing, fluffy infiltrates and occasionally nodular lesions or a spontaneous pneumothorax, but these findings must be differentiated from findings in other types of pneumonia or acute respiratory distress syndrome.
• Histologic studies confirm *P. jiroveci*. In clients with human immunodeficiency virus (HIV) infection, initial examination of a first morning sputum specimen (induced by inhaling an ultrasonically dispersed saline mist) may be sufficient; however, this technique is usually ineffective in clients without HIV infection.

Key treatments
• O_2 therapy, which may include endotracheal intubation and mechanical ventilation
• Antibiotics: co-trimoxazole (Bactrim), pentamidine (Pentam)
• Antipyretic: acetaminophen (Tylenol)

Key interventions
• Assess the client's respiratory status, and monitor ABG levels.
• Administer O_2 therapy as necessary. Encourage ambulation, deep-breathing exercises, and use of incentive spirometry.
• Administer antipyretics, as required.

Respiratory refresher (continued)

PNEUMOCYSTIS PNEUMONIA (CONTINUED)

- Monitor intake and output and daily weight. Replace fluids as necessary.
- Give antimicrobial drugs as required. Never give pentamidine I.M. Administer the I.V. form slowly over 60 minutes.
- Monitor the client for adverse reactions to antimicrobial drugs. If he's receiving co-trimoxazole, watch for nausea, vomiting, rash, bone marrow suppression, thrush, fever, hepatotoxicity, and anaphylaxis. If he's receiving pentamidine, watch for cardiac arrhythmias, hypotension, dizziness, azotemia, hypocalcemia, and hepatic disturbances.
- Provide nutritional supplements and encourage the client to eat a high-calorie, protein-rich diet. Offer small, frequent meals.

PNEUMONIA

Key signs and symptoms

- Chills, fever
- Crackles, rhonchi, pleural friction rub on auscultation
- Shortness of breath, dyspnea, tachypnea, accessory muscle use
- Sputum production that's rusty, green, or bloody with pneumococcal pneumonia; yellow-green with bronchopneumonia

Key test results

- Chest X-ray shows pulmonary infiltrates.
- Sputum study identifies organism.

Key treatments

- O_2 therapy
- Chest physiotherapy and respiratory treatments
- Antibiotics: according to organism sensitivity

Key interventions

- Monitor and record intake and output.
- Monitor laboratory studies.
- Monitor pulse oximetry and assess respiratory status.
- Encourage fluid intake of 3 to 4 qt (3 to 4 L)/day unless contraindicated, and administer I.V. fluids.

PNEUMOTHORAX AND HEMOTHORAX

Key signs and symptoms

- Diminished or absent breath sounds unilaterally
- Dyspnea, tachypnea, subcutaneous emphysema, cough
- Sharp pain that increases with exertion

Key test results

- Chest X-ray reveals pneumothorax or hemothorax.

Key treatments

- Chest tube to water-seal drainage or continuous suction

Key interventions

- Monitor and record vital signs.
- Assess respiratory status.
- Monitor chest tube function and drainage.
- Assess cardiovascular status.

PULMONARY EDEMA

Key signs and symptoms

- Dyspnea, orthopnea, tachypnea
- Productive cough (frothy, bloody sputum)

Key test results

- Chest X-ray shows diffuse haziness of the lung fields and, commonly, cardiomegaly and pleural effusions.
- Hemodynamic monitoring shows increases in pulmonary artery pressure, pulmonary artery wedge pressure, and central venous pressure as well as decreased cardiac output.

Key treatments

- O_2 therapy: possibly intubation and mechanical ventilation
- Diuretics: furosemide (Lasix), bumetanide (Bumex), metolazone (Zaroxolyn)
- Nitrates: isosorbide (Isordil), nitroglycerin
- Cardiac glycoside: digoxin (Lanoxin)
- Inotropic agents: dobutamine, inamrinone (Amrinone), milrinone
- Vasodilator: nitroprusside (Nitropress)

Key interventions

- Assess cardiovascular and respiratory status and hemodynamic variables.
- Keep the client in high Fowler's position if blood pressure tolerates; if hypotensive, maintain in a semi-Fowler's position if tolerated.

PULMONARY EMBOLISM

Key signs and symptoms

- Sudden onset of dyspnea, tachypnea, crackles

Key test results

- ABG levels show respiratory alkalosis and hypoxemia.
- Lung scan shows ventilation/perfusion ($\dot{V}/\dot{Q}$) mismatch.
- Spiral computed tomography of the chest shows central pulmonary emboli.

Key treatments

- Vena cava filter insertion or pulmonary embolectomy
- O_2 therapy, intubation, and mechanical ventilation, if necessary
- Anticoagulants: enoxaparin (Lovenox), heparin, followed by warfarin (Coumadin)
- Fibrinolytics: streptokinase (Streptase), urokinase (Abbokinase)

(continued)

Respiratory refresher (continued)

PULMONARY EMBOLISM (CONTINUED)
Key interventions
- Assess respiratory status.
- Assess cardiovascular status.
- Administer O_2.

RESPIRATORY ACIDOSIS
Key signs and symptoms
- Cardiovascular abnormalities, such as tachycardia, hypertension, atrial and ventricular arrhythmias and, in severe acidosis, hypotension with vasodilation

Key test results
- ABG measurements confirm respiratory acidosis. $Paco_2$ exceeds the normal level of 45 mm Hg and pH is usually below the normal range of 7.35 to 7.45. The client's bicarbonate level is normal in the acute stage and elevated in the chronic stage.

Key treatments
- Treatment of underlying cause
- Sodium bicarbonate in severe cases

Key interventions
- Closely monitor the client's blood pH level.
- Be alert for critical changes in the client's respiratory, central nervous system (CNS), and cardiovascular functions. Also watch closely for variations in ABG values and electrolyte status. Maintain adequate hydration.
- If acidosis requires mechanical ventilation, maintain a patent airway and provide adequate humidification. Perform tracheal suctioning regularly and vigorous chest physiotherapy if needed. Continuously monitor ventilator settings and respiratory status.

RESPIRATORY ALKALOSIS
Key signs and symptoms
- Agitation
- Cardiac arrhythmias that fail to respond to conventional treatment (severe respiratory alkalosis)
- Circumoral or peripheral paresthesia (a prickling sensation around the mouth or extremities)
- Deep, rapid breathing, possibly exceeding 40 breaths/minute (cardinal sign)
- Light-headedness or dizziness (from decreased cerebral blood flow)

Key test results
- ABG analysis confirms respiratory alkalosis and rules out respiratory compensation for metabolic acidosis. $Paco_2$ is below 35 mm Hg and pH is elevated in proportion to the fall in $Paco_2$ in the acute stage but drops toward normal in the chronic stage. Bicarbonate level is normal in the acute stage but below normal in the chronic stage.

Key treatments
- Correction of underlying cause
- Increasing CO_2 levels (for respiratory alkalosis caused by hyperventilation) by having the client breathe into a paper bag

Key interventions
- Assess neurologic, neuromuscular, and cardiovascular functions.
- Monitor ABG and serum electrolyte levels closely, watching for any variations.

SARCOIDOSIS
Key signs and symptoms
Initial signs
- Arthralgia (in the wrists, ankles, and elbows)
- Fatigue
- Malaise
- Weight loss
Respiratory
- Breathlessness
- Substernal pain
Cutaneous
- Erythema nodosum
- Subcutaneous skin nodules with maculopapular eruptions
Ophthalmic
- Anterior uveitis (common)
Musculoskeletal
- Muscle weakness
- Pain
Hepatic
- Granulomatous hepatitis (usually asymptomatic)
Genitourinary
- Hypercalciuria (excessive calcium in the urine)
Cardiovascular
- Arrhythmias (premature beats, bundle-branch block, or complete heart block)
Central nervous system
- Cranial or peripheral nerve palsies
- Basilar meningitis (inflammation of the meninges at the base of the brain)

Key test results
- A positive Kveim-Siltzbach skin test supports the diagnosis.

Key treatments
- A low-calcium diet and avoidance of direct exposure to sunlight (in clients with hypercalcemia)
- O_2 therapy
- Systemic or topical steroid, if sarcoidosis causes ocular, respiratory, CNS, cardiac, or systemic symptoms (such as fever and weight loss), hypercalcemia, or destructive skin lesions

Respiratory refresher *(continued)*

SARCOIDOSIS *(CONTINUED)*
Key interventions
• Provide a nutritious, high-calorie diet and plenty of fluids. If the client has hypercalcemia, suggest a low-calcium diet.
• Administer O_2.

SEVERE ACUTE RESPIRATORY SYNDROME
Key signs and symptoms
• Chills
• Fever
• General discomfort
• Headache
• Shortness of breath

Key test results
• Laboratory validation includes cell culture of severe acute respiratory syndrome (SARS)-associated coronavirus (SARS-CoV), detection of SARS-CoV ribonucleic acid by the reverse transcription polymerase chain reaction test, or detection of serum antibodies to SARS-CoV.

Key treatments
• Supplemental O_2 including possible mechanical ventilation
• Chest physiotherapy
• Antibiotics
• Antivirals
• High doses of corticosteroids

Key interventions
• Treat symptoms and support the client as needed.
• Maintain a patent airway.
• Follow contact and airborne precautions, including use of an N-95 respirator for all health care professionals.
• Monitor vital signs and respiratory status.

TUBERCULOSIS
Key signs and symptoms
• Low-grade fever
• Night sweats

Key test results
• Mantoux skin test is positive.
• Stains and cultures of sputum, cerebrospinal fluid, urine, abscess drainage, or pleural fluid shows heat-sensitive, non-motile, aerobic, and acid-fast bacilli.

Key treatments
• Standard and airborne precautions
• Antituberculars: isoniazid, ethambutol (Myambutol), rifampin (Rifadin), pyrazinamide

Key interventions
• Maintain infection-control precautions; provide a negative pressure room.
• Assess respiratory status.
• Provide O_2 therapy.

Lobes: 3 and 2
As a unit, the lungs are composed of three **lobes** on the right side and two lobes on the left side. The lungs regulate air exchange by a concentration gradient. In the alveoli, gases move from an area of high concentration to an area of low concentration. Because the concentration of CO_2 is greater in the alveoli, it diffuses out into the lungs and is exhaled. Because the lungs contain a greater concentration of O_2, O_2 diffuses out of the lungs and into the alveoli, to be carried to the rest of the body.

A pleur-ality of coverings
Pleura refers to the membrane covering the lungs and lining the thoracic cavity. The pleura covering the lungs is known as the *visceral pleura*, whereas the parietal pleura lines the thoracic cavity. Pleural fluid lubricates the pleura to reduce friction during respiration.

Keep abreast of diagnostic tests

Here are the most important tests used to diagnose respiratory disorders, along with common nursing interventions associated with each test.

Deep, direct visualization
In **bronchoscopy,** the physician uses a bronchoscope to directly visualize the trachea and bronchial tree. During bronchoscopy, the physician may obtain biopsies and perform deep tracheal suctioning.

After any invasive test involving the airway—such as bronchoscopy—assess respiratory status to ensure the client's safety.

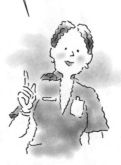

Nursing actions

Before the procedure
- Explain the procedure to the client.
- Withhold food and fluids for 6 to 12 hours, if possible.
- Make sure that written, informed consent has been obtained.
- Insert an I.V. catheter for fluid and medication administration.

During the procedure
- Administer prescribed medications.
- Monitor vital signs and cardiac rhythm.

After the procedure
- Assess respiratory status.
- Monitor vital signs and cardiac rhythm for bradycardia, which may be caused by a vasovagal response.
- Withhold food and fluids until the gag reflex returns.
- Check the cough and gag reflexes to minimize the risk of aspiration. Monitor for laryngeal edema.
- Assess sputum.
- If a biopsy was performed, monitor for hemorrhage and pneumothorax.

Looking in from the outside

A **chest X-ray** produces a radiographic picture of lung tissue. It's used to detect tumors, inflammation, air, and fluid in and around the lung. It can also be used to monitor placement of such equipment as catheters and chest tubes.

Nursing actions

- Explain the procedure to the client.
- Determine the client's ability to inhale and hold his breath.
- Make sure that the client removes jewelry before the X-ray is taken.

Dye-ing to see the lungs

In **pulmonary angiography,** the client receives an injection of a radiopaque dye through a catheter. This provides a radiographic picture of pulmonary circulation.

Nursing actions

Before the procedure
- Explain the procedure to the client.
- Note the client's allergies to iodine, seafood, and radiopaque dyes.
- Withhold food and fluids for 8 hours.

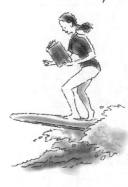

Clients who are allergic to iodine or seafood are at risk for reactions in any test involving radiopaque dyes.

- Insert an I.V. catheter for fluid, medication, and radiopaque dye administration.
- Make sure that written, informed consent has been obtained.
- Instruct the client about possible flushing of the face or burning in the throat after dye is injected.

After the procedure
- Monitor vital signs.
- Assess peripheral neurovascular status.
- Check the insertion site for bleeding.
- Avoid taking blood pressure measurements in the extremity used for dye injection for 24 hours after the procedure.

Sensitive about sputum

A **sputum study** is a laboratory test that provides a microscopic evaluation of sputum, evaluating it for culture and sensitivity, Gram stain, and acid-fast bacillus.

Nursing actions

- Explain the reason for the specimen and how the specimen will be obtained.
- Obtain an early-morning sterile specimen from suctioning or expectoration.
- Make sure that the specimen is truly sputum—not saliva—before sending the specimen to the laboratory.

Focusing on intrapleural fluid

In **thoracentesis,** a needle is used to obtain a sample of intrapleural fluid to determine the cause of infection or empyema. The client undergoing thoracentesis receives local anesthesia.

Nursing actions

Before the procedure
- Explain the procedure to the client.
- Make sure that written, informed consent has been obtained.
- Place the client in an upright position.

During the procedure
- Monitor vital signs and cardiac rhythm.
- Instruct the client not to cough or talk.
- Monitor respiratory status and pulse oximetry.

After the procedure
- Assess the client's respiratory status; assess breath sounds in all fields.
- Monitor vital signs frequently.

- Position the client on the affected side, as ordered, for at least 1 hour to seal the puncture site.
- Check the puncture site for fluid leakage.

Finding out about lung function

Pulmonary function tests (PFTs) are noninvasive tests that measure lung volume, ventilation, and diffusing capacity using a spirometer. The client is asked to breathe through a mouthpiece following specific directions. A computer then calculates the volumes.

Nursing actions

- Explain the procedure to the client.
- Instruct the client to refrain from smoking or eating a heavy meal 4 to 6 hours before testing.
- Tell the client to avoid bronchodilators or opioids for 6 hours before the procedure.

From the artery to the lab

Arterial blood gas (ABG) analysis is a laboratory test that assesses the arterial blood for tissue oxygenation, ventilation, and acid-base status.

Nursing actions

Before the procedure
- Explain the procedure to the client.
- Note the client's temperature.
- Document O_2 and assisted mechanical ventilation used.

After the procedure
- Apply pressure to the site for at least 5 minutes to prevent hematoma.
- Assess the puncture site for bleeding.
- Maintain a pressure dressing for at least 30 minutes.

Image through inhalation or injection

A **lung scan,** or ventilation/perfusion scan ($\dot{V}/\dot{Q}$ scan), uses visual inhalation or I.V. injection of radioisotopes to create an image of blood flow in the lungs.

Nursing actions

Before the procedure
- Explain the procedure to the client.
- Insert an I.V. catheter for radiopaque dye administration.

- Make sure that written, informed consent has been obtained.
- Instruct the client to remove all metal objects before the procedure.
- Determine the client's ability to lie still for about 1 hour during the procedure.

After the procedure
- Check the catheter insertion site for bleeding after the procedure.
- Monitor vital signs and pulse oximetry.

TB or not TB?

In the **Mantoux intradermal skin test,** the client receives an injection of tuberculin to detect tuberculosis (TB) antibodies.

Nursing actions

- Explain the procedure to the client.
- Document current dermatitis or rashes.
- Circle and record the test site.
- Note the date for follow-up reading (48 to 72 hours after injection).

Let's look at the larynx

Laryngoscopy uses a laryngoscope to directly visualize the larynx.

Nursing actions

Before the procedure
- Explain the procedure to the client.
- Make sure that written, informed consent has been obtained.
- Withhold food and fluids for 6 to 8 hours.
- Explain that the client will receive a sedative to promote relaxation.

After the procedure
- Assess respiratory status and pulse oximetry.
- Allay the client's anxiety.
- Withhold food and fluids until the gag reflex returns; monitor for laryngeal edema.

Little bit of lung tissue

A **lung biopsy** involves the removal of a small amount of lung tissue for histologic evaluation. Lung biopsy may be done by surgical exposure of the lung (open biopsy) or with endoscopy using a needle designed to remove a core of lung tissue.

Nursing actions
Before the procedure
- Explain the procedure to the client.
- Withhold food and fluids for 8 hours.
- Make sure that written, informed consent has been obtained.

After the procedure
- Monitor and record vital signs and pulse oximetry.
- Assess respiratory status (checking for signs of pneumothorax, air embolism, hemoptysis, and hemorrhage).
- Check the incision site for bleeding.

Taking a pulse
Pulse oximetry is a noninvasive test that measures oxygen saturation of hemoglobin with a laser device. The device is applied to the finger, ear, bridge of the nose, or forehead.

Nursing actions
- Explain the procedure to the client.
- Monitor readings intermittently or continuously.

Taking a snooze
A **sleep study test** is performed in a sleep laboratory and monitors the client's body while he sleeps. It's commonly used to diagnose obstructive sleep apnea.

Nursing actions
- Explain the procedure to the client.
- Tell the client what supplies to bring from home, such as pajamas.
- Instruct the client to limit his intake of caffeine, nicotine, and alcohol on the day of the test.

Analyzing blood, part A
A **blood chemistry test** assesses a blood sample for potassium, sodium, calcium, phosphorus, glucose, bicarbonate, blood urea

nitrogen, creatinine, protein, albumin, osmolality, and alpha$_1$-antitrypsin.

Nursing actions
- Explain the procedure to the client.
- Withhold food and fluids before the procedure, as directed.
- Check the site for bleeding after the procedure.

Analyzing blood, part B
A **hematologic study** uses a blood sample to analyze red blood cell (RBC) and white blood cell (WBC) counts, prothrombin time (PT), international normalized ratio (INR), partial thromboplastin time (PTT), erythrocyte sedimentation rate (ESR), platelet count, hemoglobin (Hb) level, and hematocrit (HCT).

Nursing actions
- Explain the procedure to the client.
- Note current drug therapy before the procedure.
- Check the venipuncture site for bleeding after the procedure.

Polish up on client care

Major respiratory disorders include acute respiratory distress syndrome (ARDS), acute respiratory failure, asbestosis, asphyxia, asthma, atelectasis, bronchiectasis, chronic bronchitis, cor pulmonale, emphysema, idiopathic pulmonary fibrosis (IPF), lung cancer, pleural effusion and empyema, pleurisy, *Pneumocystis carinii* pneumonia (PCP), pneumonia, pneumothorax and hemothorax, pulmonary edema, pulmonary embolism, respiratory acidosis, respiratory alkalosis, sarcoidosis, severe acute respiratory syndrome (SARS), and tuberculosis.

Acute respiratory distress syndrome

In ARDS, fluid builds up in the lungs and causes them to stiffen. This impairs breathing, thereby reducing the amount of O_2 in the capillaries that supply the lungs. When severe,

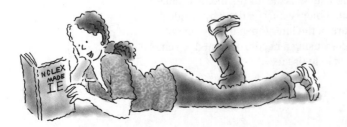

Clients with ARDS should be kept in a prone position.

the syndrome can cause an unmanageable and ultimately fatal lack of O_2. However, those who recover may have little or no permanent lung damage.

CAUSES
- Aspiration
- Decreased surfactant production
- Fat emboli
- Fluid overload
- Neurologic injuries
- O_2 toxicity
- Respiratory infection
- Pulmonary embolism
- Sepsis
- Shock
- Trauma

ASSESSMENT FINDINGS
- Agitation, confusion
- Altered level of consciousness
- Use of accessory muscles
- Tachycardia
- Hypertension or hypotension
- Cool, clammy skin
- Fatigue
- Anxiety, restlessness
- Cough
- Crackles, rhonchi, decreased breath sounds
- Cyanosis
- Dyspnea, tachypnea

DIAGNOSTIC TEST RESULTS
- ABG levels show respiratory acidosis, metabolic acidosis, and hypoxemia that doesn't respond to increased fraction of inspired oxygen (FIO_2).
- Blood culture shows infectious organism.
- Chest X-ray shows bilateral infiltrates (in early stages) and lung fields with a ground-glass appearance and, with irreversible hypoxemia, massive consolidation of both lung fields (in later stages).
- Pulse oximetry readings are decreased.
- Sputum study reveals the infectious organism.

NURSING DIAGNOSES
- Activity intolerance
- Anxiety
- Fear
- Ineffective airway clearance
- Impaired gas exchange
- Ineffective breathing pattern
- Ineffective peripheral tissue perfusion

TREATMENT
- Bed rest with prone positioning, if possible; passive range-of-motion exercises
- Chest physiotherapy, postural drainage, and suction
- Dietary changes, including restricting fluid intake or, if intubated, nothing by mouth
- Extracorporeal membrane oxygenation, if available
- O_2 therapy: intubation and mechanical ventilation using positive end-expiratory pressure (PEEP) or pressure-controlled inverse ratio ventilation
- Respiratory treatments

Drug therapy
- Anesthetic: propofol (Diprivan)
- Analgesic: morphine
- Bronchodilator: albuterol (Ventolin HFA)
- Antacid: aluminum hydroxide gel
- Antibiotics: according to infectious organism sensitivity
- Anticoagulants: heparin, enoxaparin (Lovenox), warfarin (Coumadin)
- Antianxiety agent: lorazepam (Ativan)
- Diuretics: furosemide (Lasix), ethacrynic acid (Edecrin)
- Exogenous surfactant: beractant (Survanta)
- Mucosal barrier fortifier: sucralfate (Carafate)
- Neuromuscular blocking agents: pancuronium, vecuronium
- Steroids: hydrocortisone (Solu-Cortef), methylprednisolone (Solu-Medrol)

INTERVENTIONS AND RATIONALES
- Assess respiratory, cardiovascular, and neurologic status *to detect evidence of hypoxemia, such as tachycardia, tachypnea, and irritability.*
- Monitor pulse oximetry continuously *to determine the effectiveness of therapy.*
- Monitor laboratory studies. *A drop in Hb and HCT affects the oxygen-carrying capacity of the blood. An increase in WBC count suggests an infection such as pneumonia. To detect*

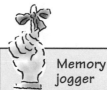

Memory jogger

To remember what happens in ARDS, use this mnemonic.

Assault to the pulmonary system

Respiratory distress

Decreased lung compliance

Severe respiratory failure

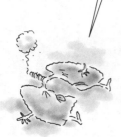

Pao$_2$ less than or equal to 50 mm Hg or Paco$_2$ greater than or equal to 50 mm Hg with a pH of 7.25 or less signals respiratory failure.

disseminated intravascular coagulation, a complication of ARDS, monitor platelet count, fibrinogen level, PT, INR, and PTT.
• Monitor and record intake and output and central venous pressure (CVP) *to determine fluid status and hemodynamic variables.*
• Monitor mechanical ventilation (high PEEP leaves the client at risk for pneumothorax) *to increase partial pressure of arterial oxygen (Pao$_2$) without raising F$_{IO_2}$, thereby reducing risk of O$_2$ toxicity,* and perform nasopharyngeal or oropharyngeal suctioning as necessary *to aid in removal of secretions.*
• Maintain bed rest, with prone positioning, if possible, *to promote oxygenation.*
• Maintain fluid restrictions *to reduce fluid volume overload.*
• Reposition the client every 2 hours *to stimulate postural drainage and mobilize secretions.*
• Provide chest physiotherapy *to promote drainage and keep airways clear.*
• Keep the client in high Fowler's position *to promote chest expansion.*
• Administer total parenteral nutrition or enteral feedings, as appropriate, *to prevent respiratory muscle impairment and maintain nutritional status.*
• Administer medications, as prescribed, *to optimize respiratory and hemodynamic status.*
• Organize nursing care with rest periods *to conserve energy and avoid overexertion and fatigue.*
• Weigh the client daily *to detect fluid retention.*
• Encourage the client to express feelings about fear of suffocation *to reduce anxiety and, therefore, O$_2$ demands.*

Teaching topics
• Explanation of the disorder and treatment plan
• Recognizing the signs and symptoms of respiratory distress
• Performing coughing and deep-breathing exercises and incentive spirometry
• Drug therapy
• Nutritional therapy and fluid restrictions if appropriate
• Importance of adequate rest
• Avoiding exposure to chemical irritants and pollutants

Acute respiratory failure

In acute respiratory failure, the respiratory system can't adequately supply the body with the O$_2$ it needs or adequately remove CO$_2$. A client is considered to be in respiratory failure when Pao$_2$ is less than or equal to 50 mm Hg or the partial pressure of arterial carbon dioxide (Paco$_2$) is greater than or equal to 50 mm Hg with a pH of less than or equal to 7.25.

Acute respiratory failure can be classified as ventilatory failure or oxygenation failure. Ventilatory failure is characterized by alveolar hypoventilation. Oxygenation failure is characterized by $\dot{V}/\dot{Q}$ ratio mismatching (blood flow to areas of the lung with reduced ventilation, or ventilation to lung tissue that's experiencing reduced blood flow) or physiologic shunting (blood moving from the right side of the heart to the left without being oxygenated).

CAUSES
• Abdominal or thoracic surgery
• ARDS
• Anesthesia
• Atelectasis
• Brain tumors
• Chronic obstructive pulmonary disease (COPD)
• Drug overdose
• Encephalitis
• Flail chest
• Guillain-Barré syndrome
• Head trauma
• Hemothorax
• Meningitis
• Multiple sclerosis
• Muscular dystrophy
• Myasthenia gravis
• Pleural effusion
• Pneumonia
• Pneumothorax
• Poliomyelitis
• Polyneuritis
• Pulmonary edema
• Pulmonary embolism
• Stroke

ASSESSMENT FINDINGS

- Adventitious breath sounds (crackles, rhonchi, wheezing, and pleural friction rub)
- Change in mentation, anxiety
- Chest pain
- Cough, sputum production, hemoptysis
- Cyanosis, diaphoresis
- Decreased respiratory excursion, accessory muscle use, retractions
- Difficulty breathing, shortness of breath, dyspnea, tachypnea, orthopnea
- Fatigue
- Nasal flaring
- Tachycardia

DIAGNOSTIC TEST RESULTS

- ABG levels show hypoxemia, acidosis, alkalosis, and hypercapnia.
- Chest X-ray shows pulmonary infiltrates, interstitial edema, and atelectasis.
- Hematology reveals increased WBC count and ESR.
- Lung scan shows $\dot{V}/\dot{Q}$ ratio mismatches.
- Sputum study identifies organism.

NURSING DIAGNOSES

- Activity intolerance
- Impaired gas exchange
- Ineffective peripheral tissue perfusion
- Ineffective airway clearance
- Anxiety
- Ineffective breathing pattern

TREATMENT

- Chest physiotherapy, postural drainage (position the client prone or supine with the foot of the bed elevated higher than the head for postural drainage), incentive spirometry
- Chest tube insertion, if pneumothorax develops from high PEEP administration
- Dietary changes, including establishing a high-calorie, high-protein diet, and restricting or encouraging fluids depending on the cause of the disorder
- O_2 therapy, intubation, and mechanical ventilation (possibly with PEEP)

Drug therapy

- Anesthetic: propofol (Diprivan)
- Antianxiety agent: lorazepam (Ativan)

- Antibiotics: according to sensitivity of causative organism
- Anticoagulant: enoxaparin (Lovenox)
- Bronchodilators: terbutaline, aminophylline, theophylline (Theochron); via nebulizer: albuterol (Proventil-HFA), ipratropium (Atrovent)
- Diuretic: furosemide (Lasix) if fluid overload is the cause
- Histamine-2 blockers: famotidine (Pepcid), ranitidine (Zantac), nizatidine (Axid)
- Neuromuscular blocking agents: pancuronium, vecuronium, atracurium
- Steroids: hydrocortisone (Solu-Cortef), methylprednisolone (Solu-Medrol)

INTERVENTIONS AND RATIONALES

- Assess respiratory status *to detect early signs of compromise and hypoxemia.*
- Monitor and record intake and output *to detect fluid volume excess, which may lead to pulmonary edema.*
- Track laboratory values. Report deteriorating ABG levels, such as a fall in Pa_{O_2} levels and rise in Pa_{CO_2} levels. *Low Hb and HCT levels reduce oxygen-carrying capacity of the blood. Electrolyte abnormalities may result from use of diuretics.*
- Monitor pulse oximetry *to detect a drop in arterial oxygen saturation (Sa_{O_2}).*
- Monitor and record vital signs. *Tachycardia and tachypnea may indicate hypoxemia.*
- Monitor and record color, consistency, and amount of sputum *to determine hydration status, effectiveness of therapy, and presence of infection.*
- During steroid therapy, monitor blood glucose level every 6 to 12 hours using a blood glucose meter *to detect hyperglycemia caused by steroid use.*
- Administer O_2 *to reduce hypoxemia and relieve respiratory distress.*
- Monitor mechanical ventilation *to prevent complications and optimize Pa_{O_2}.*
- Provide suctioning; assist with turning, coughing, and deep breathing; perform chest physiotherapy and postural drainage *to facilitate mobilization and removal of secretions.*
- Maintain bed rest *to reduce O_2 requirement.*

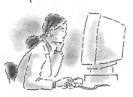

The client exhibits adventitious breath sounds and reports feeling "tired of breathing." It could be acute respiratory failure.

- Keep the client in semi-Fowler's or high Fowler's position *to promote chest expansion and ventilation.*
- Maintain diet restrictions. *Fluid restrictions and a low-sodium diet may be necessary to avoid fluid overload.*
- Administer medications, as prescribed, *to treat infection, dilate airways, and reduce inflammation.*
- Monitor chest tube system *to assess for lung re-expansion.*

Teaching topics
- Explanation of the disorder and treatment plan
- Recognizing the early signs and symptoms of respiratory difficulty
- Performing deep-breathing and coughing exercises and incentive spirometry
- Drug therapy
- Nutritional therapy
- Importance of adequate rest

Asbestosis

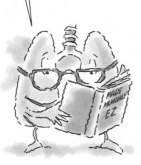

In asbestosis, my spaces are filled with and inflamed by asbestos fibers!

Asbestosis is characterized by widespread filling and inflammation of lung spaces with asbestos fibers. In asbestosis, asbestos fibers assume a longitudinal orientation in the airway, move in the direction of airflow, and penetrate respiratory bronchioles and alveolar walls. This causes diffuse interstitial fibrosis (tissue is filled with fibers).

Asbestosis can develop as long as 15 to 35 years after regular exposure to asbestos has ended. It increases the risk of lung cancer in cigarette smokers. No treatment can reverse the effects of asbestosis. Treatment focuses on relieving symptoms.

CAUSES
- Inhalation of asbestos fibers

ASSESSMENT FINDINGS
- Cor pulmonale
- Dry crackles at lung bases
- Dry cough
- Dyspnea on exertion (usually first symptom)
- Dyspnea at rest (in advanced disease)
- Finger clubbing
- Pleuritic chest pain
- Pulmonary hypertension
- Recurrent respiratory infections
- Right ventricular hypertrophy
- Tachypnea

DIAGNOSTIC TEST RESULTS
- ABG analysis reveals decreased PaO_2 and low $PaCO_2$.
- Chest X-rays show fine, irregular, and linear diffuse infiltrates; extensive fibrosis results in a "honeycomb" or "ground-glass" appearance. X-rays may also show pleural thickening and pleural calcification, with bilateral obliteration of costophrenic angles and, in later stages, an enlarged heart with a classic "shaggy" heart border.
- PFTs show decreased vital capacity, forced vital capacity, and total lung capacity and reduced diffusing capacity of the lungs.

NURSING DIAGNOSES
- Impaired gas exchange
- Ineffective breathing pattern
- Ineffective airway clearance
- Ineffective peripheral tissue perfusion
- Imbalanced nutrition: Less than body requirements
- Fatigue

TREATMENT
- Chest physiotherapy
- Fluid intake: at least 3 qt (3 L)/day unless contraindicated
- O_2 therapy or mechanical ventilation (in advanced cases)

Drug therapy
- Antibiotics: according to susceptibility of infecting organism (for treatment of respiratory tract infections)
- Cardiac glycoside: digoxin (Lanoxin)
- Diuretic: furosemide (Lasix)
- Mucolytic inhalation therapy: acetylcysteine

INTERVENTIONS AND RATIONALES
- Perform chest physiotherapy techniques, such as controlled coughing and segmental bronchial drainage, with chest percussion and vibration *to relieve respiratory symptoms.* Aerosol therapy, inhaled mucolytics, and

increased fluid intake (at least 3 qt [3 L] daily) *may also help relieve respiratory symptoms.*
• Administer diuretics and cardiac glycoside preparations for clients with cor pulmonale *to treat dyspnea, tachycardia, and dependent edema.*
• Administer O_2 by cannula or mask (1 to 2 L/minute), or by mechanical ventilation if Pao_2 can't be maintained above 40 mm Hg *to prevent complications of hypoxemia.*
• Prompt administration of antibiotics is required for respiratory infections *to prevent complications such as sepsis.*

Teaching topics
• Explanation of the disorder and treatment plan
• Drug therapy
• Avoiding chemical irritants and pollutants
• Signs and symptoms of complications
• Preventing infections by avoiding crowds, avoiding persons with infections, and receiving influenza and pneumococcal vaccines

Asphyxia

In asphyxia, interference with respiration leads to insufficient O_2 and accumulating CO_2 in the blood and tissues. Asphyxia leads to cardiopulmonary arrest and is fatal without prompt treatment.

CAUSES
• Extrapulmonary obstruction, such as tracheal compression from a tumor, strangulation, trauma, or suffocation
• Hypoventilation as a result of opioid overdose, medullary disease, hemorrhage, pneumothorax, respiratory muscle paralysis, or cardiopulmonary arrest
• Inhalation of toxic agents, such as carbon monoxide poisoning, smoke inhalation, and excessive O_2 inhalation
• Intrapulmonary obstruction, such as airway obstruction, severe asthma, foreign body aspiration, pulmonary edema, pneumonia, and near-drowning

ASSESSMENT FINDINGS
• Agitation
• Altered respiratory rate (apnea, bradypnea, occasional tachypnea)

• Anxiety
• Central and peripheral cyanosis (cherry-red mucous membranes in late-stage carbon monoxide poisoning)
• Confusion leading to coma
• Decreased breath sounds
• Dyspnea
• Fast, slow, or absent pulse
• Hypotension
• Seizures

DIAGNOSTIC TEST RESULTS
• ABG measurement indicates decreased Pao_2 (< 60 mm Hg) and increased $Paco_2$ (> 50 mm Hg).
• Chest X-rays may show a foreign body, pulmonary edema, or atelectasis.
• PFTs may indicate respiratory muscle weakness.
• Pulse oximetry reveals decreased Hb saturation of O_2.
• Toxicology tests may show drugs, chemicals, or abnormal Hb levels.

NURSING DIAGNOSES
• Decreased cardiac output
• Ineffective peripheral tissue perfusion
• Ineffective breathing pattern
• Ineffective airway clearance
• Impaired gas exchange
• Impaired spontaneous ventilation
• Risk for suffocation

TREATMENT
• Bronchoscopy (for extraction of a foreign body)
• Gastric lavage (for poisoning or overdose)
• O_2 therapy, which may include endotracheal intubation and mechanical ventilation
• Psychiatric evaluation (with overdose)

Drug therapy
• Opioid antagonist: naloxone (for opioid overdose)
• Activated charcoal
• Antidote for poisoning

INTERVENTIONS AND RATIONALES
• Assess cardiac and respiratory status *to detect early signs of compromise.*

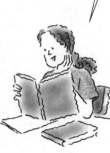

Because asbestosis can't be cured, client care focuses on relieving respiratory symptoms and controlling complications.

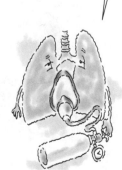

Gasp! In asphyxia, client care focuses on treating the cause and providing me with oxygen.

- Position the client upright, if his condition tolerates, *to promote lung expansion and improve oxygenation.*
- Reassure the client during treatment *to ease anxiety associated with respiratory distress.*
- Give prescribed medications *to promote ventilation and oxygenation.*
- Suction carefully, as needed, and encourage deep breathing *to mobilize secretions and maintain a patent airway.*
- Closely monitor vital signs and laboratory test results *to guide the treatment plan.*

Teaching topics
- Cause of asphyxia and treatment plan
- Need for follow-up medical or psychiatric care
- Avoiding a combination of alcohol with other central nervous system (CNS) depressants

Asthma

Asthma is a form of chronic obstructive airway disease in which the bronchial linings overreact to various stimuli, causing episodic spasms and inflammation that severely restrict the airways. Symptoms range from mild wheezing and labored breathing to life-threatening respiratory failure.

Asthma can be extrinsic or intrinsic (or a person may have both). Extrinsic (atopic) asthma is caused by sensitivity to specific external allergens. Intrinsic (nonatopic) asthma is caused by a reaction to internal, nonallergic factors.

CAUSES
Extrinsic asthma
- Allergens (pollen, dander, dust, sulfite food additives)

Intrinsic asthma
- Endocrine changes
- Exercise
- Noxious fumes
- Respiratory infection
- Stress
- Temperature and humidity

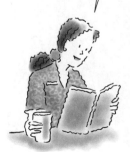

Clients with asthma should receive 3 qt (3 L) of fluids per day.

ASSESSMENT FINDINGS
- Absent or diminished breath sounds during severe obstruction
- Chest tightness
- Dyspnea
- Lack of symptoms between attacks (usually)
- Productive cough with thick mucus
- Prolonged expiration
- Tachypnea, tachycardia
- Use of accessory muscles
- Wheezing, primarily on expiration but sometimes on inspiration

DIAGNOSTIC TEST RESULTS
- ABG studies in acute severe asthma show decreased Pao_2 and decreased, normal, or increased $Paco_2$.
- Blood tests: Serum immunoglobulin E may increase from an allergic reaction; complete blood count (CBC) may reveal increased eosinophil count.
- Chest X-ray shows hyperinflated lungs with air trapping during an attack.
- PFTs during attacks show decreased forced expiratory volumes that improve with therapy and increased residual volume and total lung capacity.
- Skin tests may identify allergens.
- Pulse oximetry readings are decreased.

NURSING DIAGNOSES
- Ineffective airway clearance
- Impaired gas exchange
- Ineffective health management
- Ineffective breathing pattern
- Anxiety
- Fear

TREATMENT
- Desensitization to allergens (see *An ounce of prevention*)
- Fluids to 3 qt (3 L)/day unless contraindicated
- Intubation and mechanical ventilation if respiratory status worsens
- Oxygen therapy at 2 L/minute

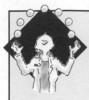

Management moments

An ounce of prevention

Because in many cases clients with asthma can use prevention techniques to avoid asthma attacks, it's important for you to educate the client about these techniques. Begin by helping the client identify attack triggers, such as exercise, stress, anxiety, and cold air. Then instruct the client to avoid these triggers. When avoiding the triggers isn't possible, tell the client to use a metered dose inhaler prophylactically to avoid an attack. Also, teach the client peak flow meter use so he can quickly identify when his respiratory status is deteriorating.

Drug therapy
- Antacid: aluminum hydroxide gel
- Antibiotics: according to sensitivity of infective organism
- Antileukotrienes: zafirlukast (Accolate), montelukast (Singulair)
- Beta-adrenergic drugs: epinephrine, salmeterol (Serevent)
- Bronchodilators: terbutaline, aminophylline, theophylline (Theochron); via metered dose inhaler: albuterol (Proventil-HFA), ipratropium (Atrovent)
- Mast cell stabilizer: cromolyn (Intal)
- Steroids: hydrocortisone (Solu-Cortef), methylprednisolone (Solu-Medrol)
- Steroids (via metered dose inhaler): beclomethasone (Beconase AQ), triamcinolone (Azmacort)
- Mucolytics: acetylcysteine, guaifenesin

INTERVENTIONS AND RATIONALES
- Administer low-flow humidified O_2 *to reduce inflammation of the airways, ease breathing, and increase Sao_2.*
- Administer medications, as prescribed, *to reduce inflammation and obstruction of airways.* Auscultate lungs for improved breath sounds. Observe for complications of drug therapy.
- Encourage the client to express feelings about fear of suffocation *to reduce anxiety. As breathlessness and hypoxemia are relieved, anxiety should be reduced.*
- Allow activity, as tolerated, with rest periods *to reduce work of breathing and reduce O_2 demands.*
- Assess respiratory status *to determine the effectiveness of therapy, such as clear breath sounds and improved airflow, PFTs, Sao_2, and ease of breathing.*
- Assist with turning, coughing, deep breathing, and breathing retraining *to mobilize and clear secretions. Pursed-lip and diaphragmatic breathing promote more effective ventilation.*
- Keep the client in high Fowler's position *to improve ventilation.*
- Maintain the client's diet and administer small, frequent feedings *to reduce pressure on the diaphragm and increase caloric intake.*
- Encourage fluids *to treat dehydration and liquefy secretions to facilitate their removal.*
- Monitor and record the color, amount, and consistency of sputum. *Changes in sputum characteristics may signal a respiratory infection.*
- Monitor and record vital signs. *Tachycardia may indicate worsening asthma or drug toxicity. Hypertension may indicate hypoxemia. Fever may signal infection.*
- Monitor laboratory studies. *An increase in WBC count may signal infection. Eosinophilia may indicate an allergic response. Drug levels may reveal toxicity.*
- Provide chest physiotherapy, postural drainage, incentive spirometry, and suction *to aid in the removal of secretions.*
- During steroid therapy, monitor blood glucose level every 6 to 12 hours using a blood glucose meter *to detect hyperglycemia caused by steroid use.*

Teaching topics
- Explanation of the disorder and treatment plan
- Identifying and avoiding triggers

Humidified O_2 reduces inflammation of asthmatic airways, eases breathing, and increases Sao_2.

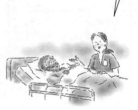

- Recognizing the early signs and symptoms of respiratory infection and hypoxia
- Keeping medications readily available in case of emergency
- Taking medications properly and using a metered dose inhaler
- Using a peak flow meter
- Performing pursed-lip, diaphragmatic breathing and coughing and deep-breathing exercises
- Avoiding exposure to chemical irritants and pollutants
- Avoiding gas-producing foods, spicy foods, and extremely hot or cold foods
- Smoking cessation
- Increasing fluid intake to 3 qt (3 L)/day unless contraindicated
- Contacting the American Lung Association

Atelectasis

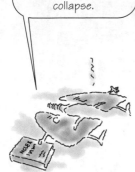

Atelectasis is the incomplete expansion of a lung, which may result in partial or complete collapse.

Atelectasis is marked by incomplete expansion of lobules (clusters of alveoli) or lung segments, which may result in partial or complete lung collapse. The collapsed areas are unavailable for gas exchange; blood that lacks O_2 passes through unchanged, thereby producing hypoxemia.

Atelectasis may be chronic or acute. It occurs to some degree in many clients undergoing upper abdominal or thoracic surgery. The prognosis depends on prompt removal of any airway obstruction, relief of hypoxia, and re-expansion of the collapsed lung.

CAUSES
- Bronchial occlusion by mucus plugs, as in clients with COPD, bronchiectasis, or cystic fibrosis or those who smoke heavily
- CNS depression
- External compression, such as from upper abdominal surgical incisions, rib fractures, pleuritic chest pain, tight dressings around the chest, or obesity
- Occlusion by foreign bodies, bronchogenic carcinoma, and inflammatory lung disease
- Prolonged immobility

ASSESSMENT FINDINGS
- Diminished or bronchial breath sounds
- Dyspnea
- Pulmonary crackles
- Pain on the affected side
- Tachypnea

In severe cases
- Anxiety
- Cyanosis
- Diaphoresis
- Hyperinflation of unaffected areas of the lung
- Peripheral circulatory collapse
- Severe dyspnea
- Substernal or intercostal retraction
- Tachycardia

DIAGNOSTIC TEST RESULTS
- Chest X-ray shows characteristic horizontal lines in the lower lung zones and, with segmental or lobar collapse, characteristic dense shadows associated with hyperinflation of neighboring lung zones (in widespread atelectasis).

NURSING DIAGNOSES
- Impaired gas exchange
- Ineffective breathing pattern
- Risk for infection
- Anxiety
- Fear
- Activity intolerance

TREATMENT
- Bronchoscopy
- Chest physiotherapy
- Surgery or radiation therapy to remove an obstructing neoplasm

Drug therapy
- Analgesic: morphine
- Antibiotics: according to causative organism (when bacterial infection is present)
- Bronchodilator: albuterol (Proventil-HFA)
- Mucolytic inhalation therapy: acetylcysteine

INTERVENTIONS AND RATIONALES
- Encourage postoperative and other high-risk clients to cough and deep breathe every 1 to 2 hours *to prevent atelectasis.*

- Teach the client how to use an incentive spirometer and encourage him to use it every 1 to 2 hours *to encourage deep inspiration through positive reinforcement.*
- Teach the splinting technique *to minimize pain during coughing exercises in postoperative clients.*
- Encourage ambulation *to prevent atelectasis.*
- Administer adequate analgesics *to control pain. Pain may inhibit the client from taking deep breaths, which leads to atelectasis.*
- During mechanical ventilation, maintain tidal volume at 8 to 10 ml/kg of the client's body weight *to ensure adequate lung expansion.* Use the sigh mechanism on the ventilator, if appropriate, *to intermittently increase tidal volume at the rate of 10 to 15 sighs/hour.*
- Reposition the client every 2 hours *to help mobilize secretions.*
- Humidify inspired air and encourage adequate fluid intake *to liquefy secretions.* Perform postural drainage and chest percussion *to promote loosening and clearance of secretions.*
- Provide suctioning as needed. Use sedatives with discretion *because they depress respirations and the cough reflex and suppress sighing.*
- Assess breath sounds and ventilatory status frequently and be alert for any changes *to prevent respiratory compromise.*
- Encourage lifestyle changes, such as stopping smoking, losing weight, or both, as needed. Refer him to appropriate support groups for help *to modify risk factors.*
- Provide reassurance and emotional support *to decrease anxiety that may affect breathing.*

Teaching topics
- Explanation of the disorder and treatment plan
- Importance of adequate fluid intake
- Performing effective incisional splinting
- Performing respiratory care such as postural drainage, coughing, deep breathing, and incentive spirometry
- Stopping smoking and losing weight if appropriate
- Performing relaxation techniques

Bronchiectasis

Bronchiectasis is marked by chronic abnormal dilation of bronchi (large air passages of the lungs) and destruction of bronchial walls.

Bronchiectasis has three forms: cylindrical (fusiform), varicose, and saccular (cystic). It can occur throughout the tracheobronchial tree or can be confined to one segment or lobe. However, it's usually bilateral and involves the basilar segments of the lower lobes.

The disorder affects people of both sexes and all ages and, once established, is irreversible. Because of the availability of antibiotics to treat acute respiratory tract infections, the incidence of bronchiectasis has dramatically decreased in the past 20 years.

CAUSES
- Inhalation of corrosive gas or repeated aspiration of gastric juices into the lungs
- Immunologic disorders such as agammaglobulinemia
- Mucoviscidosis (in cases of cystic fibrosis)
- Obstruction (by a foreign body, tumor, or stenosis) in association with recurrent infection
- Recurrent, inadequately treated bacterial respiratory tract infections, such as TB and complications of measles, pneumonia, pertussis, or influenza

ASSESSMENT FINDINGS
- Chronic cough that produces copious, foul-smelling, mucopurulent secretions, possibly totaling several cupfuls daily
- Coarse crackles during inspiration over involved lobes or segments, rhonchi, wheezing
- Exertional dyspnea
- Fatigue
- Fetid breath
- Digital clubbing
- Sinusitis
- Anorexia

DIAGNOSTIC TEST RESULTS
- Bronchoscopy helps to identify the source of secretions or the bleeding site in hemoptysis
- Chest X-rays show peribronchial thickening, areas of atelectasis, and scattered cystic changes.

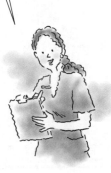

Using an incentive spirometer can help clients become involved in their own care.

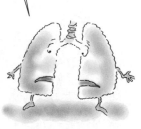

The bad news is bronchiectasis is irreversible when established. The good news is antibiotics have drastically reduced the incidence of this disorder.

- CBC detects anemia and leukocytosis.
- PFTs detect decreased vital capacity, expiratory flow, and hypoxemia.
- Sputum culture and Gram stain identify predominant organisms.

NURSING DIAGNOSES
- Imbalanced nutrition: Less than body requirements
- Impaired gas exchange
- Ineffective airway clearance
- Activity intolerance
- Ineffective breathing pattern
- Anxiety

TREATMENT
- Bronchoscopy (to mobilize secretions)
- Chest physiotherapy and incentive spirometry
- O_2 therapy

Drug therapy
- Antibiotics: according to sensitivity of causative organism
- Bronchodilator: albuterol (Proventil-HFA)
- Mucolytic: acetylcysteine

INTERVENTIONS AND RATIONALES
- Assess respiratory status *to detect early signs of decompensation*.
- Provide supportive care and help the client adjust to the permanent changes in lifestyle that irreversible lung damage necessitates *to facilitate positive coping*.
- Administer antibiotics as needed *to eradicate infection*.
- Explain all diagnostic tests to the client *to decrease anxiety*.
- Perform chest physiotherapy, including postural drainage and chest percussion designed for involved lobes, several times per day. Encourage use of incentive spirometry every 1 to 2 hours while the client is awake *to mobilize secretions*.
- Encourage increased fluid intake (unless contraindicated) *to liquefy secretions*.

Teaching topics
- Explanation of the disorder and treatment plan
- Drug therapy
- Home O_2 therapy

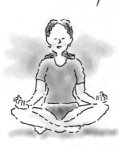

You've read about your client's breathing—now it's time to do some breathing of your own. Take a deep breath and relax—and then get back to studying.

- Instruction for family members on how to perform chest physiotherapy
- Importance of quitting smoking
- Dietary considerations and fluid intake
- Signs and symptoms of complications
- Proper disposal of secretions to prevent the spread of infection to others

Chronic bronchitis

Chronic bronchitis, a form of COPD, results from irritants and infections that increase mucus production, impair airway clearance, and cause irreversible narrowing of the small airways. This causes a severe $\dot{V}/\dot{Q}$ imbalance, leading to hypoxemia and CO_2 retention.

CAUSES
- Airborne irritants and pollutants
- Chronic respiratory infections
- Smoking

ASSESSMENT FINDINGS
- Dyspnea
- Finger clubbing, later in the disease
- Increased sputum production
- Productive cough
- Prolonged expiration
- Rhonchi, wheezes
- Use of accessory muscles
- Weight gain, edema, jugular vein distention
- Reddish-blue skin color (later in the disease)

DIAGNOSTIC TEST RESULTS
- ABG studies show decreased Pao_2 and normal or increased $Paco_2$.
- Chest X-ray shows hyperinflation and increased bronchovascular markings.
- Electrocardiogram (ECG) shows atrial arrhythmias, peaked P waves in leads II, III, and aV_F and, occasionally, right ventricular hypertrophy.
- PFTs may reveal increased residual volume, decreased vital capacity and forced expiratory volumes, and normal static compliance and diffusion capacity.
- Sputum culture may reveal many microorganisms and neutrophils.

NURSING DIAGNOSES
- Activity intolerance
- Ineffective airway clearance
- Ineffective breathing pattern
- Impaired gas exchange

TREATMENT
- Chest physiotherapy, postural drainage, and incentive spirometry
- Dietary changes, including establishing a diet high in protein, vitamin C, calories, and nitrogen, and avoiding milk
- Fluid intake up to 3 qt (3 L)/day, if not contraindicated
- Endotracheal intubation and mechanical ventilation, if respiratory status deteriorates
- O_2 therapy at 2 to 3 L/minute

Drug therapy
- Antacid: aluminum hydroxide gel
- Antibiotics: according to sensitivity of infective organism
- Bronchodilators: terbutaline, aminophylline, theophylline (Theochron); via nebulizer or metered dose inhaler: albuterol (Proventil-HFA), ipratropium (Atrovent)
- Diuretic: furosemide (Lasix) for edema
- Expectorant: guaifenesin
- Influenza and Pneumovax vaccines
- Steroids: hydrocortisone (Solu-Cortef), methylprednisolone (Solu-Medrol)
- Steroids (via nebulizer or metered dose inhaler): beclomethasone (Beconase AQ), triamcinolone (Azmacort)

INTERVENTIONS AND RATIONALES
- Administer low-flow O_2. *Because clients with chronic bronchitis have chronic hypercapnia, they have a hypoxic respiratory drive. Higher flow rates may eliminate this hypoxic respiratory drive.*
- Administer medications, as prescribed, *to relieve symptoms and prevent complications.*
- During steroid therapy, monitor blood glucose level every 6 to 12 hours using a blood glucose meter *to detect hyperglycemia caused by steroid use.*
- Allow activity, as tolerated, *to avoid fatigue and reduce O_2 demands.*
- Assess respiratory status, ABG levels, and pulse oximetry *to detect respiratory compromise, severe hypoxemia, and hypercapnia.*

- Assist with turning, coughing, and deep breathing *to mobilize secretions and facilitate removal.*
- Assist with diaphragmatic and pursed-lip breathing *to strengthen respiratory muscles.*
- Keep the client in high Fowler's position *to improve ventilation.*
- Maintain the client's diet and administer small, frequent feedings *to avoid fatigue when eating and reduce pressure on the diaphragm from a full stomach.*
- Monitor and record the color, amount, and consistency of sputum. *Changes in sputum characteristics may signal a respiratory infection.*
- Monitor and record cardiovascular status and vital signs. *Edema, jugular venous distention, tachycardia, and elevated CVP suggest right-sided heart failure. An irregular pulse may indicate an arrhythmia caused by altered ABG levels. Tachycardia and tachypnea may indicate hypoxemia.*
- Monitor laboratory studies. *Follow drug levels for evidence of toxicity. Electrolyte imbalances may occur with the use of diuretics. Reduced Hb levels and HCT affect the oxygen-carrying capacity of the blood.*
- Monitor intake and output and daily weights *to detect fluid overload associated with right-sided heart failure. Dehydration impairs the removal of secretions.*
- Provide chest physiotherapy, postural drainage, incentive spirometry, and suction *to aid in removal of secretions.*
- Weigh the client daily *to detect fluid gain caused by right-sided heart failure.*

Teaching topics
- Explanation of the disorder and treatment plan
- Drug therapy
- Pulmonary rehabilitation
- Recognizing the early signs and symptoms of respiratory infection and hypoxia
- Home O_2 and nebulizer equipment use
- Performing pursed-lip, diaphragmatic breathing, coughing, and deep-breathing, and incentive spirometer exercises
- Avoiding exposure to chemical irritants and pollutants
- Avoiding gas-producing foods, spicy foods, and extremely hot or cold foods
- Smoking cessation

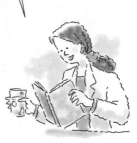

You should encourage clients with chronic bronchitis to drink 3 qt of fluids a day—unless it's contraindicated.

- Increasing fluid intake to 3 qt (3 L)/day, if not contraindicated
- Contacting the American Lung Association

Cor pulmonale

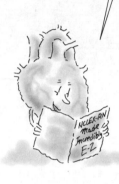

Pulmonary peril. In cor pulmonale, my right ventricle enlarges because of diseases that affect the lungs.

A chronic heart condition, cor pulmonale is hypertrophy (enlargement) of the heart's right ventricle that results from diseases affecting the function or the structure of the lungs. To compensate for the extra work needed to force blood through the lungs, the right ventricle dilates and enlarges.

Invariably, cor pulmonale follows some disorder of the lungs, pulmonary vessels, chest wall, or respiratory control center. For example, COPD produces pulmonary hypertension, which leads to right ventricular hypertrophy, which can lead to right-sided heart failure (although cor pulmonale can occur without heart failure). Because cor pulmonale generally occurs late during the course of COPD and other irreversible diseases, the prognosis is generally poor.

CAUSES
- COPD (about 25% of clients with COPD eventually develop cor pulmonale)
- Living at high altitudes (chronic mountain sickness)
- Loss of lung tissue after extensive lung surgery
- Obesity-hypoventilation syndrome (pickwickian syndrome) and upper airway obstruction
- Obstructive lung diseases such as bronchiectasis and cystic fibrosis
- Pulmonary vascular diseases, such as recurrent thromboembolism, primary pulmonary hypertension, schistosomiasis, and pulmonary vasculitis
- Respiratory insufficiency without pulmonary disease, as seen in chest wall disorders, such as kyphoscoliosis, neuromuscular incompetence resulting from muscular dystrophy and amyotrophic lateral sclerosis, polymyositis, and spinal cord lesions above C6
- Restrictive lung diseases, such as pneumoconiosis, interstitial pneumonitis, scleroderma, and sarcoidosis

ASSESSMENT FINDINGS
- Chronic productive cough
- Dyspnea on exertion
- Edema
- Fatigue
- Orthopnea
- Tachypnea
- Weakness
- Wheezing respirations

DIAGNOSTIC TEST RESULTS
- ABG analysis shows decreased Pao_2 (< 70 mm Hg).
- Blood tests show HCT greater than 50%.
- Chest X-ray shows large central pulmonary arteries and suggests right ventricular enlargement by rightward enlargement of cardiac silhouette on an anterior chest film.
- Echocardiography or angiography indicates right ventricular enlargement, and echocardiography can estimate pulmonary artery pressure (PAP).
- ECG commonly shows arrhythmias, such as premature atrial and ventricular contractions and atrial fibrillation during severe hypoxia. It may also show right bundle-branch block, right axis deviation, prominent P waves and an inverted T wave in right precordial leads, and right ventricular hypertrophy.
- PAP measurements show increased right ventricular pressure as a result of increased pulmonary vascular resistance.
- PFTs show results consistent with the underlying pulmonary disease.

NURSING DIAGNOSES
- Activity intolerance
- Excess fluid volume
- Impaired gas exchange
- Anxiety
- Ineffective breathing pattern

TREATMENT
- Diet: low salt, with restricted fluid intake
- O_2 therapy by mask or cannula in concentrations ranging from 24% to 40%, depending on Pao_2 as necessary and, in acute cases, endotracheal intubation and mechanical ventilation

Drug therapy

• Angiotensin-converting enzyme inhibitor: captopril (Capoten)
• Antibiotics (when respiratory infection is present)
• Anticoagulant: heparin
• Calcium channel blocker: diltiazem (Cardizem)
• Cardiac glycoside: digoxin (Lanoxin)
• Diuretic: furosemide (Lasix)
• Vasodilators: diazoxide, hydralazine, nitroprusside (Nitropress), prostaglandins (in primary pulmonary hypertension)

INTERVENTIONS AND RATIONALES

• Provide small, frequent feedings rather than three heavy meals *because the client may lack energy and tire easily when eating.*
• Limit the client's fluid intake to 1 to 2 qt (1 to 2 L)/day, and provide a low-sodium diet *to prevent fluid retention.*
• Monitor serum potassium levels closely if the client is receiving diuretics. *Low serum potassium levels can potentiate the risk of arrhythmias associated with cardiac glycosides.*
• Monitor digoxin level *to prevent symptoms of cardiac glycoside toxicity, such as anorexia, nausea, vomiting, and yellow halos around visual images.*
• Reposition the client every 2 hours *to prevent atelectasis and to avoid skin breakdown.*
• Provide meticulous respiratory care, including O_2 therapy and, for clients with COPD, pursed-lip breathing exercises, *to improve oxygenation.*
• Monitor ABG levels and watch for signs of respiratory failure such as a change in pulse rate; deep, labored respirations; and increased fatigue produced by exertion. *Monitoring these parameters helps detect early signs of worsening respiratory status.*

Teaching topics

• Explanation of the disorder and treatment plan
• Smoking cessation, if appropriate
• Drug therapy
• Dietary and fluid recommendations
• Importance of follow-up examinations.
• Home O_2 therapy

• How to check a radial pulse before taking a cardiac glycoside and when to report changes in pulse rate

Emphysema

Emphysema is a form of COPD in which recurrent pulmonary inflammation damages and eventually destroys the alveolar walls, creating large air spaces. This breakdown leaves the alveoli unable to recoil normally after expanding, and, upon expiration, results in bronchiolar collapse. This traps air in the lungs, leading to overdistention and reduced gas exchange.

CAUSES

• Deficiency of alpha$_1$-antitrypsin
• Smoking

ASSESSMENT FINDINGS

• Anorexia, weight loss
• Barrel chest
• Decreased breath sounds
• Dyspnea
• Finger clubbing (late in the disease)
• Hyper-resonance (with percussion over lung fields)
• Prolonged expiration
• Pursed-lip breathing
• Use of accessory muscles for breathing

DIAGNOSTIC TEST RESULTS

• ABG studies show reduced PaO_2, with normal $PaCO_2$ until late in the disease.
• Chest X-ray in advanced disease reveals a flattened diaphragm, reduced vascular markings in the lung periphery, enlarged anteroposterior chest diameter, and a vertical heart.
• CBC shows increased Hb late in disease when client has severe persistent hypoxia.
• ECG shows tall, symmetrical P waves in leads II, III, and aV_F, vertical QRS axis, and signs of right ventricular hypertrophy late in disease.
• PFTs show increased residual volume, total lung capacity, and compliance as well as decreased vital capacity, diffusing capacity, and expiratory volumes.

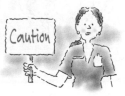

Cor pulmonale clients with underlying COPD shouldn't receive high concentrations of oxygen. It could lead to subsequent respiratory depression.

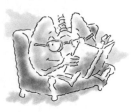

Check it out. With emphysema, PFTs show an increase in my residual volume, total capacity, and compliance.

Diaphragmatic and pursed-lip breathing strengthens respiratory muscles.

NURSING DIAGNOSES
- Ineffective breathing pattern
- Anxiety
- Activity intolerance
- Fatigue
- Impaired gas exchange
- Risk for infection

TREATMENT
- Chest physiotherapy, postural drainage, and incentive spirometry
- Dietary changes, including establishing a diet high in protein, vitamin C, calories, and nitrogen
- Fluid intake up to 3 qt (3 L)/day, if not contraindicated
- Endotracheal intubation and mechanical ventilation, if respiratory status deteriorates
- O_2 therapy at 2 to 3 L/minute; transtracheal therapy for home O_2 therapy
- Ultrasonic or mechanical nebulizer treatments
- Lung volume reduction surgery

Drug therapy
- Alpha$_1$-antitrypsin therapy
- Antacid: aluminum hydroxide gel
- Antibiotics: according to sensitivity of infective organism
- Bronchodilators: terbutaline, aminophylline, theophylline (Theocron); via nebulizer: albuterol (Proventil-HFA), ipratropium (Atrovent)
- Diuretic: furosemide (Lasix) for edema
- Expectorant: guaifenesin
- Influenza and Pneumovax vaccines
- Steroids: hydrocortisone (Solu-Cortef), methylprednisolone (Solu-Medrol)
- Steroids (via nebulizer): beclomethasone (Beconase AQ), triamcinolone (Azmacort)

INTERVENTIONS AND RATIONALES
- Administer low-flow O_2 *because emphysema clients have chronic hypercapnia, so they have a hypoxic respiratory drive. Higher flow rates may eliminate this hypoxic respiratory drive.*
- Administer medications, as prescribed, *to relieve symptoms and prevent complications.*
- Allow activity, as tolerated, *to avoid fatigue and reduce O_2 demands.*
- Assess respiratory status, ABG levels, and pulse oximetry *to detect respiratory compromise, severe hypoxemia, and hypercapnia.*

- Monitor and record cardiovascular status and vital signs. *An irregular pulse may indicate an arrhythmia caused by altered ABG levels. Tachycardia and tachypnea may indicate hypoxemia. Late in the disease, pulmonary hypertension may lead to right ventricular hypertrophy and right-sided heart failure. Jugular vein distention, edema, hypotension, tachycardia, third heart sound (S_3), a loud pulmonic component of second heart sound (S_2), heart murmurs, and hepatojugular reflux may be present.*
- Assist with turning, coughing, and deep breathing, and encourage use of incentive spirometry *to mobilize secretions and facilitate removal.*
- Assist with diaphragmatic and pursed-lip breathing *to strengthen respiratory muscles.*
- Keep the client in high Fowler's position *to improve ventilation.*
- Maintain the client's diet and administer small, frequent feedings *to avoid fatigue when eating. Small meals relieve pressure on the diaphragm and allow fuller lung movement.*
- Monitor and record the color, amount, and consistency of sputum. *Changes in sputum may signal a respiratory infection.*
- Monitor laboratory studies. *Follow drug levels for evidence of toxicity. Electrolyte imbalances may occur with the use of diuretics. Reduced Hb levels and HCT affect the oxygen-carrying capacity of the blood.*
- Monitor intake and output and daily weight *to detect fluid overload associated with right-sided heart failure. Dehydration may impair the removal of secretions.*
- Encourage fluids, unless contraindicated, *to liquefy secretions.*
- Provide chest physiotherapy and postural drainage and suction *to help remove secretions.*

Teaching topics
- Explanation of the disorder and treatment plan
- Drug therapy
- Pulmonary rehabilitation
- Recognizing the early signs and symptoms of respiratory infection and hypoxia
- Using home O_2 and nebulizer equipment properly

- Performing pursed-lip, diaphragmatic breathing, coughing and deep-breathing exercises, and incentive spirometry
- Avoiding exposure to chemical irritants and pollutants
- Avoiding gas-producing foods, spicy foods, and extremely hot or cold foods
- Smoking cessation
- Increasing fluid intake to 3 qt (3 L)/day, if not contraindicated
- Avoiding people with respiratory infections
- Receiving vaccinations
- Contacting the American Lung Association

Idiopathic pulmonary fibrosis

IPF is a chronic and usually fatal interstitial pulmonary disease. About 50% of clients with IPF will die within 5 years of the IPF diagnosis. Once thought to be a rare condition, IPF is now diagnosed with much greater frequency.

CAUSES
- Possible genetic or viral cause
- Unknown stimulus begins inflammation

ASSESSMENT FINDINGS
- Bronchial breath sounds
- Clubbing of fingertips
- Dry, hacking, paroxysmal cough
- Dyspnea
- Rapid, shallow breathing

In late cases
- Augmented S_3 and S_4 gallop
- Cyanosis
- Profound hypoxemia
- Pulmonary hypertension

DIAGNOSTIC TEST RESULTS
- ABG analysis and pulse oximetry shows hypoxemia, which may be mild in the early stages, and then becomes severe.
- Chest X-rays may show one of four distinct patterns: interstitial, reticulonodular, ground-glass, or honeycomb. Chest X-rays are helpful in identifying the presence of an abnormality, but they don't help determine disease severity. Serial X-rays may help track the progression of the disease.
- High-resolution computed tomography (CT) scans help distinguish the patterns seen on chest X-ray and help establish the diagnosis of IPF.
- Lung biopsy findings vary based on the stage of the disease. In general, the alveolar walls are swollen with chronic inflammatory infiltrates. In the late disease stages, the alveolar walls are destroyed and are replaced by honeycombing cysts.
- PFTs show reduction in vital capacity and total lung capacity and impaired diffusing capacity for carbon monoxide.

NURSING DIAGNOSES
- Impaired gas exchange
- Ineffective breathing pattern
- Fatigue
- Activity intolerance

TREATMENT
- Lung transplant: in younger, otherwise healthy clients
- O_2 therapy

Drug therapy
- Corticosteroids and cytotoxic drugs: to suppress inflammation, but are usually unsuccessful
- Interferon-gamma-1B (has shown early promise in treating the disease)

INTERVENTIONS AND RATIONALES
- Assess respiratory status.
- Monitor O_2 levels *to determine the client's oxygen needs.*
- Administer O_2 as needed *to help minimize the client's dyspnea.*
- Encourage activity to the extent the client is able *to help the client maintain his lifestyle.*
- Provide emotional support *because the client and his family will be dealing with his increasing disability, dyspnea, and probable death.*
- Set up O_2 therapy at home *because the client will require it around-the-clock.*
- Encourage good nutritional habits *because the client may find that dyspnea interferes with eating.*

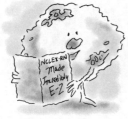

In lung cancer, unregulated cell growth and uncontrolled cell division result in the development of a neoplasm.

Teaching topics
- Explanation of the disorder and treatment plan
- Drug therapy
- Home O_2 therapy
- Dietary recommendations
- Planning of daily activities

Lung cancer

In lung cancer, unregulated cell growth and uncontrolled cell division result in the development of a neoplasm. Cancer may also affect the lungs as a result of metastasis from other organs, mainly the liver, brain, bone, kidneys, and adrenal glands.

Four histologic types of lung cancer include:

☝ squamous cell (epidermoid), a slow-growing cancer that originates from bronchial epithelium. It metastasizes late to the surrounding area, but may cause bronchial obstruction.

✌ adenocarcinoma, a moderately growing cancer located in peripheral areas of the lung. It metastasizes through the bloodstream to other organs.

🤟 large-cell anaplastic, a very fast-growing cancer associated with early and extensive metastasis. It's more common in peripheral lung tissue.

🖐 small-cell (oat cell cancer), a very fast-growing cancer that metastasizes very early through lymph vessels and the bloodstream to other organs.

CAUSES
- Tobacco use
- Exposure to environmental pollutants
- Exposure to occupational pollutants

ASSESSMENT FINDINGS
- Hypoxemia
- Hypotension
- Chest pain
- Chills, fever
- Cough, hemoptysis
- Dyspnea, wheezing

In a client with lung cancer, a chest X-ray shows the lesion or mass.

- Weakness, fatigue
- Weight loss, anorexia

DIAGNOSTIC TEST RESULTS
- Bronchoscopy reveals a positive biopsy.
- Chest X-ray shows a lesion or mass.
- Lung scan shows a mass.
- Open lung biopsy reveals a positive biopsy.
- Sputum study reveals positive cytology for cancer cells.

NURSING DIAGNOSES
- Fear
- Activity intolerance
- Anxiety
- Impaired gas exchange

TREATMENT
- Dietary changes, including establishing a high-protein, high-calorie diet and providing small, frequent meals
- Incentive spirometry
- Laser photocoagulation
- O_2 therapy, intubation and, if the condition deteriorates, mechanical ventilation
- Radiation therapy
- Resection of the affected lobe (lobectomy) or lung (pneumonectomy)

Drug therapy
- Analgesics: morphine, fentanyl (Sublimaze)
- Antiemetics: prochlorperazine, ondansetron (Zofran)
- Antineoplastics: cyclophosphamide, doxorubicin (Doxil), cisplatin (Platinol), vincristine
- Diuretics: furosemide (Lasix), ethacrynic acid (Edecrin)

INTERVENTIONS AND RATIONALES
- Assess respiratory status to detect respiratory complications. *Cyanosis may suggest respiratory failure, whereas an increase in sputum production may suggest an infection.*
- Assess the client's pain level and administer analgesics, as prescribed, *to control pain.*
- Evaluate the effects of medications *to modify treatment as needed.*
- Monitor and record vital signs. *Tachycardia and tachypnea may indicate hypoxemia. An elevated temperature suggests an infection.*

4

4

- Monitor and record intake and output *to assess fluid status.*
- Track laboratory values, and monitor for bleeding, infection, and electrolyte imbalance due to effects of chemotherapy. *A low WBC count increases the risk of infection. Low platelet count increases the risk of bleeding. Electrolyte abnormalities, especially hypercalcemia, may also occur.*
- Monitor pulse oximetry values and report a drop in O_2 saturation, *which suggests hypoxemia.*
- Administer O_2 *to maintain tissue oxygenation.*
- Encourage fluids and administer I.V. fluids *to provide hydration and liquefy secretions to facilitate removal. Drinking moistens mucous membranes.*
- Provide suctioning, and assist with turning, coughing, and deep breathing *to facilitate removal of secretions.*
- Keep the client in semi-Fowler's position *to maximize ventilation.*
- Administer total parenteral nutrition or enteral feeding, as indicated, *to optimize nutrition and bolster the immune system.*
- Administer medications, as prescribed, *to treat the cancer and provide pain relief.*
- Encourage the client to express feelings about changes in body image and a fear of dying *to reduce anxiety.*
- Provide mouth care *to improve comfort and reduce risk of stomatitis (with chemotherapy).*
- Provide skin care *to minimize adverse effects of radiation therapy.*
- Provide rest periods *to enhance tissue oxygenation.*

Teaching topics
- Explanation of the disorder and treatment plan
- Drug therapy
- Radiation therapy
- Preoperative and postoperative care
- Wound care
- Activity recommendations
- Signs and symptoms of complications
- Hospice or end-of-life issues as appropriate
- Performing deep-breathing and coughing exercises
- Following dietary recommendations and restrictions

- Measures to prevent infection, such as avoiding crowds and infected individuals, especially children with communicable disease
- Contacting the American Cancer Society

Pleural effusion and empyema

Pleural effusion is an excess of fluid in the pleural space (the thin space between the lung tissue and the membranous sac that protects it). Normally, the pleural space contains a small amount of extracellular fluid that lubricates the pleural surfaces. Increased production or inadequate removal of this fluid results in pleural effusion.

Empyema is the accumulation of pus and necrotic tissue in the pleural space. Blood (hemothorax) and chyle (chylothorax) may also collect in this space.

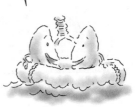

I need my space. Pleural effusion is an excess of fluid in the pleural space.

CAUSES
- Bacterial or fungal pneumonitis or empyema
- Chest trauma
- Collagen disease (lupus erythematosus and rheumatoid arthritis)
- Heart failure
- Hepatic disease with ascites
- Hypoalbuminemia
- Infection in the pleural space
- Malignancy
- Myxedema
- Pancreatitis
- Peritoneal dialysis
- Pulmonary embolism with or without infarction
- Subphrenic abscess
- TB

ASSESSMENT FINDINGS
- Decreased breath sounds
- Dyspnea
- Fever
- Malaise
- Pleuritic chest pain

DIAGNOSTIC TEST RESULTS
- Chest X-ray shows radiopaque fluid in dependent regions.
- Thoracentesis shows lactate dehydrogenase (LD) levels less than 200

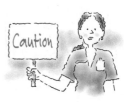

If fluid is removed too quickly during thoracentesis, the client may suffer bradycardia, hypotension, pain, pulmonary edema, or even cardiac arrest.

international units and protein levels less than 3 g/dl (in transudative effusions); ratio of protein in pleural fluid to serum greater than or equal to 0.5, LD in pleural fluid greater than or equal to 200 international units, and ratio of LD in pleural fluid to LD in serum greater than 0.6 (in exudative effusions); and acute inflammatory WBC count and microorganisms (in empyema).

• Tuberculin skin test rules out TB as the cause.

NURSING DIAGNOSES
• Hyperthermia
• Impaired gas exchange
• Risk for infection
• Activity intolerance
• Acute pain

TREATMENT
• Thoracentesis (to remove fluid) with chest tube insertion if necessary
• Thoracotomy if thoracentesis isn't effective
• O_2 therapy

Drug therapy
• Antibiotics for empyema: according to sensitivity of causative organism
• Antipyretic: acetaminophen (Tylenol)
• Analgesic: acetaminophen with oxycodone (Percocet)

INTERVENTIONS AND RATIONALES
• Explain thoracentesis to the client. Before the procedure, tell the client to expect a stinging sensation from the local anesthetic and a feeling of pressure when the needle is inserted *to allay anxiety.*
• Instruct the client to tell you immediately if he feels uncomfortable or has trouble breathing during the procedure. *Difficulty breathing may indicate pneumothorax, which requires immediate chest tube insertion.*
• Reassure the client during thoracentesis *to allay anxiety.* Advise the client to breathe normally and to avoid sudden movements, such as coughing and sighing, *to prevent improper placement of the needle.* Monitor vital signs and watch for syncope *to prevent injury.*
• Watch for respiratory distress or pneumothorax (sudden onset of dyspnea, cyanosis)

after thoracentesis *to detect complications of thoracentesis.*
• Administer O_2 *to improve oxygenation.*
• Administer antibiotics *to treat empyema.*
• Encourage the client to do deep-breathing exercises *to promote lung expansion* and use of an incentive spirometer *to promote deep breathing.*
• Provide meticulous chest tube care, and use sterile technique for changing dressings around the tube insertion site in empyema *to prevent infection at the insertion site.*
• Ensure chest tube patency by watching for bubbles in the underwater seal chamber *to prevent respiratory distress resulting from chest tube obstruction.*
• Record the amount, color, and consistency of chest tube drainage *to monitor the effectiveness of treatment.*

Teaching topics
• Explanation of the disorder and treatment plan
• Signs and symptoms of complications
• Seeking prompt medical attention for chest colds (if pleural effusion was a complication of pneumonia or influenza)
• Importance of continuing antibiotic therapy for the duration prescribed
• Chest tube care or wound care for the insertion site, if necessary, after discharge

Pleurisy

Also known as *pleuritis*, pleurisy is inflammation of the visceral and parietal pleurae, the serous membranes that line the inside of the thoracic cage and envelop the lungs.

CAUSES
• Cancer
• Chest trauma
• Dressler's syndrome
• Pneumonia
• Pulmonary infarction
• Rheumatoid arthritis
• Systemic lupus erythematosus
• TB
• Uremia
• Viruses

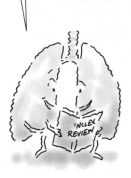

Pleurisy is an inflammation of the membranes that line the inside of the rib cage and envelop the lungs.

ASSESSMENT FINDINGS
- Dyspnea
- Pleural friction rub (a coarse, creaky sound heard during late inspiration and early expiration)
- Sharp, stabbing pain that increases with respiration

DIAGNOSTIC TEST RESULTS
- Although diagnosis generally rests on the client's history and the nurse's respiratory assessment, diagnostic tests help rule out other causes and pinpoint the underlying disorder.
- ECG rules out coronary artery disease as the source of the client's pain.
- Chest X-rays can identify pneumonia.

NURSING DIAGNOSES
- Activity intolerance
- Ineffective breathing pattern
- Acute pain
- Anxiety

TREATMENT
- Bed rest
- Thoracentesis (for pleurisy with pleural effusion)
- O_2 therapy

Drug therapy
- Analgesic: acetaminophen with oxycodone (Percocet)
- Anti-inflammatories: indomethacin (Indocin), ibuprofen (Motrin)

INTERVENTIONS AND RATIONALES
- Stress the importance of bed rest and plan your care *to allow the client as much uninterrupted rest as possible.*
- Administer antitussives and pain medication as necessary *to relieve cough and pain.*
- Encourage the client to cough and deep breathe. Teach him to apply firm pressure at the pain site during coughing exercises *to minimize pain.*

Teaching topics
- Explanation of the disorder and treament plan
- Drug therapy
- Coughing and deep-breathing exercises
- All procedures, including thoracentesis if appropriate
- Importance of regular rest periods

Pneumocystis pneumonia

The microorganism *Pneumocystis jiroveci* is part of the normal flora in most healthy people. However, in the immunocompromised client, *P. jiroveci* becomes an aggressive pathogen. *Pneumocystis* pneumonia (PCP) is an opportunistic infection caused by *P. jiroveci* and strongly associated with human immunodeficiency virus (HIV) infection.

PCP occurs in up to 90% of HIV-infected clients in the United States at some point during their lifetime. It's the leading cause of death in these clients. Disseminated infection doesn't occur. PCP is also associated with other immunocompromised conditions, including organ transplantation, leukemia, and lymphoma.

CAUSES
- *Pneumocystis jiroveci*

ASSESSMENT FINDINGS
- Hypoxemia
- Anorexia
- Dyspnea
- Generalized fatigue
- Low-grade, intermittent fever
- Nonproductive cough
- Shortness of breath
- Tachypnea
- Weight loss

DIAGNOSTIC TEST RESULTS
- ABG studies detect hypoxia and an increased alveolar-arterial gradient.
- Chest X-ray may show slowly progressing, fluffy infiltrates and occasionally nodular lesions or a spontaneous pneumothorax, but these findings must be differentiated from findings in other types of pneumonia or ARDS.
- Fiber-optic bronchoscopy confirms PCP.

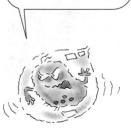

P. jiroveci is part of the normal flora in most healthy people. However, in the immunocompromised client, it becomes an aggressive pathogen.

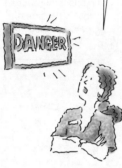

Watch out! Because of immune system impairment due to HIV, many PCP clients experience serious adverse drug reactions.

• Gallium scan may show increased uptake over the lungs even when the chest X-ray appears relatively normal.
• Histologic studies confirm *P. jiroveci*. In clients with HIV infection, initial examination of a first morning sputum specimen (induced by inhaling an ultrasonically dispersed saline mist) may be sufficient; however, this technique is usually ineffective in clients without HIV infection.

NURSING DIAGNOSES
• Ineffective protection
• Impaired gas exchange
• Risk for infection
• Anxiety
• Activity intolerance

TREATMENT
• Diet modification, including maintaining adequate nutrition
• O_2 therapy, which may include endotracheal intubation and mechanical ventilation

Drug therapy
• Antibiotics: co-trimoxazole (Bactrim), pentamidine (Pentam)
• Antipyretic: acetaminophen (Tylenol)

INTERVENTIONS AND RATIONALES
• Assess the client's respiratory status, and monitor ABG levels *to detect early signs of hypoxemia*.
• Administer O_2 therapy as necessary. Encourage the client to ambulate and to perform deep-breathing exercises, and incentive spirometry *to facilitate effective gas exchange*.
• Administer antipyretics, as required, *to relieve fever*.
• Monitor intake and output and daily weight *to evaluate fluid balance*. Replace fluids as necessary *to correct fluid volume deficit*.
• Give antimicrobial drugs as required. Never give pentamidine I.M. *because it can cause pain and sterile abscesses*. Administer the I.V. form slowly over 60 minutes *to reduce the risk of hypotension*.
• Monitor the client for adverse reactions to antimicrobial drugs. If he's receiving co-trimoxazole, watch for nausea, vomiting, rash, bone marrow suppression, thrush, fever, hepatotoxicity, and anaphylaxis. If he's receiving

In pneumonia, microorganisms enter alveolar spaces through droplet inhalation. Sounds dreadful.

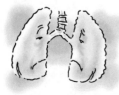

pentamidine, watch for cardiac arrhythmias, hypotension, dizziness, azotemia, hypocalcemia, and hepatic disturbances. *These measures detect problems early to avoid crisis*.
• Provide diversional activities and coordinate health care team activities *to allow adequate rest periods between procedures*.
• Provide nutritional supplements as needed. Encourage the client to eat a high-calorie, protein-rich diet. Offer small, frequent meals. *These measures ensure that the client's nutritional intake meets metabolic needs*.
• Provide a relaxing environment, eliminate excessive environmental stimuli, and allow ample time for meals *to reduce anxiety*.
• Give emotional support and help the client identify and use meaningful support systems *to promote emotional well-being*.

Teaching topics
• Explanation of the disorder and treatment plan
• Dietary recommendations
• Signs and symptoms of complications
• Practicing energy conservation techniques
• Home O_2 therapy
• Drug therapy and recognition of adverse reactions

Pneumonia

Pneumonia refers to a bacterial, viral, parasitic, or fungal infection that causes inflammation of the alveolar spaces. In pneumonia, microorganisms enter alveolar spaces through droplet inhalation, resulting in inflammation and an increase in alveolar fluid. Ventilation decreases as secretions thicken.

CAUSES
• Aspiration
• Chemical irritants
• Organisms such as *Escherichia coli, Haemophilus influenzae, Staphylococcus aureus, Pneumocystis jiroveci, Streptococus pneumoniae,* and *Pseudomonas*

ASSESSMENT FINDINGS
• Chills, fever
• Cough

- Crackles, rhonchi, pleural friction rub on auscultation
- Malaise
- Pleuritic pain
- Restlessness, confusion
- Shortness of breath, dyspnea, tachypnea, accessory muscle use
- Sputum production that's rusty, green, or bloody with pneumococcal pneumonia and yellow-green with bronchopneumonia

DIAGNOSTIC TEST RESULTS
- ABG levels show hypoxemia and respiratory alkalosis.
- Chest X-ray shows pulmonary infiltrates.
- Hematology study shows increased WBC count and ESR.
- Sputum study identifies organism.
- Pulse oximetry levels are decreased.

NURSING DIAGNOSES
- Ineffective airway clearance
- Risk for aspiration
- Impaired spontaneous ventilation
- Activity intolerance
- Impaired gas exchange
- Anxiety

TREATMENT
- Chest physiotherapy and respiratory treatments
- Dietary changes, including establishing a high-calorie, high-protein diet and forcing fluids
- Intubation and mechanical ventilation if condition deteriorates
- O_2 therapy
- Nutritional support, including enteral nutrition if client requires intubation

Drug therapy
- Antibiotics: according to organism sensitivity
- Antipyretics: aspirin, acetaminophen (Tylenol)
- Bronchodilator: albuterol (Proventil-HFA)

INTERVENTIONS AND RATIONALES
- Monitor and record intake and output. *Insensible water loss secondary to fever may cause dehydration.*
- Monitor laboratory studies. *An elevated WBC count suggests infection. Blood and sputum cultures may identify the causative agent.*

- Monitor pulse oximetry and assess respiratory status *to detect respiratory compromise.*
- Monitor and record vital signs. *An elevated temperature increases O_2 demands. Hypotension and tachycardia may suggest hypovolemic shock.*
- Monitor and record color, consistency, and amount of sputum. *Sputum amount and consistency may indicate hydration status and effectiveness of therapy. Foul-smelling sputum suggests respiratory infection.*
- Administer O_2 *to help relieve respiratory distress.*
- Maintain the client's diet *to offset hypermetabolic state due to infection.*
- Encourage fluid intake of 3 qt (3 L)/day, unless contraindicated, and administer I.V. fluids *to help liquefy secretions to aid in their removal.*
- Provide suction and assist with turning, coughing, deep breathing, and use of incentive spirometry *to promote mobilization and removal of secretions.*
- Administer chest physiotherapy and postural drainage *to facilitate removal of secretions.*
- Administer medications, as prescribed, *to treat infection and improve ventilation.*
- Encourage the client to express feelings about fear of suffocation *to reduce his anxiety.*
- Provide tissues and a bag for hygienic sputum disposal *to prevent spread of infection.*
- Provide oral hygiene *to promote comfort and improve nutrition.*

Teaching topics
- Explanation of the disorder and treatment plan
- Drug therapy
- Recognizing signs and symptoms of respiratory infections and other complications
- Avoiding exposure to people with infections
- Increasing fluid intake to 3 qt (3 L)/day

Pneumothorax and hemothorax

In pneumothorax, loss of negative intrapleural pressure results in the collapse of the

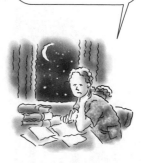

Don't stop now! Just a few more respiratory disorders to go!

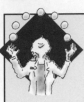

Management moments

Checking in on chest tubes

Caring for a client with a chest tube is a common subject on the NCLEX. Here are some typical nursing actions regarding chest tubes, beginning when the chest tube is in place:
• First, have the client take several deep breaths to fully inflate his lungs and help push pleural air out through the tube.
• Next, palpate his chest around the tube for subcutaneous emphysema and notify the physician of any increase.
• Routinely assess the function of the chest tube. Describe and record the amount of drainage on the intake and output sheet.

If there's a leak
• Bubbling in the water-seal chamber or air leak meter indicates that there's an air leak. If there's no air leak, the water level in this chamber will rise and fall with the client's respirations, reflecting normal pressure changes in the pleural cavity.

• If the water level fluctuates with respirations (for example, fluctuation occurs on exhalation in the client breathing spontaneously), the lung is most likely the source of the air leak.
• If the lung isn't the source of the air leak, check and tighten the connections. If the leak is in the tubing, replace the unit.

If the tube becomes dislodged
• Cover the opening immediately with petroleum gauze and apply pressure to prevent negative inspiratory pressure from sucking into the client's chest. Call the physician and continue to keep the opening closed. Then get ready to start the chest tube process all over again.
• If the chest tube becomes cracked, place the distal end of the tube in sterile water and call the physician.

---

lung. Pneumothorax may be described as spontaneous, open, or tension:
• Spontaneous pneumothorax results from the rupture of a bleb.
• Open pneumothorax occurs when an opening through the chest wall allows air to flow between the pleural space and the outside of the body.
• Tension pneumothorax results from a buildup of air in the pleural space that can't escape.

In all cases, the surface area for gas exchange is reduced, resulting in hypoxia and hypercapnia.

In hemothorax, blood accumulates in the pleural space when a rib lacerates lung tissue or an intercostal artery. This compresses the lung and limits respiratory capacity. Hemothorax can also result from rupture of large or small pulmonary vessels.

CAUSES
• Blunt chest trauma
• Central venous catheter insertion
• Penetrating chest injuries
• Rupture of a bleb
• Thoracentesis
• Thoracic surgeries
• Barotrauma

ASSESSMENT FINDINGS
• Anxiety
• Diaphoresis, pallor
• Diminished or absent breath sounds unilaterally
• Dullness on chest percussion (in the case of hemothorax and tension pneumothorax)
• Dyspnea, tachypnea, subcutaneous emphysema, cough
• Hypotension (in the case of hemothorax)
• Sharp pain that increases with exertion
• Tachycardia
• Tracheal shift, decreased chest expansion unilaterally

DIAGNOSTIC TEST RESULTS
• ABG levels show respiratory and hypoxemia.
• Chest X-ray reveals pneumothorax or hemothorax.
• Lung scan shows $\dot{V}/\dot{Q}$ ratio mismatches.
• Pulse oximetry levels are decreased.

NURSING DIAGNOSES
• Ineffective breathing pattern
• Impaired gas exchange
• Acute pain
• Anxiety
• Fear
• Ineffective peripheral tissue perfusion

TREATMENT
- Chest tube to water-seal drainage, or continuous suction (see *Checking in on chest tubes*)
- Incentive spirometry
- Occlusive dressing (for open pneumothorax)
- O_2 therapy

Drug therapy
- Analgesic: morphine I.V.

INTERVENTIONS AND RATIONALES
- Monitor and record vital signs. *Hypotension, tachycardia, and tachypnea suggest tension pneumothorax.*
- Check the chest drainage system for air leaks *that can impair lung expansion.*
- Assess respiratory status. *Dyspnea, tachypnea, diminished breath sounds, subcutaneous emphysema, and use of accessory muscles suggest accumulation of air in pleural space.*
- Monitor chest tube function and drainage. *An increase in the amount of bloody drainage suggests new bleeding or an increase in bleeding. Check tubing for kinks if there's a sudden reduction in drainage.*
- Assess cardiovascular status. *Tachycardia, hypotension, and jugular venous distention suggest tension pneumothorax.*
- Assess the client's pain level and administer medications, as prescribed, *to control pain.*
- Administer O_2 *to relieve respiratory distress caused by hypoxemia.*
- Assist with turning, coughing, deep breathing, and incentive spirometry *to enhance mobilization of secretions and prevent atelectasis.*
- Keep the client in high Fowler's position *to enhance chest expansion.*

Teaching topics
- Explanation of the disorder and treatment plan
- Deep breathing exercises and use of an incentive spirometer
- Recognizing the early signs and symptoms of recurrent pneumothorax and respiratory infection
- Avoiding heavy lifting

Pulmonary edema

Pulmonary edema is a complication of left-sided heart failure. It occurs when pulmonary capillary pressure exceeds intravascular osmotic pressure and results in increased pressure in the capillaries of the lungs and acute transudation of fluid. This leads to impaired oxygenation and hypoxia.

CAUSES
- ARDS
- Atherosclerosis
- Drug overdose: heroin, barbiturates, morphine sulfate
- Heart failure
- Hypertension
- Myocardial infarction
- Myocarditis
- Overload of I.V. fluids
- Smoke inhalation
- Valvular disease

ASSESSMENT FINDINGS
- Agitation, restlessness, intense fear
- Blood-tinged, frothy sputum
- Productive cough (frothy, bloody sputum)
- Cold, clammy skin
- Crackles over lung fields
- Dyspnea, orthopnea, tachypnea
- Jugular vein distention
- Syncope
- Tachycardia, S_3 and S_4, chest pain

DIAGNOSTIC TEST RESULTS
- ABGs show respiratory alkalosis or acidosis and hypoxemia.
- Chest X-ray shows diffuse haziness of the lung fields and, commonly, cardiomegaly and pleural effusions.
- ECG reveals tachycardia and ventricular enlargement.
- Hemodynamic monitoring shows increases in PAP, pulmonary artery wedge pressure, and CVP as well as decreased cardiac output.
- Pulse oximetry reveals hypoxia.

NURSING DIAGNOSES
- Anxiety
- Excess fluid volume
- Impaired gas exchange

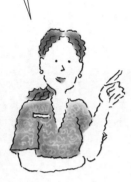

Weigh clients with pulmonary edema every day to help detect fluid retention.

TREATMENT

- O_2 therapy: possibly intubation and mechanical ventilation
- Activity changes: maintaining bed rest and implementing range-of-motion and isometric exercises
- Dietary changes: establishing a low-sodium diet and limiting oral fluids
- Hemodialysis and ultrafiltration, if available

Drug therapy

- Diuretics: furosemide (Lasix), bumetanide (Bumex), metolazone (Zaroxolyn)
- Nitrates: isosorbide (Isordil), nitroglycerin
- Analgesic: morphine sulfate I.V.
- Cardiac glycoside: digoxin (Lanoxin)
- Inotropic agents: dobutamine, inamrinone (Amrinone), milrinone
- Vasodilator: nitroprusside (Nitropress)

INTERVENTIONS AND RATIONALES

- Administer oxygen, as prescribed, *to increase alveolar oxygen concentration and enhance arterial blood oxygenation.*
- Administer medications *to improve gas exchange, improve myocardial function, and reduce anxiety.*
- Note the color, amount, and consistency of sputum. *Sputum amount and consistency may indicate hydration status. A change in color or foul-smelling sputum may indicate a respiratory infection.*
- Assess cardiovascular and respiratory status and hemodynamic variables *to detect changes in fluid balance. Tachycardia, S_3, hypotension, increased respiratory rate, and crackles indicate increased fluid volume.*
- Monitor and record intake and output. *Intake greater than output and elevated specific gravity suggest fluid retention.*
- Weigh the client daily to detect fluid retention. *Weight gain of 1 to 2 lb (0.5 to 1 kg) per day suggests a fluid gain.*
- Track laboratory values. *Blood urea nitrogen and creatinine indicate renal function. Electrolytes, hemoglobin, and hematocrit indicate fluid status.*
- Keep the client in high Fowler's position if blood pressure tolerates; if hypotensive, maintain in a semi-Fowler's position if tolerated. *Elevating the head of the bed reduces venous return to the heart and promotes chest expansion.*
- Withhold food and fluids, as directed, *to prevent aspiration.*
- Encourage the client to express feelings such as a fear of suffocation *to reduce anxiety and lessen oxygen demands.*

Teaching topics

- Elevating the head of the bed while sleeping
- Eating foods high in potassium
- Recognizing early signs of fluid overload
- Recognizing signs and symptoms of respiratory distress
- Taking medications exactly as prescribed
- Recording weight daily

Pulmonary embolism

Pulmonary embolism is the obstruction of the pulmonary arterial bed. It results from a mass (commonly a thrombus) that lodges in the main pulmonary artery or branch.

CAUSES

- Deep vein thrombosis
- Pelvic, renal, and hepatic vein thrombosis
- Right heart thrombosis
- Upper extremity thrombosis
- Bone, air, fat, amniotic fluid, or tumor cell emboli (rare)

CONTRIBUTING FACTORS

- Abdominal, pelvic, or thoracic surgery
- Atrial fibrillation
- Central venous catheter insertion
- Flat, long bone fractures
- Heart failure
- Hormonal contraceptives
- Hypercoagulability
- Malignant tumors
- Obesity
- Polycythemia vera
- Pregnancy
- Prolonged bed rest
- Sickle cell anemia
- Thrombophlebitis
- Valvular heart disease
- Venous stasis

The client has a pulmonary embolism. Interventions are likely to include administering an anticoagulant such as heparin.

ASSESSMENT FINDINGS
- Anxiety
- Chest pain
- Cough, hemoptysis
- Low-grade fever
- Hypotension
- Sudden onset of dyspnea, tachypnea, crackles
- S_3 and S_4 gallop with increased intensity of the pulmonic component of S_2
- Transient plural friction rub
- Tachycardia, arrhythmias
- Weak, rapid pulse

DIAGNOSTIC TEST RESULTS
- ABG levels show respiratory alkalosis and hypoxemia.
- D-dimer levels are elevated.
- Chest X-ray shows dilated pulmonary arteries, pneumoconstriction, and diaphragm elevation on the affected side.
- Spiral CT scan of the chest shows central pulmonary emboli.
- ECG shows tachycardia, nonspecific ST-segment changes, and right axis deviation.
- Pulmonary angiography shows location of embolism and filling defect of pulmonary artery.
- Lung scan shows $\dot{V}/\dot{Q}$ mismatch.

NURSING DIAGNOSES
- Acute pain
- Decreased cardiac output
- Anxiety
- Impaired gas exchange
- Ineffective peripheral tissue perfusion

TREATMENT
- Bed rest with active and passive range-of-motion and isometric exercises
- Vena cava filter insertion or pulmonary embolectomy
- O_2 therapy, intubation, and mechanical ventilation, if necessary

Drug therapy
- Analgesic: morphine
- Anticoagulants: enoxaparin (Lovenox), heparin, followed by warfarin (Coumadin)
- Diuretic: furosemide (Lasix) if right ventricular failure develops
- Fibrinolytics: streptokinase (Streptase), urokinase (Abbokinase)

INTERVENTIONS AND RATIONALES
- Assess respiratory status *to detect respiratory distress.*
- Assess cardiovascular status. *An irregular pulse may signal arrhythmia caused by hypoxemia. If pulmonary embolism is caused by thrombophlebitis, temperature may be elevated.*
- Monitor laboratory studies *to guide anticoagulation therapy.*
- Monitor ABG levels *for evidence of pulmonary compromise.*
- Monitor and record CVP. *CVP may rise if right-sided heart failure develops.*
- Monitor and record intake and output *to detect fluid volume overload and renal perfusion.*
- Administer O_2 *to enhance arterial oxygenation.*
- Assist with turning, coughing, and deep breathing *to mobilize secretions and clear airways.*
- Keep the client in high Fowler's position *to enhance ventilation.*
- Provide suctioning, and monitor and record color, consistency, and amount of sputum. *A productive cough and blood-tinged sputum may be present with pulmonary embolism.*
- Administer I.V. fluids, as ordered, *to maintain hydration.*
- Administer medications, as prescribed, *to enhance tissue oxygenation.*

Teaching topics
- Explanation of the disorder and treatment plan
- Drug therapy
- Recognizing signs and symptoms of respiratory distress and other complications
- Avoiding activities that promote venous thrombosis (prolonged sitting and standing, wearing constrictive clothing, crossing legs when seated, using hormonal contraceptives)
- Monitoring anticoagulation therapy

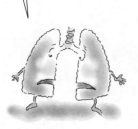

It all falls on my shoulders. If I don't eliminate enough CO_2 through ventilation, excess CO_2 accumulates in the blood and pH can drop below normal.

Respiratory acidosis

Respiratory acidosis is an acid-base disturbance characterized by excess of CO_2 in the blood (hypercapnia), indicated by a $Paco_2$ greater than 45 mm Hg. It results from reduced alveolar ventilation. It can be acute (from a sudden failure in ventilation) or chronic (as in long-term pulmonary disease).

CAUSES
- Airway obstruction or parenchymal lung disease
- CNS trauma
- Chronic metabolic alkalosis
- Drugs, such as opioids, anesthetics, hypnotics, and sedatives
- Neuromuscular diseases, such as myasthenia gravis, Guillain-Barré syndrome, and poliomyelitis

ASSESSMENT FINDINGS
- Bounding pulse
- Cardiovascular abnormalities, such as tachycardia, hypertension, atrial and ventricular arrhythmias and, in severe acidosis, hypotension with vasodilation
- Coma
- Confusion
- Diaphoresis
- Dyspnea and tachypnea with papilledema and depressed reflexes
- Fine or flapping tremor (asterixis)
- Headaches
- Hypoxemia
- Restlessness

DIAGNOSTIC TEST RESULTS
- ABG measurements confirm respiratory acidosis. $Paco_2$ exceeds the normal level of 45 mm Hg and pH is usually below the normal range of 7.35 to 7.45. The client's bicarbonate level is normal in the acute stage and elevated in the chronic stage.

NURSING DIAGNOSES
- Anxiety
- Fear
- Impaired gas exchange
- Ineffective breathing pattern
- Decreased cardiac output

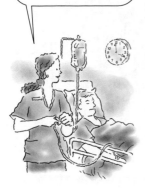

If the pH level drops below 7.15, severe CNS and cardiovascular deterioration may result. This situation requires quick administration of I.V. sodium bicarbonate.

TREATMENT
Treatment of respiratory acidosis is designed to correct the underlying cause of alveolar hypoventilation. It may include:
- endotracheal intubation and mechanical ventilation
- dialysis to remove toxic drugs
- removal of foreign body, if appropriate.

Drug therapy
- Antibiotics according to organism sensitivity, if pneumonia is present
- Bronchodilator: albuterol (Proventil-HFA)
- Sodium bicarbonate in severe cases

INTERVENTIONS AND RATIONALES
- Closely monitor the client's blood pH level *to guide the treatment plan.*
- Be alert for critical changes in the client's respiratory, CNS, and cardiovascular functions. Also watch closely for variations in ABG values and electrolyte status. Maintain adequate hydration. *These measures help prevent and detect life-threatening complications.*
- If acidosis requires mechanical ventilation, maintain a patent airway and provide adequate humidification. Perform tracheal suctioning regularly and vigorous chest physiotherapy if needed. Continuously monitor ventilator settings and respiratory status *to ensure adequate oxygenation.*
- Closely monitor clients with COPD and chronic CO_2 retention for signs of acidosis. Also, administer O_2 at low flow rates and closely monitor all clients who receive narcotics and sedatives *to prevent respiratory acidosis.*
- Instruct the client who has received a general anesthetic to turn, cough, and perform deep-breathing exercises frequently *to prevent the onset of respiratory acidosis.*
- Perform appropriate interventions for the underlying cause.

Teaching topics
- Explanation of the disorder and treatment plan
- Signs and symptoms of complications
- Home O_2 use
- Coughing and deep-breathing exercises
- Medication regimen and possible adverse reactions

Respiratory alkalosis

Respiratory alkalosis is characterized by a deficiency of CO_2 in the blood (hypocapnia), as indicated by a decrease in $Paco_2$. $Paco_2$ is below 35 mm Hg (normal level is 45 mm Hg).

This condition is caused by alveolar hyperventilation. Elimination of CO_2 by the lungs exceeds the production of CO_2 at the cellular level, leading to deficiency of CO_2 in the blood.

Uncomplicated respiratory alkalosis leads to a decrease in hydrogen ion concentration, which causes elevated blood pH.

CAUSES
Pulmonary causes
- Acute asthma
- Interstitial lung disease
- Pneumonia
- Pulmonary vascular disease

Nonpulmonary causes
- Anxiety
- Aspirin toxicity
- CNS disease (inflammation or tumor)
- Fever
- Hepatic failure
- Metabolic acidosis
- Pregnancy
- Sepsis

ASSESSMENT FINDINGS
- Agitation
- Cardiac arrhythmias that fail to respond to conventional treatment (severe respiratory alkalosis)
- Carpopedal spasms (spasms affecting the wrist and the foot)
- Circumoral or peripheral paresthesias (a prickling sensation around the mouth or extremities)
- Deep, rapid breathing, possibly exceeding 40 breaths/minute (cardinal sign)
- Light-headedness or dizziness (from decreased cerebral blood flow)
- Muscle weakness
- Seizures (severe respiratory alkalosis)
- Twitching (possibly progressing to tetany)

DIAGNOSTIC TEST RESULTS
- ABG analysis confirms respiratory alkalosis and rules out respiratory compensation for metabolic acidosis. In the acute stage, $Paco_2$ is below 35 mm Hg and pH is elevated in proportion to the fall in $Paco_2$, but pH drops toward normal in the chronic stage. Bicarbonate level is normal in the acute stage but below normal in the chronic stage.

NURSING DIAGNOSES
- Anxiety
- Impaired gas exchange
- Ineffective breathing pattern
- Ineffective peripheral tissue perfusion

TREATMENT
- Correction of underlying cause, which may include removal of ingested toxins, treatment of CNS disease, or treatment of fever or sepsis
- Increasing CO_2 levels (for respiratory alkalosis caused by hyperventilation) by having the client breathe into a paper bag

INTERVENTIONS AND RATIONALES
- Assess neurologic, neuromuscular, and cardiovascular functions *to ensure prompt recognition and treatment.*
- Monitor ABG and serum electrolyte levels closely, watching for any variations *to detect early changes and prevent complications.*
- Perform appropriate interventions for the underlying cause.

Teaching topics
- Explanation of the disorder and treatment plan
- Relaxation techniques
- Breathing into a paper bag during an acute anxiety attack

Sarcoidosis

Sarcoidosis is a multisystemic, granulomatous disorder (this means it affects many body systems and produces nodules of chronically inflamed tissue). Sarcoidosis may lead to lymphadenopathy (disease of the lymph nodes), pulmonary infiltration, and skeletal, liver, eye, or skin lesions.

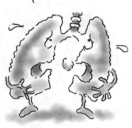

I overdo it sometimes. When I eliminate CO_2 faster than it's produced at the cellular level, it leads to respiratory alkalosis—deficiency of CO_2 in the blood—which can lead to a loss of hydrogen ions and an increase in pH.

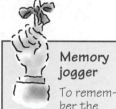

Memory jogger

To remember the significance of pH, think "percentage hydrogen," recalling that H is the symbol for hydrogen. pH refers to the balance of hydrogen ions (acids) and bicarbonate ions (base) in a solution.

When H goes up, pH goes down. Normal arterial pH is 7.35 to 7.45. In acidosis, hydrogen ions (acids) accumulate and pH goes down. In alkalosis, hydrogen ions decrease and pH goes up.

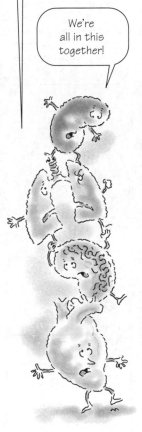

Yes, sarcoidosis is a pulmonary disorder, but it affects many body systems.

We're all in this together!

Sarcoidosis occurs most commonly in young adults (ages 20 to 40). In the United States, sarcoidosis occurs predominantly among blacks and affects twice as many women as men.

Acute sarcoidosis usually resolves within 2 years. Chronic, progressive sarcoidosis, which is uncommon, is associated with pulmonary fibrosis and progressive pulmonary disability.

CAUSES

Although the cause of sarcoidosis is unknown, the following explanations are possible:
- hypersensitivity response (possibly from a T-cell imbalance) to such agents as mycobacteria, fungi, and pine pollen
- genetic predisposition (suggested by a slightly higher incidence of sarcoidosis within the same family)
- chemicals, such as zirconium or beryllium, which can lead to illnesses resembling sarcoidosis.

ASSESSMENT FINDINGS

Initial signs
- Arthralgia (in the wrists, ankles, and elbows)
- Fatigue
- Malaise
- Weight loss

Respiratory
- Breathlessness
- Cor pulmonale (in advanced pulmonary disease)
- Cough (usually nonproductive)
- Dyspnea
- Pulmonary hypertension (in advanced pulmonary disease)
- Substernal pain

Cutaneous
- Erythema nodosum
- Subcutaneous skin nodules with maculopapular eruptions
- Extensive nasal mucosal lesions

Ophthalmic
- Anterior uveitis (common)
- Glaucoma and blindness (rare)

Lymphatic
- Lymphadenopathy
- Splenomegaly (enlarged spleen)

Musculoskeletal
- Muscle weakness
- Polyarthralgia (pain affecting many joints)
- Pain
- Punched-out lesions on phalanges

Hepatic
- Granulomatous hepatitis (usually asymptomatic)

Genitourinary
- Hypercalciuria (excessive calcium in the urine)

Cardiovascular
- Arrhythmias (premature beats, bundle-branch block, or complete heart block)
- Cardiomyopathy (rare)

Central nervous system
- Cranial or peripheral nerve palsies
- Basilar meningitis (inflammation of the meninges at the base of the brain)
- Seizures
- Pituitary and hypothalamic lesions producing diabetes insipidus

DIAGNOSTIC TEST RESULTS
- A positive Kveim-Siltzbach skin test supports the diagnosis. In this test, the client receives an intradermal injection of an antigen prepared from human sarcoidal spleen or lymph nodes from clients with sarcoidosis. If the client has active sarcoidosis, granuloma develops at the injection site in 2 to 6 weeks. This reaction is considered positive when a biopsy of the skin at the injection site shows discrete epithelioid cell granuloma.
- ABG analysis shows decreased Pao_2.
- Chest X-ray shows bilateral hilar and right paratracheal adenopathy with or without diffuse interstitial infiltrates; occasionally large nodular lesions are present in lung parenchyma.
- Lymph node, skin, or lung biopsy reveals noncaseating granulomas with negative cultures for mycobacteria and fungi.

- Negative tuberculin skin test, fungal serologies, sputum cultures for mycobacteria and fungi, and negative biopsy cultures help rule out infection.
- Other laboratory data infrequently reveal increased serum calcium, mild anemia, leukocytosis, or hyperglobulinemia.
- PFTs show decreased total lung capacity and compliance and decreased diffusing capacity.

NURSING DIAGNOSES
- Anxiety
- Impaired gas exchange
- Risk for injury
- Fear
- Acute pain
- Activity intolerance

TREATMENT
- Low-calcium diet and avoidance of direct exposure to sunlight (in clients with hypercalcemia)
- O_2 therapy
- No treatment (for asymptomatic sarcoidosis)

Drug therapy
- Systemic or topical steroid, if sarcoidosis causes ocular, respiratory, CNS, cardiac, or systemic symptoms (such as fever and weight loss), hypercalcemia, or destructive skin lesions

INTERVENTIONS AND RATIONALES
- Monitor laboratory results *that could alter client care.*
- For the client with arthralgia, administer analgesics as needed *to promote client comfort.* Record signs of progressive muscle weakness *to detect deterioration in the client's condition.*
- Provide a nutritious, high-calorie diet and plenty of fluids *to ensure that nutritional intake meets the client's metabolic needs.* If the client has hypercalcemia, suggest a low-calcium diet *to prevent complications of hypercalcemia, such as muscle weakness, heart block, hypertension, and cardiac arrest.*
- Monitor respiratory function. Note and record any bloody sputum or increase in sputum. If the client has pulmonary hypertension or end-stage cor pulmonale, check ABG values, and monitor for arrhythmias. *These measures promptly detect deterioration in the client's condition.*

- Administer O_2 as needed *to improve oxygenation.*
- During steroid therapy, monitor blood glucose level every 6 to 12 hours using a blood glucose monitor *to detect hyperglycemia caused by steroid use.*
- Assess for fluid retention, electrolyte imbalance (especially hypokalemia), moonface, hypertension, and personality change, *which are adverse effects of steroids.*
- Provide emotional support and answer all questions *to improve the client's knowledge and decrease anxiety.*

Teaching topics
- Explanation of the disorder and treatment plan
- Activity recommendations
- Dietary recommendations
- Need for compliance with prescribed steroid therapy and regular, careful follow-up examinations and treatment
- Information on community support and resource groups and the American Foundation for the Blind, if necessary

Severe acute respiratory syndrome

SARS is a viral respiratory infection that can progress to pneumonia, and eventually, death. The disease was first recognized in 2003 with outbreaks in China, Canada, Singapore, Taiwan, and Vietnam, with other countries—including the United States—reporting a smaller number of cases.

SARS is caused by the SARS-associated coronavirus (SARS-CoV). Coronaviruses are a common cause of mild respiratory illnesses in humans, but researchers believe that a virus may have mutated, allowing it to cause this potentially life-threatening disease.

CAUSES
- Close contact with an infected person

ASSESSMENT FINDINGS
- Chills
- Dry cough
- Fever
- General discomfort
- Headache

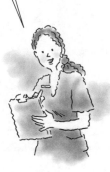

Remember that the client on long-term or high-dose steroid therapy is vulnerable to infection.

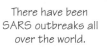

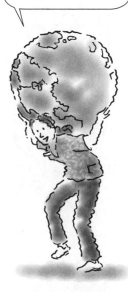

There have been SARS outbreaks all over the world.

- Myalgia
- Rigors
- Shortness of breath
- Sore throat

DIAGNOSTIC TEST RESULTS

- Detectable levels of antibodies may not be present until 21 days after the onset of illness.
- Diagnosis of severe respiratory illness is made with a fever greater than 100.4° F (38° C) or clinical findings of lower respiratory illness and a chest X-ray showing pneumonia or ARDS.
- Laboratory validation includes cell culture of SARS-CoV, detection of SARS-CoV ribonucleic acid by the reverse transcription polymerase chain reaction test, or detection of serum antibodies to SARS-CoV.

NURSING DIAGNOSES

- Impaired gas exchange
- Ineffective breathing pattern
- Fatigue
- Activity intolerance

TREATMENT

- Chest physiotherapy
- Supplemental O_2 including possible mechanical ventilation

Drug therapy

- Antibiotics to treat bacterial causes of atypical pneumonia
- Antivirals
- General benefit of drug therapy: not determined
- High doses of corticosteroids to reduce lung inflammation

INTERVENTIONS AND RATIONALES

- Treat symptoms and support the client as needed *to help increase the client's comfort.*
- Maintain a patent airway *to increase oxygenation.*
- Follow contact and airborne precautions, including the use of an N-95 respirator for all health care professionals *to help decrease the risk of transmission of illness to other clients.*
- Monitor vital signs and respiratory status *for any changes.*

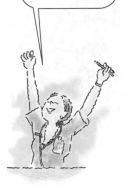

Just a few more pages of respiratory review!

- Report suspected cases of SARS to local and national health organizations *as required by law.*

Teaching topics

- Explanation of the disorder and treatment plan
- Drug therapy
- Hand washing and covering the mouth and nose when sneezing or coughing
- Not sharing eating utensils, towels, and bedding until they have been washed and disinfected
- Not going to work, school, or other public places

Tuberculosis

TB is an airborne, infectious, communicable disease that can occur acutely or chronically. In TB, alveoli become the focus of infection from inhaled droplets containing bacteria. Tubercle bacilli multiply, spread through the lymphatics, and drain into the systemic circulation. Cell-mediated immunity to the mycobacteria, which develops 3 to 6 weeks later, usually contains the infection and arrests the disease.

If the infection reactivates, the body's response characteristically leads to caseation—the conversion of necrotic tissue to a cheeselike material. The caseum may localize, undergo fibrosis, or excavate and form cavities, the walls of which are studded with multiplying tubercle bacilli. If this occurs, infected caseous debris may spread throughout the lungs by the tracheobronchial tree.

CAUSES

- *Mycobacterium tuberculosis*

ASSESSMENT FINDINGS

- Anorexia, weight loss
- Cough, yellow and mucoid sputum, hemoptysis
- Crackles
- Dyspnea
- Fatigue, malaise, irritability
- Low-grade fever
- Night sweats

- Pleuritic chest pain
- Tachycardia

NURSING DIAGNOSES
- Ineffective airway clearance
- Fatigue
- Social isolation
- Anxiety
- Imbalanced nutrition: Less than body requirements
- Impaired gas exchange

DIAGNOSTIC TEST RESULTS
- Chest X-ray shows active or calcified lesions.
- Chest CT scan or magnetic resonance imaging shows presence and extent of lung damage or supports the diagnosis.
- Hematology shows increased WBC count and ESR.
- Mantoux skin test is positive.
- Stains and cultures of sputum, cerebrospinal fluid, urine, abscess drainage, or pleural fluid show heat-sensitive, nonmotile, aerobic, and acid-fast bacilli.

TREATMENT
- Chest physiotherapy, postural drainage, and incentive spirometry
- Dietary changes, including establishing a diet high in carbohydrates, protein, vitamins B_6 and C, and calories
- Standard and airborne precautions

Drug therapy
- Antibiotic: streptomycin
- Antituberculars: isoniazid, ethambutol (Myambutol), rifampin (Rifadin), pyrazinamide

INTERVENTIONS AND RATIONALES
- Assess respiratory status *to detect respiratory complications such as pleural effusion.*
- Monitor and record vital signs and laboratory studies *to detect signs of compromise.*
- Provide a well-balanced, high-calorie diet and small, frequent meals *to increase caloric intake.*
- Perform chest physiotherapy and postural drainage *to facilitate mobilization of secretions.*

- Assist with turning, coughing, and deep-breathing and provide suction, if necessary, *to mobilize and remove secretions.*
- Administer medications, as prescribed, *to avoid development of drug-resistant organisms.*
- Maintain infection-control precautions *to reduce the spread of infectious organisms.*
- Instruct the client to cover his nose and mouth when sneezing *to reduce transmission by droplet.*
- Encourage fluids *to liquefy secretions.*
- Provide frequent oral hygiene *to promote comfort and improve appetite.*
- Provide a negative pressure room *to prevent the spread of infection.*
- Monitor and record intake and output *to assess hydration. Adequate hydration is necessary to facilitate removal of secretions.*
- Provide O_2 therapy *to improve oxygenation.*

Teaching topics
- Explanation of the disorder and treatment plan
- Preventing spread of droplets of sputum
- Drug therapy and the importance of finishing the entire course of medication (6 to 18 months)
- Signs and symptoms of complications
- Contacting the American Lung Association

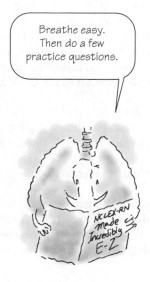

Breathe easy. Then do a few practice questions.

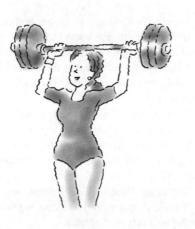

Pump up on practice questions

1. During the insertion of a rigid scope for bronchoscopy, a client experiences a vaso-vagal response. The nurse should expect:
1. the client's pupils to become dilated.
2. the client to experience bronchodilation.
3. a decrease in gastric secretions.
4. a drop in the client's heart rate.

Answer: 4. During a bronchoscopy, a vaso-vagal response may be caused by stimulating the pharynx which, in turn, may cause stimulation of the vagus nerve. The client may experience a sudden drop in the heart rate leading to syncope. Stimulation of the vagus nerve doesn't lead to mydriasis (pupillary dilation) or bronchodilation. Stimulation of the vagus nerve increases gastric secretions.

➡ *NCLEX keys*
Client needs category: Physiological integrity
Client needs subcategory: Reduction of risk potential
Cognitive level: Comprehension

2. A client with right lower lobe pneumonia is ordered chest percussion and postural drainage. When performing percussion and postural drainage, the nurse should position the client:

1. in semi-Fowler's position with the knees bent.
2. right side-lying with the foot of the bed elevated.
3. prone or supine with the foot of the bed elevated higher than the head.
4. bent at the waist leaning slightly forward.

Answer: 3. The aim of percussion and postural drainage is to mobilize pulmonary secretions so they can be effectively expectorated. In right lower lobe bronchopneumonia, the nurse should position the client with the right side up or lower lobes elevated above the upper lobes. This position would employ gravity in mobilizing pulmonary secretions. Semi-Fowler's position and being bent at the waist would hamper mobilization of secretions from the right lower lobe.

➡ *NCLEX keys*
Client needs category: Physiological integrity
Client needs subcategory: Physiological adaptation
Cognitive level: Application

3. A client with acquired immunodeficiency syndrome (AIDS) develops *Pneumocystis* pneumonia (PCP). Which nursing diagnosis has the highest priority for this client?
1. *Impaired gas exchange*
2. *Impaired oral mucous membrane*
3. *Imbalanced nutrition: Less than body requirements*
4. *Activity intolerance*

Answer: 1. Although all these nursing diagnoses are appropriate for the client with AIDS, *Impaired gas exchange* is the priority nursing diagnosis for the client with PCP. Airway, breathing, and circulation take top priority for any client.

➡ *NCLEX keys*
Client needs category: Physiological integrity
Client needs subcategory: Physiological adaptation
Cognitive level: Analysis

4. A client has chronic bronchitis. The nurse is teaching him breathing exercises. Which instruction should the nurse include in the teaching?
1. Make inhalation longer than exhalation.
2. Exhale through an open mouth.
3. Use diaphragmatic breathing.
4. Use chest breathing.

Answer: 3. In chronic bronchitis, the diaphragm is flat and weak. Diaphragmatic breathing helps to strengthen the diaphragm and maximizes ventilation. Inhalation should be no longer than exhalation to prevent collapse of the bronchioles. The client with chronic bronchitis should exhale through pursed lips to prolong exhalation, keep the bronchioles from collapsing, and prevent air trapping. Diaphragmatic breathing, not chest breathing, increases lung expansion.

➡ *NCLEX keys*

Client needs category: Physiological integrity
Client needs subcategory: Reduction of risk potential
Cognitive level: Application

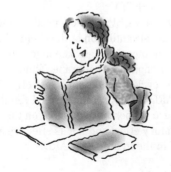

5. A client comes to the emergency department with status asthmaticus. Based on the documentation note below, the nurse suspects the client has what abnormality?

Progress notes

| 11/7/2010 1245 | Pt is confused, diaphoretic, and restless. RR 22, BP 140/90, P 110, T 98.4 F, ABG results show pH 7.6, Paco₂ 80 mm Hg, HCO₃ 24 mEg/L |
| A. Teschlog, RN |

1. Metabolic acidosis
2. Metabolic alkalosis
3. Respiratory acidosis
4. Respiratory alkalosis

Answer: 3. Because the partial pressure of arterial carbon dioxide is high at 80 mm Hg and the bicarbonate (HCO_3^-) is normal, the client has respiratory acidosis. The pH is less than 7.35 (acidemic), which eliminates respiratory and metabolic alkalosis as possibilities. Metabolic acidosis is characterized by a decreased HCO_3^- level.

➡ *NCLEX keys*

Client needs category: Physiological integrity
Client needs subcategory: Physiological adaptation
Cognitive level: Analysis

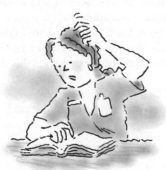

6. A client experiencing acute respiratory failure will most likely demonstrate:
1. hypocapnia, hypoventilation, hyperoxemia.
2. hypocapnia, hyperventilation, hyperoxemia.
3. hypercapnia, hyperventilation, hypoxemia.
4. hypercapnia, hypoventilation, hypoxemia.

Answer: 4. Acute respiratory failure is marked by hypercapnia (elevated arterial carbon dioxide), hypoventilation, and hypoxemia (subnormal oxygen).

➡ *NCLEX keys*

Client needs category: Physiological integrity
Client needs subcategory: Physiological adaptation
Cognitive level: Comprehension

7. A client returns to the clinic 48 hours after receiving a Mantoux skin test. The area of induration at the injection site measures 18 mm. The client hasn't previously had a reaction to this test. The nurse's first action is to:
1. move the client to a negative pressure room.
2. have the client put on a face mask.
3. prepare the client to have a chest X-ray.
4. draw a blood sample to check the client's complete blood count (CBC) for an elevated white blood cell count.

Answer: 2. A client with an initial positive reaction to a Mantoux test is at higher risk for active tuberculosis. Before taking him to another room or for a procedure such as a chest X-ray, he should be fitted with a mask to decrease the risk of disease transmission to others. Drawing blood for a CBC isn't necessary at this time.

➡ *NCLEX keys*

Client needs category: Physiological integrity

Client needs subcategory: Reduction of risk potential
Cognitive level: Application

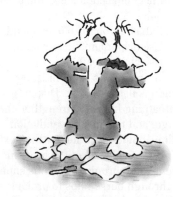

8. A client with acute respiratory distress syndrome (ARDS) is intubated and placed on mechanical ventilation. His partial pressure of arterial oxygen (Pao_2) is 60 mm Hg on 100% fraction of inspired oxygen (Fio_2). To increase his Pao_2 without raising the Fio_2, the client will most likely be placed on:
1. time-cycled ventilation.
2. volume-cycled ventilation.
3. pressure support.
4. positive end-expiratory pressure (PEEP).

Answer: 4. PEEP is widely used during mechanical ventilation of the client with ARDS. It improves gas exchange over the alveolar capillary membrane. Time- or volume-cycled ventilation is less effective with ARDS than pressure-cycled ventilation. Pressure support is dependent on the client's inspiratory effort and not as effective as PEEP in the treatment of ARDS.

➡ *NCLEX keys*

Client needs category: Physiological integrity

Client needs subcategory: Physiological adaptation
Cognitive level: Application

Client needs subcategory: Pharmacological and parenteral therapies
Cognitive level: Application

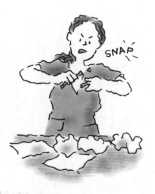

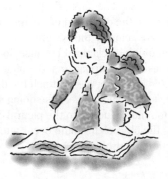

9. A client with clinically active pulmonary tuberculosis is ordered isoniazid, rifampin, pyrazinamide, and ethambutol. Which findings best indicate effectiveness of drug therapy?
1. Cavities are no longer evident on chest X-ray.
2. Tuberculin skin test is negative.
3. The client is afebrile and no longer coughing.
4. The sputum culture converts to negative.

Answer: 4. A change in sputum culture from positive to negative is the best indication of the effectiveness of antitubercular medication. Cavities disappearing from the chest X-ray aren't a reliable indicator of drug effectiveness. Tuberculin skin tests don't convert from positive to negative. Disappearance of symptoms isn't the best indicator of the treatment's effectiveness because the causative organism may still be present.

➡ *NCLEX keys*
Client needs category: Physiological integrity

10. Following pneumothorax, a client receives a chest tube attached to a three-chamber chest drainage system. During the night, the client becomes disoriented, gets out of bed, and steps on the drainage device, causing it to crack open and lose its seal. The nurse should immediately:
1. clamp the chest tube close to the client's thorax.
2. attach the chest tube directly to low wall suction.
3. place the device on a sterile field and call the physician.
4. place the end of the chest tube in a container of sterile water.

Answer: 4. When a chest drainage system cracks open, the closed system between the pleural space and the device is broken. This will allow air to move through the tubing into the pleural space, exacerbating the pneumothorax. The nurse should immediately place the distal end of the tube in sterile water, closing the system again. The tube shouldn't be clamped because doing so increases pressure against the pleural space. It's inappropriate to attach the drain directly to wall suction because doing so may cause too much suction to the pleural cavity. Calling the physician should occur after correcting the problem.

➡ *NCLEX keys*
Client needs category: Physiological integrity
Client needs subcategory: Physiological adaptation
Cognitive level: Application

Yes! You made it through another chapter. Great work!

Brush up on key concepts

The immune and hematologic systems are closely related. The immune system consists of specialized cells and structures that defend the body against invasion by harmful organisms or chemical toxins. The hematologic system also functions as an important part of the body's defenses. Blood transports the components of the immune system throughout the body. In addition, blood delivers oxygen and nutrients to all tissues and removes wastes. Both immune system cells and blood cells originate in the bone marrow.

The key components of the immune system are the lymph nodes, thymus, spleen, and tonsils. The key components of the hematologic system are blood and bone marrow. Blood components play a vital role in transporting electrolytes and regulating acid-base balance.

At any time, you can review the major points of this chapter by consulting the *Cheat Sheet* on pages 118 to 127.

Fluid movers
Lymphatic vessels consist of capillary-like structures that are permeable to large molecules. Lymphatic vessels prevent edema by moving fluid and proteins from interstitial spaces to venous circulation. They also reabsorb fats from the small intestine.

Bacteria filters
Lymph nodes are tissues that filter out bacteria and other foreign cells. They're grouped by region. Here are the groups of lymph nodes:
- cervicofacial
- supraclavicular
- axillary
- epitrochlear

- inguinal
- femoral.

Water plus
Lymph is the fluid found in interstitial spaces. Lymph is composed of water and the end products of cell metabolism.

Body guard
The **tonsils,** which are located at the back of the mouth in the oropharynx, fight off pathogens entering the mouth and nose. They're made of lymphatic tissue and produce lymphocytes.

Filters blood, kills bacteria
The **spleen** is a major lymphatic organ. Here's what it does:
- destroys bacteria
- filters blood
- serves as blood reservoir
- forms lymphocytes and monocytes
- traps formed particles.

Home of hematopoiesis
Bone marrow may be described as either red or yellow:
- Red bone marrow is a source of lymphocytes and macrophages. Hematopoiesis is carried out by red bone marrow. Hematopoiesis is the process by which erythrocytes, leukocytes, and thrombocytes are produced.
- Yellow bone marrow is red bone marrow that has changed to fat.

Getting down to the marrow
Bone marrow contains **stem cells,** which may develop into several different cell types during hematopoiesis:
- Some stem cells evolve into lymphocytes; lymphocytes may become B cells or T cells.
- Other stem cells evolve into phagocytes.

(Text continues on page 127.)

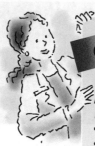

Cheat sheet

Hematologic and immunologic refresher

ACQUIRED IMMUNODEFICIENCY SYNDROME
Key signs and symptoms
- Anorexia, weight loss, recurrent diarrhea
- Disorientation, confusion, dementia
- Night sweats
- Opportunistic infections

Key test results
- CD4$^+$ T-cell count is less than 200 cells/µl.
- Enzyme-linked immunosorbent assay shows positive human immunodeficiency virus antibody titer.
- Western blot is positive.

Key treatments
- Transfusion therapy: fresh frozen plasma, platelets, and packed red blood cells (RBCs)
- Antibiotic: co-trimoxazole (Bactrim)
- Antivirals: dapsone, didanosine (Videx), ganciclovir, zidovudine (Retrovir, AZT), acyclovir (Zovirax), pentamidine (Pentam), aerosolized pentamidine (NebuPent)
- Fusion inhibitor: enfuvirtide (Fuzeon)

Combination therapy
- Nonnucleoside reverse transcriptase inhibitors: delavirdine (Rescriptor), nevirapine (Viramune)
- Nucleoside reverse transcriptase inhibitors: abacavir (Epzicon), lamivudine (Epivir), zidovudine (Retrovir, AZT)
- Protease inhibitors: indinavir (Crixivan), nelfinavir (Viracept), ritonavir (Norvir), saquinavir (Invirase)

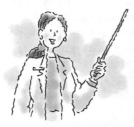

No time to study a long chapter? Just use this *Cheat sheet.*

Key interventions
- Monitor for opportunistic infections.
- Provide high-calorie, high-protein meals.
- Provide mouth care.
- Maintain standard precautions.
- Make referrals to community agencies for support.
- Monitor laboratory values.

ANAPHYLAXIS
Key signs and symptoms
- Sudden physical distress within seconds or minutes after exposure to an allergen (may include feeling of impending doom or fright, weakness, sweating, sneezing, shortness of breath, nasal pruritus, urticaria, and angioedema, followed rapidly by symptoms in one or more target organs)
- Cardiovascular symptoms (hypotension, shock, cardiac arrhythmias) that may precipitate circulatory collapse if untreated

Key test results
- Anaphylaxis can be diagnosed by the rapid onset of severe respiratory or cardiovascular symptoms after an insect sting or after ingestion or injection of a drug, vaccine, diagnostic agent, food, or food additive.

Key treatments
- Immediate injection of epinephrine 1:1,000 aqueous solution, 0.1 to 0.5 ml, repeated every 5 to 20 minutes as necessary

Key interventions
- In the early stages of anaphylaxis, give epinephrine I.M. or subcutaneously and help it move into the circulation faster by massaging the injection site. With severe reactions, give epinephrine I.V.
- Maintain airway patency. Observe for early signs of laryngeal edema (stridor, hoarseness, and dyspnea), and prepare for endotracheal intubation or tracheotomy and oxygen therapy.
- Assess for hypotension and shock, and administer volume expanders (plasma, plasma expanders, saline solution, and albumin) as needed. Maintain blood pressure with I.V. vasopressors (norepinephrine [Levophed] and dopamine). Monitor blood pressure, central venous pressure, and urine output.

ANKYLOSING SPONDYLITIS
Key signs and symptoms
- Intermittent lower back pain (the first indication), usually most severe in the morning or after a period of inactivity
- Mild fatigue, fever, anorexia, or weight loss; unilateral acute anterior uveitis; aortic insufficiency and cardiomegaly; upper lobe pulmonary fibrosis (mimics tuberculosis)
- Stiffness and limited motion of the lumbar spine
- Symptoms progress unpredictably; disease can go into remission, exacerbation, or arrest at any stage

Hematologic and immunologic refresher (continued)

ANKYLOSING SPONDYLITIS (CONTINUED)

Key test results
• Confirmation requires characteristic X-ray findings: blurring of the bony margins of joints in the early stage, bilateral sacroiliac involvement, patchy sclerosis with superficial bony erosions, eventual squaring of vertebral bodies, and "bamboo spine" with complete ankylosis.
• Typical symptoms, a family history, and the presence of HLA-B27 strongly suggest ankylosing spondylitis.

Key treatments
• Anti-inflammatory agents: aspirin, ibuprofen (Motrin), indomethacin (Indocin), sulfasalazine (Azulfidine), sulindac (Clinoril) to control pain and inflammation
• Promoting good posture, stretching and deep-breathing exercises and, in some clients, braces and lightweight supports to delay further deformity (because ankylosing spondylitis progression can't be stopped)

Key interventions
• Assess pain level and administer medications as needed.
• Apply local heat and provide massage.
• Assess mobility and degree of discomfort frequently.

APLASTIC ANEMIA

Key signs and symptoms
• Dyspnea, tachypnea
• Epistaxis
• Melena
• Palpitations, tachycardia
• Purpura, petechiae, ecchymosis, pallor

Key test results
• Bone marrow biopsy shows fatty marrow with reduction of stem cells.

Key treatments
• Transfusion of platelets and packed RBCs
• Antithymocyte globulin
• Hematopoietic growth factor: epoetin alfa (Epogen)

Key interventions
• Monitor for infection, bleeding, and bruising.
• Administer oxygen.
• Administer transfusion therapy, as prescribed.
• Maintain protective precautions.
• Avoid giving the client I.M. injections.

CALCIUM IMBALANCE

Key signs and symptoms
Hypocalcemia
• Cardiac arrhythmias
• Chvostek's sign
• Tetany
• Trousseau's sign
Hypercalcemia
• Anorexia
• Decreased muscle tone
• Lethargy
• Muscle weakness
• Nausea
• Polydipsia
• Polyuria

Key test results
• Serum ionized calcium level less than 4.5 mEq/L confirms hypocalcemia; a level greater than 5.5 mEq/L confirms hypercalcemia. (Because approximately one-half of serum calcium is bound to albumin, changes in serum protein must be considered when interpreting serum calcium levels.)
• Electrocardiogram reveals a lengthened QT interval, a prolonged ST segment, and arrhythmias in hypocalcemia; in hypercalcemia, a shortened QT interval and heart block.

Key treatments
Hypocalcemia
• Diet: adequate intake of calcium, vitamin D, and protein
• Ergocalciferol (vitamin D_2), cholecalciferol (vitamin D_3), calcitriol, dihydrotachysterol (synthetic form of vitamin D_2) for severe deficiency
• I.V. calcium gluconate or calcium chloride for acute hypocalcemia (an emergency)
Hypercalcemia
• Calcitonin
• Loop diuretics, such as ethacrynic acid (Edecrin) and furosemide (Lasix), to promote calcium excretion (thiazide diuretics contraindicated in hypercalcemia because they inhibit calcium excretion)

Key interventions
Hypocalcemia
• Monitor serum calcium levels every 12 to 24 hours. Check for Trousseau's and Chvostek's signs.
• Administer calcium gluconate slow I.V. in dextrose 5% in water (*never* in saline solution, which encourages renal calcium loss). Don't add calcium gluconate I.V. to solutions containing bicarbonate.
Hypercalcemia
• Monitor serum calcium levels. Monitor for cardiac arrhythmias.
• Increase fluid intake.
• Administer loop diuretics (not thiazide diuretics).

(continued)

Hematologic and immunologic refresher *(continued)*

CHLORIDE IMBALANCE
Key signs and symptoms
Hypochloremia
- Muscle hypertonicity (in conditions related to loss of gastric secretions)
- Muscle weakness
- Shallow, depressed breathing
- Twitching

Hyperchloremia
- Agitation
- Deep, rapid breathing
- Diminished cognitive ability
- Hypertension
- Pitting edema
- Tachycardia
- Weakness

Key test results
- Serum chloride level that's less than 98 mEq/L confirms hypochloremia; supportive values with metabolic alkalosis include a serum pH greater than 7.45 and a serum carbon dioxide level greater than 32 mEq/L.
- Serum chloride level greater than 108 mEq/L confirms hyperchloremia; with metabolic acidosis, serum pH is less than 7.35 and the serum carbon dioxide level is less than 22 mEq/L.

Key treatments
Hypochloremia
- Acidifying agent: ammonium chloride
- Diet: salty broth
- Saline solution I.V.

Hyperchloremia
- Alkalinizing agent: sodium bicarbonate I.V.
- Lactated Ringer's solution

Key interventions
- Monitor serum chloride levels frequently, particularly during I.V. therapy.
Hypochloremia
- Administer I.V. saline and medications as ordered.
Hyperchloremia
- Administer medications and I.V. fluids as ordered.

DISSEMINATED INTRAVASCULAR COAGULATION
Key signs and symptoms
- Abnormal bleeding without an accompanying history of serious hemorrhagic disorder (petechiae, hematomas, ecchymosis, cutaneous oozing)
- Oliguria
- Shock

Key test results
- Blood tests show prothrombin time (PT) greater than 15 seconds; partial thromboplastin time (PTT) greater than 60 to

80 seconds; fibrinogen levels less than 150 mg/dl; platelets less than 100,000/µl; fibrin degradation products typically greater than 100 mcg/ml; and a positive D-dimer test specific for disseminated intravascular coagulation.

Key treatments
- Anticoagulant: heparin I.V.
- Bed rest
- Transfusion therapy: fresh frozen plasma, platelets, packed RBCs

Key interventions
- Enforce complete bed rest during bleeding episodes.
- Check all I.V. and venipuncture sites frequently for bleeding. Apply pressure to injection sites for at least 10 minutes. Alert other personnel to the client's tendency to hemorrhage.
- Administer blood products as ordered.
- Monitor for transfusion reactions and signs of fluid overload.
- Monitor the results of serial blood studies (particularly hematocrit [HCT], hemoglobin [Hb], and coagulation studies).

FIBROMYALGIA SYNDROME
Key signs and symptoms
- Diffuse, dull, aching pain across the neck, shoulders, lower back, and proximal limbs
- Fatigue
- Sleep disturbances

Key test results
- The diagnosis is made mostly based on subjective information from the client.

Key treatments
- Antidepressants: amitriptyline (Elavil), nortriptyline (Aventyl)
- Duloxetine (Cymbalta), milnacipran (Savella), pregabalin (Lyrica) for pain and fatigue
- Physical therapy

Key interventions
- Provide client education for managing symptoms.
- Encourage regular, low-impact aerobic exercise.
- Recommend cognitive behavioral therapy to help the client deal with stressful situations.
- Provide regular rest periods throughout the day.

HEMOPHILIA
Key signs and symptoms
- Hematuria (bloody urine)
- Joint tenderness
- Pain and swelling in a weight-bearing joint
- Prolonged bleeding after major trauma or surgery (in mild hemophilia)
- Tarry stools
- Subcutaneous and I.M. hematomas (in moderate hemophilia)
- Spontaneous or severe bleeding after minor trauma (in severe hemophilia)

Hematologic and immunologic refresher *(continued)*

HEMOPHILIA *(CONTINUED)*
Key test results
- Factor VIII assay reveals 0% to 25% of normal factor VIII (hemophilia A).
- Factor IX assay shows deficiency (hemophilia B).

Key treatments
- Cryoprecipitate antihemophilic factor (AHF), lyophilized (dehydrated) AHF, or both (for hemophilia A)
- Factor IX concentrate (for hemophilia B)
- Analgesic: morphine
- Hormone: desmopressin (DDAVP)

Key interventions
- Monitor for signs of bleeding.
- Administer clotting factor or plasma as ordered.
- Administer analgesics. Avoid I.M. injections, aspirin, and aspirin-containing medications.
- If the client has bled into a joint, immediately elevate the painful joint as ordered.

IDIOPATHIC THROMBOCYTOPENIC PURPURA
Key signs and symptoms
- Ecchymoses
- Hemorrhage (rare)
- Mucosal bleeding from mouth, nose, or GI tract
- Petechiae
- Purpuric lesions on vital organs

Key test results
- Platelet count is less than 20,000/µl.
- Blood test shows prolonged bleeding time.
- Bone marrow study shows an increase of megakaryocytes and a decrease in circulating platelet survival time.

Key treatments
- Blood transfusion of blood and blood components
- Glucocorticoids: prednisone, methylprednisone (Solu-Cortef)
- May resolve spontaneously
- Splenectomy if unresponsive to high-dose steroids
- Vitamin K for coagulation defects

Key interventions
- Transfuse blood and blood products as needed.
- Monitor the client for petechiae, ecchymoses, and other signs of bleeding.
- Monitor platelet function and other coagulation values.
- Help the client avoid unnecessary trauma.
- Test stool for bleeding.

IRON DEFICIENCY ANEMIA
Key signs and symptoms
- Pallor
- Sensitivity to cold
- Weakness and fatigue

Key test results
- Hematology shows decreased Hb, HCT, iron, ferritin, reticulocytes, red cell indices, transferrin, and saturation; absent hemosiderin; and increased iron-binding capacity.

Key treatments
- Diet high in iron, roughage, and protein with increased fluids; avoidance of teas and coffee, which reduce absorption of iron
- Vitamins: pyridoxine (vitamin B_6), ascorbic acid (vitamin C)
- Antianemics: ferrous sulfate (Feosol), iron dextran (DexFerrum)

Key interventions
- Assess cardiovascular and respiratory status.
- Monitor stool, urine, and emesis for occult blood.
- Administer medications, as prescribed. Administer iron injection deep into muscle using Z-track technique to avoid subcutaneous irritation and discoloration from leaking drug.
- Provide mouth, skin, and foot care.

KAPOSI'S SARCOMA
Key signs and symptoms
- One or more obvious lesions in various shapes, sizes, and colors (ranging from red-brown to dark purple) that appear most commonly on the skin, buccal mucosa, hard and soft palates, lips, gums, tongue, tonsils, conjunctivae, and sclerae
- Pain (if the sarcoma advances beyond the early stages or if a lesion breaks down or impinges on nerves or organs)

Key test results
- Tissue biopsy identifies the lesion's type and stage.

Key treatments
- High-calorie, high-protein diet
- Radiation therapy
- Chemotherapy: doxorubicin, etoposide (VePesid), vinblastine, vincristine
- Antiemetic: aprepitant (Emend)

Key interventions
- Provide skin care, and assess for skin breakdown or new lesions.
- Administer pain medications. Suggest distractions, position the client for comfort, and help with relaxation techniques.
- Provide reassurance.
- Provide high-calorie, high-protein meals. Consult with the dietitian, and plan meals around the client's treatment.
- Assess for adverse reactions to radiation therapy or chemotherapy—such as anorexia, nausea, vomiting, and diarrhea—and take steps to prevent or alleviate them.
- Teach infection-prevention techniques and, if necessary, demonstrate basic hygiene measures. Maintain standard precautions.

(continued)

Hematologic and immunologic refresher (continued)

LATEX ALLERGY

Key signs and symptoms
Life-threatening reaction
- Bronchospasm
- Flushing
- Hypotension
- Oxygen desaturation
- Syncope
- Tachycardia
- Urticaria

Mild reaction
- Diarrhea
- Nausea
- Swollen lips

Key test results
- Blood test for latex sensitivity measures specific immunoglobulin E antibodies against latex.

Key treatments
- Avoiding latex exposure in clients sensitive to or with suspected sensitivity to latex
- Supportive care
- Premedication before exposure: diphenhydramine (Benadryl), prednisone, cimetidine (Tagamet)
- Postexposure medication: hydrocortisone, diphenhydramine (Benadryl), famotidine (Pepcid)

Key interventions
- Be aware of all products containing latex and avoid their use in clients with known or suspected sensitivity.
- Premedicate the client before exposure, if possible.
- If the client has a reaction to latex, ensure a patent airway, and administer oxygen.
- Encourage the client to wear a medical identification tag stating his allergy.
- Be aware that the more a latex-sensitive client is exposed to latex, the more severe his reaction will be.

LEUKEMIA

Key signs and symptoms
- Enlarged lymph nodes, spleen, and liver
- Frequent infections
- Weakness and fatigue

Key test results
- Bone marrow biopsy shows large numbers of immature leukocytes.

Key treatments
- Antimetabolites: fluorouracil, methotrexate (Trexall)
- Alkylating agents: busulfan (Myleran), chlorambucil (Leukeran)
- Antineoplastics: vinblastine, vincristine
- Antibiotic: doxorubicin
- Hematopoietic growth factor: epoetin alfa (Epogen)

Key interventions
- Monitor laboratory studies.
- Monitor for bleeding.
- Monitor for infection. Promptly report temperature over 101° F (38.3° C), and decreased white blood cell (WBC) counts so that antibiotic therapy may be initiated.
- Administer transfusion therapy, as ordered, and monitor for adverse reactions.
- Provide gentle mouth and skin care.

LYMPHOMA

Key signs and symptoms
- Predictable pattern of spread (Hodgkin's disease)
- Enlarged, nontender, firm, and movable lymph nodes in cervical regions (Hodgkin's disease)
- Less predictable pattern of spread (malignant lymphoma)
- Prominent, painless, generalized lymphadenopathy (malignant lymphoma)

Key test results
- Bone marrow aspiration and biopsy reveals small, diffuse lymphocytic or large, follicular-type cells (malignant lymphoma).
- Lymph node biopsy is positive for Reed-Sternberg cells (Hodgkin's disease).

Key treatments
- Radiation therapy
- Transfusion of packed RBCs
- Chemotherapy for Hodgkin's disease: mechlorethamine (Mustargen), vincristine, procarbazine (Matulane), doxorubicin, bleomycin (Blenoxane), vinblastine, dacarbazine (DTIC-Dome)
- Chemotherapy for malignant lymphoma: cyclophosphamide (Cytoxan), vincristine, doxorubicin

Key interventions
- Monitor for bleeding, infection, jaundice, and electrolyte imbalance.
- Provide mouth and skin care.
- Encourage fluids and administer I.V. fluids as ordered.
- Administer medications, as prescribed, and monitor for adverse effects.
- Administer transfusion therapy, as prescribed, and monitor for adverse reactions.

MAGNESIUM IMBALANCE

Key signs and symptoms
Hypomagnesemia
- Arrhythmias
- Neuromuscular irritability
- Chvostek's sign
- Mood changes
- Confusion

Hematologic and immunologic refresher (continued)

MAGNESIUM IMBALANCE (CONTINUED)
Hypermagnesemia
- Diminished deep tendon reflexes
- Weakness
- Confusion
- Heart block
- Nausea
- Vomiting

Key test results
- Serum magnesium level less than 1.5 mEq/L confirms hypomagnesemia; serum magnesium level greater than 2.5 mEq/L confirms hypermagnesemia.

Key treatments
Hypomagnesemia
- Oral or I.M. magnesium supplements
- High-magnesium diet
- Magnesium sulfate I.V. (10 to 40 mEq/L diluted in I.V. fluid) for severe deficiency
Hypermagnesemia
- Low-magnesium diet with increased fluid intake
- Loop diuretic: furosemide (Lasix)
- Magnesium antagonist: calcium gluconate (10%)
- Peritoneal dialysis or hemodialysis if renal function fails or if excess magnesium can't be eliminated

Key interventions
Hypomagnesemia
- Monitor serum electrolyte levels (including magnesium, calcium, and potassium) daily for mild deficits and every 6 to 12 hours during replacement therapy.
- Monitor intake and output. (Urine output shouldn't fall below 25 ml/hour or 600 ml/day.)
- Monitor vital signs during I.V. therapy. Infuse magnesium replacement slowly, and watch for bradycardia, heart block, and decreased respiratory rate.
Hypermagnesemia
- Assess level of consciousness, muscle activity, and vital signs.
- Monitor intake and output. Provide sufficient fluids.
- Treat abnormal serum electrolyte levels.
- Monitor cardic rhythm.

METABOLIC ACIDOSIS
Key signs and symptoms
- Central nervous system depression
- Kussmaul's respirations
- Lethargy

Key test results
- Arterial blood gas (ABG) analysis reveals pH below 7.35 and bicarbonate level less than 24 mEq/L.

Key treatments
- Treatment of underlying cause
- Sodium bicarbonate I.V. or orally for chronic metabolic acidosis

Key interventions
- Monitor vital signs, laboratory results, and level of consciousness.
- Monitor intake and output.
- Provide appropriate treatment for the underlying cause.
- Administer medications and I.V. fluids as ordered.

METABOLIC ALKALOSIS
Key signs and symptoms
- Atrial tachycardia
- Confusion
- Diarrhea
- Hypoventilation
- Twitching
- Vomiting

Key test results
- ABG analysis reveals pH greater than 7.45 and a bicarbonate level above 29 mEq/L.

Key treatments
- Treatment of underlying cause
- Acidifying agent: hydrochloric acid
- Carbonic anhydrase inhibitors: acetazolomide (Diamox)

Key interventions
- Monitor respiratory status.
- Monitor cardiac rhythm and vital signs.
- Provide appropriate treatment for underlying cause.
- Administer medication and I.V. fluids as ordered.

MULTIPLE MYELOMA
Key signs and symptoms
- Anemia, thrombocytopenia, hemorrhage
- Constant, severe bone pain
- Pathologic fractures, skeletal deformities of the sternum and ribs, loss of height

Key test results
- X-ray shows diffuse, round, punched out bone lesions; osteoporosis; osteolytic lesions of the skull; and widespread demineralization.

Key treatments
- Orthopedic devices: braces, splints, casts
- Alkylating agents: melphalan (Alkeran), cyclophosphamide (Cytoxan)
- Androgen: fluoxymesterone

(continued)

Hematologic and immunologic refresher *(continued)*

MULTIPLE MYELOMA *(CONTINUED)*
- Antibiotic: doxorubicin
- Antigout agent: allopurinol
- Antineoplastics: vinblastine, vincristine
- Glucocorticoid: prednisone

Key interventions
- Assess renal status.
- Assess pain level.
- Encourage oral fluids and administer I.V. fluids.

PERNICIOUS ANEMIA
Key signs and symptoms
- Tingling and paresthesia of hands and feet
- Weight loss, anorexia, dyspepsia

Key test results
- Bone marrow aspiration shows increased megaloblasts, few maturing erythrocytes, and defective leukocyte maturation.
- Peripheral blood smear reveals oval, macrocytic, hyperchromic erythrocytes.

Key treatments
- Vitamins: pyridoxine (vitamin B_6), ascorbic acid (vitamin C), cyanocobalamin (vitamin B_{12}), folic acid (vitamin A)

Key interventions
- Assess cardiovascular status.
- Administer medications as prescribed.
- Provide mouth care before and after meals.
- Institute fall prevention measures.

PHOSPHORUS IMBALANCE
Key signs and symptoms
Hypophosphatemia
- Anorexia
- Muscle weakness
- Paresthesia
- Tremor
Hyperphosphatemia
- Usually asymptomatic

Key test results
- Serum phosphorus level less than 1.7 mEq/L (or 2.5 mg/dl) confirms hypophosphatemia. A urine phosphorus level more than 1.3 g/24 hours supports this diagnosis.
- Serum phosphorus level exceeding 2.6 mEq/L (or 4.5 mg/dl) confirms hyperphosphatemia. Supportive values include decreased levels of serum calcium (less than 9 mg/dl) and urine phosphorus (less than 0.9 g/24 hours).

Key treatments
Hypophosphatemia
- High-phosphorus diet
- Phosphate supplements

Hyperphosphatemia
- Low-phosphorus diet
- Calcium supplement: calcium acetate (PhosLo)

Key interventions
Hypophosphatemia
- Monitor intake and output. Administer potassium phosphate slow I.V. Assess renal function, and be alert for hypocalcemia when giving phosphate supplements.
- Provide a high-phosphorus diet containing milk and milk products, kidney, liver, turkey, and dried fruits.
Hyperphosphatemia
- Monitor intake and output. If urine output falls below 25 ml/hour or 600 ml/day, notify the physician immediately.
- Assess for signs of hypocalcemia, such as muscle twitching and tetany, which commonly accompany hyperphosphatemia.
- Provide foods low in phosphorus such as vegetables.

POLYCYTHEMIA VERA
Key signs and symptoms
- Clubbing of the digits
- Dizziness
- Headache
- Hypertension
- Ruddy cyanosis of the nose
- Thrombosis of smaller vessels
- Visual disturbances (blurring, diplopia, engorged veins of fundus and retina)

Key test results
- Blood tests show increased RBC mass and normal arterial oxygen saturation in association with splenomegaly or two of the following: thrombocytosis, leukocytosis, elevated leukocyte alkaline phosphatase level, or elevated serum vitamin B_{12} or unbound B_{12} binding capacity.

Key treatments
- Phlebotomy (typically, 350 to 500 ml of blood is removed every other day until the client's HCT is reduced to the low-normal range)
- Plasmapheresis
- Chemotherapy: busulfan (Myleran), chlorambucil (Leukeran), melphalan (Alkeran)
- Antigout agent: allopurinol

Key interventions
- Monitor vital signs.
- Assess for tachycardia, clamminess, or complaints of vertigo during phlebotomy. If these effects occur, stop the procedure.
- After phlebotomy, administer 24 oz (720 ml) of juice or water.
- Administer I.V. fluids and medications as ordered.

Hematologic and immunologic refresher (continued)

POLYCYTHEMIA VERA (CONTINUED)
During myelosuppressive treatment
• Monitor complete blood count and platelet count before and during therapy.

RHEUMATOID ARTHRITIS
Key signs and symptoms
• Painful, swollen joints, crepitus, morning stiffness
• Symmetrical joint swelling (mirror image of affected joints)

Key test results
• Antinuclear antibody test is positive.
• Rheumatoid factor test is positive.

Key treatments
• Cold therapy during acute episodes
• Heat therapy to relax muscles and relieve pain for chronic disease
• Antirheumatic: hydroxychloroquine (Plaquenil)
• Glucocorticoids: prednisone, hydrocortisone (Solu-Cortef)
• Nonsteroidal anti-inflammatory drugs (NSAIDs): indomethacin (Indocin), ibuprofen (Advil, Motrin), sulindac (Clinoril), piroxicam (Feldene), flurbiprofen (Ansaid), diclofenac (Voltaren), naproxen (Naprosyn), diflunisal
• Tumor necrosis factor inhibitors: etanercept (Enbrel), adalimumab (Humira), infliximab (Remicade)

Key interventions
• Assess joints for swelling, pain, and redness.
• Monitor laboratory studies.
• Splint inflamed joints.
• Provide warm or cold therapy, as prescribed.
• Administer medications as ordered, and monitor for adverse reactions.

SCLERODERMA
Key signs and symptoms
• Pain
• Signs and symptoms of Raynaud's phenomenon, such as blanching, cyanosis, and erythema of the fingers and toes in response to stress or exposure to cold
• Stiffness
• Swelling of fingers and joints
• Taut, shiny skin over the entire hand and forearm
• Tight and inelastic facial skin, causing a masklike appearance and "pinching" of the mouth
• Renal involvement, usually accompanied by malignant hypertension, the main cause of death

Key test results
• Blood studies show slightly elevated erythrocyte sedimentation rate (ESR), positive rheumatoid factor in 25% to 35% of clients, and positive antinuclear antibody test.
• Skin biopsy may show changes consistent with the progress of the disease, such as marked thickening of the dermis and occlusive vessel changes.

Key treatments
• Palliative measures: heat therapy, rest periods
• Immunosuppressants: cyclosporine (Sandimmune), chlorambucil (Leukeran)
• Physical therapy to maintain function and promote muscle strength
• Antihypertensives: nifedipine (Procardia), amlodipine (Norvasc), losatan (Cozaar), captopril (Capoten)

Key interventions
• Assess activity ability motion restrictions, pain, vital signs, intake and output, respiratory function, and daily weight.
• Monitor blood pressure and report any increases above baseline.
• Assist with prescribed exercises.

SEPTIC SHOCK
Key signs and symptoms
Early stage
• Chills
• Oliguria
• Sudden fever (temperature over 101° F [38.3° C])
Late stage
• Altered level of consciousness
• Anuria
• Hyperventilation
• Hypotension
• Hypothermia
• Restlessness
• Tachycardia
• Tachypnea

Key test results
• Blood cultures isolate the organism.
• Blood tests show decreased platelet count and leukocytosis (15,000 to 30,000/μl), increased blood urea nitrogen and creatinine levels, decreased creatinine clearance, and abnormal PT and PTT.

Key treatments
• Removing or replacing any I.V., intra-arterial, or indwelling urinary catheters that may be the source of infection
• Oxygen therapy (may require endotracheal intubation and mechanical ventilation)
• Colloid or crystalloid infusion to increase intravascular volume
• Diuretic: furosemide (Lasix) after sufficient fluid volume has been replaced to maintain urine output above 20 ml/hour

(continued)

Hematologic and immunologic refresher (continued)

SEPTIC SHOCK (CONTINUED)
- Antibiotics: according to sensitivity of causative organism
- Vasopressor: dopamine or norepinephrine (Levophed) if fluid resuscitation fails to increase blood pressure

Key interventions
- Replace I.V., intra-arterial, or indwelling urinary catheters.
- Administer normal saline solution or lactated Ringer's solution.
- Monitor intake and output for fluid loss.
- Administer antibiotics I.V. and monitor drug levels.
- Monitor vital signs and pulse oximetry.
- Monitor respiratory, cardiovascular, and neurologic status. Assist with endotracheal intubation if necessary.
- Administer vasopressors and titrate appropriately.

SICKLE CELL ANEMIA
Key signs and symptoms
- Aching bones
- Jaundice, pallor (jaundice worsens during painful crisis)
- Unexplained dyspnea or dyspnea on exertion
- Tachycardia
- Severe pain (during sickle cell crisis)

Key test results
- Blood tests show low RBC counts, elevated WBC and platelet counts, decreased ESR, increased serum iron levels, decreased RBC survival, and reticulocytosis.
- Hb electrophoresis shows Hb S.

Key treatments
- Supplements: iron and folic acid
- I.V. fluid therapy to prevent dehydration and vessel occlusion
- Analgesic: meperidine or morphine (to relieve pain from vaso-occlusive crises)

Key interventions
- Apply warm compresses to painful areas.
- Maintain bed rest during crisis.
- Encourage fluid intake.
- Administer prescribed I.V. fluids.

SODIUM IMBALANCE
Key signs and symptoms
Hyponatremia
- Abdominal cramps
- Altered mental status
- Cold, clammy skin
- Cyanosis
- Hypotension
- Oliguria or anuria
- Seizures
- Tachycardia
Hypernatremia
- Dry, sticky mucous membranes

- Excessive weight gain
- Flushed skin
- Hypertension
- Intense thirst
- Oliguria
- Pitting edema
- Rough, dry tongue
- Tachycardia

Key test results
- Serum sodium level less than 135 mEq/L indicates hyponatremia.
- Serum sodium level greater than 145 mEq/L indicates hypernatremia.

Key treatments
Hyponatremia
- I.V. infusion of saline solution
- Potassium supplement: potassium chloride (K-Lor)
Hypernatremia
- Low-sodium diet
- Salt-free I.V. solution (such as dextrose in water), followed by infusion of 0.45% sodium chloride to prevent hyponatremia

Key interventions
Hyponatremia
- Monitor serum sodium and serum chloride levels. Monitor urine specific gravity and other laboratory results. Monitor fluid intake and output, and weigh the client daily.
- Assess for signs of fluid overload.
Hypernatremia
- Monitor serum sodium levels every 6 hours or at least daily.
- Monitor vital signs, especially for rising pulse rate.
- Assess for signs of hypervolemia, especially in the client receiving I.V. fluids.
- Monitor fluid intake and output, checking for body fluid loss.
- Weigh the client daily.

SYSTEMIC LUPUS ERYTHEMATOSUS
Key signs and symptoms
- Butterfly rash on face (rash may vary in severity from malar erythema to discoid lesions)
- Fatigue
- Migratory pain, stiffness, and joint swelling

Key test results
- Lupus erythematosus cell preparation is positive.

Key treatments
- Cytotoxic drugs: azathioprine (Imuran), methotrexate (Trexall); these drugs may delay or prevent deteriorating renal status
- Immunosuppressants: azathioprine (Imuran), cyclophosphamide (Cytoxan)

Hematologic and immunologic refresher (continued)

SYSTEMIC LUPUS ERYTHEMATOSUS (CONTINUED)
• NSAIDs: indomethacin (Indocin), ibuprofen (Motrin), sulindac (Clinoril), piroxicam (Feldene), flurbiprofen (Ansaid), diclofenac sodium (Voltaren), naproxen (Naprosyn), diflunisal

Key interventions
• Assess musculoskeletal status.
• Monitor renal status.
• Provide prophylactic skin, mouth, and perineal care.
• Maintain seizure precautions.
• Minimize environmental stress and provide rest periods.
• Administer medications, as ordered, and monitor for adverse reactions.

VASCULITIS
Key signs and symptoms
Wegener's granulomatosis
• Cough
• Fever
• Malaise
• Pulmonary congestion
• Weight loss
Temporal arteritis
• Fever
• Headache (associated with polymyalgia rheumatica syndrome)
• Jaw claudication
• Myalgia
• Visual changes
Takayasu's arteritis
• Arthralgias
• Bruits
• Loss of distal pulses
• Malaise
• Pain or paresthesia distal to affected area
• Syncope
• Weight loss

Key test results
Wegener's granulomatosis
• Tissue biopsy shows necrotizing vasculitis with granulomatous inflammation.
Temporal arteritis
• Tissue biopsy shows panarteritis with infiltration of mononuclear cells, giant cells within vessel wall, fragmentation of internal elastic lamina, and proliferation of intima.
Takayasu's arteritis
• Arteriography shows calcification and obstruction of affected vessels.
• Tissue biopsy shows inflammation of adventitia and intima of vessels and thickening of vessel walls.

Key treatments
• Removal of identified environmental antigen
• Diet: elimination of antigenic food, if identifiable; increased fluid intake (3 qt [3 L] daily), if not contraindicated
• Corticosteroid: prednisone
• Antineoplastic: cyclophosphamide (Cytoxan)

Key interventions
• Regulate environmental temperature.
• Monitor vital signs. Use a Doppler ultrasonic flowmeter, if available.
• Monitor intake and output and assess for edema.
• Monitor WBC count during cyclophosphamide therapy.

Oxygen carriers
Erythrocytes (also called **red blood cells** or **RBCs**) are formed in the bone marrow and contain hemoglobin (Hb). Oxygen binds with Hb to form oxyhemoglobin, which is then carried by erythrocytes throughout the body.

Clotting contributors
Thrombocytes (also called **platelets**) are formed in the bone marrow and function in the coagulation of blood.

Infection fighters
Leukocytes (also called **white blood cells** or **WBCs**) are formed in the bone marrow and lymphatic tissue and include granulocytes and agranulocytes. WBCs provide immunity and protection from infection by phagocytosis (engulfing, digesting, and destroying microorganisms).

Liquid partner
Plasma is the liquid portion of the blood, and its composition is water, protein (albumin and globulin), glucose, and electrolytes.

Of donors and recipients
A person's **blood type** is determined by a system of antigens located on the surface of RBCs. The four blood types are:
• A antigen
• B antigen
• AB (both A and B) antigens
• O (no antigens).

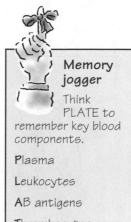

Memory jogger

Think PLATE to remember key blood components.

Plasma
Leukocytes
AB antigens
Thrombocytes
Erythrocytes

Because group O blood lacks both A and B antigens, it can be transfused in limited amounts in an emergency, regardless of the recipient's blood type, with little risk of adverse reaction. That's why people with group O blood are called universal donors. A person with AB blood type has neither anti-A nor anti-B antibodies. This person may receive A, B, AB, or O blood, which makes him a universal recipient.

In addition, the antigen Rh factor is found on the RBCs of approximately 85% of people. A person with the Rh factor is Rh positive. A person without the factor is Rh negative. A person may only receive blood from a person with the same Rh factor.

Now, some more about the immune system

In cell-mediated immunity, T cells respond directly to antigens (foreign substances such as bacteria or toxins that induce antibody formation). This response involves destruction of target cells—such as virus-infected cells and cancer cells—through secretion of lymphokines (lymph proteins). Examples of cell-mediated immunity are rejection of transplanted organs and delayed immune responses that fight disease.

About 80% of blood cells are T cells. They probably originate from stem cells in the bone marrow; the thymus gland controls their maturity. In the process, a large number of antigen-specific cells are produced.

Killer, helper, or suppressor

T cells can be killer, helper, or suppressor T cells:
• Killer cells bind to the surface of the invading cell, disrupt the membrane, and destroy it by altering its internal environment.
• Helper cells stimulate B cells to mature into plasma cells, which begin to synthesize and secrete immunoglobulin (proteins with known antibody activity).
• Suppressor cells reduce the humoral response.

Don't forget B cells

B cells act in a different way from T cells to recognize and destroy antigens. B cells are responsible for humoral or immunoglobulin-mediated immunity. B cells originate in the bone marrow and mature into plasma cells that produce antibodies (immunoglobulin molecules that interact with a specific antigen). Antibodies destroy bacteria and viruses, thereby preventing them from entering host cells.

A word about immunoglobulins

Five major classes of immunoglobulin exist:
• Immunoglobulin G (IgG) makes up about 80% of plasma antibodies. It appears in all body fluids and is the major antibacterial and antiviral antibody.
• Immunoglobulin M (IgM) is the first immunoglobulin produced during an immune response. It's too large to easily cross membrane barriers and is usually present only in the vascular system.
• Immunoglobulin A (IgA) is found mainly in body secretions, such as saliva, sweat, tears, mucus, bile, and colostrum. It defends against pathogens on body surfaces, especially those that enter the respiratory and GI tracts.
• Immunoglobulin D (IgD) is present in plasma and is easily broken down. It's the predominant antibody on the surface of B cells and is mainly an antigen receptor.
• Immunoglobulin E (IgE) is the antibody involved in immediate hypersensitivity reactions, or allergic reactions that develop within minutes of exposure to an antigen. IgE stimulates the release of mast cell granules, which contain histamine and heparin.

Keep abreast of diagnostic tests

Here are the most important tests used to diagnose hematologic and immune disorders, along with common nursing actions associated with each test.

Blood sample study #1

A **blood chemistry test** uses a blood sample to measure potassium, sodium, calcium, blood urea nitrogen (BUN), creatinine, protein, albumin, and bilirubin levels.

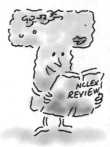

Wow! I can be a killer, helper, or suppressor!

Nursing actions
Before the procedure
- Withhold food and fluids, as directed.
- Explain the procedure to the client.

After the procedure
- Check the venipuncture site for bleeding.

Blood sample study #2
A **hematologic study** uses a blood sample to analyze WBCs, RBCs, erythrocyte sedimentation rate (ESR), Hb, and hematocrit (HCT), red cell indices, hemoglobin electrophoresis, iron and total iron binding capacity, sickle cell test, and CD4$^+$ cell count.

Nursing actions
Before the procedure
- Note the client's current drug therapy.
- Explain the procedure to the client.

After the procedure
- Check the venipuncture site for bleeding.
- Handle the specimen gently to prevent hemolysis.

Check on immune status
Immunologic studies use a small sample of blood to analyze rheumatoid factor, lupus erythematosus cell preparation, antinuclear antibodies, and serum protein electrophoresis.

Nursing actions
Before the procedure
- Note the client's current drug therapy.
- Explain the procedure to the client.

After the procedure
- Check the venipuncture site for bleeding.

HIV detector
Enzyme-linked immunosorbent assay (ELISA) uses a blood sample to detect the human immunodeficiency virus (HIV) antibody.

Nursing actions
Before the procedure
- Verify that informed consent has been obtained and documented.
- Provide the client with appropriate pretest counseling.
- Explain the procedure to the client.

After the procedure
- Check the venipuncture site for bleeding.

Confirming the diagnosis
A **Western blot test** uses a blood sample to detect the presence of specific viral proteins to confirm HIV infection.

Nursing actions
Before the procedure
- Verify that informed consent has been obtained and documented.
- Explain the procedure to the client.

After the procedure
- Check the venipuncture site for bleeding.

Small sample
A **urine test** uses a small sample of urine to analyze hemosiderin and Hb.

Nursing actions
- Explain the procedure to the client.
- Collect a random urine specimen of about 30 ml.

Radiographic snapshot
A **lymphangiography** involves an injection of radiopaque dye through a catheter, which provides a radiographic picture of the lymphatic system and the dissection of lymph vessels.

Nursing actions
Before the procedure
- Note any allergies to iodine, seafood, and radiopaque dyes.
- Explain the procedure to the client.
- Warn of possible throat irritation and flushing after injection of the dye.
- Make sure that written, informed consent has been obtained.
- Withhold food and fluids, as directed.

After the procedure
- Assess vital signs and peripheral pulses.
- Monitor the catheter insertion site for bleeding.
- Encourage fluid intake.
- Advise the client that skin, stool, and urine will have a blue discoloration for about 48 hours after the procedure.

Marrow removal
A **bone marrow examination,** also called *aspiration* or *biopsy,* involves the percutaneous removal of bone

> Postdiagnostic test monitoring, such as checking the venipuncture site, the catheter insertion site, or the site of bone marrow aspiration, is a key nursing responsibility.

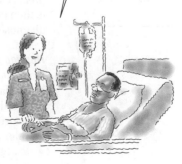

marrow and an examination of erythrocytes, leukocytes, thrombocytes, and precursor cells.

Nursing actions

Before the procedure
- Make sure that written, informed consent has been obtained.
- Explain the procedure to the client.
- Determine the client's ability to lie still during aspiration.
- Tell the client that he may experience a burning sensation as the bone marrow is aspirated.

After the procedure
- Maintain a pressure dressing at the aspiration site.
- Monitor the aspiration site for bleeding and infection.
- Maintain bed rest as ordered.

Swallow this and wait

A **Schilling test** involves administration of an oral radioactive cyanocobalamin and an intramuscular cyanocobalamin. Following this is microscopic examination of a 24-hour urine sample for cyanocobalamin (vitamin B_{12}).

Nursing actions

- Explain the procedure to the client.
- Withhold food and fluids for 12 hours before administration of the radioactive substance.
- Withhold laxatives during the test.
- Instruct the client to save all voided urine for 24 hours and keep the urine at room temperature.

What's in the stomach?

Gastric analysis involves the aspiration of stomach contents through a nasogastric (NG) tube. A fasting analysis of gastric secretions is then performed to measure acidity and to diagnose pernicious anemia.

Nursing actions

Before the procedure
- Explain the procedure to the client.
- Withhold food and fluids for 12 hours.
- Instruct the client not to smoke or chew gum for at least 8 hours before the test.
- Withhold medications that can affect gastric secretions.

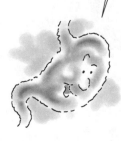

In gastric analysis, my contents are aspirated through an NG tube.

After the procedure
- Obtain vital signs.
- Assess for reactions to gastric acid stimulant, if used.

No red meats or turnips

A **fecal occult blood test** involves a microscopic analysis of Hb to detect occult blood in stool.

Nursing actions

- Explain the procedure to the client.
- Instruct the client to maintain a high-fiber diet and to refrain from eating red meats, beets, turnips, and horseradish for 48 to 72 hours.
- Explain that the test requires collection of three stool specimens.
- Withhold iron preparations, iodides, rauwolfia derivatives, indomethacin, colchicine, salicylates, steroids, and ascorbic acid for 48 hours before the test and throughout the collection period.

RBC longevity measure

Erythrocyte life span determination involves a reinjection of the client's blood that has been tagged with chromium 51. Its purpose is to measure the life span of circulating RBCs.

Nursing actions

Before the procedure
- Explain the procedure to the client.
- Inform the client that frequent blood samples will be drawn over a 2-week period.

After the procedure
- Check the venipuncture site for bleeding.
- Apply a pressure dressing to the venipuncture site.

Balancing act

The **Romberg test** is a physical test in which the client stands with his feet together, his eyes open, and his arms at either side, while the examiner stands and protects him from falling. The client is then asked to close his eyes. If he loses his balance or sways to one side, the Romberg test is positive. This is done to assess loss of balance in pernicious anemia.

Nursing actions
- Explain the procedure to the client.
- Monitor the client for imbalance.
- Prevent the client from falling.

How fast does it burst?
In the **erythrocyte fragility test,** a blood sample is used to measure the rate at which RBCs burst in varied hypotonic solutions.

Nursing actions
Before the procedure
- Explain the test to the client.

After the procedure
- Check the venipuncture site for bleeding.
- Send the specimen to the laboratory.

Bone picture
A **bone scan** is an I.V. injection of radioisotope, which creates a visual image of bone metabolism.

Nursing actions
Before the procedure
- Explain the procedure to the client.
- Ask the client about allergies.
- Determine the client's ability to lie still for approximately 1 hour.
- Advise the client to drink lots of fluids to maintain hydration and reduce the radiation dose to the bladder. (Have him do this during the interval between the injection of the tracer and the actual scanning.)

After the procedure
- Check the injection site for redness or swelling.
- Avoid scheduling any other radionuclide test for 24 to 48 hours.
- Tell the client to drink lots of fluids and to empty his bladder frequently for 24 to 48 hours.
- Provide analgesics for pain resulting from positioning on the scanning table, as needed.

Clot measure
A **coagulation study** tests a blood sample to analyze platelet function, platelet count, prothrombin time (PT), international normalized ratio, partial thromboplastin time (PTT), coagulation time, and bleeding time.

Nursing actions
- Explain the procedure to the client.
- Note the client's current drug therapy before the procedure.
- Check the venipuncture site for bleeding after the procedure.

Polish up on client care

Major hematologic and immune disorders include acquired immunodeficiency syndrome (AIDS), anaphylaxis, ankylosing spondylitis, aplastic anemia, calcium imbalance, chloride imbalance, disseminated intravascular coagulation (DIC), fibromyalgia syndrome (FMS), hemophilia, idiopathic thrombocytopenic purpura (ITP), iron deficiency anemia, Kaposi's sarcoma, latex allergy, leukemia, lymphoma, magnesium imbalance, metabolic acidosis, metabolic alkalosis, multiple myeloma, pernicious anemia, phosphorus imbalance, polycythemia vera, rheumatoid arthritis, scleroderma, septic shock, sickle cell anemia, sodium imbalance, systemic lupus erythematosus (SLE), and vasculitis.

> Most questions on the exam focus on what a nurse should do in a specific situation. Always look for the client care angle.

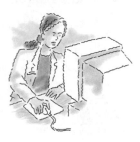

Acquired immunodeficiency syndrome

AIDS is a defect in T-cell–mediated immunity caused by HIV. AIDS places a client at significant risk for the development of potentially fatal opportunistic infections. A diagnosis of AIDS is based on laboratory evidence of HIV infection coexisting with one or more indicator diseases, such as herpes simplex virus, cytomegalovirus, mycobacteria, candidal infection, *Pneumocystis* pneumonia, Kaposi's sarcoma, wasting syndrome, or dementia.

CAUSES
- Exposure to blood containing HIV: transfusions, contaminated needles, handling of blood, in utero
- Exposure to semen and vaginal secretions containing HIV: sexual intercourse, handling of semen and vaginal secretions

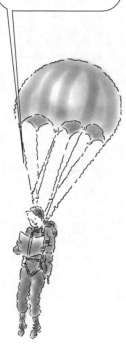

Combination therapy to treat HIV and AIDS usually includes nonnucleoside reverse transcriptase inhibitors, nucleoside reverse transcriptase inhibitors, and protease inhibitors.

• Ingestion of breast milk from an infected mother

ASSESSMENT FINDINGS
• Anorexia, weight loss, recurrent diarrhea
• Cough
• Disorientation, confusion, dementia
• Fatigue and weakness
• Fever
• Lymphadenopathy
• Malnutrition
• Night sweats
• Opportunistic infections
• Pallor
• Pain
• Shortness of breath
• Skin lesions

DIAGNOSTIC TEST RESULTS
• Blood chemistry shows increased transaminase, alkaline phosphatase, and gamma globulin levels and a decreased albumin level.
• CD4+ T-cell count is less than 200 cells/μl.
• ELISA shows positive HIV antibody titer.
• Hematology shows decreased WBCs, RBCs, and platelets.
• Western blot is positive.

NURSING DIAGNOSES
• Ineffective protection
• Hopelessness
• Social isolation
• Impaired gas exchange
• Risk for infection
• Diarrhea

TREATMENT
• Activity: as tolerated, active and passive range-of-motion exercises
• High-calorie, high-protein diet in small, frequent feedings (see *Meeting the HIV challenge*)
• Nutritional support: total parenteral nutrition (TPN), enteral feedings if necessary
• Plasmapheresis
• Respiratory treatments: chest physiotherapy, postural drainage, and incentive spirometry
• Specialized bed: air therapy bed
• Standard precautions
• Transfusion therapy: fresh frozen plasma, platelets, and packed RBCs

Drug therapy
• Antibiotic: co-trimoxazole (Bactrim)
• Antiemetic: prochlorperazine
• Antifungals: fluconazole (Diflucan), amphotericin B (Fungizone)
• Antivirals: dapsone, didanosine (Videx), ganciclovir, zidovudine (Retrovir, AZT), acyclovir (Zovirax), pentamidine (Pentam 300), aerosolized pentamidine (NebuPent)
• Interferon alfa-2a, recombinant
• Fusion inhibitor: enfuvirtide (Fuzeon)
Combination therapy
• Nonnucleoside reverse transcriptase inhibitors: delavirdine (Rescriptor), nevirapine (Viramune)
• Nucleoside reverse transcriptase inhibitors: abacavir (Epzicon), lamivudine (Epivir), zidovudine (Retrovir, AZT)
• Protease inhibitors: indinavir (Crixivan), nelfinavir (Viracept), ritonavir (Norvir), saquinavir (Invirase)

INTERVENTIONS AND RATIONALES
• Assess respiratory and neurologic systems *to detect AIDS-related dementia. Other factors, such as anemia, fever, hypoxemia, and fluid balance, can also affect neurologic status.*
• Monitor and record vital signs *to detect evidence of compromise.*
• Monitor for opportunistic infections *because early treatment may limit complications.*
• Administer oxygen *to enhance oxygenation.*
• Encourage incentive spirometry use and assist with turning, coughing, and deep breathing *to mobilize and remove secretions.*
• Encourage fluids or administer I.V. fluids *to prevent dehydration.*
• Provide high-calorie, high-protein meals *to fight opportunistic infection and maintain weight.*
• Administer TPN and enteral feedings, if necessary, *to bolster nutritional reserves and immune system.*
• Administer medications, as prescribed, *to reduce the risk of complications and halt reproduction of HIV.*
• Maintain activity, as tolerated, *to encourage independence.*
• Provide rest periods *to reduce oxygen demands and prevent fatigue.*
• Provide mouth care *to prevent infection, provide comfort, and enhance the taste of meals.*

- Maintain standard precautions *to avoid exposure to blood, body fluids, and secretions.*
- Encourage verbalization of feelings about changes in body image, a fear of dying, and social isolation *to help him cope with his chronic illness and reduce anxiety.*
- Make referrals to community agencies for support *to enhance the quality of life and independence.*
- Monitor intake and output, daily weight, and urine specific gravity *for early recognition and treatment of dehydration.*
- Monitor laboratory values *for early detection and complications. Thrombocytopenia requires precautions to prevent bleeding. Leukopenia requires precautions to protect the client from infection.*
- Provide skin care. Assess for skin lesions and breakdown *to prevent infection and guide care.*
- Assess pain level and administer analgesics *to improve comfort.*

Teaching topics
- Explanation of the disorder and treatment plan
- Drug therapy
- Lifestyle changes, such as rehabilitation, if the client is an I.V. drug user
- Safer sex practices
- Infection control (avoiding transmission of infection and avoiding opportunistic infection)
- Nutritional therapy
- Support agencies
- Refraining from donating blood

Anaphylaxis

Anaphylaxis is a dramatic and widespread acute atopic reaction. It's marked by the sudden onset of rapidly progressive urticaria and respiratory distress. A severe anaphylactic reaction may cause vascular collapse, leading to systemic shock and, sometimes, death.

CAUSES
Systemic exposure to or ingestion of sensitizing drugs or other substances such as:
- allergen extracts
- diagnostic chemicals (sulfobromophthalein, sodium dehydrocholate, and radiographic contrast media)

- enzymes (such as L-asparaginase)
- foods (legumes, nuts, berries, seafood, and egg albumin) and food additives with sulfites
- hormones
- insect venom (honeybees, wasps, hornets, yellow jackets, fire ants, mosquitoes, and certain spiders)
- local anesthetics
- penicillin and other antibiotics
- polysaccharides
- ruptured hydatid cyst (rarely)
- salicylates
- serums (usually horse serum)
- sulfonamides
- vaccines.

ASSESSMENT FINDINGS
- Sudden physical distress within seconds or minutes after exposure to an allergen (may include feeling of impending doom or fright, weakness, sweating, sneezing, shortness of breath, nasal pruritus, urticaria, and angioedema, followed rapidly by symptoms in one or more target organs)
- Cardiovascular symptoms (hypotension, shock, cardiac arrhythmias) that may precipitate circulatory collapse if untreated
- Respiratory symptoms (nasal mucosal edema, profuse watery rhinorrhea, itching, nasal congestion, sudden sneezing attacks; edema of upper respiratory tract that causes hoarseness, stridor, and dyspnea is early sign of acute respiratory failure)
- GI and genitourinary symptoms (severe stomach cramps, nausea, diarrhea, urinary urgency and incontinence)
- Persistent or delayed reaction (may occur up to 24 hours after exposure to allergen)
- Severity of reaction inversely related to interval between exposure to an allergen and onset of symptoms—the longer the interval, the less severe the reaction

DIAGNOSTIC TEST RESULTS
- Anaphylaxis can be diagnosed by the rapid onset of severe respiratory or cardiovascular symptoms after an insect sting or after ingestion or injection of a drug, vaccine, diagnostic agent, food, or food additive.
- If symptoms occur without a known allergic stimulus, other possible causes of shock (such as acute myocardial infarction,

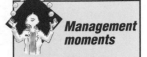

Management moments

Meeting the HIV challenge

Maintaining nutritional status is one of the great challenges in managing human immunodeficiency virus (HIV) infection. GI disturbances and muscle wasting pose ongoing problems for many clients. Drugs to increase appetite (such as dronabinol [Marinol]) and dietary supplements (such as Ensure) are commonly prescribed. Encouraging the consumption of small, frequent meals that are high in calories may also be helpful.

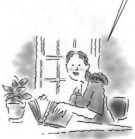

Yikes! Anaphylaxis may cause vascular collapse and lead to systemic shock and, sometimes, death.

status asthmaticus, or heart failure) need to be ruled out.

NURSING DIAGNOSES
- Risk for suffocation
- Decreased cardiac output
- Anxiety
- Impaired gas exchange
- Ineffective airway clearance

TREATMENT
- Cardiopulmonary resuscitation in case of cardiac arrest
- Endotracheal tube insertion or a tracheotomy and oxygen therapy with laryngeal edema
- Other therapy as indicated by clinical response

Drug therapy
- Immediate injection of epinephrine 1:1,000 aqueous solution, 0.1 to 0.5 ml, repeated every 5 to 20 minutes as necessary
- Other medications given after initial emergency (may include subcutaneous epinephrine, longer-acting epinephrine, corticosteroids, diphenhydramine [Benadryl] I.V. for long-term management)
- Vasopressors: norepinephrine (Levophed), and dopamine, if hypotensive

INTERVENTIONS AND RATIONALES
- In the early stages of anaphylaxis, give epinephrine I.M. or subcutaneously, and help it move into the circulation faster by massaging the injection site. With severe reactions, give epinephrine I.V. *to prevent crisis.*
- Maintain airway patency. Observe for early signs of laryngeal edema (stridor, hoarseness, and dyspnea), and prepare for endotracheal tube insertion or a tracheotomy and oxygen therapy *to prevent cerebral anoxia.*
- In case of cardiac arrest, provide cardiopulmonary resuscitation, including closed-chest heart massage and assisted ventilation; administer other therapy as indicated by clinical response and per advanced cardiac life support protocol. *These measures are necessary to prevent irreversible organ damage.*
- Assess for hypotension and shock, and administer volume expanders (plasma, plasma expanders, saline solution, and albumin) as needed. Maintain blood pressure

with I.V. vasopressors (norepinephrine and dopamine) *to prevent altered tissue perfusion.* Monitor blood pressure, central venous pressure, and urine output *to monitor response to treatment.*
- Administer other medications, such as subcutaneous epinephrine, longer-acting epinephrine, corticosteroids, and diphenhydramine I.V. for long-term management *to prevent recurrence of symptoms.*
- A client with a known history of allergies should receive a drug with a high anaphylactic potential only after cautious pretesting for sensitivity. Closely monitor the client during testing, and make sure that resuscitative equipment and epinephrine are ready *to prevent a severe reaction that may lead to cardiopulmonary arrest.*
- Closely monitor the client undergoing diagnostic tests that use radiographic contrast dyes, such as cardiac catheterization, excretory urography, and angiography, *to detect early signs of anaphylaxis.*

Teaching topics
- Explanation of the disorder and treatment plan
- Preventing anaphylaxis (avoiding exposure to known allergens, including all forms of the offending food or drug, avoiding open fields and wooded areas during the insect season in case of reaction to insect bite or sting)
- Carrying an anaphylaxis kit containing epinephrine
- Risks of delayed symptoms and need to report any recurrence of shortness of breath, chest tightness, sweating, angioedema, or other symptoms
- Wearing a medical identification bracelet identifying the client's allergies

Ankylosing spondylitis

Ankylosing spondylitis is a chronic, usually progressive inflammatory disease that primarily affects the spine and adjacent soft tissue. Generally, the disease begins in the sacroiliac joints (between the sacrum and the ileum) and gradually progresses to the lumbar, thoracic, and cervical regions of the spine. Deterioration of bone and cartilage can

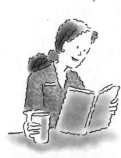

Immediately after exposure to an allergen, a client may report a feeling of impending doom or fright.

lead to fibrous tissue formation and eventual fusion of the spine or peripheral joints.

Ankylosing spondylitis affects five times as many males as females. Progressive disease is well recognized in men, but the diagnosis is commonly overlooked in women, who tend to have more peripheral joint involvement.

CAUSES
- Possible familial tendency
- Possible link to underlying infection
- Presence of histocompatibility antigen HLA-B27 and circulating immune complexes suggests immunologic activity
- Secondary ankylosing spondylitis may be associated with reactive arthritis (Reiter's syndrome), psoriatic arthritis, or inflammatory bowel disease

ASSESSMENT FINDINGS
- Intermittent lower back pain (the first indication) usually most severe in morning or after period of inactivity
- Kyphosis in advanced stages, caused by chronic stooping to relieve symptoms, and hip deformity and associated limited range of motion (ROM)
- Mild fatigue, fever, anorexia, or loss of weight; unilateral acute anterior uveitis; aortic insufficiency and cardiomegaly; upper lobe pulmonary fibrosis (mimics tuberculosis)
- Pain and limited expansion of the chest due to involvement of the costovertebral joints
- Pain or tenderness at tendon insertion sites (enthesitis), especially the Achilles or patellar tendon
- Peripheral arthritis involving the shoulders, hips, and knees
- Severe neurologic complications, such as cauda equina syndrome or paralysis, secondary to fracture of a rigid cervical spine or C1-C2 subluxation
- Stiffness and limited motion of the lumbar spine
- Symptoms that progress unpredictably; disease can go into remission, exacerbation, or arrest at any stage
- Tenderness over the site of inflammation

DIAGNOSTIC TEST RESULTS
- Confirmation requires characteristic X-ray findings: blurring of the bony margins of joints in the early stage, bilateral sacroiliac involvement, patchy sclerosis with superficial bony erosions, eventual squaring of vertebral bodies, and "bamboo spine" with complete ankylosis.
- ESR and alkaline phosphatase and creatine kinase levels may be slightly elevated. A negative rheumatoid factor helps rule out rheumatoid arthritis, which produces similar symptoms.
- Typical symptoms, a family history, and the presence of HLA-B27 strongly suggest ankylosing spondylitis.

NURSING DIAGNOSES
- Chronic pain
- Impaired physical mobility
- Activity intolerance

TREATMENT
- Promoting good posture, stretching and deep-breathing exercises and, in some clients, braces and lightweight supports to delay further deformity (because ankylosing spondylitis progression can't be stopped)
- Long-term daily exercise program (essential to delay loss of function)
- Spinal wedge osteotomy to separate and reposition vertebrae in case of severe spinal involvement (performed only on selected clients because of risk of spinal cord damage and long convalescence)
- Surgical hip replacement in case of severe hip involvement

Drug therapy
- Anti-inflammatory agents: aspirin, ibuprofen (Motrin), indomethacin (Indocin), sulfasalazine (Azulfidine), sulindac (Clinoril) to control pain and inflammation

INTERVENTIONS AND RATIONALES
- Offer support and reassurance. *Ankylosing spondylitis can be an extremely painful and crippling disease; the caregiver's main responsibility is to promote the client's comfort while preserving as much mobility as possible.*

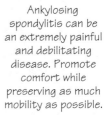

Typically, ankylosing spondylitis begins in the lower back and progresses up the spine to the neck.

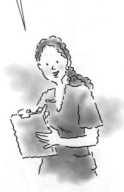

Ankylosing spondylitis can be an extremely painful and debilitating disease. Promote comfort while preserving as much mobility as possible.

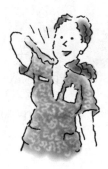

The fact that you're studying shows that you have the ability to set a goal for yourself. Give yourself credit for setting achievable goals.

Keep in mind that the client's limited ROM makes simple tasks difficult.
• Assess pain level and administer medications as needed *to decrease inflammation and pain.*
• Apply local heat and provide massage *to relieve pain.*
• Assess mobility and degree of discomfort frequently *to monitor for disease progression.*
• Teach and assist with daily exercises as needed *to maintain strength and function.* Stress the importance of maintaining good posture *to prevent kyphosis.*
• If treatment includes surgery, provide postoperative care *to prevent postoperative complications, such as wound infection, thrombophlebitis, and pneumonia.*
• Obtain referrals for a social worker, visiting nurse, and dietitian *because ankylosing spondylitis is a chronic, progressively crippling condition.*

Teaching topics
• Explanation of the disorder and treatment plan
• Avoiding physical activity that causes stress on the back, such as lifting heavy objects
• Practicing good posture (standing upright; sitting upright in a high, straight chair; and avoiding leaning over a desk)
• Sleeping in a prone position on a hard mattress and avoiding use of pillows under neck or knees
• Avoiding prolonged walking, standing, sitting, or driving
• Performing regular stretching and deep-breathing exercises and swimming regularly, if possible
• Measuring height every 3 to 4 months to detect any tendency toward kyphosis
• Contacting the local Arthritis Foundation chapter for a support group

Aplastic anemia

Aplastic anemia, also known as *pancytopenia*, results from suppression, destruction, or aplasia of the bone marrow. This damage to the bone marrow causes an inability to produce

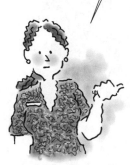

Aplastic anemia results from injury or destruction to stem cells, which are located in the bone marrow and function to produce new blood cells.

adequate amounts of erythrocytes, leukocytes, and platelets.

CAUSES
• Chemotherapy
• Drug-induced from carbamazepine (Tegretol), phenytoin (Dilantin)
• Exposure to chemicals
• Idiopathic
• Radiation
• Viral hepatitis

ASSESSMENT FINDINGS
• Anorexia
• Dyspnea, tachypnea
• Epistaxis
• Fatigue, weakness
• Gingivitis
• Headache
• Melena
• Multiple infections, fever
• Palpitations, tachycardia
• Purpura, petechiae, ecchymosis, pallor

DIAGNOSTIC TEST RESULTS
• Bone marrow biopsy shows fatty marrow with reduction of stem cells.
• Fecal occult blood test is positive.
• Hematology shows decreased granulocytes, thrombocytes, and RBCs.
• Peripheral blood smear shows pancytopenia.
• Urine chemistry reveals hematuria.

NURSING DIAGNOSES
• Anxiety
• Activity intolerance
• Risk for deficient fluid volume
• Risk for infection

TREATMENT
• High-protein, high-calorie, high-vitamin diet
• Tepid sponge baths, cooling blankets
• Transfusion of platelets and packed RBCs

Drug therapy
• Analgesics: ibuprofen (Motrin), acetaminophen (Tylenol)
• Androgen: oxymetholone (Anadrol-50)

- Antibiotics: according to the sensitivity of the infecting organism
- Antithymocyte globulin
- Hematopoietic growth factor: epoetin alfa (Epogen)
- Human granulocyte colony-stimulating factor: filgrastim (Neupogen)

INTERVENTIONS AND RATIONALES

- Assess respiratory status *to detect hypoxemia caused by low hemoglobin levels.*
- Assess vital signs *for signs of hemorrhage, infection, and activity intolerance.*
- Assess cardiovascular status *to detect arrhythmias or myocardial ischemia.*
- Monitor and record intake and output and urine specific gravity *to determine fluid balance.*
- Monitor laboratory values *to determine the effectiveness of therapy.*
- Assess stool, urine, and emesis *for occult blood loss caused by reduced platelet levels.*
- Monitor for infection, bleeding, and bruising *caused by reduced levels of WBCs and platelets.*
- Encourage fluids and administer I.V. fluids *to replace fluids lost by fever and bleeding.*
- Administer oxygen *because low hemoglobin levels reduce the oxygen-carrying capacity of the blood.*
- Assist with turning, coughing, and deep breathing *to mobilize and remove secretions.*
- Administer transfusion therapy, as prescribed, *to replace low blood components.*
- Administer medications, as ordered, *to treat the client's disorder and prevent complications.*
- Provide a high-protein, high-calorie, high-vitamin diet *to promote red blood cell production and fight infection.*
- Encourage verbalization of concerns and fears *to allay the client's anxiety.*
- Alternate rest periods with activity *to conserve energy and reduce weakness caused by anemia.*
- Provide cooling blankets and tepid sponge baths for fever *to promote comfort and reduce metabolic demands.*
- Maintain protective precautions *to prevent infection and hemorrhage.*
- Provide mouth care before and after meals *to enhance the taste of meals.*

- Provide skin care *to prevent skin breakdown due to bed rest, dehydration, and fever.*
- Initiate fall protection protocol *to reduce the risk of injury.*
- Avoid giving the client I.M. injections *to reduce the risk of hemorrhage.*

Teaching topics

- Explanation of the disorder and treatment plan
- Drug therapy
- Nutritional therapy
- Activity restrictions
- Signs and symptoms of bleeding and infection
- Wearing a medical identification bracelet
- Refraining from using over-the-counter medications without the physician's approval
- Monitoring stool for occult blood
- Using an electric razor to avoid bleeding

Calcium imbalance

Calcium plays an indispensable role in cell permeability, formation of bones and teeth, blood coagulation, transmission of nerve impulses, and normal muscle contraction.

Nearly all (99%) of the body's calcium is found in the bones. The remaining 1% exists in ionized form in serum; maintaining ionized calcium in the serum is critical to healthy neurologic function.

The parathyroid glands regulate ionized calcium and determine its resorption into bone, absorption from the GI mucosa, and excretion in urine and stool. Severe calcium imbalance requires emergency treatment, because a deficiency (hypocalcemia) can lead to tetany and seizures; an excess (hypercalcemia), to cardiac arrhythmias and coma.

CAUSES
Hypocalcemia
- Hypomagnesemia
- Hypoparathyroidism
- Inadequate intake of calcium and vitamin D
- Malabsorption or loss of calcium from the GI tract
- Overcorrection of acidosis
- Pancreatic insufficiency

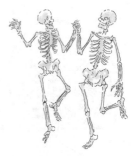

Together with phosphorus, calcium is responsible for the formation and structure of bones and teeth.

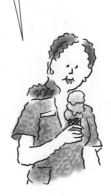

Hypocalcemia can occur when the body doesn't take in enough calcium, doesn't absorb the mineral properly, or loses excessive amounts of calcium.

- Renal failure
- Severe infections or burns

Hypercalcemia
- Hyperparathyroidism
- Hypervitaminosis D
- Multiple fractures and prolonged immobilization
- Multiple myeloma
- Other causes (milk-alkali syndrome, sarcoidosis, hyperthyroidism, adrenal insufficiency, and thiazide diuretics)
- Tumors

ASSESSMENT FINDINGS
Hypocalcemia
- Cardiac arrhythmias   *overfunction of muscle*
- Carpopedal spasm   *quivers*
- Chvostek's sign
- Perioral paresthesia
- Seizures
- Tetany
- Trousseau's sign
- Twitching

Hypercalcemia   → *underfunction of muscle*
- Anorexia
- Cardiac arrhythmias and eventual coma with severe hypercalcemia (serum levels greater than 5.7 mEq/L)
- Constipation
- Decreased muscle tone
- Dehydration
- Lethargy
- Muscle weakness
- Nausea
- Polydipsia
- Polyuria
- Vomiting

DIAGNOSTIC TEST RESULTS
- A serum ionized calcium level less than 4.5 mEq/L confirms hypocalcemia; a level greater than 5.5 mEq/L confirms hypercalcemia. (Because approximately one-half of serum calcium is bound to albumin, changes in serum protein must be considered when interpreting serum calcium levels.)
- Sulkowitch urine test shows increased urine calcium precipitation in hypercalcemia.

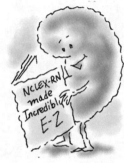

NCLEX-RN made Incredibly E-Z

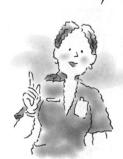

Hypercalcemia occurs when the rate of calcium entry into the extracellular fluid exceeds the rate of calcium excretion by the kidneys.

4.5-5.5 mEq/L calcium

Because nearly half of all calcium is bound to the protein albumin, serum protein abnormalities can influence total serum calcium levels.

- Electrocardiogram (ECG) reveals a lengthened QT interval, a prolonged ST segment, and arrhythmias in hypocalcemia; in hypercalcemia, a shortened QT interval and heart block.

NURSING DIAGNOSES
Hypocalcemia
- Imbalanced nutrition: Less than body requirements
- Acute pain
- Risk for imbalanced fluid volume
- Risk for infection

Hypercalcemia
- Impaired physical mobility
- Impaired urinary elimination
- Risk for injury
- Risk for imbalanced fluid volume

TREATMENT
Hypocalcemia
- Diet: adequate intake of calcium, vitamin D, and protein

Drug therapy
- Ergocalciferol (vitamin D_2), cholecalciferol (vitamin D_3), calcitriol, dihydrotachysterol (synthetic form of vitamin D_2) for severe deficiency
- I.V. calcium gluconate or calcium chloride for acute hypocalcemia (an emergency)
- Vitamin D in multivitamin preparation for mild hypocalcemia
- Vitamin D supplements to facilitate GI absorption of calcium to treat chronic hypocalcemia

Hypercalcemia
- Hydration with normal saline solution to eliminate excess serum calcium through urine excretion
- Diet: low calcium with increased oral fluid intake

Drug therapy
- Calcitonin
- Corticosteroids: prednisone, hydrocortisone (Solu-Cortef) for treating sarcoidosis, hypervitaminosis D, and certain tumors

- Loop diuretics: ethacrynic acid (Edecrin), furosemide (Lasix) to promote calcium excretion (thiazide diuretics contraindicated in hypercalcemia because they inhibit calcium excretion)
- Sodium phosphate solution administered by mouth or by retention enema (promotes calcium deposits in bone and inhibits absorption from GI tract)

INTERVENTIONS AND RATIONALES

- Assess for hypocalcemia in clients receiving massive transfusions of citrated blood and in those with chronic diarrhea, severe infections, and insufficient dietary intake of calcium and protein (especially elderly clients). *Identifying clients at risk can ensure early treatment intervention.*

Hypocalcemia

- Monitor serum calcium levels every 12 to 24 hours; a calcium level below 4.5 mEq/L requires immediate attention. When giving calcium supplements, frequently check the pH level; an alkalotic state that exceeds 7.45 pH inhibits calcium ionization. Check for Trousseau's and Chvostek's signs, which indicate hypocalcemia *to identify and rapidly treat dangerous calcium levels.*
- Administer calcium gluconate slow I.V. in dextrose 5% in water *(never in saline solution, which encourages renal calcium loss).* Don't add calcium gluconate I.V. to solutions containing bicarbonate *to avoid precipitation.*
- Assess for signs of hypercalcemia (anorexia, nausea, and vomiting), *to determine overcorrection of hypocalcemia.*
- Monitor cardiac rhythm and digoxin (Lanoxin) level, if indicated. *Calcium supplements may cause a synergistic effect.*
- Administer oral calcium supplements 1 to 1½ hours after meals or with milk *to promote absorption.*
- Provide a diet high in calcium *to help correct imbalances.*
- Provide a quiet, stress-free environment for the client with tetany *to prevent seizure activity.* Observe seizure precautions for clients with severe hypocalcemia that may lead to seizures *to prevent client injury.*
- Monitor intake and output and administer I.V. fluids as ordered

Hypercalcemia

- Monitor serum calcium levels. Monitor for cardiac arrhythmias if the serum calcium level exceeds 5.7 mEq/L *to avoid cardiovascular compromise.*
- Increase fluid intake *to dilute calcium in serum and urine and to prevent renal damage and dehydration.*
- Monitor for signs of heart failure in clients receiving normal saline solution diuresis therapy. *Infusion of large volumes of normal saline may cause fluid volume excess, leading to heart failure.*
- Administer loop diuretics (not thiazide diuretics) *to promote diuresis and rid the body of excess calcium.*
- Monitor intake and output, and check the urine for renal calculi and acidity. Provide acid-ash drinks, such as cranberry or prune juice, *because calcium salts are more soluble in acid than in alkali.*
- Monitor the client's ECG and vital signs frequently. In the client receiving cardiac glycosides, watch for signs of toxicity, such as anorexia, nausea, vomiting, and bradycardia (often with arrhythmia). *Fatal arrhythmias may result when digoxin is administered in hypercalcemia.*
- Encourage and assist with ambulation as soon as possible. Handle the client with chronic hypercalcemia gently *to prevent pathologic fractures.*
- Reposition the bedridden client frequently and assist with ROM exercises *to promote circulation and prevent urinary stasis and calcium loss from bone.*

Teaching topics

- Explanation of the disorder and treatment plan
- Drug therapy
- Nutritional therapy
- Importance of exercise to prevent injury
- Importance of calcium for normal bone formation and blood coagulation

When calcium levels are too high, the thyroid releases calcitonin. High levels of calcitonin inhibit bone resorption, which causes a decrease in the amount of calcium available from bone, thereby decreasing serum calcium levels. Calcitonin may also be administered as a drug to treat hypercalcemia.

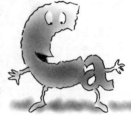

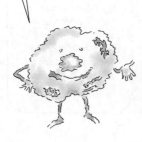

Chloride is quite an anion. It helps maintain acid-base balance and assists in carbon dioxide transport in red blood cells.

Chloride imbalance

Hypochloremia and hyperchloremia are, respectively, conditions of deficient or excessive serum levels of the anion chloride (an anion is a negatively charged ion). Chloride appears predominantly in extracellular fluid (fluid outside the cells) and accounts for two-thirds of all serum anions.

Secreted by stomach mucosa as hydrochloric acid, chloride provides an acid medium conducive to digestion and activation of enzymes. It also participates in maintaining acid-base and body water balances, influences the osmolality or tonicity of extracellular fluid, plays a role in the exchange of oxygen and carbon dioxide in red blood cells, and helps activate salivary amylase (which, in turn, activates the digestive process).

CAUSES
Hypochloremia
- Administration of dextrose I.V. without electrolytes
- Loss of hydrochloric acid in gastric secretions from vomiting, gastric suctioning, or gastric surgery
- Low dietary sodium intake
- Metabolic alkalosis
- Potassium deficiency
- Prolonged diarrhea or diaphoresis
- Sodium deficiency

Hyperchloremia
- Hyperingestion of ammonium chloride
- Ureterointestinal anastomosis, which can lead to hyperchloremia by allowing reabsorption of chloride by the bowel

ASSESSMENT FINDINGS
Hypochloremia
- Muscle hypertonicity (in conditions related to loss of gastric secretions)
- Muscle weakness
- Shallow, depressed breathing
- Tetany
- Twitching

Hyperchloremia
- Agitation
- Coma

Sodium imbalance or chloride imbalance? These two conditions commonly produce similar assessment findings, such as muscle twitching, weakness, and dyspnea.

- Deep, rapid breathing
- Diminished cognitive ability
- Dyspnea
- Hypertension
- Pitting edema
- Tachycardia
- Weakness

DIAGNOSTIC TEST RESULTS
- Serum chloride level less than 98 mEq/L confirms hypochloremia; supportive values with metabolic alkalosis include a serum pH greater than 7.45 and a serum carbon dioxide level greater than 32 mEq/L.
- Serum chloride level greater than 108 mEq/L confirms hyperchloremia; with metabolic acidosis, serum pH is less than 7.35 and the serum carbon dioxide level is less than 22 mEq/L.

NURSING DIAGNOSES
Hypochloremia
- Ineffective breathing pattern
- Risk for injury

Hyperchloremia
- Excess fluid volume
- Disturbed thought processes
- Ineffective breathing pattern

TREATMENT
Hypochloremia
- Diet: salty broth
- Saline solution I.V.

Drug therapy
- Acidifying agent: ammonium chloride

Hyperchloremia
- Lactated Ringer's solution

Drug therapy
- Alkalinizing agent: sodium bicarbonate I.V.

INTERVENTIONS AND RATIONALES
- Monitor serum chloride levels frequently, particularly during I.V. therapy, *to guide the treatment plan.*
- Monitor for signs of hyperchloremia or hypochloremia. Be alert for respiratory difficulty *to prevent respiratory distress.*

Hypochloremia

- Monitor laboratory results (serum electrolyte and arterial blood gas [ABG] levels) and fluid intake and output of clients who are vulnerable to chloride imbalance, particularly those recovering from gastric surgery *to prevent hypochloremia.*
- Watch for excessive or continuous loss of gastric secretions as well as prolonged infusion of dextrose in water without saline, *to prevent chloride imbalance.*
- Administer I.V. saline and medications as ordered *to correct chloride level.*

Hyperchloremia

- Monitor serum electrolyte levels every 3 to 6 hours. If the client is receiving high doses of sodium bicarbonate, watch for signs of overcorrection (metabolic alkalosis, respiratory depression) or lingering signs of hyperchloremia, which indicate inadequate treatment. *Frequent monitoring of electrolyte levels helps guide the treatment plan and avoids complications of chloride imbalance.*
- Administer medications and I.V. fluids as ordered *to correct chloride level.*

Teaching topics

- Explanation of the disorder and treatment plan
- Explanation of all tests and procedures
- Dietary sources of sodium, potassium, and chloride in the client experiencing hypochloremia

Disseminated intravascular coagulation

DIC, also called *consumption coagulopathy* and *defibrination syndrome,* occurs as a complication of diseases and conditions that accelerate clotting. This accelerated clotting process causes small blood vessel occlusion, organ necrosis, depletion of circulating clotting factors and platelets, and activation of the fibrinolytic system—which, in turn, can provoke severe hemorrhage.

Clotting in the microcirculation usually affects the kidneys and extremities but may occur in the brain, lungs, pituitary and adrenal glands, and GI mucosa. Other conditions,

such as vitamin K deficiency, hepatic disease, and anticoagulant therapy, may cause a similar hemorrhage.

DIC is generally an acute condition but may be chronic in cancer clients. The prognosis depends on early detection and treatment, the severity of the hemorrhage, and treatment of the underlying disease or condition.

CAUSES

- Infection (the most common cause), including gram-negative or gram-positive septicemia; viral, fungal, or rickettsial infection; and protozoal infection (falciparum malaria)
- Disorders that produce necrosis, such as extensive burns and trauma, brain tissue destruction, transplant rejection, and hepatic necrosis
- Neoplastic disease, including acute leukemia and metastatic carcinoma
- Obstetric complications, such as abruptio placentae, amniotic fluid embolism, and retained dead fetus

ASSESSMENT FINDINGS

- Abnormal bleeding without an accompanying history of a serious hemorrhagic disorder (petechiae, hematomas, ecchymosis, cutaneous oozing)
- Coma
- Dyspnea
- Nausea
- Oliguria
- Seizures
- Severe muscle, back, and abdominal pain
- Shock
- Vomiting

DIAGNOSTIC TEST RESULTS

- Blood tests show prolonged PT greater than 15 seconds; prolonged PTT greater than 60 to 80 seconds; fibrinogen levels less than 150 mg/dl; platelets less than 100,000/µl; fibrin degradation products typically greater than 100 mcg/ml; and a positive D-dimer test specific for DIC.

NURSING DIAGNOSES

- Risk for deficient fluid volume
- Ineffective peripheral tissue perfusion

DIC causes blockages in the small blood vessels, depletes the body's supply of clotting factors and platelets, and destroys fibrin.

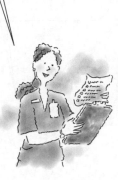

Abnormal bleeding with no accompanying hemorrhagic disorder? That sounds like DIC.

- Fatigue
- Anxiety
- Impaired gas exchange

TREATMENT
- Supportive care
- Bed rest
- Transfusion therapy: fresh frozen plasma, platelets, packed RBCs

Drug therapy
- Anticoagulant: heparin I.V.
- Thrombolytic agent: antithrombin III (Thrombate III)

INTERVENTIONS AND RATIONALES
- Don't scrub bleeding areas *to prevent clots from dislodging and causing fresh bleeding.* Use pressure, cold compresses, and topical hemostatic agents to control bleeding.
- Enforce complete bed rest during bleeding episodes. If the client is agitated, pad the side rails *to protect him from injury.*
- Check all I.V. and venipuncture sites frequently for bleeding. Apply pressure to injection sites for at least 10 minutes. Alert other personnel to the client's tendency to hemorrhage. *These measures prevent hemorrhage.*
- Monitor intake and output hourly in acute DIC, especially when administering blood products, *to monitor the effectiveness of volume replacement.*
- Administer blood products as ordered. Monitor for transfusion reactions and signs of fluid overload *to prepare for possible complications.*
- Weigh dressings and linen and record drainage *to measure the amount of blood lost.*
- Weigh the client daily, particularly in renal involvement, *to monitor for fluid volume excess.*
- Assess for bleeding from the GI and genitourinary tracts *to detect early signs of hemorrhage.* Measure the client's abdominal girth at least every 4 hours, and monitor closely for signs of shock *to detect intra-abdominal bleeding.*
- Monitor the results of serial blood studies (particularly HCT, Hb, and coagulation studies) *to guide the treatment plan.*
- Provide emotional support *to decrease anxiety.*

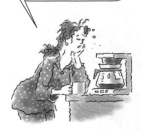

Daily fatigue and poor sleep quality? Is that the life of a health care professional or FMS?!

Teaching topics
- Explanation of the disorder and treatment plan
- Drug therapy
- Bleeding prevention

Fibromyalgia syndrome

FMS is a diffuse pain syndrome and one of the most common causes of chronic musculoskeletal pain. It's characterized by diffuse musculoskeletal pain, daily fatigue, and poor-quality sleep, along with multiple tender points on examination.

More women than men are affected, and although FMS may occur at almost any age, the peak incidence is in clients between ages 20 and 60.

The development of FMS may be multifactorial and influenced by stress (physical and mental), physical conditioning, poor-quality sleep, neuroendocrine factors, psychiatric factors and, possibly, hormonal factors.

CAUSES
- Unknown (theories include endocrine dysfunction or abnormal neurotransmitter levels)

ASSESSMENT FINDINGS
- Diffuse, dull, aching pain across the neck, shoulders, lower back, and proximal limbs that's worse in the morning
- Fatigue that occurs shortly after rising
- Irritable bowel syndrome
- Paresthesia
- Puffy hands
- Sleep disturbances
- Tension headaches

DIAGNOSTIC TEST RESULTS
- Diagnosis is based on characteristic symptoms and exclusion of other illnesses that can cause similar features.

NURSING DIAGNOSES
- Chronic pain
- Fatigue
- Activity intolerance
- Disturbed body image

TREATMENT
- Acupuncture, phototherapy, yoga, and tai chi
- Physical therapy

Drug therapy
- Antidepressants: amitriptyline (Elavil), nortriptyline (Aventyl)
- Duloxetine (Cymbalta), milnacipran (Savella), pregabalin (Lyrica)
- Opioids to control pain only in severe cases and under management of a pain specialist

INTERVENTIONS AND RATIONALES
- Encourage regular, low-impact aerobic exercise *to help improve the client's muscle conditioning, energy level, and sense of well-being.*
- Recommend cognitive behavioral therapy *to help deal with stressful situations.*
- Provide regular rest periods throughout the day *to help the client perform activities throughout the day.*

Teaching topics
- Explanation of the disorder and treatment plan
- Exercising daily
- Resting for periods throughout the day
- Developing a bedtime sleep routine
- Drug therapy
- Decreasing stress

Hemophilia

A hereditary bleeding disorder, hemophilia produces mild to severe abnormal bleeding. After a platelet plug develops at a bleeding site, the lack of clotting factor prevents a stable fibrin clot from forming. Although hemorrhaging doesn't usually happen immediately, delayed bleeding is common. Two types of hemophilia exist:
- hemophilia A or classic hemophilia (deficiency or nonfunction of factor VIII)
- hemophilia B or Christmas disease (deficiency or nonfunction of factor IX).

   Severity and prognosis of hemophilia vary with the degree of deficiency and the site of bleeding.

CAUSES
- Genetic inheritance: both types of hemophilia inherited as X-linked recessive traits

ASSESSMENT FINDINGS
- Hematemesis (bloody vomit)
- Hematomas on the extremities, torso, or both
- Hematuria (bloody urine)
- History of prolonged bleeding after surgery, dental extractions, or trauma
- Joint tenderness
- Limited ROM
- Pain and swelling in a weight-bearing joint (such as the hip, knee, or ankle)
- Signs of decreased tissue perfusion: chest pain, confusion, cool and clammy skin, decreased urine output, hypotension, pallor, restlessness, anxiety, tachycardia
- Signs of internal bleeding, such as abdominal, chest, or flank pain
- Tarry stools

Mild hemophilia
- No spontaneous bleeding
- Prolonged bleeding after major trauma or surgery (blood may ooze slowly or intermittently for up to 8 days following surgery)

Moderate hemophilia
- Occasional spontaneous bleeding
- Subcutaneous and I.M. hematomas

Severe hemophilia
- Excessive bleeding following circumcision (often the first sign of the disease)
- Large subcutaneous and deep I.M. hematomas
- Spontaneous or severe bleeding after minor trauma

DIAGNOSTIC TEST RESULTS
Hemophilia A
- PTT is prolonged.
- Factor VIII assay reveals 0% to 25% of normal factor VIII.
- Platelet count and function, bleeding time, PT, and International Normalized Ratio are normal.

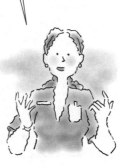

Hemophilia is inherited as an X-linked recessive trait...

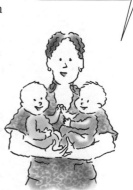

...this means that female carriers have a 50% chance of transmitting the gene to a daughter, making her a carrier, and a 50% chance of transmitting the gene to a son, who would be born with the disease.

Hemophilia B
- Baseline coagulation result is similar to that of hemophilia A, with normal factor VIII.
- Factor IX assay shows deficiency.

NURSING DIAGNOSES
- Impaired gas exchange
- Acute pain
- Parental role conflict
- Activity intolerance
- Risk for deficient fluid volume

TREATMENTS
- Bleeding prevention
- Medical treatment after head, neck, or abdominal injury
- Blood transfusion (with severe blood loss)

Drug therapy (both types)
- Hemostatic drug: aminocaproic acid (Amicar)
- Analgesic: morphine

Hemophilia A
- Cryoprecipitate antihemophilic factor (AHF), lyophilized (dehydrated) AHF, or both
- Hormone: desmopressin (DDAVP)

Hemophilia B
- Factor IX concentrate

INTERVENTIONS AND RATIONALES
- Monitor for signs of bleeding *to provide rapid intervention.*
- Provide emotional support *because hemophilia is a chronic disorder.*
- Refer new clients to a hemophilia treatment center *for education, evaluation, and development of a treatment plan.*
- Refer clients and carriers for genetic counseling *to determine risk of passing the disease to offspring.*

During bleeding episodes
- Apply pressure to cuts and during epistaxis *to stop bleeding. In many cases, pressure is the only treatment needed for surface cuts.*
- Apply cold compresses or ice bags and elevate the injured part *to control bleeding.*
- Administer sufficient clotting factor or plasma, as ordered, *to promote hemostasis.* The body uses AHF in 48 to 72 hours, so repeat infusions may be necessary.

- Administer analgesics *to control pain.* Avoid I.M. injections and aspirin and aspirin-containing medications as ordered.

If the client has bled into a joint
- Immediately elevate the painful joint *to control bleeding.*
- Begin range-of-motion exercises, if ordered, at least 48 hours after the bleeding has been controlled *to restore joint mobility.*
- Don't allow client to bear weight on the affected joint until bleeding stops and swelling subsides *to prevent deformities due to hemarthrosis.*

After bleeding episodes and surgery
- Watch for signs of further bleeding *to detect and control bleeding as soon as possible.*
- Closely monitor PTT. *Prolonged times increase risk of bleeding.*

Teaching topics
- Explanation of the disorder and treatment plan
- Signs of severe internal bleeding
- When to notify primary care provider; for example, after even a minor injury
- Wearing a medical identification bracelet
- Injury prevention
- Importance of medical follow-up
- Risk of infection such as hepatitis from blood component administration
- Bleeding prevention
- Caring for injuries
- Home administration of blood factor components, as appropriate

Idiopathic thrombocytopenic purpura

ITP—thrombocytopenia that results from immunologic platelet destruction—may be acute (postviral thrombocytopenia) or chronic (Werlhof's disease, purpura hemorrhagica, essential thrombocytopenia, and autoimmune thrombocytopenia). The prognosis for acute ITP is excellent; nearly four out of five clients recover without treatment. The prognosis for chronic ITP is good; remission lasting weeks or years are common, especially among women.

Acute ITP usually follows a viral infection, such as rubella or chicken pox. Chronic ITP is commonly liked to immunologic disorders and drug reactions.

CAUSES
• Autoimmune disorder

ASSESSMENT FINDINGS
• Ecchymoses
• Hemorrhage (rare)
• Mucosal bleeding from mouth, nose, or GI tract
• Petechiae
• Purpuric lesions on vital organs

DIAGNOSTIC TEST RESULTS
• Bleeding time is prolonged.
• Bone marrow study shows an increase in megakaryocytes and decreased circulating platelet survival time.
• Platelet antibodies may be found in vitro, but this doesn't usually help make a diagnosis of ITP.
• Platelet count is less than 20,000 µl.

NURSING DIAGNOSES
• Ineffective protection
• Anxiety
• Fear
• Risk for injury

TREATMENT
• Blood transfusion of blood and blood components
• May resolve spontaneously
• Splenectomy (if unresponsive to high-dose steroids)

Drug therapy
• Anti-RhD therapy (in clients with specific blood types)
• Glucocorticoids: prednisone, methylprednisone (Solu-Cortef)
• Immunoglobulin I.V.
• Vitamin K for coagulation defects

INTERVENTIONS AND RATIONALES
• Transfuse blood and blood products as needed *to help replace platelets and blood volume lost from bleeding.*

• Monitor the client for petechiae, ecchymoses and other signs of bleeding *to determine if he is bleeding.*
• Monitor platelet function and other coagulation values *to monitor progression or remission of disease.*
• Help the client avoid unnecessary trauma *to decrease the risk of bleeding.*
• Test stool for bleeding *because internal bleeding may not be visible.*
• Avoid administering aspirin, ibuprofen, and warfarin (Coumadin) *because these drugs interfere with platelet function and blood clotting.*

Teaching topics
• Explanation of the disorder and treatment plan
• Drug therapy
• Informing all health care professionals about diagnosis
• Avoiding trauma that could cause bleeding
• Using soft toothbrush, electric razor
• Avoiding aspirin and other medications before checking with physician
• Recognizing signs and symptoms of bleeding

Iron deficiency anemia

Iron deficiency anemia is a chronic, slowly progressing disease involving circulating RBCs. Iron deficiency results when an individual either absorbs inadequate amounts of iron or loses excessive amounts (such as through chronic bleeding). This decreased iron affects formation of hemoglobin and RBCs which, in turn, decreases the capacity of the blood to transport oxygen.

CAUSES
• Acute and chronic bleeding
• Alcohol abuse
• Certain drugs
• Gastrectomy
• Inadequate intake of iron-rich foods
• Malabsorption syndrome
• Menstruation
• Pregnancy
• Vitamin B_6 deficiency

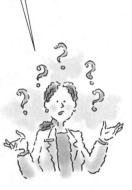

Creating question scenarios while you study can help you remember important info...

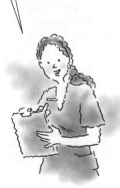

...For example, imagine that you're teaching a client with iron deficiency anemia about dietary changes. What would you teach?

ASSESSMENT FINDINGS
- Cheilosis (scaling and fissures of the lips)
- Dizziness
- Dyspnea
- Koilonychia (spoon-shaped nails)
- Pale, dry mucous membranes
- Pallor
- Palpitations
- Papillae atrophy of the tongue
- Sensitivity to cold
- Stomatitis
- Weakness and fatigue

DIAGNOSTIC TEST RESULTS
- Hematology shows decreased Hb, HCT, iron, ferritin, reticulocytes, red cell indices, transferrin, and saturation; absent hemosiderin; and increased iron-binding capacity.
- Peripheral blood smear reveals microcytic and hypochromic RBCs.

NURSING DIAGNOSES
- Activity intolerance
- Fatigue
- Imbalanced nutrition: Less than body requirements
- Impaired gas exchange

TREATMENT
- Diet: high in iron, roughage, and protein with increased fluids; avoidance of teas and coffee, which reduce absorption of iron
- Transfusion therapy with packed RBCs, if necessary
- Vitamins: pyridoxine (vitamin B_6), ascorbic acid (vitamin C)

Drug therapy
- Antianemics: ferrous sulfate (Feosol), iron dextran (DexFerrum)

INTERVENTIONS AND RATIONALES
- Monitor intake and output *to detect fluid imbalances.*
- Monitor laboratory studies *to determine the effectiveness of therapy.*
- Assess cardiovascular and respiratory status *to detect decreased activity intolerance and dyspnea on exertion.*
- Monitor and record vital signs *to determine activity intoleranc*e.

- Monitor stool, urine, and emesis for occult blood *to identify the cause of anemia.*
- Administer oxygen, as necessary, *to treat hypoxemia caused by reduced hemoglobin.*
- Provide a diet high in iron *to replace iron stores in the body.*
- Administer medications, as prescribed, *to replace iron stores in the body.* Administer iron injection deep into muscle using Z-track technique *to avoid subcutaneous irritation and discoloration from leaking drug.*
- Encourage fluids *to avoid dehydration.*
- Provide rest periods *to avoid fatigue and reduce oxygen demands.*
- Provide mouth, skin, and foot care *because the tongue or lips may be dry or inflamed and nails may be brittle.*
- Protect the client from falls caused by weakness and fatigue. *Falls may result in bleeding and bruising.*

Teaching topics
- Explanation of the disorder and treatment plan
- Nutritional therapy and supplements
- Signs and symptoms of bleeding
- Monitoring stools for occult blood
- Refraining from using hot pads and hot water bottles

Kaposi's sarcoma

Kaposi's sarcoma is a cancer of the lymphatic cell wall. It's the most common AIDS related cancer. When associated with AIDS, it progresses aggressively, involving the lymph nodes, the viscera and, possibly, GI structures.

CAUSES
- Unknown, possibly related to immunosuppression

ASSESSMENT FINDINGS
- One or more obvious lesions in various shapes, sizes, and colors (ranging from red-brown to dark purple) appearing most commonly on the skin, buccal mucosa, hard and soft palates, lips, gums, tongue, tonsils, conjunctivae, and sclerae

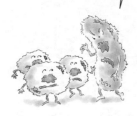

Kaposi's sarcoma is aggressive. It involves the lymph nodes, internal organs and, possibly, the digestive tract.

- Dyspnea (in cases of pulmonary involvement), wheezing, hypoventilation, and respiratory distress from bronchial blockage
- Edema from lymphatic obstruction
- Pain (if the sarcoma advances beyond the early stages or if a lesion breaks down or impinges on nerves or organs)

DIAGNOSTIC TEST RESULTS

- Computed tomography scan detects and evaluates possible metastasis.
- Tissue biopsy identifies the lesion's type and stage.

NURSING DIAGNOSES

- Ineffective protection
- Risk for infection
- Disturbed body image
- Anxiety
- Acute pain
- Social isolation

TREATMENT

- High-calorie, high-protein diet
- Radiation therapy
- I.V. fluid therapy

Drug therapy

- Chemotherapy: doxorubicin, etoposide (VePesid), vinblastine, vincristine
- Biological response modifier: interferon alfa-2b (ineffective in advanced disease)
- Antiemetic: aprepitant (Emend)

INTERVENTIONS AND RATIONALES

- Provide a referral for psychological counseling *to assist the client who's coping poorly.* Family members may also need help in coping with the client's disease and with any associated demands that the disorder places on them.
- Encourage participation in self-care decisions and self-care measures whenever possible. *Involving the client in the treatment plan helps him gain some sense of control over his situation.*
- Provide skin care, and assess for skin breakdown or new lesions *to evaluate disease progression.*
- Administer pain medications. Suggest distractions, position the client for comfort, and help with relaxation techniques *to divert pain and promote comfort.*

- Provide reassurance *to help the client adjust to changes in his appearance.*
- Monitor the client's daily weight *to evaluate if nutritional needs are being met.*
- Provide high-calorie, high-protein meals. If the client can't tolerate regular meals, provide him with frequent smaller meals. Consult with the dietitian, and plan meals around the client's treatment. *Adverse reactions to medications and the disease itself may make it difficult for the client's nutritional intake to meet metabolic needs.*
- If the client can't take food by mouth, administer I.V. fluids and parenteral nutrition *to maintain hydration and nutritional status.* Also provide antiemetics *to combat nausea and encourage nutritional intake.*
- Assess for adverse reactions to radiation therapy or chemotherapy—such as anorexia, nausea, vomiting, and diarrhea—and take steps to prevent or alleviate them. *Adverse reactions are common and can further compromise the client's condition.*
- Provide an explanation of treatments and possible adverse reactions and how to manage them *to ensure prompt intervention and treatment.* For example, during radiation therapy, instruct the client to keep irradiated skin dry *to avoid possible breakdown and subsequent infection.*
- Explain all prescribed medications, including any possible adverse effects and drug interactions, *to promote compliance with the medication regimen.*
- Teach infection-prevention techniques and, if necessary, demonstrate basic hygiene measures *to prevent infection.* Maintain standard precautions *to prevent the spread of infection to others.*
- Plan daily periods of alternating activity and rest *to help the client cope with fatigue.*
- Explain the proper use of assistive devices, when appropriate, *to ease ambulation and promote independence.*
- Refer the client to support groups offered by the social services department *to promote emotional well-being.*
- Provide information about hospice care, if indicated. *Hospice care provides much needed support to caregivers and helps the client through the dying process.*

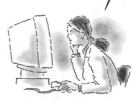

One or more obvious lesions in conjunction with an AIDS diagnosis? I think they're asking about Kaposi's sarcoma.

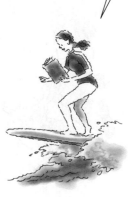

Need a diversion from the pain of studying? Take a break!

Teaching topics
- Explanation of the disorder and treatment plan
- Drug therapy
- Hospice care
- Energy-conservation techniques
- High-calorie, high-protein diet, consumed in small, frequent amounts if necessary
- Infection control measures
- Ongoing treatment and care
- Legal issues (such as advance directives and a durable power of attorney)

Latex allergy

Latex is a substance found in an increasing number of products in the work and home environment; the number of latex allergy cases is also increasing. A latex allergy is a hypersensitivity reaction to products that contain natural latex, which is derived from the sap of a rubber tree (not synthetic latex).

About 1% of the population has a latex allergy. Those who are in frequent contact with latex-containing products are at risk for developing a latex allergy. (See *Products that contain latex.*)

The more frequent the exposure, the greater the risk. Those at greatest risk are medical and dental professionals, workers in latex companies, and clients with spina bifida.

Other individuals at risk include:
- clients with a history of asthma or allergies, particularly to bananas, avocados, tropical fruits, or chestnuts
- clients with a history of multiple intra-abdominal or genitourinary surgeries
- clients who require frequent intermittent urinary catheterization.

CAUSES
- Sensitivity to latex

ASSESSMENT FINDINGS
Life-threatening reaction
- Abdominal pain
- Bronchospasm
- Flushing
- Hypotension
- Oxygen desaturation
- Palpitations

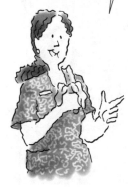

Many people enjoy bananas; unfortunately, those with latex allergies should probably stay away from them!

- Syncope
- Tachycardia
- Urticaria

Mild reaction
- Diarrhea
- Nausea
- Red, swollen, teary eyes
- Swollen lips

DIAGNOSTIC TEST RESULTS
- Blood test for latex sensitivity measures specific immunoglobulin E antibodies against latex.

NURSING DIAGNOSES
- Anxiety
- Risk for impaired gas exchange
- Risk for injury
- Disturbed body image

TREATMENT
- Avoiding latex exposure in clients sensitive to or with suspected sensitivity to latex
- Cardiopulmonary resuscitation and fluid resuscitation (for severe reaction)
- Oxygen therapy if needed
- Supportive care

Drug therapy
- Premedication before exposure: diphenhydramine (Benadryl), prednisone, cimetidine (Tagamet)
- Postexposure medication: hydrocortisone, diphenhydramine (Benadryl), famotidine (Pepcid)

INTERVENTIONS AND RATIONALES
- Use silicone products instead of latex *to decrease the risk of a reaction.*
- Be aware of all products containing latex and avoid use in a client with known or suspected sensitivity *because the more the client is exposed to latex, the greater the risk of allergy.*
- Premedicate the client before exposure, if possible, *to decrease the likelihood of a reaction.*
- Encourage the client to wear a medical identification tag stating his allergy *to help health care professionals in case of an emergency.*

Products that contain latex

Many medical and everyday items contain latex, which can be a threat to a client with a latex allergy. The most common items that contain latex are listed below.

MEDICAL PRODUCTS
- Adhesive bandages
- Airways, nasogastric tubes
- Blood pressure cuff, tubing, and bladder
- Catheters
- Catheter leg straps
- Dental dams
- Elastic bandages
- Electronic pads
- Fluid-circulating hypothermia blankets
- Handheld resuscitation bag
- Hemodialysis equipment
- I.V. catheters
- Latex or rubber gloves
- Medical vials
- Pads for crutches
- Protective sheets
- Reservoir breathing bags
- Rubber airway and endotracheal tubes
- Stethoscopes
- Tape
- Tourniquets

NONMEDICAL PRODUCTS
- Adhesive tape
- Balloons (excluding Mylar)
- Cervical diaphragms
- Condoms
- Dishwashing gloves
- Disposable diapers
- Elastic stockings
- Glue
- Latex paint
- Nipples and pacifiers
- Racquet handles
- Rubber bands
- Tires

Teaching topics
- Explanation of the disorder and treatment plan
- Avoiding products with latex
- Using silicone products when possible
- Carrying epinephrine and emergency medications
- Wearing a medical identification bracelet

Leukemia

Leukemia is characterized by an uncontrolled proliferation of WBC precursors that fail to mature. Leukemia occurs when normal hemopoietic cells are replaced by leukemic cells in bone marrow. Immature forms of WBCs circulate in the blood, infiltrating the liver, spleen, and lymph nodes. Types of leukemia include:
- acute lymphocytic
- acute myelogenous
- chronic lymphocytic
- chronic myelocytic.

CAUSES
- Altered immune system
- Exposure to chemicals
- Genetics
- Radiation
- Virus

ASSESSMENT FINDINGS
- Enlarged lymph nodes, spleen, and liver
- Epistaxis
- Fever
- Frequent infections
- Generalized pain
- Gingivitis and stomatitis
- Hematemesis
- Hypotension
- Jaundice
- Joint, abdominal, and bone pain
- Melena
- Night sweats
- Petechiae and ecchymoses
- Prolonged menses
- Tachycardia
- Weakness and fatigue

DIAGNOSTIC TEST RESULTS
- Bone marrow biopsy reveals a large number of immature leukocytes.
- Hematology shows decreased HCT, Hb, RBCs, and platelets and increased ESR, immature WBCs, and prolonged bleeding time.

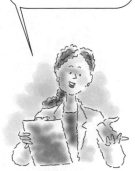

Frequent infections and easy bruising are key signs of leukemia.

Think about therapeutic communication. A client with leukemia might want to talk about body image changes. Allow him to express his feelings.

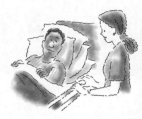

Management moments

Alleviating anxiety

Anxiety can be overwhelming for the client with leukemia. It can also aggravate complications of the disease. Therefore it's important to allow him time to verbalize his feelings and concerns about the disease and its effect on him and his family as well as his fears about death.

STRATEGIC PLANNING
Help the client and his family find coping strategies that can effectively deal with their anxiety. Make sure to allow ample time for their questions.

REST AND RELAXATION
Teaching the client relaxation techniques can help reduce anxiety. Explain that resting frequently throughout the day is also helpful. Provide comfort measures and encourage the family's participation.

KNOWLEDGE FACTOR
You can also reduce the client's anxiety level by teaching him what to expect from the disease process and his treatment plan. After a teaching session, allow plenty of time for questions. In addition, be sure to provide him and his family with uninterrupted time alone when needed.

NURSING DIAGNOSES
• Imbalanced nutrition: Less than body requirements
• Chronic pain
• Risk for infection
• Ineffective protection
• Ineffective coping

TREATMENT
• High-protein, high-vitamin, high-mineral diet, involving soft, bland foods in small, frequent feedings
• Stem cell transplant
• Transfusion of platelets, packed RBCs, and whole blood

Drug therapy
• Alkylating agents: busulfan (Myleran), chlorambucil (Leukeran)
• Antibiotic: doxorubicin
• Antimetabolites: fluorouracil, methotrexate (Trexall)
• Antineoplastics: vinblastine, vincristine
• Hematopoietic growth factor: epoetin alfa (Epogen)

INTERVENTIONS AND RATIONALES
• Monitor and record vital signs *to promptly detect deterioration in client's condition.*
• Monitor intake, output, and daily weight *because body weight may decrease as a result of fluid loss.*
• Monitor laboratory studies *to help establish blood replacement needs, assess fluid status, and detect possible infection.*
• Monitor for bleeding. *Regular assessment may help anticipate or alleviate problems.*
• Place the client with epistaxis in an upright position leaning slightly forward *to reduce vascular pressure and prevent aspiration.*
• Monitor for infection. *Damage to bone marrow may suppress WBC formation.* Promptly report temperature over 101° F (38.3° C) and decreased WBC counts so that antibiotic therapy may be initiated.
• Administer oxygen therapy. *Oxygen therapy increases alveolar oxygen concentration and enhances arterial blood oxygenation.*
• Administer oral or I.V. fluids *to maintain adequate hydration.*
• Reposition the client every 2 hours *to prevent venous stasis and skin breakdown.*
• Encourage coughing and deep breathing *to help remove secretions and prevent pulmonary complications.*

• Keep the client in semi-Fowler's position when in bed *to promote chest expansion and ventilation of basilar lung fields.*
• Provide a high-protein, high-vitamin, high-mineral diet *to provide necessary nutrition.*
• Administer TPN, if needed, *to provide the client with electrolytes, amino acids, and other nutrients tailored to his needs.*
• Administer transfusion therapy as prescribed and monitor for adverse reactions. *Transfusion reactions may occur during blood administration and may further compromise the client's condition.*
• Administer medications as prescribed *to combat disease and promote wellness.*
• Provide gentle mouth and skin care *to prevent oral mucous membrane or skin breakdown.*
• Encourage the client to express his feelings about changes in his body image and fear of dying *to reduce anxiety.* (See *Alleviating anxiety.*)
• Avoid giving the client I.M. injections and enemas and taking rectal temperature *to prevent bleeding and infection.*

Teaching topics
• Recognizing signs and symptoms of occult bleeding
• Preventing constipation
• Using an electric razor
• Refraining from using over-the-counter (OTC) medications (unless cleared by the client's physician)
• Increasing fluid intake
• Contacting the American Cancer Society

Lymphoma

Lymphoma can be classified as either Hodgkin's disease or malignant lymphoma (also called *non-Hodgkin's lymphoma*).

In Hodgkin's disease, Reed-Sternberg cells proliferate in a single lymph node and travel contiguously through the lymphatic system to other lymphatic nodes and organs. (See *Hodgkin's progress.*)

In malignant lymphoma, tumors occur throughout lymph nodes and lymphatic organs in unpredictable patterns. Malignant lymphoma may be categorized as:
• lymphocytic
• histiocytic
• mixed cell types.

CAUSES
• Environmental (Hodgkin's disease)
• Genetic (Hodgkin's disease)
• Immunologic
• Viral

ASSESSMENT FINDINGS
• Anorexia and weight loss
• Cough
• Hepatomegaly
• Malaise and lethargy
• Night sweats
• Recurrent infection
• Recurrent, intermittent fever
• Severe pruritus
• Splenomegaly

> Remember, in Hodgkin's disease, tumors follow a pattern. In malignant lymphoma, tumors occur more randomly.

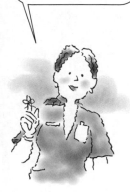

Hodgkin's progress

Hodgkin's disease occurs in four stages.

Stage I: Disease occurs in a single lymph node region or single extralymphatic organ.

Stage II: Disease occurs in two or more nodes on same side of diaphragm or in an extralymphatic organ.

Stage III: Disease spreads to both sides of diaphragm and perhaps to an extralymphatic organ, the spleen, or both.

Stage IV: Disease disseminates.

Hodgkin's disease
- Bone pain
- Dysphagia
- Dyspnea
- Edema and cyanosis of the face and neck
- Enlarged, nontender, firm, and movable lymph nodes in lower cervical regions
- Predictable pattern of spread

Malignant lymphoma
- Less predictable pattern of spread
- Prominent, painless, generalized lymph-adenopathy

DIAGNOSTIC TEST RESULTS
- Bone marrow aspiration and biopsy reveals small, diffuse lymphocytic or large, follicular-type cells (malignant lymphoma).
- Blood chemistry shows increased alkaline phosphatase (Hodgkin's disease).
- Chest X-ray reveals lymphadenopathy.
- Hematology shows decreased Hb, HCT, and platelets and increased ESR, increased immature leukocytes, and increased gamma-globulin (Hodgkin's disease).
- Lymph node biopsy is positive for Reed-Sternberg cells (Hodgkin's disease).
- Lymphangiogram shows positive lymph node involvement (Hodgkin's disease).

NURSING DIAGNOSES
- Ineffective protection
- Impaired tissue integrity
- Risk for infection
- Anxiety
- Fatigue
- Fear
- Acute pain

TREATMENT
- Diet high in protein, calories, vitamins, minerals, iron, and calcium that should consist of bland, soft foods
- Radiation therapy
- Transfusion of packed RBCs

Chemotherapy
- Hodgkin's disease: mechlorethamine (Mustargen), vincristine, procarbazine (Matulane), doxorubicin, bleomycin (Blenoxane), vinblastine, dacarbazine (DTIC-Dome)
- Malignant lymphoma: cyclophosphamide (Cytoxan), vincristine, doxorubicin

INTERVENTIONS AND RATIONALES
- Monitor and record vital signs *to allow for early detection of complications.*
- Monitor intake and output and specific gravity. *Low urine output and high specific gravity indicate hypovolemia.*
- Monitor laboratory studies. *Electrolytes, Hb, and HCT help indicate fluid status; WBC measurement may indicate bone marrow suppression.*
- Monitor for bleeding, infection, jaundice, and electrolyte imbalance *to detect complications associated with lymphoma.*
- Keep the client in semi-Fowler's position when in bed *to promote chest expansion and ventilation of basilar lung fields.*
- Administer oxygen. *Supplemental oxygen helps reduce hypoxemia.*
- Reposition the client every 2 hours *to prevent skin breakdown* and encourage coughing and deep breathing *to help remove secretions and prevent pulmonary complications.*
- Provide mouth and skin care *to prevent breakdown of oral mucous membrane and skin.*
- Provide an appropriate diet *to ensure nutritional requirements are met.*
- Encourage fluids and administer I.V. fluids as ordered *to prevent dehydration and complications associated with chemotherapy drugs.*
- Administer medications as prescribed, and monitor for adverse reactions *to prevent further complications.*
- Administer transfusion therapy as prescribed, and monitor for adverse reactions. *Transfusion reactions during blood administration may further compromise the client's condition.*
- Provide rest periods *to enhance immune function and decrease weakness caused by anemia.*
- Encourage verbalization of feelings about changes in body image and fear of dying *to allay the client's anxiety.*

Teaching topics
- Explanation of the disorder and treatment plan
- Drug therapy
- Nutritional therapy
- Infection prevention
- Recognizing early signs and symptoms of motor and sensory deficits
- Increasing fluid intake
- Using an electric razor only

- Refraining from using OTC medications (unless cleared by the client's physician)
- Contacting the American Cancer Society

Magnesium imbalance

Magnesium is the second most common cation (positively charged ion) in intracellular fluid. Its major function is to enhance neuromuscular integration. Magnesium regulates muscle contractions. By acting on the myoneural junctions (the sites where nerve and muscle fibers meet), magnesium affects the irritability and contractility of skeletal and cardiac muscles.

Magnesium also stimulates parathyroid hormone (PTH) secretion, thus regulating intracellular fluid calcium levels. Therefore, magnesium deficiency (hypomagnesemia) may result in transient hypoparathyroidism and may also interfere with the peripheral action of PTH.

In addition, magnesium activates many enzymes for proper carbohydrate and protein metabolism, aids in cell metabolism and the transport of sodium and potassium across cell membranes, and influences sodium, potassium, calcium, and protein levels.

Approximately one-third of the magnesium taken into the body is absorbed through the small intestine and is eventually excreted in urine; the remaining unabsorbed magnesium is excreted in stool.

Because many common foods contain magnesium, a dietary deficiency is rare. Hypomagnesemia generally follows impaired absorption, too-rapid excretion, or inadequate intake during TPN. It frequently coexists with other electrolyte imbalances, especially low calcium and potassium levels. Magnesium excess (hypermagnesemia) is common in clients with renal failure and excessive intake of antacids containing magnesium.

CAUSES

Hypomagnesemia usually results from impaired absorption of magnesium in the intestines or excessive excretion in the urine or stools. Hypermagnesemia results from the kidneys' inability to excrete magnesium that was either absorbed from the intestines or was infused.

Hypomagnesemia
- Chronic alcoholism
- Severe dehydration and diabetic acidosis
- Decreased magnesium intake or absorption, as in malabsorption syndrome, chronic diarrhea, or postoperative complications after bowel resection
- Hyperaldosteronism and hypoparathyroidism, which result in hypokalemia and hypocalcemia
- Hyperparathyroidism and hypercalcemia; excessive release of adrenocortical hormones; diuretic therapy
- Prolonged diuretic therapy, nasogastric suctioning, or administration of parenteral fluids without magnesium salts; starvation or malnutrition

Hypermagnesemia
- Chronic renal insufficiency
- Overcorrection of hypomagnesemia
- Overuse of magnesium-containing antacids
- Severe dehydration (resulting oliguria can cause magnesium retention)
- Use of laxatives (magnesium sulfate, milk of magnesia, and magnesium citrate solutions), especially with renal insufficiency

ASSESSMENT FINDINGS
Hypomagnesemia
- Arrhythmias
- Neuromuscular irritability
- Leg and foot cramps
- Chvostek's sign
- Mood changes
- Confusion
- Delusions
- Hallucinations
- Seizures

Hypermagnesemia
- Diminished deep tendon reflexes
- Weakness
- Flaccid paralysis
- Respiratory muscle paralysis (severe hypermagnesemia)
- Drowsiness
- Confusion
- Diminished sensorium may progress to coma
- Bradycardia
- Weak pulse

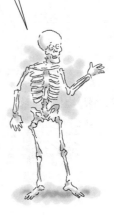

By acting on the myoneural junctions, magnesium affects the irritability and contractility of skeletal muscles...

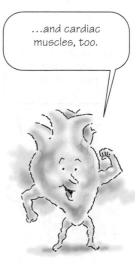

...and cardiac muscles, too.

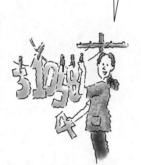

> Here are the key numbers: Serum magnesium less than 1.5 mEq/L confirms hypomagnesemia; greater than 2.5 mEq/L confirms hypermagnesemia.

- Hypotension
- Heart block
- Cardiac arrest (severe hypermagnesemia)
- Nausea
- Vomiting

DIAGNOSTIC TEST RESULTS

- Serum magnesium levels less than 1.5 mEq/L confirms hypomagnesemia.
- Serum magnesium levels greater than 2.5 mEq/L confirms hypermagnesemia.

NURSING DIAGNOSES

- Risk for injury
- Decreased cardiac output
- Impaired gas exchange
- Disturbed thought process

TREATMENT
Hypomagnesemia

- I.M. or oral magnesium supplements
- High-magnesium diet
- I.V. fluid therapy
- Magnesium sulfate I.V. (10 to 40 mEq/L diluted in I.V. fluid) for severe deficiency

Hypermagnesemia

- Low-magnesium diet with increased fluid intake
- Loop diuretic: furosemide (Lasix)
- Magnesium antagonist: calcium gluconate (10%)
- Peritoneal dialysis or hemodialysis if renal function fails or if excess magnesium can't be eliminated

INTERVENTIONS AND RATIONALES
Hypomagnesemia

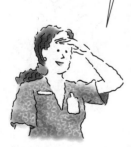

> The best treatment for hypomagnesemia is prevention. Keep a watchful eye on clients at risk for this imbalance, such as those who can't tolerate oral intake.

- Monitor serum electrolyte levels (including magnesium, calcium, and potassium) daily for mild deficits and every 6 to 12 hours during replacement therapy *to guide the treatment plan.*
- Monitor intake and output. (Urine output shouldn't fall below 25 ml/hour or 600 ml/day.) *The kidneys excrete excess magnesium, and hypermagnesemia could occur with renal insufficiency.*
- Monitor vital signs during I.V. therapy. Infuse magnesium replacement slowly, and watch for bradycardia, heart block, and decreased respiratory rate *to prevent complications that may occur with rapid infusion.*

- Provide a diet high in magnesium, such as fish and green vegetables, *to help raise magnesium level with dietary sources.*
- Assess for and report signs of hypomagnesemia in clients with predisposing diseases or conditions, especially those not permitted anything by mouth or who receive I.V. fluids without magnesium *to prevent complications associated with magnesium deficiency.*

Hypermagnesemia

- Assess level of consciousness, muscle activity, and vital signs *to detect complications of magnesium excess.*
- Monitor intake and output. Provide sufficient fluids *for adequate hydration and maintenance of renal function.*
- Treat abnormal serum electrolyte levels immediately *to prevent complications of magnesium excess.*
- Monitor cardiac rhythm *to detect arrhythmias.*
- Assess for signs of hypermagnesemia in predisposed clients. Observe closely for respiratory distress if serum magnesium levels exceed 10 mEq/L *to prevent respiratory decompensation.*

Teaching topics

- Explanation of the disorder and treatment plan
- Avoiding laxative and diuretic abuse
- Supplements (for hypomagnesemia)
- Nutritional therapy

Metabolic acidosis

Metabolic acidosis refers to a state of excess acid accumulation and deficient base bicarbonate. It's produced by an underlying pathologic disorder. Symptoms result from the body's attempts to correct the acidotic condition through compensatory mechanisms in the lungs, kidneys, and cells.

Metabolic acidosis is more prevalent among children, who are vulnerable to acid-base imbalance because their metabolic rates are faster and their ratios of water to total-body weight are lower. Severe or untreated metabolic acidosis can be fatal.

CAUSES

- Anaerobic carbohydrate metabolism
- Chronic alcoholism
- Diabetic ketoacidosis
- Diarrhea or intestinal malabsorption
- Low-carbohydrate, high-fat diet
- Malnutrition
- Renal insufficiency and failure

ASSESSMENT FINDINGS

- Central nervous system depression
- Drowsiness
- Headache
- Kussmaul's respirations
- Lethargy
- Stupor

DIAGNOSTIC TEST RESULTS

- ABG analysis reveals pH below 7.35 and bicarbonate level less than 24 mEq/L.

NURSING DIAGNOSES

- Ineffective breathing pattern
- Disturbed thought processes
- Decreased cardiac output
- Risk for injury

TREATMENT

- Treatment of the underlying cause
- Endotracheal intubation and mechanical ventilation to ensure adequate respiratory compensation (in severe cases)

Drug therapy

- Sodium bicarbonate I.V. or orally for chronic metabolic acidosis
- Insulin administration and I.V. fluid administration if diabetic ketoacidosis is the cause

INTERVENTIONS AND RATIONALES

- Monitor vital signs, laboratory results, and level of consciousness *to detect changes in health status.*
- Administer medications and I.V. fluids as ordered *to replace fluid and electrolyte losses.*
- Monitor intake and output *to assess renal function.*
- Assess for signs of excessive serum potassium—weakness, flaccid paralysis, and arrhythmias, possibly leading to cardiac arrest. After treatment, check for overcorrection

to hypokalemia *to prevent complications of potassium imbalance.*
- Initiate seizure precautions *to prevent injury.*
- Provide good oral hygiene. Use sodium bicarbonate washes *to neutralize mouth acids,* and lubricate the client's lips *to prevent skin breakdown.*
- Carefully observe clients receiving I.V. therapy or who have intestinal tubes in place as well as those suffering from shock, hyperthyroidism, hepatic disease, circulatory failure, or dehydration *to prevent metabolic acidosis.*
- Provide appropriate treatment for the underlying cause.

Teaching topics

- Explanation of the disorder and treatment plan
- Testing urine for sugar and acetone
- Encouraging strict adherence to insulin or oral antidiabetic therapy
- Medication therapy and possible adverse reactions

Metabolic alkalosis

Metabolic alkalosis is a clinical state marked by decreased amounts of acid or increased amounts of base bicarbonate. It causes metabolic, respiratory, and renal responses, producing characteristic symptoms—most notably, hypoventilation. This condition always occurs secondary to an underlying cause. With early diagnosis and prompt treatment, the prognosis is good; however, untreated metabolic alkalosis may lead to coma and death.

CAUSES

- Loss of acid from vomiting, nasogastric tube drainage, or lavage without adequate electrolyte replacement, fistulas, the use of steroids and certain diuretics (furosemide, thiazides, and ethacrynic acid), or hyperadrenocorticism
- Retention of base from excessive intake of bicarbonate of soda or other antacids (usually for treatment of gastritis or peptic ulcer), excessive intake of absorbable alkali (as in milk-alkali syndrome), administration of excessive amounts of I.V. fluids with high

You win some, you lose some. Metabolic acidosis is characterized by a gain in acid and a loss of bicarbonate in the plasma.

You lose some, you win some. Metabolic alkalosis is characterized by a loss of acid, a gain in bicarbonate, or both.

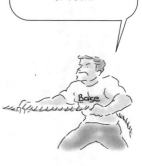

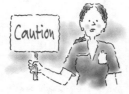

When administering ammonium chloride 0.9%, limit the infusion rate to 1¼ hours.

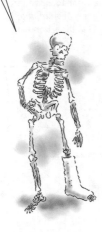

concentrations of bicarbonate or lactate, or respiratory insufficiency

ASSESSMENT FINDINGS
- Apnea
- Atrial tachycardia
- Confusion
- Cyanosis
- Diarrhea
- Hypoventilation
- Irritability
- Nausea
- Picking at bedclothes (carphology)
- Twitching
- Vomiting

DIAGNOSTIC TEST RESULTS
- ABG analysis reveals pH greater than 7.45 and a bicarbonate level above 29 mEq/L

NURSING DIAGNOSES
- Disturbed thought processes
- Decreased cardiac output
- Risk for injury
- Ineffective breathing pattern

TREATMENT
- Treatment of underlying cause

Drug therapy
- Acidifying agent: hydrochloric acid
- Potassium supplement: potassium chloride I.V.
- Carbonic anhydrase inhibitor: acetazolamide (Diamox)
- Ammonia supplement: ammonium chloride (severe or persistent metabolic alkalosis)

INTERVENTIONS AND RATIONALES
- When administering ammonium chloride 0.9%, infuse over at least 1¼ hours; *faster administration may cause hemolysis of RBCs.* Avoid overdosage *because it may cause overcorrection to metabolic acidosis.* Don't give ammonium chloride to a client with signs of hepatic or renal disease *to avoid toxicity.*
- Monitor cardiac rhythm and vital signs *to evaluate cardiovascular status. Hypotension and tachycardia may indicate electrolyte imbalance, especially hypokalemia.*
- Monitor respiratory status. *Respiratory rate usually decreases in an effort to compensate for alkalosis.*

Because multiple myeloma causes bone destruction, bone pain and fractures are assessment findings to remember for this disorder.

- Irrigate nasogastric tubes with isotonic saline solution instead of plain water *to prevent loss of gastric electrolytes.* Monitor I.V. fluid concentrations of bicarbonate or lactate *to prevent acid base imbalance.*
- Provide appropriate treatment *to address the underlying cause.*
- Administer medications and I.V. fluids as ordered.

Teaching topics
- Explanation of the disorder and treatment plan
- For clients with ulcers, recognizing signs of milk-alkali syndrome: a distaste for milk, anorexia, weakness, and lethargy
- Avoiding overuse of alkaline agents

Multiple myeloma

Multiple myeloma is the abnormal proliferation of plasma cells. These plasma cells are immature and malignant and invade the bone marrow, lymph nodes, liver, spleen, and kidneys, triggering osteoblastic activity and leading to bone destruction throughout the body.

CAUSES
- Environmental
- Genetic
- Unknown

ASSESSMENT FINDINGS
- Anemia, thrombocytopenia, hemorrhage
- Constant, severe bone pain
- Headaches
- Hepatomegaly
- Multiple infections
- Pathologic fractures, skeletal deformities of sternum and ribs, loss of height
- Renal calculi
- Splenomegaly
- Vascular insufficiency

DIAGNOSTIC TEST RESULTS
- Bence Jones protein assay is positive.
- Blood chemistry tests show increased calcium, uric acid, BUN, and creatinine.
- Bone marrow biopsy shows increased number of immature plasma cells.

- Bone scan reveals increased uptake.
- Hematology shows decreased HCT, WBCs, and platelets and increased ESR.
- Immunoelectrophoresis shows monoclonal spike.
- Urine chemistry shows increased calcium and uric acid.
- X-rays show diffuse, round, punched-out bone lesions; osteoporosis; osteolytic lesions of the skull; and widespread demineralization.

NURSING DIAGNOSES
- Chronic pain
- Impaired physical mobility
- Risk for infection
- Fear
- Anxiety
- Risk for injury

TREATMENT
- Allogenic bone marrow transplantation
- High-protein, high-carbohydrate, high-vitamin, and high-mineral diet in small, frequent feedings
- Orthopedic devices: braces, splints, casts
- Peritoneal dialysis and hemodialysis
- Radiation therapy
- Transfusion therapy: packed RBCs

Drug therapy
- Alkylating agents: melphalan (Alkeran), cyclophosphamide (Cytoxan)
- Analgesic: morphine
- Androgen: fluoxymesterone
- Antacids: magnesium hydroxide and aluminum hydroxide (Maalox), aluminum hydroxide
- Antibiotic: doxorubicin
- Antiemetic: prochlorperazine (Compazine)
- Antigout agent: allopurinol
- Antineoplastics: vinblastine, vincristine
- Diuretic: furosemide (Lasix)
- Glucocorticoid: prednisone

INTERVENTIONS AND RATIONALES
- Assess renal status *to detect renal stones and renal failure secondary to hypercalcemia.*
- Monitor and record vital signs *to allow for early detection of complications.*
- Monitor intake and output, urine specific gravity, and daily weight *to identify fluid volume excess or deficit.*

- Monitor laboratory studies. *RBCs, WBCs, Hb, HCT, and platelets may be affected by chemotherapy.*
- Assess cardiovascular and respiratory status *to detect signs of compromise.*
- Assess pain level *to determine client's response to analgesics.*
- Monitor for infection and bruising *to detect complications.*
- Provide an adequate diet *to ensure nutritional requirements are met.*
- Encourage oral fluids and administer I.V. fluids *to prevent dehydration and dilute calcium.*
- Assist with turning, coughing, and deep breathing *to mobilize and remove secretions.*
- Administer transfusion therapy as prescribed *to replace blood components.*
- Administer medications, as prescribed, and monitor for adverse effects *to prevent complications.*
- Maintain seizure precautions *to prevent injury.*
- Provide skin and mouth care *to prevent breakdown of oral mucous membrane and skin.*
- Provide rest periods between activities *to prevent fatigue.*
- Institute fall prevention measures *because the client is vulnerable to fractures.*
- Apply and maintain braces, splints, and casts *to prevent injury and reduce pain.*

Teaching topics
- Explanation of the disorder and treatment plan
- Drug therapy
- Nutritional therapy
- Exercising regularly, with particular attention to muscle-strengthening exercises
- Signs and symptoms of renal calculi, fractures, and seizures
- Avoiding lifting, constipation, and OTC medications
- Monitoring stool for occult blood
- Using braces, splints, and casts
- Contacting the American Cancer Society

Pernicious anemia

Pernicious anemia is a chronic, progressive, macrocytic anemia caused by a deficiency of intrinsic factor, a substance normally secreted

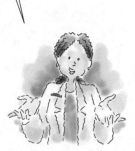

If you remember that pernicious anemia results from a lack of vitamin B_{12} absorption, then it's easy to recall that vitamins are a big part of treating the disorder.

by the stomach. Without intrinsic factor, dietary vitamin B_{12} can't be absorbed by the ileum, inhibiting normal deoxyribonucleic acid (DNA) synthesis and resulting in defective maturation of RBCs.

CAUSES
- Autoimmune disease
- Bacterial or parasitic infections
- Deficiency of intrinsic factor
- Gastric mucosal atrophy
- Genetics
- Lack of administration of vitamin B_{12} after small-bowel resection or total gastrectomy
- Malabsorption
- Prolonged iron deficiency

ASSESSMENT FINDINGS
- Constipation or diarrhea
- Depression
- Delirium
- Dyspnea
- Glossitis, sore mouth
- Mild jaundice of sclera
- Pallor
- Paralysis, gait disturbances
- Tachycardia, palpitations
- Tingling and paresthesia of hands and feet
- Weakness, fatigue
- Weight loss, anorexia, dyspepsia

DIAGNOSTIC TEST RESULTS
- Blood chemistry tests reveal increased bilirubin and lactate dehydrogenase levels.
- Bone marrow aspiration shows increased megaloblasts, few maturing erythrocytes, and defective leukocyte maturation.
- Gastric analysis shows hypochlorhydria.
- Hematology shows decreased HCT and Hb.
- Peripheral blood smear reveals oval, macrocytic, hyperchromic erythrocytes.
- Romberg test is positive.
- Schilling test is positive.
- Upper GI series shows atrophy of gastric mucosa.

NURSING DIAGNOSES
- Imbalanced nutrition: Less than body requirements
- Impaired gas exchange
- Risk for injury

- Constipation
- Diarrhea

TREATMENT
- Diet high in iron and protein that restricts highly seasoned, coarse, or extremely hot foods
- Transfusion therapy with packed RBCs
- Vitamins: pyridoxine (vitamin B_6), ascorbic acid (vitamin C), cyanocobalamin (vitamin B_{12}), folic acid (vitamin A)

Drug therapy
- Antianemics: ferrous sulfate (Feosol), iron dextran (DexFerrum)

INTERVENTIONS AND RATIONALES
- Assess cardiovascular status *to detect signs of compromise as the heart works harder to compensate for the reduced oxygen-carrying capacity of the blood.*
- Monitor and record vital signs *to allow for early detection of compromise.*
- Monitor and record amount, consistency, and color of stools *to allow for early detection and treatment of diarrhea and constipation.*
- Provide an adequate diet *to ensure adequate intake of vitamins, iron, and protein.*
- Administer medications as prescribed. *Vitamin B_{12} injections are given monthly and are lifelong.*
- Encourage activity, as tolerated, *to avoid fatigue.*
- Provide mouth care before and after meals *to provide comfort and reduce the risk of oral mucous membrane breakdown.*
- Advise the client to use soft toothbrushes *to avoid injuring mucous membranes.*
- Maintain a warm environment *to keep the client comfortable.*
- Provide foot and skin care *because sensation to feet may be reduced.*
- Institute fall prevention measures *to reduce risk of injury resulting from reduced coordination, paresthesia of the feet, and reduced thought processes.*
- Assess neurologic status *because poor memory and confusion increase the risk of injury.*
- Monitor laboratory studies *to detect effectiveness of therapy.*

Teaching topics
- Explanation of the disorder and treatment plan
- Drug therapy
- Nutritional therapy
- Recognizing the signs and symptoms of skin breakdown
- Altering activities of daily living (ADLs) to compensate for paresthesia
- Avoiding the use of heating pads and electric blankets

Phosphorus imbalance

Phosphorus exists primarily in inorganic combination with calcium in teeth and bones. In extracellular fluid, the phosphate ion supports several metabolic functions: utilization of B vitamins, acid-base homeostasis, bone formation, nerve and muscle activity, cell membrane integrity, transmission of hereditary traits, and metabolism of carbohydrates, proteins, and fats.

Renal tubular reabsorption of phosphate is inversely regulated by calcium levels—an increase in phosphorus causes a decrease in calcium. An imbalance causes hypophosphatemia or hyperphosphatemia. Incidence of hypophosphatemia varies with the underlying cause; hyperphosphatemia occurs most commonly in clients who tend to consume large amounts of phosphorus-rich foods and beverages and in those with renal insufficiency.

CAUSES
Hypophosphatemia
- Chronic diarrhea
- Deficiency of vitamin D
- Hyperparathyroidism with resultant hypercalcemia
- Hypomagnesemia
- Inadequate dietary intake, such as from malnutrition resulting from a prolonged catabolic state or chronic alcoholism
- Intestinal malabsorption

Hyperphosphatemia
- Hypervitaminosis D
- Hypocalcemia
- Hypoparathyroidism

- Overuse of phosphate enemas or laxatives with phosphates
- Renal failure

ASSESSMENT FINDINGS
Hypophosphatemia
- Anorexia
- Muscle weakness
- Osteomalacia (inadequate mineralization of bone)
- Paresthesia
- Peripheral hypoxia
- Tremor

Hyperphosphatemia
- Tetany and seizures (with hypocalcemia)
- Usually asymptomatic

DIAGNOSTIC TEST RESULTS
- Serum phosphorus level less than 1.7 mEq/L (or 2.5 mg/dl) confirms hypophosphatemia. A urine phosphorus level more than 1.3 g/24 hours supports this diagnosis.
- Serum phosphorus level exceeding 2.6 mEq/L (or 4.5 mg/dl) confirms hyperphosphatemia. Supportive values include decreased levels of serum calcium (less than 9 mg/dl) and urine phosphorus (less than 0.9 g/24 hours).

NURSING DIAGNOSES
- Imbalanced nutrition: Less than or more than body requirements
- Risk for injury
- Deficient knowledge (treatment plan)
- Diarrhea

TREATMENT
Hypophosphatemia
- High-phosphorus diet

Drug therapy
- Phosphate supplements
- Potassium phosphate I.V. (in severe deficiency)

Hyperphosphatemia
- Low-phosphorus diet
- Peritoneal dialysis or hemodialysis (in severe cases)

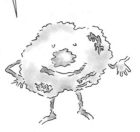

Phosphorus plays a crucial role in cell membrane integrity.

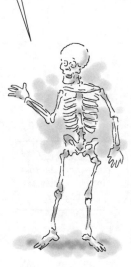

Phosphorus also plays a crucial role in bone formation.

Drug therapy
• Calcium supplement: calcium acetate (PhosLo)

INTERVENTIONS AND RATIONALES
• Carefully monitor serum electrolyte, calcium, magnesium, and phosphorus levels. Report any changes immediately *to guide treatment plan.*

Hypophosphatemia
• Monitor intake and output. Administer potassium phosphate slow I.V. *to prevent over-correction to hyperphosphatemia.* Assess renal function, and be alert for hypocalcemia when giving phosphate supplements.
• Provide a high-phosphorus diet containing milk and milk products, kidney, liver, turkey, and dried fruits *to prevent recurrence.*

Hyperphosphatemia
• Monitor intake and output. If urine output falls below 25 ml/hour or 600 ml/day, notify the physician immediately *because decreased output can seriously affect renal clearance of excess serum phosphorus.*
• Assess for signs of hypocalcemia, such as muscle twitching and tetany, which commonly accompany hyperphosphatemia *to ensure timely intervention.*
• Provide foods with low phosphorus content, such as vegetables, *to prevent recurrence.*
• Obtain dietary consultation if the condition results from chronic renal insufficiency *to aid in making sound nutritional choices that help prevent hyperphosphatemia.*

Teaching topics
• Explanation of the disorder and treatment plan
• Supplements (hypophosphatemia)
• Nutritional therapy
• Drug therapy
• Avoiding OTC drugs that contain phosphorus, such as laxatives and enemas (hyperphosphatemia)

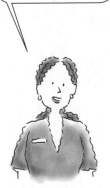

A myeloproliferative disorder, such as polycythemia vera, is characterized by proliferation of bone marrow constituents.

Polycythemia vera

Polycythemia vera is a chronic myeloproliferative disorder characterized by increased RBC mass, leukocytosis, thrombocytosis, and increased Hb concentration, with normal or increased plasma volume. It usually occurs between ages 40 and 60, most commonly among males of Jewish ancestry; it rarely affects children or blacks and doesn't appear to be familial. It may also be known as *primary polycythemia, erythremia, polycythemia rubra vera, splenomegalic polycythemia,* or *Vaquez Osler disease.*

The prognosis depends on age at diagnosis, the treatment used, and complications. Mortality is high if polycythemia is untreated or is associated with leukemia or myeloid metaplasia.

CAUSES
• Unknown (possibly due to a multipotential stem cell defect)

ASSESSMENT FINDINGS
• Clubbing of the digits
• Congestion of the conjunctiva, retina, and retinal veins
• Dizziness
• Dyspnea
• Feeling of fullness in the head
• Headache
• Hemorrhage
• Hypertension
• Ruddy cyanosis of the nose
• Thrombosis of smaller vessels
• Visual disturbances (blurring, diplopia, engorged veins of fundus and retina)
• Weight loss

DIAGNOSTIC TEST RESULTS
• Blood tests show increased RBC mass and normal arterial oxygen saturation in association with splenomegaly or two of the following: thrombocytosis, leukocytosis, elevated leukocyte alkaline phosphatase level, or elevated serum vitamin B_{12} or unbound B_{12} binding capacity.

NURSING DIAGNOSES
• Chronic pain
• Activity intolerance
• Ineffective tissue perfusion: Cardiopulmonary
• Imbalanced nutrition: Less than body requirements
• Disturbed sensory perception (visual)

TREATMENT

- Phlebotomy (typically, 350 to 500 ml of blood is removed every other day until the client's HCT is reduced to the low-normal range)
- Plasmapheresis

Drug therapy

- Chemotherapy: busulfan (Myleran), chlorambucil (Leukeran), melphalan (Alkeran)
- Myelosuppressive drugs: hydroxyurea (Hydrea), radioactive phosphorus (^{32}P)
- Antigout agent: allopurinol

INTERVENTIONS AND RATIONALES

- Monitor vital signs *to evaluate the client's tolerance of the procedure.*
- During phlebotomy, assess for tachycardia, clamminess, or complaints of vertigo. *These signs and symptoms indicate hypovolemia.*
- After phlebotomy, administer 24 oz (720 ml) of juice or water *to replace fluid volume lost during the procedure.*
- Assess for and report symptoms of iron deficiency (pallor, weight loss, weakness, glossitis). *After repeated phlebotomies, the client will develop iron deficiency, which stabilizes RBC production and reduces the need for future phlebotomies.*
- Encourage ambulation *to prevent thrombosis.*
- Monitor for complications, such as hypervolemia, thrombocytosis, and signs of an impending stroke (decreased sensation, numbness, transitory paralysis, fleeting blindness, headache, and epistaxis), *to ensure early treatment intervention.*
- Assess for signs and symptoms of bleeding *to decrease the risk of hemorrhage.*
- Administer I.V. fluids and medications *to improve the client's condition.*
- Report acute abdominal pain immediately *to avoid treatment delay.* Acute pain may signal splenic infarction, renal calculi, or abdominal organ thrombosis.

During myelosuppressive treatment

- Monitor complete blood count and platelet count before and during therapy *to evaluate effects of treatment.*

- Warn a nonhospitalized client who develops leukopenia that his resistance to infection is low; advise him to avoid crowds and watch for the symptoms of infection. *These measures help protect the client from developing life-threatening infection.*
- If leukopenia develops, maintain protective isolation *to decrease the chance of spreading infection to the client.*
- If thrombocytopenia develops, monitor for signs of bleeding *to prevent hemorrhage.*
- Watch for adverse reactions. If nausea and vomiting occur, begin antiemetic therapy and adjust the client's diet *to promote comfort.*

Teaching topics

- Explanation of the disorder and treatment plan
- Drug therapy
- Signs and symptoms of bleeding
- Importance of remaining as active as possible
- Avoiding infection
- Keeping the environment free from hazards that could cause falls
- Using a safety razor to prevent bleeding
- Measures to prevent adverse reaction to treatment such as using antiemetics to prevent nausea and vomiting
- Available community resources

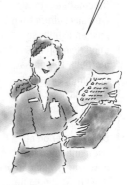

Phlebotomy is usually the first treatment for polycythemia vera. The client may have 350 to 500 ml of blood removed every other day.

Rheumatoid arthritis

Believed to be an autoimmune disorder, rheumatoid arthritis is a systemic inflammatory disease that affects the synovial lining of the joints. Antibodies first attack the synovium of the joint, causing it to become inflamed and swollen. Eventually, the articular cartilage and surrounding tendons and ligaments are affected.

Inflammation of the synovial membranes is followed by formation of pannus (granulation tissue) and destruction of cartilage, bone, and ligaments. Pannus is replaced by fibrotic tissue and calcification, which causes subluxation of the joint. The joint becomes ankylosed—or fused—leaving a very painful joint and limited ROM.

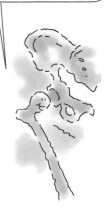

In rheumatoid arthritis, antibodies attack the synovial lining of the joints.

CAUSES
- Autoimmune disease
- Genetic transmission

ASSESSMENT FINDINGS
- Anorexia and weight loss
- Dry eyes and mucous membranes
- Enlarged lymph nodes
- Fatigue
- Fever
- Leukopenia and anemia
- Limited ROM
- Malaise
- Painful, swollen joints; crepitus; and morning stiffness
- Paresthesia of the hands and the feet
- Pericarditis
- Raynaud's phenomenon
- Splenomegaly
- Subcutaneous nodules
- Symmetrical joint swelling (mirror image of affected joints)

DIAGNOSTIC TEST RESULTS
- Antinuclear antibody (ANA) test is positive.
- Hematology shows increased ESR, WBC, platelets, and anemia.
- Rheumatoid factor test is positive.
- Serum protein electrophoresis shows elevated serum globulins.
- Synovial fluid analysis shows increased WBC count, increased volume and turbidity, and decreased viscosity and complement (C_3 and C_4 levels).
- X-rays reveal bone demineralization and soft-tissue swelling in early stages; in later stages, X-rays reveal a loss of cartilage, a narrowing of joint spaces, cartilage and bone destruction, and erosion, subluxations, and deformity.

NURSING DIAGNOSES
- Activity intolerance
- Disturbed body image
- Chronic pain
- Risk for infection
- Fatigue
- Risk for injury

TREATMENT
- Cold therapy during acute episodes
- Heat therapy to relax muscles and relieve pain for chronic disease (see *Conquering pain and stiffness*)
- Physical therapy (to forestall loss of joint function), passive ROM exercises, and observance of rest periods
- Weight control
- Well-balanced diet

Drug therapy
- Analgesic: aspirin
- Antacids: magnesium hydroxide and aluminum hydroxide (Maalox), aluminum hydroxide
- Antimetabolite: methotrexate (Rheumatrex)
- Antirheumatic: hydroxychloroquine (Plaquenil)
- Glucocorticoids: prednisone, hydrocortisone (Solu-Cortef)
- Gold therapy: gold sodium thiomalate
- Nonsteroidal anti-inflammatory drugs (NSAIDs): indomethacin (Indocin), ibuprofen (Motrin), sulindac (Clinoril), piroxicam (Feldene), flurbiprofen (Ansaid), diclofenac (Voltaren), naproxen (Naprosyn), diflunisal
- Tumor necrosis factor inhibitors: etanercept (Enbrel), adalimumab (Humira), infliximab (Remicade)

INTERVENTIONS AND RATIONALES
- Monitor vital signs *to allow for early detection of complications.*
- Monitor neuromuscular status *to determine client's capabilities.*
- Assess joints for swelling, pain, and redness *to determine the extent of disease and effectiveness of treatment.*
- Monitor laboratory studies *to detect remissions and exacerbations.*
- Administer medications as ordered and monitor for adverse reactions *to enhance the treatment regimen.* Administer medications, such as misoprostol (Cytotec), *to treat and prevent NSAID-induced gastric ulcers.*
- Provide passive ROM exercises *to prevent joint contractures and muscle atrophy.*
- Splint inflamed joints *to maintain joints in a functional position and prevent musculoskeletal deformities.*
- Provide warm or cold therapy as prescribed *to help alleviate pain.*
- Provide skin care *to prevent skin breakdown.*

- Minimize environmental stress and plan rest periods *to help the client cope with the disease.*
- Encourage verbalization of feelings about changes in body image *to help the client express doubts and resolve concerns.*

Teaching topics
- Explanation of the disorder and treatment plan
- Drug therapy
- Nutritional therapy
- Stress reduction techniques
- The need for 8 to 10 hours of sleep every night
- Avoiding cold, stress, and infection
- Performing complete skin and foot care daily
- Contacting groups such as the Arthritis Foundation

Scleroderma

Scleroderma is a diffuse connective tissue disease characterized by inflammatory and then degenerative and fibrotic changes in skin, blood vessels, synovial membranes, skeletal muscles, and internal organs (especially the esophagus, intestinal tract, thyroid, heart, lungs, and kidneys). The disease, also known as *progressive systemic sclerosis*, affects more women than men, especially between ages 30 and 50.

CAUSES
- Unknown

ASSESSMENT FINDINGS
- Pain
- Signs and symptoms of Raynaud's phenomenon, such as blanching, cyanosis, and erythema of the fingers and toes in response to stress or exposure to cold
- Slowly healing ulcerations on the tips of the fingers or toes that may lead to gangrene
- Stiffness
- Swelling of fingers and joints
- Taut, shiny skin over the entire hand and forearm
- Tight and inelastic facial skin, causing a masklike appearance and "pinching" of the mouth

- Cardiac and pulmonary fibrosis (in advanced disease)
- Renal involvement, usually accompanied by malignant hypertension, the main cause of death

DIAGNOSTIC TEST RESULTS
- Blood studies show slightly elevated ESR, positive rheumatoid factor in 25% to 35% of clients, and positive antinuclear antibody test.
- Chest X-rays show bilateral basilar pulmonary fibrosis.
- ECG reveals possible nonspecific abnormalities related to myocardial fibrosis.
- GI X-rays show distal esophageal hypomotility and stricture, duodenal loop dilation, small-bowel malabsorption pattern, and large diverticula.
- Hand X-rays show terminal phalangeal tuft resorption, subcutaneous calcification, and joint space narrowing and erosion.
- Pulmonary function studies show decreased diffusion and vital capacity.
- Skin biopsy may show changes consistent with the progress of the disease, such as marked thickening of the dermis and occlusive vessel changes.
- Urinalysis reveals proteinuria, microscopic hematuria, and casts (with renal involvement).

NURSING DIAGNOSES
- Impaired physical mobility
- Chronic pain
- Impaired skin integrity
- Activity intolerance
- Fatigue

TREATMENT
- Palliative measures: heat therapy, rest periods
- Physical therapy to maintain function and promote muscle strength
- Surgical debridement or digital sympathectomy

Drug therapy
- Immunosuppressants: cyclosporine (Sandimmune), chlorambucil (Leukeran)
- Antihypertensives: nifedipine (Procardia), amlodipine (Norvasc), losatan (Cozaar), captopril (Capoten)

> Fibrotic changes to the skin are usually the first clue to diagnosis of scleroderma.

> Treatment for scleroderma aims to preserve normal body functions and minimize complications.

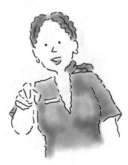

> What a shock! Septic shock is caused by bacterial infection. Without prompt treatment, it may rapidly progress to death.

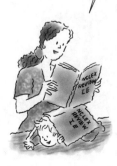

> Hypotension, altered level of consciousness, and hyperventilation may be the only signs of septic shock among infants and elderly people.

INTERVENTIONS AND RATIONALES

- Assess activity ability, pain, vital signs, intake and output, respiratory function, and daily weight *to monitor disease progression and guide the treatment plan.*
- Monitor blood pressure and report any increases above baseline. *Malignant hypertension is the main cause of death in clients diagnosed with scleroderma.*
- Avoid fingerstick blood tests *because of compromised circulation.*
- Provide emotional support. Encourage verbalization of feelings *to alleviate anxiety.*
- Assist with prescribed exercises *to help maintain mobility.*

Teaching topics

- Explanation of the disorder and treatment plan
- Drug therapy
- Signs and symptoms of impending relapse
- Methods to manage symptoms, such as tension, nervousness, insomnia, decreased ability to concentrate, and apathy
- Avoiding air conditioning and tobacco use, which may aggravate Raynaud's phenomenon
- Avoiding fatigue by pacing activities and organizing schedules to include necessary rest

Septic shock

Septic shock is usually the result of bacterial infection. It causes inadequate blood perfusion and circulatory collapse.

Septic shock occurs most commonly among hospitalized clients, especially men older than age 40 and women ages 25 to 45. It's second only to cardiogenic shock as the leading cause of shock death. About 25% of those who develop gram-negative bacteremia go into shock. Unless vigorous treatment begins promptly, preferably before symptoms fully develop, septic shock rapidly progresses to death (commonly within a few hours) in up to 80% of cases.

CAUSES

- Infection with gram-negative bacteria (in two-thirds of clients): *Escherichia coli, Klebsiella, Enterobacter, Proteus, Pseudomonas,* and *Bacteroides*

- Infection from gram-positive bacteria: *Streptococcus pneumoniae, S. pyogenes,* and *Actinomyces*

ASSESSMENT FINDINGS

Indications of septic shock vary according to the stage of the shock, the organism causing it, and the client's age.

Early stage

- Chills
- Diarrhea
- Nausea
- Oliguria
- Prostration
- Sudden fever (temperature over 101° F [38.3° C])
- Vomiting

Late stage

- Altered level of consciousness
- Anuria
- Apprehension
- Hyperventilation
- Hypotension
- Hypothermia
- Irritability
- Restlessness
- Tachycardia
- Tachypnea
- Thirst from decreased cerebral tissue perfusion

DIAGNOSTIC TEST RESULTS

- ABG analysis indicates respiratory alkalosis (low partial pressure of carbon dioxide, low or normal bicarbonate level, and high pH).
- Blood cultures isolate the organism.
- Blood tests show decreased platelet count and leukocytosis (15,000 to 30,000/µl), increased BUN and creatinine levels, decreased creatinine clearance, and abnormal PT and PTT.
- ECG shows ST-segment depression, inverted T waves, and arrhythmias resembling myocardial infarction.

NURSING DIAGNOSES

- Decreased cardiac output
- Deficient fluid volume
- Risk for injury

- Ineffective peripheral tissue perfusion
- Disturbed thought processes
- Hyperthermia

TREATMENT
- Removing or replacing any I.V., intra-arterial, or indwelling urinary catheters that may be the source of infection
- Oxygen therapy (may require endotracheal intubation and mechanical ventilation)
- Colloid or crystalloid infusion to increase intravascular volume
- Blood transfusion, if anemia is present
- Surgery to drain abscesses, if present

Drug therapy
- Antibiotics: according to sensitivity of causative organism
- Diuretic: furosemide (Lasix) after sufficient fluid volume has been replaced to maintain urine output above 20 ml/hour
- Vasopressor: dopamine or norepinephrine (Levophed) if fluid resuscitation fails to increase blood pressure

INTERVENTIONS AND RATIONALES
- Replace I.V., intra-arterial, or indwelling urinary catheters that may be a source of infection *to decrease the client's risk of infection.*
- Administer normal saline solution or lactated Ringer's solution *to support blood pressure and replace fluid.*
- Administer oxygen therapy. Assist with endotracheal intubation, if indicated, and maintain mechanical ventilation *to support organ perfusion.*
- Monitor pulmonary artery catheter readings *to monitor fluid volume status and cardiac output.* Check ABG values for adequate oxygenation or gas exchange, watching for any changes *to prevent hypoxemia.*
- Monitor intake and output for body fluid loss *to prevent dehydration.*
- Administer antibiotics I.V. *to achieve effective blood levels quickly* and monitor drug levels *to prevent toxicity.*
- Monitor vital signs and pulse oximetry *to detect changes in condition.*
- Administer vasopressors and titrate appropriately *to support blood pressure.*
- Assess for complications of septic shock: DIC (abnormal bleeding), renal failure

(oliguria, increased specific gravity), heart failure (dyspnea, edema, tachycardia, distended neck veins), GI ulcers (hematemesis, melena), and hepatic abnormalities (jaundice, hypoprothrombinemia, and hypoalbuminemia) *to prevent crisis.*
- Monitor respiratory, cardiovascular, and neurologic status. Assist with endotracheal intubation, if necessary, *to provide adequate oxygenation.*

Teaching topics
- Explanation of the disorder and treatment plan
- Drug therapy
- Risk associated with blood transfusion

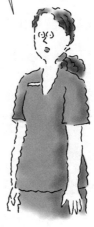

This is an example of NCLEX-induced shock.

Sickle cell anemia

Sickle cell anemia is a congenital hematologic disease that causes impaired circulation, chronic ill health, and premature death. Although it's most common in tropical Africa and in people of African descent, it also occurs in people from Puerto Rico, Turkey, India, the Middle East, and the Mediterranean.

In clients with sickle cell anemia, a change in the gene that encodes the beta chain of Hb results in a defect in HbS. When hypoxia (oxygen deficiency) occurs, the HbS in the RBCs becomes insoluble. The cells become rigid and rough, forming an elongated sickle shape and impairing circulation. Infection, stress, dehydration, and conditions that provoke hypoxia—strenuous exercise, high altitude, unpressurized aircraft, cold, and vasoconstrictive drugs—may all provoke periodic crisis. Crises can occur in different forms, including painful crisis, aplastic crisis, and acute sequestration crisis.

CAUSES
- Genetic inheritance: results from homozygous inheritance of an autosomal recessive gene that produces a defective Hb molecule (HbS); heterozygous inheritance results in sickle cell trait (people with this trait are carriers who can then pass the gene to their offspring)

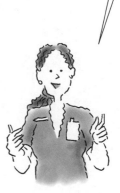

In the autosomal recessive inheritance pattern, if two carriers have offspring, each child has a one-in-four chance of developing the disease.

ASSESSMENT FINDINGS
- Aching bones
- Chronic fatigue
- Family history of the disease
- Frequent infections
- Jaundice, pallor
- Joint swelling
- Leg ulcers (especially on ankles)
- Severe localized and generalized pain
- Tachycardia
- Unexplained dyspnea or dyspnea on exertion
- Unexplained, painful erections (priapism)

Sickle cell crisis (general symptoms)
- Hematuria
- Irritability
- Lethargy
- Pale lips, tongue, palms, and nail beds
- Severe pain

Painful crisis (vaso-occlusive crisis, which appears periodically after age 5)
- Dark urine
- Low-grade fever
- Severe abdominal, thoracic, muscle, or bone pain
- Tissue anoxia and necrosis, caused by blood vessel obstruction by tangled sickle cells
- Worsening of jaundice

Aplastic crisis (generally associated with viral infection)
- Dyspnea
- Lethargy, sleepiness
- Markedly decreased bone marrow activity
- Pallor
- Possible coma
- RBC hemolysis (destruction)

Acute sequestration crisis (rare; occurs in infants ages 8 months to 2 years)
- Hypovolemic shock caused by entrapment of RBCs in spleen and liver
- Lethargy
- Liver congestion and enlargement
- Pallor
- Worsened chronic jaundice

DIAGNOSTIC TEST RESULTS
- Blood tests show low RBC counts, elevated WBC and platelet counts, decreased ESR, increased serum iron levels, decreased RBC survival, and reticulocytosis.
- Hb electrophoresis shows HbS.
- Hb levels may be low or normal.
- Stained blood smear shows sickle cells.

NURSING DIAGNOSES
- Impaired gas exchange
- Acute pain
- Risk for activity intolerance
- Fatigue
- Ineffective peripheral tissue perfusion

TREATMENT
- Application of warm compresses for pain relief
- Blood transfusion therapy if Hb levels drop
- I.V. fluid therapy to prevent dehydration and vessel occlusion

Drug therapy
- Analgesic: meperidine or morphine to relieve pain from vaso-occlusive crises
- Supplements: iron, folic acid

INTERVENTIONS AND RATIONALES
- Monitor vital signs *to identify complications.*
- Assess pain level and administer analgesics *to promote comfort.*
- Provide emotional support *to allay anxiety.*
- Refer for genetic counseling *to decrease anxiety and help understand the chances of passing the disease to offspring.*
- Refer client and family to community support groups *to help him and his family cope with his illness.*

During a crisis
- Apply warm compresses to painful areas. *Cold compresses and temperature can aggravate the condition.*
- Administer an analgesic-antipyretic, such as aspirin or acetaminophen, *for pain relief.* (Additional pain relief may be necessary during an acute crisis.)
- Maintain bed rest *to reduce workload on the heart and reduce pain.*
- Administer blood components (packed RBCs) as ordered *for aplastic crisis caused by bone marrow suppression.*
- Administer oxygen *to enhance oxygenation and reduce sickling.*

- Encourage fluid intake *to prevent dehydration, which can precipitate a crisis.*
- Administer prescribed I.V. fluids *to ensure fluid balance and renal perfusion.*
- Give antibiotics as ordered *to treat infections and avoid precipitating a crisis.*

Teaching topics

- Explanation of the disorder and treatment plan
- Supplements
- Signs and symptoms of complications
- Avoiding circulation restriction
- Importance of normal childhood immunizations
- Importance of prompt treatment for infections
- Maintaining increased fluid intake to prevent dehydration
- Preventing hypoxia

Sodium imbalance

Sodium is the major cation (positively charged ion) in extracellular fluid. Its functions include maintaining tonicity and concentration of extracellular fluid, acid-base balance (reabsorption of sodium ions and excretion of hydrogen ions), nerve conduction and neuromuscular function, glandular secretion, and water balance.

A sodium-potassium pump is constantly at work in every body cell. Potassium is the major cation in intracellular fluid. According to the laws of diffusion, a substance moves from an area of high concentration to an area of lower concentration. Sodium ions, normally most abundant outside the cells, want to diffuse inward. Potassium ions, normally outside the cells, want to diffuse outward. The sodium-potassium pump works to combat this ionic diffusion and maintain normal sodium-potassium balance.

During repolarization, the sodium-potassium pump continually shifts sodium into the cells and potassium out of the cells; during depolarization, it does the reverse.

The body requires only 2 to 4 g of sodium daily. However, most Americans consume 6 to 10 g daily (mostly sodium chloride, as table salt), excreting excess sodium through the kidneys and skin.

A low-sodium diet or excessive use of diuretics may induce hyponatremia (decreased serum sodium concentration); dehydration may induce hypernatremia (increased serum sodium concentration).

CAUSES
Hyponatremia

- Diarrhea
- Excessive perspiration or fever
- Excessive water intake
- Low-sodium diet
- Malnutrition
- Potent diuretics
- Starvation
- Suctioning
- Trauma, wound drainage, or burns
- Vomiting

Hypernatremia

- Decreased water intake
- Diabetes insipidus
- Excess adrenocortical hormones, as in Cushing's syndrome
- Severe vomiting and diarrhea with water loss that exceeds sodium loss

ASSESSMENT FINDINGS
Hyponatremia

- Abdominal cramps
- Altered mental status
- Anxiety
- Cold, clammy skin
- Cyanosis
- Headaches
- Hypotension
- Muscle twitching and weakness
- Nausea and vomiting
- Oliguria or anuria
- Renal dysfunction
- Seizures
- Tachycardia

Hypernatremia

- Agitation and restlessness
- Circulatory disorders
- Decreased level of consciousness
- Dry, sticky mucous membranes
- Dyspnea
- Excessive weight gain
- Fever
- Flushed skin

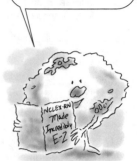

Pass the salt. The body needs sodium to maintain proper extracellular fluid osmolality, the proper concentration of fluid outside cells.

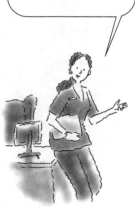

A sodium-potassium pump is constantly at work in every body cell to maintain normal sodium-potassium balance.

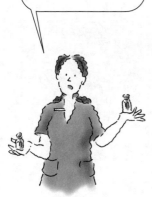

Too little sodium can cause kidney dysfunction and, in severe cases, seizures. Too much sodium can produce fluid in the lungs, circulatory disorders, and decreased level of consciousness.

- Hypertension
- Intense thirst
- Oliguria
- Pitting edema
- Pulmonary edema
- Rough, dry tongue
- Seizures
- Tachycardia

DIAGNOSTIC TEST RESULTS
- Serum sodium level less than 135 mEq/L indicates hyponatremia.
- Serum sodium level greater than 145 mEq/L indicates hypernatremia.

NURSING DIAGNOSES
Hyponatremia
- Deficient fluid volume
- Risk for injury
- Anxiety

Hypernatremia
- Excess fluid volume
- Disturbed thought processes

TREATMENT
Hyponatremia
- Antibiotic: demeclocycline (Declomycin)
- I.V. infusion of saline solution
- Potassium supplement: potassium chloride (K-Lor)

Hypernatremia
- Low-sodium diet
- Salt-free I.V. solution (such as dextrose in water), followed by infusion of 0.45% sodium chloride to prevent hyponatremia

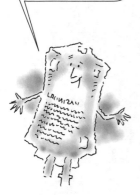

Don't overdo it. During administration of isosmolar or hyperosmolar saline solution to a client with hyponatremia, watch closely for signs of hypervolemia.

INTERVENTIONS AND RATIONALES
Hyponatremia
- Monitor serum sodium and serum chloride levels. Monitor urine specific gravity and other laboratory results. Monitor fluid intake and output, and weigh the client daily *to guide the treatment plan.*
- Assess for signs of fluid overload *to detect complications.*
- During administration of isosmolar or hyperosmolar saline solution, watch closely for signs of hypervolemia (dyspnea, crackles, engorged neck or hand veins) *to prevent respiratory distress.*

- Note conditions that may cause excessive sodium loss—diaphoresis, prolonged diarrhea or vomiting, or severe burns—*to prevent hyponatremia.*
- Refer the client receiving a maintenance dosage of diuretics to a dietitian for instruction about dietary sodium intake *to increase dietary intake of sodium and decrease the risk of hyponatremia.*

Hypernatremia
- Monitor serum sodium levels every 6 hours or at least daily *to detect changes.*
- Monitor vital signs, especially for rising pulse rate, *to detect changes.*
- Assess for signs of hypervolemia, especially in the client receiving I.V. fluids, *to guide the treatment regimen.*
- Monitor fluid intake and output, checking for body fluid loss *to prevent dehydration and accompanying hypernatremia.*
- Weigh the client daily *to monitor fluid volume status.*
- Obtain a drug history *to check for drugs that promote sodium retention.*

Teaching topics
- Explanation of the disorder and treatment plan
- Supplements
- Nutritional therapy
- Drug therapy

Systemic lupus erythematosus

SLE is an autoimmune disorder that involves most organ systems. It's chronic in nature and characterized by periods of exacerbation and remission.

In SLE, there's a depression of T-cell activity and an increase in the production of antibodies, specifically antibodies to DNA and ribonucleic acid and anti-erythrocyte, antinuclear, and antiplatelet antibodies. The immune response results in an inflammatory process involving the veins and arteries (vasculitis), which causes pain, swelling, and tissue damage in any area of the body.

CAUSES
- Autoimmune disease
- Drug-induced: procainamide, hydralazine, and phenytoin (Dilantin)
- Genetic
- Unknown
- Viral

ASSESSMENT FINDINGS
- Alopecia
- Anorexia and weight loss
- Anemia, leukopenia, and thrombocytopenia
- Butterfly rash on face (rash may vary in severity from malar erythema to discoid lesions)
- Erythema on palms
- Fatigue
- Glomerulonephritis, renal dysfunction and failure (renal involvement)
- Impaired cognitive function, psychosis, depression, seizures, peripheral neuropathies, strokes, and organic brain syndrome (central nervous system involvement)
- Low-grade fever
- Lymphadenopathy, splenomegaly, and hepatomegaly
- Migratory pain, stiffness, and joint swelling
- Oral and nasopharyngeal ulcerations
- Photosensitivity
- Pleurisy, pericarditis, myocarditis, noninfectious endocarditis, and hypertension (cardiac involvement)
- Raynaud's phenomenon

DIAGNOSTIC TEST RESULTS
- ANA test is positive.
- Blood chemistry shows decreased complement fixation.
- Hematology shows decreased Hb, HCT, WBC, and platelets and an increased ESR.
- Lupus erythematosus cell preparation is positive.
- Rheumatoid factor is positive.
- Urine chemistry shows proteinuria and hematuria.

NURSING DIAGNOSES
- Impaired physical mobility
- Ineffective breathing pattern
- Risk for infection
- Fatigue
- Imbalanced nutrition: Less than body requirements

TREATMENT
- Diet high in iron, protein, and vitamins (especially vitamin C)
- Hemodialysis or kidney transplant, if renal failure occurs
- Limited exertion and maintenance of adequate rest
- Plasmapheresis

Drug therapy
- Analgesic: aspirin
- Antianemics: ferrous sulfate (Feosol), ferrous gluconate (Fergon)
- Antirheumatic: hydroxychloroquine (Plaquenil)
- Cytotoxic drugs: azathioprine (Imuran), methotrexate (Trexall); these drugs may delay or prevent deteriorating renal status
- Glucocorticoid: prednisone
- Immunosuppressants: azathioprine (Imuran), cyclophosphamide (Cytoxan)
- NSAIDs: indomethacin (Indocin), ibuprofen (Motrin), sulindac (Clinoril), piroxicam (Feldene), flurbiprofen (Ansaid), diclofenac (Voltaren), naproxen (Naprosyn), diflunisal

INTERVENTIONS AND RATIONALES
- Assess musculoskeletal status *to determine the client's baseline functional abilities.*
- Monitor renal status. *Decreased urine output without lowered fluid intake may indicate decreased renal perfusion, a possible indication of decreased cardiac output.*
- Monitor vital signs *to promptly determine if the client's condition is deteriorating and evaluate the effectiveness of treatment. Fever can signal an exacerbation.*
- Provide prophylactic skin, mouth, and perineal care *to prevent skin and oral mucous membrane breakdown.*
- Administer medications, as ordered, and monitor for adverse reactions *to enhance the treatment regimen.*
- Maintain seizure precautions *to prevent client injury.*
- Monitor dietary intake *to help ensure adequate nutritional intake.*

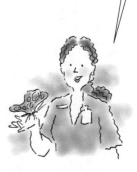

SLE can affect many different organs, but note that a butterfly rash is the signature finding.

- Minimize environmental stress and provide rest periods *to avoid fatigue and help the client to cope with illness.*
- Promote independence in ADLs *to help the client develop self-esteem.*
- Administer antiemetics *to alleviate nausea and vomiting.*
- Administer antidiarrheals, as prescribed, *to alleviate diarrhea.*
- Encourage verbalization of feelings about changes in body image and the chronic nature of the disease *to help the client voice doubts and resolve concerns.*

Teaching topics
- Explanation of the disorder and treatment plan
- Drug therapy
- Nutritional therapy
- Smoking cessation (if appropriate)
- Stress reduction techniques
- Signs and symptoms of complications
- Avoiding exposure to people with infections
- Performing daily, complete mouth care
- Avoiding OTC medications
- Avoiding exposure to sunlight
- Avoiding hair spray or hair coloring
- Avoiding hormonal contraceptives
- Using liquid cosmetics to cover rashes
- Contacting groups such as the Lupus Foundation of America

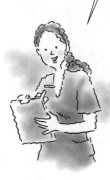

One name, many disorders. Vasculitis refers to a variety of disorders characterized by inflammation and necrosis of blood vessels.

Vasculitis

Vasculitis is a broad spectrum of disorders characterized by inflammation and necrosis of blood vessels. Its clinical effects depend on the vessels involved and reflect tissue ischemia caused by blood flow obstruction.

Prognosis is also variable. For example, hypersensitivity vasculitis is usually a benign disorder limited to the skin, but more extensive polyarteritis nodosa can be rapidly fatal.

Vasculitis can occur at any age, except for mucocutaneous lymph node syndrome, which occurs only during childhood. Vasculitis may be a primary disorder or secondary to other disorders, such as rheumatoid arthritis or SLE.

CAUSES
- Excessive levels of antigen
- High-dose antibiotic therapy
- Often associated with serious infectious disease such as hepatitis B or bacterial endocarditis

ASSESSMENT FINDINGS
A few examples of vasculitis and their specific assessment findings are listed here.

Wegener's granulomatosis
This form of vasculitis affects medium- to large-sized vessels of the upper and lower respiratory tract and kidney; may also involve small arteries and veins. Assessment findings include:
- anorexia
- cough
- fever
- malaise
- mild to severe hematuria
- pulmonary congestion
- weight loss.

Temporal arteritis
Temporal arteritis affects medium- to large-sized arteries, most commonly branches of the carotid artery; involvement may skip segments. Assessment findings include:
- fever
- headache (associated with polymyalgia rheumatica syndrome)
- jaw claudication
- myalgia
- visual changes.

Takayasu's arteritis
Also known as *aortic arch syndrome*, Takayasu's arteritis affects medium- to large-sized arteries, particularly the aortic arch and its branches and, possibly, the pulmonary artery. Assessment findings include:
- anorexia
- arthralgias
- bruits
- diplopia and transient blindness if carotid artery is involved
- heart failure (with disease progression)
- loss of distal pulses
- malaise

- nausea
- night sweats
- pain or paresthesia distal to affected area
- pallor
- stroke (with disease progression)
- syncope
- weight loss.

DIAGNOSTIC TEST RESULTS
Wegener's granulomatosis
- Tissue biopsy shows necrotizing vasculitis with granulomatous inflammation.
- Blood studies show leukocytosis, elevated ESR, IgA, and IgG; low titer rheumatoid factor; circulating immune complexes: antineutrophil cytoplasmic antibody in more than 90% of clients.
- Renal biopsy shows focal segmental glomerulonephritis.

Temporal arteritis
- Blood studies show decreased Hb and elevated ESR.
- Tissue biopsy shows panarteritis with infiltration of mononuclear cells, giant cells within vessel wall (seen in 50%), fragmentation of internal elastic lamina, and proliferation of intima.

Takayasu's arteritis
- Blood studies show decreased Hb, leukocytosis, positive lupus erythematosus cell preparation, and elevated ESR.
- Arteriography shows calcification and obstruction of affected vessels.
- Tissue biopsy shows inflammation of adventitia and intima of vessels and thickening of vessel walls.

NURSING DIAGNOSES
- Ineffective peripheral tissue perfusion
- Risk for injury
- Disturbed sensory perception (tactile)
- Hyperthermia
- Imbalanced nutrition: Less than body requirements

TREATMENT
- Removal of identified environmental antigen
- Diet: elimination of antigenic food, if identifiable; increased fluid intake (3 qt [3 L] daily), if not contraindicated

Drug therapy
- Corticosteroid: prednisone
- Antineoplastic: cyclophosphamide (Cytoxan)

INTERVENTIONS AND RATIONALES
- Assess for dry nasal mucosa in clients with Wegener's granulomatosis. Instill nose drops *to lubricate the mucosa and help diminish crusting.* Or irrigate the nasal passages with warm normal saline solution *to combat drying.*
- Regulate environmental temperature *to prevent additional vasoconstriction caused by cold.*
- Monitor vital signs. Use a Doppler ultrasonic flowmeter, if available, *to auscultate blood pressure in clients with Takayasu's arteritis, whose peripheral pulses are frequently difficult to palpate.*
- Monitor intake and output and assess for edema *to reduce the risk of hemorrhagic cystitis associated with cyclophosphamide therapy.*
- Provide emotional support to help the client and his family cope with an altered body image—the result of the disorder or its therapy. (For example, Wegener's granulomatosis may be associated with saddle nose, steroids may cause weight gain, and cyclophosphamide may cause alopecia.)
- Monitor WBC count during cyclophosphamide therapy *to prevent severe leukopenia.*

Teaching topics
- Explanation of the disorder and treatment plan
- Drug therapy
- Signs and symptoms of complications
- Importance of increasing fluids during cyclophosphamide therapy

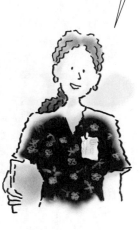

Treatment for vasculitis aims to minimize tissue damage associated with decreased blood flow.

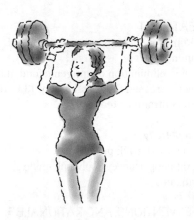

Pump up on practice questions

1. A client with major abdominal trauma needs an emergency blood transfusion. The client's blood type is AB negative. Of the blood types available, the safest type for the nurse to administer is:

  1. AB positive.
  2. A positive.
  3. B negative.
  4. O positive.

Answer: 3. Individuals with AB negative blood (AB type, Rh negative) can receive A negative, B negative, and AB negative blood. It's unsafe to give Rh-positive blood to an Rh-negative person.

➡ *NCLEX keys*

Client needs category: Physiological integrity
Client needs subcategory: Pharmacological and parenteral therapies
Cognitive level: Application

2. A nurse is preparing a client with systemic lupus erythematosus for discharge. Which instructions should the nurse include in the teaching plan?

  1. Exposure to sunlight will help control skin rashes.
  2. There are no activity limitations between flare-ups.
  3. Monitor body temperature.
  4. Corticosteroids may be stopped when symptoms are relieved.

Answer: 3. The client should monitor his temperature because fever can signal an exacerbation and should be reported to the physician. Sunlight and other sources of ultraviolet light may precipitate severe skin reactions and exacerbate the disease. Fatigue can cause a flare-up of systemic lupus erythematosus, and clients should be encouraged to pace activities and plan for rest periods. Corticosteroids must be gradually tapered because they can suppress the function of the adrenal gland. Abruptly stopping corticosteroids can cause adrenal insufficiency, a potentially life-threatening situation.

➡ *NCLEX keys*

Client needs category: Physiological integrity
Client needs subcategory: Reduction of risk potential
Cognitive level: Application

3. The nurse is administering didanosine (Videx) to a client with acquired immunodeficiency syndrome. Which intervention is most appropriate?

  1. Crushing the tablets and mixing them with fruit juice
  2. Instructing the client to swallow the tablets whole with water
  3. Telling the client to chew the tablets thoroughly before swallowing
  4. Dissolving the tablets in fruit juice

Answer: 3. Didanosine is an antiretroviral drug (reverse transcriptase inhibitor) that's given to treat human immunodeficiency virus infections. Didanosine tablets contain buffers that raise stomach pH to levels that prevent degradation of the active drug. Tablets must be chewed thoroughly before swallowing. They may also be crushed and mixed with water. They shouldn't be added to fruit juices or other acidic liquids. Tablets may be dispersed in a nonacidic liquid for administration. Didanosine tablets aren't taken whole.

➡ *NCLEX keys*

Client needs category: Physiological integrity
Client needs subcategory: Pharmacological and parenteral therapies
Cognitive level: Application

4. A client with thrombocytopenia, secondary to leukemia, develops epistaxis. The nurse should instruct the client to:
1. lie supine with his neck extended.
2. sit upright, leaning slightly forward.
3. blow his nose and then put lateral pressure on his nose.
4. hold his nose while bending forward at the waist.

Answer: 2. The upright position, leaning slightly forward, avoids increasing the vascular pressure in the nose and helps the client avoid aspirating blood. Lying supine won't prevent aspiration of the blood. Nose blowing can dislodge any clotting that has occurred. Bending at the waist increases vascular pressure in the nose and promotes bleeding rather than halting it.

➡ *NCLEX keys*
Client needs category: Physiological integrity
Client needs subcategory: Physiological adaptation
Cognitive level: Application

5. The nurse is preparing to administer iron dextran (Imferon) to a client with iron deficiency anemia. Which action is appropriate?
1. Using a 25G needle
2. Administering a Z-track injection
3. Using the same needle to draw up the solution and to administer the injection
4. Preparing the deltoid site for injection

Answer: 2. A Z-track or zig-zag technique should be used to administer an iron injection. This prevents iron from leaking into and irritating the subcutaneous tissue. A 25G needle is used for a subcutaneous injection, not for a deep I.M. injection (such as that needed to administer iron). The needle should be changed after drawing up the iron solution to avoid staining and irritating the tissues. A deep I.M. site such as the upper outer quadrant of the buttocks should be used to administer iron; the deltoid site doesn't provide enough muscle mass for an iron injection.

➡ *NCLEX keys*
Client needs category: Physiological integrity
Client needs subcategory: Pharmacological and parenteral therapies
Cognitive level: Application

6. A nurse is reviewing the laboratory report of a client who underwent a bone marrow biopsy. The finding that would most strongly support a diagnosis of acute leukemia is the presence of a large number of immature:
1. monocytes.
2. thrombocytes.
3. basophils.
4. leukocytes.

Answer: 4. Leukemia is manifested by an abnormal overproduction of immature leukocytes in the bone marrow. An increased number of monocytes may result from a viral infection. An increased number of basophils may result from an allergic reaction. A large number of thrombocytes indicates polycythemia vera.

➡ *NCLEX keys*
Client needs category: Physiological integrity
Client needs subcategory: Reduction of risk potential
Cognitive level: Comprehension

7. Which nonpharmacologic interventions should a nurse include in the care plan for a client who has moderate rheumatoid arthritis? Select all that apply.
1. Massaging inflamed joints
2. Avoiding range-of-motion (ROM) exercises
3. Applying splints to inflamed joints
4. Using assistive devices at all times
5. Selecting clothing that has Velcro fasteners
6. Applying moist heat to joints

Answer: 3, 5, 6. Supportive, nonpharmacologic measures for a client with rheumatoid arthritis include applying splints to rest inflamed joints, choosing clothes with Velcro fasteners to aid in dressing, and applying moist heat to joints to relax muscles and relieve pain. Inflamed joints should never be massaged because doing so can aggravate inflammation. A physical therapy program including ROM exercises and carefully individualized therapeutic exercises prevents loss of joint function. Assistive devices should be used only when marked loss of ROM occurs.

➡ *NCLEX keys*

Clients needs category: Physiologic integrity
Client needs subcategory: Basic care and comfort
Cognitive level: Application

8. A nurse is providing care for a client with acquired immunodeficiency syndrome (AIDS) and *Pneumocystis* pneumonia (PCP). The client is receiving aerosolized pentamidine isethionate (NebuPent). What is the best evidence that the therapy is succeeding?
1. A sudden gain in lost body weight
2. Whitening of lung fields on the chest X-ray
3. Improving client vitality and activity tolerance
4. Afebrile body temperature and development of leukocytosis

Answer: 3. Because a common manifestation of PCP is activity intolerance and loss of vitality, improvements in these areas would suggest success of pentamidine isethionate therapy. Sudden weight gain, whitening of the lung fields on chest X-ray, and leukocytosis aren't evidence of therapeutic success.

➡ *NCLEX keys*

Client needs category: Physiological integrity
Client needs subcategory: Pharmacological and parenteral therapies
Cognitive level: Application

9. A nurse is documenting her care for a client with iron deficiency anemia. Which nursing diagnosis is most appropriate?
1. *Impaired gas exchange*
2. *Deficient fluid volume*
3. *Ineffective airway clearance*
4. *Ineffective breathing pattern*

Answer: 1. Hemoglobin is responsible for oxygen transport in the body. Iron is necessary for hemoglobin synthesis. Iron deficiency anemia causes subnormal hemoglobin levels, which impair tissue oxygenation and impair gas exchange. Iron deficiency anemia doesn't cause deficient fluid volume and is less directly related to ineffective airway clearance and breathing pattern than it is to impaired gas exchange.

➡ *NCLEX keys*

Client needs category: Physiological integrity
Client needs subcategory: Physiological adaptation
Cognitive level: Comprehension

10. A nurse is administering cyanocobalamin (vitamin B_{12}) to a client with pernicious anemia, secondary to gastrectomy. Which administration route should the nurse use?
1. Topical route
2. Transdermal route
3. Enteral route
4. Parenteral route

Answer: 4. Following a gastrectomy, the client no longer has the intrinsic factor available to promote vitamin B_{12} absorption in his GI tract. Vitamin B_{12} is administered parenterally (I.M. or deep subcutaneous). Topical and transdermal administrations aren't available, and the enteral route is inappropriate in a gastrectomy.

➡ *NCLEX keys*

Client needs category: Physiological integrity
Client needs subcategory: Pharmacological and parenteral therapies
Cognitive level: Application

> Now it's time to reward yourself. Remember, it's an important part of an effective study program.

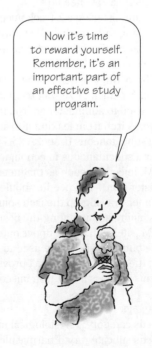

6 Neurosensory system

Brush up on key concepts

The neurosensory system serves as the body's communication network. It processes information from the outside world (through the sensory portion) and coordinates and organizes the functions of all other body systems. Major parts of the neurosensory system include the brain, spinal cord, peripheral nerves, eyes, and ears.

At any time, you can review the major points of the disorders in this chapter by consulting the *Cheat sheet* on pages 176 to 183.

The little conductor that could

The **neuron,** or nerve cell, is the basic functional unit of the neurosensory system. This highly specialized conductor cell receives and transmits electrochemical nerve impulses. From its cell body, delicate, thread-like nerve fibers called axons and dendrites extend and transmit signals. Axons carry impulses away from the cell body; dendrites carry impulses toward the cell body.

A covering called a myelin sheath protects the entire neuron. Substances known as *neurotransmitters* (acetylcholine, serotonin, dopamine, endorphins, gamma-aminobutyric acid, and norepinephrine) help conduct impulses across a synapse and into the next neuron.

House of intelligence

The **central nervous system** (CNS) includes the brain and spinal cord. These fragile structures are protected by the skull and vertebrae, cerebrospinal fluid (CSF), and three membranes: the dura mater, the pia mater, and the arachnoid membrane.

The **cerebrum,** the largest part of the brain, houses the nerve center that controls motor and sensory functions and intelligence. It's divided into hemispheres. Because motor impulses descending from the brain cross in the medulla, the right hemisphere controls the left side of the body and the left hemisphere controls the right side of the body. Several fissures divide the cerebrum into four lobes:
• frontal lobe—the site of personality, memory, reasoning, concentration, and motor control of speech
• parietal lobe—the site of sensation, integration of sensory information, and spatial relationships
• temporal lobe—the site of hearing, speech, memory, and emotion
• occipital lobe—the site of vision and involuntary eye movements.

Brain networking

The **thalamus** is a structure located deep within the brain that consists of two oval-shaped parts, one located in each hemisphere. The thalamus is referred to as the relay station of the brain because it receives input from all of the senses except olfaction (smell), analyzes that input, and then transmits that information to other parts of the brain.

The **hypothalamus,** located beneath the thalamus, controls sleep and wakefulness, temperature, respiration, blood pressure, sexual arousal, fluid balance, and emotional response.

Movement, balance, and posture

The **cerebellum,** at the base of the brain, coordinates muscle movements, maintains balance, and controls posture.

(Text continues on page 183.)

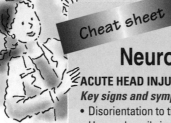

Cheat sheet

Neurosensory refresher

ACUTE HEAD INJURY

Key signs and symptoms
- Disorientation to time, place, or person
- Unequal pupil size, loss of pupillary reaction (if edema is present)

Key test results
- Computed tomography (CT) scan shows hemorrhage, cerebral edema, or shift of midline structures.
- Magnetic resonance imaging (MRI) shows hemorrhage, cerebral edema, or shift of midline structures.

Key treatments
- Cervical collar (until neck injury is ruled out)
- Anticonvulsant: phenytoin (Dilantin)
- Barbiturate: pentobarbital (Nembutal) if unable to control intracranial pressure (ICP) with diuresis
- Diuretics: mannitol, furosemide (Lasix) to combat cerebral edema
- Dopamine to maintain cerebral perfusion pressure above 50 mm Hg (if blood pressure is low and ICP is elevated)
- Glucocorticoid: dexamethasone to reduce cerebral edema
- Histamine$_2$ (H$_2$)-receptor antagonists: ranitidine (Zantac), famotidine (Pepcid), nizatidine (Axid)
- Mucosal barrier fortifier: sucralfate (Carafate)
- Posterior pituitary hormone: vasopressin if client develops diabetes insipidus

Key interventions
- Assess neurologic and respiratory status.
- Observe for signs of increasing ICP (including ICP measurements greater than 20 mm Hg for more than 10 minutes).
- Monitor and record vital signs, intake and output, hemodynamic variables, ICP measurements, cerebral perfusion pressure, specific gravity, laboratory studies, and pulse oximetry.
- Monitor for signs of diabetes insipidus (low urine specific gravity, high urine output).
- Provide rest periods between nursing activities.

AMYOTROPHIC LATERAL SCLEROSIS

Key signs and symptoms
- Awkwardness of fine finger movements
- Dysphagia

- Fatigue
- Muscle weakness in the hands and feet

Key test results
- Creatinine kinase level is elevated.
- Electromyography (EMG) shows decreased amplitude of evoked potentials.

Key treatments
- Management of symptoms
- Neuroprotective agent: riluzole (Rilutek)

Key interventions
- Monitor neurologic and respiratory status.
- Assess swallow and gag reflexes.
- Monitor and record vital signs and intake and output.
- Devise an alternate method of communication, when necessary.
- Suction the oral pharynx, as necessary.
- Assist with range-of-motion (ROM) exercises.

BELL'S PALSY

Key signs and symptoms
- Inability to close eye completely on the affected side
- Pain around the jaw or ear of affected side
- Unilateral facial weakness

Key test results
- EMG helps predict the level of expected recovery by distinguishing temporary conduction defects from a pathologic interruption of nerve fibers.

Key treatments
- Moist heat
- Corticosteroid: prednisone to reduce facial nerve edema and improve nerve conduction and blood flow
- Artificial tears to protect the cornea from injury

Key interventions
- Monitor for adverse reactions to prednisone, especially GI distress, fluid retention, and hyperglycemia.
- Apply moist heat to the affected side of the face, taking care not to burn the skin.
- Massage the client's face with a gentle upward motion two to three times daily for 5 to 10 minutes, or have him massage his face himself. When he's ready for active exercises, teach him to exercise by grimacing in front of a mirror.

> When I'm on overload, I skip directly to the Cheat sheet.

Neurosensory refresher (continued)

BELL'S PALSY (CONTINUED)
• Provide privacy during mealtimes.
• Provide emotional support. Give reassurance that recovery is likely within 1 to 8 weeks.

BRAIN ABSCESS
Key signs and symptoms
• Headache
• Chills
• Fever
• Confusion
• Drowsiness

Key test results
• Physical examination shows signs of increased ICP.
• Enhanced CT scan reveals the abscess site.
• A CT-guided stereotactic biopsy may be performed to drain and culture the abscess.

Key treatments
• Penicillinase-resistant antibiotic: nafcillin
• Surgical aspiration or drainage of the abscess

Key interventions
• Monitor neurologic status, especially cognition and mentation, speech, and sensorimotor and cranial nerve function.
• Assess and record vital signs at least once every hour.
• Monitor fluid intake and output.
• Monitor for signs of meningitis (nuchal rigidity, headaches, chills, sweats).
• Perform dressing changes as needed.
• Position the client on the operative side.
• Measure drainage from Jackson-Pratt or other types of drains.

BRAIN TUMOR
Key signs and symptoms
Frontal lobe
• Memory loss
• Personality changes
Temporal lobe
• Aphasia
• Seizures
Parietal lobe
• Motor seizures
• Sensory impairment
Occipital lobe
• Visual impairment
Cerebellum
• Impaired coordination

Key test results
• CT scan shows location and size of tumor.
• MRI shows location and size of tumor.

Key treatments
• Craniotomy
• Anticonvulsant: phenytoin (Dilantin)
• Glucocorticoid: dexamethasone
• H_2-receptor antagonists: cimetidine (Tagamet), ranitidine (Zantac), famotidine (Pepcid), nizatidine (Axid)
• Mucosal barrier fortifier: sucralfate (Carafate)
• Chemotherapy
• Radiation therapy

Key interventions
• Monitor neurologic and respiratory status.
• Assess for and treat pain.
• Assess for signs of increased ICP.
• Monitor for signs and symptoms of syndrome of inappropriate antidiuretic hormone (edema, weight gain, positive fluid balance, high urine specific gravity).
• Provide support and encourage verbalization of feelings about changes in body image and fear of dying.

CATARACT
Key signs and symptoms
• Dimmed or blurred vision
• Better vision in dim light with pupil dilated
• Yellow, gray, or white pupil

Key test results
• Ophthalmoscopy or slit-lamp examination confirms the diagnosis by revealing a dark area in the normally homogeneous red reflex.

Key treatments
• Extracapsular cataract extraction or intracapsular lens implant

Key interventions
• Provide a safe environment for the client.
• Modify the environment to help the client meet his self-care needs (for example, by placing items on the unaffected side).

CEREBRAL ANEURYSM
Key signs and symptoms
• Headache (commonly described by the client as the worst he has ever had)
• Altered level of consciousness

Key test results
• Cerebral angiogram identifies the aneurysm.
• Spiral CT angiography shows a shift of intracranial midline structures, blood in subarachnoid space.

Key treatments
• Aneurysm clipping
• Endovascular embolization

(continued)

Neurosensory refresher *(continued)*

CEREBRAL ANEURYSM *(CONTINUED)*
- Anticonvulsant: phenytoin (Dilantin)
- Calcium channel blocker: nimodipine preferred to prevent cerebral vasospasm
- Glucocorticoid: dexamethasone
- H$_2$-receptor antagonists: cimetidine (Tagamet), ranitidine (Zantac), famotidine (Pepcid), nizatidine (Axid)
- Stool softener: docusate sodium (Colace)

Key interventions
- Monitor neurologic status.
- Administer crystalloid solutions after aneurysm clipping.
- Monitor vital signs every 1 to 2 hours initially and then every 4 hours when the client becomes stable.
- Provide rest periods between nursing activities.

CONJUNCTIVITIS
Key signs and symptoms
- Excessive tearing
- Itching, burning
- Mucopurulent discharge

Key test results
- Culture and sensitivity tests identify the causative bacterial organism and indicate appropriate antibiotic therapy.

Key treatments
- Antiviral agent: oral acyclovir (Zovirax) if herpes simplex is the cause
- Corticosteroids: dexamethasone, fluorometholone (Flarex)
- Mast cell stabilizer: cromolyn (Opticrom) for allergic conjunctivitis
- Topical antibiotics: according to the sensitivity of the infective organism (if bacterial)

Key interventions
- Teach proper hand-washing technique.
- Stress the risk of spreading infection to family members by sharing washcloths, towels, and pillows. Warn against rubbing the infected eye, which can spread the infection to the other eye and to other persons.
- Apply warm compresses and therapeutic ointment or drops. Don't irrigate the eye.
- Teach the client how to instill eyedrops and ointments correctly—without touching the bottle tip to his eye or lashes.

CORNEAL ABRASION
Key signs and symptoms
- Burning
- Increased tearing
- Redness
- Pain in affected eye disproportionate to the size of the injury

Key test results
- Staining the cornea with fluorescein stain confirms the diagnosis: the injured area appears green when examined with a flashlight.

Key treatments
- Cycloplegic agent: tropicamide (Mydriacyl)
- Irrigation with saline solution
- Pressure patch (a tightly applied eye patch)
- Removal of a deeply embedded foreign body with a foreign body spud, using a topical anesthetic

Key interventions
- Assist with examination of the eye. Check visual acuity before beginning treatment.
- Irrigate the eye with normal saline solution, if foreign body is visible.
- Stress the importance of instilling prescribed antibiotic eyedrops properly and leaving the eye patch in place for 6 to 8 hours.

ENCEPHALITIS
Key signs and symptoms
- Meningeal irritation (stiff neck and back) and neuronal damage (drowsiness, coma, paralysis, seizures, ataxia, and organic psychoses)
- Sudden onset of fever
- Headache
- Vomiting

Key test results
- Blood studies identify the virus and confirm diagnosis.
- Cerebrospinal fluid (CSF) analysis identifies the virus.

Key treatments
- Oxygen therapy: endotracheal intubation and mechanical ventilation
- Nasogastric tube feedings or total parenteral nutrition
- Anticonvulsants: phenytoin (Dilantin), phenobarbital
- Analgesics and antipyretics: aspirin or acetaminophen (Tylenol) to relieve headache and reduce fever
- Diuretic: furosemide (Lasix) or mannitol to reduce cerebral swelling
- Corticosteroid: dexamethasone to reduce cerebral inflammation and edema

Key interventions
During acute phase
- Monitor neurologic function often. Observe the client's mental status and cognitive abilities.
- Maintain adequate fluid balance. Measure and record intake and output accurately.

Neurosensory refresher (continued)

ENCEPHALITIS (CONTINUED)
- Reposition the client every 2 hours and provide skin care.
- Assist with ROM exercises.
- Maintain a quiet environment. Darken the room.

GLAUCOMA
Key signs and symptoms
Acute angle-closure glaucoma
- Acute ocular pain
- Blurred vision
- Dilated pupil
- Halo vision

Chronic open-angle glaucoma
- Initially asymptomatic

Key test results
- Ophthalmoscopy shows atrophy and cupping of optic nerve head.
- Tonometry shows increased intraocular pressure.

Key treatments
Acute angle-closure glaucoma
- Cholinergic agent: pilocarpine
- Laser iridectomy or surgical iridectomy if pressure doesn't decrease with drug therapy

Chronic open-angle glaucoma
- Alpha-adrenergic agonist: brimonidine (Alphagan-P)
- Beta-adrenergic antagonist: timolol (Timoptic)

Key interventions
- Assess eye pain and administer medication as prescribed.
- Modify the environment for safety.

GUILLAIN-BARRÉ SYNDROME
Key signs and symptoms
- Muscle weakness (ascending from the legs to arms and facial muscles)

Key test results
- A history of preceding febrile illness (usually a respiratory tract infection) and typical clinical features suggest Guillain-Barré syndrome.
- CSF protein level begins to rise, peaking in 4 to 6 weeks. The CSF white blood cell count remains normal but, in severe disease, CSF pressure may rise above normal.

Key treatments
- Immune globulin I.V.
- Corticosteroid: prednisone
- Endotracheal intubation or tracheotomy if the client has difficulty clearing secretions; possibly mechanical ventilation
- I.V. fluid therapy

- Nasogastric tube feedings or parenteral nutrition
- Plasmapheresis
- Prophylaxis for deep vein thrombosis (DVT)

Key interventions
- Monitor for ascending sensory loss, which precedes motor loss. Also, monitor vital signs and level of consciousness.
- Assess and treat respiratory dysfunction. If respiratory muscles are weak, take serial vital capacity recordings. Use a respirometer with a mouthpiece or a facemask for bedside testing.
- Monitor arterial blood gas measurements.
- Assist with endotracheal tube insertion, if respiratory failure occurs.
- Reposition the client every 2 hours and provide skin care.
- Provide nasogastric feedings or parenteral nutrition as ordered.
- Monitor for signs of DVT; provide prophylactic measures.
- Provide adequate fluid intake (2 qt [2 L]/day), unless contraindicated.
- Measure and record intake and output.

HEARING LOSS
Key signs and symptoms
- Inability to understand spoken word
- Sudden deafness
- Tinnitus

Key test results
- Audiologic examination provides evidence of hearing loss.
- Weber, Rinne, and specialized audiologic tests differentiate between conductive and sensorineural hearing loss.

Key treatments
- Hearing aids
- Speech and hearing rehabilitation

Key interventions
- Speak slowly and clearly.
- Make sure all staff members are aware of disability and client's preferred communication method.
- Provide emotional support.
- Determine cause of hearing loss, if possible.

HUNTINGTON'S DISEASE
Key signs and symptoms
- Dementia (can be mild at first but eventually disrupts the client's personality)
- Gradual loss of musculoskeletal control, eventually leading to total dependence

(continued)

Neurosensory refresher *(continued)*

HUNTINGTON'S DISEASE *(CONTINUED)*
Key test results
- Positron emission tomography detects the disease.
- Deoxyribonucleic acid analysis detects the disease.

Key treatments
- Antidepressant: imipramine (Tofranil) to help control choreic movements
- Antipsychotics: chlorpromazine and haloperidol (Haldol) to help control choreic movements
- Supportive, protective treatment aimed at relieving symptoms (because Huntington's disease has no known cure)

Key interventions
- Provide physical support by attending to the client's basic needs, such as hygiene, skin care, bowel and bladder care, and nutrition. Increase this support as mental and physical deterioration make him increasingly immobile.
- Assess psychological status and provide surveillance, if the client demonstrates suicidal ideations.

MÉNIÈRE'S DISEASE
Key signs and symptoms
- Sensorineural hearing loss
- Severe vertigo
- Tinnitus

Key test results
- Audiometric studies indicate a sensorineural hearing loss and loss of discrimination and recruitment.

Key treatments
- Restriction of sodium intake to less than 2 g/day
- Anticholinergic: atropine (may stop an attack in 20 to 30 minutes)
- Antihistamine: diphenhydramine (Benadryl) for severe attack

Key interventions
- Advise the client against reading and exposure to glaring lights.
- Provide assistance when getting out of bed or walking.
- Instruct the client to avoid sudden position changes and any tasks that vertigo makes hazardous.
Before surgery
- Monitor fluid intake and output.
- Administer antiemetics as necessary, and give small amounts of fluid frequently.
After surgery
- Tell the client to expect dizziness and nausea for 1 to 2 days after surgery.

MENINGITIS
Key signs and symptoms
- Chills
- Fever
- Headache
- Malaise
- Photophobia
- Positive Brudzinski's sign (client flexes hips or knees when the nurse places her hands behind his neck and bends it forward)—a sign of meningeal inflammation and irritation
- Positive Kernig's sign (pain or resistance when the client's leg is flexed at the hip or knee while he's in a supine position)
- Stiff neck and back
- Vomiting

Key test results
- A lumbar puncture shows elevated CSF pressure, cloudy or milky white CSF, high protein level, positive Gram stain and culture that usually identifies the infecting organism (unless it's a virus) and depressed CSF glucose concentration.
- Xpert EV test, when used in combination with other laboratory tests, can differentiate bacterial from viral meningitis.

Key treatments
- Analgesics or antipyretics: acetaminophen (Tylenol), aspirin
- Antibiotics: penicillin G (Pfizerpen), ampicillin (Omnipen), or nafcillin; or tetracycline (Sumycin) if allergic to penicillin
- Anticonvulsants: phenytoin (Dilantin), phenobarbital
- Bed rest
- Diuretic: mannitol
- Hypothermia blanket
- I.V. fluid administration
- Oxygen therapy, possibly with endotracheal intubation and mechanical ventilation

Key interventions
- Monitor neurologic function often.
- Monitor fluid balance. Maintain adequate fluid intake
- Measure central venous pressure and intake and output accurately.
- Suction the client only if necessary. Limit suctioning to 10 to 15 seconds per pass of the catheter.
- Position the client carefully.
- Maintain a quiet environment and darken the room.
- Assess pain level and administer analgesics as ordered. Evaluate effectiveness of treatment.

MULTIPLE SCLEROSIS
Key signs and symptoms
- Nystagmus, diplopia, blurred vision, optic neuritis
- Weakness, paresthesia, impaired sensation, paralysis

Key test results
- CT scan eliminates other diagnoses such as brain or spinal cord tumors.
- MRI of the brain and spine shows scarring or lesions.

Neurosensory refresher *(continued)*

MULTIPLE SCLEROSIS *(CONTINUED)*
Key treatments
- Plasmapheresis (for antibody removal)
- Cholinergic: bethanechol (Urecholine)
- Glucocorticoids: prednisone, dexamethasone, corticotropin (ACTH)
- Immunosuppressants: interferon beta-1b (Betaseron), cyclophosphamide (Cytoxan), methotrexate (Trexall)
- Skeletal muscle relaxants: dantrolene (Dantrium), baclofen (Lioresal)

Key interventions
- Assess changes in motor coordination, paralysis, or muscular weakness and report changes.
- Encourage verbalization of feelings about changes in body image and provide emotional support.
- Establish a bowel and bladder program.
- Maintain activity, as tolerated (alternating rest and activity).

MYASTHENIA GRAVIS
Key signs and symptoms
- Dysphagia, drooling
- Muscle weakness and fatigability (typically, muscles are strongest in the morning but weaken throughout the day, especially after exercise)
- Profuse sweating

Key test results
- EMG shows decreased amplitude of evoked potentials.
- Neostigmine (Prostigmin) or edrophonium (Tensilon) test relieves symptoms after medication administration—a positive indication of the disease

Key treatments
- Anticholinesterase inhibitors: neostigmine (Prostigmin), pyridostigmine (Mestinon), ambenonium (Mytelase)
- Glucocorticoids: prednisone, dexamethasone, corticotropin (ACTH)
- Immunosuppressants: azathioprine (Imuran), cyclophosphamide (Cytoxan)

Key interventions
- Monitor neurologic and respiratory status.
- Assess swallow and gag reflexes.
- Monitor client for choking while eating.

OTOSCLEROSIS
Key signs and symptoms
- Progressive hearing loss
- Tinnitus

Key test results
- Audiometric testing confirms hearing loss.

Key treatments
- Stapedectomy and insertion of a prosthesis to restore partial or total hearing

Key interventions
- Develop alternative means of communication.

PARKINSON'S DISEASE
Key signs and symptoms
- Pill-rolling tremors, tremors at rest
- Masklike facial expression
- Shuffling gait, stiff joints, dyskinesia, cogwheel rigidity, stooped posture

Key test results
- EEG reveals minimal slowing of brain activity.

Key treatments
- Antidepressant: amitriptyline (Elavil)
- Antiparkinsonian agents: carbidopa-levodopa (Sinemet), benztropine (Cogentin)
- Deep brain stimulation

Key interventions
- Monitor neurologic and respiratory status.
- Reinforce gait training.
- Reinforce independence in care.

RETINAL DETACHMENT
Key signs and symptoms
- Painless change in vision (floaters and flashes of light)
- With progression of detachment, painless vision loss may be described as a "veil curtain" or "cobweb" that eliminates part of visual field

Key test results
- Indirect ophthalmoscope shows retinal tear or detachment.
- Slit-lamp examination shows retinal tear or detachment.

Key treatments
- Cryopexy
- Scleral buckling or diathermy to reattach the retina

Key interventions
- Postoperatively instruct the client to lie on his back or on his unoperated side.
- Discourage straining during defecation, bending down, and hard coughing, sneezing, or vomiting.

(continued)

Neurosensory refresher (continued)

SEIZURE DISORDER
Key signs and symptoms
- Recurring seizures

Key test results
- EEG shows continuing tendency to have seizures.

Key treatments
- Anticonvulsants: phenytoin (Dilantin), carbamazepine (Tegretol), gabapentin (Neurontin), valproic acid, clonazepam (Klonopin)
- Surgical removal of demonstrated focal lesion

Key interventions
- Keep the client safe during seizure activity. Don't restrain the client during a seizure; instead, place the client in a flat, side-lying position; maintain a patent airway, but don't force anything into the client's mouth.
- Monitor the client's medication levels.
- Monitor the client for seizure activity.
- Provide the client and his family with as much information about the seizure disorder and medication as possible.
- If the client has status epilepticus, be prepared to administer diazepam (Valium), lorazepam (Ativan), or phenytoin.

SPINAL CORD INJURY
Key signs and symptoms
- Loss of bowel and bladder control
- Paralysis below the level of the injury
- Paresthesia below the level of the injury

Key test results
- CT scan shows spinal cord edema, vertebral fracture, and spinal cord compression.
- MRI shows spinal cord edema, vertebral fracture, and spinal cord compression.

Key treatments
- Flat position, with neck immobilized in a cervical collar
- Maintenance of vertebral alignment through skull tongs and Halo vest
- Surgery for stabilization of the upper spine such as insertion of Harrington rods
- Antianxiety agent: lorazepam (Ativan)
- Glucocorticoid: methylprednisolone infusion immediately following injury
- H_2-receptor antagonists: cimetidine (Tagamet), ranitidine (Zantac), famotidine (Pepcid)
- Laxative: bisacodyl (Dulcolax)
- Mucosal barrier fortifier: sucralfate (Carafate)
- Muscle relaxant: dantrolene (Dantrium)

Key interventions
- Monitor neurologic and respiratory status.
- Assess for spinal shock and initiate prompt treatment.
- Monitor for autonomic dysreflexia (sudden extreme rise in blood pressure) in clients with spinal injury T6 or higher.
- Reposition the client every 2 hours; provide skin care.

STROKE
Key signs and symptoms
- Sudden numbness or weakness of arm or leg on one side of the body
- Sudden change in mental status; difficulty speaking or understanding
- Sudden vision disturbances
- Sudden difficulty walking, maintaining balance, or complaint of dizziness
- Sudden severe headache

Key test results
- CT scan reveals intracranial bleeding, infarct (shows up 24 hours after the initial symptoms), or shift of midline structures.
- Digital subtraction angiography reveals occlusion or narrowing of vessels.
- MRI shows intracranial bleeding, infarct, or shift of midline structures.

Key treatments
- Anticoagulants: heparin, warfarin (Coumadin), ticlopidine (Ticlid)
- Anticonvulsant: phenytoin (Dilantin)
- Glucocorticoid: dexamethasone
- Thrombolytic therapy: tissue plasminogen activator given within the first 3 hours of symptoms to restore circulation to the affected brain tissue and limit the extent of brain injury

Key interventions
- Monitor vital signs every 1 to 2 hours initially and then every 4 hours when the client becomes stable.
- Elevate the head of the bed 30 degrees.
- Monitor neurologic status every 1 to 2 hours initially and then every 4 hours when the client becomes stable.
- Administer medications and evaluate their effects.
- Provide emotional support.

TRIGEMINAL NEURALGIA
Key signs and symptoms
- Searing pain in the facial area
- Splinting of the affected area
- Holding the face immobile when talking
- Unwashed, unshaven face on affected side

Neurosensory refresher *(continued)*

TRIGEMINAL NEURALGIA *(CONTINUED)*

Key test results
• Skull X-rays, tomography, and CT scans rule out sinus or tooth infections and tumors.

Key treatments
• Anticonvulsant: carbamazepine (Tegretol) or phenytoin (Dilantin) may temporarily relieve or prevent pain
• Microsurgery for vascular decompression

Key interventions
• Observe and record the characteristics and triggers of each attack, including the client's protective mechanisms.

• Provide adequate nutrition in small, frequent meals at room temperature.
• Observe for adverse reactions to carbamazepine, especially cutaneous and hematologic reactions (erythematous and pruritic rashes, urticaria, photosensitivity, exfoliative dermatitis, leukopenia, agranulocytosis, eosinophilia, aplastic anemia, thrombocytopenia) and, possibly, urine retention and transient drowsiness.
• Advise the client to place food in the unaffected side of his mouth when chewing, to brush his teeth and rinse his mouth often, and to see a dentist twice a year to detect cavities.
• Monitor neurologic status and vital signs often after surgery.

Conjunction junction

The **brain stem** provides the connection between the spinal cord and the brain. It contains three sections:
• the midbrain—mediates pupillary reflexes and eye movements; it's also the reflex center for the third and fourth cranial nerves
• the pons—helps regulate respiration; it's also the reflex center for the fifth through eighth cranial nerves and mediates chewing, tasting, saliva secretion, and equilibrium
• the medulla oblongata—contains the vomiting, vasomotor, respiratory, and cardiac centers.

Information super-highway

The **spinal cord** functions as a two-way conductor pathway between the brain stem and the peripheral nervous system. It consists of gray matter and white matter. The gray matter is made up of cell bodies and dendrites and axons. The white matter contains ascending (sensory) and descending (motor) tracts, sending signals up to the brain and motor signals out to the muscles.

Like the post office

The **peripheral nervous system** delivers messages from the spinal cord to outlying areas of the body. The main nerves of this system are grouped into:
• 31 pairs of spinal nerves, which carry mixed impulses (motor and sensory) to and from the spinal cord
• 12 pairs of cranial nerves—olfactory, optic, oculomotor, trochlear, trigeminal, abducens,

facial, acoustic, glossopharyngeal, vagus, spinal accessory, and hypoglossal.

Involuntary actions

The **autonomic nervous system,** a subdivision of the peripheral nervous system, controls involuntary body functions, such as digestion, respiration, and cardiovascular function.

It's divided into two cooperating systems to maintain homeostasis: the sympathetic nervous system and the parasympathetic nervous system. The sympathetic nervous system coordinates activities that handle stress (the flight or fight response). The parasympathetic nervous system conserves and restores energy stores.

Blink and you'll miss it

The **eyes** are composed of both external and internal structures. External structures include the eyelids, conjunctivae (thin, transparent mucous membranes that line the lids), lacrimal apparatuses (which lubricate and protect the cornea and conjunctivae by producing and absorbing tears), extraocular muscles (which hold the eyes parallel to create binocular vision), and the eyeballs themselves.

An inside view

The eye also contains numerous **internal structures.** Some of the most important include:
• the iris—a thin, circular pigmented muscular structure in the eye that gives color to the eye and divides the space between the cornea and lens into anterior and posterior chambers

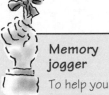

Memory jogger

To help you remember the cranial nerves (and their order) think of the mnemonic "On Old Olympus's Towering Tops, A Finn And German Viewed Some Hops."

Olfactory (CN I)

Optic (CN II)

Oculomotor (CN III)

Trochlear (CN IV)

Trigeminal (CN V)

Abducens (CN VI)

Facial (CN VII)

Acoustic (CN VIII)

Glossopharyngeal (CN IX)

Vagus (CN X)

Spinal accessory (CN XI)

Hypoglossal (CN XII)

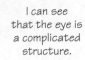

I can see that the eye is a complicated structure.

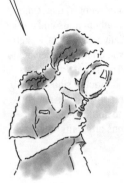

- the cornea—a smooth, transparent tissue that works with the sclera to give the eye its shape
- the pupil—the circular aperture in the iris that changes size as the iris adapts to the amount of light entering the eye
- the lens—a biconvex, avascular, colorless, and transparent structure suspended behind the iris and in front of the vitreous body, by the ciliary zonulae
- the vitreous humor— a clear, transparent, avascular, gelatinous fluid that fills the cavity (vitreous body) in the posterior portion of the eye and maintains the transparency and form of the eye
- the retina—a thin, semitransparent layer of nerve tissue that lines the eye wall and contains optic nerve fibers
- retinal cones—visual cell segments responsible for visual acuity and color discrimination under bright lights
- retinal rods—visual cell segments responsible for peripheral vision under decreased light conditions
- the optic nerve—the second cranial nerve located at the posterior portion of the eye that transmits visual impulses from the retina to the brain.

External, middle, and inner

The **ears** are composed of three sections: external, middle, and inner. The external ear includes the pinna (auricle) and external auditory canal. It's separated from the middle ear by the tympanic membrane.

The middle ear, known as the tympanum, is an air-filled cavity in the temporal bone. It contains three small bones (malleus, incus, and stapes).

The inner ear, known as the *labyrinth*, is the portion of the ear that consists of the cochlea, vestibule, and semicircular canals.

Keep abreast of diagnostic tests

Here are the most important tests used to diagnose neurosensory disorders, along with common nursing actions associated with each test.

Electrical graph

An **electroencephalogram** (EEG) records the electrical activity of the brain. Using electrodes, this noninvasive test gives a graphic representation of brain activity.

Nursing actions

- Explain the procedure to the client.
- Determine the client's ability to lie still.
- Reassure the client that electrical shock won't occur.
- Explain that the client will be subjected to stimuli, such as lights and sounds.
- Withhold medications that may interfere with the results (such as anticonvulsants, antianxiety agents, sedatives, and antidepressants) and caffeine for 24 to 48 hours before the procedure.

Brain images

A **computed tomography (CT) scan,** used to identify brain abnormalities, produces a series of tomograms translated by a computer and displayed on a monitor, which represent cross-sectional images of various layers of the brain. It can be used to identify intracranial tumors and other brain lesions. It may be performed with or without the injection of contrast dye.

Nursing actions

- Explain the procedure to the client.
- Note the client's allergies to iodine, seafood, and radiopaque dyes, if dye will be used.
- Make sure that written, informed consent has been obtained, per facility policy.
- Inform the client about possible throat irritation and facial flushing, if contrast dye is injected.
- Insert an I.V. catheter, if contrast dye is to be used.

Magnetic snapshot

Magnetic resonance imaging (MRI) provides a detailed visualization of the brain and its structures using magnetic and radio waves.

Nursing actions

- Explain the procedure to the client.
- Remove jewelry and metal objects from the client.
- Determine the client's ability to lie still.

- Administer sedation as prescribed.
- Evaluate the client for pacemaker, surgical or orthopedic clips, or shrapnel that would contraindicate the test.
- Make sure written, informed consent has been obtained per facility policy.

Upstairs artery exam
A **cerebral angiogram** examines blood flow through the arteries using dye, in conjunction with X-rays.

Nursing actions
Before the procedure
- Explain the procedure to the client.
- Note the client's allergies to iodine, seafood, or radiopaque dyes.
- Make sure that written, informed consent has been obtained per facility policy.
- Inform the client about possible throat irritation and facial flushing when the dye is injected.

After the procedure
- Monitor vital signs.
- Check the insertion site for bleeding and assess pulses distal to the site.
- Assess neurologic status.
- Encourage fluid intake if the client's condition allows.

Puncture reveals pressure
A **lumbar puncture** (LP) is the introduction of a needle into the lumbar subarachnoid space to collect CSF for analysis, measure CSF pressure, or inject radiopaque dye for a myelogram.

Nursing actions
Before the procedure
- Determine the client's ability to lie still in a flexed, lateral, recumbent position.
- Explain the procedure to the client.
- Make sure that written, informed consent has been obtained per facility policy.
- Be aware that a substantial increase in intracranial pressure (ICP) is a contraindication for having the test.

After the procedure
- Monitor neurologic status.
- Keep the client flat in bed, as directed (from 20 minutes to a few hours).
- Administer analgesics as prescribed.

- Check the puncture site for bleeding or CSF leakage.
- Encourage fluid intake if the client's condition allows.

Fluid to the lab
Cerebrospinal fluid analysis allows microscopic examination of CSF for blood, white blood cells (WBCs), immunoglobulins, bacteria, protein, glucose, and electrolytes.

Nursing actions
- Label specimens properly and send them to the laboratory immediately.
- Follow nursing interventions for an LP.

Electric flex
Electromyography (EMG) uses electrodes to graphically record the electrical activity of a muscle at rest and during contraction.

Nursing actions
Before the procedure
- Explain the procedure to the client.
- Explain that the client must flex and relax the muscles during the procedure.
- Explain that the client will feel some discomfort but not pain.

After the procedure
- Administer analgesics as prescribed.

See the spine
A **myelography** is visualization of the subarachnoid space, spinal cord, and vetebrae after injection of radiopaque dye by LP.

Nursing actions
Before the procedure
- Explain the procedure to the client.
- Note the client's allergies to iodine, seafood, and radiopaque dyes.
- Make sure that written, informed consent has been obtained per facility policy.
- Inform the client about possible throat irritation and facial flushing after dye injection.

After the procedure
- Monitor neurologic status.
- Keep the client flat in bed, as directed.
- Check the puncture site for bleeding or CSF leakage.
- Encourage fluid intake, if the client's condition allows.

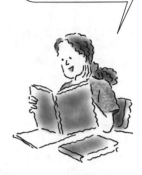

Hmmm... Contraindications count. The presence of a pacemaker rules out an MRI.

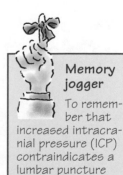

Memory jogger

To remember that increased intracranial pressure (ICP) contraindicates a lumbar puncture (LP), think:

Increased ICP—No LP.

Snooping on the skull

Skull X-rays provide a radiographic picture of the head and neck bones.

Nursing actions
- Explain the procedure to the client.
- Determine the client's ability to lie still during the procedure.

Marking blood flow in the brain

Positron emission tomography (PET) is injection of a radioisotope after visualization of the brain's oxygen uptake, blood flow, and glucose metabolism.

Nursing actions
Before the procedure
- Explain the procedure to the client.
- Determine the client's ability to remain still during the procedure.
- Withhold alcohol, tobacco, and caffeine for 24 hours before the procedure.
- Withhold medications, as directed.
- Insert an I.V. catheter.

After the procedure
- Check the injection site for bleeding.

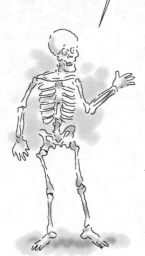

The head bone is connected to the neck bone.

Studying blood once...

A **blood chemistry test** analyzes a blood sample for potassium, sodium, calcium, phosphorus, protein, osmolality, glucose, bicarbonate, blood urea nitrogen, and creatinine.

Nursing actions
- Before the procedure, explain the reason for testing and how the specimen will be obtained.
- After the procedure, monitor the venipuncture site for bleeding.

...Studying blood twice...

A **hematologic study** is a laboratory test of a blood sample that analyzes WBCs, red blood cells, erythrocyte sedimentation rate, platelets, hemoglobin, and hematocrit.

Nursing actions
Before the procedure
- Explain the procedure to the client.
- Note current drug therapy before the procedure.

After the procedure
- Check the venipuncture site for bleeding.

...Studying blood three times

A **coagulation study** is a laboratory test of a blood sample that analyzes prothrombin time, international normalized ratio, and partial thromboplastin time.

Nursing actions
Before the procedure
- Explain the procedure to the client.
- Note current drug therapy before the procedure.

After the procedure
- Check the venipuncture site for bleeding.

Ye olde eye chart

A **visual acuity test** measures clarity of vision using a letter chart (Snellen's) placed 20′ (6 m) from the client. Acuity is expressed in a ratio that relates what a person with normal vision sees at 20′ to what the client can see at 20′.

Nursing actions
- Explain the testing procedure to the client.
- Remind the client to bring eyeglasses or contact lenses, if presently prescribed.
- Advise the examiner if the client is unable to read alphabet letters.
- Advise the examiner if the client has difficulty hearing or following directions.

All lined up?

Extraocular eye muscle testing checks for parallel alignment of the eyes, muscle strength, and cranial nerve function.

Nursing actions
- Explain the testing procedure to the client.
- Advise the examiner if the client has difficulty hearing or following directions.

Seeing on the side

A **visual field examination** tests the degree of peripheral vision of each eye.

Nursing actions
- Explain the testing procedure to the client.
- Advise the examiner if the client has difficulty hearing or following directions.

Puff to measure pressure

A **tonometry test** measures intraocular fluid pressure using an applanation tonometer or an air-puff tonometer.

Nursing actions

- Explain the testing procedure to the client.
- Ask the client to remain still.
- Depending on the method of examination, advise the client that a puff of air or the instrument may be felt on the eye.

Tick-tock test

An **auditory acuity test** assesses hearing by assessing ability to hear a whispered phrase or ticking watch.

Nursing actions

- Explain the testing procedure to the client.
- Advise the examiner if the client has difficulty following directions.

Scope inside the ear

An **otoscopic examination** uses an otoscope to visualize the tympanic membrane.

Nursing actions

- Explain the procedure to the client.
- Advise the client to hold still during the examination.
- Explain that a gentle pull will be felt on the auricle and slight pressure will be felt in the ear.

Determining degree of deafness

Audiometry measures the degree of deafness using pure-tone or speech methods.

Nursing actions

- Explain the testing procedure to the client.
- Explain that the client will need to wear earphones and will be asked to signal when a tone is heard while sitting in a soundproof room.

Polish up on client care

Major neurosensory disorders include acute head injury, amyotrophic lateral sclerosis, Bell's palsy, brain abscess, brain tumor, cataract, cerebral aneurysm, conjunctivitis, corneal abrasion, encephalitis, glaucoma, Guillain-Barré syndrome, hearing loss, Huntington's disease, Ménière's disease, meningitis, multiple sclerosis, myasthenia gravis, otosclerosis, Parkinson's disease, retinal detachment, seizure disorder, spinal cord injury, stroke, and trigeminal neuralgia.

Acute head injury

Acute head injury results from a trauma to the head, leading to brain injury or bleeding within the brain. Effects of injury may include edema and hypoxia. Manifestations of the injury can vary greatly from a mild cognitive defect to severe functional deficits.

A head injury is classified by brain injury type: fracture, hemorrhage, or trauma. Fractures can be depressed, comminuted, or linear. Hemorrhages are classified as epidural, subdural, intracerebral, or subarachnoid.

CAUSES

- Assault
- Automobile accident
- Blunt trauma
- Fall
- Penetrating trauma

ASSESSMENT FINDINGS

- Decreased level of consciousness (LOC)
- Disorientation to time, place, or person
- Otorrhea, rhinorrhea, frequent swallowing (if a CSF leak occurs)
- Paresthesia
- Unequal pupil size, loss of pupillary reaction (if edema is present)
- Pain at site of impact
- Wound at site of impact

DIAGNOSTIC TEST RESULTS

- CT scan shows hemorrhage, cerebral edema, or shift of midline structures.
- EEG may reveal seizure activity.
- ICP monitoring shows increased ICP.
- MRI shows hemorrhage, cerebral edema, or shift of midline structures.
- Skull X-ray may show skull fracture.

> Too much studying giving you a decreased LOC? Take a quick break —then come back ready to review some more!

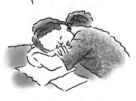

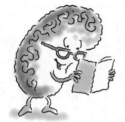

Acute head injury results from trauma to the head, leading to brain injury or bleeding within the brain. Sounds awful.

NURSING DIAGNOSES
- Ineffective tissue perfusion: Cerebral
- Decreased intracranial adaptive capacity
- Risk for injury
- Acute pain

TREATMENT
- Cervical collar (until neck injury is ruled out)
- Craniotomy: surgical incision into the cranium (may be necessary to evacuate a hematoma or evacuate contents to make room for swelling to prevent herniation)
- Oxygen therapy: intubation and mechanical ventilation, if necessary (to provide controlled hyperventilation to decrease elevated ICP)
- Restricted oral intake for 24 to 48 hours
- Ventriculostomy: insertion of a drain into the ventricles (to drain CSF in the presence of hydrocephalus, which may occur as a result of head injury; can also be used to monitor ICP)

Drug therapy
- Analgesic: codeine phosphate
- Anticonvulsant: phenytoin (Dilantin)
- Barbiturate: pentobarbital, if unable to control ICP with diuresis
- Diuretics: mannitol, furosemide (Lasix) to combat cerebral edema
- Dopamine to maintain cerebral perfusion pressure above 50 mm Hg (if blood pressure is low and ICP is elevated)
- Glucocorticoid: dexamethasone to reduce cerebral edema
- Histamine$_2$ (H$_2$)-receptor antagonists: cimetidine (Tagamet), ranitidine (Zantac), famotidine (Pepcid), nizatidine (Axid)
- Mucosal barrier fortifier: sucralfate (Carafate)
- Posterior pituitary hormone: vasopressin if client develops diabetes insipidus

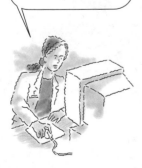

In clients with head injuries, allow a rest period between procedures to avoid increasing ICP.

INTERVENTIONS AND RATIONALES
- Assess neurologic and respiratory status *to monitor for signs of increased ICP and respiratory distress.*
- Observe for signs of increasing ICP (including ICP measurements greater than 20 mm Hg for more than 10 minutes) *to avoid treatment delay and prevent neurologic compromise.*

- Minimize stimuli if ICP is unstable *to avoid increases in ICP.*
- Monitor and record vital signs and intake and output, hemodynamic variables, ICP measurements, cerebral perfusion pressure, specific gravity, laboratory studies, and pulse oximetry *to detect early signs of compromise.*
- Assess for CSF leak as evidenced by otorrhea or rhinorrhea. *CSF leak increases the risk of infection.*
- Assess and treat pain. *Pain may cause anxiety and increase ICP.*
- Assess cough and gag reflex *to prevent aspiration.*
- Monitor for signs of diabetes insipidus (low urine specific gravity, high urine output) *to maintain hydration.*
- Administer I.V. fluids *to maintain hydration.*
- Administer oxygen and maintain position and patency of endotracheal tube, if present, *to maintain airway and hyperventilate the client to lower ICP.*
- Assist with turning, coughing, and deep breathing *to prevent pooling of secretions.*
- Provide suctioning only as necessary *to prevent increase in ICP.*
- Maintain position, patency, and low suction of nasogastric (NG) tube *to prevent vomiting.*
- Maintain seizure precautions *to maintain client safety.*
- Administer medications as prescribed *to decrease ICP and pain.*
- Provide rest periods between nursing activities *to avoid increase in ICP.*
- Encourage verbalization of feelings about changes in body image *to allay anxiety.*
- Provide appropriate sensory input and stimuli with frequent reorientation *to foster awareness of the environment.*
- Provide a means of communication, such as a communication board, *to prevent anxiety.*
- Provide eye, skin, and mouth care *to prevent tissue damage.*
- Reposition every 2 hours or maintain in a rotating bed if condition allows *to prevent skin breakdown.*

Teaching topics
- Explanation of the head injury and its implications

- Recognizing the signs and symptoms of decreased LOC
- Treatment measures
- Medication use and possible adverse effects
- Recognizing the signs of seizures and safety precautions to take during a seizure
- Adhering to fluid restrictions
- Contacting the National Head Injury Foundation

Amyotrophic lateral sclerosis

ALS, commonly known as *Lou Gehrig's disease*, is a progressive, degenerative disorder that leads to decreased motor function in the upper and lower motor neuron systems. In ALS, certain nerve cells degenerate, resulting in distorted or blocked nerve impulses. Nerve cells die and muscle fibers have atrophic changes resulting in progressive motor dysfunction. The disease affects males three times more often than females.

CAUSES
- Genetic predisposition
- Nutritional deficiency related to a disturbance in enzyme metabolism
- Slow-acting virus
- Unknown

ASSESSMENT FINDINGS
- Atrophy of tongue
- Awkwardness of fine finger movements
- Dysphagia
- Dyspnea
- Fasciculations of face
- Fatigue
- Muscle weakness of hands and feet
- Nasal quality of speech
- Spasticity

DIAGNOSTIC TEST RESULTS
- Creatinine kinase level is elevated.
- EMG shows decreased amplitude of evoked potentials.

NURSING DIAGNOSES
- Ineffective health maintenance
- Impaired physical mobility
- Ineffective airway clearance
- Ineffective breathing pattern
- Anxiety
- Fear

TREATMENT
- Management of symptoms

Drug therapy
- Anticholinergic: dicyclomine (Bentyl)
- Anticonvulsant: gabapentin (Neurontin)
- Antispasmodics: baclofen (Lioresal), lorazepam (Ativan)
- Investigational agents: thyrotropin-releasing hormone, interferon
- Neuroprotective agent: riluzole (Rilutek)

INTERVENTIONS AND RATIONALES
- Monitor neurologic and respiratory status *to detect decreases in neurologic and respiratory functioning*.
- Assess swallow and gag reflexes *to decrease the risk of aspiration*.
- Monitor and record vital signs and intake and output *to determine baseline and detect changes from baseline assessment*.
- Administer medications as prescribed *to help the client achieve maximum potential*.
- Devise an alternate method of communication, when necessary, *to help the client communicate and decrease the client's anxiety and frustration*.
- Encourage verbalization of feelings and help maintain independence for as long as possible *to decrease anxiety and promote self-esteem*.
- Suction the oral pharynx, as necessary, *to stimulate cough and clear the airways*.
- Maintain the client's diet *to improve nutritional status*.
- Provide emotional support *to decrease fear*.
- Assist with range-of-motion (ROM) exercises *to help maintain joint and muscle function*.

Teaching topics
- Explanation of the disorder and its implications
- Supportive treatment measures
- Medication use and possible adverse reactions

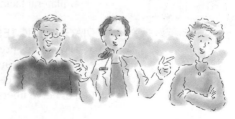

Teach family members of a client with ALS about a living will and options for long-term care.

- Maintaining tucked chin position while eating or drinking
- Using tonsillar suction tip to clear oral pharynx
- Using prosthetic devices to assist with activities of daily living (ADLs)
- Long-term care and end-of-life issues
- Contacting the Amyotrophic Lateral Sclerosis Association

Bell's palsy

Bell's palsy is inflammation around the seventh cranial (facial) nerve that produces unilateral facial weakness or paralysis. Onset is rapid. Although it affects all age-groups, it occurs most commonly in persons younger than age 60. In 80% to 90% of clients, it subsides spontaneously, with complete recovery in 1 to 8 weeks; however, recovery may be delayed in older adults. If recovery is partial, contractures may develop on the paralyzed side of the face. Bell's palsy may recur on the same or opposite side of the face.

CAUSES
- Blockage of the seventh cranial nerve, resulting from viral infection, hemorrhage, tumor, meningitis, or local trauma

ASSESSMENT FINDINGS
- Flattening of the forehead and nasolabial fold on the affected side
- Eye rolls upward and tears excessively when the client attempts to close it
- Inability to close eye completely on the affected side
- Pain around the jaw or ear of the affected side
- Ringing in the ears
- Taste distortion on the anterior portion of the tongue on the affected side
- Unilateral facial weakness

DIAGNOSTIC TEST RESULTS
- EMG helps predict the level of expected recovery by distinguishing temporary conduction defects from a pathologic interruption of nerve fibers.

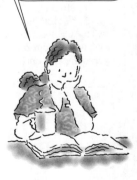

There are two facial nerves, one on each side. Bell's palsy occurs when one of those nerves becomes swollen and pinched.

NURSING DIAGNOSES
- Acute pain
- Disturbed sensory perception (gustatory)
- Disturbed body image
- Imbalanced nutrition: Less than body requirements
- Situational low self-esteem

TREATMENT
- Electrotherapy after the 14th day of prednisone therapy to help prevent facial muscle atrophy
- Moist heat
- Facial sling

Drug therapy
- Corticosteroid: prednisone to reduce facial nerve edema and improve nerve conduction and blood flow
- Antiviral: acyclovir (Zovirax) (may be helpful in treating the viral infection that may have caused nerve swelling)
- Artificial tears to protect the cornea from injury
- Analgesics: acetaminophen(Tylenol), ibuprofen (Motrin)

INTERVENTIONS AND RATIONALES
- Monitor for adverse reactions to prednisone, especially GI distress, fluid retention, and hyperglycemia. If GI distress is troublesome, a concomitant antacid usually provides relief *to prevent further complications*.
- Apply moist heat to the affected side of the face, taking care not to burn the skin, *to reduce pain*.
- Massage the client's face with a gentle upward motion two to three times daily for 5 to 10 minutes, or have him massage his face himself. When he's ready for active exercises, teach him to exercise by grimacing in front of a mirror *to help maintain muscle tone*.
- Provide privacy during mealtimes *to reduce embarrassment*.
- Apply a facial sling *to improve lip alignment*.
- Encourage frequent and complete mouth care, being careful to remove residual food that collects between the cheeks and gums *to prevent breakdown of oral mucosa*.

* Provide emotional support. Give reassurance that recovery is likely within 1 to 8 weeks *to allay anxiety.*

Teaching topics
* Explanation of the disorder and treatment measures
* Medication use and possible adverse effects
* Protecting the eye by covering it with an eye patch, especially when outdoors
* Keeping warm, avoiding exposure to dust and wind, and covering face when exposure is unavoidable
* Performing facial exercises

Brain abscess

Brain abscess is a free or encapsulated collection of pus that usually occurs in the temporal lobe, cerebellum, or frontal lobes. Brain abscess is rare. Although it can occur at any age, it's most common in people ages 10 to 35 and is rare in older adults.

An untreated brain abscess is usually fatal; with treatment, the prognosis is only fair.

CAUSES
* Infection, especially otitis media, sinusitis, dental abscess, and mastoiditis
* Subdural empyema
* Physical trauma

ASSESSMENT FINDINGS
* Headache
* Chills
* Fever
* Malaise
* Confusion
* Drowsiness

Temporal lobe abscess
* Auditory-receptive dysphasia
* Central facial weakness
* Hemiparesis

Cerebellar abscess
* Dizziness
* Coarse nystagmus
* Gaze weakness on lesion side
* Tremor
* Ataxia

Frontal lobe abscess
* Expressive dysphasia
* Hemiparesis with unilateral motor seizure
* Drowsiness
* Inattention
* Mental function impairment
* Seizures

DIAGNOSTIC TEST RESULTS
* Physical examination shows signs of increased ICP.
* Enhanced CT scan reveals the abscess site.
* Arteriography highlights the abscess by a halo appearance.
* A CT-guided stereotactic biopsy may be performed to drain and culture the abscess.
* Culture and sensitivity of drainage identifies the causative organism.

NURSING DIAGNOSES
* Decreased intracranial adaptive capacity
* Disturbed thought process
* Impaired physical mobility
* Risk for injury

TREATMENT
* Endotracheal (ET) intubation and mechanical ventilation
* I.V. therapy
* Surgical aspiration or drainage of the abscess

Drug therapy
* Diuretic: mannitol
* Corticosteroid: dexamethasone
* Penicillinase-resistant antibiotic: nafcillin
* Anticonvulsants: phenytoin (Dilantin), phenobarbital

INTERVENTIONS AND RATIONALES
* Provide intensive care and monitoring *to monitor ICP and provide necessary life support.*
* Monitor neurologic status, especially cognition and mentation, speech, and sensorimotor and cranial nerve function *to detect early signs of increased ICP.* (See *Using the Glasgow Coma Scale,* page 192.)
* Assess and record vital signs at least once every hour *to detect trends that may signify increasing ICP, such as increasing systolic*

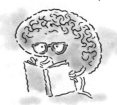

Location, location, location. Effects of a brain abscess depend on which part of me is affected.

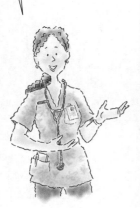

Early increases in intracranial pressure can be detected by using the Glasgow Coma Scale.

Using the Glasgow Coma Scale

The Glasgow Coma Scale is used to assess a client's level of consciousness. It was designed to help predict a client's survival and recovery after a head injury. The scale scores three observations: eye opening response, best motor response, and best verbal response. Each response receives a point value. If the client is alert, can follow simple commands, and is completely oriented to person, place, and time, his score will total 15 points. If the client is comatose, his score will total 7 or less. A score of 3, the lowest possible score, indicates brain death.

OBSERVATION	RESPONSE	SCORE
Eye response	Opens spontaneously	4
	Opens to verbal command	3
	Opens to pain	2
	No response	1
Best motor response	Follows commands	6
	Localizes pain	5
	Flexion withdrawal	4
	Abnormal flexion	3
	Abnormal extension	2
	No response	1
Verbal response	Is oriented and converses	5
	Is disoriented but converses	4
	Uses inappropriate words	3
	Makes incomprehensible sounds	2
	No response	1
Total score		Ranges between 3 and 15

blood pressure, widening pulse pressure, and slowing heart rate.
• Monitor fluid intake and output *because fluid overload could contribute to cerebral edema.*
• Explain the procedure or surgery to the client and if indicated, answer all questions *to allay anxiety.*
• Monitor vital signs and intake and output *to detect any complications.*
• Monitor for signs of meningitis (nuchal rigidity, headaches, chills, sweats) *to avoid treatment delay.*
• Perform dressing changes as needed *to prevent bacterial growth.*
• Position the client on the operative side *to promote drainage and prevent reaccumulation of the abscess.*
• Measure drainage from Jackson-Pratt drain or other types of drains *to assess* effectiveness of the drains and detect signs of hemorrhage (blood accumulating in drain).
• Reposition every 2 hours; provide skin care *to prevent pressure ulcers*, and position *to preserve function and prevent contractures.*
• Encourage ambulation as soon as possible *to prevent complications of immobility and encourage independence.*
• Administer medication *to promote health.*

Teaching topics
• Explanation of the disorder and treatment plan
• Medication use and possible adverse effects
• Need for treatment of otitis media, mastoiditis, dental abscess, and other infections to prevent brain abscess

Brain tumor

A brain tumor is an abnormal mass found in the brain resulting from unregulated cell growth and division. These tumors can either infiltrate and destroy surrounding tissue or be encapsulated and displace brain tissue. The presence of the lesion causes compression of blood vessels, producing ischemia, edema, and increased ICP.

Symptoms and manifestations vary depending on the location of the tumor in the brain. The tumor can be primary (originating in the brain tissue) or secondary (metastasizing from another area of the body). Tumors are classified according to the tissue of origin, such as gliomas (composed of neuroglial cells), meningiomas (originating in the meninges), and astrocytomas (composed of astrocytes).

CAUSES
- Environmental
- Genetic

ASSESSMENT FINDINGS
- Deficits in cerebral function
- Headache

Frontal lobe
- Aphasia
- Memory loss
- Personality changes

Temporal lobe
- Aphasia
- Seizures

Parietal lobe
- Motor seizures
- Sensory impairment

Occipital lobe
- Homonymous hemianopsia (defective vision or blindness affecting the right halves or the left halves of the visual field of the two eyes)
- Visual hallucinations
- Visual impairment

Cerebellum
- Impaired coordination
- Impaired equilibrium

DIAGNOSTIC TEST RESULTS
- CT scan shows location and size of tumor.
- MRI shows location and size of tumor.

NURSING DIAGNOSES
- Anxiety
- Risk for injury
- Disturbed sensory perception (kinesthetic)
- Acute pain
- Fear

TREATMENT
- Craniotomy
- High-calorie diet
- Radiation therapy
- Chemotherapy

Drug therapy
- Anticonvulsant: phenytoin (Dilantin)
- Antineoplastics: vincristine, lomustine (CeeNU), carmustine (BiCNU)
- Diuretics: mannitol, furosemide (Lasix) if increased ICP
- Glucocorticoid: dexamethasone
- H$_2$-receptor antagonists: cimetidine (Tagamet), ranitidine (Zantac), famotidine (Pepcid), nizatidine (Axid)
- Mucosal barrier fortifier: sucralfate (Carafate)

INTERVENTIONS AND RATIONALES
- Monitor neurologic and respiratory status *to determine baseline and deviations from baseline assessment.*
- Assess for and treat pain *to provide adequate comfort.*
- Assess for signs of increased ICP *to facilitate early intervention and prevent neurologic complications.*
- Monitor and record vital signs and intake and output, ICP measurements, and laboratory studies *to determine baseline and detect early deviations from baseline assessment.*
- Monitor for signs and symptoms of syndrome of inappropriate antidiuretic hormone (edema, weight gain, positive fluid balance, high urine specific gravity) *to facilitate early intervention and prevent increased ICP through fluid restriction and I.V. infusion of normal saline solution.*

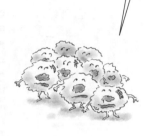

A brain tumor is an abnormal mass found in the brain resulting from unregulated cell growth and division.

- Reposition the client every 2 hours *to maintain skin integrity*.
- Maintain the client's diet *to promote healing*.
- Administer I.V. fluids and encourage oral fluids *to maintain hydration*.
- Administer oxygen *to prevent ischemia*.
- Administer enteral nutrition or total parenteral nutrition (TPN), as indicated, *to meet nutritional needs*.
- Limit environmental noise. *Auditory stimuli can contribute to increased ICP*.
- Provide support and encourage verbalization of feelings about changes in body image and a fear of dying *to decrease anxiety*.
- Monitor arterial blood gas (ABG) levels. *Hypercapnia results in vasodilation, increased cerebral blood volume, and increased ICP*.
- Maintain normothermia and control shivering. *Shivering causes isometric muscle contraction, which can increase ICP*.
- Provide rest periods. *Cerebral blood flow increases during rapid eye-movement sleep*.
- Maintain seizure precautions and administer anticonvulsants, as ordered. *Seizures increase intrathoracic pressure, decrease cerebral venous outflow, and increase cerebral blood volume, thereby increasing ICP*.

Teaching topics
- Explanation of the disorder and treatment plan
- Medication use and possible adverse effects
- Recognizing decreased LOC
- Maintaining a safe, quiet environment
- Discussing quality-of-life decisions
- Arranging for hospice care, if appropriate

Cataract

A cataract occurs when the normally clear, transparent crystalline lens in the eye becomes opaque. With age, lens fibers become more densely packed, making the lens less transparent and giving the lens a yellowish hue. These changes result in vision loss.

A cataract usually develops first in one eye but, in many cases, is often followed by the development of a cataract in the other eye.

CAUSES
- Aging
- Anterior uveitis
- Blunt or penetrating trauma
- Diabetes mellitus
- Hypoparathyroidism
- Long-term steroid treatment
- Radiation exposure
- Ultraviolet light exposure

ASSESSMENT FINDINGS
- Dimmed or blurred vision
- Disabling glare
- Distorted images
- Better vision in dim light with pupil dilated
- Yellow, gray, or white pupil

DIAGNOSTIC TEST RESULTS
- Ophthalmoscopy or slit-lamp examination confirms the diagnosis by revealing a dark area in the normally homogeneous red reflex.

NURSING DIAGNOSES
- Impaired physical mobility
- Risk for injury
- Disturbed sensory perception (visual)

TREATMENT
- Extracapsular cataract extraction or intracapsular lens implant

INTERVENTIONS AND RATIONALES
- Provide a safe environment for the client. *Orienting the client to his surroundings reduces the risk of injury*.
- Modify the environment to help the client meet his self-care needs by placing items on the unaffected side *to discourage movement or positions that would apply pressure to the operative site or cause increased intraocular pressure*.
- Provide sensory stimulation (such as large print or tapes) *to help compensate for vision loss*.

Teaching topics
- Explanation of the disorder and treatment plan
- Medication use and possible adverse effects
- Returning for a checkup the day after surgery

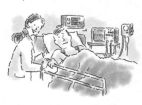

It's clear. Postoperative client teaching is an important part of cataract care.

- Protecting the eye from injury by wearing an eye shield
- How to instill eyedrops
- Notifying the physician immediately if sharp eye pain occurs
- Maintaining activity restrictions

Cerebral aneurysm

A cerebral aneurysm is an outpouching of a cerebral artery that results from weakness of the middle layer of an artery. It usually results from a congenital weakness in the structure of the artery and remains asymptomatic until it ruptures.

Cerebral aneurysms are classified by size or shape, such as saccular, berry, and dissecting. Saccular aneurysms, the most common, occur at the base of the brain at the juncture where the large arteries bifurcate.

CAUSES
- Atherosclerosis
- Congenital weakness
- Head trauma

ASSESSMENT FINDINGS
- Asymptomatic until aneurysm ruptures
- Decreased LOC
- Diplopia, ptosis, blurred vision
- Fever
- Headache (commonly described by the client as the worst he's ever had)
- Hemiparesis
- Nuchal rigidity
- Seizure activity
- Altered LOC

DIAGNOSTIC TEST RESULTS
- Cerebral angiogram identifies the aneurysm.
- Spiral CT angiography shows a shift of intracranial midline structures and blood in subarachnoid space.
- LP (contraindicated with increased ICP) shows increased CSF pressure, protein level, and WBCs and grossly bloody and xanthochromic CSF.
- MRI shows shift of intracranial midline structures and blood in subarachnoid space.

NURSING DIAGNOSES
- Anxiety
- Ineffective tissue perfusion: Cerebral
- Decreased intracranial adaptive capacity
- Acute pain

TREATMENT
- Aneurysm and seizure precautions
- Aneurysm clipping
- Endovascular embolization
- Bed rest
- I.V. therapy
- Oxygen therapy (intubation and mechanical ventilation with hyperventilation, if increased ICP)

Drug therapy
- Analgesic: codeine sulfate
- Anticonvulsant: phenytoin (Dilantin)
- Antihypertensives: hydralazine, nitroprusside (Nitropress), labetalol (Trandate), metoprolol (Lopressor), esmolol (Brevibloc)
- Calcium channel blocker: nimodipine (preferred drug to prevent cerebral vasospasm)
- Glucocorticoid: dexamethasone
- H_2-receptor antagonist: cimetidine (Tagamet), ranitidine (Zantac), famotidine (Pepcid), nizatinide (Axid)
- Possibly dopamine to maintain systolic blood pressure at 140 to 160 mm Hg
- Mucosal barrier fortifier: sucralfate (Carafate)
- Stool softener: docusate sodium (Colace)

INTERVENTIONS AND RATIONALES
- Monitor neurologic status *to screen for changes in the client's condition.* (See *On the lookout for subarachnoid hemorrhage complications,* page 196.)
- Maintain a quiet environment *to reduce increased ICP.*
- Administer diuretics *to prevent or treat increased ICP.*
- Administer crystalloid solutions after aneurysm clipping *to maintain adequate fluid volume and cerebral perfusion, thus decreasing the risk of vasospasm.*
- Administer oxygen (may require intubation and mechanical ventilation) *to maintain oxygenation and cerebral perfusion.*
- Keep the head of the bed elevated at approximately 30 degrees, per neurosurgeon's order, *to reduce increased ICP.*

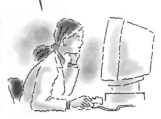

Let's see... precautions to prevent complications in clients with cerebral aneurysm? Keep the lights low. No stress.

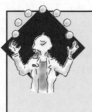

Management moments

On the lookout for subarachnoid hemorrhage complications

Because the mortality rate is high for clients who experience subarachnoid hemorrhages as a result of cerebral aneurysm rupture, prompt recognition of changes and rapid treatment are essential. When caring for a client at risk for subarachnoid hemorrhage, be sure to follow these guidelines:
• Perform neurologic assessment frequently. Monitor for subtle changes in level of consciousness or an increase in headache, which may indicate further bleeding. If changes occur, notify the physician immediately.
• Maintain the client on bed rest with the head of bed elevated 0 to 30 degrees.
• Avoid engaging the client in any activities that can increase intracranial pressure.
• Keep the lights dim and minimize other stimuli.
• Space nursing care to avoid overstimulation.

• Monitor for Cushing's triad (bradycardia, systolic hypertension, and wide pulse pressure), *a sign of impending hemorrhage.*
• Monitor vital signs every 1 to 2 hours initially and then every 4 hours when the client becomes stable *to detect early signs of complications.*
• Provide rest periods between nursing activities *to reduce increased ICP.*
• Maintain seizure precautions and administer anticonvulsants, as ordered. *Seizures increase intrathoracic pressure, decrease cerebral venous outflow, and increase cerebral blood volume, thereby increasing ICP.*
• Reposition the client every 2 hours and provide skin care *to prevent pressure ulcers.*
• Maintain adequate nutrition *to facilitate tissue healing and meet metabolic needs.*
• Administer stool softeners to prevent constipation and straining at defecation *to prevent increased ICP.*

Teaching topics
• Explanation of the disorder and treatment plan
• Medication use and possible adverse effects
• End-of-life care and organ donation issues
• Recognizing decreasing LOC
• Minimizing environmental stress
• Altering ADLs to compensate for neurologic deficits
• Preventing constipation

Conjunctivitis

Conjunctivitis is inflammation of the conjunctiva, the delicate membrane that lines the eyelids and covers the exposed surface of the eyeball. It may result from infection, allergy, or chemical reactions.

Conjunctivitis is common. Bacterial and viral conjunctivitis is highly contagious but is also self-limiting after a couple weeks' duration. Chronic conjunctivitis may result in degenerative changes to the eyelids.

CAUSES
Bacterial
• *Staphylococcus aureus*
• *Streptococcus pneumoniae*
• *Neisseria gonorrhoeae*
• *N. meningitidis*

Chlamydial
• *Chlamydia trachomatis* (inclusion conjunctivitis)

Viral
• Adenovirus types 3, 7, and 8
• Herpes simplex virus, type 1

Other causes
• Allergic reactions to pollen, grass, topical medications, air pollutants, and smoke
• Fungal infections (rare)
• Occupational irritants (acids and alkalies)

Encourage the client with conjunctivitis to practice meticulous hygiene. The disorder can be highly contagious.

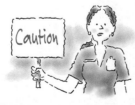

Caution

- Parasitic diseases caused by *Phthirus pubis* or *Schistosoma haematobium*
- Rickettsial diseases (Rocky Mountain spotted fever)

ASSESSMENT FINDINGS
- Excessive tearing
- Hyperemia (engorgement) of the conjunctiva, sometimes accompanied by discharge and tearing
- Itching, burning
- Mucopurulent discharge

DIAGNOSTIC TEST RESULTS
- Culture and sensitivity tests identify the causative bacterial organism and indicate appropriate antibiotic therapy.

NURSING DIAGNOSES
- Risk for infection
- Disturbed sensory perception (visual)
- Disturbed body image

TREATMENT
- Cold compresses to relieve itching for allergic conjunctivitis
- Warm compresses to treat bacterial or viral conjunctivitis

Drug therapy
- Antiviral agent: oral acyclovir (Zovirax) if herpes simplex is the cause
- Corticosteroids: dexamethasone, fluorometholone (Flarex)
- Mast cell stabilizer: cromolyn (Opticrom) for allergic conjunctivitis
- Topical antibiotics according to sensitivity of infective organism (if bacterial)

INTERVENTIONS AND RATIONALES
- Teach proper hand-washing technique *because certain forms of conjunctivitis are highly contagious.*
- Stress the risk of spreading infection to family members by sharing washcloths, towels, and pillows. Warn against rubbing the infected eye, which can spread the infection to the other eye and to other persons. *These measures prevent the spread of infection.*
- Apply warm compresses and therapeutic ointment or drops. Don't irrigate the eye; *this spreads infection.*

- Remind the client to wash his hands before he uses the medication, and use clean washcloths or towels frequently *so he doesn't infect his other eye.*
- Teach the client to instill eyedrops and ointments correctly—without touching the bottle tip to his eye or lashes *to prevent the spread of infection.*
- Stress the importance of safety glasses for the client who works near chemical irritants *to prevent further episodes of conjunctivitis.*
- Notify public health authorities if cultures show *N. gonorrhoeae. Public health authorities track sexually transmitted diseases.*

Teaching topics
- Explanation of the disease process and treatment options
- Proper hand washing
- Preventing the spread of infection
- Eyedrop instillation

Corneal abrasion

A corneal abrasion is a scratch on the surface epithelium of the cornea, the dome-shaped transparent structure in front of the eye. This common type of eye injury is often caused by a foreign body, such as a cinder or piece of dirt or by improper use of a contact lens.

CAUSES
- Improper use of contact lenses
- Trauma caused by a foreign body (such as a cinder or a piece of dust, dirt, or grit)

ASSESSMENT FINDINGS
- Burning
- Change in visual acuity (depending on the size and location of the injury)
- Increased tearing
- Pain in affected eye disproportionate to the size of the injury
- Redness
- Sensation of "something in the eye"

DIAGNOSTIC TEST RESULTS
- Staining the cornea with fluorescein stain confirms the diagnosis: the injured area appears green when examined with a flashlight.

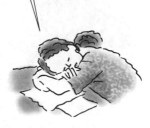

Corneal abrasions are common in people who fall asleep wearing hard contact lenses.

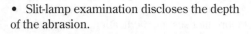

A pressure patch may be applied in corneal abrasion to prevent further corneal irritation if the client blinks.

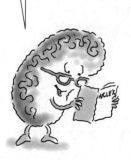

- Slit-lamp examination discloses the depth of the abrasion.

NURSING DIAGNOSES
- Acute pain
- Risk for infection
- Disturbed sensory perception (visual)

TREATMENT
- Irrigation with saline solution
- Pressure patch (a tightly applied eye patch)
- Removal of a deeply embedded foreign body with a foreign body spud, using a topical anesthetic

Drug therapy
- Antibiotic: sulfisoxazole (Gantrisin)
- Cycloplegic agent: tropicamide (Mydriacyl)

INTERVENTIONS AND RATIONALES
- Assist with examination of the eye. Check visual acuity before beginning treatment *to assess visual loss from injury.*
- Irrigate the eye with normal saline solution if the foreign body is visible, *to wash away the foreign body without damaging the eye.*
- Instruct the client with an eye patch to leave the patch in place for 6 to 8 hours *to protect the eye from further corneal irritation when the client blinks.*
- Warn the client with an eye patch that wearing a patch alters depth perception, so advise caution in everyday activities, such as climbing stairs or stepping off a curb, *to prevent injury.*
- Reassure the client that the corneal epithelium usually heals in 24 to 48 hours *to allay anxiety.*
- Stress the importance of instilling prescribed antibiotic eyedrops properly and leaving the eye patch in place for 6 to 8 hours. *An untreated corneal infection can lead to ulceration and permanent loss of vision.*
- Emphasize the importance of safety glasses, if appropriate, *to protect workers' eyes from flying fragments.*

Teaching topics
- Explanation of the disorder and treatment plan

- Eyedrop instillation
- Proper contact use

Encephalitis

Encephalitis is a severe inflammation and swelling of the brain, usually caused by a mosquito-borne or, in some areas, a tick-borne virus. Transmission may also occur through ingestion of infected goat's milk and accidental injection or inhalation of the virus. Eastern equine encephalitis may produce permanent neurologic damage and is commonly fatal.

With encephalitis, intense lymphocytic infiltration of brain tissues and the leptomeninges causes cerebral edema, degeneration of the brain's ganglion cells, and diffuse nerve cell destruction.

CAUSES
- Exposure to virus

ASSESSMENT FINDINGS
- Coma (following the acute phase of illness)
- Meningeal irritation (stiff neck and back) and neuronal damage (drowsiness, coma, paralysis, seizures, ataxia, organic psychoses)
- Sensory alterations
- Sudden onset of fever
- Headache
- Vomiting

DIAGNOSTIC TEST RESULTS
- Blood studies identify the virus and confirm the diagnosis.
- CSF analysis identifies the virus.
- LP discloses CSF pressure is elevated and, despite inflammation, the fluid is commonly clear. WBC and protein levels in CSF are slightly elevated, but the glucose level remains normal.
- EEG reveals abnormalities such as generalized slowing of waveforms.
- CT scan may be ordered to rule out cerebral hematoma.

NURSING DIAGNOSES
- Disturbed thought processes
- Hyperthermia

Encephalitis may produce only mild effects or it may cause permanent neurologic damage and death.

- Impaired physical mobility
- Risk for injury

TREATMENT
- Oxygen therapy: ET intubation and mechanical ventilation
- I.V. fluids
- NG tube feedings or TPN

Drug therapy
- Anticonvulsants: phenytoin (Dilantin), phenobarbital
- Antiviral: acyclovir (Zovirax), which is effective only against herpes encephalitis and is only effective if administered before the onset of coma
- Analgesics and antipyretics: aspirin or acetaminophen (Tylenol) to relieve headache and reduce fever
- Diuretic: furosemide (Lasix) or mannitol to reduce cerebral swelling
- Corticosteroid: dexamethasone to reduce cerebral inflammation and edema
- Laxative: bisacodyl (Dulcolax)
- Sedative: lorazepam (Ativan) for restlessness
- Stool softener: docusate sodium (Colace)

INTERVENTIONS AND RATIONALES
During acute phase
- Monitor neurologic status often. Observe the client's mental status and cognitive abilities. *If the tissue within the brain becomes edematous, changes will occur in the client's mental status and cognitive abilities.*
- Maintain adequate fluid balance *to prevent dehydration*, but avoid fluid overload, *which may increase cerebral edema*. Measure and record intake and output accurately *to assess fluid status*.
- Assist with ET intubation and maintain ventilator settings *to provide adequate oxygenation*.
- Administer acyclovir by slow I.V. infusion only. The client must be well-hydrated and the infusion given over 1 hour *to avoid kidney damage*. Watch for adverse drug effects, such as nausea, diarrhea, pruritus, and difficulty breathing *to prevent complications*. Check the infusion site often *to avoid infiltration and phlebitis*.
- Reposition the client every 2 hours and provide skin care *to prevent skin breakdown*.

- Assist with ROM exercises *to maintain joint mobility*.
- Maintain adequate nutrition *to keep up with increased metabolic needs and promote healing*. It may be necessary to give the client small, frequent meals or to supplement these meals with NG tube or parenteral feedings *to meet nutritional needs*.
- Administer a stool softener or mild laxative *to prevent constipation and minimize the risk of increased ICP from straining during defecation*.
- Provide good mouth care *to prevent breakdown of the oral mucous membrane*.
- Maintain a quiet environment *to promote comfort and decrease stimulation that can cause ICP to rise*. Darken the room *to decrease photophobia and headache*.
- Provide emotional support and reassurance *because the client is apt to be frightened by the illness and frequent diagnostic tests*.

Teaching topics
- Explanation of the disease and its effects
- Treatment and rehabilitation options
- Medication use and possible adverse effects

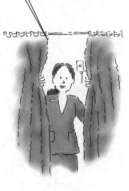

Encephalitis makes a client extremely sensitive to light—keep his room cool and dark.

Glaucoma

Glaucoma is increased intraocular pressure that causes damage to the optic nerve. It can result in visual field loss and, if left untreated, can lead to blindness.

Glaucoma is either open-angle or angle-closure. In open-angle glaucoma, increased intraocular pressure is caused by overproduction of, or obstructed outflow of, aqueous humor (a fluid in the front of the eye). In angle-closure glaucoma, there's an obstructed outflow of aqueous humor due to anatomically narrow angles.

CAUSES
- Diabetes mellitus
- Long-term steroid treatment
- Previous eye trauma or surgery
- Uveitis
- Risk factors
- Family history of glaucoma
- Race (higher incidence in Blacks)

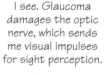

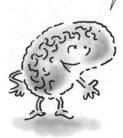

I see. Glaucoma damages the optic nerve, which sends me visual impulses for sight perception.

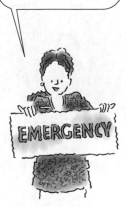

Angle-closure glaucoma is an emergency, requiring immediate treatment. If drugs don't lower intraocular pressure sufficiently, surgery follows.

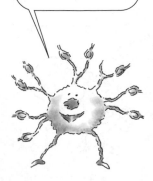

Time is on my side. The nerve damage in Guillain-Barré syndrome is usually temporary.

ASSESSMENT FINDINGS
Acute angle-closure glaucoma
- Acute ocular pain
- Blurred vision
- Dilated pupil
- Halo vision
- Increased intraocular pressure
- Nausea and vomiting

Chronic open-angle glaucoma
- Atrophy and cupping of optic nerve head
- Increased intraocular pressure
- Initially asymptomatic
- Narrowed field of vision
- Possible asymmetrical involvement

DIAGNOSTIC TEST RESULTS
- Gonioscopy reveals if angle is open or closed.
- Ophthalmoscopy shows atrophy and cupping of optic nerve head.
- Perimetry shows decreased field of vision.
- Tonometry shows increased intraocular pressure.

NURSING DIAGNOSES
- Anxiety
- Risk for injury
- Disturbed sensory perception (visual)
- Acute pain
- Fear

TREATMENT
Acute angle-closure glaucoma
- Immediate treatment to lower intraocular pressure
- Laser iridectomy or surgical iridectomy if pressure doesn't decrease with drug therapy

Drug therapy
Acute angle-closure glaucoma
- Cholinergic: pilocarpine

Chronic open-angle glaucoma
- Alpha-adrenergic agonist: brimonidine (Alphagan-P)
- Beta-adrenergic antagonist: timolol (Timoptic)

INTERVENTIONS AND RATIONALES
- Assess eye pain and administer medication as prescribed to promote comfort.

- Provide a safe environment. Orient the client to his surroundings to reduce the risk of injury.
- Modify the environment for safety to meet the client's self-care needs.
- Limit activities that increase intraocular pressure to help reduce complications.
- Encourage verbalization of feelings about changes in body image to aid acceptance of visual loss.

Teaching topics
- Explanation of the disorder and treatment plan
- Medication use and possible adverse effects
- How to instill eyedrops
- Monitoring eye for discharge, watering, blurred or cloudy vision, halos, flashes of light, and floaters

Guillain-Barré syndrome

Guillain-Barré syndrome is an acute, rapidly progressive, and potentially fatal form of polyneuritis (inflammation of several peripheral nerves at once) that causes muscle weakness and mild distal sensory loss.

Recovery is spontaneous and complete in about 95% of clients, although mild motor or reflex deficits in the feet and legs may persist. The prognosis is best when symptoms clear between 15 and 20 days after onset.

This disorder is also known as infectious polyneuritis, Landry-Guillain-Barré syndrome, and acute idiopathic polyneuritis.

CAUSES
- Cell-mediated immune response with an attack on peripheral nerves in response to a virus
- Demyelination of the peripheral nerves
- Respiratory infection

ASSESSMENT FINDINGS
- Dysphagia (difficulty swallowing) or dysarthria (poor speech caused by impaired muscular control)
- Facial diplegia (affecting like parts on both sides of the face; possibly accompanied by ophthalmoplegia [ocular paralysis])

- Hypertonia (excessive muscle tone) and areflexia (absence of reflexes)
- Muscle weakness (ascending from the legs to arms and facial muscles)
- Paresthesia
- Stiffness and pain in the form of a severe "charley horse"
- Weakness of the muscles supplied by cranial nerve XI, the spinal accessory nerve, including the muscles that affect shoulder movement and head rotation (less common finding)

DIAGNOSTIC TEST RESULTS
- A history of preceding febrile illness (usually a respiratory tract infection) and typical clinical features suggest Guillain-Barré syndrome.
- CSF protein level begins to rise, peaking in 4 to 6 weeks. The CSF WBC count remains normal but, in severe disease, CSF pressure may rise above normal.
- Blood studies reveal a complete blood count that shows leukocytosis with the presence of immature forms early in the illness, but blood study results soon return to normal.
- EMG may show repeated firing of the same motor unit rather than widespread sectional stimulation.
- Nerve conduction velocities are slowed soon after paralysis develops. Diagnosis must rule out similar diseases such as acute polio-myelitis.

NURSING DIAGNOSES
- Impaired physical mobility
- Ineffective breathing pattern
- Risk for injury

TREATMENT
- ET intubation or tracheotomy if the client has difficulty clearing secretions; possible mechanical ventilation
- NG tube feedings or parenteral nutrition
- I.V. fluid therapy
- Specialty bed or support surfaces
- Plasmapheresis
- Prophylaxis for deep vein thrombosis (DVT)

Drug therapy
- Corticosteroid: prednisone
- Antiarrhythmics: propranolol (Inderal), atropine
- Immune globulin I.V.

INTERVENTIONS AND RATIONALES
- Monitor for ascending sensory loss, which precedes motor loss. Also, monitor vital signs and LOC *to detect complications.*
- Assess and treat respiratory dysfunction *to prevent respiratory arrest.* If respiratory muscles are weak, take serial vital capacity recordings. Use a respirometer with a mouth-piece or a face mask for bedside testing *to ensure accurate measurement.*
- Monitor ABG measurements *to assess oxy-genation.*
- Auscultate breath sounds *to detect early changes in respiratory function*, and encourage coughing and deep breathing *to mobilize secretions and prevent atelectasis.*
- Assist with ET tube insertion if respiratory failure occurs *to prevent organ damage from anoxia.*
- Reposition the client every 2 hours and provide skin care *to prevent skin breakdown and pressure ulcer development.*
- Provide foam, gel, or alternating-pressure pads at points of contact *to prevent skin breakdown.*
- Perform passive ROM exercises within the client's pain limits. Remember that the proximal muscle groups of the thighs, shoulders, and trunk will be the most tender and cause the most pain on passive movement and turning. *Passive ROM exercises maintain joint function.*
- Provide gentle stretching and active assistance exercises when the client's condition stabilizes *to strengthen muscles and maintain joint function.*
- Assess the client for signs of dysphagia (coughing, choking, "wet"-sounding voice, increased presence of rhonchi after feeding, drooling, delayed swallowing, regurgitation of food, and weakness in cranial nerve V, VII,

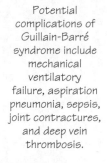

Potential complications of Guillain-Barré syndrome include mechanical ventilatory failure, aspiration pneumonia, sepsis, joint contractures, and deep vein thrombosis.

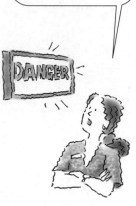

Inspect the patient's legs regularly for signs of DVT, a common complication.

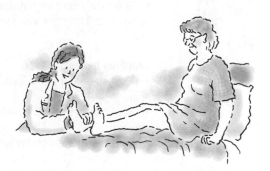

IX, X, XI, or XII). *These measures help prevent aspiration.*
• Elevate the head of the bed, position the client upright and leaning forward when eating, feed semisolid food, and check the mouth for food pockets *to minimize aspiration.*
• Encourage the client to eat slowly and remain upright for 15 to 20 minutes after eating *to prevent aspiration.*
• Provide NG feedings or parenteral nutrition, as ordered, *to prevent aspiration and ensure that nutritional needs are met.*
• Monitor for postural hypotension. Monitor blood pressure and pulse rate during tilting periods, and if necessary, apply toe-to-groin elastic bandages or an abdominal binder *to prevent postural hypotension.*
• Inspect the client's legs regularly for signs of DVT (localized pain, tenderness, erythema, edema, Homans' sign). *DVT is a common complication of Guillain-Barré syndrome.*
• Apply antiembolism stockings and give prophylactic anticoagulants as needed *to prevent DVT.*
• Provide eye and mouth care every 4 hours *to prevent corneal damage and breakdown of the oral mucosa.*
• Protect the corneas with isotonic eyedrops and conical eye shields *to prevent corneal injury.*
• Provide adequate fluid intake (2 qt [2 L]/day), unless contraindicated, *to prevent dehydration, constipation, and renal calculi formation.*
• Measure and record intake and output *to monitor fluid balance.*
• Offer prune juice and a high-bulk diet *to prevent and relieve constipation.* If necessary, give daily or alternate-day suppositories (glycerin or bisacodyl) or Fleet enemas *to relieve constipation.*
• Refer the client for physical therapy, occupational therapy, and speech therapy, as needed.

Teaching topics
• Explanation of the disorder and treatment plan
• Medication use and possible adverse effects
• Physical therapy and rehabilitation needs

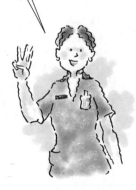

There are three major types of hearing loss.

• Nutritional therapy
• Supportive agencies to assist with home care

Hearing loss

Hearing loss results from a mechanical or nervous impediment to the transmission of sound waves. Hearing loss may be partial or total. There are three major forms of hearing loss:
• conductive loss—interrupted passage of sound from the external ear to the junction of the stapes and oval window
• sensorineural loss—impaired cochlea or eighth cranial nerve dysfunction, causing failure of transmission of sound impulses within the inner ear or brain
• mixed loss—combined dysfunction of conduction and sensorineural transmission.

Sudden deafness refers to sudden hearing loss in a person with no prior hearing impairment. This condition is considered a medical emergency because prompt treatment may restore full hearing.

Noise-induced hearing loss, which may be transient or permanent, usually follows prolonged exposure to loud noises (85 to 90 dB) or brief exposure to extremely loud noises (greater than 90 dB).

Presbycusis, an otologic effect of aging, results from a loss of hair cells in the organ of Corti. This disorder causes progressive, symmetrical, bilateral sensorineural hearing loss, usually of high-frequency tones.

Minor decreases in hearing are common after age 20. Some deafness due to nerve damage occurs in one of every five people by age 55.

CAUSES
• Acute infections
• Blood dyscrasias, such as leukemia and hypercoagulation
• Brain tumor
• Head trauma
• Loud noises
• Metabolic disorders (diabetes mellitus, hypothyroidism)

- Multiple sclerosis
- Ototoxic drugs (loop diuretics, aminogly-cosides)

ASSESSMENT FINDINGS
- Gradual loss of perception of certain frequencies (around 4,000 Hz)
- Inability to understand spoken words
- Sudden deafness (in sudden hearing loss)
- Tinnitus

DIAGNOSTIC TEST RESULTS
- Audiologic examination provides evidence of hearing loss.
- Weber, Rinne, and specialized audiologic tests differentiate between conductive and sensorineural hearing loss.

NURSING DIAGNOSES
- Anxiety
- Ineffective health maintenance
- Disturbed sensory perception
- Disturbed body image

TREATMENT
- Hearing aids
- Overnight rest, for noise-induced hearing loss
- Reduce exposure to loud noises
- Speech and hearing rehabilitation

INTERVENTIONS AND RATIONALES
- Speak slowly and clearly and avoid shouting *to help the client understand your voice.*
- Make sure all staff members are aware of the disability and the client's preferred communication method *to help communicate with the client.*
- Provide emotional support.
- Determine cause of hearing loss, if possible *to help minimize further hearing loss.*
- Stand directly in front of the client with the light on your face *so that the client can read your lips.*
- Approach the client within his vision range and use visual cues to get his attention *because the client will depend more on visual cues.*
- Monitor drug levels in the client receiving ototoxic drugs *to minimize the risk of hearing loss.*

Teaching topics
- Explanation of the disorder and treatment plan
- Using protective devices to minimize exposure to loud noises
- Using and caring for a hearing aid

Huntington's disease

Huntington's disease is a hereditary disease in which degeneration in the cerebral cortex and basal ganglia causes chronic progressive chorea (involuntary and irregular movements) and cognitive deterioration, ending in dementia. Huntington's disease usually strikes people between ages 25 and 55 (the average age is 35). Death usually results 10 to 15 years after onset from suicide, heart failure, or pneumonia. The disorder is also called *Huntington's chorea, hereditary chorea, chronic progressive chorea,* and *adult chorea.*

CAUSES
- Genetic transmission: autosomal dominant trait (Either sex can transmit and inherit the disease. Each child of a parent with this disease has a 50% chance of inheriting it; however, a child who doesn't inherit it can't pass it on to his own children.)

ASSESSMENT FINDINGS
- Choreic movements: rapid, often violent and purposeless that become progressively severe and may include mild fidgeting, tongue smacking, dysarthria (indistinct speech), athetoid movements (slow, sinuous, writhing movements, especially of the hands), and torticollis (twisting of the neck)
- Dementia (can be mild at first but eventually disrupts the client's personality)
- Gradual loss of musculoskeletal control, eventually leading to total dependence
- Personality changes, such as obstinacy, carelessness, untidiness, moodiness, apathy, loss of memory and, possibly, paranoia (in later stages of dementia)

DIAGNOSTIC TEST RESULTS
- PET detects the disease.
- Deoxyribonucleic acid analysis detects the disease.

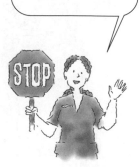

Slow down. Allow the client with Huntington's disease extra time to express himself.

- CT scan reveals brain atrophy.
- MRI demonstrates brain atrophy.
- Molecular genetics may detect the gene for Huntington's disease in people at risk while they're still asymptomatic.

NURSING DIAGNOSES
- Impaired physical mobility
- Ineffective health maintenance
- Risk for injury
- Anxiety
- Fear

TREATMENT
- Supportive, protective treatment aimed at relieving symptoms (because Huntington's disease has no known cure)

Drug therapy
- Antipsychotics: chlorpromazine, haloperidol (Haldol) to help control choreic movements
- Antidepressant: imipramine (Tofranil) to help control choreic movements

INTERVENTIONS AND RATIONALES
- Provide physical support by attending to the client's basic needs, such as hygiene, skin care, bowel and bladder care, and nutrition. Increase this support as mental and physical deterioration make him increasingly immobile. *These measures help prevent complications of immobility.*
- Assist in designing a behavioral plan that deals with the disruptive and aggressive behavior and impulse control problems. Reinforce positive behaviors, and maintain consistency with all caregiving. *These interventions consistently limit the client's negative behaviors.*

> In Ménière's disease, an increase in the amount of fluid in the labyrinth increases pressure in the inner ear and leads to a disruption in the sense of balance.

- Offer emotional support to the client and his family *to relieve anxiety and enhance coping.* Keep in mind the client's dysarthria, and allow him extra time to express himself, *thereby decreasing frustration.*
- Assess psychological status and provide surveillance if the client demonstrates suicidal ideation *to keep the client safe.*
- Provide assistive devices *to help with ambulation.*
- Refer the client and his family to appropriate community organizations.

Teaching topics
- Explanation of the disease process and treatment plan
- Medication use and possible adverse effects
- Family participation in the client's care
- Importance of genetic counseling
- End-of-life and hospice information
- Contact information for the Huntington's Disease Association

Ménière's disease

Ménière's disease is a dysfunction in the labyrinth (the part of the ear that produces balance) that produces severe vertigo, sensorineural hearing loss, and tinnitus. It usually affects adults, men slightly more often than women, between ages 30 and 60. After multiple attacks over several years, this disorder leads to residual tinnitus and hearing loss.

This disorder may also be called *endolymphatic hydrops.*

CAUSES
- Autonomic nervous system dysfunction that produces a temporary constriction of blood vessels supplying the inner ear
- Overproduction or decreased absorption of endolymph, which causes endolymphatic hydrops or endolymphatic hypertension, with consequent degeneration of the vestibular and cochlear hair cells

ASSESSMENT FINDINGS
- Sensorineural hearing loss
- Severe vertigo
- Tinnitus

- Feeling of fullness or blockage in the ear
- Severe nausea
- Vomiting
- Sweating
- Giddiness
- Nystagmus

DIAGNOSTIC TEST RESULTS
- Electronystagmography, electrocochleography, a CT scan, MRI, and X-rays of the internal meatus may be necessary for differential diagnosis.
- Audiometric studies indicate a sensorineural hearing loss and loss of discrimination and recruitment.

NURSING DIAGNOSES
- Impaired physical mobility
- Risk for injury
- Disturbed sensory perception (auditory)
- Anxiety

TREATMENT
- Restriction of sodium intake to less than 2 g/day
- Surgery to destroy the affected labyrinth: only if medical treatment fails; destruction of the labyrinth permanently relieves symptoms causing irreversible hearing loss

Drug therapy
- Anticholinergic: atropine (may stop an attack in 20 to 30 minutes)
- Cardiac stimulant: epinephrine
- Diuretic to prevent excess fluid in the labyrinth (long-term management)
- Antihistamine: diphenhydramine (Benadryl) for severe attack
- Antihistamines: meclizine (Antivert), dimenhydrinate (Dramamine) for milder attacks (may also be administered as part of prophylactic therapy)
- Sedatives: phenobarbital, diazepam (Valium) as part of prophylactic therapy

INTERVENTIONS AND RATIONALES
- Advise the client against reading and exposure to glaring lights *to reduce dizziness.*
- Provide assistance when getting out of bed or walking *to prevent injury.*
- Instruct the client to avoid sudden position changes and any tasks that vertigo makes

hazardous *because an attack can begin quite rapidly.*

Before surgery
- Monitor fluid intake and output *to assess fluid balance.*
- Administer antiemetics as necessary, and give small amounts of fluid frequently *to prevent vomiting.*

After surgery
- Record intake and output carefully *to monitor fluid status and direct the treatment plan.*
- Tell the client to expect dizziness and nausea for 1 to 2 days after surgery *to relieve anxiety.*
- Administer prophylactic antibiotics and antiemetics as required *to decrease the chance of infection and combat nausea.*

Teaching topics
- Explanation of the disease process and treatment options
- Measures to combat dizziness such as rising slowly from a sitting or lying position

Meningitis

Meningitis is an inflammation of the brain and the spinal cord meninges, usually resulting from a bacterial infection. Such inflammation may involve all three meningeal membranes: the dura mater, arachnoid, and pia mater.

The prognosis is good and complications are rare, especially if the disease is recognized early and the infecting organism responds to antibiotics. The prognosis is poorer for infants and elderly people. Mortality is high in untreated meningitis.

CAUSES
- Bacterial infection (may occur secondary to bacteremia [especially from pneumonia, empyema, osteomyelitis, and endocarditis], sinusitis, otitis media, encephalitis, myelitis, or brain abscess)
- Head trauma (may follow a skull fracture, a penetrating head wound, LP, or ventricular shunting procedure)

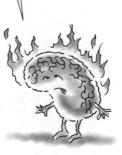

Blame it on bacteria. In meningitis, the brain and the spinal cord meninges become inflamed, usually as a result of bacterial infection.

- Virus (in aseptic viral meningitis, which is usually mild and self-limiting)
- Fungal or protozoal infection (less common)

ASSESSMENT FINDINGS
- Chills
- Coma
- Confusion
- Deep stupor
- Delirium
- Exaggerated deep tendon reflexes
- Fever
- Headache
- Increased ICP
- Irritability
- Malaise
- Opisthotonos (a spasm in which the back and extremities arch backward so that the body rests on the head and heels)
- Petechial, purpuric, or ecchymotic rash on the lower part of the body (meningococcal meningitis)
- Photophobia
- Positive Brudzinski's sign (client flexes hips or knees when the nurse places her hands behind his neck and bends it forward)—a sign of meningeal inflammation and irritation
- Positive Kernig's sign (pain or resistance when the client's leg is flexed at the hip or knee while he's in a supine position)
- Seizures
- Stiff neck and back
- Twitching
- Visual alterations (diplopia—two images of a single object)
- Vomiting

DIAGNOSTIC TEST RESULTS
- An LP shows elevated CSF pressure, cloudy or milky white CSF, high protein level, positive Gram stain and culture that usually identifies the infective organism (unless it's a virus) and depressed CSF glucose concentration.
- Chest X-rays may reveal pneumonitis or lung abscess, tubercular lesions, or granulomas secondary to fungal infection.
- Sinus and skull films may help identify the presence of cranial osteomyelitis, paranasal sinusitis, or skull fracture.

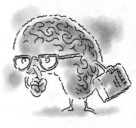

Shhh. Auditory stimuli can contribute to increased ICP. Plus, as you can see, I'm studying.

- WBC count reveals leukocytosis.
- CT scan rules out cerebral hematoma, hemorrhage, or tumor.
- X-pert EV test, when used in combination with other laboratory tests, can differentiate bacterial from viral meningitis.

NURSING DIAGNOSES
- Decreased intracranial adaptive capacity
- Hyperthermia
- Risk for injury
- Acute pain
- Disturbed thought processes

TREATMENT
- Bed rest
- Hypothermia blanket
- I.V. fluid administration
- Oxygen therapy, possibly with ET intubation and mechanical ventilation

Drug therapy
- Antibiotics: penicillin G (Pfizerpen), ampicillin (Omnipen), or nafcillin; or tetracycline (Sumycin) if allergic to penicillin
- Diuretic: mannitol
- Anticonvulsants: phenytoin (Dilantin), phenobarbital
- Analgesics or antipyretics: acetaminophen (Tylenol), aspirin
- Laxative: bisacodyl (Dulcolax)
- Stool softener: docusate sodium (Colace)

INTERVENTIONS AND RATIONALES
- Monitor neurologic function often to detect early signs of increased ICP, such as plucking at the bedcovers, vomiting, seizures, and a change in motor function and vital signs. *Detecting early signs of increased ICP prevents treatment delay.*
- Monitor fluid balance. Maintain adequate fluid intake *to avoid dehydration without causing fluid overload, which may lead to cerebral edema.*
- Measure central venous pressure and intake and output accurately *to determine fluid volume status.*
- Suction the client only if necessary. Limit suctioning to 10 to 15 seconds per pass of the catheter. *Suctioning stimulates coughing and Valsalva's maneuver; Valsalva's maneuver increases intrathoracic pressure,*

decreases cerebral venous drainage, and increases cerebral blood volume, resulting in increased ICP.

- Monitor for adverse reactions to I.V. antibiotics and other drugs *to prevent complications such as anaphylaxis.*
- Position the client carefully *to prevent joint stiffness and neck pain.*
- Reposition the client every 2 hours and provide skin care *to prevent skin breakdown.*
- Assist with ROM exercises *to prevent contractures.*
- Provide small, frequent meals or supplement meals with NG tube or parenteral feedings *to maintain adequate nutrition and elimination.*
- Administer a mild laxative or stool softener *to prevent constipation and minimize the risk of increased ICP resulting from straining during defecation.*
- Provide mouth care regularly *to prevent breakdown of the oral mucosa and promote client comfort.*
- Maintain a quiet environment and darken the room *to prevent increased ICP and to decrease photophobia.*
- Provide reassurance and support *to decrease anxiety.*
- Assess pain level and administer analgesics as ordered *to control pain.* Evaluate effectiveness of treatment.
- Follow strict aseptic technique when treating clients with head wounds or skull fractures *to prevent meningitis.*

Teaching topics
- Explanation of the disorder and treatment plan
- Medication use and possible adverse effects
- Preventing meningitis (teach clients with chronic sinusitis or other chronic infections the importance of proper medical treatment)
- Recognizing signs of meningitis
- Contagion risks; notifying anyone who came in close contact with the client

Multiple sclerosis

Multiple sclerosis is a neurodegenerative disease caused by degeneration of the myelin sheath in neurons of the brain and spinal cord. It results in patches of sclerotic tissue that impair the ability of the nervous system to conduct motor nerve impulses.

CAUSES
- Autoimmune response
- Environmental or genetic factors
- Slow-acting or latent viral infection
- Unknown

ASSESSMENT FINDINGS
- Ataxia
- Feelings of euphoria
- Heat intolerance
- Inability to sense or gauge body position
- Intention tremor
- Nystagmus, diplopia, blurred vision, optic neuritis
- Scanning speech
- Urinary incontinence or retention
- Weakness, paresthesia, impaired sensation, paralysis

DIAGNOSTIC TEST RESULTS
- CSF analysis shows increased immunoglobulin G, protein, and WBCs or it may be normal.
- CT scan eliminates other diagnoses such as brain or spinal cord tumors.
- MRI of the brain and spine shows scarring or lesions.

NURSING DIAGNOSES
- Ineffective airway clearance
- Impaired physical mobility
- Imbalanced nutrition: Less than body requirements
- Risk for injury
- Anxiety

TREATMENT
- A high-calorie, high-vitamin, gluten-free, and low-fat diet
- Increased intake of fluids
- Physical therapy
- Plasmapheresis (for antibody removal)
- Speech therapy

Drug therapy
- Cholinergic: bethanechol (Urecholine)
- Glucocorticoids: prednisone, dexamethasone, corticotropin (ACTH)

Management moments

Teaching tips for MS

Teaching the client how to live with multiple sclerosis (MS) is important in managing his care. Begin by teaching the client and his family about the chronic course of MS. Emphasize the need to avoid stress, infections, and fatigue and to maintain independence by developing new ways of performing daily activities.

FAMILY FUNCTION

• Teach the family to assist with physical therapy, such as active, resistive, and stretching exercises to maintain muscle tone and joint mobility, decrease spasticity, and improve coordination.
• Tell them that massages and relaxing baths can increase the client's comfort.
• Explain that bath water shouldn't be too hot because it may temporarily intensify otherwise subtle symptoms.
• Encourage the family and client to establish a daily routine to maintain optimal functioning. Activity should be regulated by the client's tolerance. The client should be encouraged to have regular rest periods to prevent fatigue.

• Immunosuppressants: interferon beta-1b (Betaseron), cyclophosphamide (Cytoxan), methotrexate (Trexall)
• Skeletal muscle relaxants: dantrolene (Dantrium), baclofen (Lioresal)

INTERVENTIONS AND RATIONALES

• Assess changes in motor coordination, paralysis, or muscular weakness and report changes *to facilitate early intervention.*
• Assess respiratory status at least every 4 hours *to detect early signs of compromise.*
• Maintain the client's diet *to decrease the risk of constipation.*
• Encourage fluid intake *to decrease the risk of urinary tract infection.*
• Administer medications, as prescribed, *to improve or maintain the client's condition and functional status.*
• Encourage verbalization of feelings about changes in body image and provide emotional support *to promote acceptance of muscular impairment.*
• Maintain active and passive exercises *to maintain ROM and prevent musculoskeletal degeneration.*
• Establish a bowel and bladder program *to decrease the risk of constipation and urinary retention.*
• Maintain activity, as tolerated (alternating rest and activity), *to improve muscle tone and enhance self-esteem.*

• Protect the client from falls *to prevent injury.*
• Monitor the client's neuromuscular status and voiding pattern *to facilitate early interventions for urinary retention.*

Teaching topics

• Explanation of the disorder and treatment plan
• Medication use and possible adverse effects
• Reducing stress
• Recognizing the signs and symptoms of exacerbation
• Maintaining a sense of independence
• Avoiding temperature extremes, especially heat
• Contacting the National Multiple Sclerosis Society (See *Teaching tips for MS*)

Myasthenia gravis

A neuromuscular disorder, myasthenia gravis is marked by weakness of voluntary muscles. The client experiences sporadic, progressive weakness and abnormal fatigue of voluntary skeletal muscles.

Myasthenia gravis is characterized by a disturbance in transmission of nerve impulses at neuromuscular junctions.

This transmission defect results from a deficiency in release of acetylcholine or a deficient number of acetylcholine receptor sites.

CAUSES
- Autoimmune disease
- Excessive cholinesterase
- Insufficient acetylcholine

ASSESSMENT FINDINGS
- Diplopia, ptosis, strabismus
- Dysarthria
- Dysphagia, drooling
- Impaired speech
- Masklike expression
- Muscle weakness and fatigue (typically, muscles are strongest in the morning but weaken throughout the day, especially after exercise)
- Profuse sweating
- Respiratory distress

DIAGNOSTIC TEST RESULTS
- EMG shows decreased amplitude of evoked potentials.
- Neostigmine (Prostigmin) or edrophonium (Tensilon) test relieves symptoms after medication administration—a positive indication of the disease.
- Thymus scan reveals hyperplasia or thymoma.

NURSING DIAGNOSES
- Impaired gas exchange
- Impaired physical mobility
- Impaired verbal communication
- Risk for injury
- Anxiety

TREATMENT
- A high-calorie diet with soft foods
- Plasmapheresis (in severe exacerbations)

Drug therapy
- Anticholinesterase inhibitors: neostigmine (Prostigmin), pyridostigmine (Mestinon), ambenonium (Mytelase)
- Glucocorticoids: prednisone, dexamethasone, corticotropin (ACTH)
- Immunosuppressants: azathioprine (Imuran), cyclophosphamide (Cytoxan)

INTERVENTIONS AND RATIONALES
- Monitor neurologic and respiratory status. *Respiratory muscle weakness may be severe enough in myasthenic crisis to require an emergency airway and mechanical ventilation.*
- Assess swallow and gag reflexes *to prevent aspiration and determine the extent of the neurologic deficit.*
- Monitor the client for choking while eating *to prevent aspiration of food particles.*
- Monitor and record vital signs and intake and output *to prevent fluid overload or deficit and facilitate early intervention for deterioration of respiratory status.*
- Administer medications, as prescribed, *to relieve symptoms.*
- Maintain the client's diet; encourage small, frequent meals *to conserve energy and meet nutritional needs.*
- Encourage verbalization of feelings about changes in body image and about difficulty in communicating verbally *to reduce the tendency to suppress or repress feelings about neuromuscular loss.*
- Determine the client's activity tolerance and assist in ADLs *to conserve energy and avoid fatigue.*
- Provide rest periods *to reduce the body's oxygen demands and prevent fatigue.*
- Provide oral hygiene *to promote comfort and enhance appetite.*
- Improve environmental safety *to prevent falls.*

Teaching topics
- Explanation of the disorder and treatment plan
- Medication use and possible adverse effects
- Reducing stress
- Recognizing the signs and symptoms of respiratory distress
- Recognizing the signs and symptoms of myasthenic crisis
- Adhering to activity limitations
- Contacting the Myasthenia Gravis Foundation

Otosclerosis

Otosclerosis is an overgrowth of the ear's spongy bone around the oval window and stapes footplate. This overgrowth curtails

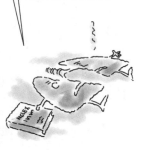

Heads up. Respiratory muscle weakness in myasthenic crisis may require an emergency airway and mechanical ventilation.

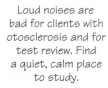

Loud noises are bad for clients with otosclerosis and for test review. Find a quiet, calm place to study.

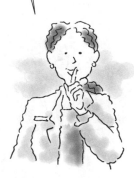

movement of the stapes in the oval window, preventing sound from being transmitted to the cochlea and resulting in conductive hearing loss.

CAUSES
• Familial tendency

ASSESSMENT FINDINGS
• Progressive hearing loss
• Tinnitus

DIAGNOSTIC TEST RESULTS
• Audiometric testing confirms hearing loss.

NURSING DIAGNOSES
• Anxiety
• Impaired verbal communication
• Disturbed sensory perception (auditory)

TREATMENT
• Hearing aid (air conduction aid with molded ear insert receiver)
• Stapedectomy and insertion of a prosthesis to restore partial or total hearing

Drug therapy
• Antibiotics postoperatively to prevent infection

INTERVENTIONS AND RATIONALES
• Monitor vital signs and dressing post-operatively for signs of bleeding *to detect complications.*
• Develop alternative means of communication *to decrease anxiety and communicate effectively with the client.*

Teaching topics
• Explanation of the disorder and treatment plan
• Medication use and possible adverse effects
• Using a hearing aid
• Avoiding loud noises and sudden pressure changes until healing is complete
• Avoiding (for at least 1 week) blowing the nose to prevent contaminated air and bacteria from entering the eustachian tube
• Protecting the ears against cold
• Avoiding activities that provoke dizziness
• Changing external ear dressings

Parkinson's disease

Parkinson's disease is a progressive, degenerative disorder of the CNS associated with dopamine deficiency. This lack of dopamine impairs the area of the brain responsible for control of voluntary movement. As a result, most symptoms relate to problems with posture and movement.

CAUSES
• Cerebral vascular disease
• Dopamine deficiency
• Drug-induced effect
• Imbalance of dopamine and acetylcholine in basal ganglia
• Repeated head trauma
• Unknown

ASSESSMENT FINDINGS
• Pill-rolling tremors, tremors at rest
• Difficulty in initiating voluntary activity
• Dysphagia, drooling
• Fatigue
• Masklike facial expression
• Shuffling gait, stiff joints, dyskinesia, cogwheel rigidity, stooped posture
• Small handwriting

DIAGNOSTIC TEST RESULTS
• CT scan is normal.
• EEG reveals minimal slowing of brain activity.

NURSING DIAGNOSES
• Activity intolerance
• Impaired physical mobility
• Imbalanced nutrition: Less than body requirements
• Disturbed body image
• Fear
• Anxiety

TREATMENT
• A high-residue, high-calorie, high-protein diet composed primarily of soft foods
• Physical therapy
• Stereotactic neurosurgery: thalamotomy or pallidotomy
• Deep brain stimulation

Because Parkinson's disease affects movement, client care includes preventing falls and other safety issues.

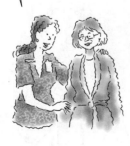

Drug therapy

- Anticholinergic: trihexyphenidyl
- Antidepressant: amitriptyline (Elavil)
- Antiparkinsonian agents: carbidopa-levodopa (Sinemet), benztropine (Cogentin)
- Antispasmodic: dantrolene (Dantrium)
- Antiviral agent: amantadine (Symmetrel) (used early on to reduce tremors and rigidity)
- Dopamine receptor agonist: bromocriptine (Parlodel)
- Enzyme inhibiting agent: selegiline (Eldepryl)

INTERVENTIONS AND RATIONALES

- Monitor neurologic and respiratory status *to detect change in status and possible need for change in treatment.*
- Monitor and record vital signs and intake and output *to detect complications.*
- Monitor the client at mealtimes *to decrease the risk of aspiration.*
- Position the client *to prevent contractures and maintain skin integrity.*
- Administer medications as prescribed *to improve functioning.* (Elderly clients may need smaller doses of antiparkinsonian drugs because of reduced tolerance. Be alert for and report orthostatic hypotension, irregular pulse, blepharospasm, and anxiety or confusion.)
- Encourage verbalization of feelings about changes in body image *to reduce anxiety and depression.*
- Promote daily ambulation *to promote independence.*
- Provide active and passive ROM exercises *to maintain mobility.*
- Maintain the client's diet *to decrease constipation.*
- Provide skin care daily *to maintain skin integrity.*
- Provide oral hygiene *to promote self-care and improve nutritional intake.*
- Reinforce gait training *to improve mobility.*
- Reinforce independence in care *to maintain self-esteem.*

Teaching topics

- Explanation of the disorder and treatment plan
- Medication use and possible adverse effects
- Physical therapy
- Nutritional therapy
- Recognizing early signs and symptoms of respiratory distress
- Alternating rest periods with activity
- Promoting a safe environment (shuffling gait and rigidity make clients very prone to falls, so encourage family members to remove obstacles and throw rugs)
- Preventing choking or aspiration
- Contacting the American Parkinson Disease Association for information about local support groups

Retinal detachment

Retinal detachment is the separation of the retina (a thin, semitransparent layer of nerve tissue that lines the eye wall) from the choroid (the middle vascular coat of the eye between the retina and the sclera). It occurs when the retina develops a hole or tear and the vitreous humour seeps between the retina and choroid. If left untreated, retinal detachment can lead to vision loss.

CAUSES

- Aging
- Diabetic neovascularization
- Familial tendency
- Hemorrhage
- Inflammatory process
- Myopia
- Trauma
- Tumor

ASSESSMENT FINDINGS

- Painless change in vision (floaters and flashes of light)
- Photopsia (recurrent flashes of light)
- With progression of detachment, painless vision loss may be described as a "veil curtain" or "cobweb" that eliminates part of visual field

DIAGNOSTIC TEST RESULTS

- Indirect ophthalmoscope shows retinal tear or detachment.
- Slit-lamp examination shows retinal tear or detachment.
- Ultrasound shows retinal tear or detachment in presence of cataract.

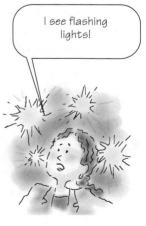

I see flashing lights!

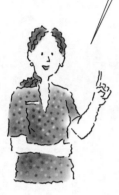

Speaking of seeing, make sure that you have good lighting. It'll help you study longer and more comfortably.

NURSING DIAGNOSES
- Anxiety
- Risk for injury
- Disturbed sensory perception (visual)

TREATMENT
- Complete bed rest and restriction of eye movement to prevent further detachment
- Cryopexy, if there's a hole in the peripheral retina
- Laser therapy, if there's a hole in the posterior portion of the retina
- Scleral buckling or diathermy to reattach the retina

INTERVENTIONS AND RATIONALES
- Assess visual status and functional vision in unaffected eye *to determine self-care needs.*
- Postoperatively instruct the client to lie on his back or on his unoperated side *to reduce intraocular pressure on the affected side.*
- Discourage straining during defecation, bending down, and hard coughing, sneezing, or vomiting *to avoid activities that can increase intraocular pressure.*
- Provide assistance with ADLs *to minimize frustration and strain.*
- Assist with ambulation, as needed, *to help the client remain independent and to prevent injury.*
- Orient client to his environment *to reduce the risk of injury.*

Teaching topics
- Explanation of the disorder and treatment plan
- Use of eye shields while playing sports
- Need for eye rest
- Keeping walkways free of clutter to prevent falls

Seizure disorder

Seizure disorder is a condition of the brain marked by a susceptibility to recurrent seizures, paroxysmal events associated with abnormal electrical discharges of neurons in the brain.

Seizure disorder affects 1% to 2% of the population. However, 80% of patients have good seizure control if they strictly adhere to the prescribed treatment regimen.

CAUSES
In about one-half of the cases of seizure disorder, the cause is unknown. Other possible causes include:
- alcohol withdrawal
- anoxia after respiratory or cardiac arrest
- birth trauma (inadequate oxygen supply to the brain)
- brain tumor
- hypoglycemia
- infectious disease, such as meningitis, encephalitis, or brain abscess
- ingestion of toxins
- inherited disorder such as phenylketonuria
- stroke.

ASSESSMENT FINDINGS
- Recurring seizures (see *Differentiating among seizure types*)

DIAGNOSTIC TEST RESULTS
- EEG shows continuing tendency to have seizures. A negative EEG doesn't rule out seizure disorder because the paroxysmal abnormalities may occur intermittently.
- Other tests that may be performed to rule out other diagnoses include serum glucose, LP, and cerebral angiography.

NURSING DIAGNOSES
- Disturbed body image
- Risk for injury
- Risk for impaired gas exchange
- Anxiety

TREATMENT
- Surgical removal of demonstrated focal lesion
- Strict ketogenic diet: can help with remission for some clients who don't respond to other treatment

Drug therapy
- For status epilepticus: diazepam (Valium), lorazepam (Ativan), phenytoin
- Phenytoin (Dilantin), carbamazepine (Tegretol), gabapentin (Neurontin) for generalized tonic-clonic seizures

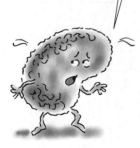

Argh! Look out for those abnormal electrical discharges by those pesky neurons!

Differentiating among seizure types

The hallmark of seizure disorder is recurring seizures, which can be classified as partial or generalized. Some clients may be affected by more than one type of seizure.

PARTIAL SEIZURES (FOCAL, LOCAL SEIZURES)

Arising from a localized area in the brain, partial seizures cause specific symptoms. Categories of partial seizures include simple partial seizures (consciousness is intact), complex partial seizures (some loss of consciousness occurs), and partial seizures in which seizure activity may be spread to the entire brain, thereby causing a generalized seizure.

Simple partial seizures

A simple partial seizure can be present in several ways depending upon the focal point of the seizure in the brain.
- motor symptoms (jerking of the thumb or the cheek)
- somatosensory symptoms (visual, vestibular, gustatory, olfactory, or auditory hallucinations or sensations)
- autonomic symptoms (such as tachycardia, sweating, and pupillary dilation)
- psychic symptoms (which rarely occur without some changes in consciousness such as feelings of déjà-vu or dreamy states).

Complex partial seizures

Consciousness becomes impaired with a complex partial seizure. This type of seizure begins as a simple partial seizure in which the consciousness isn't impaired and evolves to an impairment of consciousness. The same symptoms that present during a simple partial seizure are still seen as the seizure develops into a complex partial seizure.

Partial seizures evolving to generalized tonic-clonic seizures

A partial seizure can be either a simple partial or a complex partial seizure that progresses to a generalized seizure. An aura may precede the progression. Loss of consciousness occurs immediately or within 1 to 2 minutes of the start of the progression.

GENERALIZED SEIZURES (CONVULSIVE OR NONCONVULSIVE)

As the term suggests, generalized seizures cause a general electrical abnormality within the brain. They include several distinct types.

Absence (petit mal) seizures

An absence seizure occurs commonly in children, but it may also affect adults. It usually begins with a brief change in the level of consciousness, indicated by blinking or rolling of the eyes, or a blank stare, and slight mouth movements. Typically, the seizure lasts 1 to 10 seconds. The impairment is so brief that the patient (or parent) is sometimes unaware of it. If not properly treated, these seizures can recur as often as 100 times per day and may result in learning difficulties.

Myoclonic seizures

A myoclonic seizure is marked by brief bilateral muscular jerks of the body extremities. They may occur in a rhythmic manner and may be accompanied by brief loss of consciousness.

Generalized tonic-clonic (grand mal) seizures

Typically, a generalized tonic-clonic seizure begins with a loud cry, precipitated by air rushing from the lungs through the vocal cords. The client falls to the ground, losing consciousness. The body stiffens (tonic phase) and then alternates between episodes of muscle spasm and relaxation (clonic phase). Tongue biting, incontinence, labored breathing, apnea, and subsequent cyanosis may also occur. The seizure stops in 2 to 5 minutes, when abnormal electrical conduction of the neurons is completed. The client then regains consciousness but is somewhat confused and may have difficulty talking. If he can talk, he may complain of drowsiness,

(continued)

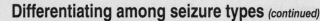

Differentiating among seizure types (continued)

fatigue, headache, muscle soreness, and arm or leg weakness. He may fall into a deep sleep after the seizure.

Atonic seizures (drop attacks)
Characterized by a general loss of postural tone and a temporary loss of consciousness, an atonic seizure occurs in young children. It's sometimes called a "drop attack" because it causes the child to fall.

• Thiamine I.V. in chronic alcoholism or withdrawal
• Valproic acid and clonazepam (Klonopin) generally used for absence seizures

INTERVENTIONS AND RATIONALES
• Keep the client safe during seizure activity. *The client is at an increased risk for injury during a seizure.*
• Don't restrain the client during a seizure; instead, place the client in a flat, side-lying position. *This helps prevent aspiration during the seizure.*
• Maintain a patent airway, but don't force anything into the client's mouth *because this can injure the client.*
• When administering phenytoin I.V., use a large vein and monitor vital signs *because it can have serious cardiovascular effects.*
• Monitor the client's medication levels *because many anticonvulsants have narrow therapeutic ranges.*
• Monitor the client for seizure activity.

Teaching topics
• Explanation of the disorder and treatment plan
• Medication regimen and adverse effects
• Monitoring of medication levels
• Caring for clients during a seizure
• Avoiding alcohol and illicit drugs
• Referring to the Epilepsy Foundation of America

Spinal cord injury

Spinal cord injuries usually result from traumatic force on the vertebral column. Necrosis and scar tissue form in the area of the traumatized cord. Damage to the spinal cord results in sensory and motor deficits. The client may experience partial or full loss of function of any or all extremities and bodily functions.

CAUSES
• Congenital anomalies
• Penetrating wounds
• Infections
• Trauma resulting from situations, such as an automobile accident, diving into shallow water, or fall
• Tumors

ASSESSMENT FINDINGS
• Absence of reflexes below the level of the injury
• Flaccid muscle
• Loss of bowel and bladder control
• Neck pain
• Numbness and tingling
• Paralysis below the level of the injury
• Paresthesia below the level of the injury
• Respiratory distress

DIAGNOSTIC TEST RESULTS
• CT scan shows spinal cord edema, vertebral fracture, and spinal cord compression.
• MRI shows spinal cord edema, vertebral fracture, and spinal cord compression.
• Spinal X-rays reveal vertebral fracture.

NURSING DIAGNOSES
• Impaired physical mobility
• Posttrauma syndrome
• Powerlessness
• Anxiety
• Fear
• Disturbed body image

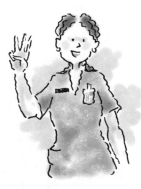

Don't stop now! Only three more disorders to go.

TREATMENT

- Flat position, with neck immobilized in a cervical collar
- Maintenance of vertebral alignment through skull tongs, Halo vest
- Specialized rotation bed
- Surgery for stabilization of the upper spine such as insertion of Harrington rods

Drug therapy

- Antianxiety agent: lorazepam (Ativan)
- Glucocorticoid: methylprednisolone infusion immediately following injury
- H_2-receptor antagonists: cimetidine (Tagamet), ranitidine (Zantac), famotidine (Pepcid)
- Laxative: bisacodyl (Dulcolax)
- Mucosal barrier fortifier: sucralfate (Carafate)
- Muscle relaxant: dantrolene (Dantrium)

INTERVENTIONS AND RATIONALES

- Monitor neurologic and respiratory status *to determine baseline and detect early complications.*
- Assess for spinal shock *to detect early changes in the client's condition* and initiate prompt treatment.
- Monitor and record vital signs and intake and output, laboratory studies, and pulse oximetry *to detect early changes in the client's condition.*
- Monitor for autonomic dysreflexia (sudden extreme rise in blood pressure) in clients with spinal injury at level T6 or higher *to prevent life-threatening complications.*
- Administer fluids *to maintain hydration.*
- Administer oxygen, as needed, *to maintain oxygenation to cells.*
- Provide suctioning, if necessary, and encourage coughing and deep breathing *to maintain patent airway.*
- Administer medications, as prescribed, *to maintain or improve the client's condition.*
- Encourage verbalization of feelings about changes in body image, changes in sexual expression and function, and altered mobility *to reduce anxiety and depression.*
- Reposition the client every 2 hours using the logrolling technique (only if the client is stabilized and not in a specialty bed) *to prevent pressure ulcers.*

- Provide skin care *to maintain skin integrity.*
- Keep the tool available to open Halo vest in the case of cardiac arrest *to maintain client safety.*
- Maintain body alignment *to maintain joint function and prevent musculoskeletal degeneration.*
- Initiate bowel and bladder retraining *to avoid stimuli that could trigger dysreflexia.*
- Provide passive ROM exercises *to maintain joint mobility and muscle tone.*
- Apply antiembolism stockings *to maintain venous circulation and prevent thromboembolism.*
- Provide sexual counseling *to encourage questions and avoid misunderstandings.*
- Provide emotional support *to decrease anxiety and fear.*

Teaching topics

- Explanation of the disorder and treatment plan
- Medication use and possible adverse effects
- Nutritional therapy
- Exercising regularly to strengthen muscles
- Recognizing the signs and symptoms of autonomic dysreflexia, urinary tract infection, and upper respiratory infection
- Continuing a bowel and bladder program
- Maintaining acidic urine with cranberry juice
- Consuming adequate fluids: 3 qt (3 L)/day
- Using assistive devices with proper body mechanics for ADLs
- Maintaining skin integrity
- Using a wheelchair and proper transfer techniques such as moving the strong part of the client's body to the chair first
- Maintaining a sense of independence
- Contacting the National Spinal Cord Injury Association

Stroke

A stroke, previously known as a *cerebrovascular accident*, results from a sudden impairment of cerebral circulation in one or more of the blood vessels supplying the brain. A stroke interrupts or diminishes oxygen supply and commonly causes serious damage or necrosis in brain tissues.

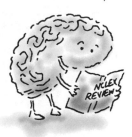

A stroke results from a sudden impairment of cerebral circulation in one or more of the blood vessels supplying the brain. Not cool.

The sooner circulation returns to normal after stroke, the better the client's chances for a complete recovery. However, about half of those who survive a stroke remain permanently disabled and experience a recurrence within weeks, months, or years.

CAUSES
- Cerebral arteriosclerosis
- Embolism
- Hemorrhage
- Hypertension
- Thrombosis
- Vasospasm

ASSESSMENT FINDINGS
Stroke symptoms depend on the artery affected. (See *Location, location, location.*)

Generalized symptoms
- Sudden numbness or weakness of the arm or leg on one side of the body
- Sudden change in mental status; difficulty speaking or understanding
- Sudden vision disturbances
- Sudden difficulty walking, maintaining balance, or dizziness
- Sudden severe headache

DIAGNOSTIC TEST RESULTS
- CT scan reveals intracranial bleeding, infarct (shows up 24 hours after the initial symptoms), or shift of midline structures.
- Digital subtraction angiography reveals occlusion or narrowing of vessels.
- EEG shows focal slowing in area of lesion.
- MRI shows intracranial bleeding, infarct, or shift of midline structures.

NURSING DIAGNOSES
- Ineffective tissue perfusion: Cerebral
- Risk for aspiration
- Risk for injury
- Disturbed body image
- Anxiety
- Fear

TREATMENT
- Active and passive ROM and isometric exercises
- Bed rest until blood pressure stabilizes
- Low-sodium diet
- Physical therapy

Drug therapy
- Analgesic: codeine sulfate or codeine phosphate (if nothing-by-mouth status) to reduce headache
- Anticoagulants: heparin, warfarin (Coumadin), ticlopidine (Ticlid)
- Anticonvulsant: phenytoin (Dilantin)
- Diuretics: mannitol, furosemide (Lasix)
- Glucocorticoid: dexamethasone
- H_2-receptor antagonists: cimetidine (Tagamet), ranitidine (Zantac), famotidine (Pepcid), nizatidine (Axid)
- Thrombolytic therapy: tissue plasminogen activator given within the first 3 hours of the start of symptoms of an ischemic stroke to restore circulation to the affected brain tissue and limit the extent of brain injury

INTERVENTIONS AND RATIONALES
- Monitor neurologic status every 1 to 2 hours initially and then every 4 hours when the client becomes stable *to screen for changes in LOC and neurologic status.*
- Monitor vital signs every 1 to 2 hours initially and then every 4 hours when the client becomes stable *to detect early signs of decreased cerebral perfusion pressure or increased ICP.*
- Elevate the head of bed 30 degrees *to facilitate venous drainage and reduce cellular edema.*
- Maintain the client's diet *to promote nutritional status and healing.*
- Administer I.V. fluids and monitor intake and output *to prevent volume overload or deficit.*
- Take client's temperature at least every 4 hours. *Hyperthermia causes increased ICP; hypothermia causes reduced cerebral perfusion pressure.*
- Monitor hemoglobin and hematocrit and report anomalies *to prevent tissue ischemia.*
- Assess respiratory status at least every 4 hours *for signs of aspiration or respiratory depression.*
- Administer medications and evaluate their effects *to improve or maintain the client's condition.*

Location, location, location

Clinical features of stroke vary with the artery affected (and, consequently, the portion of the brain the artery supplies), the severity of damage, and the extent of collateral circulation that develops to help the brain compensate for decreased blood supply.

Typical arteries affected and their associated signs and symptoms are described here.

MIDDLE CEREBRAL ARTERY
Injury to the middle cerebral artery causes aphasia, dysphagia, visual field cuts, and hemiparesis on the affected side (more severe in the face and arm than in the leg).

CAROTID ARTERY
If the carotid artery is affected, the client may develop weakness, paralysis, numbness, sensory changes, and visual disturbances on the affected side; altered level of consciousness, bruits, headaches, aphasia, and ptosis.

VERTEBROBASILAR ARTERY
A stroke affecting the vertebrobasilar artery may lead to weakness on the affected side, numbness around the lips and mouth, visual field cuts, diplopia, poor coordination, dysphagia, slurred speech, dizziness, amnesia, and ataxia.

ANTERIOR CEREBRAL ARTERY
If the anterior cerebral artery becomes affected, the client may develop confusion, weakness and numbness (especially in the leg) on the affected side, incontinence, loss of coordination, impaired motor and sensory functions, and personality changes.

POSTERIOR CEREBRAL ARTERIES
If the posterior cerebral arteries are affected, the client may develop visual field cuts, sensory impairment, dyslexia, coma, and cortical blindness. Usually, paralysis is absent.

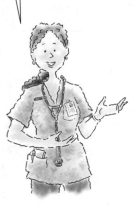

Stroke care shifts focus. When the emergency has passed, care turns to rehab and recovery.

• Provide oral suction, as needed, *to keep the client's airway clear.*
• Administer oxygen *to promote cerebral tissue oxygenation.*
• Assist the client with coughing and deep breathing *to mobilize secretions.*
• Administer enteral nutrition or TPN depending on the client's condition *to facilitate tissue healing and meet metabolic needs.*
• Apply antiembolism stockings *to promote venous return and prevent thromboembolism formation.*
• Maintain seizure precautions and administer anticonvulsants as ordered. *Seizures increase intrathoracic pressure, decrease cerebral venous outflow, and increase cerebral blood volume, thereby increasing ICP.*
• Provide passive ROM exercises *to prevent venous thrombosis and contractures.*
• Reposition the client every 2 hours and provide skin care *to prevent pressure ulcers.*
• Provide means of communication *to promote understanding and decrease anxiety.*
• Maintain routine bowel and bladder function and administer diuretics, as ordered, *to promote fluid mobilization.*
• Encourage expression of feelings about changes in body image and about difficulty in communicating verbally *to promote reduced anxiety and expression of feelings.*
• Maintain a quiet environment *to prevent increases in ICP.*
• Protect the client from falls and injury and provide a safe environment *to reduce the risk of injury.*
• Provide emotional support *to decrease anxiety and fear.*

Teaching topics
• Explanation of the disorder and treatment plan
• Medication use and possible adverse effects
• Physical therapy and rehabilitation options
• Nutritional therapy and speech therapy
• Monitoring blood pressure
• Recognizing signs and symptoms of stroke
• Minimizing environmental stress
• Communicating effectively (for an aphasic client)
• Using devices to assist in ADLs
• Reducing stress
• Contacting the American Heart Association and the National Stroke Association

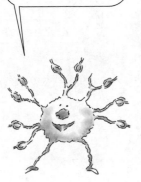

Who says I'm not sensitive? In trigeminal neuralgia, pain may be triggered by touching a sensitive area on the face or even by temperature changes.

Trigeminal neuralgia

Trigeminal neuralgia is a painful disorder of one or more branches of the fifth cranial (trigeminal) nerve that produces paroxysmal attacks of excruciating facial pain. Attacks are precipitated by stimulation of a trigger zone, a hypersensitive area of the face.

It occurs mostly in people older than age 40, in women more commonly than men, and on the right side of the face more often than the left. Trigeminal neuralgia can subside spontaneously, with remissions lasting from several months to years. The disorder is also called *tic douloureux*.

CAUSES

Although the cause remains undetermined, trigeminal neuralgia may:
• reflect an afferent reflex phenomenon located centrally in the brain stem or more peripherally in the sensory root of the trigeminal nerve
• be related to compression of the nerve root by posterior fossa tumors, middle fossa tumors, or vascular lesions (subclinical aneurysm), although such lesions usually produce simultaneous loss of sensation
• occasionally be a manifestation of multiple sclerosis or herpes zoster.

Triggers

• Light touch to a sensitive area of the face (trigger zone)
• Exposure to hot or cold
• Eating, smiling, or talking
• Drinking hot or cold beverages

ASSESSMENT FINDINGS

• Searing pain in the facial area
• Splinting of the affected area
• Holding the face immobile when talking
• Unwashed, unshaven face on the affected side

DIAGNOSTIC TEST RESULTS

• Skull X-rays, tomography, and CT scan rule out sinus or tooth infections and tumors.

NURSING DIAGNOSES

• Acute pain
• Powerlessness
• Anxiety

Offer the client with trigeminal neuralgia small, frequent meals at room temperature. Temperature extremes may cause an attack.

TREATMENT

• Percutaneous radio frequency procedure, which causes partial root destruction and relieves pain
• Microsurgery for vascular decompression
• Percutaneous electrocoagulation of nerve rootlets, under local anesthesia

Drug therapy

• Anticonvulsant: carbamazepine (Tegretol) or phenytoin (Dilantin) may temporarily relieve or prevent pain

INTERVENTIONS AND RATIONALES

• Observe and record the characteristics and triggers of each attack, including the client's protective mechanisms *to gain information for developing the treatment plan.*
• Provide adequate nutrition in small, frequent meals at room temperature *to ensure nutritional needs are met. Temperature extremes may cause an attack.*
• Observe for adverse reactions to carbamazepine, especially cutaneous and hematologic reactions (erythematous and pruritic rashes, urticaria, photosensitivity, exfoliative dermatitis, leukopenia, agranulocytosis, eosinophilia, aplastic anemia, thrombocytopenia) and, possibly, urine retention and transient drowsiness. *Identifying adverse reactions early helps to limit complications.*
• Watch for adverse reactions to phenytoin, including ataxia, skin eruptions, gingival hyperplasia, and nystagmus. *Early detection of adverse reactions limits complications with early intervention.*
• After resection of the first division of the trigeminal nerve, instruct the client to avoid rubbing his eyes and using aerosol spray. Advise him to wear glasses or goggles outdoors and to blink often *to prevent injury.*
• After surgery to sever the second or third division, instruct the client to avoid hot foods and drinks, *which could burn his mouth.* Also advise him to chew carefully *to avoid biting his mouth.*
• Advise the client to place food in the unaffected side of his mouth when chewing, to brush his teeth often, and to see a dentist twice per year to detect cavities. *Cavities in the area of the severed nerve won't cause pain.*

- After surgery, monitor neurologic status and vital signs often *to detect early signs of postoperative complications*.
- Reinforce natural avoidance of stimulation (air, heat, cold) of trigger zones (lips, cheeks, gums) *to prevent further episodes*.

Teaching topics

- Disease process and treatment options
- Avoiding triggers of an attack such as temperature extremes

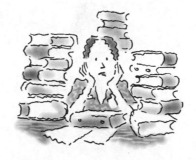

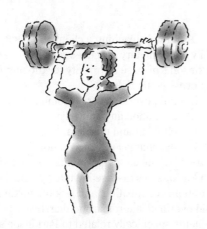

Pump up on practice questions

1. A nurse is caring for a client with dysphasia. Most likely, the client has experienced damage to the:

1. frontal lobe.
2. parietal lobe.
3. occipital lobe.
4. temporal lobe.

Answer: 4. The portion of the cerebrum that controls speech is the temporal lobe. Injury to the frontal lobe causes personality changes, difficulty speaking, and disturbances in memory, reasoning, and concentration. Injury to the parietal lobe causes sensory alterations and problems with spatial relationships. Damage to the occipital lobe causes vision disturbances.

➡ *NCLEX keys*
Client needs category: Physiological integrity
Client needs subcategory: Physiological adaptation
Cognitive level: Application

2. A client is hospitalized with a possible diagnosis of Guillain-Barré syndrome. When collecting history data from the client, the nurse should ask:

1. "Do you bruise easily?"
2. "Have you had an upper respiratory tract infection recently?"
3. "Have you been out of the country during the past 4 months?"
4. "Has anyone in your family ever had Guillain-Barré syndrome?"

Answer: 2. About 60% to 70% of clients with Guillain-Barré syndrome experience upper respiratory or GI viral infection 1 to 4 weeks before symptoms begin. The exact cause of Guillain-Barré syndrome is unknown, but it may be a cell-mediated immune response that attacks the peripheral nerves in response to a virus. The major pathologic effect is segmental demyelination of the peripheral nerves, which destroys the myelin sheath of the nerve. Guillain-Barré syndrome doesn't affect the clotting cascade, isn't related to exposure during foreign travel, and isn't a hereditary disorder.

➡ *NCLEX keys*
Client needs category: Physiological integrity
Client needs subcategory: Physiological adaptation
Cognitive level: Application

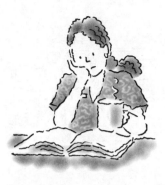

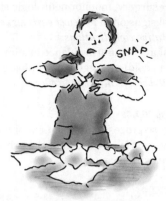

3. A nurse is caring for a client who underwent surgical repair of a detached retina of the right eye. Which interventions should the nurse perform? Select all that apply.
1. Place the client in a prone position.
2. Approach the client from the left side.
3. Encourage deep breathing and coughing.
4. Discourage bending down.
5. Orient the client to his environment.
6. Administer a stool softener.

Answer: 2, 4, 5, 6. The nurse should approach the client from the left side—the unaffected side—to avoid startling the client. She should also discourage the client from bending down, deep breathing, hard coughing and sneezing, and other activities that can increase intraocular pressure. The client should be oriented to his environment to reduce the risk of injury. Stool softeners should be administered to discourage straining during defecation. The client should lie on his back or on the unaffected side to reduce intraocular pressure on the affected eye.

➡ *NCLEX keys*
Client needs category: Physiological integrity
Client needs subcategory: Reduction of risk potential
Cognitive level: Application

4. A nurse is teaching a client and his family about dietary practices related to Parkinson's disease. A priority for the nurse to address is the risk of:
1. fluid overload and drooling.
2. aspiration and anorexia.
3. choking and diarrhea.
4. dysphagia and constipation.

Answer: 4. The eating problems associated with Parkinson's disease include dysphagia, aspiration, constipation, and risk of choking. Fluid overload, anorexia, and diarrhea aren't problems specifically related to Parkinson's disease. Drooling occurs with Parkinson's disease but doesn't take priority.

➡ *NCLEX keys*
Client needs category: Physiological integrity
Client needs subcategory: Reduction of risk potential
Cognitive level: Analysis

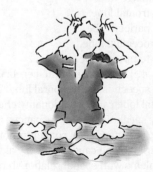

5. In some clients with multiple sclerosis (MS), plasmapheresis diminishes symptoms by removing:
1. catecholamines.
2. antibodies.
3. plasma proteins.
4. lymphocytes.

Answer: 2. In plasmapheresis, antibodies are removed from a client's plasma. Antibodies attack the myelin sheath of the neuron causing MS symptoms. Plasmapheresis isn't for the purpose of removing catecholamines, plasma proteins, or lymphocytes.

➡ *NCLEX keys*
Client needs category: Physiological integrity
Client needs subcategory: Physiological adaptation
Cognitive level: Comprehension

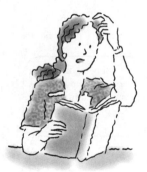

6. A client undergoes a surgical clipping of a cerebral aneurysm. To prevent vasospasm, the nurse should anticipate administering:
1. diuretics such as furosemide (Lasix).
2. blood products such as cryoprecipitate.
3. the calcium channel blocker nifedipine (Procardia).
4. volume expanders such as crystalloids.

Answer: 4. To prevent vasospasm following repair of a cerebral aneurysm, treatment focuses on increasing cerebral perfusion. This increase can be accomplished by giving volume expanders such as crystalloids. Diuretics would decrease cerebral perfusion by reducing volume. Cryoprecipitate isn't used as a volume expander. Nimodipine, not nifedipine, is the calcium channel blocker indicated for use in cerebral vasospasm treatment and prevention.

➡ *NCLEX keys*
Client needs category: Physiological integrity
Client needs subcategory: Reduction of risk potential
Cognitive level: Application

7. A client is diagnosed with a brain tumor. Palliative care is all that can be offered to the client. In addressing the client and family, it would be most therapeutic for the nurse to say:
1. "I'm sorry. I wish there was more we could do."
2. "Be optimistic. Others have survived equally as grave situations."
3. "I understand this situation is distressing and I want to help."
4. "Be thankful you and your family have each other for support during this time."

Answer: 3. Initially, the client and family may be in shock and disbelief. They need the nurse's understanding, support, and offer of help. Apologizing communicates pity. Telling the client and his family to be optimistic gives false hope. Telling them to be thankful they have each other for support communicates detachment.

➡ *NCLEX keys*
Client needs category: Psychosocial integrity
Client needs subcategory: None
Cognitive level: Application

8. A nurse is teaching a client with a T4 spinal cord injury and paralysis of the lower extremities how to independently transfer from bed to a wheelchair. When transferring, it's important for the client to move:

1. the upper and lower body simultaneously into the wheelchair.
2. his upper body to the wheelchair first.
3. his feet to the wheelchair pedals and then his hands to the wheelchair arms.
4. his feet to the floor and then his buttocks to the wheelchair seat.

Answer: 2. The proper technique in transferring from a bed to a wheelchair when there is paralysis of the lower extremities is to move the strong part of the body to the chair first. The client should move his upper body to the wheelchair first and then move his legs from the bed to the wheelchair. Other techniques are less safe and can endanger the client.

➡ *NCLEX keys*
Client needs category: Physiological integrity
Client needs subcategory: Basic care and comfort
Cognitive level: Application

9. A client who recently underwent cranial surgery develops syndrome of inappropriate antidiuretic hormone (SIADH). The nurse should anticipate that the client will:

1. experience edema and weight gain.
2. produce excessive amounts of urine.
3. need vigorous fluid replacement therapy.
4. have a low urine specific gravity.

Answer: 1. SIADH is an abnormally high release of antidiuretic hormone causing water retention, which leads to edema and weight gain. Urine output is low, fluid is restricted rather than replaced, and the urine specific gravity is high.

➡ *NCLEX keys*
Client needs category: Physiological integrity
Client needs subcategory: Reduction of risk potential
Cognitive level: Application

10. A nurse is providing care for a client following surgery to remove a cataract from the right eye. In which position should the nurse place the client?

1. Right-side lying
2. Prone
3. Supine
4. Trendelenburg's

Answer: 3. Positioning the client on his back or unoperative side prevents pressure on the operative eye. Operative side-lying or prone position may put external pressure on the affected eye. Trendelenburg's position may increase intraocular pressure.

➡ *NCLEX keys*
Client needs category: Physiological integrity
Client needs subcategory: Physiological adaptation
Cognitive level: Application

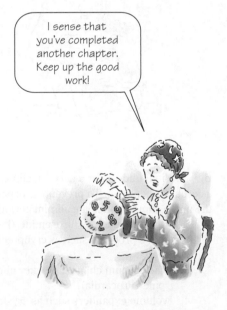

I sense that you've completed another chapter. Keep up the good work!

7 Musculoskeletal system

Brush up on key concepts

The musculoskeletal system has two main functions: to provide support and to produce movement. In addition, the musculoskeletal system protects internal tissues and organs, produces red blood cells (RBCs) in the bone marrow, and stores mineral salts such as calcium.

At any time, you can review the major points of this chapter by consulting the *Cheat sheet* on pages 224 to 227.

Mr. Bones
The **skeleton** consists of 206 bones, which work with the muscles to support and protect internal organs. The skeleton stores calcium, magnesium, and phosphorus. The bone marrow is the soft material found in the center of bones and is responsible for RBC production.

The movement machine
The **skeletal muscles,** which are attached to the bones by tendons, provide body movement and posture by tightening and shortening. The muscles begin contracting when stimulated by a motor neuron. They derive energy for contraction from the hydrolysis of adenosine triphosphate to adenosine diphosphate and phosphate.

The skeletal muscles relax with the breakdown of acetylcholine by cholinesterase. Even then, however, they retain some contraction to maintain muscle tone.

Bones to bones and bones to muscles
Ligaments and **tendons** are tough bands of collagen fibers. Ligaments connect bones to bones and encircle joints to add strength and stability. Tendons connect muscles to bones.

Where bones meet
A **joint** is the articulation of two bone surfaces. Joints provide stabilization and permit locomotion. The degree of joint movement is called range of motion (ROM).

Friction reduction
The **synovium** is the membrane that lines a joint's inner surfaces. In conjunction with cartilage, the synovium reduces friction in joints through its production of synovial fluid.

Shock absorber
Cartilage is a specialized tissue that serves as a smooth surface for articulating bones and protects underlying tissue. It absorbs shock to joints and serves as padding to reduce friction. Cartilage atrophies with limited ROM or in the absence of weight-bearing bursae (small sacs of synovial fluid).

Keep abreast of diagnostic tests

Here are the most important tests used to diagnose musculoskeletal disorders, along with common nursing actions associated with each test.

Muscle picture
Electromyography (EMG) uses electrodes to create a graphic recording of the muscle at rest and during contraction.

Nursing actions
• Explain the procedure to the client.
• Explain that the client will be asked to flex and relax his muscles during the procedure.

(Text continues on page 227.)

Musculoskeletal refresher

ARM AND LEG FRACTURES
Key signs and symptoms
- Loss of limb function
- Acute pain
- Deformity

Key test results
- Anteroposterior and lateral X-rays of the suspected fracture as well as X-rays of the joints above and below it confirm the diagnosis.

Key treatments
- Closed reduction (restoring displaced bone segments to their normal position)
- Immobilization with a splint, a cast, or traction
- Open reduction during surgery to reduce and immobilize the fracture with rods, plates, and screws when closed reduction is impossible, usually followed by application of a plaster cast
- Analgesics: morphine, acetaminophen, oxycodone (Percocet)

Key interventions
- Monitor vital signs and be especially alert for a rapid pulse, decreased blood pressure, pallor, and cool, clammy skin.
- Administer I.V. fluids as needed.
- Assess for and treat pain with analgesics, as needed.
- If the fracture requires long-term immobilization with traction, reposition the client often. Assist with active range-of-motion (ROM) exercises to the unaffected extremities. Encourage deep breathing and coughing.
- Make sure that the immobilized client receives adequate fluid intake. Watch for signs of renal calculi, such as flank pain, nausea, and vomiting.
- Provide cast care.
- Encourage and assist with ambulation as soon as possible. Demonstrate how to use crutches properly.
- Refer the client for physical therapy.

CARPAL TUNNEL SYNDROME
Key signs and symptoms
- Numbness, burning, or tingling in affected arm

- Pain in affected arm and hand
- Weakness

Key test results
- A blood pressure cuff inflated above systolic pressure on the forearm for 1 to 2 minutes provokes pain and paresthesia along the distribution of the median nerve.
- Electromyography detects a median nerve motor conduction delay of more than 5 msec.

Key treatments
- Resting the hands by splinting the wrist in neutral extension for 1 to 2 weeks (if a definite link has been established between the client's occupation and the development of carpal tunnel syndrome, he may have to seek other work)
- Corticosteroid injections: betamethasone (Celestone), hydrocortisone
- Nonsteroidal anti-inflammatory drugs (NSAIDs): indomethacin (Indocin), ibuprofen (Motrin), naproxen (Naprosyn)
- Surgical decompression of the nerve by resecting the entire transverse carpal tunnel ligament or by using endoscopic surgical techniques

Key interventions
- Administer NSAIDs as needed.
- Encourage the client to perform hand exercises as much as possible.
- Assist with eating and bathing.
- After surgery, monitor vital signs and regularly check the color, sensation, pulse, and motion of the affected hand.

COMPARTMENT SYNDROME
Key signs and symptoms
- Loss of distal pulse
- Severe or increased pain in the affected area with stretching or muscle elevation that's unrelieved by opioids
- Tense, swollen muscle

Key test results
- Intracompartment pressure is elevated, as indicated by a blood pressure machine.

> The musculoskeletal system has two main functions: provide support and produce movement.

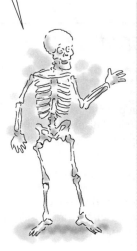

Musculoskeletal refresher (continued)

COMPARTMENT SYNDROME (CONTINUED)

Key treatments
- Fasciotomy
- Positioning the affected extremity lower than the heart
- Removal of dressings or constrictive coverings from the area

Key interventions
- Monitor the affected extremity and perform neurovascular checks.
- Perform dressing changes after fasciotomy and assess drainage.

GOUT

Key signs and symptoms
- Inflamed, painful joints

Key test results
- Blood studies show serum uric acid level above normal. The urine uric acid level is usually higher in secondary gout than in primary gout.
- Arthrocentesis reveals the presence of monosodium urate monohydrate crystals or needlelike intracellular crystals of sodium urate in the synovial fluid.

Key treatments
- Antigout drug: allopurinol (Zyloprim)
- Antilipidemic: fenofibrate (Tricor)
- Uricosuric drug: probenecid (Probalan)
- Corticosteroids: betamethasone (Celestone), hydrocortisone, prednisone
- NSAIDs: indomethacin (Indocin), naproxen (Naprosyn)
- Diet changes (avoiding purines and alcohol, achieving and maintaining optimum weight, increasing fluid intake)

Key interventions
- Encourage bed rest, but use a bed cradle.
- Assess for and treat pain, as needed, especially during acute attacks.
- Apply hot or cold packs to inflamed joints.
- Administer anti-inflammatory medication and other drugs.
- Encourage increased oral fluids (up to 2 qt [2 L]/day).
- Monitor serum uric acid levels regularly.

HERNIATED NUCLEUS PULPOSUS

Key signs and symptoms
Lumbosacral disk herniation
- Acute pain in the lower back that radiates across the buttock and down the leg
- Pain on ambulation

- Weakness, numbness, and tingling of the foot and leg
Cervical disk herniation
- Neck pain that radiates down the arm to the hand
- Neck stiffness
- Weakness of the affected upper extremities
- Weakness, numbness, and tingling of the hand

Key test results
- Myelogram shows spinal cord compression.
- X-ray shows narrowing of disk space.
- Magnetic resonance imaging identifies spinal canal compression by the herniated disk and damage to the intervertebral disk.

Key treatments
- Corticosteroid: cortisone
- NSAIDs: indomethacin (Indocin), ibuprofen (Motrin), sulindac (Clinoril), piroxicam (Feldene), flurbiprofen (Ansaid), diclofenac sodium (Voltaren), naproxen (Naprosyn), diflunisal
- Surgery: laminectomy or diskectomy

Key interventions
- Monitor neurovascular status.
- Reposition the client every 2 hours using the logrolling technique.

HIP FRACTURE

Key signs and symptoms
- Shorter appearance and outward rotation of affected leg resulting in limited or abnormal ROM
- Edema and discoloration of surrounding tissue
- Pain in affected hip and leg that's exacerbated by movement

Key test results
- Computed tomography scan (for complicated fractures) pinpoints abnormalities.
- X-ray reveals a break in the continuity of the bone.

Key treatments
- Abductor splint or trochanter roll between legs to prevent loss of alignment
- Surgical immobilization or joint replacement

Key interventions
- Monitor neurovascular and respiratory status. Assess for compromised circulation, hemorrhage, and neurologic impairment in the affected extremity and pneumonia in the bedridden client.
- Provide active and passive ROM and isometric exercises for unaffected limbs.
- Provide a trapeze.

(continued)

Musculoskeletal refresher *(continued)*

OSTEOARTHRITIS
Key signs and symptoms
- Crepitation
- Joint stiffness
- Pain that's relieved by resting the joints

Key test results
- Arthroscopy reveals bone spurs and narrowing of joint space.
- X-rays show joint deformity, narrowing of joint space, and bone spurs.

Key treatments
- Cold therapy
- Heat therapy
- NSAIDs: indomethacin (Indocin), ibuprofen (Motrin), sulindac (Clinoril), piroxicam (Feldene), flurbiprofen (Ansaid), diclofenac (Voltaren), naproxen (Naprosyn), diflunisal

Key interventions
- Assess musculoskeletal status.
- Assess for adverse reactions to aspirin and NSAIDs, especially signs of increased bleeding or bruising tendency.

OSTEOMYELITIS
Key signs and symptoms
- Pain in afffected bone
- Tenderness
- Swelling

Key test results
- Blood cultures identify the causative organism.
- Erythrocyte sedimentation rate and C-reactive protein (CRP) are elevated. Note that CRP appears to be a better diagnostic tool.

Key treatments
- Immobilization of the affected bone by plaster cast, traction, or bed rest
- Antibiotics: large doses of I.V. antibiotics, usually a penicillinase-resistant penicillin, such as nafcillin, or a cephalosporin, such as cefazolin, after blood cultures are taken

Key interventions
- Use strict sterile technique when changing dressings and irrigating wounds.
- Assess vital signs and wound appearance daily, and monitor for new pain.
- Monitor circulation in affected extremity.
- Monitor the cast for signs of drainage. If a wet spot appears on the cast, circle it with a marking pen and note the time of appearance (on the cast). Be aware of how much drainage is expected. Check the circled spot at least every 4 hours. Watch for any enlargement.

OSTEOPOROSIS
Key signs and symptoms
- Deformity
- Kyphosis
- Pain
- Pathologic fracture

Key test results
- X-rays show typical degeneration in the lower thoracic and lumbar vertebrae. The vertebral bodies may appear flattened and may look denser than normal. Loss of bone mineral becomes evident in later stages.
- Bone mineral density is 2.5 standard deviations or more below the normal reference range (−2.5 or less).

Key treatments
- Physical therapy
- Hormonal agents: conjugated estrogen (Premarin), parathyroid hormone
- Antiresorption drugs: calcium, vitamin D, calcitonin (Calcimar)
- Antihypercalcemic: etidronate (Didronel)
- Biphosphonates: alendronate (Fosomax), ibandronate (Boniva)

Key interventions
- Provide a safe environment and institute fall prevention measures.
- Encourage the client to perform weight-bearing or resistance exercises as able.
- Provide a balanced diet high in such nutrients as vitamin D, calcium, and protein.
- Administer analgesics and heat.
- Treat fractures.

RHABDOMYOLYSIS
Key signs and symptoms
- Dark urine
- Fever
- Muscle pain
- Myalgia
- Nausea
- Vomiting
- Weakness

Key test results
- Creatine kinase levels 100 times normal or greater suggest rhabdomyolysis.
- A positive serum or urine myoglobin test indicates rhabdomyolysis.

Musculoskeletal refresher (continued)

RHABDOMYOLYSIS (CONTINUED)

Key treatments
- Early aggressive hydration
- Diuretics: furosemide (Lasix), ethacrynic acid, bumetanide, mannitol
- Bicarbonate
- Dialysis, if kidney failure is present

Key interventions
- I.V. fluids help minimize damage to the kidneys.
- Monitor the client's intake and output.
- Carefully monitor the client's kidney function tests, electrolyte levels, and daily weight.
- Notify the physician immediately if the client has dark or decreased urine.

- Instruct the client that the procedure may cause some minor discomfort but isn't painful.
- Avoid administration of stimulants, including caffeine and sedatives, 24 hours before the procedure.
- Administer analgesics, as prescribed, after the procedure.

Direct view of a joint

Arthroscopy is a relatively simple surgical procedure, performed under local anesthesia, that allows for direct visualization of a joint.

Nursing actions
Before the procedure
- Administer prophylactic antibiotics, as prescribed.
- Explain the procedure, skin preparation, and use of local anesthetics to the client.

After the procedure
- Apply a pressure dressing to the injection site.
- Monitor neurovascular status.
- Apply ice to the affected joint.
- Limit weight bearing or joint use until allowed by the physician.
- Administer analgesics, as prescribed.

Fluid removal

In **arthrocentesis**, synovial fluid is removed from a joint using a needle.

Nursing actions
Before the procedure
- Administer prophylactic antibiotics, as prescribed.
- Explain the procedure to the client.

After the procedure
- Maintain a pressure dressing on the aspiration site.
- Monitor neurovascular status.
- Apply ice to the affected area.
- Limit weight bearing or joint use until allowed by the physician.
- Administer analgesics, as prescribed.

Bone image

A **bone scan** is used to reveal bone abnormalities. It involves the injection of a radioisotope, which (in conjunction with a scanner) allows a visual image of bone metabolism.

Nursing actions
- Explain the procedure to the client.
- Determine the client's ability to lie still during the scan.
- Make sure that written, informed consent has been obtained before the procedure.
- Advise the client that a radioisotope will be injected I.V.
- Explain to the client that he'll be required to drink several glasses of fluid during the waiting period to enhance excretion of any radioisotope that isn't absorbed by bone tissue.

Vertebrae visual

A **myelogram** involves the injection of radiopaque dye into the spine during a lumbar puncture. This dye allows fluoroscopic visualization of the subarachnoid space, spinal cord, and vertebral bodies.

Nursing actions
Before the procedure
- Explain the procedure to the client.

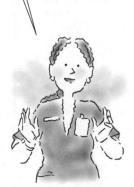

A myelogram—evaluation of the subarachnoid space—requires a lumbar puncture. Inspect the insertion site, and monitor neurologic status.

- Make sure that written, informed consent has been obtained before the procedure.
- Note the client's allergies to iodine, seafood, and radiopaque dyes.
- Inform the client about possible throat irritation and flushing of the face from the dye injection.

After the procedure
- Maintain bed rest. (Assist the client to the bathroom, if necessary.)
- Inspect the insertion site for bleeding.
- Monitor neurologic status.
- Encourage fluid intake.

Solving for X
An **X-ray** is a noninvasive procedure that provides a radiographic image for examination of bones and joints.

Nursing actions
- Use caution when moving a client with a suspected fracture.
- Explain the procedure to the client.
- Make sure that the client isn't pregnant (to prevent possible fetal damage from radiation exposure).

Lab exam #1
A **blood chemistry test** is a laboratory test that analyzes a blood sample for potassium, sodium, calcium, phosphorus, glucose, bicarbonate, blood urea nitrogen, creatinine, protein, albumin, osmolality, creatine kinase, serum aspartate aminotransferase, aldolase, rheumatoid factor, complement fixation, lupus erythematosus cell preparation, antinuclear antibody, anti-deoxyribonucleic acid, and C-reactive protein (CRP).

Nursing actions
- Explain the procedure to the client.
- Withhold food and fluid before the procedure, if appropriate.
- Monitor the venipuncture site for bleeding after the procedure.

Lab exam #2
A **hematologic study** analyzes a blood sample for white blood cells (WBCs), RBCs, platelets, prothrombin time, international normalized ratio, partial thromboplastin time, erythrocyte sedimentation rate (ESR), hemoglobin (Hb), and hematocrit (HCT).

Nursing actions
- Explain the procedure to the client.
- Note current drug therapy to anticipate possible interference with test results.
- Assess the venipuncture site for bleeding after the procedure.

Polish up on client care

Major musculoskeletal disorders include arm and leg fractures, carpal tunnel syndrome, compartment syndrome, gout, herniated nucleus pulposus, hip fracture, osteoarthritis, osteomyelitis, osteoporosis, and rhabdomyolysis.

Arm and leg fractures

A bone fracture is a break in the continuity of the bone. Fractures of the arms and legs usually result from trauma and commonly cause substantial muscle, nerve, and other soft-tissue damage. The prognosis varies with the extent of disability or deformity, the amount of tissue and vascular damage, the adequacy of reduction and immobilization, and the client's age, health, and nutritional status.

Children's bones usually heal rapidly and without deformity. Bones of adults in poor health or with impaired circulation may never heal properly. Severe open fractures, especially of the femoral shaft, may cause substantial blood loss and life-threatening hypovolemic shock.

CAUSES
- Bone tumors
- Trauma
- Osteoporosis

ASSESSMENT FINDINGS
- Discoloration around site of injury
- Loss of limb function
- Acute pain
- Swelling

Memory jogger

When assessing for fractures, remember the 5 Ps:

Pain

Pallor

Pulse loss

Paresthesia

Paralysis.

The last three are distal to the fracture site.

- Deformity
- Crepitus

DIAGNOSTIC TEST RESULTS
- Anteroposterior and lateral X-rays of the suspected fracture as well as X-rays of the joints above and below it confirm the diagnosis.

NURSING DIAGNOSES
- Acute pain
- Impaired physical mobility
- Anxiety
- Risk for injury

TREATMENT
Initial care
- Splinting the limb above and below the suspected fracture
- Cold pack application
- Elevation of the extremity to reduce edema and pain
- Direct pressure to control bleeding in severe fractures that cause blood loss
- Rapid fluid replacement to prevent hypovolemic shock, if blood loss has occurred as a result of the fracture

Fracture care
- Closed reduction (restoring displaced bone segments to their normal position)
- Immobilization with a splint, a cast, or traction
- Open reduction during surgery to reduce and immobilize the fracture using rods, plates, and screws when closed reduction is impossible, usually followed by application of a plaster cast
- Skin or skeletal traction (if splint or a cast fails to maintain the reduction)
- Surgery to repair soft-tissue damage
- Thorough debridement of the wound

Drug therapy
- Analgesics: morphine, acetaminophen, oxycodone (Percocet)
- Prophylactic antibiotics: cefazolin, cefotetan (Cefotan)
- Tetanus prophylaxis: tetanus toxoid

INTERVENTIONS AND RATIONALES
- Monitor for signs of shock in the client with a severe open fracture of a large bone such as the femur. *Open fractures can cause increased blood loss, leading to hypovolemic shock.*
- Monitor vital signs and be especially alert for a rapid pulse, decreased blood pressure, pallor, and cool, clammy skin—*all of which may indicate that the client is in shock.*
- Administer I.V. fluids as needed *to replace fluid loss.*
- Monitor neurovascular status of the affected extremity *to detect vascular compromise.*
- Offer reassurance. *With any fracture, the client is likely to be frightened and in pain.*
- Assess for and treat pain with analgesics as needed *to promote comfort.*
- If the client is immobile, reposition him every 2 hours and provide skin care *to increase comfort and prevent pressure ulcers.*
- Assist with active ROM exercises of the unaffected extremities *to prevent muscle atrophy.*
- Encourage deep breathing and coughing *to avoid hypostatic pneumonia.*
- Make sure that the immobilized client receives adequate fluid intake and watch for signs of renal calculi, such as flank pain, nausea, and vomiting
- Provide cast care *to prevent skin breakdown.*
- Encourage and assist with ambulation as soon as possible *to prevent complications of immobility such as renal calculi.* Demonstrate how to use crutches properly *to prevent injury.*
- Refer the client for physical therapy *to restore limb mobility.*

Teaching topics
- Cast care
- Use of assistive devices
- Explanation of the disorder and treatment plan
- Medication use and possible adverse effects
- Physical therapy or rehabilitation options

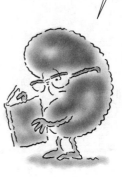

Leave no stone unturned. Immobilized clients are at risk for renal calculi.

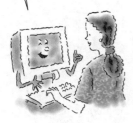

Any strenuous use of the hands, including taking the exam, aggravates carpal tunnel syndrome.

Carpal tunnel syndrome

Carpal tunnel syndrome is the compression of the median nerve at the wrist, within the carpal tunnel. This nerve—along with blood vessels and flexor tendons—passes through to the fingers and thumb. Compression neuropathy causes sensory and motor changes in the median distribution of the hand. Carpal tunnel is the most common of the nerve entrapment syndromes.

Carpal tunnel syndrome usually occurs in women between ages 30 and 60 and poses a serious occupational health problem. Assembly-line workers, packers, typists, and persons who repeatedly use poorly designed tools are most likely to develop this disorder. Any strenuous use of the hands—sustained grasping, twisting, or flexing—aggravates this condition.

CAUSES
- Flexor tenosynovitis (commonly associated with rheumatic disease)
- Nerve compression
- Physical trauma
- Rheumatoid arthritis

ASSESSMENT FINDINGS
- Atrophic nails
- Numbness, burning, or tingling in affected arm
- Pain in affected arm and hand
- Shiny, dry skin
- Weakness

DIAGNOSTIC TEST RESULTS
- Physical examination reveals decreased sensation to light touch or pinpricks in the affected fingers. Thenar muscle atrophy occurs in about half of all cases of carpal tunnel syndrome. The client exhibits a positive Tinel's sign (tingling over the median nerve on light percussion). He also responds positively to Phalen's wrist-flexion test, in which holding the forearms vertically and allowing both hands to drop into complete flexion at the wrists for 1 minute reproduces symptoms of carpal tunnel syndrome.
- A blood pressure cuff inflated above systolic pressure on the forearm for 1 to 2 minutes provokes pain and paresthesia along the distribution of the median nerve.
- EMG detects a median nerve motor conduction delay of more than 5 msec.

NURSING DIAGNOSES
- Impaired physical mobility
- Chronic pain
- Disturbed sensory perception (kinesthetic, tactile)

TREATMENT
- Resting the hands by splinting the wrist in neutral extension for 1 to 2 weeks (if a definite link has been established between the client's occupation and the development of carpal tunnel syndrome, he may have to seek other work)
- Correction of underlying disorder
- Surgical decompression of the nerve by resecting the entire transverse carpal tunnel ligament or by using endoscopic surgical techniques (neurolysis, or releasing of nerve fibers, may also be necessary)

Drug therapy
- Nonsteroidal anti-inflammatory drugs (NSAIDs): indomethacin (Indocin), ibuprofen (Motrin), naproxen (Naprosyn)
- Corticosteroid injections: betamethasone (Celestone), hydrocortisone

INTERVENTIONS AND RATIONALES
- Administer NSAIDs as needed *to reduce inflammation and pain.*
- Encourage the client to perform hand exercises *to maintain ROM.*
- Assist with eating and bathing. *Mobility may be limited with carpal tunnel syndrome.*
- Assess the client's degree of physical immobility *to evaluate the effectiveness of the current treatment plan.*
- After surgery, monitor vital signs and regularly check the color, sensation, pulse, and motion of the affected hand *to detect signs of compromised circulation.*

Teaching topics
- Explanation of the disease process and treatment options
- Applying the splint and removing it to perform gentle ROM exercises daily

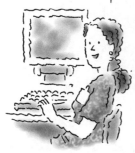

Poorly designed keyboards are commonly the culprits in cases of carpal tunnel syndrome.

- ROM exercises
- Importance of taking NSAIDs with food or antacids to avoid stomach upset
- Reinforcing that maximum effects of drug therapy may not be seen for 2 to 4 weeks
- Contacting an occupational counselor

Compartment syndrome

Compartment syndrome is increased pressure within a muscle and its surrounding structures that results in pain and circulation impairment. Tissue damage occurs after 30 minutes; after 4 hours, irreversible damage may occur.

If compartment syndrome is suspected, pressure within muscles is assessed by sticking a needle into a muscle. The needle is attached to an I.V. bag with tubing and a stopcock. Elevated pressure, as indicated by a blood pressure machine, indicates compartment syndrome.

CAUSES
- Application of a dressing or cast that's too tight
- Burns
- Closed fracture injury
- Crushing injuries
- Muscle swelling after exercise

ASSESSMENT FINDINGS
- Decreased movement, strength, and sensation
- Loss of distal pulse
- Numbness and tingling distal to the involved muscle
- Severe or increased pain in the affected area with stretching or muscle elevation that's unrelieved by opioids
- Paralysis
- Tense, swollen muscle
- Decreased or absent pulse

DIAGNOSTIC TEST RESULTS
- Intracompartment pressure is elevated, as indicated by a blood pressure machine.

NURSING DIAGNOSES
- Impaired physical mobility
- Acute pain

- Risk for peripheral neurovascular dysfunction

TREATMENT
- Fasciotomy
- Positioning the affected extremity lower than the heart
- Removal of dressings or constrictive coverings from the area

Drug therapy
- Opioid analgesics

INTERVENTIONS AND RATIONALES
- Monitor vital signs *to detect early changes and prevent complications.*
- Monitor the affected extremity and perform neurovascular checks *to detect signs of impaired circulation.*
- Maintain the extremity in a position lower than the heart *to ensure adequate circulation and to reduce pressure.*
- Assess for and treat pain and anxiety *because stress may lead to vasoconstriction.*
- Perform dressing changes after fasciotomy and assess drainage *to evaluate and promote wound healing.*

Teaching topics
- Explanation of the disorder and treatment plan
- Medication use and possible adverse effects
- Activity restrictions
- Wound care
- Signs and symptoms of complications

Gout

Gout is a metabolic disease marked by urate deposits in the joints, which cause painfully arthritic joints. It can strike any joint but favors those in the feet and legs. *Primary gout* (originating from a metabolic cause that's genetic or inborn) usually occurs in men older than age 30 and in postmenopausal women. *Secondary gout* (originating from drug therapy or from a metabolic cause that isn't genetic or inborn) occurs in elderly clients.

Gout follows an intermittent course and may leave clients free from symptoms for

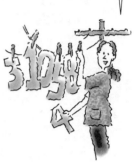

Numbers to know for compartment syndrome: Tissue damage after 30 minutes. Permanent damage after 4 hours.

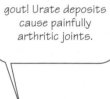

Shout about gout! Urate deposits cause painfully arthritic joints.

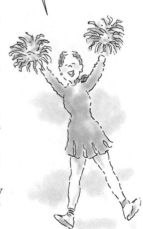

years between attacks. Gout can lead to chronic disability or incapacitation and, rarely, severe hypertension and progressive renal disease. The prognosis is good with treatment.

CAUSES
- Genetic predisposition
- Increased uric acid

ASSESSMENT FINDINGS
- Hypertension
- Back pain
- Inflamed, painful joints

DIAGNOSTIC TEST RESULTS
- Arthrocentesis reveals the presence of monosodium urate monohydrate crystals or needlelike intracellular crystals of sodium urate in synovial fluid taken from an inflamed joint or a tophus.
- Blood studies show serum uric acid level above normal. The urine uric acid level is usually higher in secondary gout than in primary gout.
- X-ray examination results are normal initially. X-rays show damage of the articular cartilage and subchondral bone in chronic gout and outward displacement of the overhanging margin from the bone contour.

NURSING DIAGNOSES
- Chronic pain
- Impaired physical mobility
- Risk for injury
- Fear

TREATMENT
- Bed rest
- Immobilization and protection of the inflamed joints
- Local application of heat and cold
- Diet changes (avoiding purines and alcohol, achieving and maintaining optimum weight, increasing fluid intake)

Drug therapy
- Antigout drug: allopurinol (Zyloprim)
- Uricosuric drug: probenecid (Probalan)
- Alkalinizing drug: sodium bicarbonate
- Corticosteroids: betamethasone (Celestone), hydrocortisone, prednisone

- NSAIDs: indomethacin (Indocin), naproxen (Naprosyn)
- Antilipemic: fenofibrate (Tricor)

INTERVENTIONS AND RATIONALES
- Encourage bed rest but use a bed cradle *to keep bedcovers off extremely sensitive, inflamed joints.*
- Assess for and treat pain, as needed, especially during acute attacks, *to promote comfort.*
- Apply hot or cold packs to inflamed joints *to promote comfort.*
- Administer anti-inflammatory medication and other drugs *to decrease inflammation and increase excretion of uric acid.*
- Monitor for GI disturbances with colchicine administration *to prevent complications.*
- Encourage increased oral fluids (up to 2 qt [2 L]/day) *to prevent renal calculi formation.*
- Monitor serum uric acid levels regularly *to evaluate the effectiveness of the treatment plan.*
- Stress the importance of having serum uric acid levels checked periodically *to help ensure compliance.*
- Advise the client receiving allopurinol, probenecid, and other drugs to immediately report adverse effects, such as drowsiness, dizziness, nausea, vomiting, urinary frequency, and dermatitis, *to prevent complications.*
- Warn the client taking probenecid to avoid aspirin and other salicylates *because their combined effect causes urate retention.*

Teaching topics
- Explanation of the disorder and treatment plan
- Medication use and possible adverse effects
- Adequate fluid intake
- Avoiding alcohol, especially beer and wine
- Sparing use of purine-rich foods, such as anchovies, liver, sardines, kidneys, sweetbreads, and lentils
- Losing weight, if obese

Herniated nucleus pulposus

Herniated nucleus pulposus is the rupture of an intervertebral disk, which causes a protrusion of the nucleus pulposus (the soft, central portion of a spinal disk) into the spinal canal. This protrusion compresses the spinal cord or nerve roots, causing pain, numbness, and loss of motor function. Commonly known as a *herniated disk*, herniated nucleus pulposus can be further described as lumbosacral (affecting the lumbar vertebrae L4 and L5 and the sacral vertebra S1) or cervical (affecting the cervical vertebrae C5, C6, and C7).

CAUSES
- Back or neck strain
- Congenital bone deformity
- Degeneration of disk
- Heavy lifting
- Trauma
- Weakness of ligaments

ASSESSMENT FINDINGS
Lumbosacral disk herniation
- Acute pain in the lower back that radiates across the buttock and down the leg
- Pain on ambulation
- Weakness, numbness, and tingling of the foot and leg

Cervical disk herniation
- Atrophy of biceps and triceps
- Neck pain that radiates down the arm to the hand
- Neck stiffness
- Straightening of normal lumbar curve with scoliosis away from the affected side
- Weakness of affected upper extremities
- Weakness, numbness, and tingling of the hand

DIAGNOSTIC TEST RESULTS
- Magnetic resonance imaging identifies spinal cord compression caused by a herniated disk and damage to the intervertebral disk.
- Cerebrospinal fluid analysis shows increased protein.
- Deep tendon reflexes are depressed or absent in the upper extremities or Achilles' tendon.
- EMG shows spinal nerve involvement.
- Lasègue's sign is positive.
- Myelogram shows spinal cord compression.
- X-ray shows narrowing of disk space.

NURSING DIAGNOSES
- Impaired physical mobility
- Posttrauma syndrome
- Acute pain
- Anxiety
- Fear

TREATMENT
- Bed rest with active and passive ROM and isometric exercises
- Diet that includes increased fiber and fluids
- Heating pad and moist, hot compresses
- Surgery: laminectomy or diskectomy
- Orthopedic devices, including back brace and cervical collar
- Transcutaneous electrical nerve stimulation
- Physical therapy

Drug therapy
- Analgesic: oxycodone hydrochloride (OxyContin)
- Chemonucleolysis using chymopapain
- Corticosteroid: cortisone
- Muscle relaxants: diazepam (Valium), cyclobenzaprine (Flexeril)
- NSAIDs: indomethacin (Indocin), ibuprofen (Motrin), sulindac (Clinoril), piroxicam (Feldene), flurbiprofen (Ansaid), diclofenac sodium (Voltaren), naproxen (Naprosyn), diflunisal
- Stool softener: docusate sodium (Colace)

INTERVENTIONS AND RATIONALES
- Monitor neurovascular status *to determine baseline and detect early changes.*
- Monitor and record vital signs, intake and output, and results of laboratory studies *to detect changes in the client's condition.*
- Maintain the client's diet; increase fluid intake *to maintain hydration.*
- Keep the client in semi-Fowler's position with moderate hip and knee flexion *to promote comfort.*
- Administer medications, as prescribed, *to maintain or improve the client's condition.*
- Assess for and treat pain with analgesics *to promote comfort.*
- Encourage the client to express his fears and feelings about changes in his body

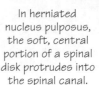

In herniated nucleus pulposus, the soft, central portion of a spinal disk protrudes into the spinal canal.

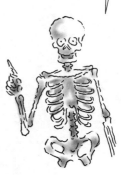

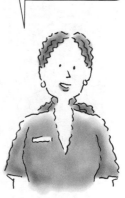

Treatment for herniated nucleus pulposus ranges from bed rest to surgery. Provide emotional support and reinforcement during the treatment and recovery period.

image and his disability *to help him resolve his feelings*.
• Provide skin and back care *to promote comfort and prevent skin breakdown*.
• Reposition the client every 2 hours using the logrolling technique *to prevent injury*.
• Maintain bed rest and body alignment *to maintain joint function and prevent neuromuscular deformity*.
• Maintain traction, braces, and cervical collar *to prevent further injury and to promote healing*.
• Promote independence in activities of daily living (ADLs) *to maintain self-esteem*.

Teaching topics
• Explanation of the disorder and treatment plan
• Medication use and possible adverse effects
• Exercising regularly, with special attention to exercises that strengthen and stretch the muscles
• Avoiding lifting, sleeping prone, climbing stairs, and riding in a car
• Avoiding flexion, extension, or rotation of the neck, if cervical
• Using one pillow for support while sleeping
• Using a back brace or cervical collar
• Physical therapy options

Hip fracture

A fracture occurs when too much stress is placed on the bone. As a result, the bone breaks and local tissue becomes injured, causing muscle spasm, edema, hemorrhage, compressed nerves, and ecchymosis.

Sites of hip fractures include intracapsular (within the capsule of the femur), extracapsular (outside the capsule of the femur), intertrochanteric (within the trochanter), or subtrochanteric (below the trochanter).

CAUSES
• Bone tumors
• Cushing's syndrome
• Immobility
• Malnutrition
• Multiple myeloma

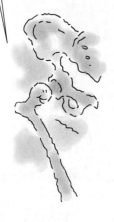

A hip fracture occurs when too much stress is placed on the bone. See what happens when you go out on a limb!

• Osteomyelitis
• Osteoporosis
• Steroid therapy
• Trauma

ASSESSMENT FINDINGS
• Shorter appearance and outward rotation of affected leg, resulting in limited or abnormal ROM
• Edema and discoloration of surrounding tissue
• History of a fall or other trauma to the bones
• Pain in the affected hip and leg that's exacerbated by movement

DIAGNOSTIC TEST RESULTS
• Computed tomography scan (for complicated fractures) pinpoints abnormalities.
• Hematology shows decreased Hb and HCT.
• X-ray reveals a break in continuity of bone.

NURSING DIAGNOSES
• Risk for activity intolerance
• Risk for impaired skin integrity
• Ineffective role performance
• Acute pain
• Fear

TREATMENT
• Abductor splint or trochanter roll between legs to prevent loss of alignment
• Isometric exercises, such as tensing and relaxing the muscles of the leg
• Physical therapy to teach the client non–weight-bearing transfers and to work with changes in weight-bearing status
• Skin traction: Buck's or Russell's
• Surgical immobilization or joint replacement

Drug therapy
• Analgesics: opioid or nonopioid

INTERVENTIONS AND RATIONALES
• Monitor neurovascular and respiratory status. Assess for compromised circulation, hemorrhage, and neurologic impairment in the affected extremity and pneumonia in the bedridden client *to detect changes and prevent complications*.

Management moments

Preventing hip fracture complications in elderly clients

Hip fractures are a leading cause of disability among elderly clients. They're one of many events that may permanently change the client's level of functioning and independence. Many clients who survive a hip fracture never return to their prefracture ambulatory status.

Fractures in the older person are typically related to falls, osteoporosis, and other skeletal disorders. The most common site of fracture is the head of the femur, with women experiencing a higher incidence than men. Older adults' bones fracture more easily because they're more brittle. They also heal more slowly, increasing the risk of immobility complications.

FOILING FRACTURE COMPLICATIONS

Complications can delay or prevent rehabilitation and may require that the client be admitted to a long-term care facility. These complications may include:
• pneumonia
• venous thrombosis
• pressure ulcers
• voiding dysfunction.

Nursing care should be aimed at preventing complications, using the following interventions:
• Keep the client's skin clean and dry.
• Turn the client often, and consider using an alternating pressure mattress to prevent skin breakdown.
• Provide good nutrition to promote healing and to increase resistance to infection. Encourage the older person to eat as much of his meals as possible. Offer high-protein, high-calorie snacks.
• As soon as the physician permits, help the client ambulate. Reassure him that the repaired hip is safe to use. Plan progress in small steps. At the first session, have him walk to a nearby chair, as prescribed. Then gradually increase the distance by having him walk in the hallway. The client's early involvement in physical therapy is vital to successful recovery.

• Monitor and record vital signs, intake and output, and results of laboratory studies *to detect early changes in the client's condition.*
• Maintain the client's diet; increase fluid intake *to maintain hydration.*
• Keep the client in a flat position with the foot of the bed elevated 25 degrees when in traction *to prevent further injury.*
• Keep the legs abducted *to prevent dislocation of the hip joint.*
• Administer medications, as prescribed, *to improve or maintain the client's condition.*
• Provide skin care, and reposition the client every 2 hours *to maintain skin integrity and prevent pressure ulcers.* (See *Preventing hip fracture complications in elderly clients.*)

• Encourage coughing, deep breathing, and incentive spirometry *to maintain a patent airway.*
• Keep the hip extended *to prevent further injury and maintain circulation.*
• Promote independence in ADLs *to promote self-esteem.*
• Provide active and passive ROM and isometric exercises for unaffected limbs *to maintain joint mobility.*
• Provide a trapeze *to promote independence in self-care.*
• Provide diversional activities *to promote self-esteem.*
• Apply antiembolism stockings *to promote venous circulation and prevent deep vein thrombosis.*
• Provide emotional support *to decrease anxiety.*

Teaching topics
- Explanation of the disorder and treatment plan
- Medication use and possible adverse reactions
- Physical therapy and rehabilitation options
- Avoiding putting weight on the affected limb
- Performing skin and foot care daily

Osteoarthritis

Also known as *degenerative joint disease*, osteoarthritis is degeneration of cartilage in weight-bearing joints, such as the spine, knees, and hips. It occurs when cartilage softens with age, narrowing the joint space. The narrowed joint space allows bones to rub together, causing pain and limiting joint movement.

Osteoarthritis can be primary or secondary. Primary osteoarthritis, a normal part of aging, results from metabolic, genetic, chemical, and mechanical factors. Secondary osteoarthritis usually follows an identifiable cause, such as obesity and congenital deformity, and leads to degenerative changes.

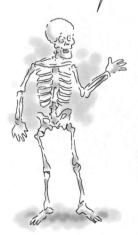

Don't get soft on me. In osteoarthritis, cartilage softens, narrowing the joint space and allowing bones to rub together.

CAUSES
- Congenital abnormalities
- Joint trauma
- Obesity

ASSESSMENT FINDINGS
- Crepitation
- Enlarged, edematous joints
- Heberden's nodes
- Increased pain in damp, cold weather
- Joint stiffness
- Limited ROM
- Pain that's relieved by resting the joints
- Smooth, taut, shiny skin

DIAGNOSTIC TEST RESULTS
- Arthroscopy reveals bone spurs and narrowing of joint space.
- Hematology shows increased ESR.
- X-rays show joint deformity, narrowing of joint space, and bone spurs.

NURSING DIAGNOSES
- Activity intolerance
- Impaired physical mobility
- Chronic pain

TREATMENT
- Canes or walkers
- Cold therapy
- Low-calorie diet if the client isn't at optimal weight
- Heat therapy
- Isometric exercises

Drug therapy
- Analgesic: aspirin
- NSAIDs: indomethacin (Indocin), ibuprofen (Motrin), sulindac (Clinoril), piroxicam (Feldene), flurbiprofen (Ansaid), diclofenac (Voltaren), naproxen (Naprosyn), diflunisal

INTERVENTIONS AND RATIONALES
- Assess musculoskeletal status *to determine baseline and detect changes.*
- Monitor and record vital signs and intake and output *to evaluate hydration.*
- Assess for and treat pain *to promote comfort.*
- Maintain the client's diet *to promote nutrition and healing.*
- Keep joints extended *to prevent contractures and maintain joint mobility.*
- Assess for adverse reactions to aspirin and NSAIDs, especially signs of increased bleeding or bruising tendency. *Doing so facilitates early intervention for adverse drug effects.*
- Encourage verbalization of feelings about changes in body image *to encourage acceptance of changes.*
- Provide skin care *to promote skin integrity.*
- Provide rest periods *to conserve energy.*
- Provide moist compresses (heat therapy), as prescribed, *to promote comfort.*
- Teach proper body mechanics *to prevent injury.*
- Provide passive ROM exercises or encourage active ROM exercises *to maintain joint mobility.*

Teaching topics

- Explanation of the disorder and treatment plan
- Medication use and possible adverse reactions
- Avoiding certain exercises (jogging, jumping, lifting)
- Identifying ways to reduce physical stress (weight loss, muscle strengthening)
- Performing complete skin and foot care daily
- Contacting the Arthritis Foundation

Osteomyelitis

Osteomyelitis is a pyogenic (pus-producing) bone infection. It may be chronic or acute and commonly results from a combination of local trauma—usually quite trivial but resulting in hematoma formation—and an acute infection originating elsewhere in the body. Although osteomyelitis commonly remains localized, it can spread through the bone to the marrow, cortex, and periosteum (the membrane that covers the bone).

Acute osteomyelitis is usually a blood-borne disease that most commonly affects rapidly growing children. Chronic osteomyelitis (rare) is characterized by multiple draining sinus tracts and metastatic lesions.

Osteomyelitis occurs more commonly in children than in adults—particularly in boys—usually as a complication of an acute, localized infection. The most common sites in children are the lower end of the femur and the upper end of the tibia, humerus, and radius. In adults, the most common sites are the pelvis and vertebrae, generally the result of contamination associated with surgery or trauma.

CAUSES

- Exposure to disease-causing organisms

ASSESSMENT FINDINGS

- Pain in affected bone
- Tenderness
- Swelling
- Erythema

DIAGNOSTIC TEST RESULTS

- Blood cultures identify the causative organism.
- ESR and CRP are elevated. Note that CRP appears to be a better diagnostic tool.
- WBC count shows leukocytosis.

NURSING DIAGNOSES

- Impaired tissue integrity
- Impaired physical mobility
- Activity intolerance
- Acute pain

TREATMENT

- Early surgical drainage to relieve pressure buildup and sequestrum formation (Sequestrum is dead bone that has separated from sound bone.)
- High-protein diet with extra vitamin C
- Immobilization of the affected bone by plaster cast, traction, or bed rest
- I.V. fluids

Drug therapy

- Antibiotics: large doses of I.V. antibiotics, usually a penicillinase-resistant penicillin, such as nafcillin, or a cephalosporin, such as cefazolin, after blood cultures are taken
- Analgesics: ibuprofen (Motrin), acetaminophen and oxycodone (Percocet), morphine sulfate (MS Contin)

INTERVENTIONS AND RATIONALES

- Use strict sterile technique when changing dressings and irrigating wounds *to prevent infection.*
- If the client is in skeletal traction, provide pin care *to prevent infection.*
- Administer I.V. fluids, as necessary, *to maintain adequate hydration.*
- Provide a diet high in protein and vitamin C *to promote healing.*
- Assess vital signs and wound appearance daily, and monitor for new pain, *which may indicate a secondary infection.*
- Support the affected limb with firm pillows. Keep the limb level with the body—don't let it sag—*to prevent injury.*
- Reposition the client every 2 hours and provide skin care *to prevent skin breakdown.*

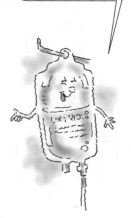

Antibiotic treatment for osteomyelitis usually includes large doses of a penicillinase-resistant penicillin and may begin even before the diagnosis is confirmed.

- Provide cast care. Support the cast with firm pillows and "petal" the edges with pieces of adhesive tape or moleskin to smooth rough edges *to prevent skin breakdown, which may lead to infection*.
- Monitor circulation in the affected extremity *to detect circulatory compromise*.
- Monitor the cast for signs of drainage. If a wet spot appears on the cast, circle it with a marking pen and note the time of appearance (on the cast). Be aware of how much drainage is expected. Check the circled spot at least every 4 hours. Watch for any enlargement. *These measures help to detect early signs of hemorrhage.*
- Provide safety measures *to prevent injury*.
- Monitor for sudden pain, crepitus, or deformity. Watch for sudden malposition of the limb *to detect fracture*.
- Provide emotional support and appropriate diversions *to reduce anxiety*.

Teaching topics
- Explanation of the disorder and treatment plan
- Medication use and possible adverse reactions
- Wound care
- Recognizing signs of infection
- Need for follow-up examinations
- Seeking prompt treatment for possible sources of recurrence—blisters, boils, styes, and impetigo

Osteoporosis

In osteoporosis, a metabolic bone disorder, the rate of bone resorption accelerates while the rate of bone formation slows down, causing a loss of bone mass. Bones affected by this disease lose calcium and phosphate salts and, thus, become porous, brittle, and abnormally vulnerable to fracture.

Osteoporosis may be primary or secondary to an underlying disease. Primary osteoporosis is commonly called senile or postmenopausal osteoporosis because it most commonly develops in elderly, postmenopausal women.

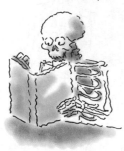

In osteoporosis, bones deteriorate faster than the body can replace them.

CAUSES
- Decreased hormonal function
- Negative calcium balance

ASSESSMENT FINDINGS
- May be asymptomatic
- Pathologic fracture
- Deformity
- Kyphosis
- Pain

DIAGNOSTIC TEST RESULTS
- Bone biopsy shows thin and porous, but otherwise normal-looking bone.
- Dual- or single-photon absorptiometry allows measurement of bone mass, which helps to assess the extremities, hips, and spine.
- Bone mineral density is 2.5 standard deviations or more below the normal reference range (–2.5 or less).
- Serum calcium, phosphorus, and alkaline phosphatase are all within normal limits, but parathyroid hormone may be elevated.
- X-rays show typical degeneration in the lower thoracic and lumbar vertebrae. The vertebral bodies may appear flattened and may look denser than normal. Loss of bone mineral becomes evident in later stages.

NURSING DIAGNOSES
- Impaired physical mobility
- Risk for injury
- Chronic pain

TREATMENT
- Physical therapy
- Supportive devices for weakened vertebrae
- Balanced diet high in vitamin D, calcium, and protein

Drug therapy
- Analgesics: aspirin, indomethacin (Indocin)
- Hormonal agents: conjugated estrogen (Premarin), parathyroid hormone
- Antiresorption drugs: calcium, vitamin D, calcitonin (Calcimar)

- Antihypercalcemic drug: etidronate (Didronel)
- Biphosphonates: alendronate (Fosamax), ibandronate (Boniva), risedronate (Actonel)

INTERVENTIONS AND RATIONALES

- Assess the client's fragility, stressing careful positioning, ambulation, and prescribed exercises, *to prevent injury*.
- Monitor the client's skin daily for redness, warmth, and new sites of pain, *which may indicate new fractures*. Encourage activity; help the client walk several times daily *to slow progress of the disease*.
- Treat fractures *to prevent deformities*.
- Encourage the client to perform weight-bearing or resistance exercises as able. *These measures help slow disease progression*.
- Provide a balanced diet high in such nutrients as vitamin D, calcium, and protein *to support skeletal metabolism*.
- Administer analgesics and heat *to relieve pain*.
- Advise the client to sleep on a firm mattress *to promote comfort* and avoid excessive bed rest *to slow disease progression*.
- Provide a safe environment and institute fall prevention measures *to prevent injury*.

Teaching topics

- Explanation of the disorder and treatment plan
- Medication use and possible adverse effects
- Using good body mechanics while lifting
- Importance of regular exercise, including weight-bearing and resistance exercises
- Importance of reporting new pain sites immediately, especially after trauma, no matter how slight
- Proper technique for self-examination of the breasts if receiving estrogen therapy
- Need for regular gynecologic examinations and reporting abnormal bleeding promptly while receiving estrogen therapy

Rhabdomyolysis

Rhabdomyolysis is the breakdown of muscle fibers that results in the release of muscle fiber content into the circulation. Myoglobin is released into the bloodstream, and then is filtered by the kidneys. Myoglobin may occlude the structure of the kidney, causing damage, such as acute tubular necrosis or kidney failure. Necrotic skeletal muscle may cause massive fluid shifts from the bloodstream into the muscle, reducing the relative fluid volume of the body and leading to shock and reduced blood flow to the kidneys.

Predisposing factors include trauma, ischemia polymyositis, and drug overdose. Toxins and environmental, infectious, and metabolic factors may induce it. Rhabdomyolysis accounts for 8% to 15% of cases of acute renal failure.

CAUSES

Any condition that causes damage to skeletal muscle, such as:
- blunt trauma
- burns
- excessive exercise
- falls
- heatstroke
- infections
- near electrocution
- prolonged immobilization
- snakebite.

ASSESSMENT FINDINGS

- Dark urine
- Fatigue
- Fever
- Joint pain
- Muscle pain (especially in the thighs, calves, or lower back)
- Myalgia
- Nausea
- Vomiting
- Weakness
- Weight gain

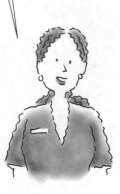

Changes in the diet and activity of the client with osteoporosis may help avoid fractures.

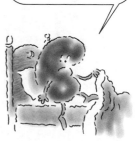

Reduced blood flow? Kidney damage and failure? I think I better head to bed!

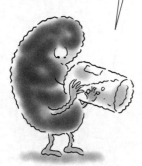

Is this what they mean by early and aggressive hydration?

DIAGNOSTIC TEST RESULTS
• A positive serum or urine myoglobin test indicates rhabdomyolysis.
• Creatine kinase levels 100 times normal or greater suggest rhabdomyolysis.

NURSING DIAGNOSES
• Risk for injury
• Fatigue
• Excess fluid volume
• Impaired urinary elimination

TREATMENT
• Dialysis, if kidney failure is present
• Early aggressive hydration
• Kidney transplant (severe cases)

Drug therapy
• Bicarbonate with sufficient urinary output to help prevent dissociation of myoglobin
• Diuretics: furosemide (Lasix), ethacrynic acid, bumetanide, mannitol

INTERVENTIONS AND RATIONALES
• Administer aggressive I.V. fluids *to help minimize damage to the kidneys.*
• Monitor the client's intake and output *to monitor changes in urine output that could indicate kidney failure.*
• Carefully monitor the client's kidney function tests, electrolyte levels, and daily weight *to monitor for renal failure.*
• Notify the physician immediately if the client has dark or decreased urine *because this is a sign of worsening rhabdomyolysis.*
• Auscultate breath sounds and monitor for signs of pulmonary edema *to assess for fluid overload.*

Teaching topics
• Explanation of the disorder and treatment plan
• Drug therapy

Pump up on practice questions

1. A client with a sports injury undergoes a diagnostic arthroscopy of his left knee. After the procedure, the nurse assesses the client's leg. Which assessment factors are the priority?
　　1. Wound and integumentary assessments
　　2. Mobility assessment
　　3. Vascular and integumentary assessments
　　4. Circulatory and neurologic assessments

Answer: 4. Following a procedure on an extremity, nursing assessment should focus on neurovascular status of the extremity. Swelling of the extremity can impair neurologic and circulatory function of the leg. After the neurovascular stability of the extremity has been established, the nurse can address the other concerns of skin integrity, mobility, and pain.

➡ *NCLEX keys*
Client needs category: Physiological integrity
Client needs subcategory: Reduction of risk potential
Cognitive level: Application

2. A client undergoes a lumbar puncture for a myelogram. Shortly after the procedure, he reports a severe headache. What should the nurse do?

1. Increase the client's fluid intake.
2. Administer prescribed antihypertensives.
3. Offer roll lenses to the client.
4. Place cooling packs over the lumbar puncture site.

Answer: 1. Headache following a lumbar puncture is usually caused by cerebrospinal fluid (CSF) leakage. Increased fluid intake will help restore CSF volume. Antihypertensives don't address the problem. Roll lenses reduce light irritation to the eyes and ice may reduce site pain, but neither intervention addresses the problem of reduced CSF volume, which caused the headache.

➦ *NCLEX keys*

Client needs category: Physiological integrity
Client needs subcategory: Reduction of risk potential
Cognitive level: Analysis

3. While examining the hands of a client with osteoarthritis, the nurse notes Heberden's nodes on the second (pointer) finger. Identify the area on the finger where the nurse observed the node.

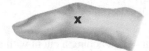

Answer: Heberden's nodes appear on the distal interphalangeal joints. These bony and cartilaginous enlargements are usually hard and painless and typically occur in middle-aged and elderly clients with osteoarthritis.

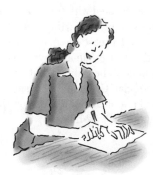

➦ *NCLEX keys*

Client needs category: Physiological integrity
Client needs subcategory: Physiological adaptation
Cognitive level: Application

Time to give your bones a break. Take a brief stretch and then jump right in to this practice test.

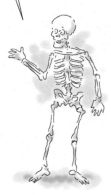

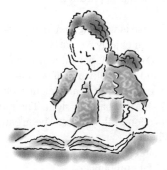

4. A client with osteoarthritis develops coagulopathy secondary to long-term nonsteroidal anti-inflammatory drug (NSAID) use. The coagulopathy is most likely the result of:
1. impaired vitamin K synthesis.
2. blocked prothrombin conversion.
3. decreased platelet adhesiveness.
4. factor VIII destruction.

Answer: 3. NSAIDs reduce platelet adhesiveness and can impair coagulation. They don't impair vitamin K synthesis, block prothrombin conversion, or destroy factor VIII.

➡ *NCLEX keys*
Client needs category: Physiological integrity
Client needs subcategory: Physiological adaptation
Cognitive level: Analysis

5. A nurse is teaching a client with osteoarthritis about lifestyle changes. The nurse knows the client understands the teaching when she states that she will:
1. avoid exercise.
2. restrict caffeine.
3. abstain from alcohol.
4. lose weight.

Answer: 4. Osteoarthritis (degenerative joint disease) is a disorder caused by wear and tear on the joints. Excess body weight is a risk factor associated with the development and progression of osteoarthritis. Weight reduction can decrease the manifestations of osteoarthritis. Certain aggravating exercises may need to be avoided, but exercise can be beneficial. Caffeine isn't associated with clinical manifestations of osteoarthritis. Alcohol intake isn't prohibited.

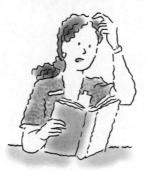

➡ *NCLEX keys*
Client needs category: Physiological integrity
Client needs subcategory: Physiological adaptation
Cognitive level: Application

6. A client with a sports injury undergoes a diagnostic arthroscopy of his left knee. After the procedure, the nurse assesses the client's leg. Which are the priority nursing assessment factors?
1. Wound and skin
2. Mobility and sensation
3. Vascular and integumentary
4. Circulatory and neurologic

Answer: 4. After a procedure on an extremity, nursing assessment should focus on neurovascular status of the extremity. Swelling of the extremity can impair neurologic and circulatory function of the leg. After the neurovascular status of the extremity has been established, the nurse can address the other concerns of skin, mobility, and pain.

➡ *NCLEX keys*
Client needs category: Physiological integrity
Client needs subcategory: Reduction of risk potential
Cognitive level: Application

7. A nurse is walking in a local park and witnesses an elderly woman fall. The woman reports severe pain, has difficulty moving her left leg, and is unable to bear weight on the affected leg. The nurse notices her left leg appears shorter than her right. The nurse suspects a femoral fracture. The greatest risk to the client is:
1. infection.
2. fat embolus.
3. neurogenic shock.
4. hypovolemia.

Answer: 4. The greatest risk to the client with a femoral fracture is hypovolemia from hemorrhage, which may be covert and can be fatal if not detected. Infection and fat emboli are potential complications less frequently seen in femoral fracture. Neurogenic shock isn't directly associated with femoral fracture.

➡ NCLEX keys

Client needs category: Physiological integrity
Client needs subcategory: Reduction of risk potential
Cognitive level: Comprehension

8. A client is undergoing rehabilitation following a fracture. As part of his regimen, the client performs isometric exercises. Which action provides the best evidence that the client understands the proper technique?
1. Exercising of bilateral extremities simultaneously
2. Periodic monitoring of his heart rate
3. Forced resistance against stable objects
4. Swinging of limbs through full range of motion

Answer: 3. Isometric exercises involve applying pressure against a stable object, such as pressing the hands together or pushing an arm against a wall. Exercising extremities simultaneously isn't a characteristic of isometrics. Heart rate monitoring is associated with aerobic exercise. Limb swinging isn't isometric.

➡ NCLEX keys

Client needs category: Physiological integrity
Client needs subcategory: Physiological adaptation
Cognitive level: Application

9. The nurse is doing preoperative teaching with a client who's admitted for hip replacement surgery. Which statement by the client indicates the need for further preoperative teaching?
1. "I'll begin gait training within 48 hours."
2. "I'll rest in bed for 2 to 3 hours after surgery."
3. "I need to turn, cough, and breathe deeply every 2 hours."
4. "I should do muscle strengthening exercises in both legs."

Answer: 2. After total joint replacement, few clients can get up 2 to 3 hours after surgery, although most are out of bed within 24 hours of surgery. The other options indicate that the client understands the nurse's preoperative teaching.

➡ NCLEX keys

Client needs category: Physiological integrity
Client needs subcategory: Basic care and comfort
Cognitive level: Analysis

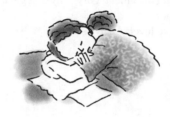

10. A trauma client reports tingling and severe pain in his cast right leg. When the nurse inspects the exposed toes, she notes cyanosis. What should the nurse do?
1. Apply a heating pad.
2. Elevate the extremity.
3. Notify the physician immediately.
4. Ask the client to wiggle his toes.

Answer: 3. The nurse should notify the physician immediately. Severe pain, tingling, and cyanosis are signs that the client's circulation is impaired by the cast, causing tissue ischemia. The cast should be removed immediately to relieve the pressure and prevent tissue damage. Applying a heating pad, elevating the extremity, and asking the client to wiggle his toes would delay treatment, further compromising the client's condition.

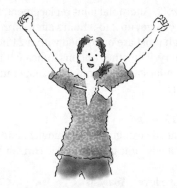

▶▶ *NCLEX keys*
Client needs category: Physiological integrity
Client needs subcategory: Physiological
adaptation
Cognitive level: Analysis

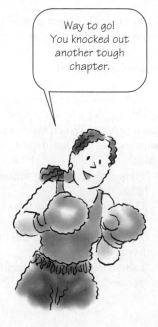

Way to go!
You knocked out
another tough
chapter.

8 Gastrointestinal system

Brush up on key concepts

The GI system is the body's food processing complex. The GI tract is basically a hollow, muscular tube through which food is digested. In addition, accessory organs, such as the liver and pancreas, contribute substances that are vital to digestion.

At any time, you can review the major points of this chapter by consulting the *Cheat sheet* on pages 246 to 252.

The breakdown begins

The digestive process begins in the **mouth,** where a mechanical (tongue and teeth) and chemical (saliva) combination begins to break down food.

Straight to the stomach

The **esophagus** transfers food from the oropharynx (behind the palate) to the stomach. The esophagus contains two structures, the epiglottis and the cardiac sphincter, that direct food into the stomach. The epiglottis closes to prevent food from entering the trachea, while the cardiac sphincter closes to prevent reflux of gastric contents.

Creating chyme

The **stomach** is a hollow muscular pouch that secretes pepsin, mucus, and hydrochloric acid for digestion. In the stomach, food mixes with gastric juices to become chyme, which the stomach stores before parceling it into the small intestine. The stomach also secretes the intrinsic factor necessary for absorption of vitamin B_{12}.

Digestion central

The **small intestine** consists of the duodenum, jejunum, and ileum. Nearly all digestion takes place in the small intestine, which contains digestive agents, such as bile and pancreatic secretions. The small intestine is also lined with villi, which contain capillaries and lymphatics that transport nutrients from the small intestine to the body.

Absorb, synthesize, and store

The **large intestine** consists of the ascending colon, transverse colon, descending colon, sigmoid colon, and rectum. It absorbs fluid and electrolytes, synthesizes vitamin K, and stores fecal material.

Not just bile

The **liver** is the largest organ in the body. Its many functions include:
• producing and conveying bile
• metabolizing carbohydrates, fats, and proteins
• synthesizing coagulation factors VII, IX, and X and prothrombin
• storing copper, iron, and vitamins A, D, E, K, and B_{12}
• detoxifying chemicals, excreting bilirubin, and producing and storing glycogen.

Pear-shaped storage

The **gallbladder** is a hollow, pear-shaped organ that stores bile and then delivers it through the cystic duct to the common bile duct.

Enzymes and hormones

The **pancreas** secretes three digestive enzymes: amylase, lipase, and trypsin. It also secretes the hormones insulin, glucagon, and somatostatin from the islets of Langerhans into the blood. In addition, the pancreas secretes large amounts of sodium bicarbonate, which is used to neutralize the acid in chyme.

(Text continues on page 252.)

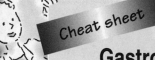

Gastrointestinal refresher

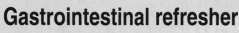

APPENDICITIS

Key signs and symptoms
- Anorexia
- Generalized abdominal pain that localizes in the right lower abdomen (McBurney point)
- Nausea and vomiting
- Sudden cessation of pain (indicates rupture)

Key test results
- Hematologic studies reveal moderately elevated white blood cell (WBC) count.
- Abdominal computed tomography (CT) scan identifies appendicitis or periappendical abcesses.

Key treatments
- Appendectomy

Key interventions
- Assess GI status and pain.
- Maintain nothing-by-mouth status until bowel sounds return postoperatively and then advance diet as tolerated.
- Monitor dressings for drainage and the incision for infection postoperatively.

CHOLECYSTITIS

Key signs and symptoms
- Episodic colicky pain in epigastric area that radiates to the back and shoulder
- Indigestion or chest pain after eating fatty or fried foods
- Nausea, vomiting, and flatulence

Key test results
- Blood chemistry reveals increased alkaline phosphatase, bilirubin, direct bilirubin transaminase, amylase, lipase, aspartate aminotransferase (AST), and lactate dehydrogenase (LD) levels.
- Cholangiogram shows calculi in the biliary tree.

Key treatments
- Laparoscopic cholecystectomy or open cholecystectomy
- Analgesics: meperidine (Demerol), morphine

Key interventions
- Assess abdominal status and pain.

- Provide postoperative care. (Monitor dressings for drainage; if open cholecystectomy, monitor and record T-tube drainage, monitor the incision for signs of infection, get the client out of bed as soon as possible, and encourage use of patient-controlled analgesia [PCA].)
- Maintain the position, patency, and low suction of the nasogastric (NG) tube if present.

CIRRHOSIS

Key signs and symptoms
- Abdominal pain (possibly because of an enlarged liver)
- Anorexia
- Fatigue
- Jaundice
- Nausea
- Vomiting
- Weakness

Key test results
- Liver biopsy, the definitive test for cirrhosis, detects destruction and fibrosis of hepatic tissue.
- Liver enzyme levels are elavated.
- CT scan with I.V. contrast reveals enlarged liver, identifies liver masses, and visualizes hepatic blood flow and obstruction, if present.

Key treatments
- Blood transfusions
- Schlerotherapy or gastric intubation and esophageal balloon tamponade for bleeding esophageal varices (Sengstaken-Blakemore method, esophagogastric tube method, Minnesota tube method)
- Transjugular intrahepatic portal-systemic shunting (TIPS procedure) as a last resort for clients with bleeding esophageal varicies and portal hypertension
- I.V. therapy using colloid volume expanders or crystalloids
- Vasoconstrictor: vasopressin for esophageal varices
- Diuretics: furosemide (Lasix), spironolactone (Aldactone) for edema (diuretics require careful monitoring; fluid and electrolyte imbalance may precipitate hepatic encephalopathy)

> Want a 5-minute review? Check out our Cheat sheet.

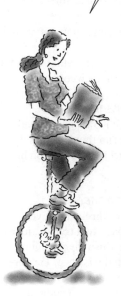

Gastrointestinal refresher (continued)

CIRRHOSIS (CONTINUED)
• Vitamin K: phytonadione for bleeding tendencies caused by hypoprothrombinemia

Key interventions
• Assess respiratory status frequently. Position the client to facilitate breathing.
• Check skin, gums, stool, and emesis regularly for bleeding.
• Observe the client closely for signs of behavioral or personality changes—especially increased stupor, lethargy, hallucinations, and neuromuscular dysfunction.
• Monitor ammonia levels and assess neurologic status.
• Carefully evaluate the client before, during, and after paracentesis.

COLORECTAL CANCER
Key signs and symptoms
• Abdominal cramping
• Change in bowel habits and shape of stools
• Diarrhea and constipation
• Blood in the stools
• Weight loss

Key test results
• Colonoscopy identifies and locates the mass.
• Digital rectal examination reveals the mass.
• Biopsy is positive for cancer cells.

Key treatments
• Radiation therapy
• Surgery depending on tumor location
• Antineoplastics: doxorubicin, 5-fluorouracil
• Analgesics: morphine, hydromorphone (Dilaudid)

Key interventions
• Administer postoperative care if indicated (monitor vital signs and intake and output; make sure the NG tube is kept patent; monitor dressing for drainage; assess the wound for infection; assist with turning, coughing, deep breathing, and incentive spirometry. Assess pain level and medicate for pain as necessary or guide the client in use of PCA).

CROHN'S DISEASE
Key signs and symptoms
• Abdominal cramps and spasms after meals
• Chronic diarrhea with blood
• Pain in right lower quadrant

Key test results
• Colonoscopy identifies pattern of disease.

• Upper GI series shows classic string sign: segments of stricture separated by normal bowel.

Key treatments
• Colectomy with ileostomy in many clients with extensive disease of the large intestine and rectum
• Antibiotics: ciprofloxacin (Cipro), metronidazole (Flagyl)
• Anticholinergics: propantheline, dicyclomine (Bentyl)
• Antidiarrheal: diphenoxylate with atropine (Lomotil)
• Anti-inflammatory agents: mesalamine (Apriso), sulfasalazine (Azulfidine)
• Immunosuppressants: mercaptopurine (6-MP) (Purinethol), azathioprine (Imuran), prednisone

Key interventions
• Assess GI status (note excessive abdominal distention) and fluid balance, and monitor stools for blood.
• Minimize stress and encourage verbalization of feelings.
• If surgery is necessary, provide postoperative care (monitor vital signs; monitor dressings for drainage; monitor ileostomy drainage and perform ileostomy care as needed; assess the incision for signs of infection; assist with turning, coughing, and deep breathing; get the client out of bed on the first postoperative day if stable).

DIVERTICULAR DISEASE
Key signs and symptoms
• Anorexia
• Change in bowel habits
• Flatulence
• Left lower quadrant pain or midabdominal pain that radiates to the back
• Nausea

Key test results
• Sigmoidoscopy shows a thickened wall in the diverticula.

Key treatments
• Colon resection (for diverticulitis refractory to medical treatment)
• High-fiber, low-fat diet for diverticulosis after pain subsides or liquid diet for mild diverticulitis or diverticulosis before pain subsides; avoidance of dietary irritants, such as nuts or popcorn
• Temporary colostomy possible for perforation, peritonitis, obstruction, or fistula that accompanies diverticulitis
• Analgesic: meperidine (Demerol)

(continued)

Gastrointestinal refresher *(continued)*

DIVERTICULAR DISEASE *(CONTINUED)*
• Antibiotics: gentamicin, tobramycin, clindamycin (Cleocin) for mild diverticulitis
• Anticholinergic: propantheline
• Bulk-forming laxative: psyllium (Metamucil)
• Stool softener: docusate sodium (Colace) for diverticulosis or mild diverticulitis

Key interventions
• Assess abdominal distention and bowel sounds.
• Prepare the client for surgery if necessary (administer cleaning enemas, osmotic purgative, oral and parenteral antibiotics).
• Provide postoperative care (watch for signs of infection; perform meticulous wound care; watch for signs of postoperative bleeding; assist with turning, coughing, and deep breathing; teach ostomy self-care).

ESOPHAGEAL CANCER
Key signs and symptoms
• Dysphagia
• Substernal pain
• Weight loss

Key test results
• Endoscopic examination of the esophagus, punch and brush biopsies, and an exfoliative cytologic test confirm esophageal tumors.

Key treatments
• Gastrostomy or jejunostomy to help provide adequate nutrition
• Radiation therapy
• Radical surgery to excise the tumor and resect either the esophagus alone or the stomach and the esophagus
• Antineoplastic: porfimer (Photofrin)

Key interventions
• Before surgery, answer the client's questions and let him know what to expect after surgery (gastrostomy tubes, closed chest drainage, NG suctioning).
• After surgery, monitor vital signs and watch for unexpected changes. If surgery included an esophageal anastomosis, keep the client flat on his back.
• Promote adequate nutrition, and assess the client's nutritional and hydration status.
• If the client has a gastrostomy tube, give food slowly, using gravity to adjust the flow rate. The prescribed amount usually ranges from 200 to 500 ml. Offer him something to chew before each feeding.
• Provide emotional support for the client and his family.

GASTRIC CANCER
Key signs and symptoms
• Anorexia
• Epigastric fullness and pain
• Nausea and vomiting
• Pain after eating that isn't relieved by antacids
• Weight loss

Key test results
• Gastric analysis shows positive cancer cells and achlorhydria.
• Gastroscopy biopsy is positive for cancer cells.

Key treatments
• Gastric surgery: gastroduodenostomy, gastrojejunostomy, partial gastric resection, total gastrectomy
• Antineoplastics: carmustine (BiCNU), 5-fluorouracil
• Vitamin supplements: folic acid (Folvite), cyanocobalamin (vitamin B_{12}) for clients who have undergone total gastrectomy

Key interventions
• Assess GI status postoperatively.
• Maintain the position, patency, and low suction of the NG tube (without irrigating or repositioning the NG tube because it may put pressure on the suture line).
• Provide emotional support and support client coping mechanisms.

GASTRITIS
Key signs and symptoms
• Abdominal cramping
• Epigastric discomfort
• Hematemesis
• Indigestion
• Nausea and vomiting

Key test results
• Upper GI endoscopy with biopsy confirms the diagnosis when performed within 24 hours of bleeding.

Key treatments
• I.V. fluid therapy
• NG lavage to control bleeding
• Histamine-2 (H_2) receptor antagonists: cimetidine (Tagamet), ranitidine (Zantac), famotidine (Pepcid), nizatidine (Axid) (may block gastric secretions)

Key interventions
• Administer antiemetics and I.V. fluids.
• Monitor fluid intake and output and electrolyte levels.
• Provide a bland diet. Monitor the client for recurrent symptoms as food is reintroduced.

Gastrointestinal refresher (continued)

GASTRITIS (CONTINUED)
- Offer small, frequent meals. Eliminate foods that cause gastric upset.
- If surgery is necessary, prepare the client preoperatively and provide appropriate postoperative care.
- Administer antacids and other prescribed medications.
- Provide emotional support to the client.

GASTROENTERITIS
Key signs and symptoms
- Abdominal discomfort
- Diarrhea
- Nausea

Key test results
- Stool culture identifies the causative bacteria, parasites, or amoebae.

Key treatments
- I.V. fluid and electrolyte replacement
- Antidiarrheals: diphenoxylate with atropine, loperamide (Imodium)

Key interventions
- Administer I.V. fluids and medications.
- Encourage clear liquids and electrolyte replacement.
- Monitor intake and output. Watch for signs of dehydration, such as dry skin and mucous membranes, fever, and sunken eyes.

GASTROESOPHAGEAL REFLUX
Key signs and symptoms
- Dysphagia
- Heartburn (burning sensation in the upper abdomen)

Key test results
- Barium swallow fluoroscopy indicates reflux.
- Esophagoscopy shows reflux.
- Endoscopy allows visualization and confirmation of pathologic changes in the mucosa.

Key treatments
- Positional therapy to help relieve symptoms by decreasing intra-abdominal pressure
- Antacid: aluminum hydroxide administered 1 hour and 3 hours after meals and at bedtime
- GI stimulants: metoclopramide (Reglan), bethanechol (Urecholine)
- H_2-receptor antagonists: cimetidine (Tagamet), ranitidine (Zantac), famotidine (Pepcid), nizatidine (Axid)
- Proton pump inhibitors: esomeprazole (Nexium), omeprazole (Prilosec)

Key interventions
- Help the client make dietary adjustments as appropriate.
- Have the client sleep in reverse Trendelenburg's position (with the head of the bed elevated 6" to 12" [15 to 30 cm]).
- Instruct the client to avoid lying down after eating.
- Advise the client to avoid alcohol and tobacco.

After surgery using a thoracic approach
- Carefully watch and record chest tube drainage and respiratory status.
- If needed, give chest physiotherapy and oxygen.
- Place the client with an NG tube in semi-Fowler's position.

HEPATITIS
Key signs and symptoms
During preicteric phase (usually 1 to 5 days)
- Fatigue
- Right upper quadrant pain
- Weight loss
- Vomiting
- Joint pain

During icteric phase (usually 1 to 2 weeks)
- Fatigue
- Jaundice
- Pruritus
- Weight loss
- Clay-colored stools

During posticteric or recovery phase (usually 2 to 12 weeks, sometimes longer in clients with hepatitis B, C, or E)
- Decreased hepatomegaly
- Decreased jaundice
- Fatigue

Key test results
- Blood chemistry analysis shows increased alanine amino-transferase, AST, alkaline phosphatase, LD, bilirubin, and erythrocyte sedimentation rate.
- Serologic tests identify hepatitis A virus, hepatitis B virus, hepatitis C virus, and delta antigen, if present.

Key treatments
- Vitamins and minerals: vitamin K, vitamin C (ascorbic acid), vitamin B complex (mega-B)
- Antivirals: ribavirin (Rebetol), lamivudine (Epivir-HBV)
- Interferon alfa-2a (Roferon-A) or interferon alfa-2b (Intron A)

Key interventions
- Assess GI status and watch for bleeding and fulminant hepatitis.

(continued)

Gastrointestinal refresher *(continued)*

HEPATITIS *(CONTINUED)*
• Maintain standard precautions.
• Encourage hepatitis B vaccination of family members and those in close contact with the client.

HIATAL HERNIA
Key signs and symptoms
• Dysphagia
• Regurgitation
• Sternal pain after eating

Key test results
• Barium swallow reveals protrusion of the hernia.
• Chest X-ray shows protrusion of abdominal organs into the thorax.
• Esophagoscopy shows incompetent cardiac sphincter.

Key treatments
• Bland diet of small, frequent meals and decreased intake of caffeine and spicy foods
• Anticholinergic: propantheline
• H_2-receptor antagonists: cimetidine (Tagamet), ranitidine (Zantac), famotidine (Pepcid)

Key interventions
• Assess respiratory status.
• Avoid flexion at the waist when positioning the client.

INTESTINAL OBSTRUCTION
Key signs and symptoms
• Abdominal distention
• Cramping pain
• Diminished or absent bowel sounds
• Vomiting fecal material

Key test results
• Abdominal X-ray shows increased amount of gas in bowel.
• Abdominal CT scan shows obstruction.

Key treatments
• Bowel resection with or without anastomosis if other treatment fails
• GI decompression using NG, Miller-Abbott, or Cantor tube
• Fluid and electrolyte replacement

Key interventions
• Monitor GI status. Assess and record bowel sounds and abdominal distention once per shift.
• Measure and record the client's abdominal girth.
• Maintain the position, patency, and low intermittent suction of NG and GI decompression tubes.

• Administer postoperative care if indicated (monitor vital signs and intake and output; monitor dressings for drainage; assess the wound for infection; assist with turning, coughing, and deep breathing; medicate for pain as necessary or guide the client in use of postoperative PCA).

IRRITABLE BOWEL SYNDROME
Key signs and symptoms
• Abdominal bloating
• Constipation, diarrhea, or both
• Heartburn
• Lower abdominal pain
• Nausea
• Passage of mucus
• Pasty, pencil-like stools

Key test results
• Sigmoidoscopy may disclose spastic contractions.

Key treatments
• Dietary changes: avoidance of foods that trigger symptoms; increased fiber intake
• Stress management
• Antispasmodic: propantheline
• Antidiarrheal: diphenoxylate with atropine (Lomotil)

Key interventions
• Help the client deal with stress, and warn against dependence on sedatives or antispasmodics.
• Provide nutritional counseling.

PANCREATITIS
Key signs and symptoms
• Abdominal tenderness and distention
• Abrupt onset of severe pain in the epigastric area that radiates to the shoulder, substernal area, back, and flank
• Aching, burning, stabbing, or pressing pain
• Nausea and vomiting
• Tachycardia

Key test results
• Blood chemistry analysis shows increased amylase, lipase.
• Cullen's sign is positive.
• Grey Turner's sign is positive.
• Abdominal CT scan reveals an enlarged pancreas.
• Ultrasonography reveals cysts, bile duct inflammation, and dilation.

Key treatments
• Bed rest
• I.V. fluids (vigorous replacement of fluids and electrolytes)

Gastrointestinal refresher (continued)

PANCREATITIS (CONTINUED)
- Transfusion therapy with packed red blood cells
- Analgesic: meperidine (Demerol) (morphine contraindicated)
- Antidiabetic: insulin (possible infusion to stabilize blood glucose levels)
- Corticosteroid: hydrocortisone
- Potassium supplement: I.V. potassium chloride

Key interventions
- Monitor abdominal, cardiac, and respiratory status (as the disease progresses, watch for respiratory failure, tachycardia, and worsening GI status).
- Assess fluid balance and monitor intake and ouput.
- Perform bedside glucose monitoring.
- Administer I.V. fluids.
- Keep the client in bed and reposition every 2 hours.

PEPTIC ULCER
Key signs and symptoms
- Anorexia
- Hematemesis
- Left epigastric pain 1 to 2 hours after eating
- Relief of pain after administration of antacids

Key test results
- Barium swallow shows ulceration of the gastric mucosa.
- Endoscopy shows the location of the ulcer.
- *Helicobacter pylori* test detects *H. pylori* antibodies.

Key treatments
- Endoscopy therapy for bleeding peptic ulcer
- If severe GI hemorrhage, gastric surgery that may include gastroduodenostomy, gastrojejunostomy, partial gastric resection, and total gastrectomy
- Saline lavage by NG tube until clear return (if bleeding present)
- Antibiotics if *H. pylori* is present: amoxicillin (Amoxil), metronidazole (Flagyl)
- H_2-receptor antagonists: cimetidine (Tagamet), ranitidine (Zantac), nizatidine (Axid), famotidine (Pepcid)
- Combination treatment: if *H. pylori* is present, two antibiotics with acid suppression or cytoprotective agent (Prevpac, Helidac)
- Proton pump inhibitors: omeprazole (Prilosec), esomeprazole (Nexium)
- Cytoprotective agents: sucralfate (Carafate), bismuth subsalicylate (Pepto-Bismol)

Key interventions
- Assess GI status.
- Assess cardiovascular status.

- Maintain the position, patency, and low suction of the NG tube if gastric decompression is ordered.
- Provide postoperative care if necessary (don't reposition the NG tube; irrigate it gently if ordered; medicate for pain as needed and ordered; monitor dressings for drainage; assess bowel sounds; get the client out of bed as tolerated).
- Recommend dietary changes to avoid acidic or spicy foods and caffeine.
- Advise client to avoid tobacco and alcohol.

PERITONITIS
Key signs and symptoms
- Abdominal resonance and tympany on percussion
- Abdominal rigidity and distention
- Constant, diffuse, and intense abdominal pain
- Decreased or absent bowel sounds
- Decreased urine output
- Fever
- Point tenderness
- Shallow respirations
- Weak, rapid pulse

Key test results
- WBC count is elevated.
- Abdominal X-ray may show free air in the abdomen under the diaphragm.
- CT of abdomen may detect abdominal fluid and areas of inflammation.

Key treatments
- Surgical intervention when the client's condition stabilized to treat the cause (For example, if the client has a perforated appendix, then an appendectomy is indicated.); drains placed for drainage of infected material
- Antibiotics: gentamicin, clindamycin (Cleocin), ofloxacin, meropenem (Merrem)
- Antipyretic: acetaminophen (Tylenol)
- Analgesic: meperidine (Demerol)

Key interventions
- Assess abdominal and respiratory status and fluid balance.
- Monitor and record vital signs and temperature, intake and output, laboratory studies, central venous pressure, daily weight, and urine specific gravity.
- Provide routine postoperative care (monitor vital signs and intake and output, including drainage from drains; assist with turning, incentive spirometry, coughing, and deep breathing; and get the client out of bed on the first postoperative day, if his condition allows).

(continued)

Gastrointestinal refresher (continued)

ULCERATIVE COLITIS

Key signs and symptoms
- Abdominal cramping
- Bloody, purulent, mucoid, watery stools (15 to 20 per day)
- Hyperactive bowel sounds
- Weight loss

Key test results
- Barium enema shows ulcerations.
- Sigmoidoscopy shows ulceration and hyperemia.

Key treatments
- Colectomy or pouch ileostomy
- Total parenteral nutrition (TPN) if necessary to rest the GI tract
- Anticholinergics: propantheline, dicyclomine (Bentyl)

- Antidiarrheals: diphenoxylate with atropine (Lomotil), loperamide (Imodium)
- Antiemetic: prochlorperazine
- Anti-inflammatory agents: 5-ASA compounds such as sulfasalizine, hydrocortisone
- Immunomodulators: azathioprine (Imuran), methotrexate (Trexall)

Key interventions
- Assess GI status and fluid balance.
- Monitor the number, amount, and character of stools.
- Administer I.V. fluids and TPN.
- Maintain the position, patency, and low suction of the NG tube.

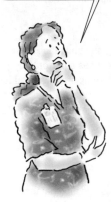

Visualize. Imagine that you're caring for a real-life client and performing each nursing action. It will make information more meaningful and help you remember.

Keep abreast of diagnostic tests

Here are the most important tests used to diagnose GI disorders, along with common nursing interventions associated with each test.

Barium upstairs

A **barium swallow test** involves fluoroscopic examination of the pharynx and esophagus.

Nursing actions
- Explain the procedure to the client.
- Before the procedure, withhold food and fluids for at least 8 hours and assess the client's ability to swallow.
- After the procedure, encourage intake of fluids unless contraindicated and administer laxatives as prescribed.

Barium in the middle

An **upper GI series** uses an X-ray to examine the esophagus, stomach, duodenum, and other portions of the small bowel after the client swallows barium.

Nursing actions
Before the procedure
- Explain the procedure to the client.

- Withhold food and fluids for at least 8 hours.
- Withhold medications that interfere with gastric motion for 12 to 24 hours before the test.
- Administer I.V. fluids, cathartics, and enemas, as prescribed.
After the procedure
- Inform the client that his stools will be light-colored for several days.
- Administer cathartics, fluids, and enemas, as prescribed.

Barium below

A **lower GI series,** also known as a *barium enema,* uses an X-ray to examine the large intestine.

Nursing actions
Before the procedure
- Explain the procedure to the client.
- Withhold food and fluids for at least 8 hours.
- Administer bowel preparation (laxatives and enemas), as prescribed.
After the procedure
- Encourage intake of fluids unless contraindicated.
- Administer enemas and laxatives, as prescribed.
- Monitor color and consistency of stools.

Viewing the stomach directly

Endoscopy uses an endoscope to view the esophagus and stomach, obtain specimens, and provide treatment, if necessary.

Nursing actions

Before the procedure
- Explain the procedure to the client.
- Withhold food and fluids for at least 8 hours.
- Make sure that written, informed consent has been obtained.
- Obtain baseline vital signs.
- Administer sedatives as prescribed.

After the procedure
- Assess gag and cough reflexes.
- Assess vasovagal response.
- Withhold food and fluids until the gag reflex returns.

Blood search

A **fecal occult blood test** analyzes stools for the presence of blood.

Nursing actions

- Explain the test to the client.
- Instruct the client to avoid red meat for 3 days before the test.
- Provide a container for the specimen.
- Document administration of aspirin, anti-coagulants, vitamin C, and anti-inflammatory drugs.

Fat search

A **fecal fat test** analyzes stools for the presence of fat.

Nursing actions

- Explain the procedure to the client.
- Instruct the client to abstain from alcohol and to maintain a high-fat diet (100 g/day) for 3 days before and during the 72-hour stool collection.
- Provide a container for the specimen.
- Refrigerate the specimen until they're sent to the laboratory.
- Document current medications.

From colon to canal

Proctosigmoidoscopy uses a lighted scope to view the sigmoid colon, rectum, and anal canal.

Nursing actions

Before the procedure
- Explain the procedure to the client.
- Administer bowel preparation as prescribed.
- Make sure that written, informed consent has been obtained.

After the procedure
- Document iron intake.
- Check the client for bleeding.
- Monitor the client's vital signs.
- Assess the client for signs and symptoms of such complications as a perforated bowel (abdominal tenderness, rigidity, distention).

Detailing the biliary duct

Cholangiography uses dye injection to produce a radiographic picture of the biliary duct system.

Nursing actions

Before the procedure
- Explain the procedure to the client.
- Encourage a low-residue, high-fat diet 1 day before the examination.
- Make sure that written, informed consent has been obtained.
- Withhold food and fluids after midnight.
- Note the client's allergies to iodine, seafood, and radiopaque dyes.
- Inform the client about possible throat irritation and flushing of the face.

After the procedure
- Check the injection site for bleeding.
- Monitor the client's vital signs.
- Administer fluids to flush the dye out through the kidneys.

Liver image

A **liver scan** produces an image of blood flow in the liver using an injection of a radioisotope.

Nursing actions

Before the procedure
- Explain the procedure to the client.
- Determine the client's ability to lie still during the procedure.
- Check the client for possible allergies.
- Make sure that written, informed consent has been obtained.

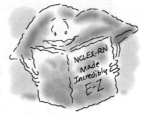

A biliary duct, also called a *bile duct*, is a duct by which bile passes from the liver or gallbladder to the duodenum.

After the procedure
- Assess the client for signs of delayed allergic reaction to the radioisotope, such as itching and hives.

Acid analysis
A **gastric analysis** measures the acidity of gastric secretions aspirated through a nasogastric (NG) tube.

Nursing actions
Before the procedure
- Explain the procedure to the client.
- Withhold food and fluids after midnight.
- Instruct the client not to smoke for 8 to 12 hours before the test.
- Withhold medications that can affect gastric secretions for 24 hours before the procedure.

After the procedure
- Obtain vital signs.
- Note reactions to the gastric acid stimulant, if used.

Organ echo
Ultrasonography uses echoes from sound waves to visualize body organs.

Nursing actions
- Assess the client's ability to lie still during the procedure.
- Explain the procedure to the client.

Blood study 1
Blood chemistry tests are used to analyze the client's blood. Samples may be obtained to analyze potassium, sodium, calcium, phosphorus, glucose, bicarbonate, blood urea nitrogen, creatinine, protein, albumin, osmolality, amylase, lipase, alkaline phosphatase, ammonia, bilirubin, lactate dehydrogenase (LD), aspartate aminotransferase (AST), serum alanine aminotransferase (ALT), hepatitis-associated antigens, and carcinoembryonic antigen (CEA).

Nursing actions
- Explain the procedure to the client.
- Note current drug therapy.
- Check the venipuncture site for bleeding.

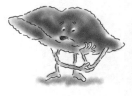

Ouch!
Liver biopsy involves percutaneous removal of liver tissue with a needle. Afterward, watch for signs of shock and pneumothorax.

Blood study 2
A **hematologic study** analyzes a blood sample for red blood cells (RBCs), white blood cells (WBCs), platelets, prothrombin time (PT), International Normalized Ratio (INR), partial thromboplastin time (PTT), hemoglobin (Hb), hematocrit (HCT), fibrin split products (FSPs), and erythrocyte sedimentation rate (ESR).

Nursing actions
- Explain the procedure to the client.
- Note current drug therapy.
- Check the venipuncture site for bleeding.

Tissue removal
A **liver biopsy,** which is used to diagnose such disorders as cirrhosis and cancer, involves percutaneous removal of liver tissue with a needle.

Nursing actions
Before the procedure
- Explain the procedure to the client.
- Withhold food and fluids after midnight.
- Make sure that written, informed consent has been obtained.
- Assess baseline clotting studies and vital signs.
- Instruct the client to exhale and hold his breath during insertion of the needle.

After the procedure
- Check the insertion site for bleeding.
- Monitor the client's vital signs.
- Observe the client for signs of shock (hypotension, tachycardia, oliguria) and pneumothorax (decreased breath sounds on the affected side, tachypnea, shortness of breath).
- Position the client on his right lateral side for hemostasis.

Lighting the large intestine
Colonoscopy uses a lighted scope to directly visualize the large intestine and obtain specimens.

Nursing actions
Before the procedure
- Explain the procedure to the client.
- Make sure that written, informed consent has been obtained.

- Provide a clear liquid diet 48 hours before the test.
- Administer a bowel preparation the day before the test.
- Explain that the client will feel cramping and the sensation of needing to have a bowel movement.
- Explain the use of air to distend the bowel lumen.

After the procedure
- Monitor for gross rectal bleeding.
- Assess for signs of colon perforation (abdominal distention, pain, rigidity).
- Withhold food and fluids for 2 hours.
- Check for blood in stools if polyps were removed.

Detailing ducts
Endoscopic retrograde cholangiopancreatography (ERCP) is radiographic examination of the hepatobiliary tree and pancreatic ducts using a contrast medium and a lighted scope.

Nursing actions
Before the procedure
- Explain the procedure to the client.
- Make sure that written, informed consent has been obtained.
- Withhold food and fluids after midnight.
- Check for allergies to iodine or seafood.

After the procedure
- Monitor for respiratory depression.
- Monitor for urine retention.
- Assess the client's gag reflex and withhold food until it returns.
- Assess for procedure-induced pancreatitis (abdominal pain, nausea, vomiting).

Tracking the bile trail
Percutaneous transhepatic cholangiography is fluoroscopic examination of the biliary ducts. It involves injection of a contrast medium.

Nursing actions
Before the procedure
- Explain the procedure to the client.
- Inform the client that the X-ray table will be tilted and rotated during the procedure
- Make sure that written, informed consent has been obtained.

- Check for allergies to iodine or seafood.
- Check PT, INR, and PTT.
- Type and crossmatch the client's blood.
- Withhold food and fluids after midnight.

After the procedure
- Make sure the client rests for at least 6 hours on his side.
- Check for bleeding at the injection site.
- Monitor vital signs.
- Withhold food and fluids for 2 hours.

Polish up on client care

Major GI disorders include appendicitis, cholecystitis, cirrhosis, colorectal cancer, Crohn's disease, diverticular disease, esophageal cancer, gastric cancer, gastritis, gastroenteritis, gastroesophageal reflux, hepatitis, hiatal hernia, intestinal obstruction, irritable bowel syndrome, pancreatitis, peptic ulcer, peritonitis, and ulcerative colitis.

Appendicitis

Appendicitis is an inflammation of the appendix. Although the appendix has no known function, it regularly fills with and empties itself of food. Appendicitis occurs when the appendix becomes inflamed from ulceration of the mucosa or from obstruction of the lumen.

CAUSES
- Barium ingestion
- Fecal mass
- Stricture
- Viral infection

ASSESSMENT FINDINGS
- Anorexia
- Constipation
- Generalized abdominal pain that becomes localized in the right lower abdomen (McBurney point)
- Lying in knee-bent position
- Malaise
- Nausea and vomiting
- Sudden cessation of pain (indicates rupture)

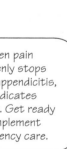

When pain suddenly stops during appendicitis, it indicates rupture. Get ready to implement emergency care.

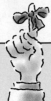

Memory jogger

Cholecystitis occurs most commonly in overweight women older than age 40 who haven't gone through menopause. To remember risk factors associated with cholecystitis, think of the 4 Fs.

Female

Fertile

Forty

Fat

DIAGNOSTIC TEST RESULTS
- Hematology shows moderately elevated WBC count.
- An abdominal X-ray shows rigid lower quadrant density.
- Abdominal computed tomography (CT) scan identifies appendicitis or periappendicial abscesses.

NURSING DIAGNOSES
- Imbalanced nutrition: Less than body requirements
- Acute pain
- Risk for infection

TREATMENT
- Appendectomy, open or laproscopic
- I.V. fluids to prevent dehydration

Drug therapy
- Analgesics: meperidine (Demerol), morphine (administered only when diagnosis is confirmed)
- Prophylactic antibiotics (if rupture occurs): cefotetan, cefoxitin

INTERVENTIONS AND RATIONALES
- Assess GI status and pain. *Sudden cessation of pain preoperatively may indicate appendix rupture.*
- Monitor and record vital signs and intake and output *to determine fluid volume.*
- Administer medications as ordered *to maintain or improve the client's condition.*
- Maintain nothing-by-mouth status until bowel sounds return postoperatively and then advance diet as tolerated *to promote healing and meet metabolic needs.*
- Assist the client with incentive spirometry, turning, coughing, and deep breathing *to mobilize secretions and promote lung expansion.*
- Monitor dressings for drainage and the incision for infection postoperatively *to detect early signs of infection and prevent complications.*

Teaching topics
- Explanation of the disorder and treatment plan
- Completing follow-up medical care
- Following activity restrictions
- Recognizing the signs and symptoms of infection

Cholecystitis

Cholecystitis is acute or chronic inflammation of the gallbladder most commonly associated with cholelithiasis (presence of gallstones). It occurs when an obstruction, such as calculi or edema, prevents the gallbladder from contracting when fatty foods enter the duodenum.

CAUSES
- Cholelithiasis
- Estrogen therapy
- Infection of the gallbladder
- Neoplasm of the common bile duct
- Major surgery
- Obesity
- Trauma

ASSESSMENT FINDINGS
- Abdominal pain
- Belching
- Clay-colored stools
- Dark amber urine
- Ecchymosis
- Episodic colicky pain in the epigastric area that radiates to the back and shoulder
- Fever
- Indigestion or chest pain after eating fatty or fried foods
- Jaundice
- Murphy's sign (tenderness over the gallbladder that increases on inspiration)
- Nausea, vomiting, and flatulence
- Pruritus
- Steatorrhea

DIAGNOSTIC TEST RESULTS
- Blood chemistry reveals increased alkaline phosphatase, bilirubin, direct bilirubin transaminase, amylase, lipase, AST, and LD levels.
- Cholangiogram shows calculi in the biliary tree.
- Gallbladder series shows calculi in the biliary tree.
- Hematology shows increased WBC count.
- Liver scan shows obstruction of the biliary tree.

- Ultrasound shows bile duct distention and calculi.
- ERCP reveals the presence of ductal stones.

NURSING DIAGNOSES

- Acute pain
- Deficient fluid volume
- Imbalanced nutrition: Less than body requirements
- Risk for infection

TREATMENT

- Small, frequent meals of a low-fat, low-calorie diet high in carbohydrates, protein, and fiber with restricted intake of gas-forming foods or no foods or fluids, as directed
- Extracorporeal shock wave lithotripsy
- Incentive spirometry
- Laparoscopic cholecystectomy or open cholecystectomy

Drug therapy

- Analgesics: meperidine (Demerol), morphine
- Antibiotics: ceftazidime (Fortaz), clindamycin (Cleocin), gentamicin
- Anticholinergics: propantheline, dicyclomine (Bentyl)
- Antiemetic: prochlorperazine
- Antipruritic: diphenhydramine (Benadryl)

INTERVENTIONS AND RATIONALES

- Assess abdominal status and pain *to determine baseline and detect changes in the client's condition.*
- Monitor and record vital signs, intake and output, laboratory studies, and urine specific gravity *to assess fluid and electrolyte balance.*
- Administer I.V. fluids *to provide the client with the necessary fluids and electrolytes.*
- Administer medications as prescribed *to treat infection, decrease pain, and promote comfort.*
- Provide postoperative care (monitor dressings for drainage; if open cholecystectomy, monitor and record T-tube drainage, monitor incision for signs of infection, get the client out of bed as soon as possible, and encourage use of patient-controlled analgesia [PCA]) *to maintain the client's condition and prevent postoperative complications.*

- Assist with turning, incentive spirometry, coughing, and deep breathing *to mobilize secretions and promote lung expansion.*
- Maintain the position, patency, and low suction of the NG tube (if present) *to prevent nausea and vomiting.*
- Keep the client in semi-Fowler's position *to promote comfort and facilitate GI emptying.*
- Provide skin, nares, and mouth care *to promote client comfort and prevent tissue breakdown.*
- Provide analgesics *to promote comfort.*
- Maintain a quiet environment *to promote rest.*

Teaching topics

- Explanation of the disorder and treatment plan
- Dietary modifications
- Medication use and possible adverse effects
- Using PCA
- Completing daily skin care
- Recognizing the signs and symptoms of infection
- Limiting activity as necessary

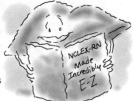

In cirrhosis, drug therapy requires special caution because the cirrhotic liver can't detoxify harmful substances efficiently.

Cirrhosis

Cirrhosis is a chronic hepatic disease characterized by diffuse destruction of hepatic cells, which are replaced by fibrous cells. Necrotic tissue leads to fibrosis. Cirrhosis alters liver structure and normal vasculature, impairs blood and lymph flow, and eventually causes hepatic insufficiency. Cirrhosis is irreversible.

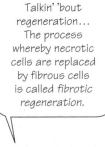

Talkin' 'bout regeneration... The process whereby necrotic cells are replaced by fibrous cells is called fibrotic regeneration.

CAUSES

- Alcoholism and resulting malnutrition
- Autoimmune disease, such as sarcoidosis, or chronic inflammatory bowel disease
- Exposure to hepatitis (types A, B, C, and D; viral hepatitis) or toxic substances

ASSESSMENT FINDINGS

- Abdominal pain (possibly because of an enlarged liver)
- Anorexia
- Constipation
- Diarrhea
- Fatigue
- Jaundice

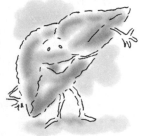

- Indigestion
- Muscle cramps
- Nausea
- Vomiting
- Weakness

DIAGNOSTIC TEST RESULTS

- Liver biopsy, the definitive test for cirrhosis, detects hepatic tissue destruction and fibrosis.
- Liver enzyme levels are elevated.
- CT scan with I.V. contrast medium reveals enlarged liver, identifies liver masses, and visualizes hepatic blood flow and obstruction, if present.
- Magnetic resonance imaging can further assess hepatic nodules.
- Esophagogastroduodenoscopy reveals bleeding esophageal varices, stomach irritation or ulceration, or duodenal bleeding and irritation.
- Blood studies reveal decreased platelets and decreased levels of Hb and HCT, albumin, serum electrolytes (sodium, potassium, chloride, magnesium), and folate.
- Blood studies reveal elevated levels of globulin, ammonia, total bilirubin, alkaline phosphatase, AST, ALT, and LD and increased thymol turbidity, and γ-glutamyltransferase.
- Urine studies show increased levels of bilirubin and urobilinogen.
- Stool studies reveal decreasing urobilinogen levels.

NURSING DIAGNOSES

- Imbalanced nutrition: Less than body requirements
- Risk for injury
- Ineffective breathing pattern

TREATMENT

- Blood transfusions
- Fluid restriction (usually to 1,500 ml/day)
- Schlerotherapy or gastric intubation and esophageal balloon tamponade for bleeding esophageal varices (Sengstaken-Blakemore method, esophagogastric tube method, Minnesota tube method)
- I.V. therapy using colloid volume expanders or crystalloids
- Oxygen therapy (may require endotracheal (ET) intubation and mechanical ventilation)

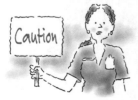

Watch ammonia levels in the client with cirrhosis; elevated ammonia levels may lead to encephalopathy.

Caution

- Paracentesis to reduce abdominal pressure from ascites
- Transjugular intrahepatic portal-systemic shunting (TIPS procedure) as a last resort for clients with bleeding esophageal varices and portal hypertension
- Sodium restriction (usually up to 500 mg/day)
- Low-protein diet
- Surgical intervention: peritoneovenous shunt

Drug therapy

- Antiemetic: ondansetron (Zofran)
- Vasoconstrictor: vasopressin for esophageal varices
- Diuretics: furosemide (Lasix), spironolactone (Aldactone) for edema (diuretics require careful monitoring; fluid and electrolyte imbalance may precipitate hepatic encephalopathy)
- Vitamin K: phytonadione for bleeding tendencies caused by hypoprothrombinemia
- Beta-adrenergic blocker: propranolol (Inderal) to decrease pressure from varices
- Laxative: lactulose to reduce serum ammonia levels

INTERVENTIONS AND RATIONALES

- Assess respiratory status frequently *because abdominal distention may interfere with lung expansion.* Position the client *to facilitate breathing.*
- Check skin, gums, stools, and emesis regularly for bleeding *to recognize early signs of bleeding and prevent hemorrhage.*
- Apply pressure to injection sites *to prevent bleeding.*
- Warn the client against taking aspirin, straining during defecation, and blowing his nose or sneezing too vigorously *to avoid bleeding.* Suggest using an electric razor and a soft toothbrush. *These measures also prevent bleeding.*
- Observe the client closely for signs of behavioral or personality changes—especially increased stupor, lethargy, hallucinations, and neuromuscular dysfunction. *Behavioral or personality changes may indicate increased ammonia levels.*
- Watch for asterixis, *a sign of developing hepatic encephalopathy.*

- Monitor ammonia levels and assess neurologic status *to determine the effectiveness of lactulose therapy.*
- Weigh the client and measure his abdominal girth daily, inspect the ankles and sacrum for dependent edema, and accurately record intake and output *to assess fluid retention.*
- Carefully evaluate the client before, during, and after paracentesis *because this drastic loss of fluid may induce shock.*
- Avoid using soap when bathing the client; instead, use lubricating lotion or moisturizing agents *to prevent skin breakdown associated with edema and pruritus.*
- Handle the client gently, and turn and reposition him often *to keep skin intact.*
- Encourage rest and good nutrition *to help the client conserve energy and decrease metabolic demands on the liver.*
- Encourage frequent, small meals *to ensure that nutritional needs are met.*

Teaching topics
- Explanation of the disorder and treatment plan
- Medication use and possible adverse effects
- Importance of avoiding infections and abstaining from alcohol
- Contacting Alcoholics Anonymous
- Avoiding activities that increase intra-abdominal pressure, such as heavy lifting, vigorous coughing, and straining during a bowel movement
- Avoiding alcohol
- Avoiding over-the-counter medications that may affect the liver such as acetaminophen

Colorectal cancer

Colorectal cancer is a malignant tumor of the colon or rectum. It may be primary or metastatic. It begins when unregulated cell growth and uncontrolled cell division develop into a neoplasm. Adenocarcinomas then infiltrate and cause obstruction, ulcerations, and hemorrhage.

CAUSES
- Aging
- Chronic constipation

- Chronic ulcerative colitis
- Diverticulosis
- Familial polyposis
- Low-fiber, high-carbohydrate diet

ASSESSMENT FINDINGS
- Abdominal cramping
- Abdominal distention
- Anorexia
- Blood in the stools
- Change in bowel habits and shape of stools
- Diarrhea and constipation
- Fecal oozing
- Melena
- Pallor
- Palpable mass
- Rectal bleeding
- Vomiting
- Weakness
- Weight loss

DIAGNOSTIC TEST RESULTS
- Barium enema locates mass.
- Biopsy is positive for cancer cells.
- CEA is positive.
- Colonoscopy identifies and locates the mass.
- Digital rectal examination reveals the mass.
- Fecal occult blood test is positive.
- Lower GI series shows location of mass.
- Hematology shows decreased levels of Hb and HCT.
- Sigmoidoscopy identifies and locates mass.

NURSING DIAGNOSES
- Anxiety
- Deficient fluid volume
- Acute pain
- Fear

TREATMENT
- Radiation therapy
- Surgery depending on tumor location (see *The lowdown on location*, page 260)

Drug therapy
- Analgesics: morphine, hydromorphone (Dilaudid)
- Antiemetics: prochlorperazine, ondansetron (Zofran)

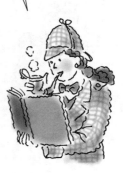

Hmmm. A change in bowel habits, abdominal cramping, and a mass detected by colonoscopy. Sounds like colorectal cancer.

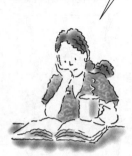

Patient-controlled analgesia allows the client to control I.V. delivery of an analgesic, usually morphine.

The lowdown on location

Surgery for colorectal cancer depends on the location of the tumor:
• If the tumor is in the cecum and ascending colon, surgery is a right hemicolectomy. This surgery may include resection of the terminal segment of the ileum, cecum, ascending colon, and right half of the transverse colon with corresponding mesentery.
• If the tumor is in the proximal and middle transverse colon, surgery is a right colectomy that includes the transverse colon and mesentery, or segmental resection of the transverse colon and associated midcolic vessels.
• If the tumor is in the sigmoid colon, surgery is limited to the sigmoid colon and mesentery.
• If the tumor is in the upper rectum, surgery is an anterior or low anterior resection.
• If the tumor is in the lower rectum, surgery is an abdominoperineal resection and permanent sigmoid colostomy.

• Antineoplastics: doxorubicin, 5-fluorouracil
• Folic acid derivative: leucovorin

INTERVENTIONS AND RATIONALES
• Assess GI status *to determine baseline and detect changes in the client's condition.*
• Monitor and record vital signs and intake and output, laboratory studies, and daily weight *to assess fluid and electrolyte status.*
• Monitor and record the color, consistency, amount, and frequency of stools *to detect early changes and bleeding.*
• Monitor for bleeding, infection, and electrolyte imbalance *to detect early changes and prevent complications.*
• Maintain the client's diet *to meet metabolic needs and promote healing.*
• Keep the client in semi-Fowler's position *to promote emptying of the GI tract.*
• Administer total parenteral nutrition (TPN) *to improve nutritional status when the client can't consume adequate calories through the GI tract.*
• Administer postoperative care, if indicated (monitor vital signs and intake and output; make sure the NG tube is kept patent; monitor dressings for drainage; assess the wound for infection; assist with turning, coughing, deep breathing, and incentive spirometry) *to prevent complications and promote healing.*

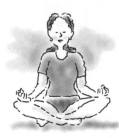

Crohn's disease is a chronic disorder. Client care involves long-term concerns such as reducing stress.

• Assess pain level and medicate for pain as necessary or guide the client with use of PCA *to promote comfort.*
• Encourage the client to express his feelings about changes in body image and a fear of dying and support coping mechanisms *to increase potential for further adaptive behavior.*
• Provide skin and mouth care *to maintain tissue integrity.*
• Provide rest periods *to promote healing and conserve energy.*
• Provide postchemotherapeutic and postradiation nursing care *to promote healing and prevent complications.*
• Monitor dietary intake *to determine nutritional adequacy.*
• Administer antiemetics and antidiarrheals, as prescribed, *to prevent further fluid loss.*

Teaching topics
• Explanation of the disorder and treatment plan
• Medication use and possible adverse effects
• Performing ostomy self-care if indicated
• Monitoring changes in bowel elimination
• Self-monitoring for infection
• Alternating rest periods with activity
• Contacting the United Ostomy Association and the American Cancer Society

Crohn's disease

Crohn's disease is a chronic inflammatory disease of the small intestine, usually affecting the terminal ileum. It also sometimes affects the large intestine, usually in the ascending colon. It's slowly progressive with exacerbations and remissions.

CAUSES
- Immune factors
- Unknown

CONTRIBUTING FACTORS
- Family history

ASSESSMENT FINDINGS
- Abdominal cramps and spasms after meals
- Chronic diarrhea
- Fever
- Flatulence
- Nausea
- Pain in right lower quadrant
- Weight loss

DIAGNOSTIC TEST RESULTS
- Abdominal X-ray shows a congested, thickened, fibrosed, narrowed intestinal wall.
- Barium enema shows lesions in the terminal ileum.
- Colonoscopy identifies pattern of disease.
- Fecal fat test shows increased fat.
- Fecal occult blood test is positive.
- Proctosigmoidoscopy shows ulceration.
- Upper GI series shows classic string sign: segments of stricture separated by normal bowel.

NURSING DIAGNOSES
- Anxiety
- Diarrhea
- Imbalanced nutrition: Less than body requirements
- Acute pain

TREATMENT
- Colectomy with ileostomy in many clients with extensive disease of the large intestine and rectum
- Small, frequent meals of a diet high in protein, calories, and carbohydrates and low in fat, fiber, and residue with bland foods and restricted intake of milk and gas-forming foods or no food or fluids
- TPN to rest the bowel

Drug therapy
- Analgesics: meperidine (Demerol), morphine
- Antianemics: ferrous sulfate, ferrous gluconate (Fergon)
- Antibiotics: ciprofloxacin (Cipro), metronidazole (Flagyl)
- Anticholinergics: propantheline, dicyclomine (Bentyl)
- Antidiarrheal: diphenoxylate with atropine
- Antiemetic: prochlorperazine
- Anti-inflammatory agents: 5-ASA (Apriso), sulfasalazine (Azulfidine)
- Immunosuppressants: mercaptopurine (6-MP) (Purinethol), azathioprine (Imuran), prednisone
- Potassium supplements: potassium chloride (K-Lor) administered with food, potassium gluconate (Kaon)

INTERVENTIONS AND RATIONALES
- Assess GI status (note excessive abdominal distention) and monitor stools for blood *to determine baseline and detect changes in the client's condition.*
- Monitor and record vital signs and intake and output, laboratory studies, daily weight, urine specific gravity, and fecal occult blood *to detect bleeding and dehydration.*
- Monitor the number, amount, and character of stools *to detect deterioration in GI status.*
- Administer TPN *to rest the bowel and promote nutritional status.*
- Administer medications, as prescribed, *to maintain or improve the client's condition.*
- Maintain the client's diet; withhold food and fluids as necessary *to minimize GI discomfort.*
- Minimize stress and encourage verbalization of feelings *to allay the client's anxiety.* (See *Coping with Crohn's.*)
- Provide skin and perianal care *to prevent skin breakdown.*
- If surgery is necessary, provide postoperative care (monitor vital signs; monitor dressings for drainage; monitor ileostomy drainage and perform ileostomy care as needed; assess

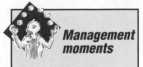

Management moments

Coping with Crohn's

Clients with Crohn's disease may have difficulty coping with their illness. Acute episodes of the disease are exhausting and, in many cases, incapacitating. The client may be unable to work. Therefore, it's important to take the following actions:
- Spend time with the client in a private environment.
- Encourage him to verbalize his feelings.
- Help the client find ways to cope with his disease when he returns home. For example, suggest he purchase a commode if getting to the bathroom during an acute episode is a problem.
- Help the client to identify successful coping mechanisms to deal with stress.
- Discuss the importance of avoiding fatigue and getting adequate rest.

the incision for signs of infection; assist with turning, coughing, and deep breathing; get the client out of bed on the first postoperative day if stable) *to promote healing and prevent complications.*

Teaching topics

• Explanation of the disorder and treatment plan
• Medication use and possible adverse effects
• Performing ileostomy self-care
• Avoiding laxatives and aspirin
• Performing perianal care daily
• Reducing stress
• Recognizing the signs and symptoms of rectal hemorrhage and intestinal obstruction

Diverticular disease

Occuring most commonly in people older than age 40, diverticular disease has two clinical forms: diverticulosis and diverticulitis. Diverticulosis occurs when the intestinal mucosa protrudes through the muscular wall. The common sites for diverticula are in the descending and sigmoid colon, but they may develop anywhere from the proximal end of the pharynx to the anus.

Diverticulitis is an inflammation of the diverticula that may lead to infection, hemorrhage, or obstruction.

CAUSES

• Chronic constipation
• Congenital weakening of the intestinal wall
• Low intake of roughage and fiber
• Straining during defecation

ASSESSMENT FINDINGS

• Anorexia
• Bloody stools
• Change in bowel habits
• Constipation and diarrhea
• Fever
• Flatulence
• Left lower quadrant pain or midabdominal pain that radiates to the back
• Nausea
• Rectal bleeding

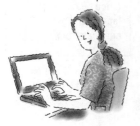

Common sites for diverticula are the descending and sigmoid colon.

DIAGNOSTIC TEST RESULTS

• Barium enema (contraindicated in acute diverticulitis) shows inflammation, narrow lumen of the bowel, and diverticula.
• Hematologic study shows increased WBC count and ESR.
• Sigmoidoscopy shows a thickened wall in the diverticula.

NURSING DIAGNOSES

• Constipation
• Diarrhea
• Acute pain

TREATMENT

• Generally no treatment for asymptomatic diverticulosis
• Colon resection (for diverticulitis refractory to medical treatment)
• High-fiber, low-fat diet for diverticulosis after pain subsides or liquid diet for mild diverticulitis or diverticulosis before pain subsides; avoidance of dietary irritants, such as nuts or popcorn
• Temporary colostomy possible for perforation, peritonitis, obstruction, or fistula that accompanies diverticulitis

Drug therapy

• Analgesic: meperidine (Demerol)
• Antibiotics: gentamicin, tobramycin, clindamycin (Cleocin) for mild diverticulitis
• Anticholinergic: propantheline
• Bulk-forming laxative: psyllium (Metamucil)
• Stool softener: docusate sodium (Colace) for diverticulosis or mild diverticulitis

INTERVENTIONS AND RATIONALES

• Assess abdominal distention and bowel sounds *to determine baseline and detect changes in the client's condition.*
• Monitor and record vital signs, intake and output, and laboratory studies *to assess fluid status.*
• Assess pain level, administer analgesics *to promote comfort* and evaluate their effect.
• Monitor stools for occult blood *to detect bleeding.*

- Maintain the client's diet *to improve nutritional status and promote healing.*
- Maintain position, patency, and low suction of the NG tube *to prevent nausea and vomiting.*
- Keep the client in semi-Fowler's position *to promote comfort and GI emptying.*
- Prepare the client for surgery if necessary (administer cleaning enemas, osmotic purgative, and oral and parenteral antibiotics), *to avoid wound contamination from bowel contents during surgery.*
- Provide postoperative care (watch for signs of infection; perform meticulous wound care; watch for signs of postoperative bleeding; assist with turning, coughing, and deep breathing; teach ostomy self-care) *to promote healing and prevent complications.*
- Administer TPN *to improve nutritional status when the client can't receive nutrition through the GI tract.*
- Administer medications as prescribed *to maintain or improve the client's condition.*

Teaching topics
- Explanation of the disorder and treatment plan
- Medication use and possible adverse effects
- Decreasing constipation
- Following dietary recommendations and restrictions
- Avoiding corn and nuts and fruits and vegetables with seeds
- Monitoring stools for bleeding

Esophageal cancer

Esophageal cancer attacks the esophagus, the muscular tube that runs from the back of the throat to the stomach. Cells in the lining of the esophagus start to multiply rapidly and form a tumor that may spread to other parts of the body.

Nearly always fatal, esophageal cancer usually develops in men over age 60. This disease occurs worldwide, but incidence varies geographically. It's most common in Japan, China, the Middle East, and parts of South Africa.

CONTRIBUTING FACTORS
- Excessive use of alcohol
- Nutritional deficiency
- Reflux esophagitis
- Smoking

ASSESSMENT FINDINGS
- Dysphagia
- Substernal pain
- Weight loss

DIAGNOSTIC TEST RESULTS
- Endoscopic examination of the esophagus, punch and brush biopsies, and an exfoliative cytologic test confirm esophageal tumors.
- X-rays of the esophagus with barium swallow and motility studies reveal structural and filling defects and reduced peristalsis.

NURSING DIAGNOSES
- Imbalanced nutrition: Less than body requirements
- Impaired swallowing
- Risk for aspiration
- Anxiety
- Fear

TREATMENT
- Endoscopic laser treatment and bipolar electrocoagulation to help restore swallowing by vaporizing cancerous tissue
- Esophageal dilation
- Gastrostomy or jejunostomy to help provide adequate nutrition
- Radiation therapy
- Radical surgery to excise the tumor and resect either the esophagus alone or the stomach and the esophagus

Drug therapy
- Antineoplastic: porfimer (Photofrin)
- Analgesics: morphine (MS Contin), fentanyl (Duragesic-25)

INTERVENTIONS AND RATIONALES
- Before surgery, answer the client's questions and let him know what to expect after surgery (gastrostomy tubes, closed chest drainage, NG suctioning) *to allay his anxiety.*
- After surgery, monitor vital signs and watch for unexpected changes *to detect early*

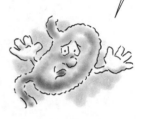

Esophageal cancer is usually advanced when diagnosed; surgery and other treatments can only relieve symptoms.

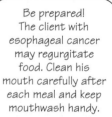

Be prepared! The client with esophageal cancer may regurgitate food. Clean his mouth carefully after each meal and keep mouthwash handy.

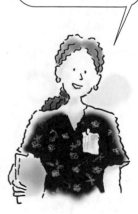

signs of complications and avoid treatment delay. If surgery included an esophageal anastomosis, keep the client flat on his back *to avoid tension on the suture line.*

• Promote adequate nutrition, and assess the client's nutritional and hydration status *to determine the need for supplementary parenteral feedings.*

• Place the client in Fowler's position for meals *to avoid aspiration of food.*

• Provide high-calorie, high-protein, pureed food as needed *to meet increased metabolic demands and prevent aspiration.*

• If the client has a gastrostomy tube, give food slowly (usually 200 to 500 ml), using gravity to adjust the flow rate, *to prevent abdominal discomfort.*

• Provide emotional support for the client and his family *to help them cope with terminal illness.*

Teaching topics

• Explanation of the disorder and treatment plan

• Medication use and possible adverse effects

• Dietary modifications

• Avoiding aspiration pneumonia

• Caring for the gastrostomy tube

• Contacting the American Cancer Society and local support groups

Gastric cancer

Gastric cancer is cancer of the GI tract that's classified according to gross appearance (polypoid, ulcerating, ulcerating and infiltrating, or diffuse). It may be primary or metastatic. Its precise cause is unknown, but it's commonly associated with gastritis, gastric atrophy, and other conditions. About one-half of gastric cancers occur in the pyloric area of the stomach.

CAUSES

• Unknown

CONTRIBUTING FACTORS

• Achlorhydria

• Chronic gastritis

• Family history of gastric cancer

• High intake of salted and smoked foods

• Low intake of vegetables and fruits

• Gastroesophageal reflux disease

• High alcohol consumption

• Smoking

• Obesity

• High-fat diet

ASSESSMENT FINDINGS

• Anorexia

• Epigastric fullness and pain

• Fatigue

• Hematemesis

• Indigestion

• Malaise

• Melena

• Nausea and vomiting

• Pain after eating that isn't relieved by antacids

• Regurgitation

• Shortness of breath

• Syncope

• Weakness

• Weight loss

DIAGNOSTIC TEST RESULTS

• CEA test is positive.

• Fecal occult blood test is positive.

• Gastric analysis shows positive cancer cells and achlorhydria.

• Gastroscopy biopsy is positive for cancer cells.

• Upper GI series reveals a gastric mass.

• Hematology shows decreased levels of Hb and HCT.

• Gastric hydrochloric acid level is decreased.

NURSING DIAGNOSES

• Anxiety

• Ineffective tissue perfusion: GI

• Risk for deficient fluid volume

• Acute pain

• Fear

TREATMENT

• Gastric surgery: gastroduodenostomy, gastrojejunostomy, partial gastric resection, total gastrectomy

• TPN

• High-calorie diet

• Radiation therapy

> In gastric cancer, pain after eating isn't relieved by antacids and weight loss is common.

Drug therapy
- Analgesics: meperidine (Demerol), morphine
- Antiemetic: prochlorperazine
- Antineoplastics: carmustine (BiCNU), 5-fluorouracil
- Vitamin supplements: folic acid (Folvite), cyanocobalamin (vitamin B_{12}) for clients who have undergone total gastrectomy

INTERVENTIONS AND RATIONALES
- Assess GI status postoperatively *to monitor the client for dumping syndrome (weakness, nausea, flatulence, and palpitations 30 minutes after a meal).*
- Monitor and record vital signs, intake and output, laboratory studies, and daily weight *to determine baseline and early changes in the client's condition.*
- Assess pain level, provide analgesics, and evaluate their effect *to promote comfort.*
- Monitor the consistency, amount, and frequency of stools *to detect GI compromise.*
- Monitor the color of stools *to detect bleeding and prevent hemorrhage.*
- Maintain the client's diet *to promote nutritional balance.*
- Maintain the position, patency, and low suction of the NG tube (without irrigating or repositioning the NG tube because it may put pressure on the suture line) *to prevent complications, nausea, and vomiting.*
- Monitor incision site for redness and purulent drainage *to detect infection.*
- Administer TPN for 1 week or longer if gastric surgery is extensive *to meet metabolic needs and promote wound healing.*
- Administer medications, as prescribed, *to maintain or improve the client's condition.*
- Provide emotional support and support client coping mechanisms *to increase the potential for adaptive behavior.*
- Provide skin and mouth care *to prevent skin breakdown and damage to the oral mucosa and improve nutritional intake.*
- Provide rest periods *to conserve energy.*

Teaching topics
- Explanation of disorder and treatment plan
- Medication use and possible adverse effects
- Avoiding exposure to people with infections
- Alternating rest periods with activity

- Monitoring temperature
- Recognizing the signs and symptoms of wound infection
- Recognizing the signs and symptoms of ulceration
- Completing skin care daily
- Contacting the American Cancer Society and local suport groups

Gastritis

Gastritis is an inflammation of the gastric mucosa (the stomach lining). It may be acute or chronic:
- Acute gastritis produces mucosal reddening, edema, hemorrhage, and erosion.
- Chronic gastritis is common among elderly people and people with pernicious anemia. In chronic atrophic gastritis, all stomach mucosal layers are inflamed.

CAUSES
Acute gastritis
- Chronic ingestion of irritating foods, spicy foods, or alcohol
- Drugs, such as aspirin and other nonsteroidal anti-inflammatory drugs (NSAIDs) (in large doses), cytotoxic agents, caffeine, corticosteroids, antimetabolites, phenylbutazone, and indomethacin
- Endotoxins released from infecting bacteria, such as staphylococci, *Escherichia coli,* and *Salmonella.*
- *Helicobacter pylori* infection
- Ingestion of poisons, especially DDT, ammonia, mercury, carbon tetrachloride, and corrosive substances

Chronic gastritis
- Alcohol ingestion
- Cigarette smoke
- Environmental irritants
- Peptic ulcer disease

ASSESSMENT FINDINGS
- Abdominal cramping
- Epigastric discomfort
- Hematemesis
- Indigestion
- Nausea and vomiting

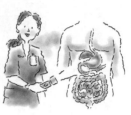

Gastritis is an inflammation of the gastric mucosa that produces abdominal cramping, epigastric discomfort, and indigestion.

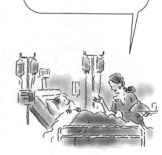

Of course we have a special diet for the client with gastritis. Smaller, more frequent portions of bland food. Bon appetit!

DIAGNOSTIC TEST RESULTS
- Fecal occult blood test can detect occult blood in vomitus and stools if the client has gastric bleeding.
- Blood studies show low Hb level and HCT when significant bleeding has occurred.
- Upper GI endoscopy with biopsy confirms the diagnosis when performed within 24 hours of bleeding.
- Upper GI series may be performed to exclude serious lesions.

NURSING DIAGNOSES
- Risk for deficient fluid volume
- Imbalanced nutrition: Less than body requirements
- Acute or chronic pain (depending on the type of gastritis)

TREATMENT
- Angiography with vasopressin infused in normal saline solution (when gastritis causes massive bleeding)
- Blood transfusion
- I.V. fluid therapy
- NG lavage to control bleeding
- Oxygen therapy if necessary
- Partial or total gastrectomy (rare)
- Vagotomy and pyloroplasty (limited success when conservative treatments have failed)

Drug therapy
- Antibiotics: according to sensitivity of infecting organism (if the cause is bacterial)
- Antidote: according to the ingested poison (if the cause is poisoning)
- Antiemetics: prochlorperazine, ondansetron (Zofran)
- Histamine-2 (H_2) receptor antagonists: cimetidine (Tagamet), ranitidine (Zantac), famotidine (Pepcid), nizatidine (Axid) (may block gastric secretions)

INTERVENTIONS AND RATIONALES
- Administer antiemetics and I.V. fluids *to prevent dehydration and electrolyte imbalance.*
- Monitor fluid intake and output and electrolyte levels *to detect early signs of dehydration and electrolyte loss.*

- Provide a bland diet *to prevent recurrence.* Monitor the client for recurrent symptoms as food is reintroduced.
- Offer small, frequent meals *to reduce irritating gastric secretions.* Eliminate foods that cause gastric upset *to prevent gastric irritation.*
- If surgery is necessary, prepare the client preoperatively and provide appropriate postoperative care *to decrease preoperative anxiety and prevent intraoperative and postoperative complications.*
- Administer antacids and other prescribed medications *to promote gastric healing.*
- Provide emotional support to the client *to help him manage his symptoms.*

Teaching topics
- Explanation of the disorder and treatment plan
- Medication use and possible adverse effects
- Contacting support groups for smoking cessation
- Dietary modifications, such as avoiding spicy foods and foods and beverages containing caffeine

Gastroenteritis

Gastroenteritis is an irritation and inflammation of the digestive tract characterized by diarrhea, nausea, vomiting, and abdominal cramping. It occurs in all age-groups and is usually self-limiting in adults.

In the United States, gastroenteritis ranks second to the common cold as a cause of lost work time and fifth as the cause of death among young children. It also can be life-threatening in elderly and debilitated persons. It's a major cause of morbidity and mortality in developing nations.

This disorder is also called *intestinal flu, traveler's diarrhea, viral enteritis,* and *food poisoning.*

CAUSES
- Amoebae, especially *Entamoeba histolytica*
- Bacteria (responsible for acute food poisoning): *Staphylococcus aureus, Salmonella,*

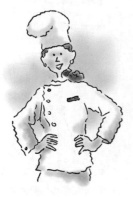

What's the recipe for preventing gastroenteritis? Clean utensils and cook food thoroughly. Refrigerate perishable foods. Wash hands with warm water and soap before handling foods.

Shigella, Clostridium botulinum, Escherichia coli, Clostridium perfringens
• Drug reactions (especially antibiotics)
• Enzyme deficiencies
• Food allergens
• Ingestion of toxins: plants or toadstools (mushrooms)
• Parasites: *Ascaris, Enterobius, Trichinella spiralis*
• Viruses (may be responsible for traveler's diarrhea): adenovirus, echovirus, or coxsackievirus

ASSESSMENT FINDINGS
• Abdominal discomfort
• Diarrhea
• Nausea and vomiting

DIAGNOSTIC TEST RESULTS
• Stool culture identifies causative bacteria, parasites, or amoebae.
• Blood culture identifies causative organism.

NURSING DIAGNOSES
• Diarrhea
• Risk for deficient fluid volume
• Acute pain

TREATMENT
• Increased fluid intake
• I.V. fluid and electrolyte replacement
• Nutritional support

Drug therapy
• Antibiotic therapy according to the sensitivity of the causative organism
• Antidiarrheals: diphenoxylate with atropine, loperamide (Imodium)
• Antiemetics: prochlorperazine, trimethobenzamide (Tigan) (These medications should be avoided in clients with viral or bacterial gastroenteritis.)

INTERVENTIONS AND RATIONALES
• Administer I.V. fluids and medications; correlate dosages, routes, and times appropriately with the client's meals and activities; for example, give antiemetics 30 to 60 minutes before meals *to prevent the onset of symptoms.*

• Encourage clear liquids and electrolyte replacement *to prevent dehydration.*
• Instruct the client to avoid milk and milk products, *which may exacerbate the condition.*
• Monitor intake and output. Watch for signs of dehydration, such as dry skin and mucous membranes, fever, and sunken eyes, *to prevent complications of dehydration.*
• Stress hand washing to client and visitors.

Teaching topics
• Explanation of the disorder and treatment plan
• Increased fluid intake
• Cleaning utensils thoroughly; avoiding drinking water or eating raw fruit or vegetables when visiting a foreign country; eliminating flies and roaches in the home
• Thoroughly cooking foods, especially pork; refrigerating perishable foods
• Washing hands with warm water and soap before handling food, especially after using the bathroom

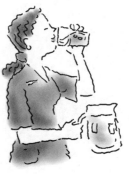

Drink up. Increased fluid intake helps relieve gastroenteritis.

Gastroesophageal reflux

Gastroesophageal reflux refers to the backflow, or reflux, of gastric and duodenal contents past the lower esophageal sphincter and into the esophagus. Reflux may or may not cause symptoms or pathologic changes. Persistent reflux may cause reflux esophagitis (inflammation of the esophageal mucosa). The prognosis varies with the underlying cause.

CAUSES
• Pressure within the stomach that exceeds lower esophageal sphincter pressure

CONTRIBUTING FACTORS
• Any action that decreases lower esophageal sphincter pressure, such as smoking cigarettes and ingesting food, alcohol, anticholinergics (atropine, belladonna, propantheline), and other drugs (morphine, diazepam, meperidine)
• Any condition or position that increases intra-abdominal pressure
• Hiatal hernia (especially in children)

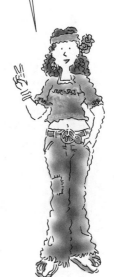

Get back. In gastroesophageal reflux, duodenal contents get back to where they don't belong—into the esophagus.

- Long-term NG intubation (more than 5 days)
- Pyloric surgery (alteration or removal of the pylorus), which allows reflux of bile or pancreatic juice

ASSESSMENT FINDINGS
- Dysphagia
- Heartburn (burning sensation in the upper abdomen)

Atypical symptoms
- Asthma
- Atypical chest pain
- Chronic cough
- Laryngitis
- Sore throat

DIAGNOSTIC TEST RESULTS
- Barium swallow fluoroscopy indicates reflux.
- Esophageal pH probe reveals a low pH, which indicates reflux.
- Esophagoscopy shows reflux.
- Acid perfusion (Bernstein) test shows that reflux is the cause of symptoms.
- Endoscopy allows visualization and confirmation of pathologic changes in the mucosa.
- Biopsy allows visualization and confirmation of pathologic changes in the mucosa.

NURSING DIAGNOSES
- Risk for aspiration
- Chronic pain
- Deficient knowledge (disease process and treatment plan)

TREATMENT
- Low-fat, high-fiber diet with no caffeine or carbonated beverages
- Oxygen therapy
- Positional therapy to help relieve symptoms by decreasing intra-abdominal pressure
- Surgery: fundoplication (the fundus of the stomach is sutured in place around the lower esophagus)

Drug therapy
- Antacid: aluminum hydroxide administered 1 hour and 3 hours after meals and at bedtime

- GI stimulants: metoclopramide (Reglan), bethanechol (Urecholine)
- H_2-receptor antagonists: cimetidine (Tagamet), ranitidine (Zantac), famotidine (Pepcid), nizatidine (Axid)
- Proton pump inhibitors: esomeprazole (Nexium), omeprazole (Prilosec)

INTERVENTIONS AND RATIONALES
- Help the client make dietary adjustments, as appropriate, *to ensure compliance.*
- Have the client sleep in reverse Trendelenburg's position (with the head of the bed elevated 6″ to 12″ [15 to 30 cm]) *to reduce intra-abdominal pressure.*
- Instruct the client to avoid lying down after eating *to decrease chance of acid reflux.*
- Advise the client to avoid alcohol and tobacco *to decrease chance of acid reflux.*
- After surgery, assess the incisions for signs of infection. Carefully watch and record chest tube drainage and respiratory status.
- If needed, give chest physiotherapy and oxygen *to mobilize secretions and prevent hypoxemia.*
- Place the client with an NG tube in semi-Fowler's position *to help prevent reflux.*
- Offer reassurance and emotional support *to help the client cope with pain and discomfort.*

Teaching topics
- Explanation of the disorder and treatment plan
- Medication use and possible adverse effects
- Positional therapy
- Dietary modification
- Weight loss (if indicated)
- Lifestyle modification, such as smoking and alcohol cessation

Hepatitis

Hepatitis is the inflammation of liver tissue that causes inflammation of hepatic cells, hypertrophy, and proliferation of Kupffer's cells and bile stasis. Hepatitis is typically caused by one of five viruses: hepatitis A, B, C, D, or E.

CAUSES

- Hepatitis A: contaminated food, milk, water, feces (most commonly foodborne)
- Hepatitis B: parenteral (needle sticks), blood, sexual contact, secretions
- Hepatitis C: blood or serum (blood transfusion, exposure to contaminated blood), sexual contact
- Hepatitis D: similar to causes of type B virus
- Hepatitis E: fecal-oral route

ASSESSMENT FINDINGS

Assessment findings are consistent for the different types of hepatitis, but signs and symptoms progress over several stages.

During preicteric phase (usually 1 to 5 days)

- Anorexia
- Constipation and diarrhea
- Fatigue
- Fever
- Headache
- Hepatomegaly
- Vomiting

- Joint pain
- Malaise
- Nasal discharge
- Nausea and vomiting
- Pharyngitis
- Pruritus
- Right upper quadrant pain
- Splenomegaly
- Weight loss

During icteric phase (usually 1 to 2 weeks)

- Clay-colored stools
- Dark urine
- Fatigue
- Hepatomegaly
- Jaundice
- Pruritus
- Splenomegaly
- Weight loss

During posticteric or recovery phase (usually 2 to 12 weeks, sometimes longer in clients with hepatitis B, C, or E)

- Decreased hepatomegaly
- Decreased jaundice

Management moments

Recognizing fulminant hepatitis

A rare but severe form of hepatitis, fulminant hepatitis rapidly causes massive liver necrosis. It usually occurs in clients with hepatitis B, D, or E. Although mortality is extremely high (more than 80% of clients lapse into deep coma), clients who survive may recover completely.

ASSESSMENT

In a client with viral hepatitis, suspect fulminant hepatitis if you assess:
- confusion
- somnolence
- ascites
- edema
- rapidly rising bilirubin level
- markedly prolonged prothrombin time
- elevated ammonia level.

As the disease progresses quickly to the terminal phase, the client may experience

cerebral edema, brain stem compression, GI bleeding, sepsis, respiratory failure, cardiovascular collapse, and renal failure.

EMERGENCY ACTIONS

If you suspect fulminant hepatitis, you should:
- notify the physician immediately
- provide supportive care, such as maintaining fluid volume, supporting ventilation through mechanical means, controlling bleeding, and correcting hypoglycemia
- restrict protein intake
- expect to administer oral lactulose or neomycin and, possibly, massive doses of glucocorticoids
- prepare the client for a liver transplant if necessary and if he meets the criteria.

- Fatigue
- Improved appetite

DIAGNOSTIC TEST RESULTS
- Blood chemistry analysis shows increased ALT, AST, alkaline phosphatase, LD, bilirubin, and ESR.
- Serologic tests identify hepatitis A, B, or C and delta antigen, if present.
- Hematologic studies show increased PT and FSPs.
- Stool specimen reveals hepatitis A virus (in hepatitis A cases).
- Urine chemistry shows increased urobilinogen.

NURSING DIAGNOSES
- Deficient fluid volume
- Imbalanced nutrition: Less than body requirements
- Chronic pain
- Anxiety

TREATMENT
- High-calorie, high-carbohydrate, moderate-protein, low-fat diet in small, frequent meals
- Rest

Drug therapy
- Antiemetic: prochlorperazine
- Antivirals: ribavirin (Rebetol), lamivudine (Epivir-HBV)
- Interferon: alfa-2a (Roferon-A) and alfa-2b (Intron A)
- Vitamins and minerals: vitamin K, vitamin C (ascorbic acid), vitamin B complex (mega-B)

INTERVENTIONS AND RATIONALES
- Assess GI status and watch for bleeding and fulminant hepatitis *to detect early complications.* (See *Recognizing fulminant hepatitis*, page 269.)
- Monitor and record vital signs, intake and output, and laboratory studies *to detect early signs of deficient fluid volume.*

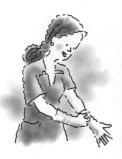

Maintaining standard precautions affects your safety and the client's safety; it's an important topic to cover.

Standard precautions

Standard precautions apply to blood; all body fluids, secretions, and excretions (except sweat), regardless of whether they contain visible blood; nonintact skin; and mucous membranes.

HAND WASHING
Wash hands after touching blood, body fluids, secretions, excretions, and contaminated items, whether or not gloves are worn. Wash hands immediately after gloves are removed, between client contacts, and when otherwise indicated to avoid transfer of microorganisms to other clients or environments. It may be necessary to wash hands between tasks and procedures on the same client to prevent cross-contamination of different body sites.

GLOVES
Wear gloves when touching blood, body fluids, secretions, excretions, or contaminated items. Put on clean gloves just before touching mucous membranes and nonintact skin. Remove gloves promptly after use and wash hands.

MASK, EYE PROTECTION, FACE SHIELD
Wear a mask, eye protection, and a face shield to protect the mucous membranes of your eyes, nose, and mouth during procedures and client care activities that are likely to generate splashes of blood, body fluids, secretions, or excretions.

GOWN
Wear a gown to protect skin and prevent soiling of clothing during procedures and client care activities that are likely to generate splashes of blood, body fluids, secretions, or excretions.

- Administer medications, as prescribed, *to maintain or improve the client's condition.*
- Maintain standard precautions. *Hand washing prevents the spread of pathogens to others.* (See *Standard precautions.*)
- Provide rest periods *to conserve the client's energy and reduce metabolic demands.*
- Encourage small, frequent meals *to improve the client's nutritional status.*
- Change the client's position every 2 hours *to reduce the risk of skin breakdown.*
- Monitor for signs of bleeding *to prevent hemorrhage.*
- Encourage hepatitis B vaccination of family members and those in close contact with the client.

Teaching topics

- Explanation of the disorder and treatment plan
- Medication use and possible adverse effects
- Avoiding exposure to people with infections
- Avoiding alcohol
- Maintaining good personal hygiene
- Refraining from donating blood
- Increasing fluid intake to 3,000 ml/day (approximately 12 8-oz glasses)
- Abstaining from sexual intercourse until serum liver studies are within normal limits
- Importance of hepatitis B vaccination of family and close contacts

Hiatal hernia

A hiatal hernia, also known as an *esophageal hernia*, is a protrusion of the stomach through the diaphragm into the thoracic cavity.

CAUSES

- Congenital weakness
- Increased abdominal pressure
- Unknown

CONTRIBUTING FACTORS

- Aging
- Obesity
- Pregnancy
- Trauma

ASSESSMENT FINDINGS

- Cough
- Dysphagia
- Dyspnea
- Feeling of fullness
- Pyrosis
- Regurgitation
- Sternal pain after eating
- Tachycardia
- Vomiting

DIAGNOSTIC TEST RESULTS

- Barium swallow reveals protrusion of the hernia.
- Chest X-ray shows protrusion of abdominal organs into the thorax.
- Esophagoscopy shows incompetent cardiac sphincter.

NURSING DIAGNOSES

- Anxiety
- Imbalanced nutrition: Less than body requirements
- Chronic pain

TREATMENT

- Antireflux surgical repair if complications develop
- Bland diet of small, frequent meals and decreased intake of caffeine and spicy foods
- Weight loss, if necessary

Drug therapy

- Anticholinergic: propantheline
- H_2-receptor antagonists: cimetidine (Tagamet), ranitidine (Zantac), famotidine (Pepcid)

INTERVENTIONS AND RATIONALES

- Assess respiratory status *to detect early signs of respiratory distress.*
- Monitor and record vital signs, intake and output, and daily weight *to determine baseline and detect early signs of nutritional deficit.*
- Administer oxygen *to help relieve respiratory distress.*
- Avoid flexion at the waist in positioning the client *to promote comfort.*
- Maintain the client's diet *to maintain and improve nutritional status.*

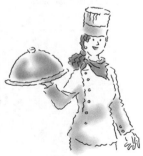

When planning meals for clients with hiatal hernia, make them small, frequent, and bland.

- Maintain position, patency, and low suction of the NG tube *to prevent nausea and vomiting.*
- Keep the client in semi-Fowler's position *to promote comfort.*
- Administer medications, as prescribed, *to improve GI function.*

Teaching topics

- Explanation of the disorder and treatment plan
- Medication use and possible adverse effects
- Eating small, frequent meals
- Avoiding carbonated beverages and alcohol
- Remaining upright for 2 hours after eating
- Avoiding constrictive clothing
- Avoiding lifting, bending, straining, and coughing
- Sleeping with upper body elevated to reduce gastric reflux

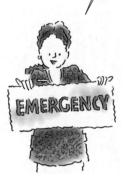

Complete intestinal blockage is life-threatening. It must be treated within hours.

Intestinal obstruction

An intestinal obstruction is the blockage of the intestinal lumen, causing gas, fluid, and digested substances to accumulate near the obstruction and increasing peristalsis in the area of the obstruction. Water and electrolytes are then secreted into the blocked bowel, causing inflammation and inhibiting absorption.

CAUSES

- Adhesions
- Diverticulitis
- Fecal impaction
- Hernia
- Inflammation (Crohn's disease)
- Intussusception
- Mesenteric thrombosis
- Paralytic ileus
- Tumors
- Volvulus

Withhold food and fluids from the client with intestinal obstruction.

ASSESSMENT FINDINGS

- Abdominal distention
- Constipation
- Cramping pain
- Diminished or absent bowel sounds
- Fever
- Nausea
- Vomiting fecal material
- Weight loss

DIAGNOSTIC TEST RESULTS

- Abdominal ultrasound shows distended bowel.
- Abdominal X-ray shows increased amount of gas in bowel.
- Abdominal CT scan shows obstruction.
- Blood chemistry shows decreased sodium and potassium levels.
- Hematologic study shows increased WBC count.

NURSING DIAGNOSES

- Ineffective tissue perfusion: GI
- Imbalanced nutrition: Less than body requirements
- Acute pain

TREATMENT

- Bowel resection with or without anastomosis if other treatment fails
- GI decompression using NG, Miller-Abbott, or Cantor tube
- Withholding food and fluids
- Fluid and electrolyte replacement

Drug therapy

- Analgesics: meperidine (Demerol), morphine
- Antibiotic: gentamicin

INTERVENTIONS AND RATIONALES

- Monitor GI status. Assess and record bowel sounds once per shift *to determine GI status.*
- Monitor and record vital signs, intake and output, and laboratory studies *to detect early signs of deficient fluid volume.*
- Withhold food and fluids *to prevent nausea and vomiting.*
- Monitor and record the frequency, color, and amount of stools *to assess and determine resolution of obstruction.*
- Measure and record the client's abdominal girth *to determine the presence of distention.*
- Administer I.V. fluids *to maintain hydration.*
- Maintain position, patency, and low intermittent suction of the NG or GI decompression tube *to prevent nausea and vomiting and resolve the obstruction, if possible.*

- Keep the client in semi-Fowler's position *to promote comfort*.
- Administer postoperative care if indicated (monitor vital signs and intake and output; monitor dressings for drainage; assess the wound for infection; assist with turning, coughing, and deep breathing; medicate for pain as necessary or guide the client in the use of postoperative PCA) *to promote healing and detect early postoperative complications*.
- Administer medications, as prescribed, *to maintain or improve the client's condition*.

Teaching topics
- Explanation of the disorder and treatment plan
- Medication use and possible adverse effects
- Avoiding constipation-causing foods
- Monitoring the frequency and color of stools
- Recognizing the signs and symptoms of diverticulitis
- Contacting the American Ostomy Association, if appropriate

Irritable bowel syndrome

Irritable bowel syndrome is marked by chronic symptoms of abdominal pain, alternating constipation and diarrhea, and abdominal distention. This disorder is extremely common; a substantial portion of clients, however, never seek medical attention.

This disorder may also be referred to as *spastic colon* or *spastic colitis*.

CAUSES
- Unknown

CONTRIBUTING FACTORS
- Diverticular disease
- Family history
- Irritants (caffeine, alcohol)
- Smoking
- Stress

ASSESSMENT FINDINGS
- Abdominal bloating
- Constipation, diarrhea, or both
- Dyspepsia
- Faintness
- Heartburn
- Lower abdominal pain
- Nausea
- Passage of mucus
- Pasty, pencil-like stools
- Weakness

DIAGNOSTIC TEST RESULTS
- Barium enema may reveal colonic spasm and tubular appearance of the descending colon. It also rules out other disorders, such as diverticula, tumors, and polyps.
- Manometry reveals changes in interluminal pressure.
- Sigmoidoscopy may disclose spastic contractions.
- Stool examination for occult blood, parasites, and pathogenic bacteria is negative.

NURSING DIAGNOSES
- Constipation
- Diarrhea
- Chronic pain

TREATMENT
- Dietary changes: avoidance of foods that trigger symptoms; increased fiber intake
- Increasing fluid intake to at least eight 8-oz glasses per day
- Stress management
- Heat application

Drug therapy
- Sedatives: alprazolam (Xanax), lorazepam (Ativan)
- Antiflatulent: simethicone
- Antispasmodic: propantheline
- Antidiarrheal: diphenoxylate with atropine

INTERVENTIONS AND RATIONALES
- Help the client deal with stress, and warn against dependence on sedatives or antispasmodics *because stress may be the underlying cause of irritable bowel syndrome*.
- Encourage regular checkups. For clients older than age 40, emphasize the need for a yearly flexible sigmoidoscopy and rectal examination. *Irritable bowel syndrome is*

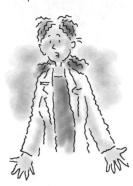

Want one good reason not to get stressed out about the exam? Stress contributes to the development of irritable bowel syndrome.

associated with a higher-than-normal incidence of diverticulitis and colon cancer.

• Provide nutritional counseling *to help the client adjust his diet.*

Teaching topics
• Explanation of the disorder and treatment plan
• Medication use and possible adverse effects
• Dietary modifications
• Avoiding alcohol
• Managing stress
• Smoking cessation (smoking can increase GI motility)

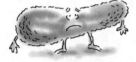

Treatment for pancreatitis includes a bland diet, bed rest, and I.V. fluids to replace fluids and electrolytes.

Pancreatitis

Pancreatitis is inflammation of the pancreas. In acute pancreatitis, pancreatic enzymes are activated in the pancreas rather than the duodenum, resulting in tissue damage and autodigestion of the pancreas.

In chronic pancreatitis, chronic inflammation results in fibrosis and calcification of the pancreas, obstruction of the ducts, and destruction of the secreting acinar cells.

CAUSES
• Alcoholism
• Bacterial or viral infection
• Biliary tract disease
• Blunt trauma to pancreas or abdomen
• Drug-induced: steroids, thiazide diuretics, hormonal contraceptives
• Duodenal ulcer
• Hyperlipidemia
• Hyperparathyroidism

Keep the client with pancreatitis in bed and turn him frequently to prevent pressure ulcers.

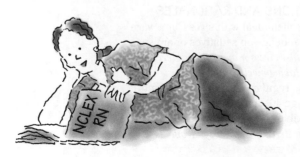

ASSESSMENT FINDINGS
• Abdominal tenderness and distention
• Abrupt onset of severe pain in epigastric area that radiates to the shoulder, substernal area, back, and flank
• Aching, burning, stabbing, or pressing pain
• Decreased or absent bowel sounds
• Dyspnea
• Fever
• Hypotension
• Jaundice
• Nausea and vomiting
• Pain upon eating
• Knee-chest position, fetal position, or leaning forward for comfort
• Steatorrhea
• Tachycardia
• Weight loss

DIAGNOSTIC TEST RESULTS
• Arteriography reveals fibrous tissue and calcification of pancreas.
• Blood chemistry analysis shows increased amylase, lipase.
• Elevated LD, glucose, AST, and lipid levels and decreased calcium and potassium levels.
• CT scan shows enlarged pancreas.
• Cullen's sign is positive.
• ERCP reveals biliary obstruction.
• Fecal fat test is positive.
• Glucose tolerance test shows decreased tolerance.
• Grey Turner's sign is positive.
• Abdominal CT scan reveals an enlarged pancreas.
• Hematology shows increased WBC count and decreased levels of Hb and HCT.
• Ultrasonography reveals cysts, bile duct inflammation, and dilation.
• Urine chemistry shows increased amylase.

NURSING DIAGNOSES
• Deficient fluid volume
• Imbalanced nutrition: Less than body requirements
• Acute or chronic pain
• Ineffective breathing pattern

TREATMENT
- Bland, low-fat, high-protein diet of small, frequent meals with restricted intake of caffeine, alcohol, and gas-forming foods; as disease progresses, nothing by mouth
- Bed rest
- I.V. fluids (vigorous replacement of fluids and electrolytes)
- NG suction to relieve nausea and vomiting and provide decompression
- Sequential compression device to prevent blood clot formation
- Surgical intervention to treat underlying cause if appropriate
- Transfusion therapy with packed RBCs

Drug therapy
- Analgesic: meperidine (Demerol) (morphine contraindicated)
- Anticholinergics: propantheline, dicyclomine (Bentyl)
- Antidiabetic: insulin (possible infusion to stabilize blood glucose levels)
- Antiemetic: prochlorperazine
- Calcium supplement: calcium gluconate
- Corticosteroid: hydrocortisone
- Digestant: pancrelipase (Pancrease)
- H_2-receptor antagonists: cimetidine (Tagamet), ranitidine (Zantac), famotidine (Pepcid), nizatidine (Axid)
- Cytoprotective agent: sucralfate (Carafate)
- Potassium supplement: I.V. potassium chloride
- Sedatives: lorazepam (Ativan), alprazolam (Xanax)

INTERVENTIONS AND RATIONALES
- Monitor abdominal, cardiac, and respiratory status (as the disease progresses, watch for respiratory failure, tachycardia, and worsening GI status) *to determine baseline and detect early changes and signs of complications.*
- Assess fluid balance and monitor intake and output *to detect excess or deficient fluid volume.*
- Monitor and record vital signs, laboratory studies, central venous pressure (CVP), daily weight, and urine specific gravity *to detect signs of worsening condition.*
- Monitor urine and stools for color, character, and amount *to detect bleeding.*

- Withhold food and fluids *to rest the pancreas and prevent nausea and vomiting.*
- Perform bedside glucose monitoring *to assess for hyperglycemia.*
- Administer oxygen and maintain ET and mechanical ventilation, if necessary, *to improve oxygenation* and provide suctioning, as needed, *to stabilize secretions.*
- Administer I.V. fluids *to treat or prevent hypovolemic shock and restore electrolyte balance.*
- Maintain position, patency, and low suction of the NG tube *to prevent nausea and vomiting.*
- Keep the client in semi-Fowler's position, if the client's blood pressure allows, *to promote comfort and lung expansion.*
- Administer TPN. *TPN is necessary to meet the client's metabolic needs. In severe cases, reintroduction of food may be associated with pancreatic abscess.*
- Keep the client in bed and reposition every 2 hours *to prevent pressure ulcers.*
- Administer medications, as prescribed, *to improve or maintain the client's condition.*
- Provide skin, nares, and mouth care *to prevent tissue damage.*
- Provide a quiet, restful environment *to conserve energy and decrease metabolic demands.*

Teaching topics
- Explanation of the disorder and treatment plan
- Medication use and possible adverse effects
- Avoiding alcohol
- Monitoring blood glucose levels frequently
- Monitoring stools for steatorrhea
- Recognizing the signs and symptoms of infection
- Recognizing the signs and symptoms of increased blood glucose levels
- Adhering to activity limitations
- Modifying risk factors

Peptic ulcer

Peptic ulcers are breaks in the continuity of the esophageal, gastric, or duodenal mucosa. They may occur in any part of the GI tract that comes in contact with gastric substances, hydrochloric acid, and pepsin. The ulcers may be found in the esophagus, stomach, duodenum, or (after gastroenterostomy) jejunum.

CAUSES
- Alcohol abuse
- Drug-induced: salicylates, steroids, NSAIDs, reserpine
- Gastritis
- *H. pylori* infection
- Smoking
- Stress
- Zollinger-Ellison syndrome

ASSESSMENT FINDINGS
- Anorexia
- Hematemesis
- Left epigastric pain 1 to 2 hours after eating
- Melena
- Nausea and vomiting
- Relief of pain after administration of antacids
- Weight loss

DIAGNOSTIC TEST RESULTS
- Barium swallow shows ulceration of the gastric mucosa.
- Fecal occult blood test is positive.
- Gastric analysis is normal.
- *H. pylori* test detects *H. pylori* antibodies.
- Hematologic study shows decreased levels of Hb and HCT (if bleeding is present).
- Serum gastrin level is normal or increased.
- Endoscopy shows the location of the ulcer.

NURSING DIAGNOSES
- Anxiety
- Imbalanced nutrition: Less than body requirements
- Acute pain
- Risk for deficient fluid volume

TREATMENT
- Endoscopy therapy for bleeding peptic ulcer
- If severe GI hemorrhage, gastric surgery that may include gastroduodenostomy, gastrojejunostomy, partial gastric resection, and total gastrectomy
- Diet that avoids extremes in temperature, caffeine, and foods that cause pain (acidic or spicy)
- Photocoagulation to control bleeding

- Saline lavage by NG tube until clear return (if bleeding present)
- Transfusion therapy with packed RBCs (if bleeding is present and levels of Hb and HCT are low)
- Avoiding tobacco and alcohol

Drug therapy
- Antacids: magnesium and aluminum hydroxide (Maalox), aluminum hydroxide gel
- Antibiotics (if *H. pylori* is present): amoxicillen (Amoxil), metronidazole (Flagyl)
- Anticholinergics: propantheline, dicyclomine (Bentyl)
- Combination treatment (if *H. pylori* is present): two antibiotics with acid suppressor or cytoprotective agent (Prevpac, Helidac)
- H_2-receptor antagonists: cimetidine (Tagamet), ranitidine (Zantac), nizatidine (Axid), famotidine (Pepcid)
- Vasoconstrictor: vasopressin to manage bleeding
- Proton pump inhibitor: omeprazole (Prilosec), esomeprazole (Nexium)
- Cytoprotective agents: sucralfate, bismuth subsalicylate (Pepto-Bismol)
- Prostaglandin: misoprostol (Cytotec) to protect the stomach lining

INTERVENTIONS AND RATIONALES
- Assess GI status *to monitor for signs of bleeding.*
- Assess cardiovascular status *to detect early signs of GI hemorrhage.*
- Monitor and record vital signs, intake and output, laboratory studies, fecal occult blood studies, and gastric pH *to detect signs of bleeding.*
- Monitor the consistency, color, amount, and frequency of stools *to detect early signs of GI bleeding.*
- Maintain the client's diet, as tolerated, *to meet metabolic needs and promote healing.*
- Maintain the position, patency, and low suction of the NG tube if gastric decompression is ordered, *to prevent nausea and vomiting.*
- Administer medications, as prescribed, *to maintain or improve the client's condition.*
- Provide nose and mouth care *to maintain tissue integrity.*

• Provide postoperative care if necessary (don't reposition the NG tube; irrigate it gently if ordered; medicate for pain as needed and ordered; monitor dressings for drainage; assess bowel sounds; get client out of bed as tolerated) *to detect early complications and promote healing.*
• Recommend dietary changes *to avoid acidic or spicy foods and caffeine.*
• Advise client to avoid tobacco and alcohol.

Teaching topics
• Explanation of the disorder and treatment plan
• Medication use and possible adverse effects
• Reducing stress
• Performing relaxation techniques
• Following dietary recommendations and restrictions such as avoiding caffeine, alcohol, and spicy and fried foods
• Following postoperative care and restrictions
• Smoking cessation

Peritonitis

Peritonitis is inflammation of the peritoneal cavity. It occurs when irritants in the perito-neal area cause inflammatory edema, vascular congestion, and hypermotility of the bowel.

CAUSES
• Bacterial invasion
• Chemical invasion
• Trauma

ASSESSMENT FINDINGS
• Abdominal resonance and tympany on percussion
• Abdominal rigidity and distention
• Anorexia
• Constant, diffuse, and intense abdominal pain
• Decreased or absent bowel sounds
• Decreased peristalsis
• Decreased urine output
• Fever
• Malaise
• Nausea
• Point tenderness
• Shallow respirations
• Weak, rapid pulse

DIAGNOSTIC TEST RESULTS
• WBC count is elevated.
• Abdominal X-ray may show free air in the abdomen under the diaphragm.
• Hematologic study shows increased WBC count and low Hb level and HCT if blood loss has occurred.
• Peritoneal aspiration is positive for blood, pus, bile, bacteria, or amylase.
• CT of abdomen may detect abdominal fluid and areas of inflammation.

NURSING DIAGNOSES
• Anxiety
• Acute pain
• Deficient fluid volume

TREATMENT
• Withholding food or fluid
• Surgical intervention when the client's condition stabilized to treat the cause (For example, if the client has a perforated appendix, appendectomy is indicated.); drains placed for drainage of infected material

Drug therapy
• Analgesic: meperidine (Demerol)
• Antibiotics: gentamicin, clindamycin (Cleocin), ofloxacin, meropenem (Merrem)
• Antipyretic: acetaminophen (Tylenol)

INTERVENTIONS AND RATIONALES
• Assess abdominal and respiratory status and fluid balance *to detect and assess signs of deficient fluid volume.*
• Monitor and record vital signs and temper-ature, intake and output, laboratory studies, CVP, daily weight, and urine specific gravity *to detect signs of deficient fluid volume.*
• Assess pain level and provide analgesics *to promote comfort.*
• Measure and record the client's abdominal girth *to assess for abdominal distention.*
• Withhold food and fluids *to prevent nausea and vomiting.*
• Administer I.V. fluids *to maintain hydration and electrolyte balance.*
• Provide routine postoperative care (monitor vital signs and intake and output, including drainage from drains; assist with turning, incentive spirometry, coughing, and

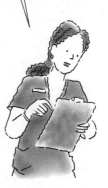

Withhold food and fluids from the client with acute peritonitis. Provide TPN.

deep breathing; and get the client out of bed on the first postoperative day, if his condition allows) *to promote healing and prevent and detect early complications.*
• Maintain position, patency, and low suction of the NG tube *to prevent nausea and vomiting.*
• Keep the client in semi-Fowler's position *to promote comfort and prevent pulmonary complications.*
• Administer TPN *to meet the client's metabolic needs.*
• Administer medications, as prescribed, *to treat infection and control pain.*

Teaching topics
• Explanation of the disorder and treatment plan
• Medication use and possible adverse effects
• Recognizing the signs and symptoms of infection
• Recognizing the signs and symptoms of GI obstruction
• Performing ostomy self-care if indicated

Ulcerative colitis

Ulcerative colitis causes damage to the large intestine's mucosal and submucosal layers.

Ulcerative colitis is an inflammatory disorder of the colon. It's typically a chronic condition and causes damage to the large intestine's mucosal and submucosal layers.

CAUSES
• Genetics
• Idiopathic cause
• Allergies
• Autoimmune disease
• Viral and bacterial infections

ASSESSMENT FINDINGS
• Dehydration
• Nausea and vomiting
• Abdominal cramping
• Abdominal distention
• Abdominal tenderness
• Anorexia
• Bloody, purulent, mucoid, watery stools (15 to 20 per day)
• Cachexia
• Debilitation
• Fever
• Hyperactive bowel sounds
• Weakness
• Weight loss

DIAGNOSTIC TEST RESULTS
• Barium enema shows ulcerations.
• Blood chemistry shows decreased potassium level and increased osmolality.
• Hematology shows increased WBC count and decreased Hb level and HCT.
• Sigmoidoscopy shows ulceration and hyperemia.
• Stool specimen is positive for blood and mucus.
• Urine chemistry displays increased urine specific gravity.

NURSING DIAGNOSES
• Diarrhea
• Deficient fluid volume
• Imbalanced nutrition: Less than body requirements
• Chronic pain

TREATMENT
• Colectomy or pouch ileostomy
• High-protein, high-calorie, low-residue diet, with bland foods in small, frequent meals and restricted intake of milk and gas-forming foods or no food or fluids
• TPN, if necessary, to rest the GI tract
• Transfusion therapy with packed RBCs

Drug therapy
• Analgesic: meperidine (Demerol)
• Antianemics: ferrous sulfate (Feosol), ferrous gluconate (Fergon)
• Anticholinergics: propantheline, dicyclomine (Bentyl)
• Antidiarrheals: diphenoxylate with atropine, loperamide (Imodium)
• Antiemetic: prochlorperazine
• Anti-inflammatory agents: 5-ASA compounds such as sulfasalazine, hydrocortisone
• Immunomodulators: azathioprine (Imuran), methotrexate (Trexall)
• Potassium supplements: potassium chloride (K-Lor), potassium gluconate (Kaon)
• Sedative: lorazepam (Ativan)

INTERVENTIONS AND RATIONALES

- Assess GI status and fluid balance *to determine deficient fluid volume.*
- Monitor and record vital signs, intake and output, laboratory studies, daily weight, urine specific gravity, calorie count, and fecal occult blood studies *to determine deficient fluid volume.*
- Assess pain level and provide analgesics *to promote comfort.*
- Monitor the number, amount, and character of stools *to determine status of nutrient absorption.*
- Maintain the client's diet; withhold food and fluids as necessary *to prevent nausea and vomiting.*
- Administer I.V. fluids and TPN *to maintain hydration and improve nutritional status.*
- Maintain the position, patency, and low suction of the NG tube *to prevent nausea and vomiting.*
- Keep the client in semi-Fowler's position *to promote comfort.*
- Administer medications, as prescribed, *to maintain or improve the client's condition.*
- Provide skin, mouth, nares, and perianal care *to promote comfort and prevent skin breakdown.*

Teaching topics

- Explanation of the disorder and treatment plan
- Medication use and possible adverse effects
- Monitoring weight
- Reducing stress and performing relaxation techniques
- Recognizing the early signs and symptoms of rectal hemorrhage and intestinal obstruction
- Contacting the United Ostomy Association and the National Foundation of Ileitis and Colitis

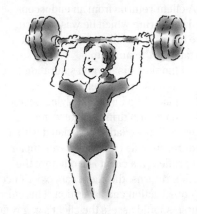

Pump up on practice questions

Feeling full of information on GI disorders? Take this practice test.

1. A nurse is caring for a client with a hiatal hernia. The client complains of abdominal pain and sternal pain after eating. The pain makes it difficult for him to sleep. Which instructions should the nurse recommend when teaching this client? Select all that apply.

1. Avoid constrictive clothing.
2. Lie down for 30 minutes after eating.
3. Decrease intake of caffeine and spicy foods.
4. Eat three meals per day.
5. Sleep in semi-Fowler's position.
6. Maintain a normal body weight.

Answer: 1, 3, 5, 6. To reduce gastric reflux, the nurse should instruct the client to avoid constrictive clothing, caffeine, and spicy foods; sleep with his upper body elevated; lose weight, if obese; remain upright for 2 hours after eating; and eat small, frequent meals.

➨ NCLEX keys

Client needs category: Physiological integrity
Client needs subcategory: Basic care and comfort
Cognitive level: Application

2. A client returns from an endoscopic procedure during which he was sedated. Before offering the client food, it's most important for the nurse to:

　　1.　monitor his oxygen saturation levels.
　　2.　assess his gag reflex.
　　3.　place him in the side-lying position.
　　4.　have him drink sips of water.

Answer: 2. The sedation associated with a procedure, such as endoscopy, can impair the gag reflex. If a client is fed before the gag reflex returns, the client can experience airway obstruction and aspiration. Therefore, the nurse should assess the client's gag reflex before offering the client food. Monitoring hemoglobin saturation levels is important after an endoscopic procedure but its results won't support feeding the client. In this situation, the side-lying position isn't necessary. Having the client drink water isn't the proper method of assessing for a gag reflex.

➡ *NCLEX keys*

Client needs category: Physiological integrity
Client needs subcategory: Reduction of risk potential
Cognitive level: Application

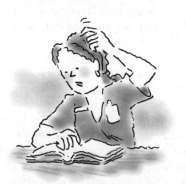

3. A client with a history of hiatal hernia reports to the nurse that he has trouble sleeping because of abdominal pain. It would be most beneficial to the client if the nurse instructed him to sleep:

　　1.　with his upper body elevated.
　　2.　in the prone position.
　　3.　flat or in a side-lying position.
　　4.　with his lower body slightly elevated.

Answer: 1. Upper body elevation can reduce the gastric reflux associated with hiatal hernia. Lying prone, flat, on the side, or with the lower body slightly elevated won't benefit the client.

➡ *NCLEX keys*

Client needs category: Physiological integrity
Client needs subcategory: Basic care and comfort
Cognitive level: Analysis

4. A client with peptic ulcer disease secondary to chronic nonsteroidal anti-inflammatory drug (NSAID) use is prescribed misoprostol (Cytotec). The nurse would be most accurate in informing the client that the drug:

　　1.　reduces gas formation.
　　2.　increases the speed of gastric emptying.
　　3.　protects the stomach's lining.
　　4.　increases lower esophageal sphincter pressure.

Answer: 3. Misoprostol is a synthetic prostaglandin that, like prostaglandin, protects the gastric mucosa. NSAIDs decrease prostaglandin production and predispose the client to peptic ulceration. Cytotec is prescribed to clients with peptic ulcer disease who are also taking NSAIDs. Misoprostol doesn't reduce gas formation, improve emptying of the stomach, or increase lower esophageal sphincter pressure.

➡ *NCLEX keys*

Client needs category: Physiological integrity
Client needs subcategory: Pharmacological and parenteral therapies
Cognitive level: Application

5. A nurse is reviewing the diagnostic data of a client suspected of having gastric cancer. What laboratory finding is the nurse most likely to find?

　　1.　Elevated levels of hemoglobin and hematocrit
　　2.　Negative fecal occult blood test
　　3.　Subnormal gastric hydrochloric acid level
　　4.　Negative carcinoembryonic antigen (CEA) test

Answer: 3. One manifestation of gastric cancer is achlorhydria, an absence of free hydrochloric acid in the stomach. In gastric cancer, a subnormal hemoglobin level and hematocrit is most likely; fecal occult blood test is most likely to be positive. The CEA test would most likely be positive in gastric cancer.

➡ *NCLEX keys*

Client needs category: Health promotion and maintenance
Client needs subcategory: None
Cognitive level: Analysis

6. A physician orders gastric decompression for a client with small bowel obstruction. The nurse should plan for the suction to be:
   1. low pressure and intermittent.
   2. low pressure and continuous.
   3. high pressure and intermittent.
   4. high pressure and continuous.

Answer: 1. Gastric decompression is typically low pressure and intermittent. High pressure and continuous gastric suctioning predisposes the gastric mucosa to injury and ulceration.

➡ *NCLEX keys*

Client needs category: Physiological integrity
Client needs subcategory: Reduction of risk potential
Cognitive level: Application

7. A client with Crohn's disease has a serum potassium level of 3.1 mEq/dl. The client is prescribed 30 mEq of oral potassium chloride (K-lor) twice daily. The nurse should plan to give the supplement:
   1. with food or after the client eats.
   2. on an empty stomach.
   3. along with no other medications.
   4. 2 hours before or after eating.

Answer: 1. Supplemental potassium can be irritating to the esophagus and stomach and is best tolerated with or shortly after meals. It's typically appropriate to give oral potassium at the same time other medications are being administered.

➡ *NCLEX keys*

Client needs category: Physiological integrity
Client needs subcategory: Pharmacological and parenteral therapies
Cognitive level: Application

8. A nurse is evaluating the effectiveness of dietary instructions in a client with diverticulitis. Regular consumption of which food would indicate that the client hasn't understood the instructions?
   1. Fiber
   2. Bananas
   3. Cucumbers
   4. Milk products

Answer: 3. In diverticulitis, vegetables with seeds are prohibited in the diet because the seeds can lodge in diverticula and cause flare-ups. Fiber and residue are recommended in the diet. Bananas and milk products aren't contraindicated.

➡ *NCLEX keys*

Client needs category: Physiological integrity
Client needs subcategory: Reduction of risk potential
Cognitive level: Analysis

9. A client with a history of peptic ulcer disease develops a fever of 101° F (38.3° C). Which accompanying sign most strongly indicates the client has peritonitis?
   1. Leukopenia
   2. Hyperactive bowel sounds
   3. Abdominal rigidity
   4. Polyuria

Answer: 3. Abdominal rigidity is a classic sign of peritonitis. The client would more

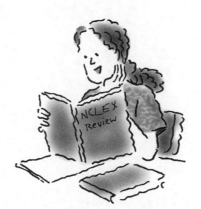

likely have leukocytosis, hypoactive bowel sounds, and decreased urine output.

➡ *NCLEX keys*
Client needs category: Physiological integrity
Client needs subcategory: Reduction of risk potential
Cognitive level: Analysis

10.   Daily abdominal girth measurements are prescribed for a client with liver dysfunction and ascites. To increase accuracy, the nurse should use which landmark?
   1.   Xiphoid process
   2.   Umbilicus
   3.   Iliac crest
   4.   Symphysis pubis
Answer: 2. The proper technique for abdominal girth measurement involves circumventing the abdomen with a tape measure using the umbilicus as a landmark. Using the xiphoid process, iliac crest, or symphysis pubis would give inaccurate measurements.

➡ *NCLEX keys*
Client needs category: Physiological integrity
Client needs subcategory: Reduction of risk potential
Cognitive level: Application

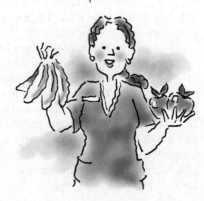

All that talk about the GI system makes me hungry. Remember that healthy eating promotes good studying.

9 Endocrine system

Brush up on key concepts

The endocrine system consists of chemical transmitters called hormones and specialized cell clusters called glands.

At any time, you can review the major points of this chapter by consulting the *Cheat sheet* on pages 284 to 288.

Thermostat central

The **hypothalamus** controls temperature, respiration, blood pressure, thirst, hunger, and water balance. Its functions affect the emotional states. The hypothalamus also produces hypothalamic-stimulating hormones, which affect the inhibition and release of pituitary hormones.

Heavy on the hormones

The **pituitary gland** is composed of anterior and posterior lobes. Together these lobes produce various hormones that affect the body.

The anterior lobe secretes:
• **follicle-stimulating hormone,** which stimulates graafian follicle growth and estrogen secretion in women and sperm maturation in men
• **luteinizing hormone,** which induces ovulation and the development of the corpus luteum in women and stimulates testosterone secretion in men
• **adrenocorticotropic hormone (ACTH),** also called corticotropin, which stimulates secretion of hormones from the adrenal cortex
• **thyroid-stimulating hormone (TSH),** which regulates the secretory activity of the thyroid gland
• **growth hormone (GH),** which is an insulin antagonist that stimulates the growth of cells, bones, muscle, and soft tissue.

The posterior lobe secretes:
• **vasopressin** (antidiuretic hormone, also called ADH), which helps the body retain water
• **oxytocin,** which stimulates uterine contractions during labor and milk secretion in lactating women.

Growth gland

The **thyroid gland** accelerates growth and cellular reactions, including basal metabolic rate (BMR). It's controlled by the pituitary gland's secretion of TSH.

The thyroid gland produces thyrocalcitonin, triiodothyronine (T_3), and thyroxine (T_4), which are necessary for growth and development.

Coping with calcium

The **parathyroid gland** secretes parathyroid hormone (parathormone), which regulates calcium and phosphorus levels and promotes the resorption of calcium from bones.

Androgen, estrogen, and others

The **adrenal glands** are composed of the adrenal cortex and the adrenal medulla. The adrenal cortex secretes three major hormones:
• **glucocorticoids** (cortisol, cortisone, and corticosterone), which mediate the stress response, promote sodium and water retention and potassium secretion, and suppress ACTH secretion
• **mineralocorticoids** (aldosterone and deoxycorticosterone), which promote sodium and water retention and potassium secretion
• **sex hormones** (androgens, estrogens, and progesterone), which develop and maintain secondary sex characteristics and libido.

The adrenal medulla secretes two hormones:
• **norepinephrine,** which regulates generalized vasoconstriction

(Text continues on page 288.)

Cheat sheet

Endocrine refresher

ACROMEGALY AND GIGANTISM

Key signs and symptoms
Acromegaly
- Enlarged supraorbital ridge
- Thickened ears and nose
- Paranasal sinus enlargement
- Thickening of the tongue

Gigantism
- Abrupt excessive growth in all parts of the body

Key test results
- Plasma human growth hormone (hGH) levels measured by radioimmunoassay typically are elevated. However, because hGH secretion is pulsatile, the results of random sampling may be misleading. Insulin-like growth factor-I (somatomedin-C) levels offer a better screening alternative.

Key treatments
- Surgery to remove the affecting tumor (transsphenoidal hypophysectomy)
- Thyroid hormone replacement therapy after surgery: levothyroxine (Synthroid)
- Corticosteroid: cortisone
- Dopamine agonist: bromocriptine (Parlodel)
- Somatotropic hormone: octreotide (Sandostatin)

Key interventions
- Provide emotional support.
- Perform or assist with range-of-motion exercises.
- Be aware of inexplicable mood changes. Reassure the family that these mood changes result from the disease and can be modified with treatment.
- After surgery, monitor vital signs and neurologic status.
- Monitor blood glucose levels.
- Monitor intake and output hourly, watching for large increases.
- Encourage the client to ambulate on the first or second day after surgery.

ADDISON'S DISEASE

Key signs and symptoms
- Hypoglycemia
- Orthostatic hypotension
- Weakness and lethargy
- Weight loss

Key test results
- Blood chemistry analysis reveals decreased hematocrit; decreased hemoglobin, cortisol, glucose, sodium, chloride, and aldosterone levels; and increased blood urea nitrogen and potassium levels.
- Fasting blood glucose analysis reveals hypoglycemia.
- Urine chemistry test shows decreased 17-ketosteroids (17-KS) and 17-hydroxycorticosteroids (17-OHCS).
- Adrenocorticotropic hormone (ACTH) (Cortrosyn) stimulation test reveals decreased cortisol response.

Key treatments
- In adrenal crisis, I.V. hydrocortisone given promptly along with 3 to 5 L of saline solution
- Glucocorticoids: cortisone, hydrocortisone
- Mineralocorticoid: fludrocortisone
- Dextrose, 50%, to treat hypoglycemia

Key interventions
- Be prepared to administer I.V. hydrocortisone and saline solution promptly if the client is in adrenal crisis.
- Administer I.V. fluids.
- Instruct the client to avoid sitting or standing.
- Monitor glucose levels.
- Weigh the client daily.

CUSHING'S SYNDROME

Key signs and symptoms
- Amenorrhea
- Hypertension
- Mood swings
- Muscle wasting
- Weight gain, especially truncal obesity, buffalo hump, and moonface

Key test results
- Blood chemistry analysis shows increased cortisol, aldosterone, sodium, corticotropin, and glucose levels and a decreased potassium level.
- Dexamethasone suppression test shows no decrease in 17-OHCS.

Only have time for a quick review? Check out the Cheat sheet.

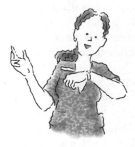

Endocrine refresher (continued)

CUSHING'S SYNDROME (CONTINUED)
- Magnetic resonance imaging shows pituitary or adrenal tumors.
- Urine chemistry shows increased 17-OHCS and 17-KS, decreased urine specific gravity, and glycosuria.

Key treatments
- Hypophysectomy or bilateral adrenalectomy
- Adrenal suppressants: metyrapone (Metopirone), ketoconazole (Nizoral), etomidate (Amidate)
- Antidiabetic agents: insulin or oral antidiabetic agents, such as chlorpropamide (Diabinese), glyburide (DiaBeta, Micronase), glipizide (Glucotrol), rosiglitazone (Avandia)

Key interventions
- Perform postoperative care.
- Assess for edema.
- Limit water intake.
- Weigh the client daily.

DIABETES INSIPIDUS
Key signs and symptoms
- Polydipsia (excessive thirst, consumption of 4 to 40 L/day)
- Polyuria (greater than 5 L/day)

Key test results
- Urine chemistry analysis shows urine specific gravity less than 1.004, osmolality 50 to 200 mOsm/kg, decreased urine pH, and decreased sodium and potassium levels.

Key treatments
- I.V. therapy: hydration (when first diagnosed, intake and output must be matched milliliter to milliliter to prevent dehydration), electrolyte replacement
- Antidiuretic hormone replacement: vasopressin

Key interventions
- Assess fluid balance.
- Monitor and record vital signs, intake and output (urine output should be measured every hour when first diagnosed), urine specific gravity (check every 1 to 2 hours when first diagnosed), and laboratory studies.
- Administer I.V. fluids.

DIABETES MELLITUS
Key signs and symptoms
- Polydipsia
- Polyphagia
- Polyuria
- Weight loss

Key test results
- Blood chemistry analysis shows increased glucose, potassium, chloride, ketone, cholesterol, and triglyceride levels; decreased carbon dioxide level, and pH less than 7.4.
- Fasting blood glucose level is increased (greater than or equal to 126 mg/dl).
- Two-hour postprandial blood glucose level shows hyperglycemia (greater than 200 mg/dl).

Key treatments
- Antidiabetic agents: insulins and oral agents, such as chlorpropamide (Diabinese), glyburide (DiaBeta, Micronase), glipizide (Glucotrol), rosiglitazone (Avandia), ritagliptin (Januvia), piaglitazone (Actose), metformin (Glucophage), exenatide (Byetta)

Key interventions
- Assess acid-base and fluid balance.
- Monitor for signs of hypoglycemia (vagueness, slow cerebration, dizziness, weakness, pallor, tachycardia, diaphoresis, seizures, and coma), ketoacidosis (acetone breath, dehydration, weak or rapid pulse, Kussmaul's respirations), and hyperosmolar coma (polyuria, thirst, neurologic abnormalities, stupor).
- Treat hypoglycemia; immediately give carbohydrates in the form of fruit juice, hard candy, or honey. If the client is unconscious, administer glucagon or dextrose I.V.
- Administer I.V. fluids, insulin and, usually, potassium replacement for ketoacidosis or hyperosmolar coma.
- Monitor wound healing.
- Maintain the client's diet.
- Provide meticulous skin and foot care. Clients with diabetes are at increased risk for infection from impaired leukocyte activity.
- Foster independence.

GOITER
Key signs and symptoms
- Single or multinodular, firm, irregular enlargement of the thyroid gland
- Dizziness or syncope with distended head and jugular veins and dyspnea when the client raises his arms above his head (Pemberton's sign)
- Dysphagia
- Dyspnea

Key test results
- Laboratory tests reveal high or normal thyroid-stimulating hormone (TSH) levels, low serum thyroxine (T_4) concentrations, and increased iodine 131 uptake.
- Ultrasound of thyroid reveals nodules.

(continued)

Endocrine refresher *(continued)*

GOITER *(CONTINUED)*
Key treatments
- Subtotal thyroidectomy
- Thyroid hormone replacement: levothyroxine (Synthroid)

Key interventions
- Measure the client's neck circumference. Also check for the development of hard nodules in the gland.
- Provide preoperative teaching and postoperative care, if subtotal thyroidectomy is indicated.
- Administer iodine supplements.

HYPERTHYROIDISM
Key signs and symptoms
- Atrial fibrillation
- Bruit or thrill over thyroid
- Diaphoresis
- Palpitations
- Tachycardia

Key test results
- Blood chemistry analysis shows increased triiodothyronine (T_3), T_4, and free thyroxine levels and decreased TSH and cholesterol levels.
- Radioactive iodine uptake (RAIU) is increased.

Key treatments
- Radiation therapy
- Thyroidectomy
- Iodine preparations: potassium iodide (SSKI), radioactive iodine

Key interventions
- Monitor cardiovascular status.
- Instruct the client to avoid stimulants, such as caffeine-containing drugs and foods.
- Administer I.V. fluids.
- Provide postoperative nursing care.

HYPOTHYROIDISM
Key signs and symptoms
- Dry, flaky skin and thinning nails
- Fatigue
- Hypothermia
- Menstrual disorders
- Mental sluggishness
- Weight gain or anorexia

Key test results
- Blood chemistry analysis shows decreased T_3, T_4, free thyroxine, and sodium levels and increased TSH and cholesterol levels.
- RAIU is decreased.

Key treatments
- Thyroid hormone replacement: levothyroxine (Synthroid), liothyronine (Cytomel)

Key interventions
- Avoid sedation; administer one-half to one-third the normal dose of sedatives or opiods. Clients taking warfarin (Coumadin) with levothyroxine may require lower doses of warfarin.
- Check for constipation and edema.
- Encourage fluid intake.

METABOLIC SYNDROME
Key signs and symptoms
- Abdominal obesity (waist of greater than 40" in males, 35" in females)
- Blood pressure greater than 130/85 mm Hg
- Fasting blood glucose level greater than 100 mg/dl

Key test results
- Most diagnostic procedures are nonspecific, but may show hypertension, diabetes, hyperlipidemia, and hyperinsulinemia.

Key treatments
- Lifestyle modifications, focusing on weight reduction and exercise
- Medications for weight loss: orlistat (Xenical), sibutramine (Meridia)
- Antilipemics: simvastatin (Zocor), pravastatin (Pravachol)
- Gastric bypass for appropriate candidates

Key interventions
- Monitor the client's blood pressure, blood glucose, blood cholesterol, and insulin levels.
- Encourage lifestyle modifications related to improving diet and increasing exercise.
- Schedule follow-up appointments with health care professionals.

PANCREATIC CANCER
Key signs and symptoms
- Dull, intermittent epigastric pain (early in disease)
- Continuous pain that radiates to the right upper quadrant or dorsolumbar area; may be colicky, dull, or vague and unrelated to activity or posture
- Anorexia
- Rapid, profound weight loss
- Palpable mass in the subumbilical or left hypochondrial region

Key test results
- Percutaneous fine-needle aspiration biopsy of the pancreas may detect tumor cells.

Endocrine refresher (continued)

PANCREATIC CANCER (CONTINUED)

- Ultrasound or computed tomography scan identifies pancreatic mass.
- Blood studies reveal increased serum bilirubin levels, increased serum amylase and lipase levels, prolonged prothrombin time, elevated alkaline phosphatase (with biliary obstruction) levels, and elevated aspartate aminotransferase and alanine aminotransferase levels (when liver cell necrosis is present).
- Fasting blood glucose studies may indicate hyperglycemia or hypoglycemia.

Key treatments

- Blood transfusion
- I.V. fluid therapy
- Whipple's operation or pancreatoduodenectomy (excision of the head of the pancreas along with the encircling loop of the duodenum)
- Antineoplastic combinations: fluorouracil, streptozocin (Zanosar), ifosfamide (Ifex), and doxorubicin; gemcitabine and erlitinib (Tarceva)
- Insulin after pancreatic resection to provide adequate exogenous insulin supply
- Opioid analgesics: morphine, meperidine (Demerol), and codeine, which can lead to biliary tract spasm and increase common bile duct pressure (used only when other methods fail)
- Pancreatic enzyme: pancrelipase (Pancrease)

Key interventions

- Monitor fluid balance, abdominal girth, metabolic state, and weight daily.
- Replace nutrients I.V., orally, or by nasogastric tube. Impose dietary restrictions, such as a low-sodium or fluid retention diet as required. Maintain a 2,500 calorie diet for the client.
- Administer pain medication, antibiotics, and antipyretics, as necessary.
- Monitor for signs of hypoglycemia or hyperglycemia; administer glucose or an antidiabetic agent as necessary. Monitor blood glucose levels.
- Provide emotional support.

Before surgery
- Give blood transfusions, vitamin K , antibiotics, and gastric lavage, as necessary.

After surgery
- Administer an oral pancreatic enzyme at mealtimes, if needed.

PHEOCHROMOCYTOMA

Key signs and symptoms

- Abdominal pain
- Feeling of impending doom
- Headache
- Nausea
- Persistent or paroxysmal hypertension
- Tachycardia

Key test results

- A 24-hour urine specimen shows increased urinary excretion of total free catecholamine and their metabolites, vanillylmandelic acid, and metanephrine.

Key treatments

- Surgical removal or tumor
- Alpha-adrenergic blocker before surgery
- I.V. fluids, plasma volume expanders, and blood transfusions postoperatively
- I.V. phentolamine or nitroprusside (acute hypertensive crisis)

Key interventions

- Carefully monitor the client's blood pressure and vital signs.
- Instruct the client to avoid food high in vanillin (coffee, nuts, chocolate) for 2 days before 24-urine test.
- Provide a quiet room after surgery to decrease excitement, which can trigger a hypertensive crisis.
- If autosomal dominant transmission of pheochromocytoma is suspected, inform the client's family of the need for evaluation.

THYROID CANCER

Key signs and symptoms

- Dyspnea
- Enlarged thyroid gland
- Hoarseness
- Painless, firm, irregular, and enlarged thyroid nodule or mass

Key test results

- Blood chemistry analysis shows increased calcitonin, serotonin, and prostaglandin levels.
- RAIU shows a "cold," or nonfunctioning, nodule.
- Thyroid biopsy shows cytology positive for cancer cells.

Key treatments

- Radiation therapy
- Radioactive iodine therapy
- Thyroidectomy (total or subtotal); total thyroidectomy and radical neck excision

(continued)

Endocrine refresher (continued)

THYROID CANCER (CONTINUED)
Key interventions
- Monitor respiratory status for signs of airway obstruction.
- Assess the client's ability to swallow.
- Provide postoperative thyroidectomy care.

THYROIDITIS
Key signs and symptoms
- Thyroid enlargement
- Fever
- Pain
- Tenderness and reddened skin over the gland

Key test results
Note: Precise diagnosis depends on the type of thyroiditis.
- In autoimmune thyroiditis, high titers of thyroglobulin and microsomal antibodies may be present in serum.
- In subacute granulomatous thyroiditis, tests may reveal elevated erythrocyte sedimentation rate, increased thyroid hormone levels, and decreased thyroidal RAIU.
- In chronic infective and noninfective thyroiditis, varied findings occur, depending on the underlying infection or other disease.

Key treatments
- Partial thyroidectomy to relieve tracheal or esophageal compression in Riedel's thyroiditis
- Thyroid hormone replacement: levothyroxine (Synthroid) for accompanying hypothyroidism

Key interventions
- Monitor vital signs and examine the client's neck for unusual swelling, enlargement, or redness.
- If the neck is swollen, measure and record the circumference daily.
After thyroidectomy
- Monitor vital signs every 15 to 30 minutes until the client's condition stabilizes. Stay alert for signs of tetany secondary to accidental parathyroid injury during surgery. Keep 10% calcium gluconate available for I.M. use, if needed.
- Assess dressings frequently for excessive bleeding.
- Monitor for signs of airway obstruction, such as difficulty talking and increased swallowing; keep tracheotomy equipment handy.

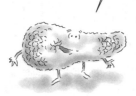

Power to the pancreas!

- **epinephrine,** which regulates instantaneous stress reaction and increases metabolism, blood glucose levels, and cardiac output.

Endo and exo
The **pancreas** is an accessory gland of digestion. In its **exocrine function,** it secretes digestive enzymes (amylase, lipase, and trypsin). Amylase breaks down starches into smaller carbohydrate molecules. Lipase breaks down fats into fatty acids and glycerol. Trypsin breaks down proteins. Note that exocrine glands discharge secretions through a duct; the pancreas secretes enzymes into the duodenum through the pancreatic duct.

In its **endocrine function,** the pancreas secretes hormones from the islets of Langerhans (insulin, glucagon, and somatostatin). Insulin regulates fat, protein, and carbohydrate metabolism and lowers blood glucose levels by promoting glucose transport into cells. Glucagon increases blood glucose levels by promoting hepatic glyconeogenesis. Somatostatin inhibits the release of insulin, glucagon, and somatotropin. Note that endocrine glands discharge secretions into the blood or lymph.

Keep abreast of diagnostic tests

Below are the major diagnostic tests for assessing endocrine disorders as well as common nursing actions associated with each test.

Draw blood and test, part 1
Blood chemistry tests are used to analyze blood samples for levels of potassium, sodium, calcium, phosphorus, glucose, bicarbonate, blood urea nitrogen (BUN), creatinine, protein, albumin, osmolality, amylase, lipase, alkaline phosphatase, lactate dehydrogenase, aldosterone, cortisol, ketones, cholesterol, triglycerides, and carbon dioxide.

Nursing actions
- Explain the procedure to the client.
- Check the venipuncture site for bleeding.

Draw blood and test, part 2
A **hematologic study** analyzes a blood sample for red blood cells (RBCs), white

blood cells (WBCs), platelets, prothrombin time, international normalized ratio, partial thromboplastin time, hemoglobin (Hb) levels, and hematocrit (HCT).

Nursing actions
- Explain the procedure to the client.
- Note current drug therapy.
- Check the venipuncture site for bleeding.

Fast and test
The **fasting blood glucose test** measures plasma glucose levels following a minimum 8-hour fast.

Nursing actions
- Explain the procedure to the client.
- Withhold food and fluids for at least 8 hours before the fasting sample is drawn.
- Withhold insulin until the test is completed.

Eat carbs and test
In a **2-hour postprandial glucose test,** a blood sample is used to analyze the body's insulin response to carbohydrate ingestion.

Nursing actions
- Explain the procedure to the client.
- List any medications that might interfere with the test.
- Note pregnancy, trauma, or infectious disease.
- Provide the client with a 100 g carbohydrate diet before the test and then ask him to fast for 2 hours.
- Instruct the client to avoid tobacco, caffeine, alcohol, and exercise after the meal.

Carb absorption assessment
The **glucose tolerance test** (GTT) uses blood samples and urine specimens to measure carbohydrate absorption.

Nursing actions
- Explain the procedure to the client.
- List any medications that might interfere with the test.
- Note pregnancy, trauma, or infectious disease.
- Provide the client with a high-carbohydrate diet for 3 days.

- Instruct the client to fast for 10 to 16 hours before the test.
- Advise the client not to use tobacco, drink coffee or alcohol, or exercise strenuously for 8 hours before or during the test.
- Withhold any medications that may interfere with testing.
- Draw a fasting blood sample and have the client provide a urine specimen at the same time.
- Administer the test dose of oral glucose and record the time of administration.
- Request laboratory collection of serum glucose samples and urine specimens at 30, 60, 120, and 180 minutes.
- Refrigerate samples and specimens and assess the client for hypoglycemia.

Months of blood glucose levels
Glycosylated hemoglobin (HbA$_{1C}$) testing uses a blood sample to measure glycosylated Hb levels. This provides information about average blood glucose levels during the preceding 2 to 3 months. This test is used to evaluate the long-term effectiveness of diabetes therapy.

Nursing actions
- Explain the procedure to the client.
- Explain to the client that this test is used to evaluate diabetes therapy.
- Tell the client that he need not restrict food or fluids and instruct him to maintain his prescribed medication and diet regimen.

Checking for cortisol
The **ACTH (corticotropin) stimulation test** analyzes blood samples for cortisol aned measures the ability of the adrenal cortex to respond to ACTH.

Nursing actions
- Explain the procedure to the client.
- List any medications that might interfere with the test.
- Know that this test is contraindicated in pregnant clients.
- Monitor 24-hour I.V. infusion of corticotropin after the baseline serum sample is drawn.

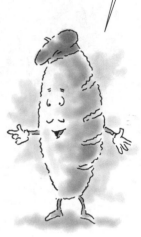

Oui! In the 2-hour postprandial test, a blood sample is used to determine the body's insulin response to carbs like me!

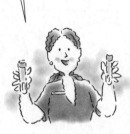

Blood and urine testing reveal volumes of information on endocrine disorders.

Blood analysis (with drug)

The **dexamethasone suppression test,** which involves administration of dexamethasone, is used to measure the response of the adreanal glands to ACTH.

Nursing actions

- Explain the procedure to the client.
- On the first day, give the client 1 mg of dexamethasone at 11 p.m.
- On the next day, collect blood samples at 4 p.m. and 11 p.m.
- Monitor the venipuncture site; if a hematoma develops, apply warm soaks.
- List any medications that might interfere with the test.
- Collect urine specimens as ordered for 3 days.

Urine analysis (24-hour collection)

The **24-hour urine test for 17-ketosteroids (17-KS) and 17-hydroxycorticosteroids (17-OHCS)** is a quantitative laboratory analysis of urine collected over 24 hours to determine hormone precursors.

Nursing actions

- Explain the procedure to the client.
- Withhold all medications for 48 hours before the test.
- Instruct the client to void and note the time (collection of urine starts with the next voiding).
- Place the urine container on ice.
- Measure each voided urine collection.
- If done on an outclient basis, instruct the client about how to collect the 24-hour specimen.
- List any medications that might interfere with the test.

The sella turcica is located in a depression at the base of the skull and contains the pituitary gland.

Epinephrine exam

The **urine vanillylmandelic acid test** is a quantitative analysis of urine collected over 24 hours to determine the end products of catecholamine metabolism (epinephrine and norepinephrine).

Nursing actions

- Explain the procedure to the client.
- List any medications, previous tests, and medical conditions that might interfere with the test.

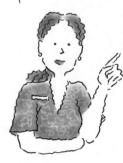

- Restrict foods that contain vanilla, coffee, tea, citrus fruits, bananas, nuts, and chocolate for 3 days before test.
- Hold any medications that might interfere with testing, such as antihypertensives and aspirin.
- Instruct the client to void and note the time (collection of urine starts with the next voiding).
- Place the urine container on ice.
- Measure each voided urine.

Oxygen in, calories used

The **BMR test** is an indirect, noninvasive measurement of BMR. The test measures oxygen consumed by the body during a given time and evaluates caloric expenditure in a 24-hour period.

Nursing actions

- Explain the procedure to the client.
- List medications taken before the procedure.
- Note environmental and emotional stressors.

Inspecting the abdomen

Computed tomography (CT) scan allows visualization of the sella turcica and abdomen.

Nursing actions

- Explain the procedure to the client.
- Note the client's allergies to iodine, seafood, and radiopaque dyes.
- Instruct the client to fast for 4 hours before the procedure.
- Ensure informed consent has been obtained per facility policy.

Echo exam

Ultrasonography allows visualization of the thyroid, pelvis, and abdomen through the use of reflected sound waves.

Nursing actions

- Explain the procedure to the client.
- Assess whether the client can lie still during the procedure.

Taking thyroid tissue

A **closed percutaneous thyroid biopsy** uses the percutaneous, sterile aspiration of a small amount of thyroid tissue for histologic evaluation.

Nursing actions
Before the procedure
- Explain the procedure to the client.
- Withhold food and fluids after midnight.
- Obtain the client's written, informed consent.

After the procedure
- Maintain bed rest for 24 hours.
- Monitor vital signs.
- Assess for esophageal or tracheal puncture and bleeding or respiratory distress caused by hematoma or edema.

Thyroid function test
A **thyroid uptake,** also called **radioactive iodine uptake** or **RAIU,** measures the amount of radioactive iodine taken up by the thyroid gland in 24 hours. This measurement gives the physician an indication of thyroid function.

Nursing actions
- Explain the procedure to the client.
- Instruct the client not to ingest iodine-rich foods for 24 hours before the test.
- Discontinue all thyroid and cough medications 7 to 10 days before the test.

Radiograph of the 'roid
A **thyroid scan** gives visual imaging of radioactivity distribution in the thyroid gland. The physician uses these results to assess size, shape, position, and anatomic function of the thyroid.

Nursing actions
Before the procedure
- Explain the procedure to the client.
- If iodine[123] (^{123}I) or ^{131}I is to be used, tell the client to fast after midnight the night before the test. Fasting isn't required if an I.V. injection of isotope technetium (^{99m}Tc) pertechnetate is used.
- Hold any medications that may interfere with the procedure.
- Instruct the client to stop consuming iodized salt, iodinated salt substitutes, and seafood 1 week before the procedure.
- Imaging follows oral administration (^{123}I or ^{131}I) by 24 hours and I.V. injection (^{99m}Tc pertechnetate) by 20 to 30 minutes.

- Remove dentures, jewelry, and other materials that may interfere with imaging.
After the procedure
- Tell the client he may resume his usual medications and diet.

Artery assessment
Arteriography gives a fluoroscopic examination of the arterial blood supply to the parathyroid, adrenal, and pancreatic glands.

Nursing actions
Before the procedure
- Explain the procedure to the client.
- Check for written, informed consent.
- Note the client's allergies to iodine, seafood, and radiopaque dyes.
- Withhold food and fluids after midnight.
After the procedure
- Monitor vital signs.
- Check the insertion site for bleeding and assess pulses distal to the site.

Counting calcium
Urine calcium (Sulkowitch's test) analyzes urine to measure the amount of calcium being excreted.

Nursing actions
- Explain the procedure to the client.
- If hypercalcemia is indicated, collect a single urine specimen *before* a meal.
- If hypocalcemia is indicated, collect a single urine specimen *after* a meal.

Memory jogger

To recall interventions for Sulkowitch's test, remember that hyper- comes before hypo- alphabetically. Then remember to collect a urine specimen before a meal for hypercalcemia and after for hypocalcemia.

Polish up on client care

Major endocrine disorders include acromegaly and gigantism, Addison's disease, Cushing's syndrome, diabetes insipidus, diabetes mellitus, goiter, hyperthyroidism, hypothyroidism, metabolic syndrome, pancreatic cancer, pheochromocytoma, and thyroid cancer.

Acromegaly and gigantism

Acromegaly and gigantism are marked by hormonal dysfunction and startling skeletal overgrowth. Both are chronic, progressive

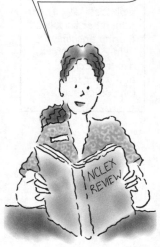

It's a question of timing. Acromegaly may occur any time after adolescence, when the arms and legs have stopped growing. Gigantism begins in childhood or adolescence when the arms and legs are still growing.

Think about therapeutic communication. The client needs help coping with his body image as well as mood changes brought on by the disorder.

diseases that occur when the pituitary gland produces too much GH, causing excessive growth. Acromegaly develops slowly; gigantism develops abruptly.

Acromegaly occurs after epiphyseal closure, causing bone thickening and transverse growth and visceromegaly (enlargement of the viscera). In other words, acromegaly may occur any time after adolescence, when the arms and legs have stopped growing. Signs of this disorder include swelling and enlargement of the arms, legs, and face.

Gigantism begins before epiphyseal closure and causes proportional overgrowth of all body tissues. In other words, gigantism begins in childhood or adolescence when the arms and legs are still growing. That's why these clients may attain giant proportions.

CAUSES
- Oversecretion of human growth hormone (hGH)
- Tumors of the anterior pituitary gland (which lead to oversecretion of hGH)

ASSESSMENT FINDINGS
Acromegaly
- Gradual development
- Enlarged supraorbital ridge
- Head enlargement
- Thickened ears and nose
- Marked prognathism (projection of the jaw) that may interfere with chewing
- Laryngeal hypertrophy
- Paranasal sinus enlargement
- Thickening of the tongue
- Oily skin
- Diaphoresis
- Severe headache
- Bitemporal hemianopia
- Loss of visual acuity
- Blindness may occur

Gigantism
- Abrupt, excessive growth in all parts of the body; height increases as much as 6″ (15.2 cm) per year; infants and children up to three times the normal height for their age; adults taller than 6′ 8″ (203 cm)

DIAGNOSTIC TEST RESULTS
- Plasma hGH levels measured by radio-immunoassay typically are elevated. However, because hGH secretion is pulsatile, the results of random sampling may be misleading. Insulin-like growth factor-I (somatomedin-C) levels offer a better screening alternative.
- Glucose normally suppresses hGH secretion; therefore, a glucose infusion that doesn't suppress the hormone level to below the accepted normal value of 2 ng/ml, when combined with characteristic clinical features, strongly suggests hyperpituitarism.
- Skull X-rays, a CT scan, arteriography, and magnetic resonance imaging (MRI) determine the presence and extent of the pituitary lesion.

NURSING DIAGNOSES
- Disturbed body image
- Chronic pain
- Impaired physical mobility
- Fatigue
- Activity intolerance
- Decreased cardiac output

TREATMENT
- Surgery to remove the affecting tumor (transsphenoidal hypophysectomy)
- Pituitary radiation therapy

Drug therapy
- Thyroid hormone replacement therapy after surgery: levothyroxine (Synthroid)
- Corticosteroid: cortisone
- Dopamine agonist: bromocriptine (Parlodel)
- Somatotropic hormone: octreotide (Sandostatin)

INTERVENTIONS AND RATIONALES
- Provide emotional support *to help the client cope with his body image. Grotesque body changes characteristic of this disorder can cause severe psychological stress.*
- Administer prescribed medications *to improve the client's condition.*

- Perform or assist with range-of-motion (ROM) exercises *to promote maximum joint mobility.*
- Evaluate muscular weakness, especially in the client with late-stage acromegaly. Check the strength of his grasp *to monitor for disease progression.* If it's weak, help with tasks such as cutting food.
- Provide skin care. Avoid using an oily lotion *because the skin is already oily.*
- Monitor blood glucose levels *to detect early signs of hyperglycemia.* Monitor for signs of hyperglycemia (fatigue, polyuria, polydipsia) *to avoid treatment delay.*
- Be aware of inexplicable mood changes. Reassure the family that these mood changes result from the disease and can be modified with treatment *to help the family cope with the client's illness.*
- Before surgery, reinforce what the surgeon has told the client, if possible, and provide a clear and honest explanation of the scheduled operation *to allay the client's fears and anxiety.*
- If the client is a child, explain to his parents that such surgery prevents permanent soft-tissue deformities but won't correct bone changes that have already taken place.
- Arrange for counseling, if necessary, *to help the child and parents cope with permanent defects.*
- After surgery, monitor vital signs and neurologic status *to detect signs of an increase in intracranial pressure due to intracranial bleeding or cerebral edema.*
- Monitor blood glucose levels. *hGH levels usually fall rapidly after surgery, removing an insulin antagonist effect in many clients and possibly precipitating hypoglycemia.*
- Monitor intake and output hourly, watching for large increases. *Transient diabetes insipidus, which sometimes occurs after surgery for hyperpituitarism, can cause such increases in urine output.*
- If the transsphenoidal approach is used, a large nasal pack should be kept in place for several days. Because the client must breathe through his mouth, provide good mouth care *to prevent breakdown of the oral mucosa.*

- The surgical site is packed with a piece of tissue generally taken from a mid-thigh donor site. Monitor for cerebrospinal fluid (CSF) leaks from the packed site. Look for increased external nasal drainage or drainage into the nasopharynx. CSF leaks may necessitate additional surgery to repair the leak. *These measures detect complications quickly and avoid treatment delays.*
- Encourage the client to ambulate on the first or second day after surgery *to prevent complications of immobility.*

Teaching topics
- Explanation of the disorder and treatment plan
- Receiving follow-up checkups (there's a slight chance that the tumor that caused his condition could recur)
- Medication use and possible adverse effects, including continuing hormone replacement therapy following surgery (warn against stopping the hormones suddenly)
- Wearing a medical identification bracelet at all times and bringing his hormone replacement schedule with him whenever he returns to the facility

Addison's disease

Addison's disease, also known as *adrenal hypofunction,* occurs when the adrenal gland fails to secrete sufficient mineralocorticoids, glucocorticoids, and androgens.

Addisonian crisis (adrenal crisis) is a critical deficiency of mineralocorticoids and glucocorticoids. It generally occurs in clients who have chronic adrenal insufficiency and follows acute stress, sepsis, trauma, surgery, or omission of steroid therapy. Addisonian crisis is a medical emergency that necessitates immediate, vigorous treatment.

CAUSES
- Autoimmune disease
- Histoplasmosis
- Idiopathic atrophy of adrenal glands
- Metastatic lesions from lung cancer

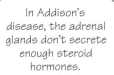

A client with acromegaly should be periodically screened for colon polyps—incidence of polyps increases with chronic hGH elevation.

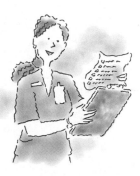

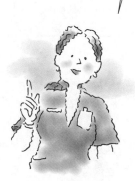

In Addison's disease, the adrenal glands don't secrete enough steroid hormones.

- Pituitary hypofunction
- Surgical removal of adrenal glands
- Trauma
- Tuberculosis

ASSESSMENT FINDINGS
- Anorexia, diarrhea, and nausea
- Bronzed skin pigmentation on nipples, scars, and buccal mucosa
- Decreased pubic and axillary hair
- Dehydration and thirst
- Depression and personality changes
- Hypotension
- Hypoglycemia
- Orthostatic hypotension
- Weakness and lethargy
- Weight loss

DIAGNOSTIC TEST RESULTS
- Blood chemistry analysis reveals decreased HCT; decreased Hb, cortisol, glucose, sodium, chloride, and aldosterone levels; and increased BUN and potassium levels.
- BMR is decreased.
- Electrocardiogram demonstrates prolonged PR and QT intervals.
- Fasting blood glucose analysis reveals hypoglycemia.
- Urine chemistry shows decreased 17-KS and 17-OHCS.
- Abdominal X-ray may show adrenal calcification.
- Abdominal CT scan may show adrenal calcification, enlargement, or atrophy.
- ACTH (Cortrosyn) stimulation test reveals decreased cortisol response.

NURSING DIAGNOSES
- Deficient fluid volume
- Imbalanced nutrition: Less than body requirements
- Risk for infection

TREATMENT
- High-carbohydrate, high-protein, high-sodium, low-potassium diet in small, frequent feedings before steroid therapy; high-potassium and low-sodium diet while on steroid therapy
- In adrenal crisis, I.V. hydrocortisone administered promptly along with 3 to 5 L of normal saline solution

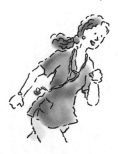

For adrenal crisis, take emergency action— I.V. hydrocortisone with 3 to 5 L of saline solution.

Drug therapy
- Antacids: magnesium and aluminum hydroxide (Maalox), aluminum hydroxide gel
- Glucocorticoids: cortisone, hydrocortisone
- Mineralocorticoid: fludrocortisone
- Vasopressor: norepinephrine (Levophed)
- Dextrose, 50%, to treat hypoglycemia

INTERVENTIONS AND RATIONALES
- Be prepared to administer I.V. hydrocortisone and saline solution promptly if the client is in adrenal crisis *to reverse shock and hyponatremia.*
- Monitor cardiac rhythm during adrenal crisis or electrolyte imbalance *to detect arrhythmias.*
- Assess fluid balance (and increase in fluid intake in hot weather) *to prevent addisonian crisis, which may be precipitated by salt or fluid loss in hot weather and during exercise.*
- Monitor and record vital signs, intake and output, urine specific gravity, and laboratory studies *to assess for deficient fluid volume.*
- Maintain the client's diet *to promote nutritional balance.*
- Administer I.V. fluids *to maintain hydration and prevent addisonian crisis.*
- Weigh the client daily *to determine nutritional status and detect fluid loss.*
- Administer medications, as prescribed, *to maintain or improve the client's condition.*
- Instruct the client to avoid sitting or standing *to avoid orthostatic hypotension.*
- Encourage fluid intake *to improve fluid status and prevent addisonian crisis.*
- Monitor glucose levels t*o check response to glucocorticoids.*
- Assist with activities of daily living *to conserve energy and decrease metabolic demands.*
- Maintain a quiet environment *to conserve energy and decrease metabolic demands.*

Teaching topics
- Explanation of the disorder and treatment plan
- Medication use and possible adverse effects
- Recognizing the signs and symptoms of adrenal crisis (profound weakness, fatigue, nausea, vomiting, hypotension, dehydration and, occasionally, high fever followed by hypothermia)

- Carrying injectable dexamethasone
- Avoiding over-the-counter drugs unless approved by the physician
- Avoiding strenuous exercise, particularly in hot weather

Cushing's syndrome

Cushing's syndrome, also known as *hyper-cortisolism,* is characterized by hyperactivity of the adrenal cortex. It results in excessive secretion of glucocorticoids, particularly cortisol. An increase in mineralocorticoids and sex hormones may also occur.

CAUSES
- Adenoma or carcinoma of the adrenal cortex
- Adenoma or carcinoma of the pituitary gland
- Excessive or prolonged administration of glucocorticoids or corticotropin
- Exogenous secretion of corticotropin by malignant neoplasms in the lungs or gallbladder
- Hyperplasia of the adrenal glands
- Hypothalamic stimulation of the pituitary gland

ASSESSMENT FINDINGS
- Acne
- Amenorrhea
- Decreased libido
- Ecchymosis
- Edema
- Enlarged clitoris
- Fragile skin
- Gynecomastia
- Hirsutism
- Hyperglycemia
- Hypertension
- Mood swings
- Muscle wasting
- Pain in joints
- Poor wound healing
- Purple striae on abdomen
- Recurrent infections
- Weakness and fatigue
- Weight gain, particularly truncal obesity, buffalo hump, and moonface

DIAGNOSTIC TEST RESULTS
- Blood chemistry analysis shows increased cortisol, aldosterone, sodium, corticotropin, and glucose levels and a decreased potassium level.
- CT scan shows pituitary or adrenal tumors.
- Dexamethasone suppression test shows no decrease in 17-OHCS.
- GTT shows hyperglycemia.
- Hematology shows increased WBC and RBC counts and decreased eosinophil count.
- MRI shows pituitary or adrenal tumors.
- Ultrasonography shows pituitary or adrenal tumors.
- Urine chemistry shows increased 17-OHCS and 17-KS, decreased urine specific gravity, and glycosuria.
- X-ray shows pituitary or adrenal tumor and osteoporosis.

NURSING DIAGNOSES
- Risk for activity intolerance
- Disturbed body image
- Deficient fluid volume
- Impaired skin integrity

TREATMENT
- Hypophysectomy or bilateral adrenalectomy
- Glucose level monitoring
- Low-sodium, low-carbohydrate, low-calorie, high-potassium, high-protein diet
- Radiation therapy
- Potassium supplements: potassium chloride (K-Lor), potassium gluconate (Kaon)

Drug therapy
- Adrenal suppressants: metyrapone (Metopirone), ketoconazole (Nizoral), etomidate (Amidate)
- Antidiabetic agents: insulin or oral antidiabetic agents, such as chlorpropamide (Diabinese), glyburide (DiaBeta, Micronase), glipizide (Glucotrol), rosiglitazone (Avandia)
- Diuretics: furosemide (Lasix), ethacrynic acid (Edecrin)

The signs of Cushing's syndrome are distinctive. Let's see...rapidly developing fatty tissue in the face, neck, and trunk and purple streaks on the skin.

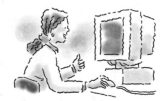

INTERVENTIONS AND RATIONALES

- Perform postoperative care *to prevent complications.*
- Assess fluid balance *to detect fluid deficit or overload.*
- Monitor and record vital signs, intake and output, urine specific gravity, capillary blood glucose levels, urine glucose and ketones, and laboratory studies. *Changed parameters may indicate altered fluid or electrolyte status.*
- Assess for edema *to detect signs of excess fluid volume.*
- Apply antiembolism stockings *to promote venous return and prevent thromboembolism formation.*
- Maintain the client's diet *to maintain nutritional status.*
- Maintain standard precautions *to protect the client from infection.*
- Provide meticulous skin care and reposition the client every 2 hours *to prevent skin breakdown.*
- Limit water intake *to prevent excess fluid volume.*
- Weigh the client daily *to detect fluid retention.*
- Administer medications, as prescribed, *to maintain or improve the client's condition.*
- Provide emotional support and encourage the client to express his feelings about changes in body image and sexual function *to help him cope effectively.*
- Provide rest periods *to prevent fatigue.*
- Provide postradiation nursing care *to prevent complications.*

Teaching topics

- Explanation of the disorder and treatment plan
- Medication use and possible adverse effects, including recognizing signs of inadequate steroid dosage (fatigue, weakness, dizziness) and overdosage (severe edema, weight gain) and avoiding discontinuing steroid dosage
- Recognizing the signs and symptoms of infection and fluid retention
- Avoiding exposure to people with infections
- Self-monitoring for infection
- Carrying a medical identification card and immediately reporting infections, which necessitate increased steroid dosage

Diabetes insipidus

Diabetes insipidus stems from a deficiency of ADH (vasopressin) secreted by the posterior lobe of the pituitary gland. Decreased ADH reduces the ability of distal and collecting renal tubules in the kidneys to concentrate urine, resulting in excessive urination, excessive thirst, and excessive fluid intake.

CAUSES

- Brain surgery
- Head injury
- Idiopathy
- Meningitis
- Trauma to the posterior lobe of the pituitary gland
- Tumor of the posterior lobe of the pituitary gland

ASSESSMENT FINDINGS

- Dehydration
- Fatigue
- Headache
- Hypotension
- Muscle weakness and pain
- Polydipsia (excessive thirst, consumption of 4 to 40 L/day)
- Polyuria (greater than 5 L/day)
- Tachycardia
- Weight loss

DIAGNOSTIC TEST RESULTS

- Blood chemistry shows decreased ADH by radioimmunoassay and increased potassium, sodium, and osmolality levels.
- Urine chemistry analysis shows urine specific gravity less than 1.004, osmolality 50 to 200 mOsm/kg, decreased urine pH, and decreased sodium and potassium levels.

NURSING DIAGNOSES

- Deficient fluid volume
- Impaired oral mucous membrane
- Risk for imbalanced body temperature

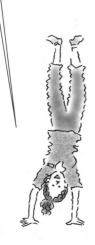

Because diabetes insipidus commonly affects fluid balance, monitoring fluid status is a key element of client care.

TREATMENT

- I.V. therapy: hydration (when first diagnosed, intake and output must be matched milliliter to milliliter to prevent dehydration), electrolyte replacement
- Regular diet with restriction of foods that exert a diuretic effect

Drug therapy

- ADH replacement: vasopressin
- ADH stimulant: carbamazepine (Tegretol)
- Antidiabetic agent: chlorpropamide (Diabenese) (promotes renal response to ADH)

INTERVENTIONS AND RATIONALES

- Assess fluid balance *to avoid dehydration*.
- Monitor and record vital signs, intake and output (urine output should be measured every hour when first diagnosed), urine specific gravity (check every 1 to 2 hours when first diagnosed), and laboratory studies *to assess for deficient fluid volume*.
- Maintain the client's diet *to maintain nutritional balance*.
- Encourage fluid intake *to keep intake equal to output and prevent dehydration*.
- Administer I.V. fluids *to replace fluid and electrolyte loss*.
- Maintain the patency of the indwelling urinary catheter *to allow accurate measuring of urine output*.
- Administer medications, as prescribed, *to enable the client to concentrate urine and prevent dehydration*.
- Weigh the client daily *to detect fluid loss*.

Teaching topics

- Explanation of the disorder and treatment plan
- Medication use and possible adverse effects
- Recognizing the signs and symptoms of dehydration
- Increasing fluid intake in hot weather
- Carrying medications at all times

Diabetes mellitus

Diabetes mellitus is a chronic disorder resulting from a disturbance in the production, action, and rate of insulin use. There are several types of diabetes mellitus.

Type 1 (insulin-dependent diabetes mellitus) usually develops in childhood. Type 2 (non–insulin-dependent diabetes mellitus) usually develops after age 30; however, it's becoming more prevalent in children and young adults. Gestational diabetes mellitus occurs with pregnancy. Secondary diabetes is induced by trauma, surgery, pancreatic disease, or medications and can be treated as type 1 or type 2.

CAUSES

- Autoimmune disease
- Blockage of insulin supply
- Failure of body to produce insulin
- Hyperpituitarism
- Hyperthyroidism
- Infection

CONTRIBUTING FACTORS

- Cushing's syndrome
- Exposure to chemicals
- Genetics
- Medications
- Pregnancy
- Receptor defect in normally insulin-responsive cells
- Obesity
- Stress
- Surgery
- Trauma

ASSESSMENT FINDINGS

- Acetone breath
- Anorexia
- Atrophic muscles
- Blurred vision
- Dehydration
- Fatigue
- Flushed, warm, smooth, shiny skin
- Kussmaul's respirations
- Mottled extremities
- Multiple infections and boils
- Pain
- Paresthesia
- Peripheral and visceral neuropathies
- Polydipsia
- Polyphagia
- Polyuria

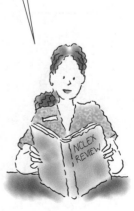

In diabetes mellitus, the body produces little or no insulin or resists the insulin it does produce.

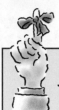

- Poor wound healing
- Retinopathy
- Sexual dysfunction
- Weakness
- Weight loss

DIAGNOSTIC TEST RESULTS
- Blood chemistry analysis shows increased glucose, potassium, chloride, ketone, cholesterol, and triglyceride levels; decreased carbon dioxide level; and pH less than 7.4.
- Fasting blood glucose level is increased (greater than or equal to 126 mg/dl).
- HbA$_{1c}$ is increased to 7 or above.
- GTT shows hyperglycemia.
- Two-hour postprandial blood glucose test shows hyperglycemia (greater than 200 mg/dl).
- Urine chemistry shows increased glucose and ketone levels.

NURSING DIAGNOSES
- Imbalanced nutrition: More than body requirements
- Risk for deficient fluid volume
- Risk for impaired skin integrity
- Anxiety

TREATMENT
- Dietary modifications
- Exercise
- Pancreas transplantation

Drug therapy
- Antidiabetic agents: insulins and oral agents, such as chlorpropamide (Diabinese), glyburide (DiaBeta, Micronase), glipizide (Glucotrol), rosiglitazone (Avandia), ritagliptin (Januvia), piaglitazone (Actose), metformin (Glucophage), exenatide (Byetta)
- Vitamin and mineral supplements (see *Treating diabetes*)

INTERVENTIONS AND RATIONALES
- Assess acid-base and fluid balance *to monitor for signs of hyperglycemia.*
- Monitor for signs of hypoglycemia (vagueness, slow cerebration, dizziness, weakness, pallor, tachycardia, diaphoresis, seizures, and coma), ketoacidosis (acetone breath, dehydration, weak or rapid pulse, Kussmaul's respirations), and hyperosmolar coma (polyuria, thirst, neurologic abnormalities, stupor) *to*

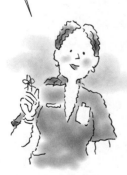

ensure early intervention and prevent complications.
- Treat hypoglycemia; immediately give carbohydrates in the form of fruit juice, hard candy, or honey. If the client is unconscious, administer glucagon or dextrose I.V. *to prevent neurologic complications.*
- Administer I.V. fluids, insulin and, usually, potassium replacement for ketoacidosis or hyperosmolar coma *to reduce the risk of potentially life-threatening complications.*
- Monitor and record vital signs, intake and output, capillary blood glucose levels, and laboratory studies *to assess fluid and electrolyte balance.*
- Monitor wound healing *to assess for infection.*
- Maintain the client's diet *to prevent complications of diabetes, such as hyperglycemia and hypoglycemia.*
- Encourage fluid intake *to maintain the client's hydration.*
- Administer medications as prescribed. *Diabetic control requires a dynamic balance between diet, the antidiabetic agent, and exercise.*
- Encourage the client to express feelings about his diet, medication regimen, and body image changes *to facilitate coping mechanisms.*
- Encourage exercise, as tolerated, *to prevent long-term complications of diabetes.*
- Weigh the client weekly *to determine nutritional status.*
- Provide meticulous skin and foot care. Clients with diabetes are at increased risk for infection from impaired leukocyte activity. *These health care practices minimize the risk of infection and promote early detection of health problems.*
- Maintain a warm and quiet environment *to provide rest and reduce metabolic demands.*
- Foster independence *to promote self-esteem.*
- Assess the client's compliance to diet, exercise, and medication regimens *to help develop appropriate interventions.*

Teaching topics
- Explanation of the disorder and treatment plan
- Medication use and possible adverse effects

Management moments

Treating diabetes

Effective treatment for diabetes optimizes blood glucose levels and decreases complications. In type 1 diabetes, treatment includes insulin replacement, meal planning, and exercise. Current forms of insulin replacement include single-dose, mixed-dose, split–mixed-dose, and multiple-dose regimens. The multiple-dose regimen may use an insulin pump.

INSULIN ACTION

Insulin may be rapid-acting (Humalog), fast-acting (Regular), intermediate-acting (NPH), long-acting (insulin glargine [Lantas]), or a premixed combination of fast-acting and intermediate-acting. Insulin may be derived from pork or human sources. Purified human insulin is used commonly today.

PERSONALIZED MEAL PLAN

Treatment for both types of diabetes also requires a meal plan to meet nutritional needs, to control blood glucose levels, and to help the client reach and maintain his ideal body weight. In type 1 diabetes, the calorie allotment may be high, depending on the client's growth stage and activity level. Weight reduction is a goal for the obese client with type 2 diabetes.

OTHER TREATMENTS

Exercise is also useful in managing type 2 diabetes because it increases insulin sensitivity, improves glucose tolerance, and promotes weight loss. In addition, clients with type 2 diabetes may need oral antidiabetic drugs to stimulate endogenous insulin production and increase insulin sensitivity at the cellular level.

THINKING LONG-TERM

Treatment for long-term complications may include dialysis or kidney transplantation for renal failure, photocoagulation for retinopathy, and vascular surgery for large vessel disease. Pancreas transplantation is also an option.

- Dietary modifications
- Understanding the importance of routine follow-up care
- Exercising regularly
- Recognizing the signs and symptoms of hyperglycemia and hypoglycemia and how to treat it
- Self-monitoring for infection, skin breakdown, changes in peripheral circulation, poor wound healing, and numbness in extremities
- Adjusting diet and insulin for changes in work, exercise, trauma, infection, fever, and stress
- Administering antidiabetic agents and using the insulin pump
- Monitoring capillary blood glucose levels
- Daily skin and foot care
- Avoiding alcohol and tobacco use
- Adhering to the treatment regimen to prevent complications
- Contacting the American Diabetes Association and local support groups

Goiter

A goiter is an enlargement of the thyroid gland that isn't caused by inflammation or a neoplasm. This condition is commonly referred to as nontoxic or simple goiter and classified as endemic or sporadic. With appropriate treatment, the prognosis is good for either type.

Endemic goiter usually results from inadequate dietary intake of iodine associated with such factors as iodine-depleted soil and malnutrition. Endemic goiter affects females more than males, especially during adolescence and pregnancy, when the demand on the body for thyroid hormone increases.

Sporadic goiter follows ingestion of certain drugs or foods. It doesn't affect one specific population segment more than others.

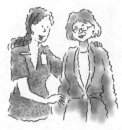

As with many endocrine disorders, therapeutic care requires helping the client with goiter cope with a change in body image.

CAUSES
- Insufficient thyroid gland production
- Depletion of glandular iodine
- Ingestion of goitrogenic foods (rutabagas, cabbage, soybeans, peanuts, peaches, peas, strawberries, spinach, radishes)
- Use of goitrogenic drugs (propylthiouracil, methimazole, iodides, lithium)

ASSESSMENT FINDINGS
- Single or multinodular, firm, irregular enlargement of the thyroid gland
- Dizziness or syncope with distended head and jugular veins and dyspnea when the client raises his arms above his head (Pemberton's sign)
- Dysphagia
- Respiratory distress
- Dyspnea

DIAGNOSTIC TEST RESULTS
- Test to rule out Graves' disease, Hashimoto's thyroiditis, and thyroid carcinoma.
- Laboratory tests reveal high or normal TSH, low serum T_4 concentrations, and increased iodine ^{131}I uptake.
- Thyroid scan and uptake identify enlarged thyroid.
- Ultrasound of thyroid reveals nodule.

NURSING DIAGNOSES
- Risk for suffocation
- Risk for injury
- Disturbed body image

TREATMENT
- Subtotal thyroidectomy

Drug therapy
- Thyroid hormone replacement: levothyroxine (Synthroid)
- Small doses of iodine (Lugol's or potassium iodide solution)
- Radioactive iodine

INTERVENTIONS AND RATIONALES
- Measure the client's neck circumference *to check for progressive thyroid gland enlargement*. Also check for the development of hard nodules in the gland, *which may indicate carcinoma*.
- Administer iodine supplements *to increase body's iodine level*.
- Provide preoperative teaching and postoperative care if subtotal thyroidectomy is indicated. *These measures allay the client's anxiety and prevent postoperative complications.*

Teaching topics
- Explanation of the disorder and treatment plan
- Medication use and possible adverse effects
- Understanding the importance of iodized salt
- Taking medications
- Recognizing the symptoms of thyrotoxicosis (increased pulse rate, palpitations, diarrhea, sweating, tremors, agitation, shortness of breath) and how to respond when symptoms occur

Hyperthyroidism

Hyperthyroidism is the increased synthesis of thyroid hormone. It can result from overactivity (Graves' disease) or a change in the thyroid gland (toxic nodular goiter).

CAUSES
- Autoimmune disease
- Genetic
- Infection
- Pituitary tumors
- Psychological or physiologic stress
- Thyroid adenomas

ASSESSMENT FINDINGS
- Anxiety and mood swings
- Atrial fibrillation
- Bruit or thrill over thyroid
- Diaphoresis
- Diarrhea
- Dyspnea
- Exophthalmos
- Fine hand tremors
- Flushed, smooth skin
- Heat intolerance
- Hyperhidrosis
- Increased hunger
- Increased systolic blood pressure
- Insomnia

- Palpitations
- Tachycardia
- Tachypnea
- Weakness
- Weight loss

DIAGNOSTIC TEST RESULTS
- Blood chemistry analysis shows increased T_3, T_4, and free thyroxine levels and decreased TSH and cholesterol levels.
- RAIU is increased.
- Thyroid scan shows nodules.

NURSING DIAGNOSES
- Decreased cardiac output
- Risk for imbalanced body temperature
- Risk for injury
- Imbalanced nutrition: Less than body requirements

TREATMENT
- High-protein, high-carbohydrate, high-calorie diet; restricting stimulants such as caffeine
- Radiation therapy
- Thyroidectomy

Drug therapy
- Adrenergic-blocking agents: propranolol (Inderal), reserpine (Serpalan)
- Antithyroid agents: methimazole (Tapazole), propylthiouracil
- Cardiac glycoside: digoxin (Lanoxin)
- Glucocorticoids: cortisone, hydrocortisone
- Iodine preparations: potassium iodide (SSKI), radioactive iodine
- Sedative: lorazepam (Ativan)
- Vitamins: thiamine (vitamin B_1), ascorbic acid (vitamin C)

INTERVENTIONS AND RATIONALES
- Monitor cardiovascular status *to detect signs of hyperthyroidism, such as tachycardia, increased blood pressure, palpitations, and atrial arrhythmias. Presence of these signs may require a change in the treatment regimen.*
- Assess fluid balance *to determine signs of deficient fluid volume.*
- Monitor and record vital signs, intake and output, and laboratory studies *to detect early changes and guide treatment.*

- Maintain the client's diet *to promote adequate nutrition.*
- Instruct the client to avoid stimulants, such as caffeine-containing drugs and foods, *to reduce or eliminate arrhythmias.*
- Administer I.V. fluids *to promote hydration.*
- Administer medications as prescribed *to maintain or improve the client's condition.*
- Provide postoperative nursing care *to promote healing and prevent complications.*
- Provide rest periods *to reduce metabolic demands.*
- Provide a quiet, cool environment *to promote comfort. Hypermetabolism causes intolerance.*
- Provide skin and eye care *to prevent complications.*
- Provide emotional support and encourage the client to express his feelings about changes in body image *to reduce anxiety and facilitate coping mechanisms.*
- Provide postradiation nursing care *to prevent complications associated with treatment.*

Teaching topics
- Explanation of the disorder and treatment plan
- Medication use and possible adverse effects
- Recognizing the signs and symptoms of thyroid storm and hypothyroidism
- Avoiding alcohol and tobacco use
- Adhering to activity limitations
- Avoiding exposure to people with infections
- Self-monitoring for infection

Hypothyroidism

Hypothyroidism, which affects women more commonly than men, occurs when the thyroid gland fails to produce sufficient thyroid hormone. This deficiency in thyroid hormone causes an overall decrease in metabolism.

CAUSES
- Hashimoto's thyroiditis
- Malfunction of pituitary gland
- Overuse of antithyroid drugs
- Thyroidectomy
- Use of radioactive iodine

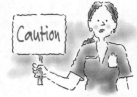

Avoid sedation. Give clients with hypothyroidism one-half to one-third the normal dose of sedatives or opioids.

ASSESSMENT FINDINGS
- Coarse hair and alopecia
- Cold intolerance
- Constipation
- Decreased diaphoresis
- Dry, flaky skin and thinning nails
- Edema
- Fatigue
- Hypersensitivity to opioids, barbiturates, and anesthetics
- Hypothermia
- Menstrual disorders
- Mental sluggishness
- Thick tongue and swollen lips
- Weight gain or anorexia

DIAGNOSTIC TEST RESULTS
- Blood chemistry analysis shows decreased T_3, T_4, and sodium levels and increased TSH and cholesterol levels.
- RAIU is decreased.

NURSING DIAGNOSES
- Activity intolerance
- Disturbed body image
- Decreased cardiac output
- Fatigue

TREATMENT
- High-fiber, high-protein, low-calorie diet

Drug therapy
- Stool softener: docusate sodium (Colace)
- Thyroid hormone replacement: levothyroxine (Synthroid), liothyronine (Cytomel)

INTERVENTIONS AND RATIONALES
- Avoid sedation: administer one-half to one-third the normal dose of sedatives or opioids *to prevent complications.* Clients taking warfarin (Coumadin) with levothyroxine may require lower doses of warfarin *because levothyroxine enhances the effects of warfarin.*
- Assess fluid balance *to determine deficient or excess fluid volume.*
- Check for constipation and edema *to detect early changes.*
- Monitor and record vital signs, intake and output, and laboratory studies *to determine fluid status.*

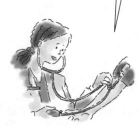

Blood pressure greater than 130/85 mm Hg can signal metabolic syndrome.

- Maintain the client's diet *to facilitate nutritional balance.*
- Encourage fluid intake *to maintain hydration.*
- Administer medications, as prescribed, *to maintain or improve the client's condition.*
- Encourage the client to express feelings of depression *to promote coping.*
- Encourage physical activity and mental stimulation *to enhance self-esteem.*
- Provide a warm environment *to promote comfort because the client with hypothyroidism may be sensitive to cold.*
- Turn the client every 2 hours and provide skin care *to prevent skin breakdown.*
- Provide frequent rest periods *because clients with hypothyroidism are easily fatigued.*

Teaching topics
- Explanation of the disorder and treatment plan
- Medication use and possible adverse effects
- Exercising regularly
- Recognizing the signs and symptoms of myxedema coma (progressive stupor, hypoventilation, hypoglycemia, hyponatremia, hypotension, hypothermia)
- Self-monitoring for constipation
- Seeking additional protection and limiting exposure during cold weather
- Avoiding sedatives
- Completing skin care daily

Metabolic syndrome

Metabolic syndrome, also called *syndrome X* or *insulin resistance syndrome,* is a cluster of conditions characterized by abdominal obesity, high blood glucose (type 2 diabetes mellitus), insulin resistance, high blood cholesterol and triglycerides, and high blood pressure. More than 22% of people in the United States meet three or more of these criteria, raising their risk of heart disease and stroke and placing them at high risk for dying of myocardial infarction.

Abdominal obesity is a strong predictor of metabolic syndrome because abdominal fat tends to be more resistant to insulin than fat in other areas. This increases the release of free fatty acid into the portal system, resulting in decreased high-density lipoprotein (HDL) and increased low-density lipoprotein (LDL) and triglyceride levels.

CAUSES
• Unknown, but there may be genetic predisposition

ASSESSMENT FINDINGS
• Abdominal obesity (waist of greater than 40" (101.6 cm) in males, 35" (89 cm) in females)
• Blood pressure greater than 130/85 mm Hg
• Fasting blood glucose level greater than 100 mg/dl
• Fatigue

DIAGNOSTIC TEST RESULTS
• Most diagnostic procedures are nonspecific, but may show hypertension, diabetes, hyperlipidemia, and hyperinsulinemia.

NURSING DIAGNOSES
• Fatigue
• Imbalanced nutrition: More than body requirements
• Risk for injury
• Disturbed body image
• Activity intolerance

TREATMENTS
• Diet high in vegetables, fruits, whole grains, and fish and low in saturated fat
• Gastric bypass: clients with a body mass index greater than 40 kg/m^2 or 35 kg/m^2 if obesity-related medical conditions present
• Lifestyle modifications, focusing on weight reduction and exercise
• Reduction of HbA$_{1c}$ level

Drug therapy
• Antilipemics: simvastatin (Zocor), pravastatin (Pravachol) to decrease LDL levels and triglycerides and to increase HDL levels
• Insulin or antidiabetic agents (if the client has hyperglycemia)
• Medications for weight loss: orlistat (Xenical), sibutramine (Meridia)

INTERVENTIONS AND RATIONALES
• Monitor the client's blood pressure, blood glucose, blood cholesterol, and insulin levels *to keep within normal limits.*
• Encourage lifestyle modifications related to improving diet and increasing exercise. *Studies have shown that lifestyle modifications have the most impact in treating metabolic syndrome.*
• Schedule follow-up appointments with health care professionals *to increase client compliance.*
• Use a positive attitude with the client and promote his active participation *to encourage successful lifestyle changes*
• If the client is scheduled for a gastric bypass, provide information and emotional support.

Teaching topics
• Explanation of the disorder and treatment plan
• Medication regimen and adverse effects
• Dietary changes
• Developing an exercise routine
• Contacting a nutritionist for further dietary teaching
• Keeping all follow-up appointments

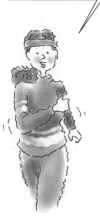

Metabolic syndrome can be treated by making sure you add some exercise into your routine!

Pancreatic cancer

Pancreatic cancer progresses rapidly and is deadly. Treatment is rarely successful because the disease has usually widely metastasized by the time it's diagnosed. Therapeutic care means helping the client and family come to terms with the end of life.

Pancreatic tumors are almost always adenocarcinomas and most arise in the head of the pancreas. Rarer tumors are those of the body and tail of the pancreas and islet cell tumors. The two main tissue types are cylinder cell and large, fatty, granular cell.

CONTRIBUTING FACTORS
• Tobacco
• Foods high in fat and protein
• Food additives
• Industrial chemicals, such as beta-naphthalene, benzidine, and urea

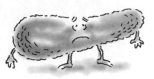

When I get cancer, it usually results in death. In most clients, the disease has widely metastasized by the time it's diagnosed.

ASSESSMENT FINDINGS
- Dull, intermittent epigastric pain (early in disease)
- Continuous pain that radiates to the right upper quadrant or dorsolumbar area and that may be colicky, dull, or vague and unrelated to activity or posture
- Anorexia
- Nausea
- Vomiting
- Diarrhea
- Jaundice
- Rapid, profound weight loss
- Palpable mass in the subumbilical or left hypochondrial region

DIAGNOSTIC TEST RESULTS
- Percutaneous fine-needle aspiration biopsy of the pancreas may detect tumor cells.
- Laparotomy with a biopsy allows definitive diagnosis.
- Ultrasound or CT scan identifies a pancreatic mass.
- Angiography reveals the vascular supply of a tumor.
- MRI shows tumor size and location.
- Blood studies reveal increased serum bilirubin levels, increased serum amylase and lipase levels, prolonged prothrombin time, elevated alkaline phosphatase levels (with biliary obstruction), elevated aspartate aminotransferase and alanine aminotransferase levels (when liver cell necrosis is present).
- Fasting blood glucose studies may indicate hyperglycemia or hypoglycemia.
- Plasma insulin immunoassay shows measurable serum insulin in the presence of islet cell tumors.
- Stool studies may show occult blood if ulceration in the GI tract or ampulla of Vater has occurred.
- Tumor markers for pancreatic cancer, including carcinoembryonic antigen, alpha-fetoprotein, carbohydrate antigen 19-9, and serum immunoreactive elastase I, are elevated.

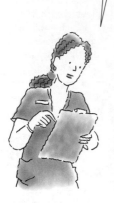

A client with pancreatic cancer may experience hypoglycemia or hyperglycemia. Administer glucose or an antidiabetic agent as necessary.

NURSING DIAGNOSES
- Acute pain
- Chronic pain
- Imbalanced nutrition: Less than body requirements
- Grieving
- Fear
- Anxiety

TREATMENT
- Blood transfusion
- I.V. fluid therapy
- Total pancreatectomy (surgical removal of the pancreas)
- Cholecystojejunostomy (surgical anastomosis of the gallbladder and the jejunum)
- Choledochoduodenostomy (surgical anastomosis of the common bile duct to the duodenum)
- Choledochojejunostomy (surgical anastomosis of the common bile duct to the jejunum)
- Whipple's operation or pancreatoduodenectomy (excision of the head of the pancreas along with the encircling loop of the duodenum)
- Gastrojejunostomy (surgical creation of an anastomosis between the stomach and the jejunum)
- Radiation therapy

Drug therapy
- Antineoplastic combinations: fluorouracil, streptozocin (Zanosar), ifosfamide (Ifex), and doxorubicin; gemcitabine and erlitinib (Tarceva)
- Antibiotic: cefotetan to prevent infection and relieve symptoms
- Anticholinergic: propantheline to decrease GI tract spasm and motility and reduce pain and secretions
- Histamine$_2$-receptor antagonists: cimetidine (Tagamet), ranitidine (Zantac), famotidine (Pepcid), nizatidine (Axid)
- Diuretic: furosemide (Lasix) to mobilize extracellular fluid from ascites
- Insulin after pancreatic resection to provide adequate exogenous insulin supply
- Opioid analgesics: morphine, meperidine (Demerol), and codeine, which can lead to biliary tract spasm and increase common bile duct pressure (used when other methods fail)

- Pancreatic enzyme: pancrelipase (Pancrease)
- Vitamin K: phytonadione
- Stool softener: docusate sodium (Colace)
- Laxative: bisacodyl (Dulcolax)

INTERVENTIONS AND RATIONALES

- Monitor fluid balance, abdominal girth, metabolic state, and weight daily *to determine fluid volume status.*
- Administer an oral pancreatic enzyme at mealtimes if needed.
- Replace nutrients I.V., orally, or by nasogastric tube *to combat weight loss.* Impose dietary restrictions, such as a low-sodium or fluid retention diet, as required, *to combat weight gain (due to ascites).* Maintain a 2,500-calorie diet for the client *to meet increased nutritional needs.*
- Administer laxatives, stool softeners, and cathartics as required; modify diet; and increase fluid intake *to prevent constipation.*
- Administer pain medication, antibiotics, and antipyretics, as necessary.
- Monitor for signs of hypoglycemia or hyperglycemia; administer glucose or an antidiabetic agent as necessary *to prevent complications of hypoglycemia or hyperglycemia.* Monitor blood glucose levels *to detect early signs of hypoglycemia or hyperglycemia.*
- Provide meticulous skin care *to avoid pruritus and necrosis.*
- Monitor for signs of upper GI bleeding; test stools and vomitus for occult blood and keep a flow sheet of Hb and HCT values *to prevent hemorrhage.*
- Apply antiembolism stockings and assist in ROM exercises *to prevent thrombosis.* If thrombosis occurs, elevate the client's legs *to promote venous return* and give an anticoagulant or aspirin, as required, *to decrease blood viscosity and prevent further thrombosis.*
- Provide emotional support to help the family and patient cope with his poor prognosis.

Before surgery

- Provide total parenteral nutrition and I.V. fat emulsions *to correct deficiencies and maintain positive nitrogen balance.*
- Give blood transfusions *to combat anemia,* vitamin K *to overcome prothrombin deficiency,* antibiotics *to prevent postoperative infection,* and gastric lavage *to maintain gastric decompression,* as necessary.
- Teach the client about expected postoperative procedures and expected adverse effects of radiation and chemotherapy *to allay anxiety.*

After surgery

- Monitor and report complications, such as fistula, pancreatitis, fluid and electrolyte imbalance, infection, hemorrhage, skin breakdown, nutritional deficiency, hepatic failure, renal insufficiency, and diabetes, *to ensure early detection and treatment of complications.*
- Treat adverse effects of chemotherapy symptomatically *to promote comfort and prevent complications.*
- Administer an oral pancreatic enzyme at mealtimes, if needed, *to aid digestion.*

Teaching topics

- Explanation of the disorder and treatment plan
- Medication use and possible adverse effects
- Wound care if appropriate
- Hospice options and end-of-life issues
- Contacting the American Cancer Society and local support groups

Pheochromocytoma

Pheochromocytoma is a chromaffin-cell tumor of the adrenal medulla that secretes an excess of the catecholamines epinephrine and norepinephrine, resulting in severe hypertension, increased metabolism, and hyperglycemia. This disorder is potentially

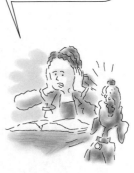

Don't forget: If the place where you're studying isn't conducive to effective learning, find a new place to study.

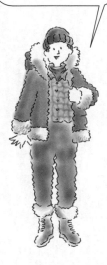

Pheochromocytoma episodes can occur with a change in body temperature. Now, where is that campfire...?

fatal, but the prognosis is generally good with treatment. However, pheochromocytoma-induced kidney damage is irreversible.

Symptomatic episodes may recur as seldom as once every 2 months or as often as 25 times per day. Episodes may occur spontaneously or may follow certain precipitating events, such as postural changes, exercise, laughing, smoking, induction of anesthesia, urination, or a change in environmental or body temperature.

CAUSES
- Inherited autosomal dominant trait in some clients
- Unknown in most clients

ASSESSMENT FINDINGS
- Abdominal pain
- Diaphoresis
- Feeling of impending doom
- Headache
- Nausea
- Palpitations
- Persistent or paroxysmal hypertension
- Tachycardia
- Tremor

DIAGNOSTIC TEST RESULTS
- A 24-hour urine specimen shows increased urinary excretion of total free catecholamine and their metabolites, vanillylmandelic acid, and metanephrine.

NURSING DIAGNOSES
- Fatigue
- Risk for injury
- Disturbed body image
- Activity intolerance

TREATMENT
- I.V. fluids, plasma volume expanders, and blood transfusions postoperatively
- I.V. phentolamine or nitroprusside (acute hypertensive crisis)
- Surgical removal of tumor (treatment of choice)

Drug therapy
- Alpha-adrenergic blocker: before surgery
- Phenoxybenzamine and propranolol if surgery isn't possible

INTERVENTIONS AND RATIONALES
- Carefully monitor the client's blood pressure and vital signs *because transient hypertensive attacks are possible.*
- Instruct the client to avoid food high in vanillin (coffee, nuts, chocolate) for 2 days before 24-urine test *to avoid interfering with laboratory results.*
- Provide a quiet room after surgery *to decrease excitement, which can trigger a hypertensive crisis.*
- Monitor the client's blood glucose levels *because he may present with hyperglycemia in addition to pheochromocytoma.*
- Postoperatively, monitor for abdominal distension and bowel sounds *to detect return of bowel function.*
- If autosomal dominant transmission of pheochromocytoma is suspected, inform the client's family of the need for evaluation.

Teaching topics
- Explanation of the disorder and treatment plan
- Medication regimen and adverse effects
- Complying with medication regimen before surgery
- Surgical treatment plan

Thyroid cancer

Thyroid cancer is a malignant, primary tumor of the thyroid. It doesn't affect thyroid hormone secretion.

CAUSES
- Chronic overstimulation of the pituitary gland
- Chronic overstimulation of the thymus gland
- Neck radiation

Management moments

Caring for the thyroidectomy client

Keep these crucial points in mind when caring for the client who has undergone thyroidectomy.
• Keep the client in Fowler's position to promote venous return from the head and neck and to decrease oozing into the incision.
• Watch for signs of respiratory distress (tracheal collapse, tracheal mucus accumulation, and laryngeal edema).
• Note that vocal cord paralysis can cause respiratory obstruction, with sudden stridor and restlessness.
• Keep a tracheotomy tray at the client's bedside for 24 hours after surgery and be prepared to assist with emergency tracheotomy if necessary.

• Assess for signs of hemorrhage.
• Assess for hypocalcemia (tingling and numbness of the extremities, muscle twitching, cramps, laryngeal spasm, and positive Chvostek's and Trousseau's signs), which may occur when parathyroid glands are damaged.
• Keep calcium gluconate available for emergency I.V. administration.
• Be alert for signs of thyroid storm (tachycardia, hyperkinesis, fever, vomiting, and hypertension).

ASSESSMENT FINDINGS
• Dysphagia
• Dyspnea
• Enlarged thyroid gland
• Hoarseness
• Painless, firm, irregular, and enlarged thyroid nodule or mass
• Palpable cervical lymph nodes

DIAGNOSTIC TEST RESULTS
• Blood chemistry analysis shows increased calcitonin, serotonin, and prostaglandin levels.
• RAIU shows a "cold," or nonfunctioning, nodule.
• Thyroid biopsy shows cytology positive for cancer cells.
• Thyroid function test is normal.

NURSING DIAGNOSES
• Anxiety
• Ineffective coping
• Chronic pain
• Ineffective breathing pattern

TREATMENT
• High-protein, high-carbohydrate, high-calorie diet with supplemental feedings

• Radiation therapy
• Radioactive iodine therapy
• Thyroidectomy (total or subtotal); total thyroidectomy and radical neck excision

Drug therapy
• Antiemetics: prochlorperazine, ondansetron (Zofran)
• Chemotherapy: chlorambucil (Leukeran), doxorubicin, vincristine
• Thyroid hormone replacements: levothyroxine (Synthroid), liothyronine (Cytomel)

INTERVENTIONS AND RATIONALES
• Monitor respiratory status for signs of airway obstruction. *A tracheotomy set should be kept at the bedside because swelling may cause airway obstruction.*
• Assess the client's ability to swallow *to maintain a patent airway.*
• Provide postoperative thyroidectomy care *to promote healing and prevent postoperative complications.* (See *Caring for the thyroidectomy client.*)
• Monitor and record vital signs, intake and output, and laboratory studies *to determine baseline and detect early changes that may*

occur with hemorrhage, airway obstruction, or hypocalcemia.
• Administer medications as prescribed *to maintain or improve the client's condition.*
• Maintain the client's diet *to improve nutritional status.*
• Provide emotional support and encourage the client to express his feelings *to facilitate coping mechanisms.*
• Provide postchemotherapy and postradiation nursing care *to prevent and treat complications associated with therapy.*

Teaching topics
• Explanation of the disorder and treatment plan
• Medication use and possible adverse effects
• Recognizing the signs and symptoms of respiratory distress, infection, myxedema coma, and difficulty swallowing
• Contacting the American Cancer Society and local support groups

Thyroiditis

Thyroiditis is inflammation of the thyroid gland. It may occur in various forms: autoimmune thyroiditis (long-term inflammatory disease; also known as *Hashimoto's thyroiditis*), subacute granulomatous thyroiditis (self-limiting inflammation), Riedel's thyroiditis (rare, invasive fibrotic process), and miscellaneous thyroiditis (acute suppurative, chronic infective, and chronic noninfective).

> After thyroidectomy, watch for signs of airway obstruction, such as difficulty talking and increased swallowing; keep tracheotomy equipment handy.

> WARNING!

CAUSES
• Antibodies to thyroid antigens
• Bacterial invasion
• Mumps, influenza, coxsackievirus, or adenovirus infection

ASSESSMENT FINDINGS
• Thyroid enlargement
• Fever
• Pain
• Tenderness and reddened skin over the gland

DIAGNOSTIC TEST RESULTS
• Precise diagnosis depends on the type of thyroiditis:
   – *autoimmune*—high titers of thyroglobulin and microsomal antibodies present in serum
   – *subacute granulomatous*—elevated erythrocyte sedimentation rate, increased thyroid hormone levels, decreased thyroidal RAIU
   – *chronic infective and noninfective*—varied findings, depending on underlying infection or other disease.

NURSING DIAGNOSES
• Risk for infection
• Acute pain
• Disturbed body image
• Ineffective breathing pattern

TREATMENT
• Partial thyroidectomy to relieve tracheal or esophageal compression in Riedel's thyroiditis

Drug therapy
• Thyroid hormone replacement: levothyroxine (Synthroid) for accompanying hypothyroidism
• Analgesic and anti-inflammatory agent: indomethacin (Indocin) for mild subacute granulomatous thyroiditis
• Beta-adrenergic blocker: propranolol (Inderal) for transient thyrotoxicosis

INTERVENTIONS AND RATIONALES
• Monitor vital signs and examine the client's neck for unusual swelling, enlargement, or redness *to detect disease progression and signs of airway occlusion.*
• Refer the client to speech therapy to evaluate swallowing ability *to prevent aspiration.*
• Measure and record neck circumference daily *to monitor progressive enlargement.*
• Monitor for signs of thyrotoxicosis (nervousness, tremor, weakness), which commonly occur in subacute thyroiditis *to initiate rapid treatment.*

After thyroidectomy

• Monitor vital signs every 15 to 30 minutes until the client's condition stabilizes. Stay alert for signs of tetany secondary to accidental parathyroid injury during surgery. Keep 10% calcium gluconate available for I.M. use, if needed. *These measures help prevent serious postoperative complications.*
• Assess dressings frequently for excessive bleeding *to detect signs of hemorrhage.*
• Monitor for signs of airway obstruction, such as difficulty talking and increased swallowing; keep tracheotomy equipment handy. *The airway may become obstructed because of postoperative edema; tracheotomy equipment should be handy to avoid treatment delay if the airway becomes obstructed.*

Teaching topics

• Explanation of the disorder and treatment plan
• Medication use and possible adverse effects, including understanding the need for lifelong thyroid hormone replacement therapy if permanent hypothyroidism occurs
• Watching for and reporting signs of hypothyroidism (lethargy, restlessness, sensitivity to cold, forgetfulness, dry skin)—especially if he has Hashimoto's thyroiditis, which commonly causes hypothyroidism
• Recognizing the need to watch for signs of hyperthyroidism, such as nervousness and palpitations

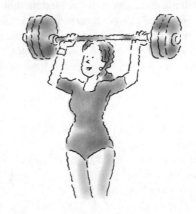

Pump up on practice questions

1. The nurse is assessing a client with hypothyroidism and finds the client has a temperature of 94° F (34.4° C) and exhibits hypotension and hypoventilation. Based on these findings, which nursing diagnosis is most appropriate for this client?
   1. *Impaired gas exchange*
   2. *Hypothermia*
   3. *Disturbed thought processes*
   4. *Deficient fluid volume*
Answer: 1. Hypothermia, hypotension, and hypoventilation are manifestations of myxedema coma, a potentially life-threatening complication of hypothyroidism. *Impaired gas exchange* is the most significant nursing diagnosis because a client with myxedema coma may suffer from hypoventilation, bradypnea, and respiratory failure caused by respiratory muscle weakness and coma. Ensuring and maintaining a patent airway always takes precedence. *Hypothermia* occurs in a client in

myxedema coma due to decreased metabolism. *Disturbed thought processes* may result from reduced cerebral perfusion secondary to reduced cardiac output. *Deficient fluid volume* may result from impaired free water clearance.

➡ *NCLEX keys*
Client needs category: Physiological integrity
Client needs subcategory: Physiological adaptation
Cognitive level: Analysis

2. A client comes to the clinic because she has experienced a weight loss of 20 lb (9.1 kg) over the past month, even though her appetite has been "ravenous" and she hasn't changed her activity level. She's diagnosed with Graves' disease. What other signs and symptoms support the diagnosis of Graves' disease? Select all that apply.
1. Rapid, bounding pulse
2. Bradycardia
3. Heat intolerance
4. Mild tremors
5. Nervousness
6. Constipation
Answer: 1, 3, 4, 5. Graves' disease, or *hyperthyroidism,* is a hypermetabolic state that's associated with rapid, bounding pulses; heat intolerance; tremors; and nervousness. Bradycardia and constipation are signs and symptoms of hypothyroidism.

➡ *NCLEX keys*
Client needs category: Health promotion and maintenance
Client needs subcategory: None
Cognitive Level: Analysis

3. In interpreting a radioactive iodine uptake test, a nurse should know that:
1. uptake increases in hyperthyroidism and decreases in hypothyroidism.
2. uptake decreases in hyperthyroidism and increases in hypothyroidism.
3. uptake increases in both hyperthyroidism and hypothyroidism.
4. uptake decreases in both hyperthyroidism and hypothyroidism.
Answer: 1. Iodine is necessary for the synthesis of thyroid hormones. In hyperthyroidism, more iodine is taken up by the thyroid so more thyroid hormones may be synthesized. In hypothyroidism, less iodine is taken up because fewer thyroid hormones are synthesized.

➡ *NCLEX keys*
Client needs category: Health promotion and maintenance
Client needs subcategory: None
Cognitive level: Comprehension

4. A client is diagnosed with hyperthyroidism. The nurse should expect clinical manifestations similar to:
1. hypovolemic shock.
2. adrenergic stimulation.
3. benzodiazepine overdose.
4. Addison's disease.
Answer: 2. Hyperthyroidism is a hypermetabolic state characterized by such signs as tachycardia, systolic hypertension, and anxiety—all seen in adrenergic (sympathetic) stimulation. Manifestations of hypovolemic shock, benzodiazepine overdose, and Addison's disease are more similar to a hypometabolic state.

➡ *NCLEX keys*
Client needs category: Physiological integrity
Client needs subcategory: Physiological adaptation
Cognitive level: Analysis

5. A client with a history of mitral valve replacement and chronic warfarin (Coumadin) usage is diagnosed with hypothyroidism and prescribed levothyroxine (Synthroid). The nurse should expect the need for the warfarin:
1. dosage to be decreased.
2. dosage to be increased.

3.   frequency to be decreased.
4.   frequency to be increased.

Answer: 1. Levothyroxine enhances the effects of warfarin; therefore, the warfarin dosage would need to be decreased.

➡ *NCLEX keys*
Client needs category: Physiological integrity
Client needs subcategory: Pharmacological and parenteral therapies
Cognitive level: Application

6.   A client with thyroid cancer undergoes a thyroidectomy. After surgery, the client develops peripheral numbness and tingling and muscle twitching and spasms. The nurse should expect to administer:
1.   thyroid supplements.
2.   antispasmodics.
3.   barbiturates.
4.   I.V. calcium.

Answer: 4. Removing the thyroid gland can cause hyposecretion of parathormone leading to calcium deficiency; indicated by numbness, tingling, and muscle spasms. Treatment includes calcium administration. Thyroid supplements will be necessary following thyroidectomy but aren't specifically related to the identified problem. Antispasmodics don't treat the problem's cause. Barbiturates aren't indicated.

➡ *NCLEX keys*
Client needs category: Physiological integrity
Client needs subcategory: Pharmacological and parenteral therapies
Cognitive level: Application

7.   A client with intractable asthma develops Cushing's syndrome. This complication can most likely be attributed to chronic use of:
1.   prednisone.
2.   theophylline.
3.   metaproterenol.
4.   cromolyn (Intal).

Answer: 1. Cushing's syndrome results from excessive glucocorticoids. This excess can occur from frequent or chronic use of corticosteroids such as prednisone. Theophylline, metaproterenol, and cromolyn don't cause Cushing's syndrome.

➡ *NCLEX keys*
Client needs category: Physiological integrity
Client needs subcategory: Pharmacological and parenteral therapies
Cognitive level: Application

8.   During treatment of a client in addisonian crisis, it's most appropriate for the nurse to administer I.V.:
1.   insulin.
2.   normal saline solution.
3.   dextrose 5% in half-normal saline solution.
4.   dextrose 5% in water.

Answer: 2. A client in addisonian crisis has hyponatremia. It's most appropriate to administer normal saline solution. Hydrocortisone, glucose, and vasopressors are also used to treat addisonian crisis. Administering dextrose 5% in half-normal saline solution, dextrose 5% in water, or insulin would be inappropriate for this client.

➡ *NCLEX keys*
Client needs category: Physiological integrity
Client needs subcategory: Pharmacological and parenteral therapies
Cognitive level: Application

9.   A client with type 1 diabetes mellitus is learning foot care. The nurse should include which teaching point?
1.   "It's OK to go barefoot at home."
2.   "Trim your toenails with scissors regularly."
3.   "Wear tight-fitting shoes without socks."
4.   "Wear cotton socks and apply foot powder to your feet to keep them dry."

Answer: 4. The nurse should instruct the client to apply foot powder and to wear cotton socks and properly fitting shoes. The nurse should also instruct the client to avoid going barefoot to prevent injury and avoid using scissors to trim his nails.

➡ *NCLEX keys*

Client needs category: Physiological integrity
Client needs subcategory: Reduction of risk potential
Cognitive level: Application

10. Which nursing diagnosis is most likely for a client with an acute episode of diabetes insipidus?

1. *Imbalanced nutrition: More than body requirements*
2. *Deficient fluid volume*
3. *Impaired gas exchange*
4. *Ineffective tissue perfusion*

Answer: 2. Diabetes insipidus causes a pronounced loss of intravascular volume. The most prominent risk to the client is *Deficient fluid volume.* Nutrition, as exchange, and tissue perfusion are also at risk beause of diabetes insipidus but this risk is a result of the fluid volume deficit caused by diabetes insipidus.

➡ *NCLEX keys*

Client needs category: Physiological integrity
Client needs subcategory: Reduction of risk potential
Cognitive level: Application

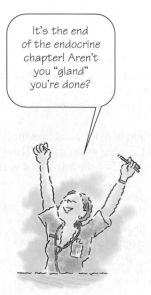

It's the end of the endocrine chapter! Aren't you "gland" you're done?

10 Genitourinary system

Brush up on key concepts

The genitourinary system is the body's water treatment plant. This system filters waste products from the body and expels them as urine. It does this by continuously exchanging water and solutes, such as hydrogen, potassium, chloride, bicarbonate, sulfate and phosphate, across cell membranes. The genitourinary system also encompasses the female and male reproductive systems.

At any time, you can review the major points of this chapter by consulting the *Cheat sheet* on pages 314 to 319.

Urinary system

Here's a brief review of urinary system components.

Fluid facts
Urine is produced by a complex process centered in the kidneys. By removing water from the body in the form of urine, the kidneys also help regulate blood pressure.

Here's how urine is formed:
• Blood from the renal artery is filtered across the glomerular capillary membrane in the Bowman's capsule.
• Filtration requires adequate intravascular volume and adequate cardiac output.
• Antidiuretic hormone and aldosterone control the reabsorption of water and electrolytes.
• Composition of formed filtrate is similar to blood plasma without proteins.
• Formed filtrate moves through the tubules of the nephron, which reabsorb and secrete electrolytes, water, glucose, amino acids, ammonia, and bicarbonate.
• What's left is excreted as urine.

Urine producers
The kidneys are two bean-shaped organs that produce urine and maintain fluid and acid-base balance. To help maintain acid-base balance, the kidneys secrete hydrogen ions, reabsorb sodium and bicarbonates, acidify phosphate salts, and produce ammonia.

The kidneys have four main components:
• the cortex, which makes up the outer layer of the kidney and contains the glomeruli, the proximal tubules of the nephron, and the distal tubules of the nephron
• the medulla, which makes up the inner layer of the kidney and contains the loops of Henle and the collecting tubules
• the renal pelvis, which collects urine from the calices
• the nephron, which makes up the functional unit of the kidney and contains Bowman's capsule, the glomerulus, and the renal tubule, which consists of the proximal convoluted tubule and collecting segments.

Blood pressure control
Regulation of fluid volume by the **kidneys** affects blood pressure. The renin-angiotensin system is activated by decreased blood pressure and can be altered by renal disease.

Transport tubule
The **ureter,** which transports urine from the kidney to the bladder, is a tubule that extends from the renal pelvis to the bladder floor.

Storage sac
The **bladder,** a muscular, distendable sac, can contain up to 1 L of urine at a single time.

(Text continues on page 319.)

Cheat sheet

Genitourinary refresher

ACUTE POSTSTREPTOCOCCAL GLOMERULONEPHRITIS
Key signs and symptoms
- Azotemia
- Hematuria
- Fatigue
- Oliguria
- Edema

Key test results
- Blood tests show elevated serum creatinine and blood urea nitrogen (BUN) levels.
- 24-hour urine specimen shows low creatinine clearance and impaired glomerular filtration.
- Elevated antistreptolysin-O titers (in 60% to 80% of clients), elevated streptozyme and anti-Dnase B titers, and low serum complement levels verify recent streptococcal infection.
- Urinalysis typically reveals proteinuria and hematuria. Red blood cells (RBCs), white blood cells, and mixed cell casts are common findings in urinary sediment.

Key treatments
- Antibiotic: penicillin (Pen-Vee K)
- Bed rest during acute phase
- Diuretics: metolazone (Zaroxolyn), furosemide (Lasix)
- Antihypertensives: hydralazine (mild to moderate hypertension), labetalol (severe hypertension)
- Fluid restriction
- High-calorie, low-sodium, low-potassium, low-protein diet during acute phase

Key interventions
- Monitor vital signs and electrolyte values. Monitor intake and output and daily weight. Assess renal function daily through serum creatinine and BUN levels and urine creatinine clearance. Watch for signs of acute renal failure (oliguria, azotemia, and acidosis).
- Provide good nutrition, use good hygienic technique, and prevent contact with infected people.
- Encourage bed rest during the acute phase.

ACUTE RENAL FAILURE
Key signs and symptoms
- Urine output less than 400 ml/day for 1 to 2 weeks followed by diuresis (3 to 5 L/day) for 2 to 3 weeks
- Weight gain

Key test results
- Creatinine clearance is low.
- Glomerular filtration rate is 20 to 40 ml/minute (renal insufficiency); 10 to 20 ml/minute (renal failure); less than 10 ml/minute (end-stage renal disease).
- Blood chemistry analysis shows increased potassium, phosphorus, magnesium, BUN, creatinine, and uric acid levels and decreased calcium, carbon dioxide, and sodium levels.

Key treatments
- Hemodialysis or continuous venovenous hemo-filtration
- Low-protein, increased-carbohydrate, moderate-fat, and moderate-calorie diet with potassium, sodium, and phosphorus intake regulated according to serum levels
- Inotropic agent: dopamine
- Diuretics: furosemide (Lasix), metolazone (Zaroxolyn)

Key interventions
- Monitor fluid balance, respiratory, cardiovascular, and neurologic status.
- Monitor and record vital signs and intake and output, central venous pressure, daily weight, urine specific gravity, and laboratory studies.
- Monitor for arrhythmias.
- Maintain the client's diet.

ACUTE TUBULAR NECROSIS
Key signs and symptoms
- Anemia
- Azotemia
- Decreased urine output
- Hyperkalemia
- Hypertension
- Pulmonary edema (in late stages)

Key test results
- Urinary test reveal urinary sediment with RBCs and casts, a low specific gravity, and high sodium level.

Key treatments
- Identification and removal of nephrotoxic substance
- Fluid management
- Transfusion of RBCs for anemia
- 50% glucose, regular insulin, and sodium bicarbonate for hyperkalemia

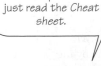
I cannot tell a lie. Sometimes I skip the chapter and just read the Cheat sheet.

Genitourinary refresher *(continued)*

ACUTE TUBULAR NECROSIS *(CONTINUED)*
Key interventions
- Maintain fluid balance, especially being alert for fluid overload.
- Carefully monitor intake and output and daily weight.
- Use sterile technique for dressing and catheter care.
- Monitor laboratory results, including electrolytes and hemoglobin and hematocrit.
- Monitor the client for complications, including acidosis and pulmonary edema.
- Provide good skin care.

BENIGN PROSTATIC HYPERPLASIA
Key signs and symptoms
- Decreased force and amount of urine
- Urgency, frequency, and burning on urination
- Enlarged prostate gland (as felt on digital rectal examination)

Key test results
- Cystoscopy shows enlarged prostate gland, obstructed urine flow, and urinary stasis.

Key treatments
- Alpha-blockers: terazosin (Hytrin), doxazosin (Cardura), tamsulosin (Flomax), alfuzosin (Uroxatral)
- Encouraging fluids
- Transurethral resection of the prostate (TURP) or prostatectomy

Key interventions
- Encourage fluid intake.

BLADDER CANCER
Key signs and symptoms
- Urinary frequency
- Hematuria
- Urinary urgency

Key test results
- Cystoscopy reveals a mass.

Key treatments
- Surgery, depending on the location and progress of the tumor

Key interventions
- Provide postoperative care. (Closely monitor urine output; observe for hematuria [reddish tint to gross bloodiness] or infection [cloudy, foul smelling, with sediment]; maintain continuous bladder irrigation if indicated; assist with turning, coughing, and deep breathing.)
- Provide emotional support and encourage the client to express feelings about a fear of dying.
- Encourage fluid intake.

BREAST CANCER
Key signs and symptoms
- Supraclavicular or axillary lymph node lump or enlargement on palpation
- Painless lump or mass in the breast or thickening of breast tissue detected on self-examination
- Skin or nipple changes
- Lump or mass in the breast or thickening of breast tissue

Key test results
- Fine-needle aspiration and excisional biopsy provide histologic cells that confirm diagnosis.
- Mammography or ultrasonography detects a tumor.

Key treatments
- Bone marrow and peripheral stem cell therapy for advanced breast cancer
- Surgery: lumpectomy, skin-sparing mastectomy, partial mastectomy, total mastectomy, and modified radical mastectomy
- Chemotherapy: cyclophosphamide (Cytoxan), methotrexate (Trexall), fluorouracil
- Hormonal therapy: tamoxifen, toremifene (Fareston), diethylstilbestrol, megestrol (Megace)

Key interventions
- Provide routine postoperative care.
- Provide emotional support and comfort measures.
- Assess pain level and administer analgesics as ordered, and monitor their effectiveness.
- Monitor for treatment-related complications, such as nausea, vomiting, anorexia, leukopenia, thrombocytopenia, GI ulceration, and bleeding.

CERVICAL CANCER
Key signs and symptoms
- Preinvasive: absence of symptoms
- Invasive: abnormal vaginal discharge (yellowish, blood-tinged, and foul-smelling); postcoital pain and bleeding; irregular bleeding

Key test results
- Colposcopy determines the source of the abnormal cells seen on Papanicolaou test.
- Cone biopsy, performed if endocervical curettage is positive, identifies malignant cells.

Key treatments
- Preinvasive: conization, cryosurgery
- Invasive: radiation therapy (internal, external, or both); radical hysterectomy

Key interventions
- Provide emotional support and comfort measures.
- Assess pain level and administer pain medication, as needed, and note its effectiveness.
- Watch for complications related to therapy.

(continued)

Genitourinary refresher (continued)

CHLAMYDIA
Key signs and symptoms
In women
- Dyspareunia
- Mucopurulent discharge
- Pelvic pain

In men
- Dysuria
- Erythema
- Tenderness of the meatus
- Urethral discharge
- Urinary frequency

Key test results
- Antigen detection methods (the diagnostic tests of choice), including enzyme-linked immunosorbent assay and direct fluorescent antibody test, identify chlamydial infection, although tissue cell cultures are more sensitive and specific.

Key treatments
- Antibiotics: doxycycline (Vibramycin), azithromycin (Zithromax)
- For pregnant women with chlamydial infections, azithromycin in a single dose

Key interventions
- Maintain standard precautions.
- Check neonates of infected mothers for signs of chlamydial infection. Obtain appropriate specimens for diagnostic testing.

CHRONIC GLOMERULONEPHRITIS
Key signs and symptoms
- Edema
- Hematuria
- Hypertension

Key test results
- Kidney biopsy identifies the underlying disease and provides data needed to guide therapy.
- Blood studies reveal rising BUN and serum creatinine levels.
- Urinalysis reveals proteinuria, hematuria, cylindruria, and RBC casts.

Key treatments
- Dialysis
- Kidney transplant
- Antihypertensive: metoprolol (Lopressor)

Key interventions
- Provide supportive care.
- Monitor vital signs, intake and output, and daily weight.
- Assess for signs of fluid, electrolyte, and acid-base imbalances.
- Administer medications and provide good skin care.

CHRONIC RENAL FAILURE
Key signs and symptoms
- Azotemia
- Decreased urine output
- Heart failure
- Lethargy
- Pruritus
- Weight gain

Key test results
- Blood chemistry analysis shows increased BUN, creatinine, phosphorus and lipid levels and decreased calcium, carbon dioxide, and albumin levels.

Key treatments
- Fluid restriction
- Low-protein, low-sodium, low-potassium, low-phosphorus, high-calorie, and high-carbohydrate diet
- Peritoneal dialysis and hemodialysis
- Antacid: aluminum hydroxide gel
- Antiemetic: prochlorperazine
- Calcium supplement: calcium carbonate (Os-Cal)
- Cation exchange resin: sodium polystyrene sulfonate (Kayexalate)
- Diuretic: furosemide (Lasix)

Key interventions
- Monitor renal, respiratory, and cardiovascular status and fluid balance.
- Assess dialysis access for bruit and thrill.
- Maintain standard precautions.
- Restrict fluids.

CYSTITIS
Key signs and symptoms
- Dark, odoriferous urine
- Urinary frequency
- Urinary urgency

Key test results
- Urine culture and sensitivity analysis positively identifies organisms *(Escherichia coli, Proteus vulgaris,* and *Streptococcus faecalis).*

Key treatments
- Increased intake of fluids and vitamin C
- Antibiotics: co-trimoxazole (Bactrim), levofloxacin (Levaquin), ciprofloxacin (Cipro)

Key interventions
- Monitor renal status.
- Encourage increased fluid intake (cranberry or orange juice) to 3 qt (3 L)/day.

Genitourinary refresher (continued)

GONORRHEA

Key signs and symptoms
- Dysuria (painful urination)
- Purulent urethral or cervical discharge
- Itching, burning, and a red and edematous meatus

Key test results
- A culture from the site of infection (urethra, cervix, rectum, or pharynx) usually establishes the diagnosis by isolating the organism.

Key treatments
- Antibiotics: ceftriaxone (Rocephin), doxycycline (Vibramycin), erythromycin (E-mycin)
- Prophylactic antibiotics: 1% silver nitrate or erythromycin (EryPed) eyedrops to prevent infection in neonates

Key interventions
- Before treatment, establish whether the client has any drug sensitivities, and watch closely for adverse effects during therapy.
- Maintain standard precautions.
- Check neonates of infected mothers for signs of infection. Take specimens for culture from the neonate's eyes, pharynx, and rectum.
- Provide education on disorder and medication use.

HERPES SIMPLEX

Key signs and symptoms
- Blisters or lesions on any part of the mouth accompanied by erythema and edema
- Dysuria (with genital herpes)
- Flulike symptoms

Key test results
- Isolation of the virus from local lesions and a histologic biopsy confirm diagnosis.

Key treatments
- Antiviral agents: idoxuridine (Herplex), trifluridine (Viroptic), vidarabine (Vira-A)
- 5% acyclovir (Zovirax) ointment (possible relief to clients with genital herpes or to immunosuppressed clients with *Herpesvirus hominis* skin infections; I.V. acyclovir to help treat more severe infections)

Key interventions
- Maintain standard precautions. For clients with extensive cutaneous, oral, or genital lesions, institute contact precautions.
- Administer pain medications and prescribed antiviral agents as ordered.
- Provide supportive care, as indicated, such as oral hygiene, nutritional supplementation, and antipyretics for fever.

NEUROGENIC BLADDER

Key symptoms
- Altered micturition
- Incontinence

Key test results
- Voiding cystourethrography evaluates bladder neck function, vesicoureteral reflux, and continence.

Key treatments
- Indwelling urinary catheter insertion

Key interventions
- Teach the client how to perform Credé's and Valsalva maneuvers.
- Provide catheter care.
- Monitor for signs of infection (fever, cloudy or foul-smelling urine).

OVARIAN CANCER

Key signs and symptoms
- Abdominal distention
- Pelvic discomfort
- Urinary frequency
- Weight loss
- Pelvic mass

Key test results
- Abdominal ultrasonography, computed tomography (CT) scan, or X-ray may delineate tumor size.

Key treatments
- Resection of the involved ovary (conservative treatment)
- Total abdominal hysterectomy and bilateral salpingo-oophorectomy with tumor resection, omentectomy, and appendectomy (aggressive treatment)
- Antineoplastics: carboplatin (Paraplatin), chlorambucil (Leukeran), cyclophosphamide (Cytoxan), dactinomycin (Cosmegen), doxorubicin (Doxil), fluorouracil, cisplatin (Platinol), paclitaxel (Taxol), topotecan (Hycamtin)
- Analgesics: morphine, fentanyl (Duragesic-25)

Key interventions
Before surgery
- Thoroughly explain all preoperative tests, the expected course of treatment, and surgical and postoperative procedures.
After surgery
- Monitor vital signs frequently.
- Monitor fluid intake and output.
- Check the dressing regularly for excessive drainage or bleeding, and watch for signs of infection.

(continued)

Genitourinary refresher (continued)

OVARIAN CANCER (CONTINUED)
- Encourage coughing and deep breathing.
- Reposition the client often and encourage her to walk shortly after surgery.
- Provide emotional support and enlist the help of a social worker, chaplain, and other members of the health care team.

PROSTATE CANCER
Key signs and symptoms
- Decreased size and force of urinary stream
- Difficulty and frequency of urination
- Urine retention
- Palpable firm nodule in gland or diffuse induration in posterior lobe revealed on digital rectal examination

Key test results
- Carcinoembryonic antigen is elevated.
- Prostate-specific antigen is increased.

Key treatments
- Radiation implant
- Radical prostatectomy (for localized tumors without metastasis) or TURP (to relieve obstruction in metastatic disease)
- Luteinizing hormone-releasing hormone agonists: goserelin (Zoladex), leuprolide (Lupron)
- Estrogen therapy: diethylstilbestrol

Key interventions
- Monitor renal and fluid status.
- Monitor for signs of infection.
- Assess pain level and note the effectiveness of analgesia.
- Maintain the client's diet.
- Maintain the patency of the urinary catheter and note drainage.
- Provide emotional support and encourage the client to express feelings about the changes in body image and fear of sexual dysfuncion.

RENAL CALCULI
Key signs and symptoms
- Mild to severe flank pain

Key test results
- Noncontrast helical CT scan identifies calculi (criterion standard)
- I.V. pylegram or excretory urography reveals calculi.
- Kidney-ureter-bladder X-rays reveal calculi.

Key treatments
- Diet: for calcium calculi, acid-ash with limited intake of calcium and milk products; for oxalate calculi, alkaline-ash with limited intake of foods high in oxalate (cola, tea); for uric acid calculi, alkaline-ash with limited intake of foods high in purine
- Extracorporeal shock wave lithotripsy
- Surgery to remove the calculus if other measures aren't effective (type of surgery dependent on location of the calculus)

Key interventions
- Monitor urine for evidence of renal calculi. Strain all urine and save all solid material for analysis.
- Encourage increased fluid intake to 3 qt (3 L)/day.
- If surgery was performed, check dressings regularly for bloody drainage, and report excessive amounts of bloody drainage to the physician; use sterile technique to change the dressing; maintain nephrostomy tube or indwelling urinary catheter if indicated; and monitor the incision site for signs of infection.

SYPHILIS
Key signs and symptoms
Primary syphilis
- Chancres on the genitalia, anus, fingers, lips, tongue, nipples, tonsils, or eyelids
Secondary syphilis
- Symmetrical mucocutaneous lesions
- Malaise
- Anorexia
- Weight loss
- Slight fever

Key test results
- Fluorescent treponemal antibody-absorption test identifies antigens of *Treponema pallidum* in tissue, ocular fluid, cerebrospinal fluid, tracheobronchial secretions, and exudates from lesions. This is the most sensitive test available for detecting syphilis in all stages. When reactive, it remains so permanently.
- Venereal Disease Research Laboratory (VDRL) slide test and rapid plasma reagin test detect nonspecific antibodies. Both tests, if positive, become reactive within 1 to 2 weeks after the primary lesion appears or 4 to 5 weeks after the infection begins.

Key treatments
- Antibiotics: penicillin G benzathine (Permapen); if allergic to penicillin, erythromycin or tetracycline

Key interventions
- Check for a history of drug sensitivity before administering the first dose of penicillin.
- Instruct the client to seek VDRL testing after 3, 6, 12, and 24 months. A client treated for latent or late syphilis should receive blood tests at 6-month intervals for 2 years.

TESTICULAR CANCER
Key signs and symptoms
• Firm, painless, smooth testicular mass, varying in size and sometimes producing a sense of testicular heaviness
In advanced stages
• Ureteral obstruction
• Abdominal mass
• Weight loss
• Fatigue
• Pallor

Key test results
• Biopsy of the mass identifies histologic verification of cancer cells.

Key treatments
• Surgery: orchiectomy (testicle removal; most surgeons remove the testicle but not the scrotum to allow for a prosthetic implant)
• High-calorie diet provided in small, frequent feedings
• I.V. fluid therapy

• Antineoplastics: bleomycin (Blenoxane), carboplatin (Paraplatin), cisplatin (Platinol), dactinomycin (Cosmegen), etoposide (VePesid), ifosfamide (Ifex), vinblastine
• Analgesics: morphine, fentanyl (Duragesic-25)
• Antiemetics: metoclopramide (Reglan), ondansetron (Zofran)

Key interventions
Before orchiectomy
• Provide emotional support.
After orchiectomy
• For the first day after surgery, apply an ice pack to the scrotum and provide analgesics.
• Check for excessive bleeding, swelling, and signs of infection.
During chemotherapy
• Give antiemetics as needed.
• Encourage small, frequent meals.
• Monitor for signs of myelosuppression.

Tube to the outside
The **urethra,** extending from the bladder to the urinary meatus, transports urine from the bladder to the exterior of the body.

Semen secretor
The **prostate gland** surrounds the male urethra. It contains ducts that secrete the alkaline portion of seminal fluid.

Female and male reproductive systems

Here's a brief review of the female and male reproductive systems, including external and internal genitalia.

FEMALE EXTERNAL GENITALIA
External female genitalia include the mons pubis, labia, clitoris, vaginal vestibule, perineal body, urethral meatus, and paraurethral glands.

Protecting the pelvic bone
The **mons pubis** provides an adipose cushion over the anterior symphysis pubis, protects the pelvic bones, and contributes to the rounded contour of the female body.

Protecting the vulval cleft
The **labia majora** are two folds that converge at the mons pubis and extend to the posterior commissure. They consist of connective tissue, elastic fibers, veins, and sebaceous glands, and they protect components of the vulval cleft.

Lubricating the vulva
The **labia minora** are within the labia majora and consist of connective tissue, sebaceous and sweat glands, nonstriated muscle fibers, nerve endings, and blood vessels. They unite to form the fourchette, the vaginal vestibule, and serve to lubricate the vulva, which adds to sexual enjoyment and fights bacteria.

Nerve center
The **clitoris**—located in the anterior portion of the vulva above the urethral opening—is made up of erectile tissue, nerves, and blood vessels and, homologous to the penis, provides sexual pleasure. The clitoris consists of:
• the glans
• the body
• two crura.

The vestibule

The **vaginal vestibule** extends from the clitoris to the posterior fourchette and consists of:

- the vaginal orifice
- the hymen—a thin, vascularized mucous membrane at the vaginal orifice
- the fossa navicularis—a depressed area between the hymen and fourchette
- Bartholin's glands—two bean-shaped glands on either side of the vagina that secrete mucus during sexual stimulation.

Episiotomy site

The **perineal body** (the area between the vagina and the anus) is the site of episiotomy during childbirth.

Urine passage

The **urethral meatus** is located $3/8''$ to $1''$ (1 to 2.5 cm) below the clitoris.

Mucus producers

The **paraurethral glands** (Skene's glands) are located on both sides of the urethral opening. Their function is to produce mucus.

FEMALE INTERNAL GENITALIA

Internal female genitalia include the vagina, uterus, fallopian tubes, and ovaries.

Copulatory and birth passage

The **vagina** is a vascularized musculomembranous tube extending from the external genitals to the uterus.

An environment for growth

Hollow and pear-shaped, the **uterus** is a muscular organ divided by a slight constriction (isthmus) into an upper portion (body or corpus) and a lower portion (cervix); the body or corpus has three layers (perimetrium, myometrium, and endometrium). The uterus receives support from broad, round, uterosacral ligaments and provides an environment for fetal growth and development.

Fertilization site

The **fallopian tubes** are about $4\frac{1}{2}''$ (12 cm) long and consist of four layers (peritoneal, subserous, muscular, mucous) divided into four portions (interstitial, isthmus, ampulla, fimbria). The fallopian tubes:

- transport ovum from the ovary to the uterus
- provide a nourishing environment for zygotes
- serve as the site of fertilization.

Ovulation site

The **ovaries** are two almond-shaped glandular structures resting below and behind the fallopian tubes on either side of the uterus. They produce sex hormones (estrogen, progesterone, androgen) and serve as the site of ovulation.

ACCESSORY FEMALE REPRODUCTIVE ORGANS

The **breasts** consist of glandular, fibrous, and adipose tissue. Stimulated by secretions from the hypothalamus, anterior pituitary, and ovaries, they provide nourishment to an infant, transfer maternal antibodies during breast-feeding, and enhance sexual pleasure.

MALE EXTERNAL GENITALIA

External male genitalia include the penis and scrotum.

Erectile tissue

The **penis,** consisting of the body (shaft) and glans, has three layers of erectile tissue—two corpora cavernosa and one corpus spongiosum. The penis deposits spermatozoa in the female reproductive tract and provides sexual pleasure.

Protective pouch

The **scrotum** is a pouchlike structure composed of skin, fascial connective tissue, and smooth-muscle fibers that houses the testes and protects spermatozoa from high body temperature.

MALE INTERNAL GENITALIA

Internal male genitalia produce and transport semen and seminal fluid.

Sperm producers

The **testes** or testicles, two oval-shaped glandular organs inside the scrotum, function to produce spermatozoa and testosterone.

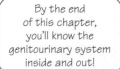

By the end of this chapter, you'll know the genitourinary system inside and out!

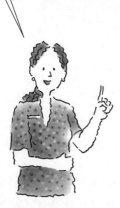

Sperm storage
The **epididymides** serve as the initial section of the testes' excretory duct system and store spermatozoa as they mature and become motile.

Sperm conduit
The **vas deferens,** which connects the epididymal lumen and the prostatic urethra, serves as a conduit for spermatozoa.

Seminal passage
The **ejaculatory ducts**—located between the seminal vesicles and the urethra—serve as passageways for semen and seminal fluid.

Excretory duct
The **urethra,** which extends from the bladder through the penis to the external urethral opening, serves as the excretory duct for urine and semen.

Motility aids
The **seminal vesicles** are two pouchlike structures between the bladder and the rectum that secrete a viscous fluid that aids in spermatozoa motility and metabolism.

Lubricating gland
The **prostate gland,** located just below the bladder, is considered homologous to Skene's glands in females. It produces an alkaline fluid that enhances spermatozoa motility and lubricates the urethra during sexual activity.

Peas in a pod
The **bulbourethral glands** (or Cowper's glands) are two pea-sized glands opening into the posterior portion of the urethra. They secrete a thick alkaline fluid that neutralizes acidic secretions in the female reproductive tract, thus prolonging spermatozoa survival.

Keep abreast of diagnostic tests

Here are the major diagnostic tests for assessing genitourinary disorders as well as common nursing actions associated with each test.

Urine specimen study #1
Urinalysis involves an examination of urine for color, appearance, pH, urine specific gravity, protein, glucose, ketones, red blood cells (RBCs), white blood cells (WBCs), and casts.

Nursing actions
• Instruct the client to wash the perineal area.
• Obtain first morning urine specimen.

Urine specimen study #2
A **urine culture and sensitivity test** examines a urine specimen for the presence of bacteria.

Nursing actions
• Explain the procedure to the client.
• Provide a container for specimen collection.
• Instruct the client to clean the perineal area and urinary meatus with bacteriostatic solution and collect a midstream specimen in a sterile container.

A day's worth of kidney function
A **24-hour urine collection** is used to analyze urine specimens collected over 24 hours to assess kidney function.

Nursing actions
• Explain the procedure to the client.
• Instruct the client to void and note the time collection starts with the next voiding.
• Place the urine container on ice.
• Measure each voided urine specimen and place it in the collection container.
• Instruct the client to void at the end of the 24-hour period.

First blood sample study
Blood chemistry tests are used to analyze blood samples for potassium, sodium, calcium, phosphorus, glucose, bicarbonate, blood urea nitrogen (BUN), creatinine, protein, albumin, osmolality, magnesium, uric acid, and carbon dioxide levels.

Nursing actions
• Explain the procedure to the client.
• Withhold food and fluids before the procedure, as directed.
• Monitor the venipuncture site for bleeding.

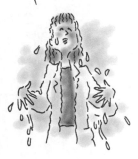

Drowning in too much information? Take a break and come back to it later.

Second blood sample study

A **hematologic study** analyzes a blood sample for WBCs, RBCs, erythrocyte sedimentation rate, platelets, prothrombin time (PT), international normalized ratio, partial thromboplastin time (PTT), hemoglobin (Hb) levels, and hematocrit (HCT).

Nursing actions
- Explain the procedure to the client.
- Check the venipuncture site for bleeding.

Picture this

A **kidney-ureter-bladder (KUB) X-ray** provides a radiographic picture of the kidneys, ureters, and bladder.

Nursing actions
- Explain the procedure to the client.
- Schedule the X-ray before other examinations requiring contrast medium.
- Ensure that the client removes metallic belts.

Scope the whole system

Excretory urography, also known as an I.V. pyelogram (IVP), produces a fluoroscopic examination of the kidneys, ureters, and bladder.

Nursing actions
Before the procedure
- Explain the procedure to the client.
- Note any allergies to iodine, seafood, and radiopaque dyes.
- Withhold food and fluids after midnight.
- Administer laxatives as prescribed.
- Make sure that written, informed consent has been obtained.
- Inform the client that he may experience a transient burning sensation and metallic taste when the contrast is injected.
After the procedure
- Instruct the client to drink at least 1 qt (1 L) of fluids.

Bladder inspection

In **cystoscopy,** a cytoscope is used to directly visualize the bladder. During the procedure, the bladder is usually distended with fluid to enhance visualization.

Nursing actions
Before the procedure
- Explain the procedure to the client.
- Withhold food and fluids.
- Make sure that written, informed consent has been obtained.
- Administer enemas and medications, as prescribed.
After the procedure
- Monitor vital signs and intake and output.
- Administer analgesics and sitz baths, as prescribed.
- Check the client's urine for blood clots.
- Encourage fluids.

Examining arteries

Renal angiography provides a radiographic examination of the renal arterial supply by injecting dye into the vascular system.

Nursing actions
Before the procedure
- Explain the procedure to the client.
- Note any allergies to iodine, seafood, and radiopaque dyes.
- Make sure that written, informed consent has been obtained.
- Withhold food and fluids after midnight.
- Instruct the client to void immediately before the procedure.
- Administer enemas as prescribed.
After the procedure
- Monitor vital signs and pulses below the catheter insertion site per facility protocol.
- Inspect the catheter insertion site for bleeding or hematoma formation.
- Encourage fluids.

Blood flow photo

A **renal scan** involves injecting a radioisotope to allow visual imaging of blood flow distribution to the kidneys.

Nursing actions
Before the procedure
- Explain the procedure to the client.
- Note any allergies.

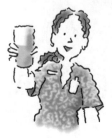

Remember that after many genitourinary tests, such as excretory urography, cytoscopy, and renal angiography, you need to encourage fluids.

- Make sure that written, informed consent has been obtained.

After the procedure
- Assess the client for signs of delayed allergic reaction, such as itching and hives.
- Wear gloves when caring for incontinent clients and double-bag linens.

Taking kidney tissue
A **renal biopsy** is the percutaneous removal of a small amount of renal tissue for histologic evaluation.

Nursing actions
Before the procedure
- Explain the procedure to the client.
- Assess baseline clotting studies and vital signs.
- Withhold food and fluids after midnight.
- Make sure that written, informed consent has been obtained.

After the procedure
- Monitor and record vital signs, Hb levels, and HCT.
- Check the biopsy site for bleeding.

Dye and shoot
In **cystourethrography,** a radiopaque dye and an X-ray are used to provide visualization of the bladder and ureters.

Nursing actions
- Explain the procedure to the client.
- Note any allergies to iodine, seafood, and radiopaque dyes before the procedure.
- Make sure that a written, informed consent has been obtained.
- Advise the client about voiding requirements during the procedure.
- Monitor voiding after the procedure.

Bladder pressure measure
Cystometrogram (CMG) graphs the pressure exerted while the bladder fills.

Nursing actions
- Explain the procedure to the client.
- Advise the client about voiding requirements during the procedure.
- Monitor voiding after the procedure.

Seeing with sound waves
In **renal ultrasound** sound waves allow visualization of the kidneys and bladdder.

Nursing actions
- Explain the procedure to the client.
- Instruct the client to drink 1 qt (1 L) of fluid 1 hour before the procedure.

Polish up on client care

Major genitourinary disorders include acute poststreptococcal glomerulonephritis (APSGN), acute renal failure (ARF), acute tubular necrosis (ATN), benign prostatic hyperplasia (BPH), bladder cancer, breast cancer, cervical cancer, chlamydia, chronic glomerulonephritis, chronic renal failure, cystitis, gonorrhea, herpes simplex, neurogenic bladder, ovarian cancer, prostate cancer, renal calculi, syphilis, and testicular cancer.

Acute poststreptococcal glomerulonephritis

APSGN is a bilateral inflammation of the glomeruli, the kidney's blood vessels, that follows a streptococcal infection of the respiratory tract or, less commonly, a skin infection such as impetigo.

CAUSES
- Trapped antigen-antibody complexes (produced as an immunologic mechanism in response to streptococci) in the glomerular capillary membranes, inducing inflammatory damage and impeding glomerular function

ASSESSMENT FINDINGS
- Azotemia
- Edema
- Fatigue
- Lethargy
- Headache
- Fever
- Hematuria

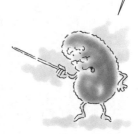

Because disorders that affect me affect fluid balance, client care commonly involves monitoring and adjusting the client's fluid status.

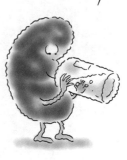

I get it! Acute poststreptococcal glomerulonephritis is a relatively common inflammation of my blood vessels.

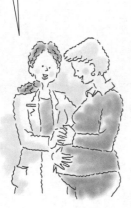

Encourage pregnant women with a history of APSGN to have frequent medical evaluations because they're at increased risk for chronic renal failure.

- Malaise
- Hypertension
- Pallor
- Oliguria
- Signs and symtoms of source of streptococcal infection, such as sore throat, dyspnea, and cough

DIAGNOSTIC TEST RESULTS

- Blood tests show elevated serum creatinine and BUN levels.
- 24-hour urine specimen shows low creatinine clearance and impaired glomerular filtration.
- Elevated antistreptolysin-O titers (in 60% to 80% of clients), elevated streptozyme and anti-Dnase B titers, and low serum complement levels verify recent streptococcal infection.
- Renal biopsy may confirm the diagnosis in a client with APSGN or may be used to assess renal tissue status (rarely done).
- Renal ultrasonography may show normal or slightly enlarged kidneys.
- Throat culture may show group A beta-hemolytic streptococci.
- Urinalysis typically reveals proteinuria and hematuria. RBCs, WBCs, and mixed cell casts are common findings in urinary sediment.

NURSING DIAGNOSES

- Impaired urinary elimination
- Excess fluid volume
- Risk for injury

TREATMENT

- Bed rest during acute phase
- Fluid restriction
- Low-sodium, low-protein, low-potassium, high-calorie diet during acute phase
- Dialysis (occasionally necessary)

Drug therapy

- Antibiotic: penicillin (Pen-Vee K)
- Diuretics: metolazone (Zaroxolyn), furosemide (Lasix)
- Antihypertensives: hydralazine (mild to moderte hypertension), labetalol (severe hypertension)

INTERVENTIONS AND RATIONALES

- Monitor vital signs and electrolyte values. Monitor fluid intake and output and daily weight. Assess renal function daily through serum creatinine and BUN levels and urine creatinine clearance. Watch for signs of acute renal failure (oliguria, azotemia, acidosis). *These measures detect early signs of complications and help guide the treatment plan.*
- Consult the dietitian *to provide a diet low in protein, sodium, potassium, and fluids.*
- Provide good nutrition, use good hygienic technique, and prevent contact with infected people *to protect the debilitated client from secondary infection.*
- Encourage bed rest during the acute phase with the client gradually resuming normal activities as symptoms subside *to prevent fatigue.*
- Provide emotional support for the client and family. If the client is on dialysis, explain the procedure fully. *These measures may help ease the client's anxiety.*

Teaching topics

- Explanation of the disorder and treatment plan
- Medication use and possible adverse effects
- The importance of immediately reporting signs of infection, such as fever and sore throat (for the client with a history of chronic upper respiratory tract infections)
- The importance of follow-up examinations to detect chronic renal failure
- The need for regular blood pressure, urinary protein, and renal function assessments during the convalescent months to detect recurrence
- What to expect (after APSGN, gross hematuria may recur during nonspecific viral infections; abnormal urinary findings may persist for years)
- The possibility of orthostatic hypotension when taking diuretics and the need to change position slowly
- The need for frequent medical evaluations in pregnant clients with a history of APSGN (pregnancy further stresses the kidneys, increasing the risk of chronic renal failure)

Acute renal failure

ARF is a sudden interruption of renal function resulting from obstruction, poor circulation, or kidney disease. With treatment, this condition is usually reversible; however, if left untreated, it may progress to end-stage renal disease or death.

ARF is classified as prerenal (results from conditions that diminish blood flow to the kidneys), intrarenal (results from damage to the kidneys, usually from acute tubular necrosis), or postrenal (results from bilateral obstruction of urine flow).

CAUSES
- Acute glomerulonephritis
- ATN
- Anaphylaxis
- BPH
- Blood transfusion reaction
- Burns
- Cardiopulmonary bypass
- Collagen diseases
- Congenital deformity
- Dehydration
- Diabetes mellitus
- Heart failure, cardiogenic shock, endocarditis, malignant hypertension
- Hemorrhage
- Hypotension
- Nephrotoxins: antibiotics, X-ray dyes, pesticides, anesthetics
- Renal calculi
- Septicemia
- Trauma
- Tumor

ASSESSMENT FINDINGS
- Anorexia, nausea, vomiting
- Circumoral numbness, tingling extremities
- Costovertebral pain
- Diarrhea or constipation
- Edema
- Epistaxis
- Hand tremor
- Fatigue
- Headache
- Hypertension
- Irritability, restlessness
- Lethargy, drowsiness, stupor, coma
- Pallor, ecchymosis
- Stomatitis
- Thick, tenacious sputum
- Urine output less than 400 ml/day for 1 to 2 weeks followed by diuresis (3 to 5 L/day) for 2 to 3 weeks
- Weight gain

DIAGNOSTIC TEST RESULTS
- Arterial blood gas (ABG) analysis shows metabolic acidosis.
- Blood chemistry analysis shows increased potassium, phosphorus, magnesium, BUN, creatinine, and uric acid levels and decreased calcium, carbon dioxide, and sodium levels.
- Creatinine clearance is low.
- Excretory urography shows decreased renal perfusion and function.
- Glomerular filtration rate is 20 to 40 ml/minute (renal insufficiency); 10 to 20 ml/minute (renal failure); less than 10 ml/minute (end-stage renal disease).
- Hematology shows decreased levels of Hb, HCT, and erythrocytes; and increased PT and PTT.
- Urine chemistry shows albuminuria, proteinuria, and increased sodium level; casts, RBCs, and WBCs; and urine specific gravity greater than 1.025, then fixed at less than 1.010.
- Renal ultrasound may identify obstruction in urinary tract.

NURSING DIAGNOSES
- Decreased cardiac output
- Excess fluid volume
- Ineffective tissue perfusion: Renal
- Anxiety

TREATMENT
- Hemodialysis or continuous venovenous hemofiltration
- Low-protein, increased-carbohydrate, moderate-fat, and moderate-calorie diet with potassium, sodium, and phosphorus intake regulated according to serum levels
- Fluid intake restricted to amount needed to replace fluid loss
- Transfusion therapy with packed RBCs administered over 1 to 3 hours as tolerated

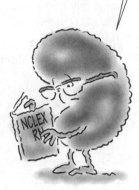

If conservative measures fail to control renal failure, hemodialysis or peritoneal dialysis may be necessary.

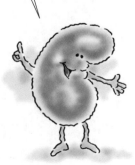

Everyone depends on me. If I fail to function, it can threaten many body systems.

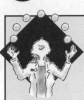

Management moments

Coping with sudden changes

The sudden life changes associated with acute renal failure may leave the client feeling anxious and afraid. Therefore, using therapeutic conversation to allow the client to express his feelings is essential. Provide the client with an environment that's relaxed and pleasant to encourage this expression. Also, allow for rest periods to minimize the client's fatigue.

EDUCATION IS KEY

Educating the client about his illness and treatment plan will help allay anxiety. Here are tips to keep in mind about your client teaching:
- Stress that following the medical regimen is essential.
- Spend uninterrupted time teaching the client, and allow plenty of time for questions.
- Provide the client and his family with written instructions when possible.
- Be sure to incorporate the client's cultural diversity in his treatment plan to aid compliance.

Obtain a dietary consult. Encourage the client and his family to discuss their needs with the dietitian, and encourage the family to bring in favorite foods that meet the client's new dietary requirements.

Drug therapy
- Alkalinizing agent: sodium bicarbonate
- Antacid: aluminum hydroxide gel
- Antibiotic: cefazolin (Ancef)
- Anticonvulsant: phenytoin (Dilantin)
- Antiemetic: prochlorperazine
- Antipyretic: acetaminophen (Tylenol)
- Inotropic agent: dopamine
- Cation exchange resin: sodium polystyrene sulfonate
- Diuretics: furosemide (Lasix), metolazone (Zaroxolyn)

INTERVENTIONS AND RATIONALES
- Monitor fluid balance, respiratory, cardiovascular, and neurologic status *to detect fluid overload, a complication of acute renal failure.*
- Monitor and record vital signs and intake and output, central venous pressure, daily weight, urine specific gravity, and laboratory studies *to detect early signs of fluid overload.*
- Monitor for arrhythmias *to assess for complications of fluid and electrolyte imbalance.*
- Assess for presence of dependent or generalized edema, *which may indicate fluid overload.*
- Maintain the client's diet *to promote nutritional status.*
- Restrict fluids *to prevent fluid volume excess.*

- Administer I.V. fluids *to correct electrolyte imbalance and maintain hydration.*
- Keep the client in semi-Fowler's position *to facilitate lung expansion.*
- Administer total parenteral nutrition or enteral nutrition, if indicated, *to promote nutritional status.*
- Administer medications, as prescribed, *to maintain or improve the client's condition.*
- Encourage the client to express feelings about changes in body image *to facilitate coping mechanisms.* (See *Coping with sudden changes.*)
- Maintain a quiet environment *to reduce metabolic demands.*
- Assist the client with turning, coughing, and deep breathing *to mobilize secretions and promote lung expansion.*
- Provide skin and mouth care *to promote comfort and prevent tissue breakdown.*
- Provide treatment for the underlying cause of ARF as directed.

Teaching topics
- Explanation of the disorder and treatment plan
- Medication use and possible adverse effects
- Avoiding over-the-counter medications
- Dietary modifications
- Maintaining a quiet environment

Acute tubular necrosis

ATN accounts for about 75% of all cases of acute renal failure and is the most common cause of ARF in critically ill patients. ATN injures the tubular segment of the nephron, causing renal failure and uremic syndrome. Mortality ranges from 40% to 70%, depending on complications from underlying diseases.

CAUSES
- Chemical agents
- Dehydration
- Hemorrhage
- Ischemic or nephrotoxic injury
- Nephrotoxic drugs
- Severe hypotension
- Shock
- Surgery
- Transfusion reaction
- Trauma

ASSESSMENT FINDINGS
- Acidosis
- Anemia
- Azotemia
- Confusion
- Decreased urine output
- Fever
- Hyperkalemia
- Hypertension
- Oliguria
- Poor wound healing (in late stages)
- Pulmonary edema (in late stages)

DIAGNOSTIC TEST RESULTS
- An electrocardiogram shows arrhythmias and widening QRS segment, disappearing P waves, and tall, peaked T waves (with hyperkalemia).
- Blood studies show elevated BUN and creatinine levels, anemia, metabolic acidosis, and hyperkalemia.
- Urinary tests reveal urinary sediment with RBCs and casts, a low specific gravity, and high sodium level.

NURSING DIAGNOSES
- Risk for infection
- Impaired tissue integrity
- Impaired urinary elimination
- Excess fluid volume

TREATMENT
- Administering large amounts of fluid to flush nephrotoxic agent through kidneys (early treatment)
- Fluid management with fluid restriction as needed
- Identification and removal of nephrotoxic substance
- Transfusion of RBCs for anemia administered over 1 to 3 hours as tolerated

DRUG THERAPY
- 50% glucose, regular insulin, and sodium bicarbonate for hyperkalemia
- Diuretics (early stages) to increase urine output

INTERVENTIONS AND RATIONALES
- Maintain fluid balance, and be especially alert for fluid overload.
- Carefully monitor intake and output and daily weight *to detect early signs of fluid overload.*
- Monitor for arrhythmias *to assess for complications of fluid and electrolyte imbalances.*
- Maintain the client's diet *to promote nutritional status.*
- Restrict fluids *to prevent fluid volume excess.*
- Administer medications, as prescribed, *to maintain or improve the client's condition.*
- Provide treatment for the underlying cause of ATN as directed.
- Use sterile technique for dressing and catheter care *because of increased risk of infection.*
- Monitor laboratory results, including electrolytes and hemoglobin and hematocrit *because of the risk of electrolyte imbalances and anemia.*
- Monitor the client for complications, including acidosis and pulmonary edema.
- Provide good skin care *to promote comfort and prevent tissue breakdown.*

Teaching topics
- Explanation of the disorder and treatment plan
- Medication regimen and adverse effects
- Avoiding over-the-counter medications
- Dietary modifications

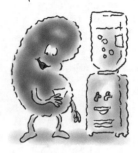

I won't let ATN ruin my day! I'm doing my part to stay hydrated!

Don't go overboard! Maintain fluid balance in a client with ATN.

Benign prostatic hyperplasia

BPH is enlargement of the prostate gland that causes compression of the urethra and possible urinary obstruction.

CAUSES
- Unknown

CONTRIBUTING FACTORS
- Aging

ASSESSMENT FINDINGS
- Decreased force and amount of urine
- Dribbling
- Dysuria
- Enlarged prostate (as felt on digital rectal examination)
- Hesitancy
- Nocturia
- Urgency, frequency, and burning on urination
- Urinary tract infection (UTI)
- Urine retention

DIAGNOSTIC TEST RESULTS
- BPH screening test indicates severity of symptoms.
- CMG shows abnormal pressure recordings.
- Cystoscopy shows enlarged prostate gland, obstructed urine flow, and urinary stasis.
- Excretory urography shows urethral obstruction, and hydronephrosis.
- Prostate-specific antigen (PSA) levels are low.
- Urinary flow rate determination shows small volume, prolonged flow pattern, low peak flow.
- Urine chemistry analysis shows bacteria, hematuria, alkaline pH, and increased urine specific gravity.

NURSING DIAGNOSES
- Sexual dysfunction
- Impaired urinary elimination
- Urinary retention

TREATMENT
- Encouraging fluids
- Transurethral resection of the prostate (TURP) or prostatectomy

Drug therapy
- Alpha-adrenergic blockers: tamsulosin (Flomax), terazosin (Hytrin), doxazosin (Cardura), alfuzosin (Uroxatral)
- Analgesic: oxycodone hydrochloride (Tylox)
- Sedative: lorazepam (Ativan)
- Antibiotic: co-trimoxazole (Bactrim)
- Urinary antiseptic: phenazopyridine

INTERVENTIONS AND RATIONALES
- Assess fluid balance *to determine fluid deficit or overload.*
- Monitor and record vital signs and intake and output. *Accurate intake and output are essential to detect urine retention if the client doesn't have an indwelling urinary catheter in place.*
- Monitor for UTI *to assess for complications.*
- Encourage fluid intake *to improve hydration.*
- Administer medications, as prescribed, *to maintain or improve the client's condition.*
- Encourage the client to express feelings about changes in body image and fear of sexual dysfunction *to help pinpoint fears, establish trust, and facilitate coping.*
- Maintain the position and patency of the indwelling urinary catheter to straight drainage *to avoid urine reflux.*
- Maintain activity, as tolerated, *to promote independence.*
- Provide routine postoperative care *to prevent complications.*
- Postoperatively, monitor continuous bladder irrigation and urine color *to assess bleeding.*

Teaching topics
- Recognizing the signs and symptoms of urine retention
- Adhering to medical follow-up

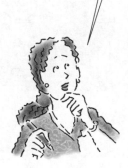

Relate assessment findings to how the disorder affects the body. BPH can compress the urethra. Decreased force and amount of urination is a key sign.

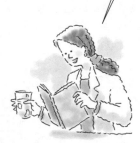

Drinking fluids is important for BPH clients—and for you. Staying hydrated will help keep your body in shape for studying.

Bladder cancer

Bladder cancer is a malignant tumor that invades the mucosal lining of the bladder. It may metastasize to the ureters, prostate gland, vagina, rectum, and periaortic lymph nodes.

CAUSES
- Chronic bladder irritation
- Cigarette smoking
- Drug-induced from cyclophosphamide (Cytoxan)
- Excessive intake of coffee, phenacetin, sodium, saccharin, sodium cyclamate
- Exposure to industrial chemicals
- Radiation

ASSESSMENT FINDINGS
- Anuria
- Chills
- Dysuria
- Fever
- Flank or pelvic pain
- Urinary frequency
- Hematuria
- Peripheral edema
- Urinary urgency

DIAGNOSTIC TEST RESULTS
- Computed tomography (CT) scan may identify a mass.
- Cystoscopy reveals a mass.
- Cytologic examination is positive for malignant cells.
- Excretory urography shows a mass or an obstruction.
- Hematology shows decreased RBC count, Hb levels, and HCT.
- KUB X-ray shows mass or obstruction.
- Urine chemistry shows hematuria.

NURSING DIAGNOSES
- Functional urinary incontinence
- Chronic pain
- Impaired urinary elimination
- Anxiety
- Fear

TREATMENT
- Transfusion therapy with packed RBCs
- Radiation therapy
- Biological therapy: interferon alfa, rituxan (Rituximab)
- Surgery, depending on location and progress of tumor (see *Bladder cancer treatment options*)

Drug therapy
- Analgesics: meperidine (Demerol), morphine
- Antispasmodic: phenazopyridine
- Sedative: lorazepam (Ativan)

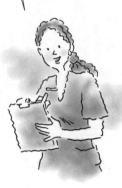

Postoperative pointer: With bladder cancer clients, be sure to monitor urine for signs of hematuria or infection.

Bladder cancer treatment options

Treatment options for bladder cancer depend on the client's lifestyle, other health problems, and mental outlook.

TUMOR THAT HASN'T INVADED MUSCLE
With transurethral resection, superficial bladder tumors are removed cytoscopically by transurethral resection and electrically by fulguration. The procedure is effective only if the tumor hasn't invaded muscle. Additional tumors may develop, and fulguration may need repeating every 3 months for years.

SUPERFICIAL TUMOR
Intravesical chemotherapy is commonly used to treat superficial bladder tumors (especially when tumors are in several sites). This treatment washes the bladder with drugs that fight cancer, usually thiotepa, doxorubicin, and mitomycin.

INFILTRATING TUMOR
Radical cystectomy is the choice for infiltrating bladder tumors or for superficial cancer that involves a large part of the bladder. In this procedure, the bladder is removed and a urinary diversion is created.

REMOVAL OF A SECTION
Segmental bladder resection removes a full-thickness section of the bladder. It's only used if the tumor isn't located near the bladder neck or ureteral orifices.

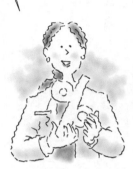

Check out this stat: 70% of breast cancer cases occur in women older than age 50.

• Systemic, regional, or intravesical chemotherapy based on type and stage of cancer

INTERVENTIONS AND RATIONALES

• Monitor renal status *to determine baseline and detect early changes*.
• Monitor and record vital signs and intake and output. *Accurate intake and output are essential for correct fluid replacement therapy*.
• Provide postoperative care *to promote healing and prevent complications*. (Closely monitor urine output; observe for hematuria [reddish tint to gross bloodiness] or infection [cloudy, foul smelling, with sediment]; maintain continuous bladder irrigation if indicated; assist with turning, coughing, and deep breathing.)
• Maintain the client's diet *to improve nutrition and meet metabolic demands*.
• Encourage fluid intake *to prevent dehydration*.
• Administer I.V. fluids *to maintain hydration*.
• Assess pain level, provide analgesics, and evaluate their effectiveness *to promote comfort*.
• Administer medications, as prescribed, *to maintain or improve the client's condition*.
• Provide emotional support and encourage the client to express feelings about a fear of dying *to encourage adequate coping mechanisms*.
• Provide postchemotherapeutic care (watch for myelosuppression, chemical cystitis, and skin rash) and postradiation nursing care *to prevent complications associated with treatment*.

Teaching topics
• Explanation of the disorder and treatment plan
• Medication use and possible adverse effects
• Wound and ostomy care, if appropriate
• Contacting the American Cancer Society
• Contacting community agencies and resources for supportive services
• Skin care after radiation therapy such as avoiding cold packs to the area

Breast cancer

Breast cancer is the most common cancer in women. Although the disease may develop any time after puberty, 70% of cases occur in women older than age 50. Breast cancer can also occur in men but the incidence is rare. Breast cancer is generally classified by the tissue of origin and the location of the lesion; for example:
• Adenocarcinoma, the most common form of breast cancer, arises from the epithelial tissues.
• Intraductal cancer develops within the ducts.
• Intrafiltrating cancer arises in the parenchymal tissue.
• Inflammatory cancer (rare) grows rapidly and causes the overlying skin to become edematous, inflamed, and indurated.
• Lobular cancer involves the lobes of the glandular tissue.
• Medullary or circumscribed cancer is a tumor that grows rapidly.

CAUSES
• Exact cause unknown (scientists have discovered specific genes linked to breast cancer, which confirms that the disease can be inherited from a person's mother or father)
• Family history of breast cancer
• First pregnancy after age 35

CONTRIBUTING FACTORS
• Heavy alcohol and tobacco use
• Being a premenopausal woman older than age 40
• Benign breast disease
• Early onset menses or late menopause
• Endometrial or ovarian cancer
• Estrogen therapy
• High-fat diet
• Previous history of breast cancer
• Nulligravida (never pregnant)
• Obesity
• Radiation exposure

ASSESSMENT FINDINGS
• Supraclavicular or axillary lymph node lump or enlargement on palpation

- Clear, milky, or bloody discharge from the nipple
- Edema in the affected arm
- Erythema
- Nipple retraction
- Painless lump or mass in the breast or thickening of breast tissue detected on self-examination
- Skin or nipple changes

DIAGNOSTIC TEST RESULTS

- Chest X-rays can pinpoint chest metastasis.
- Fine-needle aspiration and excisional biopsy provide histologic cells that confirm diagnosis.
- Hormonal receptor assay pinpoints whether the tumor is estrogen- or progesterone-dependent.
- Magnetic resonance imaging can detect a tumor, even a small one.
- Mammography or ultrasonograpy detects a tumor.
- Scans of the bone, brain, liver, and other organs can detect distant metastasis.
- Ultrasonography distinguishes between a fluid-filled cyst and a solid mass.

NURSING DIAGNOSES

- Disturbed body image
- Anxiety
- Fear
- Chronic pain

TREATMENT

- High-protein diet
- Bone marrow and peripheral stem cell therapy for advanced breast cancer
- Radiation therapy
- Surgery: lumpectomy, skin-sparing mastectomy, partial mastectomy, total mastectomy, or modified radical mastectomy, and quandrantectomy
- Transfusion therapy if needed

Drug therapy

- Analgesic: morphine
- Antiemetics: aprepitant (Emend), prochlorperazine
- Chemotherapy: cyclophosphamide (Cytoxan), methotrexate (Trexall), fluorouracil

- Hormonal therapy: tamoxifen, toremifene (Fareston), diethylstilbestrol, megestrol (Megace)

INTERVENTIONS AND RATIONALES

- Assess the client's feelings about her illness, and determine what she knows about breast cancer and what her expectations are *to help identify her needs and aid in developing a care plan.*
- Encourage the client to ask questions about her illness and treatment options *to reduce anxiety and promote autonomy.*
- Provide routine postoperative care *to prevent postoperative complications.*
- Provide emotional support and comfort measures *to promote relaxation and relieve anxiety.*
- Assess pain level and administer analgesics as ordered, and monitor their effectiveness *to promote client comfort.*
- Monitor for treatment-related complications, such as nausea, vomiting, anorexia, leukopenia, thrombocytopenia, GI ulceration, and bleeding, *to ensure that measures are taken to prevent further complications.*
- Monitor the client's weight and nutritional intake *to detect evidence of malnutrition.* Encourage a high-protein diet. Dietary supplements may be necessary *to meet increased metabolic demands.*
- Assess the client's and family's ability to cope and provide emotional support. *Counseling may be necessary to help them cope with the fear of death and dying.*

Teaching topics

- Explanation of the disorder and treatment plan
- Medication use and possible adverse effects
- Treatment options
- Managing adverse reactions to treatment
- Importance of immediately reporting signs of infection to the physician
- Breast self-examination
- Availability of community support services
- Contacting the American Cancer Society

> Assess the client's and family's ability to cope. Counseling may be necessary, especially if the breast cancer is terminal.

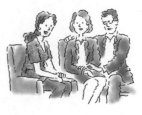

Cervical cancer

The third most common cancer of the female reproductive system, cervical cancer is cancerous cells that affect the cervix and is classified as either preinvasive or invasive. Preinvasive cancers range from minimal cervical dysplasia, in which the lower third of the epithelium contains abnormal cells, to carcinoma in situ, in which the full thickness of the epithelium contains abnormally proliferating cells.

CAUSES
• Unknown

CONTRIBUTING FACTORS
• Frequent intercourse at a young age (younger than 16)
• History of human papillomavirus or other bacterial or viral venereal infections
• Multiple pregnancies
• Multiple sex partners
• Untreated chronic cervicitis

ASSESSMENT FINDINGS
Preinvasive
• Absence of symptoms

Invasive
• Abnormal vaginal discharge (yellowish, blood-tinged, and foul-smelling)
• Gradually increasing flank pain
• Leakage of feces (with metastasis to the rectum with fistula development)
• Leakage of urine (with metastasis into the bladder with formation of a fistula)
• Postcoital pain and bleeding; irregular bleeding

DIAGNOSTIC TEST RESULTS
• Colposcopy determines the source of the abnormal cells seen on the Papanicolaou (Pap) test.
• Cone biopsy, performed if endocervical curettage is positive, identifies malignant cells.
• Lymphangiograpy, cystography, and major organ and bone scans can detect metastasis.

NURSING DIAGNOSES
• Anxiety
• Fear
• Impaired tissue integrity
• Chronic pain

TREATMENT
Preinvasive
• Conization, cryosurgery
• Hysterectomy (rare)
• Laser destruction
• Total excisional biopsy

Invasive
• Pelvic exoneration (rare)
• Radiation therapy (internal, external, or both)
• Radical hysterectomy

Drug therapy
Chemotherapy is usually ineffective in treating cervical cancer. When used, it consists of hydroxyurea (Hydrea) in combination with radiation treatment.

INTERVENTIONS AND RATIONALES
• Encourage the client to use relaxation techniques *to promote comfort during diagnostic procedures.*
• Provide emotional support and comfort measures *to help alleviate anxiety.*
• Watch for complications related to therapy *to ensure that measures can be instituted to prevent or alleviate complications.*
• Assess pain level and administer pain medication, as needed, and note its effectiveness *to promote comfort.*
• Maintain diet *to promote recovery.*

Teaching topics
• Explanation of the disorder and treatment plan
• Medication use and possible adverse effects
• Treatment options
• Postexcisional biopsy care (expecting discharge or spotting for about 1 week; avoiding douching, using tampons, or engaging in sexual intercourse during this time; reporting signs of infection)
• Follow-up Pap tests and pelvic examinations
• Contact information for American Cancer Society and local support groups

Chlamydia

Chlamydia refers to a group of infections linked to one organism: *Chlamydia trachomatis*. Chlamydia infection causes urethritis in men and urethritis and cervicitis in women. Untreated, chlamydial infections can lead to such complications as acute epididymitis, salpingitis, pelvic inflammatory disease (PID) and, eventually, sterility. Chlamydial infections are the most common sexually transmitted diseases (STDs) in the United States.

CAUSES
• Exposure to *C. trachomatis* through sexual contact

ASSESSMENT FINDINGS
In women
• Cervical erosion
• Dyspareunia
• Mucopurulent discharge
• Pelvic pain

In men
• Dysuria
• Erythema
• Pruritus
• Tenderness of the meatus
• Urethral discharge
• Urinary frequency

DIAGNOSTIC TEST RESULTS
• A swab from the site of infection (urethra, cervix, or rectum) establishes a diagnosis of urethritis, cervicitis, salpingitis, endometritis, or proctitis.
• A culture of aspirated material establishes a diagnosis of epididymitis.
• Antigen detection methods (the diagnostic tests of choice), including enzyme-linked immunosorbent assay and direct fluorescent antibody test, identify chlamydial infection, although tissue cell cultures are more sensitive and specific.

NURSING DIAGNOSES
• Impaired urinary elimination
• Chronic pain
• Deficient knowledge (disease transmission)
• Ineffective sexual patterns
• Situational low self-esteem

TREATMENT
The only treatment available for chlamydial infection is drug therapy.

Drug therapy
• Antibiotics: doxycycline (Vibramycin), azithromycin (Zithromax)
• For pregnant women with chlamydial infections, azithromycin in a single dose

INTERVENTIONS AND RATIONALES
• Maintain standard precautions *to prevent the spread of infection*.
• Make sure that the client understands the dosage requirements of any prescribed medications for this infection *to ensure compliance with the treatment regimen*.
• If required in your state, report all cases of chlamydial infection to the appropriate local public health authorities, who will conduct follow-up notification of the client's sexual contacts. *These measures help ensure that an infected sexual contact will receive medical care to treat the infection.*
• Suggest that the client and his sexual partners receive testing for human immuno-deficiency virus (HIV). *Unsafe sex practices, which lead to chlamydial infection, also place the client at risk for contracting HIV.*
• Check neonates of infected mothers for signs of chlamydial infection *to ensure prompt recognition and treatment of infection*. Obtain appropriate specimens for diagnostic testing *to confirm the diagnosis of chlamydial infection*.

Teaching topics
• Explanation of the disorder and treatment plan
• Medication use and possible adverse effects
• Safer sex practices
• Importance of taking all of the medication, even after symptoms subside
• Avoiding contact with eyes after touching discharge
• Proper hand-washing technique
• Importance of follow-up medical care

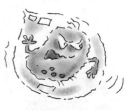

What a little microorganism can do! Chlamydia is a group of infections linked to *C. trachomatis*.

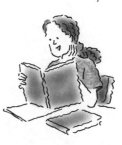

Because signs of chlamydial infection occur late in the course of illness, transmission usually occurs unknowingly.

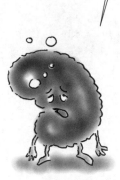

By the time chronic glomerulonephritis is diagnosed, the client usually can't be cured and must rely on dialysis or a kidney transplant.

Chronic glomerulonephritis

A slowly progressive disease, chronic glomerulonephritis is characterized by inflammation of the glomeruli (the kidney's blood vessels), which results in sclerosis, scarring and, eventually, renal failure.

By the time it produces symptoms, chronic glomerulonephritis is usually irreversible.

CAUSES
- Burns
- Hemolytic transfusion reaction
- Nephrotoxic drugs
- Renal disorders
- Septicemia
- Systemic disorders (lupus erythematosus, Goodpasture's syndrome, and diabetes mellitus)

ASSESSMENT FINDINGS
- Edema
- Hematuria
- Hypertension
- Uremic symptoms (in the late stages of the disease)

DIAGNOSTIC TEST RESULTS
- Kidney biopsy identifies underlying disease and provides data needed to guide therapy.
- Blood studies reveal rising BUN and serum creatinine levels.
- Urinalysis reveals proteinuria, hematuria, cylindruria, and RBC casts.
- X-ray or ultrasonography shows small kidneys.

NURSING DIAGNOSES
- Impaired urinary elimination
- Excess fluid volume
- Risk for injury

TREATMENT
- Dialysis
- Low-sodium, high-calorie diet with adequate protein
- Kidney transplant

Drug therapy
- Antibiotics (for symptomatic UTIs)
- Antihypertensive: metoprolol (Lopressor)
- Diuretic: furosemide (Lasix)

INTERVENTIONS AND RATIONALES
- Provide supportive care *to encourage the client to cope with chronic disease.*
- Monitor vital signs, intake and output, and daily weight *to evaluate fluid retention.*
- Assess for signs of fluid, electrolyte, and acid-base imbalances *to ensure early treatment and prevent complications.*
- Consult a dietitian *to plan low-sodium, high-calorie meals with adequate protein.*
- Administer medications and provide good skin care *to combat pruritus and edema.*
- Provide good oral hygiene *to prevent breakdown of the oral mucosa.*

Teaching topics
- Explanation of the disorder and treatment plan
- Medication use and possible adverse effects
- Reporting signs of infection, particularly UTI, and avoiding contact with people who have infections
- Importance of follow-up examinations to assess renal function
- Importance of dietary modifications

Chronic renal failure

Chronic renal failure is progressive, irreversible destruction of the kidneys, leading to loss of renal function. It may result from a rapidly progressing disease of sudden onset that destroys the nephrons and causes irreversible kidney damage.

CAUSES
- Congenital abnormalities
- Dehydration
- Diabetes mellitus
- Exacerbations of nephritis
- Hypertension
- Nephrotoxins
- Recurrent UTI
- Systemic lupus erythematosus (SLE)
- Urinary tract obstructions

ASSESSMENT FINDINGS
- Azotemia
- Bone pain
- Brittle nails and hair

- Decreased urine output
- Ecchymosis
- Heart failure
- Lethargy
- Muscle twitching
- Paresthesia
- Pruritus
- Seizures
- Stomatitis
- Weight gain

DIAGNOSTIC TEST RESULTS
- ABG analysis shows metabolic acidosis.
- Blood chemistry analysis shows increased BUN, creatinine, phosphorus, and lipid levels and decreased calcium, carbon dioxide, and albumin levels.
- Hematology shows decreased Hb levels, HCT, and platelet count.
- Urine chemistry analysis shows proteinuria, increased WBC count, sodium level, and decreased and then fixed urine specific gravity.

NURSING DIAGNOSES
- Decreased cardiac output
- Excess fluid volume
- Ineffective tissue perfusion (renal)

TREATMENT
- Fluid restriction
- Low-protein, low-sodium, low-potassium, low-phosphorus, high-calorie, and high-carbohydrate diet
- Peritoneal dialysis and hemodialysis (see *Types of dialysis,* page 336.)
- Transfusion therapy with packed RBCs and platelets

Drug therapy
- Alkalinizing agent: sodium bicarbonate
- Antacid: aluminum hydroxide gel
- Antianemics: ferrous sulfate (Feosol), iron dextran (INFeD), epoetin alfa (recombinant human erythropoietin, Epogen)
- Antiarrhythmic: procainamide (Procan)
- Antibiotic: cefazolin
- Antiemetic: prochlorperazine
- Antipyretic: acetaminophen (Tylenol)

- Beta-adrenergic blocker: dopamine
- Calcium supplement: calcium carbonate (Os-Cal)
- Cation exchange resin: sodium polystyrene sulfonate
- Cardiac glycoside: digoxin (Lanoxin)
- Diuretic: furosemide (Lasix)
- Stool softener: docusate sodium (Colace)
- Vitamins: pyridoxine (vitamin B_6), ascorbic acid (vitamin C)

INTERVENTIONS AND RATIONALES
- Monitor renal, respiratory, and cardiovascular status and fluid balance. *An increase in hemodynamic status and vital signs may indicate fluid overload caused by lack of kidney function.*
- Assess dialysis access for bruit and thrill *to ensure patency and detect complications.*
- Monitor and record vital signs, intake and output, electrocardiogram values, daily weight, laboratory studies, and stools for occult blood *to assess baseline and detect early changes in the client's condition.*
- Maintain standard precautions *to prevent the spread of infection.*
- Maintain the client's diet *to promote nutritional status.*
- Restrict fluids *to prevent fluid overload.*
- Administer medications, as prescribed, *to improve or maintain the client's condition.*
- Encourage the client to express feelings about chronicity of illness *to encourage coping.*
- Provide tepid baths *to promote comfort and reduce skin irritation.*
- Maintain a cool and quiet environment *to reduce metabolic demands.*
- Provide skin and mouth care using plain water *to promote comfort.*

Teaching topics
- Explanation of the disorder and treatment plan
- Medication use and possible adverse effects
- Dietary modifications
- Dialysis access care

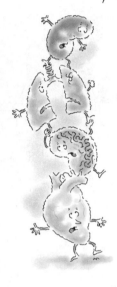

Yikes! Chronic renal failure produces major changes in all the client's body systems.

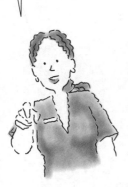

Advise the client to take diuretics in the morning so he won't have to disrupt his sleep to void.

Types of dialysis

The two types of dialysis used to treat chronic renal failure are hemodialysis and peritoneal dialysis.

REMOVING WASTE

Hemodialysis removes toxic wastes and other impurities from the blood. Blood is removed from the body through a surgically created access site, pumped through a filtration unit to remove toxins, and then returned to the body. The extracorporeal dialyzer works through osmosis, diffusion, and filtration. Hemodialysis is performed by specially trained nurses.

Nursing actions
• Monitor the venous access site for bleeding. If bleeding is excessive, maintain pressure on the site.
• Don't use the arm for blood pressure monitoring, I.V. catheter insertion, or venipuncture.
• At least four times daily, auscultate the access site for bruits and palpate for thrills.

USING THE BODY

Peritoneal dialysis removes toxins from the blood but, unlike hemodialysis, it uses the client's peritoneal membrane as a semipermeable dialyzing membrane. Hypertonic dialyzing solution is instilled through a catheter inserted into the peritoneal cavity. Then by diffusion, excessive concentrations of electrolytes and uremic toxins in the blood move across the peritoneal membrane and into the dialysis solution. Next, by osmosis, excessive water in the blood does the same.

After appropriate dwelling time, the dialysis solution is drained, taking toxins and wastes with it. The client is trained to perform this procedure.

Nursing actions
• Check the client's weight, and report any gain.
• Using sterile technique, change the catheter dressing every 24 hours and whenever it becomes wet or soiled.
• Calculate the client's fluid balance at the end of each dialysis session. Include oral and I.V. fluid intake as well as urine output and wound drainage. Record and report any significant imbalance, either positive or negative.

Cystitis

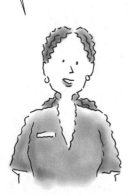

Cystitis is usually easy to cure, but reinfection and residual bacterial flare-up during treatment are possible.

Cystitis is the inflammation of the urinary bladder. It's usually related to a superficial infection that doesn't extend to the bladder mucosa.

CAUSES
• Diabetes mellitus
• Incorrect sterile technique during catheterization
• Incorrect perineal care
• Kidney infection
• Obstruction of the urethra
• Pregnancy
• Radiation
• Sexual intercourse
• Stagnation of urine in the bladder

ASSESSMENT FINDINGS
• Burning or pain on urination
• Dark, odoriferous urine
• Dribbling
• Dysuria
• Flank tenderness or suprapubic pain
• Lower abdominal discomfort
• Low-grade fever
• Nocturia
• Urge to bear down on urination
• Urinary frequency
• Urinary urgency

DIAGNOSTIC TEST RESULTS
• Cystoscopy shows obstruction or deformity.
• Urine chemistry analysis shows hematuria, pyuria, and increased protein, leukocytes, and urine specific gravity.
• Urine culture and sensitivity analysis positively identifies organisms (*Escherichia coli, Proteus vulgaris,* or *Streptococcus faecalis*).

NURSING DIAGNOSES
• Impaired urinary elimination
• Urge urinary incontinence
• Acute pain

TREATMENT

- Increased intake of fluids and vitamin C

Drug therapy

- Antibiotics: co-trimoxazole (Bactrim), levofloxacin (Levaquin), ciprofloxacin (Cipro)
- Antipyretic: acetaminophen (Tylenol)
- Urinary antiseptic: phenazopyridine

INTERVENTIONS AND RATIONALES

- Monitor renal status *to determine baseline and detect changes.*
- Monitor and record vital signs, intake and output, and laboratory studies *to assess client's status and detect early complications.*
- Maintain the client's diet *to promote nutrition.*
- Encourage increased fluid intake (cranberry or orange juice) to 3 qt (3 L)/day *because dilute urine lessens the irritation to the bladder mucosa and lowering urine pH with orange juice and cranberry juice consumption helps diminish bacterial growth.*
- Administer medications, as prescribed, *to maintain or improve the client's condition.*
- Perform sitz baths and perineal care *to relieve perineal or suprapubic discomfort.*
- Encourage voiding every 2 to 3 hours. *Frequent bladder emptying decreases bladder irritation and prevents stasis of urine.*
- Encourage female clients to wear cotton underwear *to decrease irritation.*

Teaching topics

- Explanation of the disorder and treatment plan
- Medication use and possible adverse effects
- Avoiding coffee, tea, alcohol, and carbonated beverages
- Increasing fluid intake to 3 qt (3 L)/day, using orange juice and cranberry juice
- Voiding every 2 to 3 hours and after intercourse
- Performing perineal care correctly
- Avoiding bubble baths, vaginal deodorants, and tub baths

Gonorrhea

A common STD, gonorrhea is an infection of the genitourinary tract (especially the urethra and cervix) and, occasionally, the rectum, pharynx, and eyes. Untreated gonorrhea can spread through the blood to the joints, tendons, meninges, and endocardium; in females, it can also lead to chronic PID and sterility.

After adequate treatment, the prognosis in both males and females is excellent, although reinfection is common. Gonorrhea is especially prevalent among young people and people with multiple partners, particularly those between ages 19 and 25.

CAUSES

- Exposure to *Neisseria gonorrhoeae* through sexual contact

ASSESSMENT FINDINGS

- Dysuria (painful urination)
- Purulent urethral or cervical discharge
- Redness and swelling
- Itching, burning, and a red and edematous meatus

DIAGNOSTIC TEST RESULTS

- A culture from the site of infection (urethra, cervix, rectum, or pharynx) usually establishes the diagnosis by isolating the organism.
- A Gram stain showing gram-negative diplococci supports the diagnosis and may be sufficient to confirm gonorrhea in males.

NURSING DIAGNOSES

- Chronic pain
- Ineffective sexuality patterns
- Deficient knowledge (disorder and treatment)

TREATMENT

- Moist heat to affected joints, if gonococcal arthritis is present

Drug therapy

- Antibiotics: ceftriaxone (Rocephin), doxycycline (Vibramycin), erythromycin

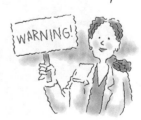

Emphasize to the client with gonorrhea that he may be infectious even if no symptoms of the disease are present.

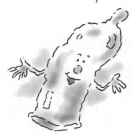

Effective treatment of all STDs includes thorough client teaching.

• Prophylactic antibiotics: 1% silver nitrate or erythromycin (EryPed) eyedrops to prevent infection in neonates

INTERVENTIONS AND RATIONALES
• Before treatment, establish whether the client has any drug sensitivities, and watch closely for adverse effects during therapy *to prevent severe adverse reactions.*
• Warn the client that, until cultures prove negative, he's still infectious and can transmit gonococcal infection *to prevent the spread of infection to others.*
• Maintain standard precautions *to prevent the spread of infection.*
• Apply moist heat *to ease pain in affected joints* (for arthritis).
• Urge the client to inform sexual contacts of his infection *so that they can seek treatment, even if cultures are negative.*
• Check neonates of infected mothers for signs of infection. Take specimens for culture from the neonate's eyes, pharynx, and rectum. *These measures ensure prompt recognition and treatment of infection in the neonate.*
• Report all cases of gonorrhea in children to child abuse authorities *to provide protection to the child.*

Teaching topics
• Explanation of the disorder and treatment plan
• Medication use and possible adverse effects
• Safer sex practices
• How disease is transmitted
• Importance of continuing antibiotic therapy for the duration prescribed

Herpes simplex

A recurrent viral infection, herpes simplex is caused by two types of *Herpesvirus hominis* (HVH), a widespread infectious agent:
• Herpes virus Type 1, which is transmitted by oral and respiratory secretions, affects the skin and mucous membranes and commonly produces cold sores and fever blisters.
• Herpes virus Type 2 primarily affects the genital area and is transmitted by sexual

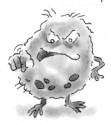

After the first infection with *H. hominis*, the person carries the virus permanently and is vulnerable to recurrent herpes infection.

contact. Cross-infection may result from orogenital sex.

CAUSES
• Exposure to herpes virus Type 2 through sexual contact
• Contact with herpes virus Type 1 through oral or respiratory secretions

ASSESSMENT FINDINGS
• Appetite loss
• Blisters or lesions on any part of the mouth accompanied by erythema and edema
• Conjunctivitis (herpetic keratoconjunctivitis or herpes of the eye)
• Fever
• Flulike symptoms
• Increased salivation
• Swelling of the lymph nodes under the jaw

Genital herpes
• Fever, swollen lymph nodes
• Fluid-filled blisters
• Dysuria

DIAGNOSTIC TEST RESULTS
• Isolation of the virus from local lesions and a histologic biopsy confirms the diagnosis.
• Blood studies reveal a rise in antibodies and moderate leukocytosis.

NURSING DIAGNOSES
• Impaired urinary elimination
• Acute or chronic pain
• Impaired oral mucous membrane

TREATMENT
Symptomatic and supportive treatment

Drug therapy
• Analgesic-antipyretic agent: acetaminophen (Tylenol) to reduce fever and relieve pain
• A drying agent, such as calamine lotion, to relieve pain of genital lesions
• Antiviral agents: idoxuridine (Herplex), trifluridine (Viroptic), and vidarabine (Vira-A)
• 5% acyclovir (Zovirax) ointment (possible relief to clients with genital herpes or to immunosuppressed clients with HVH skin infections; I.V. acyclovir to help treat more severe infections)

INTERVENTIONS AND RATIONALES

- Maintain standard precautions. For clients with extensive cutaneous, oral, or genital lesions, institute contact precautions *to prevent the spread of infection.*
- Administer pain medications and prescribed antiviral agents as ordered *to relieve pain and treat infection.*
- Provide supportive care, as indicated, such as oral hygiene, nutritional supplementation, and antipyretics for fever. *These measures enhance the client's well-being.*
- Abstain from direct client care if you have herpetic whitlow (an HVH finger infection that commonly affects health care workers) *to prevent the spread of infection.*

Teaching topics

- Explanation of the disorder and treatment plan
- Medication use and possible adverse effects
- Avoiding infecting others
- Importance of annual Pap test in women with genital herpes

Neurogenic bladder

Neurogenic bladder refers to all types of bladder dysfunction caused by an interruption of normal bladder innervation. Subsequent complications include incontinence, residual urine retention, UTI, calculus formation, and renal failure. A neurogenic bladder may be described as spastic (resulting from an upper motor neuron lesion) or flaccid (resulting from a lower motor neuron lesion).

This disorder is also known as *neuromuscular dysfunction of the lower urinary tract, neurologic bladder dysfunction,* and *neuropathic bladder.*

CAUSES

- Acute infectious diseases such as Guillain-Barré syndrome
- Cerebral disorder (stroke, brain tumor [meningioma and glioma], Parkinson's disease, multiple sclerosis, dementia)
- Chronic alcoholism
- Collagen diseases such as SLE
- Disorders of peripheral innervation
- Distant effects of cancer such as primary oat cell carcinoma of the lung
- Heavy metal toxicity
- Herpes zoster
- Metabolic disturbances (hypothyroidism, porphyria, or uremia)
- Sacral agenesis
- Spinal cord disease or trauma
- Vascular diseases such as atherosclerosis

ASSESSMENT FINDINGS

- Altered micturition
- Overflow incontinence, diminished anal sphincter tone, greatly distended bladder with an accompanying feeling of bladder fullness (flaccid neurogenic bladder)
- Hydroureteronephrosis (distention of both the ureter and the renal pelvis and calices)
- Incontinence
- Involuntary or frequent scanty urination without a feeling of bladder fullness, possible spontaneous spasms of the arms and legs, increased anal sphincter tone (spastic neurogenic bladder)
- Vesicoureteral reflux (passage of urine from the bladder back into a ureter)

DIAGNOSTIC TEST RESULTS

- Voiding cystourethrography evaluates bladder neck function, vesicoureteral reflux, and continence.
- Urodynamic studies help evaluate how urine is stored in the bladder, how well the bladder empties, and the rate of movement of urine out of the bladder during voiding.
- Retrograde urethrography reveals the presence of strictures and diverticula.

NURSING DIAGNOSES

- Impaired urinary elimination
- Urge urinary incontinence
- Urinary retention

TREATMENT

- Credé's maneuver (application of manual pressure over the lower abdomen) to evacuate the bladder

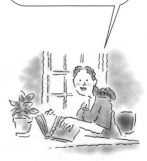

Neurogenic bladder refers to all types of bladder problems caused by disruption of normal nerve impulses to the bladder.

If urine output is considerable, empty the catheter bag more frequently than once every 8 hours. Bacteria can multiply in standing urine and migrate up the catheter and into the bladder.

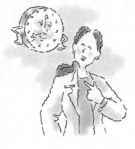

- Valsalva maneuver to promote complete emptying of the bladder
- Indwelling urinary catheter insertion
- Surgical repair if the client has structural impairment
- Surgical insertion of an artificial urinary sphincter

Drug therapy
- Urinary tract stimulants: bethanechol (Urecholine), phenoxybenzamine to facilitate bladder emptying
- Antimuscarinic agents: propantheline, flavoxate (Urispas), dicyclomine to facilitate urine storage

INTERVENTIONS AND RATIONALES
- Teach the client how to perform Credé's and Valsalva maneuvers *to evaluate the bladder.*
- Provide catheter care *to prevent infection.*
- Provide emotional support *to encourage coping.*
- Monitor for signs of infection (fever, cloudy or foul-smelling urine) *to ensure early treatment intervention and prevent complications.*
- If a urinary diversion procedure will be performed, arrange for consultation with an enterostomal therapist, and coordinate the care *to help the client cope with his change in body image.*
- Initiate a bladder program *to regulate voiding and prevent incontinence and infection.*

Teaching topics
- Explanation of the disorder and treatment plan
- Medication use and possible adverse effects
- Evacuation techniques as necessary (Credé's method, intermittent self-catheterization techniques)
- Preventing and identifying infection

Ovarian cancer

Ovarian cancer attacks the ovaries, the organs in women that produce the hormones estrogen and progesterone. After cancers of the lung, breast, and colon, primary ovarian cancer ranks as the most common cause of cancer deaths among American women. In women with previously treated breast cancer, metastatic ovarian cancer is more common than cancer at any other site. Incidence of ovarian cancer is highest in women of upper socioeconomic levels between ages 20 and 54.

The prognosis varies with the histologic type and stage of the disease but is generally poor because ovarian tumors produce few early signs and are usually advanced at diagnosis. About 40% of women with ovarian cancer survive for 5 years.

CONTRIBUTING FACTORS
- Age at menopause
- Celibacy
- Exposure to asbestos, talc, and industrial pollutants
- Familial tendency and history of breast or uterine cancer
- Fertility drugs
- High-fat diet
- Infertility

ASSESSMENT FINDINGS
- Abdominal discomfort, dyspepsia, and other mild GI disturbances
- Abdominal distention
- Constipation
- Pelvic discomfort
- Pelvic mass
- Urinary frequency
- Weight loss

DIAGNOSTIC TEST RESULTS
- Abdominal ultrasonography, CT scan, or X-ray may delineate tumor size.
- Chest X-ray may reveal distant metastasis and pleural effusions.
- Barium enema (especially in clients with GI symptoms) may reveal obstruction and size of tumor.
- Lymphangiography may show lymph node involvement.
- Mammography may rule out primary breast cancer.
- Liver scan in clients with ascites may rule out liver metastasis.
- Blood tests, such as ovarian carcinoma antigen, carcinoembryonic antigen (CEA),

and human chorionic gonadotropin, reveal presence of cancer.
- Exploratory laparotomy, including lymph node evaluation and tumor resection, confirms diagnosis and staging.

NURSING DIAGNOSES
- Ineffective protection
- Excess fluid volume
- Imbalanced nutrition: Less than body requirements
- Anxiety
- Fear
- Acute pain

TREATMENT
Conservative treatment
Occasionally, in girls or young women with a unilateral encapsulated tumor who wish to maintain fertility, the following conservative approach may be appropriate:
- resection of the involved ovary.
- biopsies of the omentum and the uninvolved ovary
- peritoneal washings for cytologic examination of pelvic fluid
- careful follow-up, including periodic chest X-rays to rule out lung metastasis

Aggressive treatment
Ovarian cancer usually requires more aggressive treatment, including:
- total abdominal hysterectomy and bilateral salpingo-oophorectomy with tumor resection, omentectomy, and appendectomy.
- lymph node biopsies with lymphadenectomy, tissue biopsies, and peritoneal washings

Drug therapy
- Antineoplastics: carboplatin (Paraplatin), chlorambucil (Leukeran), cyclophosphamide (Cytoxan), dactinomycin (Cosmegen), doxorubicin (Doxil), fluorouracil, cisplatin (Platinol), paclitaxel (Taxol), topotecan (Hycamtin)
- Analgesics: morphine, fentanyl (Duragesic-25)
- Antipyretics: aspirin, acetaminophen (Tylenol)
- Immunotherapy: bacille Calmette-Guérin vaccine

INTERVENTIONS AND RATIONALES
Before surgery
- Thoroughly explain all preoperative tests, the expected course of treatment, and surgical and postoperative procedures *to allay anxiety.*
- In premenopausal women, explain that bilateral oophorectomy artificially induces early menopause, so they may experience hot flashes, headaches, palpitations, insomnia, depression, and excessive perspiration *to help the client cope with changes in body image that occur as a result of surgery.*

After surgery
- Monitor vital signs frequently *to detect early signs of postoperative complications, such as fluid volume deficit.*
- Assess pain level, administer analgesics, and evaluate effect *to promote comfort.*
- Monitor fluid intake and output *to detect fluid volume excess or deficit.*
- Check the dressing regularly for excessive drainage or bleeding, and watch for signs of infection. *These measures detect early signs of complications and prevent treatment delay.*
- Provide abdominal support *to promote comfort,* and watch for abdominal distention, *which may indicate the presence of ascites.*
- Encourage coughing and deep breathing *to mobilize secretions and prevent postoperative pneumonia.*
- Reposition the client often *to prevent skin breakdown,* and encourage her to walk shortly after surgery *to prevent complications of immobility.*
- Monitor and treat adverse effects of radiation and chemotherapy *to prevent complications.*
- Provide emotional support and enlist the help of a social worker, chaplain, and other members of the health care team *to provide additional supportive care.*

Teaching topics
- Explanation of the disease process and treatment options
- Medication use and possible adverse effects
- Preventing and reporting infection
- Managing adverse reactions to chemotherapy

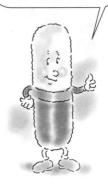

Flulike symptoms may last 12 to 24 hours after administration of immunotherapy — give aspirin or acetaminophen for fever, keep the client well covered with blankets, and provide warm liquids to relieve chills.

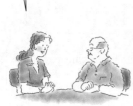

Because prostate cancer can lead to sexual dysfunction, client care may include providing information about changes in sexual activity.

Prostate cancer

Prostate cancer is a malignant tumor of the prostate gland, which can obstruct urine flow when encroaching on the bladder neck. It commonly metastasizes to bone, lymph nodes, the brain, and the lungs.

CAUSES
- No known etiology

CONTRIBUTING RISK FACTORS
- Family history
- Age
- Race
- Vasectomy
- Increased dietary fat

ASSESSMENT FINDINGS
- Decreased size and force of urine stream
- Difficulty and frequency of urination
- Hematuria
- Urine retention
- Palpable firm nodule in gland or diffuse induration in posterior lobe revealed on digital rectal examination

DIAGNOSTIC TEST RESULTS
- CEA is elevated.
- Serum acid phosphatase level is increased.
- Radioimmunoassay for acid phosphatase is increased.
- PSA is increased.
- Transurethral ultrasound studies show mass or obstruction.
- Prostate biopsy has cytology positive for cancer cells.
- Excretory urogram shows mass or obstruction.

NURSING DIAGNOSES
- Chronic pain
- Sexual dysfunction
- Impaired urinary elimination
- Anxiety
- Fear

TREATMENT
- High-protein diet with restrictions on caffeine and spicy foods
- Radiation implant
- Radical prostatectomy (for localized tumors without metastasis) or TURP (to relieve obstruction in metastatic disease)

Drug therapy
- Analgesics: oxycodone (Tylox), meperidine (Demerol), morphine
- Antiemetics: prochlorperazine (Compazine), ondansetron (Zofran)
- Antineoplastics: doxorubicin, cisplatin (Platinol)
- Corticosteroid: prednisone
- Estrogen therapy: diethylstilbestrol
- Immunosuppressant: cyclophosphamide (Cytoxan)
- Luteinizing hormone-releasing hormone agonists: goserelin (Zoladex), leuprolide (Lupron)
- Nonsteroidal anti-inflammatory drugs: indomethacin (Indocin), ibuprofen (Motrin)
- Stool softener: docusate sodium (Colace)

INTERVENTIONS AND RATIONALES
- Monitor renal and fluid status *to determine baseline and detect early changes.*
- Monitor and record vital signs, fluid intake and output, and laboratory studies. *Accurate intake and output are essential for correct fluid replacement therapy.*
- Maintain adequate hydration *to promote urination.*
- Monitor for signs of infection *to assess for complications.*
- Assess pain level and note the effectiveness of analgesia *to promote comfort.*
- Administer medications, as prescribed, *to maintain or improve the client's condition.*
- Maintain the client's diet *to maintain nutritional level and meet increased metabolic demands.*
- Maintain the patency of the urinary catheter and note drainage *to ensure urine drainage.*
- Provide emotional support and encourage the client to express feelings about the changes in body image and fear of sexual dysfunction *to encourage coping and adaptation.*
- Encourage ambulation *to prevent complications of immobility.*

• Provide postoperative, postchemotherapeutic, and postradiation nursing care *to prevent complications.*

Teaching topics
• Explanation of the disorder and treatment plan
• Medication use and possible adverse effects
• Managing changes in sexual activity
• Avoiding prolonged sitting, standing, and walking
• Avoiding the strain of exercise and lifting
• Urinating frequently
• Avoiding coffee and cola beverages
• Decreasing fluid intake during evening hours
• Performing perineal exercises
• Completing catheter care as directed
• Self-monitoring for bloody urine, pain, burning, frequency, decreased urine output, and loss of bladder control
• Contacting the American Cancer Society
• Contacting community agencies and resources for supportive services

Renal calculi

Renal calculi, also known as *kidney stones,* are crystalline substances that vary in size. Under normal circumstances, calculi are dissolved and excreted in the urine. However, larger calculi can cause great pain and may become lodged in the ureter.

CAUSES
• Urinary stasis
• Urinary tract obstruction

CONTRIBUTING FACTORS
• Chemotherapy
• Dehydration
• Diet high in calcium, vitamin D, milk, protein, oxalate, alkali
• Excessive vitamin C intake
• Genetics
• Gout
• Hypercalcemia
• Hyperparathyroidism
• Idiopathic origin
• Immobility

• Leukemia
• Polycythemia vera
• UTI

ASSESSMENT FINDINGS
• Chills and fever
• Cool, moist skin
• Costovertebral tenderness
• Diaphoresis
• Dysuria
• Mild to severe flank pain
• Frequency of urination
• Nausea and vomiting
• Pallor
• Renal colic
• Syncope
• Urgency of urination

DIAGNOSTIC TEST RESULTS
• Noncontrast helical CT scan identifies calculi (criterion standard).
• IVP or excretory urography identifies calculi.
• 24-hour urine collection shows increased uric acid, oxalate, calcium, phosphorus, and creatinine levels.
• Blood chemistry analysis shows increased calcium, phosphorus, creatinine, BUN, uric acid, protein, and alkaline phosphatase levels.
• Cystoscopy visualizes stones.
• KUB X-ray reveals calculi.
• Urine chemistry analysis shows pyuria, proteinuria, hematuria, presence of WBCs, and increased urine specific gravity.

NURSING DIAGNOSES
• Acute pain
• Risk for infection
• Impaired urinary elimination

TREATMENT
• Diet: for calcium calculi, acid-ash with limited intake of calcium and milk products; for oxalate calculi, alkaline-ash with limited intake of foods high in oxalate (cola, tea); for uric acid calculi, alkaline-ash with limited intake of foods high in purine
• Extracorporeal shock wave lithotripsy to shatter calculi
• Increased fluid intake to 3 qt (3 L)/day
• Moist heat to flank; hot baths

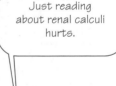

Just reading about renal calculi hurts.

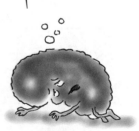

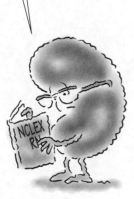

Small is better sometimes. Small calculi may pass naturally with vigorous hydration. Larger calculi may be removed by surgery or other means.

- Percutaneous nephrostolithotomy
- Surgery to remove the calculus if other measures aren't effective (type of surgery dependent on the location of the calculus)

Drug therapy
- Acidifiers: ammonium chloride
- Alkalinizing agents: potassium acetate, sodium bicarbonate
- Analgesics: meperidine (Demerol), morphine
- Antibiotics: cefazolin (Ancef), cefoxitin
- Antiemetic: prochlorperazine

INTERVENTIONS AND RATIONALES
- Monitor renal status *to determine baseline and detect complications.*
- Assess pain level and effectiveness of analgesia *to promote comfort.*
- Monitor and record vital signs, intake and output, daily weight, urine specific gravity, laboratory studies, and urine pH *to assess renal status.*
- Monitor urine for evidence of renal calculi. Strain all urine and save all solid material for analysis *to facilitate spontaneous passage of calculi.*
- Encourage increased fluid intake to 3 qt (3 L/day *to moisten mucous membranes and dilute chemicals within the body*).
- Maintain the client's diet *to promote adequate nutrition.*
- Administer medications, as prescribed, *to maintain and improve the client's condition.*
- Apply warm soaks to flank *to promote comfort.*
- If surgery was performed, check dressings regularly for bloody drainage and report excessive amounts of bloody drainage to the physician; use sterile technique to change the dressing; maintain nephrostomy tube or indwelling urinary catheter if indicated; monitor incision for signs of infection *to promote healing and detect complications.*

Teaching topics
- Explanation of the disorder and treatment plan
- Medication use and possible adverse effects

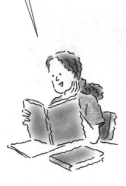

Syphilis begins in the mucous membranes and quickly becomes systemic, spreading to nearby lymph nodes and the bloodstream.

- Increasing fluid intake, especially during hot weather, illness, and exercise
- Increasing fluids at night and voiding frequently
- Voiding whenever urge is felt
- Testing urine pH

Syphilis

A chronic, infectious STD, syphilis begins in the mucous membranes and quickly becomes systemic, spreading to nearby lymph nodes and the bloodstream. This disease, when untreated, is characterized by progressive stages: primary, secondary, latent, and late (formerly called *tertiary*).

In the United States, incidence of syphilis is highest among urban populations, especially in persons ages 15 to 39, drug users, and those infected with HIV.

CAUSES
- Exposure to the spirochete *Treponema pallidum* through sexual contact
- Transmission from an infected mother to her fetus

ASSESSMENT FINDINGS
Primary syphilis
- Chancres on the genitalia, anus, fingers, lips, tongue, nipples, tonsils, or eyelids

Secondary syphilis
- Symmetrical mucocutaneous lesions
- General lymphadenopathy
- Headache
- Malaise
- Anorexia
- Weight loss
- Nausea
- Vomiting
- Sore throat
- Slight fever

DIAGNOSTIC TEST RESULTS
- Dark-field examination identifies *T. pallidum* from a lesion. This method is most effective when moist lesions are present, as in primary, secondary, and prenatal syphilis.

• Fluorescent treponemal antibody-absorption test identifies antigens of *T. pallidum* in tissue, ocular fluid, cerebrospinal fluid (CSF), tracheobronchial secretions, and exudates from lesions. This is the most sensitive test available for detecting syphilis in all stages. When reactive, it remains so permanently.

• Venereal Disease Research Laboratory (VDRL) slide test and rapid plasma reagin test detect nonspecific antibodies. Both tests, if positive, become reactive 1 to 2 weeks after the primary lesion appears or 4 to 5 weeks after the infection begins.

• CSF examination identifies neurosyphilis when the total protein level is above 40 mg/100 ml, VDRL slide test is reactive, and CSF cell count exceeds five mononuclear cells/μl.

NURSING DIAGNOSES

• Ineffective sexuality patterns
• Impaired skin integrity
• Deficient knowledge (disease process and treatment plan)

TREATMENT
Drug therapy

• Antibiotics: penicillin G benzathine (Permapen); if allergic to penicillin, then erythromycin or tetracycline

INTERVENTIONS AND RATIONALES

• Maintain standard precautions when assessing the client, collecting specimens, and treating lesions *to prevent the spread of infection.*

• Check for a history of drug sensitivity before administering the first dose of penicillin *to prevent anaphylaxis.*

• In secondary syphilis, keep lesions clean and dry. If they're draining, dispose of contaminated materials properly *to prevent the spread of infection.*

• In late syphilis, provide supportive care *to relieve the client's symptoms during prolonged treatment.*

• In cardiovascular syphilis, check for signs of decreased cardiac output (decreased urine output, hypoxia, and decreased sensorium) and pulmonary congestion *to prevent shock and respiratory distress.*

• In neurosyphilis, regularly check level of consciousness, mood, and coherence. Watch for signs of ataxia. *These measures detect neurologic complications early and prevent treatment delay.*

• Instruct clients to seek VDRL testing after 3, 6, 12, and 24 months *to detect possible relapse.* A client treated for latent or late syphilis should receive blood tests at 6-month intervals for 2 years *to detect possible relapse.*

• Report all cases of syphilis to local public health authorities. Urge the client to inform sexual partners of his infection *so that they can also receive treatment.*

• Refer the client and his sexual partners for HIV testing. *High-risk behaviors that caused the client to contract syphilis also place the client at risk for HIV.*

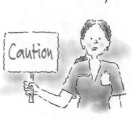

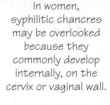

In women, syphilitic chancres may be overlooked because they commonly develop internally, on the cervix or vaginal wall.

Teaching topics

• Explanation of the disorder and treatment plan
• Medication use and possible adverse effects
• Importance of completing the course of therapy even after symptoms subside
• Safer sex practices and avoidance of spread of infection
• Follow-up VDRL testing

Testicular cancer

Testicular cancer affects the testes or testicles, the two oval-shaped glandular organs inside the scrotum that produce spermatozoa and testosterone. Malignant testicular tumors primarily affect young to middle-aged men. Testicular tumors in children are rare.

Most testicular tumors originate in gonadal cells. About 40% are seminomas—uniform, undifferentiated cells resembling primitive gonadal cells. The remainder are nonseminomas—tumor cells showing various degrees of differentiation.

The prognosis varies with the cell type and disease stage. When treated with surgery and radiation, almost all clients with localized disease survive beyond 5 years.

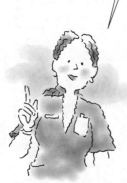

Cancer of the testicle can usually be cured easily; however, if not treated early, it can metastasize through the lymph nodes.

CONTRIBUTING FACTORS
• Age (incidence peaks between ages 20 and 40)
• Higher incidence in men with cryptorchidism and in men whose mothers used diethylstilbestrol during pregnancy

ASSESSMENT FINDINGS
• Firm, painless, smooth testicular mass, varying in size and sometimes producing a sense of testicular heaviness
• Transillumination distinguishes between a tumor (which doesn't transilluminate) and a hydrocele or spermatocele (which does)
• Nodal involvement detected on inguinal exploration (examination of the groin)

In advanced stages
• Ureteral obstruction
• Abdominal mass
• Cough
• Hemoptysis
• Shortness of breath
• Weight loss
• Fatigue
• Pallor
• Lethargy

DIAGNOSTIC TEST RESULTS
• CT scan can detect metastasis.
• Scrotal ultrasonography can differentiate between a cyst and solid mass.
• Chest X-ray may show pulmonary metastasis.
• Excretory urography may reveal ureteral deviation resulting from para-aortic node involvement.
• Serum alpha-fetoprotein and beta-human chorionic gonadotropin levels—indicators of testicular tumor activity—provide a baseline for measuring response to therapy and determining the prognosis.
• Biopsy of the mass identifies histologic verification of cancer cells.

NURSING DIAGNOSES
• Disturbed body image
• Fear
• Sexual dysfunction

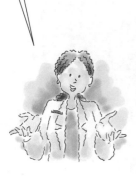

If the client receives vinblastine, assess for neurotoxicity (peripheral paresthesia, jaw pain, and muscle cramps). If he receives cisplatin, check for ototoxicity.

TREATMENT
• Radiation therapy
• Surgery: orchiectomy (testicle removal; most surgeons remove the testicle but not the scrotum to allow for a prosthetic implant)
• Retroperitoneal lymph node dissection (dissection of lymph nodes posterior to the peritoneum)
• Bone marrow transplantation (follows chemotherapy and radiation therapy in clients with unresponsive tumors)
• High-calorie diet provided in small, frequent feedings
• I.V. fluid therapy

Drug therapy
• Diuretics: furosemide (Lasix), mannitol
• Antineoplastics: bleomycin (Blenoxane), carboplatin (Paraplatin), cisplatin (Platinol), dactinomycin (Cosmegen), etoposide (VePesid), ifosfamide (Ifex), vinblastine
• Analgesics: morphine, fentanyl (Duragesic-25)
• Antiemetics: metoclopramide (Reglan), ondansetron (Zofran)
• Hormone replacement therapy (after bilateral orchiectomy)

INTERVENTIONS AND RATIONALES
• Develop a treatment plan that addresses the client's psychological and physical needs *to enhance the client's well-being.*

Before orchiectomy
• Reassure the client that sterility and impotence need not follow unilateral orchiectomy, that synthetic hormones can restore hormonal balance, and that most surgeons don't remove the scrotum. In many cases, a testicular prosthesis can correct anatomic disfigurement. *These interventions can help allay the client's anxiety.*
• Provide emotional support *to decrease anxiety.*

After orchiectomy

- For the first day after surgery, apply an ice pack to the scrotum *to reduce swelling* and provide analgesics *to promote comfort*.
- Check for excessive bleeding, swelling, and signs of infection *to detect early signs of complications and prevent treatment delay*.
- Provide a scrotal athletic supporter *to minimize pain during ambulation*.
- Assess pain level and evaluate analgesic effects *to promote comfort*.

During chemotherapy

- Give antiemetics, as needed, *to treat or prevent nausea and vomiting*.
- Encourage small, frequent meals *to maintain oral intake despite anorexia*.
- Establish a mouth care regimen *to prevent breakdown of the oral mucosa* and check for stomatitis *to detect early signs and avoid treatment delay*.
- Monitor for signs of myelosuppression *so precautions can be taken to avoid infection*.
- Encourage increased fluid intake and provide I.V. fluids, a potassium supplement, and diuretics *to prevent renal damage*.

Teaching topics

- Explanation of the disease process and treatment options
- Preventing and reporting infection
- Managing adverse reactions to chemotherapy and radiation

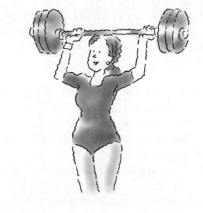

Pump up on practice questions

1. A client with bladder cancer undergoes surgical removal of the bladder with construction of an ileal conduit. What assessments by the nurse indicate that the client is developing complications? Select all that apply.

1. Urine output greater than 30 ml/hour
2. Dusky appearance of the stoma
3. Stoma protrusion from the skin
4. Mucus shreds in the urine collection bag
5. Edema of the stoma during the first 24 hours after surgery
6. Sharp abdominal pain with rigidity

Answer: 2, 3, 6. A dusky appearance of the stoma indicates decreased blood supply; a healthy stoma should appear beefy-red. Protrusion indicates prolapse of the stoma, and sharp abdominal pain with rigidity indicates peritonitis. A urine output greater than 30 ml/hour is a sign of adequate renal perfusion and is a normal finding. Because mucous membranes are used to create the conduit, mucus in the urine is expected. Stomal edema is a normal finding during the first 24 hours after surgery.

➡ NCLEX keys
Client needs category: Physiological integrity
Client needs subcategory: Reduction of risk potential
Cognitive level: Analysis

2. A client with fever and urinary urgency is asked to provide a urine specimen for culture and sensitivity analysis. The nurse should instruct the client to collect the specimen from the:
1. first stream of urine from the bladder.
2. middle stream of urine from the bladder.
3. final stream of urine from the bladder.
4. full volume of urine from the bladder.

Answer: 2. The midstream specimen is recommended because it's less likely to be contaminated with microorganisms from the external genitalia than other specimens. It isn't necessary to collect a full volume of urine for a urine culture and sensitivity.

➡ NCLEX keys
Client needs category: Physiological integrity
Client needs subcategory: Reduction of risk potential
Cognitive level: Application

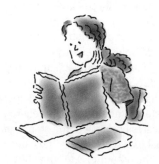

3. A client is diagnosed with cystitis. The nurse recommends the client drink cranberry juice. What assessment parameter should the nurse consider to determine if this recommendation has been effective?
1. Urine specific gravity
2. White blood cell (WBC) count
3. pH
4. Protein

Answer: 3. Because cranberry juice is an acid-ash food that lowers the urine pH, monitoring urine pH would be most useful in evaluating the effectiveness of the intervention. Urine specific gravity, WBC count, and protein level won't pinpoint the effectiveness of acid-ash food.

➡ NCLEX keys
Client needs category: Physiological integrity
Client needs subcategory: Physiological adaptation
Cognitive level: Application

4. A client with dysuria is prescribed phenazopyridine (Pyridium). The nurse should teach the client to expect urine to be:
1. greater in volume.
2. orange in color.
3. pungent in odor.
4. concentrated in consistency.

Answer: 2. Phenazopyridine causes the urine to have an orange color. Phenazopyridine doesn't cause higher urine volume, a pungent urine odor, or concentrated urine.

➡ NCLEX keys
Client needs category: Physiological integrity
Client needs subcategory: Physiological adaptation
Cognitive level: Application

5. The nurse is instructing a client with oxalate renal calculi. Which foods should the nurse urge the client to eliminate from his diet?
1. Citrus fruits, molasses, and dried apricots
2. Milk, cheese, and ice cream
3. Sardines, liver, and kidney
4. Spinach, rhubarb, and asparagus

Answer: 4. To reduce the formation of oxalate calculi, urge the client to avoid foods high in oxalate, such as spinach, rhubarb, and asparagus. Other oxalate-rich foods to avoid include tomatoes, beets, chocolate, cocoa, Ovaltine, nuts, celery, and parsley. Citrus fruits, molasses, dried apricots, milk, cheese, ice cream, sardines, and organ meats don't produce oxalate and need not be omitted from the client's diet.

➡ *NCLEX keys*

Client needs category: Physiological integrity
Client needs subcategory: Basic care and comfort
Cognitive level: Analysis

6. A nurse is instructing the client about recommended daily fluid consumption. The nurse should tell the client to drink approximately:
1. 4 cups per day.
2. 8 cups per day.
3. 12 cups per day.
4 16 cups per day.

Answer: 3. A client with renal calculi should drink 3 L of fluid per day. This amount is equivalent to 12 cups.

➡ *NCLEX keys*

Client needs category: Physiological integrity
Client needs subcategory: Reduction of risk potential
Cognitive level: Application

7. A client with chronic renal failure reports pruritus. Which instruction should the nurse include in this client's teaching plan?
1. Rub the skin vigorously with a towel.
2. Take frequent baths.
3. Apply alcohol-based emollients to the skin.
4. Keep fingernails short and clean.

Answer: 4. Calcium-phosphate deposits in the skin may cause pruritus. Scratching leads to excoriation and breaks in the skin that increase the client's risk of infection. The nurse should tell the client to keep his fingernails short and clean to reduce the risk of infection. Vigorous rubbing with a towel can cause skin irritation, leading to further itching or breaks in the skin. Frequent bathing can dry the skin, which contributes to itching. Emollients without alcohol should be used to soothe the skin and help it retain moisture.

➡ *NCLEX keys*

Client needs category: Physiological integrity
Client needs subcategory: Reduction of risk potential
Cognitive level: Application

8. A client in acute renal failure becomes severely anemic and the physician prescribes two units of packed red blood cells (RBCs). The nurse should plan to administer each unit:
1. as quickly as the client can tolerate the infusions.
2. over 30 minutes to an hour.
3. between 1 and 4 hours.
4. up to 4 hours but no longer.

Answer: 3. It's standard practice to infuse a unit of packed RBCs between 1 to 4 hours.

➡ *NCLEX keys*

Client needs category: Physiological integrity
Client needs subcategory: Pharmacological and parenteral therapies
Cognitive level: Application

9. A nurse is teaching a client with chronic renal failure about foods to avoid. It would be most accurate for the nurse to teach the client to avoid:
1. yogurt and milk.
2. whole grain breads.
3. fresh fruits and vegetables.
4. beef and pork.

Answer: 4. Proteins are typically restricted in clients with chronic renal failure because of their metabolites. The diet should be high in both calories and carbohydrates.

➡ *NCLEX keys*

Client needs category: Physiological integrity
Client needs subcategory: Physiological adaptation
Cognitive level: Application

10. A client with bladder cancer receives local radiation therapy and experiences a dry skin reaction. When teaching the client about skin care, the nurse should instruct the client to avoid:
1. lubrication.
2. cleansers.
3. cold packs.
4. cotton garments.

Answer: 3. Cold packs over the area of a dry reaction to radiation therapy are contraindicated because they reduce capillary circulation to the site and hamper healing. Lubrication, cleansers, and cotton garments aren't unconditionally contraindicated.

➡ *NCLEX keys*
Client needs category: Physiological integrity
Client needs subcategory: Reduction of risk potential
Cognitive level: Application

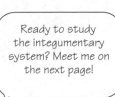

Ready to study the integumentary system? Meet me on the next page!

Brush up on key concepts

The skin, hair, and nails make up the integumentary system, which serves as protection for the body's inner organs. It also helps regulate body temperature through the sweat glands.

At any time, you can review the major points of this chapter by consulting the *Cheat sheet* on pages 352 and 353.

Outer defense layer
The **skin** provides the first line of defense against microorganisms. It's composed of three layers:

☝ the **epidermis** (outer layer), which contains keratinocytes and melanocytes, acts as a protective barrier against the environment

✌ the **dermis** (middle layer), a collagen layer that supports the epidermis, contains nerves and blood vessels, and is the origin of hair, nails, sebaceous glands, eccrine sweat glands, and apocrine sweat glands

🤟 the **hypodermis** (third layer), which is composed of loose connective tissue filled with fatty cells, provides heat, insulation, shock absorption, and a nutritional reservoir (also known as subcutaneous tissue).

Additional protection
Hair also provides protection and coverage for most of the body, with the exception of the palms, lips, soles of the feet, nipples, penis and labia.

Taking care of the tips
The **nails,** protecting the tips of the fingers and toes, are composed of dead cells filled with keratin.

Oil and sweat
The integumentary system also contains three types of glands:
• **sebaceous (oil) glands,** which lubricate the hair and the epidermis and are stimulated by sex hormones
• **eccrine sweat glands,** which regulate body temperature through water secretion
• **apocrine sweat glands,** which are located in the axilla, nipple, anal, and pubic areas and secrete odorless fluid. (Decomposition of this fluid by bacteria causes odor.)

Keep abreast of diagnostic tests

Here are the major diagnostic tests for assessing integumentary disorders as well as common nursing actions associated with each test.

Testing blood for this...
A **blood chemistry test** analyzes a blood sample for potassium, sodium, calcium, phosphorus, ketones, glucose, osmolality, chloride, blood urea nitrogen, and creatinine.

Nursing actions
• Explain the procedure to the client.
• Withhold food and fluids before the procedure, as directed.
• Check the venipuncture site for bleeding after the procedure.

...And for that
Hematologic studies analyze a blood sample for red blood cells (RBCs), white blood cells (WBCs), erythrocyte sedimentation rate, platelets, prothrombin time, international normalized ratio, partial thromboplastin time, hemoglobin (Hb), and hematocrit (HCT).

(Text continues on page 354.)

Cheat sheet

Integumentary refresher

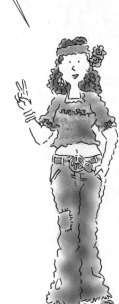

> Groovy.
> If I don't have time to study the whole chapter, I can just review the *Cheat sheet.*

ATOPIC DERMATITIS

Key signs and symptoms
- Erythematous lesions that eventually become scaly and lichenified
- Excessive dry skin
- Hyperpigmentation
- Skin eruptions

Key test results
- Serum immunoglobulin E levels are commonly elevated but this finding isn't diagnostic.

Key treatments
- Antihistamines: diphenhydramine (Benadryl), hydroxyzine (Vistaril)
- Corticosteroid: hydrocortisone

Key interventions
- Help the client set up an individual schedule and plan for daily skin care.
- Instruct the client to bathe in plain water. (He may have to limit bathing, according to the severity of the lesions.) Tell him to bathe with a special nonfatty soap and tepid water (96° F [35.6° C]), to avoid using any soap when lesions are acutely inflamed, and to limit baths or showers to 5 to 7 minutes.
- For scalp involvement, advise the client to shampoo frequently and apply corticosteroid solution to the scalp afterward.

BURNS

Key signs and symptoms
- Superficial partial-thickness: erythema, edema, pain, blanching
- Deep dermal partial-thickness: pain, oozing, fluid-filled vesicles; erythema; shiny, wet subcutaneous layer after vesicles rupture
- Full-thickness: eschar, edema, little or no pain; deeply charred subcutaneous tissue, muscle, and bone

Key test results
- Visual examination is used to estimate the extent of the burn (determined by Rule of Nines and Lund-Browder chart).

Key treatments
- I.V. therapy: hydration and electrolyte replacement, using a fluid replacement formula such a the Parkland formula
- Biological dressings
- Analgesic: morphine
- Antianxiety agent: lorazepam (Ativan)
- Antibiotic: gentamicin
- Anti-infectives: mafenide (Sulfamylon), silver sulfadiazine (Silvadene), silver nitrate, povidone-iodine (Betadine)
- Antitetanus: tetanus toxoid
- Colloid: albumin 5% (Albuminar 5%)

Key interventions
- Monitor respiratory status.
- Assess fluid status.
- Assess pain level, administer analgesics, and evaluate their effect.
- Administer I.V. fluids.
- Administer oxygen.
- Provide wound care.
- Administer total parenteral or enteral feedings.
- Maintain protective precautions.

HERPES ZOSTER

Key signs and symptoms
- Neuralgia
- Severe, deep pain
- Unilaterally clustered skin vesicles along peripheral sensory nerves on trunk, thorax, or face

Key test results
- Skin study identifies organism.
- Visual examination shows vesicles along peripheral sensory nerves.

Key treatments
- Analgesics: acetaminophen (Tylenol), codeine
- Antianxiety agents: lorazepam (Ativan), hydroxyzine (Vistaril)
- Anti-inflammatory agent: triamcinolone
- Antipruritic: diphenhydramine (Benadryl)
- Antiviral agents: acyclovir (Zovirax), valacyclovir (Valtrex), famciclovir (Famvir)

Integumentary refresher (continued)

HERPES ZOSTER (CONTINUED)
Key interventions
- Monitor neurologic status.
- Assess pain and note the effectiveness of analgesics.
- Prevent scratching and rubbing of affected areas.

PRESSURE ULCERS
Key signs and symptoms
- Suspected deep tissue injury: Intact skin or blood blister
- Stage 1: Nonblanchable erythema of intact skin
- Stage 2: Partial-thickness skin loss involving the epidermis and dermis
- Stage 3: Full-thickness skin loss involving damage or necrosis of subcutaneous tissue that may extend down to, but not through, underlying fascia
- Stage 4: Full-thickness skin loss with extensive destruction, tissue necrosis
- Unstageable: Full-thickness tissue loss with slough or eschar at the base of the wound

Key test results
- Visual inspection reveals pressure ulcer; measurement helps determine staging.

Key treatments
- High-protein, high-calorie diet in small frequent feedings; parenteral or enteral feedings if the client is unable or unwilling to take adequate nutrients orally
- Topical wound care according to facility protocol
- Wound debridement; tissue flap

Key interventions
- Assess skin integrity and watch for signs of infection.
- Monitor the bedridden client for possible changes in skin color, turgor, temperature, and sensation.
- Reposition the client every 2 hours.
- Use a bed cradle or another device.
- Provide meticulous skin care and check bony prominences.
- Maintain the client's diet and encourage oral fluid intake.

PSORIASIS
Key signs and symptoms
- Itching
- Lesions (red and usually forming well-defined patches)
- Pustules

Key test results
- Skin biopsy is positive for the disorder.

Key treatments
- Antipsoriatic agent: calcipotriene (Dovonex)
- Corticosteroid ointment: hydrocortisone
- Ultraviolet light to retard cell production; may be used in conjunction with psoralen (PUVA therapy)

Key interventions
- Teach the client about his prescribed therapy; provide written instructions.
- Monitor for adverse reactions, especially allergic reactions to anthralin, atrophy and acne from steroids, and burning, itching, nausea, and squamous cell epitheliomas from PUVA therapy.
- Initially, evaluate the client on methotrexate weekly, then monthly for red blood cell, white blood cell, and platelet counts. Liver biopsy may be performed.
- Caution the client receiving PUVA therapy to stay out of the sun on the day of treatment and to protect his eyes with sunglasses that screen UVA for 24 hours after treatment. Tell him to wear goggles during exposure to this light.

SKIN CANCER
Key signs and symptoms
- Change in color, size, or shape of preexisting lesion
- Irregular, circular bordered lesion with hues of tan, black, or blue (melanoma)
- Small, red, nodular lesion that begins as an erythematous macule or plaque with indistinct margins (squamous cell carcinoma)
- Waxy nodule with telangiectasis (basal cell epithelioma)

Key test results
- Skin biopsy shows cytology positive for cancer cells.

Key treatments
- Chemosurgery with zinc chloride
- Cryosurgery with liquid nitrogen
- Curettage and electrodesiccation
- Antimetabolite: fluorouracil

Key interventions
- Assess lesions.
- Administer medications, as prescribed.
- Provide postchemotherapy and postradiation nursing care.
- Provide emotional support and encourage the client to express feelings about changes in body image and a fear of dying.

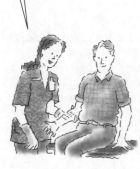

Check it out. Checking the test site for infection and bleeding is a common nursing responsibility with skin tests.

Want the skinny on atopic dermatitis? It's characterized by intense itching. Scratching the skin intensifies itching, resulting in red, weeping lesions.

Nursing actions
- Explain the procedure to the client.
- Check the venipuncture site for bleeding after the procedure.

Tissue punch test
A **skin biopsy,** also known as a *punch biopsy,* uses a circular punch instrument to remove a small amount of skin tissue for histologic evaluation.

Nursing actions
- Explain the procedure to the client.
- Make sure that written, informed consent has been obtained.
- Check the site for bleeding and infection.

Allergy exam
Skin testing uses a patch, scratch, or intradermal technique (injection administered at a 15-degree angle) to administer an allergen to the skin's surface or into the dermis. The skin can then be analyzed for reaction.

Nursing actions
- Explain the procedure to the client.
- Keep the area dry.
- Record the site, date, and time of test.
- Inspect the site for erythema, papules, vesicles, edema, and induration.
- Record the date and time for follow-up site reading.

Scrape and study
A **skin scraping** involves scraping a small sample of skin, nails, or hair for evaluation under a microscope.

Nursing actions
- Explain the procedure to the client.
- Check the scraping site for bleeding and infection.

Under the microscope
A **skin study** is a microscopic examination of skin that includes gram stain, culture and sensitivity, cytology, and immunofluorescence.

Nursing actions
- Explain the procedure to the client.
- Follow laboratory procedure guidelines.

- Note current antibiotic therapy.

Ultraviolet inspection
Wood's light test uses ultraviolet (UV) light to directly examine the skin.

Nursing actions
- Explain the procedure to the client.

Polish up on client care

Major integumentary disorders include atopic dermatitis, burns, herpes zoster, pressure ulcers, psoriasis, and skin cancer.

Atopic dermatitis

Atopic dermatitis is a chronic skin disorder characterized by superficial skin inflammation and intense itching. It may also be called *atopic eczema* or *infantile eczema*.

Atopic dermatitis may be associated with other atopic diseases, such as bronchial asthma and allergic rhinitis. It usually develops in infants and toddlers between ages 1 month and 1 year, commonly in those with strong family histories of atopic disease. In many cases, these children acquire other atopic disorders as they grow older.

Typically, this form of dermatitis flares and subsides repeatedly before finally resolving during adolescence. However, it can persist into adulthood.

CONTRIBUTING FACTORS
- Chemical irritants
- Food allergies
- Genetic predisposition
- Immune dysfunction (possibly linked to elevated serum immunoglobulin [Ig] E levels or defective T-cell function)
- Infections (with *Staphylococcus aureus*)

ASSESSMENT FINDINGS
- Characteristic location of lesions: areas of flexion and extension such as the neck, antecubital fossa (behind the elbow), popliteal

folds (posterior surface of the knee), and behind the ears
• Erythematous lesions that eventually become scaly and lichenified
• Excessive dry skin
• Hyperpigmentation
• Skin eruptions

DIAGNOSTIC TEST RESULTS
• Serum IgE levels are commonly elevated but this finding isn't diagnostic.

NURSING DIAGNOSES
• Impaired skin integrity
• Disturbed body image
• Anxiety

TREATMENT
• Washing lesions with water and little soap
• Environmental control of offending allergens

Drug therapy
• Antihistamines: diphenhydramine (Benadryl), hydroxyzine (Vistaril)
• Corticosteroid: hydrocortisone

INTERVENTIONS AND RATIONALES
• Warn that drowsiness is possible with the use of antihistamines to relieve daytime itching *to prevent injury*.
• If nocturnal itching interferes with sleep, suggest methods for inducing natural sleep, such as drinking a glass of warm milk, *to prevent overuse of sedatives*.
• Administering antihistamines at bedtime may also be useful *because antihistamines relieve itching and cause drowsiness*.
• Help the client set up an individual schedule and plan for daily skin care *to help the client cope with the chronic condition and promote compliance*.
• Instruct the client to bathe in plain water. (He may have to limit bathing, according to the severity of the lesions.) Tell him to bathe with a nonfatty soap and tepid water (96° F [35.6° C]), to avoid using any soap when lesions are acutely inflamed, and to limit baths or showers to 5 to 7 minutes. *These measures prevent worsening of the condition*.

• For scalp involvement, advise the client to shampoo frequently and apply corticosteroid solution to the scalp afterward *to improve skin integrity*.
• Advise the client to keep fingernails short *to limit excoriation and secondary infections caused by scratching*.
• Instruct the client to lubricate the skin after a shower or bath *to prevent excessive dryness*.
• Apply occlusive dressings (such as plastic film) over a corticosteroid cream intermittently as necessary *to help clear lichenified skin*.
• Provide emotional support. Help the client accept his altered body image, and encourage him to verbalize his feelings. *Coping with disfigurement is extremely difficult, especially for children and adolescents*.

Teaching topics
• Explanation of the disorder and treatment plan
• Medication use and possible adverse effects
• Understanding factors that exacerbate the condition (fabric, detergents, stress)
• Skin care
• Wearing clothing made of cotton

Burns

A burn is the destruction of skin that causes loss of intracellular fluid and electrolytes. A burn is characterized by the extent (area) and depth of the burn. Most burns are a combination of thicknesses:
• A superficial partial-thickness burn (previously known as a *first-degree burn*) involves only the epidermal layer.
• A deep dermal partial-thickness burn (previously known as a *second-degree burn*) involves the epidermal and dermal layers.
• A full-thickness burn (previously known as *third-* and *fourth-degree burns*) involves epidermal, dermal, subcutaneous layers, and nerve endings, muscle, and bone.

Number 9...Number 9
The Rule of Nines is a method used to estimate the size of a burned area. In this method, a person's skin area is divided into several sections, each representing

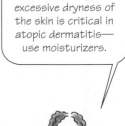

Preventing excessive dryness of the skin is critical in atopic dermatitis—use moisturizers.

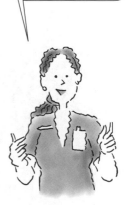

Remember your therapeutic role. Be careful not to show any anxiety or revulsion when looking at a client with impaired skin integrity.

9% (or multiples of 9%) of the total body area. By observing the size and location of a burn and assigning the appropriate body percentage, the nurse can roughly determine what percentage of a client's body has been burned. determine what percentage of a client's body has been burned.

Lund-Browder

The Lund-Browder chart is another method of estimating body surface area that's been burned. This method accounts for changes in body proportion that occur with age. Its greater accuracy can be used to help determine a client's exact fluid replacement requirements after a burn injury.

CAUSES
- Chemical: acids, alkalies, vesicants
- Electrical: lightning, electrical wires
- Mechanical: friction
- Radiation: X-ray, sun, nuclear
- Thermal: flame, frostbite, scald

ASSESSMENT FINDINGS
- Superficial partial-thickness: erythema, edema, pain, blanching
- Deep dermal partial-thickness: pain; oozing, fluid-filled vesicles; erythema; shiny, wet subcutaneous layer after vesicles rupture
- Full-thickness: eschar, edema, little or no pain, deeply charred subcutaneous tissue, muscle, and bone
- Tachycardia
- Dyspnea (if burn involves the chest or airway)

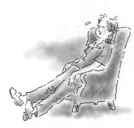

Don't BURN out on NCLEX. If you stick with your study schedule, you'll get there.

DIAGNOSTIC TEST RESULTS
- 24-hour urine collection shows decreased creatinine clearance and negative nitrogen balance.
- Arterial blood gas analysis shows metabolic acidosis.
- Blood chemistry test shows increased potassium level and decreased sodium, albumin, complement fixation, immunoglobulin levels.
- Hematologic studies show increased Hb and HCT and decreased fibrinogen and platelets and WBC count.
- Urine chemistry studies show hematuria and myoglobinuria.
- Visual examination is used to estimate extent of burn (determined by Rule of Nines and Lund-Browder chart).

NURSING DIAGNOSES
- Deficient fluid volume
- Acute pain
- Risk for infection
- Disturbed body image
- Impaired skin integrity

TREATMENT
- Biological dressings
- Diet high in protein, fat, calories and carbohydrates with small, frequent feedings
- Early excisional therapy
- Escharotomy (surgical excision of burned tissue)
- I.V. therapy: hydration and electrolyte replacement, using a fluid replacement formula such as the Parkland formula
- Protective isolation to protect client from infection
- Splints to maintain proper joint position and prevent contractures
- Transfusion therapy of fresh frozen plasma, platelets, packed RBCs, and plasma
- Hydrotherapy

Drug therapy
- Analgesic: morphine
- Antacids: magnesium and aluminum hydroxide, aluminum hydroxide gel
- Antianxiety agent: lorazepam (Ativan)
- Antibiotic: gentamicin
- Anti-infectives: mafenide (Sulfamylon), silver sulfadiazine (Silvadene), silver nitrate, povidone-iodine (Betadine)
- Antitetanus: tetanus toxoid
- Colloid: albumin 5% (Albuminar 5%)
- Diuretic: mannitol
- Histamine antagonists: cimetidine (Tagamet), ranitidine (Zantac), famotidine (Pepcid), nizatidine (Axid)
- Mucosal barrier fortifier: sucralfate (Carafate)
- Vitamins: phytonadione, cyanocobalamin (vitamin B_{12})

INTERVENTIONS AND RATIONALES

- Monitor respiratory status. *Upper airway injury is common with burns to the face, neck, and chest. Edema may narrow airways.*
- Assess fluid status. *Hypovolemia is indicated by decreased level of consciousness, urine output less than 30 ml/hour, blood pressure less than 90/60 mm Hg, heart rate greater than 100 beats/minute, dry mucous membranes, and delayed capillary refill.*
- If the client underwent skin grafting, keep pressure off the donor side *to maintain blood flow to the site and promote wound healing.*
- Monitor for signs of infection *to determine if the treatment plan must be altered.*
- Assess pain level, administer analgesics, and evaluate their effect *to promote comfort.*
- Monitor and record vital signs, fluid intake and output, laboratory studies, hemodynamic variables, stool for occult blood, specific gravity, calorie count, daily weight, wound status, neurovascular checks, and pulses *to detect complications.*
- Assess bowel sounds *to determine motility of the GI tract.*
- Administer I.V. fluids *to maintain hydration and replace fluid loss.*
- Administer oxygen *to meet cellular demands.*
- Provide wound care *to promote healing.*
- Provide suctioning; assist with turning, coughing, and deep breathing; and perform chest physiotherapy and postural drainage *to maintain patent airway.*
- Administer total parenteral nutrition or enteral feedings *to meet the client's increased metabolic demands.*
- Administer medications, as ordered, *to maintain or improve the client's condition.*
- Provide emotional support and encourage the client to express feelings about disfigurement, immobility from scarring, and a fear of dying *to encourage coping mechanisms.*
- Provide treatments: range-of-motion (ROM) exercises, Hubbard tank (for immersing the client), bed cradle, splints, and Jobst clothing *to maintain ROM and prevent complications.*
- Elevate the affected extremities *to promote venous drainage and decrease edema.*
- Maintain a warm environment during acute period *to regulate body temperature.*
- Maintain protective precautions *to prevent transmission of infection to the client.*
- Provide skin and mouth care *to promote comfort.*

Teaching topics

- Explanation of the disorder and treatment plan
- Medication use and possible adverse effects
- Wound care
- Following dietary recommendations and restrictions
- Avoiding restrictive clothing
- Using splints and Jobst clothing
- Contacting community agencies and resources

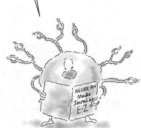

Each nerve emanates from the spine and sends signals to a skin area called a dermatome.

Herpes zoster

Herpes zoster, also known as *shingles*, is an acute viral infection of nerve structures caused by varicella zoster; affected areas include the spinal and cranial sensory ganglia and posterior gray matter of the spinal cord. Herpes zoster produces localized vesicular skin lesions confined to a dermatome and severe neurologic pain in peripheral areas innervated by nerves arising in the inflamed root ganglia.

CAUSES

- Cytotoxic drug-induced immunosuppression
- Debilitating disease
- Exposure to varicella zoster
- Hodgkin's disease

ASSESSMENT FINDINGS

- Anorexia
- Edematous skin
- Erythema
- Fever
- Headache
- Malaise
- Neuralgia
- Paresthesia
- Pruritus
- Severe, deep pain
- Unilaterally clustered skin vesicles along peripheral sensory nerves on trunk, thorax, or face

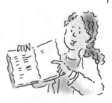

Chickenpox-like vesicles are the key sign of herpes zoster.

DIAGNOSTIC TEST RESULTS
- Skin study identifies organism.
- Visual examination shows vesicles along peripheral sensory nerves.

NURSING DIAGNOSES
- Acute pain
- Risk for infection
- Impaired skin integrity

TREATMENT
- No specific treatment; primary goal is to relieve itching and pain

Drug therapy
- Analgesics: acetaminophen (Tylenol), codeine
- Anti-inflammatory agent: triamcinolone
- Antianxiety agents: lorazepam (Ativan), hydroxyzine (Vistaril)
- Antipruritic: diphenhydramine (Benadryl)
- Antiviral agents: acyclovir (Zovirax), famciclovir (Famvir), valacyclovir (Valtrex); must be administered within 24 hours of initial outbreak
- Corticosteroid: hydrocortisone
- Nerve blocker: lidocaine (Xylocaine)

INTERVENTIONS AND RATIONALES
- Monitor neurologic status *to determine baseline and detect changes.*
- Assess pain and note the effectiveness of analgesics *to promote comfort and evaluate the need for a change in the current treatment plan.*
- Monitor and record vital signs, laboratory results (blood glucose levels may be elevated if the client is receiving corticosteroids), and cranial nerve function *to assess baseline and detect changes.*
- Administer medications, as directed, *to maintain or improve the client's condition.*
- Provide emotional support and encourage the client to express feelings about changes in physical appearance and recurrent nature of the illness *to help him adapt to his illness.*
- Prevent scratching and rubbing of affected areas *to prevent infection.*

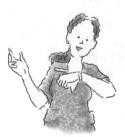

Every 2 hours: that's how often you need to reposition a client to avoid pressure ulcers.

Teaching topics
- Explanation of the disorder and treatment plan
- Medication use and possible adverse effects
- Recognizing the signs and symptoms of hearing loss
- Avoiding wool and synthetic clothing
- Wearing lightweight, loose cotton clothing
- Keeping blisters intact

Pressure ulcers

Pressure ulcers are localized areas of cellular necrosis that occur most often in skin and subcutaneous tissue over bony prominences. These ulcers may be superficial, caused by local skin irritation with subsequent surface maceration, or deep, originating in underlying tissue. Deep lesions often go undetected until they penetrate the skin but, by then, they have usually caused subcutaneous damage.

CAUSES
- Pressure, particularly over bony prominences

ASSESSMENT FINDINGS
Signs and symptoms of pressure ulcers occur in six stages. Unstageable pressure ulcers can't be staged until the base of the ulcer is exposed.

Suspected deep tissue injury
- Purple or maroon discoloration
- Intact skin or blood blister

Stage 1
- Nonblanchable erythema of intact skin
- Skin discoloration
- Warmth and hardness

Stage 2
- Blister
- Partial-thickness skin loss involving the epidermis and dermis
- Shallow crater

Stage 3
- Deep crater with or without undermining of adjacent tissue

- Full-thickness skin loss involving damage or necrosis of subcutaneous tissue that may extend down to, but not through, underlying fascia

Stage 4
- Damage to muscle, bone, tendon, or joint
- Full-thickness skin loss with extensive destruction
- Tissue necrosis

Unstageable
- Full-thickness tissue loss with slough or eschar at the base of the wound

DIAGNOSTIC TEST RESULTS
- Visual inspection reveals pressure ulcer; measurement helps determine staging.
- Wound culture and sensitivity identify infecting organism.

NURSING DIAGNOSES
- Impaired physical mobility
- Imbalanced nutrition: Less than body requirements
- Impaired skin integrity

TREATMENT
- High-protein, high-calorie diet with adequate vitamin C intake in small frequent feedings; parenteral or enteral feedings if the client is unable or unwilling to take adequate nutrients orally
- Topical wound care according to facility's protocol
- Wound debridement; tissue flap
- Special therapy bed

INTERVENTIONS AND RATIONALES
- Assess skin integrity and watch for signs of infection *to detect complications.*
- Monitor the bedridden client for possible changes in skin color, turgor, temperature and sensation *to prevent further skin breakdown.*
- Reposition the client every 2 hours *to prevent pressure ulcers.* (See *Preventing pressure ulcers,* page 360.)
- Use a bed cradle or another device *to avoid skin breakdown.*
- Provide meticulous skin care and check bony prominences *to reduce the chances of pressure ulcer development.*

- Maintain the client's diet and encourage oral fluid intake *to promote wound healing.*
- Provide wound care *to promote healing.*
- Provide ROM exercises *to promote joint mobility.*

Teaching topics
- Explanation of the disorder and treatment plan
- Wound care
- Avoiding prolonged periods of immobility
- Performing meticulous skin care
- Changing positions frequently when bedridden
- Recognizing the signs of skin breakdown
- Recognizing the signs and symptoms of infection

Psoriasis

Psoriasis, a chronic, recurrent disease, is marked by epidermal proliferation. Lesions appear as erythematous papules and plaques covered with silver scales and vary widely in severity and distribution.

Although this disorder commonly affects young adults, it may strike at any age, including infancy. Psoriasis is characterized by recurring partial remissions and exacerbations.

CONTRIBUTING FACTORS
- Genetic predisposition

ASSESSMENT FINDINGS
- Arthritic symptoms
- Characteristic location of lesions: scalp, chest, elbows, knees, back, buttocks
- Itching
- Lesions (red and usually forming well-defined patches)
- Pain
- Patches, consisting of silver scales that flake off or thicken and cover the lesions
- Pustules

DIAGNOSTIC TEST RESULTS
- Skin biopsy is positive for the disorder.
- Blood studies reveal elevated serum uric acid level in severe cases, due to accelerated nucleic acid degradation, but indications of gout are absent.

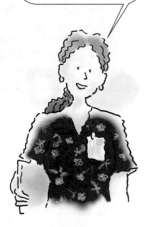

Psoriasis is marked by epidermal proliferation; in other words, the skin's outermost layer becomes overgrown.

Management moments

Preventing pressure ulcers

As a health care provider, you play a key role in maintaining the client's skin integrity, promoting comfort by averting dryness and itching, and preventing pressure ulcers, a major complication. Because your client's skin condition largely depends on his overall health, you'll need to help him maintain optimal nutrition and hydration. You may also need to provide additional guidance in personal hygiene and in protecting his skin from harsh environmental conditions.

PUTTING THE PRESSURE ON

As their name implies, pressure ulcers result when pressure—applied with great force for a short period of time or with less force over a long period of time—impairs circulation, depriving tissues of oxygen and nutrients. If left untreated, ischemic areas can progress to tissue breakdown and infection.

    Most pressure ulcers develop over bony prominences, where friction and shearing force combine with pressure to breakdown skin and underlying tissues.

MAKING THE DIFFERENCE

Preventing pressure ulcers is crucial, especially in older adults, because ulcers take long to heal, thereby increasing the client's risk of infection and other complications.

    To help prevent pressure ulcers, follow these steps:
- Turn or reposition the client every 1 to 2 hours unless contraindicated.
- Lift the client rather than sliding him because sliding increases friction and shear.
- Use pillows to position your client.
- Avoid placing your client directly on his trochanter.
- Except for brief periods, avoid raising the head of the bed more than 30 degrees to prevent shearing pressure.
- As appropriate, perform active and passive range-of-motion exercises to relieve pressure and promote circulation.
- Use support surfaces as necessary.
- Place the client in a special therapy bed.

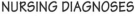

If studying is making you stressed...it's time to take a break!

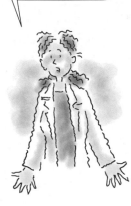

NURSING DIAGNOSES
- Impaired skin integrity
- Risk for infection
- Disturbed body image
- Acute pain

TREATMENT
- Tar, wet dressings, or oatmeal baths
- UV light to retard cell production; may be used in conjunction with psoralen (PUVA therapy)

Drug therapy
- Antipsoriatic agent: calcipotriene (Dovonex)
- Corticosteroid ointment: hydrocortisone
- Corticosteroid: intralesional steroid injections
- Anti-hypocalcemic agent: calcitriol (Rocaltrol)
- Antineoplastic agent: methotrexate (Trexall)

INTERVENTIONS AND RATIONALES
- Teach the client about his prescribed therapy; provide written instructions *to promote compliance and avoid confusion.*
- Monitor for adverse reactions, especially allergic reactions to anthralin, atrophy and acne from steroids, and burning, itching, nausea, and squamous cell epitheliomas from PUVA *to prevent complications.*
- Initially, evaluate the client on methotrexate weekly, then monthly for RBC, WBC, and platelet counts *because cytotoxins may cause hepatic or bone marrow toxicity.* Liver biopsy may be done *to assess the effects of methotrexate.*
- Caution the client receiving PUVA therapy to stay out of the sun on the day of treatment and to protect his eyes with sunglasses that screen UVA for 24 hours after treatment. Tell him to wear goggles during exposure to this light. *These measures protect the client from injury caused by excessive UVA exposure.*

• Provide emotional support and help the client learn to cope with stressful situations *because stressful situations tend to exacerbate psoriasis.*

Teaching topics

• Explanation of the disorder and treatment plan
• Medication use and possible adverse effects
• Correctly applying prescribed ointments, creams, and lotions; a steroid cream, for example, should be applied in a thin film and rubbed gently into the skin until the cream disappears
• Avoiding occlusive dressings over anthralin
• Using mineral oil, then soap and water, to remove anthralin
• Avoiding scrubbing his skin vigorously
• Using a soft brush to remove scales
• Contacting the National Psoriasis Foundation and local support group

Skin cancer

Skin cancer is a malignant primary tumor of the skin. There are three types:
• Basal cell epithelioma is a tumor commonly caused by prolonged exposure to the sun.
• Melanoma is a neoplasm that arises from melanocytes. Melanoma spreads through the lymph and vascular systems and metastasizes to the lymph nodes, skin, liver, lungs, and central nervous system.
• Squamous cell carcinoma is a slow-growing cancer that causes airway obstruction, cough, and sputum production.

CAUSES
• Chemical irritants
• Friction or chronic irritation
• Immunosuppressive drugs
• Infrared heat or light
• Precancerous lesions: leukoplakia, nevi, senile keratoses
• Radiation
• UV rays

CONTRIBUTING FACTORS
• Heredity

ASSESSMENT FINDINGS
• Change in color, size, or shape of preexisting lesion
• Irregular, circular bordered lesion with hues of tan, black, or blue (melanoma)
• Local pain
• Oozing, bleeding, crusting lesion
• Pruritus
• Small, red, nodular lesion that begins as an erythematous macule or plaque with indistinct margins (squamous cell carcinoma)
• Waxy nodule with telangiectasis (basal cell epithelioma)

DIAGNOSTIC TEST RESULTS
• Skin biopsy shows cytology positive for cancer cells.

NURSING DIAGNOSES
• Anxiety
• Disturbed body image
• Impaired oral mucous membrane
• Fear

TREATMENT
• Chemosurgery with zinc chloride
• Cryosurgery with liquid nitrogen
• Curettage and electrodesiccation
• Radiation therapy

Drug therapy
• Alkylating agents: carmustine (BiCNU), dacarbazine (DTIC-Dome)
• Antiemetics: aprepitant (Emend), ondansetron (Zofran)
• Antimetabolite: fluorouracil
• Antineoplastics: hydroxyurea (Hydrea), vincristine
• Immunotherapy for melanoma: bacille Calmette-Guérin vaccine

INTERVENTIONS AND RATIONALES
• Monitor skin punch biopsy site *for bleeding.*
• Assess lesions. *Regular assessment prevents recurrence.*
• Monitor and record vital signs *to determine baseline and detect changes.*
• Administer medications, as prescribed, *to maintain and improve the client's condition.*
• Provide emotional support and encourage the client to express feelings about changes in body image and a fear of dying *to help him accept changes in body image.*

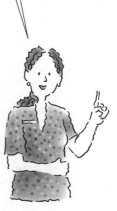

Remember, a change in color, size, or shape of a skin lesion may indicate a cancerous growth.

- Provide postchemotherapy and postradiation nursing care *to promote healing.*

Teaching topics
- Explanation of the disorder and treatment plan
- Medication use and possible adverse effects
- Avoiding contact with chemical irritants
- Using sun block and layered clothing when outdoors
- Self-monitoring for lesions and moles that don't heal or that change characteristics
- Removing moles that are subject to chronic irritation
- Contacting the Skin Cancer Foundation
- Contacting community agencies and resources and a local support group

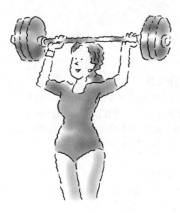

Pump up on practice questions

1.   The condition of a client with extensive third-degree burns begins to deteriorate. The nurse is aware that which type of shock may occur as a result of inadequate circulating blood volume that occurs with a burn injury?
1. Cardiogenic
2. Distributive
3. Hypovolemic
4. Septic

Answer: 3. Burns and the resulting low circulating fluid volume can cause hypovolemic shock. Cardiogenic shock occurs with inadequate pumping action of the heart. Distributive shock is caused by changes in blood vessel tone. Septic shock is a type of distributive shock.

➡ *NCLEX keys*
Client needs category: Physiological integrity
Client needs subcategory: Physiological adaptation
Cognitive level: Analysis

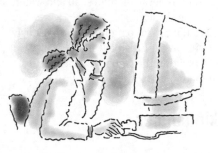

2.   A client undergoes a circular skin punch biopsy to confirm a diagnosis of skin cancer. Immediately following the procedure, the nurse should observe the site for:
1. infection.
2. dehiscence.
3. hemorrhage.
4. swelling.

Answer: 3. The nurse's main concern following a circular skin punch biopsy is to monitor for bleeding. Dehiscence is more likely in larger wounds such as surgical wounds of the abdomen or thorax. Infection is a later possible consequence of a skin punch biopsy and swelling is a normal reaction associated with any event that traumatizes the skin.

➡ *NCLEX keys*
Client needs category: Physiological integrity
Client needs subcategory: Reduction of risk potential
Cognitive level: Application

3. A client undergoes hypersensitivity testing with the intradermal technique. When the nurse administers the allergen, at what angle should the needle be inserted?
1. 0 degrees
2. 15 degrees
3. 45 degrees
4. 90 degrees

Answer: 2. The proper angle for intradermal injections is 15 degrees. There are no injections requiring a 0 degree insertion. The subcutaneous angle is 45 degrees and the intramuscular angle is 90 degrees.

➡ *NCLEX keys*
Client needs category: Health promotion and maintenance
Client needs subcategory: None
Cognitive level: Application

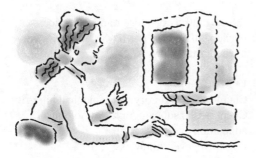

4. What is the best method for preventing hypovolemic shock in a client admitted with severe burns?
1. Administering dopamine
2. Applying medical antishock trousers
3. Infusing I.V. fluids
4. Infusing fresh frozen plasma

Answer: 3. During the early postburn period, large amounts of plasma fluid extravasates into interstitial spaces. Restoring the fluid loss is necessary to prevent hypovolemic shock; this is best accomplished with crystalloid and colloid solutions. Fresh frozen plasma is expensive and carries a slight risk of disease transmission. Medical antishock trousers would be applied to treat—not prevent—shock. Dopamine causes vasoconstriction and elevates blood pressure but it doesn't prevent hypovolemia in burn clients.

➡ *NCLEX keys*
Client needs category: Physiological integrity
Client needs subcategory: Physiological adaptation
Cognitive level: Application

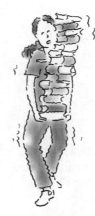

5. The Wood's light would be used during what phases of the nursing process?
1. Assessment and implementation
2. Planning and implementation
3. Diagnosis and implementation
4. Assessment and evaluation

Answer: 4. The Wood's light is used to assess for certain skin conditions and to evaluate the treatment of those conditions. It's a diagnostic tool, not a treatment device.

➡ *NCLEX keys*
Client needs category: Health promotion and maintenance
Client needs subcategory: None
Cognitive level: Application

6. The skin lesions evident in herpes zoster are similar to those seen in:
1. impetigo.
2. syphilis.
3. varicella.
4. rubella.

Answer: 3. Varicella (chickenpox) characteristically has vesicles as the hallmark lesion. Impetigo has pustules. Syphilis's primary lesion is the chancre and in rubella the lesion is a maculopapular rash.

➡ *NCLEX keys*
Client needs category: Physiological integrity
Client needs subcategory: Physiological adaptation
Cognitive level: Comprehension

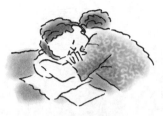

7. A client with widespread herpes zoster is placed on I.V. hydrocortisone. The nurse should monitor the client for:
1. hyperkalemia.
2. hypercalcemia.
3. hyperglycemia.
4. hypermagnesemia.

Answer: 3. Corticosteroids are known to elevate the blood glucose level and tend to lower serum potassium and calcium levels. Their effect on magnesium isn't substantial.

➡ *NCLEX keys*
Client needs category: Physiological integrity
Client needs subcategory: Pharmacological and parenteral therapies
Cognitive level: Application

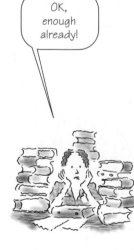

OK, enough already!

8. A client is admitted to a burn intensive care unit with extensive full-thickness burns. What should be the nurse's initial concern?
1. Fluid status
2. Risk for infection
3. Body image
4. Level of pain

Answer: 1. In early burn care, the client's greatest need has to do with fluid resuscitation because of large-volume fluid loss through the damaged skin. Infection, body image, and pain are definite concerns in the nursing care of a burn client but are less urgent than fluid management in the early phase of burn care.

➡ *NCLEX keys*
Client needs category: Physiological integrity
Client needs subcategory: Physiological adaptation
Cognitive level: Analysis

9. A triage nurse in the emergency department admits a 50-year-old male client with second-degree burns on the anterior and posterior portions of both legs. Based on the Rule of Nines, what percentage of his body is burned? Record your answer using a whole number.

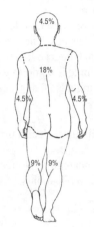

Answer: 36. The anterior and posterior portions of one leg are 18%. If both legs are burned, the total is 36%.

➡ *NCLEX keys*
Client needs category: Physiological integrity
Client needs subcategory: Physiological adaptation
Cognitive level: Analysis

10. A nurse is caring for a client with a new donor site that was harvested to treat a burn. The nurse should position the client to:
1. allow ventilation of the site.
2. make the site dependent.
3. avoid pressure on the site.
4. keep the site fully covered.

Answer: 3. A universal concern in the care of donor sites for burn care is to keep the site away from sources of pressure. Ventilation of the site and keeping the site fully covered are practices in some institutions but aren't hallmarks of donor site care. Placing the site in a position of dependence isn't a justified aspect of donor site care.

➡ *NCLEX keys*
Client needs category: Physiological integrity
Client needs subcategory: Physiological adaptation
Cognitive level: Analysis

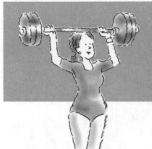

Pump up on more practice questions

1. A client experiences abdominal pain and exhibits blood in his stools and emesis. He's scheduled to undergo several diagnostic tests. The nurse may allow the client to eat normally if he is scheduled for:
1. an endoscopy.
2. a fecal occult blood test.
3. an endoscopic retrograde cholang-iopancreatography.
4. a barium swallow.

Answer: 2. The client may eat normally when a fecal occult blood test is scheduled; however, for endoscopic tests, an upper GI series, or a barium swallow, the client should have nothing by mouth before the test.

➡ *NCLEX keys*

Client needs category: Physiological integrity
Client needs subcategory: Reduction of risk potential
Cognitive level: Application

2. A nurse is providing teaching for a client with hiatal hernia. The nurse asks the client which foods he regularly consumes. What answer indicates the need for more teaching on this topic?
1. Milk products
2. Small meals
3. Fatty foods
4. Soft drinks

Answer: 4. Carbonated beverages stimulate belching and gastric reflux, causing lower esophageal irritation and associated pain of hiatal hernia. Milk products, fatty foods, and small meals aren't prohibited in the diet of a client with hiatal hernia.

➡ *NCLEX keys*

Client needs category: Physiological integrity
Client needs subcategory: Reduction of risk potential
Cognitive level: Analysis

3. A client experiences an exacerbation of ulcerative colitis. Test results reveal elevated serum osmolality and urine specific gravity. What's the most likely explanation for these test results?
1. Renal insufficiency
2. Hypoaldosteronism
3. Diabetes insipidus
4. Deficient fluid volume

Answer: 4. Ulcerative colitis causes watery diarrhea. The client will lose large volumes of fluid causing hemoconcentration and an elevated serum osmolality and urine specific gravity. Renal insufficiency, hypoaldosteronism and diabetes insipidus aren't associated with ulcerative colitis.

➡ *NCLEX keys*

Client needs category: Physiological integrity
Client needs subcategory: Reduction of risk potential
Cognitive level: Analysis

4. A client with Crohn's disease asks her nurse which food she should eat. What should the nurse recommend?
1. Celery
2. Peanut butter
3. Honey
4. Fudge

Answer: 3. The dietary recommendations for regional enteritis are foods high in protein, carbohydrates, and calories and low in fat, residue, and fiber. Honey is a high-calorie carbohydrate. Celery isn't recommended because it's high in residue and fiber. Peanut butter isn't recommended because it's high in fat. Fudge is typically high-fat and shouldn't be recommended.

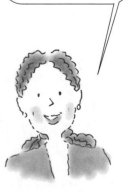

Pump up for the big test with these 30 adult health practice questions. Go for it!

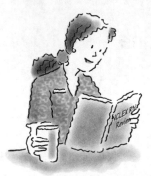

➡ *NCLEX keys*
Client needs category: Physiological integrity
Client needs subcategory: Reduction of risk potential
Cognitive level: Application

5. A client is diagnosed with acute diverticulitis. He's ordered gentamicin I.V. When administering gentamicin, the nurse should expect to give it:
1. I.V. push over 1 minute.
2. I.V. push over 2 minutes.
3. I.V. piggy back over 15 to 20 minutes.
4. I.V. piggy back over 30 to 60 minutes.

Answer: 4. Because of the risk for nephrotoxicity, aminoglycosides such as gentamicin should be administered slowly by intermittent infusion. The recommended length of time for administration is 30 to 60 minutes. I.V. boluses or pushes should be avoided.

➡ *NCLEX keys*
Client needs category: Physiological integrity
Client needs subcategory: Pharmacological and parenteral therapies
Cognitive level: Application

6. A nurse is assessing the abdomen of a client who was admitted to the emergency department with suspected appendicitis. Identify the area of the abdomen the nurse should palpate last.

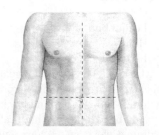

Answer: An acute attack of appendicitis localizes as pain and tenderness in the lower right quadrant, midway between the umbilicus and the crest of the ilium. This area should be palpated last to determine if pain is also present in other areas of the abdomen.

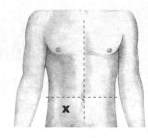

➡ *NCLEX keys*
Client needs category: Health promotion and maintenance
Client needs subcategory: None
Cognitive level: Application

7. A nurse is seeking to meet the nutritional needs of a client with acute peritonitis. The nurse should administer:
1. nasal enteral feedings.
2. gastric enteral feedings.
3. oral feedings.
4. parenteral feedings.

Answer: 4. To avoid introduction of nutritional products into the abdominal cavity through a perforation of the GI tract, the client with peritonitis is typically fed using the parenteral route either with total parenteral nutrition or peripheral parenteral nutrition. Feedings through a nasal cannula or gastric tube, or by the oral route are avoided.

➡ *NCLEX keys*
Client needs category: Physiological integrity
Client needs subcategory: Pharmacological and parenteral therapies
Cognitive level: Application

8. The client appears comfortable. However, a pulse oximetry alarm is sounding, and his oxygen saturation reads 80%. What should the nurse do first?
1. Check the client for a pulse.
2. Check the client for a pulse and auscultate breath sounds.
3. Check the temperature of the client's feet to determine if his toes are cold.
4. Check whether the heart rate reported by the pulse oximetry unit matches the client's actual heart rate.

Answer: 4. Always check a match between the heart rate reported on the pulse oximetry unit and the client's actual heart rate to determine if the equipment is functioning properly. Before checking pulse or breath sounds, ask the client how he's feeling. Cold toes could affect pulse oximetry but only if the probe is attached to the client's toes.

➡ *NCLEX keys*

Client needs category: Physiological integrity
Client needs subcategory: Reduction of risk potential
Cognitive level: Application

9. After an arteriogram for a suspected abdominal aortic aneurysm, a client reports itching skin. The nurse notes red blotches on the client's trunk. How should the nurse respond initially?
   1. Notify the physician.
   2. Administer an antihistamine.
   3. Check vital signs.
   4. Plan to monitor the blotches closely.

Answer: 3. An arteriogram involves administration of a radiopaque dye. Some clients are hypersensitive to the dye and exhibit related manifestations or pruritus and urticaria. More severe manifestations can also occur, including hypotension and dyspnea. Therefore, it's important to initially monitor vital signs. Notifying the physician, administering an antihistamine, and monitoring the red blotches have lesser priority.

➡ *NCLEX keys*

Client needs category: Physiological integrity
Client needs subcategory: Physiological adaptation
Cognitive level: Application

10. A client develops recurrent urolithiasis. What mineral will most likely be restricted in the client's diet?
   1. Phosphorus
   2. Calcium
   3. Magnesium
   4. Sodium

Answer: 2. In most cases, renal calculi are heavily composed of calcium; therefore, calcium-restricted diets are ordered in recurrent urolithiasis. Phosphorus, magnesium and sodium aren't typically restricted in the diet of the client with urolithiasis.

➡ *NCLEX keys*

Client needs category: Physiological integrity
Client needs subcategory: Reduction of risk potential
Cognitive level: Application

11. A client required a chest tube for treatment of a pneumothorax sustained in a motor vehicle accident. Several days have passed since the accident, and the physician wants to remove the chest tube. Before removing the tube, which intervention should the nurse perform?
   1. Premedicate the client 1 hour before the procedure to ensure the client's comfort during the procedure.
   2. Have one unit of packed red blood cells available for immediate transfusion.
   3. Clamp the tube for 2 hours before its removal.
   4. Have the client sign a consent form for the removal.

Answer: 1. Clients who are having procedures performed in the critical care unit should be given an analgesic 1 hour before the procedure. The procedure shouldn't be performed until the medication has taken effect. There's no reason to have blood available for this procedure. The tube should be clamped only if the physician has ordered it to be done. The consent would have been given when the chest tube was inserted.

➡ *NCLEX keys*

Client needs category: Physiological integrity
Client needs subcategory: Basic care and comfort
Cognitive level: Application

12. A 26-year-old client with chronic renal failure plans to receive a kidney transplant. The physician tells the client he's a poor candidate for transplant because of chronic uncontrolled hypertension and diabetes mellitus. Now, the client tells the nurse, "I want to go off dialysis. I'd rather not live than be on this treatment for the rest of my life." How should the nurse respond?

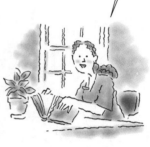

Are you feeling more confident by practicing more questions? Bring on the exam!

1. "We all have days when we don't feel like going on."
2. "You're feeling upset about the news you got about the transplant."
3. "The treatments are only three times a week. You can live with that."
4. "Whatever decision you make, we will support you."

Answer: 2. In reflecting the client's implied feelings, the nurse is promoting communication. Using platitudes such as "We all have days when we don't feel like going on" fails to address the individual client's needs. Reminding the client of the treatment frequency isn't addressing the client's needs. Offering support is therapeutic but doesn't address the client's expressed need to discuss the decision to go off dialysis.

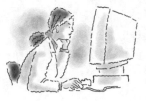

➡ **NCLEX keys**

Client needs category: Psychosocial integrity
Client needs subcategory: None
Cognitive level: Application

13. A client experiences urinary retention from benign prostatic hyperplasia and undergoes a transurethral resection of the prostate. Following the procedure, the client receives continuous bladder irrigation. The nurse notices that the drainage from the catheter has stopped. How should the nurse respond?
1. Replace the existing catheter.
2. Increase the infusion rate.
3. Attempt to dislodge a clot.
4. Notify the urologist.

Answer: 3. Most likely, the apparatus is blocked by a blood clot, which the nurse may remove by either gentle aspiration of the clot from the catheter or irrigation through the out-port. It's probably unnecessary to replace the apparatus. Increasing the flow may cause bladder distention and pain. Calling the physician isn't an appropriate initial nursing response because the nurse has the autonomy to solve this problem without calling the physician first.

➡ **NCLEX keys**

Client needs category: Physiological integrity
Client needs subcategory: Physiological adaptation
Cognitive level: Application

14. A nurse is caring for a client who has had extensive abdominal surgery and is in critical condition. The nurse notes that the complete blood count shows an 8 g/dl hemoglobin and a 30% hematocrit. Dextrose 5% in half-normal saline solution is infusing through a triple-lumen central venous access device at 125 ml/hour. The physician orders include:

Gentamicin 80 mg I.V. piggyback in 50 ml D_5W over 30 minutes.
Ranitidine (Zantac) 50 mg I.V. in 50 ml D_5W piggyback over 30 minutes.
One unit of 250 ml of packed red blood cells (RBCs) over 3 hours.
Flush the nasogastric tube with 30 ml normal saline every 2 hours.

How many milliliters should the nurse document as the intake for the 8-hour shift? Record your answer using a whole number.

_____ ml

Answer: 1,470. Use the following information to help solve the equation:

Regular I.V. at 125 ml/hour × 8 hours = 1,000 ml
Gentamicin piggyback = 50 ml
Ranitidine piggyback = 50 ml
Packed RBCs = 250 ml
Nasogastric flushes 30 ml × 4 = 120 ml
Total = 1,470 ml.

➡ **NCLEX keys**

Client needs category: Physiological integrity
Client needs subcategory: Basic care and comfort
Cognitive level: Analysis

15. A nurse is instructing a client regarding skin tests for hypersensitivity reactions. The nurse should teach the client to:
1. keep skin test areas moist with a mild lotion.
2. stay out of direct sunlight until tests are read.
3. wash the sites daily with a mild soap.
4. have the sites read on the correct date.

Answer: 4. An important facet of evaluating skin tests is to read the skin test results at the proper time. Evaluating the skin test too late or too early will give inaccurate and unreliable results. The sites should be kept dry. There's no requirement to wash the sites with soap, and direct sunlight isn't prohibited.

➡ NCLEX keys

Client needs category: Health promotion and maintenance
Client needs subcategory: None
Cognitive level: Application

16. A client is admitted to the hospital with an acute exacerbation of asthma. Auscultation reveals almost absent breath sounds. Thirty minutes after administering albuterol by nebulizer, the nurse auscultates diffuse inspiratory and expiratory wheezes throughout all lung fields. This finding most likely represents:

1. increased airflow.
2. no change in airflow.
3. decreased airflow.
4. no correlation with airflow.

Answer: 1. Changes in breath sounds provide a general indication of response to treatment. Nearly absent breath sounds or no breath sounds indicate severe airflow obstruction. A noisy chest is a sign that air is flowing through the air passages even though they're partially obstructed.

➡ NCLEX keys

Client needs category: Physiological integrity
Client needs subcategory: Physiological adaptation
Cognitive level: Application

17. A client is scheduled to perform a 24-hour urine test beginning at 8 a.m. on the first day and ending at 8 a.m. on the second day. The nurse should instruct the client to:

1. discard the second-day 8 a.m. sample.
2. discard the first and last samples.
3. discard the first-day 8 a.m. sample.
4. retain all samples collected.

Answer: 3. In a 24-hour urine test, the first sample is discarded and the last sample is retained.

➡ NCLEX keys

Client needs category: Health promotion and maintenance
Client needs subcategory: None
Cognitive level: Application

18. A nurse is planning to administer levothyroxine (Synthroid) to an adult client.

Which vital signs measurements indicate that the nurse should consider withholding the dose and consulting the physician?

1. Temperature 97.8° F (36.6° C), pulse 88 beats/minute, respirations 22 breaths/minute, blood pressure 110/70 mm Hg
2. Temperature 98.4° F (36.9° C), pulse 54 beats/minute, respirations 16 breaths/minute, blood pressure 100/56 mm Hg
3. Temperature 99° F (37.2° C), pulse 110 beats/minute, respirations 20 breaths/minute, blood pressure 136/88 mm Hg
4. Temperature 98.8° F (37.1°C), pulse 72 beats/minute, respirations 12 breaths/minute, blood pressure 118/72 mm Hg

Answer: 3. Levothyroxine can cause tachycardia, indicated here by a pulse rate of 110 beats/minute. Tachycardia is an indication of thyroid toxicity.

➡ NCLEX keys

Client needs category: Physiological integrity
Client needs subcategory: Pharmacological and parenteral therapies
Cognitive level: Application

19. A client is receiving treatment for Cushing's syndrome. A reduction in which laboratory measurement would provide an indication that treatment is successful?

1. Serum potassium levels
2. Urine sodium levels
3. Gastric pH
4. Serum glucose levels

Answer: 4. Cushing's syndrome causes hyperglycemia, which may require exogenous insulin administration. Because Cushing's syndrome causes hypokalemia and hypernatremia, a drop in serum potassium and urine sodium levels wouldn't indicate improvement. Cushing's syndrome causes increased gastric acid secretion so a reduction in gastric pH is an undesirable finding.

➡ NCLEX keys

Client needs category: Physiological integrity
Client needs subcategory: Physiological adaptation
Cognitive level: Analysis

Stay focused. You're almost done

20. A client scheduled for a gastroscopy has had nothing by mouth since midnight. The procedure is scheduled for 8 a.m. At 6:30 a.m., the nurse collects a capillary blood glucose sample that registers 40 mg/dl on the glucose monitor. The client is alert, has clear speech, and states, "I don't feel like my sugar is too low." Initially the nurse should:

1. document the finding and withhold the client's morning insulin.
2. repeat the capillary blood glucose test.
3. give the client an oral simple sugar.
4. administer dextrose 50 g I.V. immediately.

Answer: 2. Because the client is asymptomatic for hypoglycemia yet the capillary blood glucose reading is significantly subnormal, an error may have occurred in obtaining the result. The nurse should repeat the test. Because the blood glucose reading is so low, responding to the reading has precedence over documenting findings. Because of the inconsistency between the 40 mg/dl reading and the absence of symptoms, rechecking the value should precede administering glucose.

➡ *NCLEX keys*
Client needs category: Physiological integrity
Client needs subcategory: Physiological adaptation
Cognitive level: Application

21. A client who receives immunosuppressive drugs for systemic lupus erythematosus develops a fever. The nurse should:

1. administer prescribed antipyretics.
2. place the client in isolation.
3. apply cooling measures immediately.
4. help identify the cause.

Answer: 4. Immunosuppressive drugs impair the client's immunocompetence and predispose him to infection. Fever is a manifestation of infection; therefore, it's most important to discover the cause of the fever as soon as possible. Antipyretics should be withheld until cultures have been obtained. Isolation isn't indicated unless the absolute neutrophil count is less than 1,000. Cooling measures may be indicated but don't have priority over organism identification.

➡ *NCLEX keys*
Client needs category: Physiological integrity
Client needs subcategory: Reduction of risk potential
Cognitive level: Application

22. Which clinical finding distinguishes rheumatoid arthritis from osteoarthritis and gouty arthritis?

1. Crepitus with range of motion
2. Symmetry of joint involvement
3. Elevated serum uric acid levels
4. Dominance in weight-bearing joints

Answer: 2. Rheumatoid arthritis is bilateral and symmetrical; in contrast, osteoarthritis and gouty arthritis are unilateral. Crepitus is most associated with osteoarthritis. Elevated serum uric acid levels are seen in gouty arthritis; weight-bearing joint dominance occurs in osteoarthritis.

➡ *NCLEX keys*
Client needs category: Physiological integrity
Client needs subcategory: Physiological adaptation
Cognitive level: Comprehension

23. A client undergoes screening for sexually transmitted diseases. The results of an enzyme-linked immunosorbent assay (ELISA) are positive. The client asks the nurse to explain the meaning of test results. How should the nurse respond?

1. "Test results indicate that the human immunodeficiency virus is in your blood."
2. "These test results are early evidence of acquired immunodeficiency syndrome."
3. "Test results suggest that you have contracted a viral sexually transmitted disease. The specific disease needs to be identified."
4. "Test results indicate the possibility that you have contracted the human immunodeficiency virus."

Answer: 4. ELISA is a screening test for presence of the human immunodeficiency virus (HIV). A positive result implies exposure to HIV, but confirmation requires a Western blot analysis.

➡ *NCLEX keys*
Client needs category: Physiological integrity
Client needs subcategory: Reduction of risk potential
Cognitive level: Application

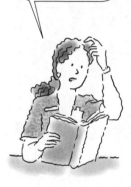

On second thought, maybe it's time for a study break.

24. The nurse is caring for a client who fractured the head of his femur in a fall and underwent internal fixation of his fractured left femur. Which assessment finding requires immediate intervention?

1. Rapid capillary refill in the left foot
2. Petechiae on the neck and upper chest
3. Abduction of the legs
4. Edema of the left foot that improves with elevation of the left leg

Answer: 2. Fat embolism occurs after long bone fractures such as a femur fracture. This forces bone marrow fat globules into the client's venous circulation. If the fat emboli are small, the client may have only vague symptoms, such as slight fever and disorientation. If the embolus is large, or if multiple emboli exist, the client may experience tachycardia, dyspnea, accessory muscle use, wheezing, and petechiae on the neck, upper chest, shoulders, axillae, and buccal membranes. Rapid capillary refill in the left foot shows that circulation in the left leg wasn't compromised by the injury. The leg should be positioned in abduction, not adduction, to prevent dislocation. Edema is normal in an affected foot after surgery.

➡ *NCLEX keys*
Client needs category: Physiological integrity
Client needs subcategory: Reduction of risk potential
Cognitive level: Analysis

25. A client with a history of severe penicillin hypersensitivity is about to undergo arthrocentesis. The orthopedic surgeon orders a broad-spectrum antibiotic for prophylactic purposes. Which antibiotic is most likely to be ordered?

1. Ampicillin and sulbactam
2. Erythromycin
3. Cefazolin
4. Gentamicin

Answer: 2. Erythromycin is a broad-spectrum antibiotic commonly used as a substitute in persons with penicillin allergy. Ampicillin is a penicillin and shouldn't be given to clients with penicillin hypersensitivity. Cefazolin is a cephalosporin. Persons allergic to penicillin can have sensitivity to cephalosporins. Gentamicin is a narrow-spectrum antibiotic and isn't suitable for prophylaxis.

➡ *NCLEX keys*
Client needs category: Physiological integrity
Client needs subcategory: Reduction of risk potential
Cognitive level: Analysis

26. A client is scheduled for a myelogram, which requires administration of an I.V. radiopaque dye. The nurse informs the client that during the procedure he may experience:

1. chest tightness.
2. burning at the I.V. site.
3. flushing of the face.
4. increased salivation.

Answer: 3. A typical response to I.V. radiopaque dye is the sensation of flushing of the face. Chest tightness is associated with a hypersensitive reaction and isn't an expected response. Neither burning at the I.V. site nor increased salivation is associated with administration of radiopaque dye.

➡ *NCLEX keys*
Client needs category: Health promotion and maintenance
Client needs subcategory: None
Cognitive level: Comprehension

27. A client with herniated nucleus pulposus of the lumbar spine is scheduled for a laminotomy. The nurse is providing preoperative teaching. How should the nurse instruct the client to get out of bed after the procedure?

1. Pulling himself up using an over-the-bed trapeze
2. Logrolling to a side-lying position
3. Twisting to a sitting position
4. Avoiding use of abdominal muscles

Answer: 2. Following back surgery such as a laminotomy, it's best for the client to initially get out of bed by logrolling to his side. Using an over-the-bed trapeze or twisting may put strain on the surgical site. When repositioning, the client should actually tighten his abdominal muscles.

➡ *NCLEX keys*
Client needs category: Physiological integrity
Client needs subcategory: Reduction of risk potential
Cognitive level: Application

28. To prevent dislocation in a client on the first postoperative day after a right total hip replacement, the nurse should avoid positioning him:
1. with the right leg externally rotated.
2. in the left lateral decubitus position.
3. with the legs adducted.
4. in semi-Fowler's position.

Answer: 3. To prevent dislocation following a total hip replacement, leg adduction should be avoided. Instead, the legs should be abducted. External rotation of the affected leg is appropriate as well as sitting at a 45-degree angle.

➡ *NCLEX keys*
Client needs category: Physiological integrity
Client needs subcategory: Reduction of risk potential
Cognitive level: Application

29. A client with Parkinson's disease is receiving carbidopa-levodopa (Sinemet). Decrease in the frequency of which clinical manifestation of the disorder best indicates the drug's effectiveness?
1. Tremors
2. Swallowing
3. Seizures
4. Lacrimation

Answer: 1. A common sign of Parkinson's disease is tremors. Successful therapy with carbidopa-levodopa should result in diminution of tremors. Increased swallowing and lacrimation aren't manifestations of Parkinson's disease. Seizures aren't associated with Parkinson's disease.

➡ *NCLEX keys*
Client needs category: Physiological integrity
Client needs subcategory: Pharmacological and parenteral therapies
Cognitive level: Application

30. The nurse is caring for a client who experienced a myocardial infarction 3 days ago. As the nurse walks into the client's room, the client slumps over and is unresponsive. The nurse checks the client's pulse and finds none. What rhythm should the nurse expect to find on the client's electrocardiogram?

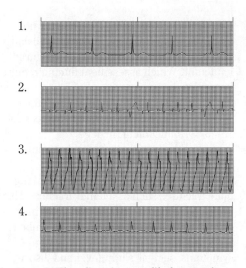

1.

2.

3.

4.

Answer: 3. The client is most likely experiencing ventricular tachycardia, as illustrated in strip #3. Strip #1 shows sinus bradycardia. The client may complain of light-headedness, but he would still have a pulse. Strip #2 shows sinus tachycardia with premature ventricular contractions. This rhythm won't cause the client's symptoms. Strip #4 shows atrial fibrillation, which may cause an irregular pulse, but the client would still have a pulse.

➡ *NCLEX keys*
Client needs category: Physiological integrity
Client needs subcategory: Reduction of risk potential
Cognitive level: Analysis

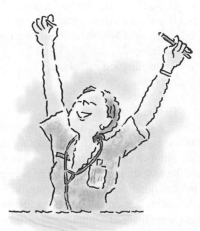

Part III   Psychiatric care

12 Essentials of psychiatric nursing

Brush up on key concepts

Effective client care of all kinds requires consideration of both psychological and physiologic aspects of health. A client who seeks medical help for chest pain, for example, may also need to be assessed for anxiety or depression. As a nurse, you'll need a fundamental understanding of communication techniques as well as an understanding of psychiatric disorders.

At anytime, you can review the major points of the essentials of psychiatric nursing by consulting the *Cheat sheet* on pages 376 and 377.

The key to any relationship

Therapeutic communication is the foundation for developing a nurse-client relationship. It's the primary intervention in psychiatric nursing. Therapeutic communication requires awareness of both the client's verbal and nonverbal messages.

To uncover and investigate the client's inner thoughts, personal problems, and emotions, the nurse must establish trust and help the client feel safe and respected. A therapeutic relationship helps the client feel understood, become comfortable discussing problems, and find better ways to meet his emotional needs and develop satisfying relationships.

You got your ears on?

Listening intently to the client enables the nurse to hear and analyze everything the client is saying, alerting the nurse to the client's communication patterns.

Connect the dots

Succinct **rephrasing** of key client statements helps ensure the nurse's understanding and emphasizes important points in the client's message. For example, the nurse might say, "You're feeling angry and you say it's because of the way your friend treated you yesterday."

Keep the door open

Using **broad openings** and **general statements** to initiate conversations encourages the client to talk about any subject that comes to mind. These openings allow the client to focus the conversation and demonstrate the nurse's willingness to interact. An example of this technique is: "Tell me what's on your mind."

Polish the rough edges

Asking the client to **clarify** a confusing or vague message demonstrates the nurse's desire to understand what the client is saying. It can also elicit precise information crucial to the client's recovery. An example of clarifying is: "I'm not sure I understood what you said."

A sharper focus

In the technique called **focusing,** the nurse assists the client in redirecting attention toward something specific. It fosters the client's self-control and helps avoid vague generalizations, thereby enabling the client to accept responsibility for facing problems. "Let's go back to what we were just talking about," is one example of this technique.

It's golden

Refraining from comment can have several benefits. **Silence** gives the client time to talk, think, and gain insight into problems. It also permits the nurse to gather more information. The nurse must use this technique judiciously, however, to avoid giving the impression of disinterest or judgment.

Valuable assistance

When used correctly, the technique of **suggesting collaboration** gives the client the

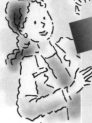

Cheat sheet

Essentials of psychiatric nursing refresher

KEY CONCEPTS
Therapeutic communication
• Requires awareness of the client's verbal and nonverbal messages
• Involves establishing trust and helping the client feel safe and respected
• Listening intently—allows the nurse to analyze what the patient is saying and alerts the nurse to communication patterns
• Rephrasing—involves rephrasing what the client says to ensure the nurse's understanding
• Broad openings and general statements—give the client an opening to focus the conversation and demonstrate the nurse's willingness to talk
• Clarification—helps the nurse resolve confusing or vague messages and demonstrates to the client a willingness to understand
• Focusing—involves redirecting the client's attention to something specific
• Silence—gives the client time to talk, think, and gain insight into problems; gives the nurse a chance to gather more information

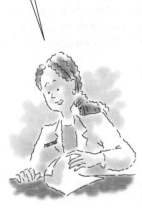

It's okay to look at this Cheat sheet.

KEY ASSESSMENTS
Client history
• Client's chief complaint or concern
• History of the present illness
• Past psychiatric illness
• Personal or developmental history
• Family history
• Social history
• Cultural considerations

Physical examination
• General appearance
• Behavior
• Mood
• Thought processes and cognitive function
• Coping mechanisms
• Potential for self-destructive behavior

KEY PSYCHOLOGICAL TESTS
• Mini–Mental Status Examination—measures orientation, registration, recall, calculation, language, and motor skills

• Cognitive Capacity Screening Examination—measures orientation, memory, calculation, and language
• Global Deterioration Scale—assesses and stages primary degenerative dementia, based on orientation, memory, and neurologic function
• Functional Dementia Scale—measures orientation, affect, and the ability to perform activities of daily living
• Beck Depression Inventory—helps diagnose depression, determine its severity, and monitor the client's response during treatment
• Eating Attitudes Test—detects patterns that suggest an eating disorder
• Minnesota Multiphasic Personality Inventory—helps assess personality traits and ego function in adults and adolescents
• Michigan Alcoholism Screen Test—24-item timed test; score of 5 or better classifies the client as an alcoholic
• CAGE Questionnaire—four questions in which two or three positive responses indicate alcoholism
• Cocaine Addiction Severity Test and Cocaine Assessment Profile—evaluate for cocaine abuse

KEY TREATMENTS
• Individual therapy—uses three phrases to establish a structured relationship between the nurse and client in attempt to achieve change in the client
• Milieu therapy—uses the hospital environment to promote self-esteem and learning of new skills and behaviors so the client can live outside of the institutional setting
• Biological therapies—used for disturbances thought to be caused by chemical imbalances or by disease-causing organisms; includes psychoactive drugs and electroconvulsive therapy
• Cognitive behavioral therapy—employs strategies, such as role playing and thought substitution, to modify the beliefs and attitudes that influence a client's feelings and behaviors

Essentials of psychiatric nursing refresher (continued)

KEY TREATMENTS (CONTINUED)

• Reality therapy—focuses on assisting the client to love and be loved and feel worthwhile and feel that others are worthwhile
• Family therapy—involves the entire family to improve family function
• Group therapy—includes an advanced practice nurse–therapist and six to eight clients and aims to increase self-awareness, change maladaptive behaviors, and improve interpersonal relationships

• Crisis intervention—short-term therapy to address an unbearable situation
• Hypnosis—induces deep relaxation by altering the client's state of consciousness; used for anxiety disorders, pain, repressed traumatic events, and addictive disorders

---

opportunity to explore the pros and cons of a suggested approach. It must be used carefully to avoid directing the client. An example of this technique is: "Perhaps we can meet with your parents to discuss the matter."

A two-way street

In the technique called **sharing impressions,** the nurse attempts to describe the client's feelings and then seeks corrective feedback from the client. This allows the client to clarify any misperceptions and gives the nurse a better understanding of the client's true feelings. For example, the nurse might say, "Tell me if my perception of what you're telling me agrees with yours."

Brush up on assessment

Because a nurse is commonly the health care provider who develops the closest long-term relationship with a client, the nurse is commonly most capable of assessing the emotional and mental health care needs of the client and identifying the appropriate interventions.

During the assessment stage, the nurse determines a client's psychological and physiologic status by assessing:
• client's history
• client's physical status (including mental status examination)
• laboratory and diagnostic tests.

Gathering data #1: Getting history

A complete **client history** provides information about:
• client's chief complaint or concern
• history of the present illness
• past psychiatric illness
• personal or developmental history
• family history
• social history
• cultural considerations that may affect the client's outcome.

Gathering data #2: Getting physical

The **physical examination** provides objective data that will help confirm or rule out assessments made during the health history interview.

In addition to the routine physical examination, the nurse should assess the client's:
• general appearance — helps indicate the client's emotional and mental status. The nurse should specifically note his dress and grooming.
• behavior — the nurse should note the client's demeanor and overall attitude as well as any extraordinary behavior.
• mood — ask the client to describe his current feelings in concrete terms and to suggest possible reasons for these feelings. Be sure to note inconsistencies between body language and mood.
• thought processes and cognitive function — the client's orientation to time, place, or person can indicate confusion or disorientation. The presence of delusions, hallucinations, obsessions, compulsions, fantasies, and day-dreams should be noted.

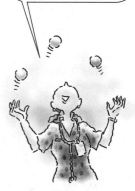

Consider all aspects of the client's functioning: biological, psychological, and social.

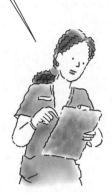

Every therapeutic relationship calls for sensitive and attentive communication.

• coping mechanisms — a client who is faced with a stressful situation may adopt excessive coping or defense mechanisms, which operate on an unconscious level to protect the ego. Examples include denial, regression, displacement, projection, reaction formation, and fantasy.
• potential for self-destructive behavior — a client who has lost touch with reality may cut or mutilate body parts to focus on physical pain, which may be less overwhelming than emotional distress.

Keep abreast of diagnostic tests

Diagnosing psychiatric disorders differs from diagnosing other medical disorders. (See *The authority*.) While many medical tests involve instrumentation and physical analyses, psychological testing focuses on questioning and observing the client.

Performing diagnostic tests on a client with a suspected psychiatric disorder may assist with accurate diagnosis, can reveal underlying physiologic disorders, establishes normal renal and hepatic function, and monitors for therapeutic medication levels.

Blood study #1
A **blood chemistry test** assesses a blood sample for potassium, sodium, calcium, phosphorus, glucose, bicarbonate, blood urea nitrogen, creatinine, protein, albumin,

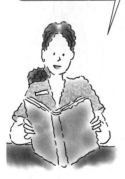

The DSM is updated regularly... make sure your information is up-to-date!

osmolality, amylase, lipase, alkaline phosphatase, ammonia, bilirubin, lactate dehydrogenase, aspartate aminotransferase, and alanine aminotransferase.

Nursing actions
• Explain the procedure to the client.
• Withhold food and fluids before the procedure, as directed.
• Check the venipuncture site for bleeding after the procedure.

Blood study #2
A **hematologic study** uses a blood sample to analyze red blood cells, white blood cells, prothrombin time, international normalized ratio, partial thromboplastin time, erythrocyte sedimentation rate, platelets, hemoglobin, and hematocrit.

Nursing actions
• Explain the procedure to the client.
• Note current drug therapy before the procedure.
• Check the venipuncture site for bleeding after the procedure.

Blood study #3
The **dexamethasone suppression test,** which involves administration of dexamethasone, is used to analyze a blood sample for serum cortisol.

Nursing actions
• Explain the procedure to the client.
• On the first day, give the client 1 mg of dextramethasone at 11 p.m.

The authority

Published by the American Psychiatric Association, the *Diagnostic and Statistical Manual of Mental Disorders (DSM)* is a standard interdisciplinary psychiatric diagnostic system designed to be used by all members of the mental health care team. The manual includes a complete description of psychiatric disorders and other conditions and describes diagnostic criteria that must be met to support each diagnosis.

The current manual is the fourth edition, text revision, commonly known as *DSM-IV-TR*. The *DSM* is updated periodically, and new information regularly replaces old.

- On the next day, collect blood samples at 4 p.m. and 11 p.m.
- Monitor the venipuncture site; if hematoma develops, apply warm soaks.
- List any medications that might interfere with the test.

AIDS-related blood study #1

Enzyme-linked immunosorbent assay uses a blood sample to detect the human immunodeficiency virus (HIV)-1 antibody (acquired immunodeficiency syndrome [AIDS] can cause psychiatric complications).

Nursing actions
- Explain the procedure to the client.
- Verify that informed consent has been obtained and documented.
- Provide the client with appropriate pretest counseling.
- After the procedure, check the venipuncture site for bleeding.

AIDS-related blood study #2

A **Western blot test** uses a blood sample to detect the presence of specific viral proteins to confirm HIV infection.

Nursing actions
- Explain the procedure to the client.
- Verify that informed consent has been obtained and documented.
- After the procedure, check the venipuncture site for bleeding.

Drug detection

Toxicology screening uses a urine specimen to detect unknown drugs.

Nursing actions
- Explain the procedure to the client.
- Make sure that written, informed consent has been obtained.
- Witness the procurement of the urine specimen and process according to the facility's protocol.

Brain meter-reading

An **electroencephalogram** records the electrical activity of the brain. Using electrodes, this noninvasive test gives a graphic representation of brain activity.

Nursing actions
- Explain the procedure to the client.
- Determine the client's ability to lie still.
- Reassure the client that electrical shock won't occur.
- Warn the client that he will be subjected to stimuli, such as lights and sounds.
- Withhold medications and caffeine for 24 to 48 hours before the procedure, as directed.

Dye job

A **computed tomography (CT) scan,** used to identify brain abnormalities, produces a finely detailed image of the brain and its structures. It may be performed with or without the injection of contrast dye.

Nursing actions
- Explain the procedure to the client.
- Note the client's allergies to iodine, seafood, and radiopaque dyes.
- Allay the client's anxiety.
- Ensure that signed, informed consent has been obtained per facility policy.
- Inform the client about possible throat irritation and flushing of the face, if contrast dye is injected.

Mental picture

Magnetic resonance imaging uses electromagnetic energy to create a detailed visualization of the brain and its structures.

Nursing actions
- Explain the procedure to the client.
- Be aware that clients with pacemakers, surgical and orthopedic clips, or shrapnel shouldn't be scanned.
- Remove jewelry and metal objects from the client.
- Determine the client's ability to lie still.
- Check that informed consent or other pretesting forms are completed as required by facility policy.
- Administer sedation, as prescribed.

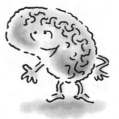

Computed tomography is used to identify brain abnormalities because it produces a finely detailed image of the brain.

Brain metabolism test

Positron emission tomography involves injection of a radioisotope, allowing visualization of the brain's oxygen uptake, blood flow, and glucose metabolism.

Nursing actions
- Explain the procedure to the client.
- Determine the client's ability to lie still during the procedure.
- Withhold alcohol, tobacco, and caffeine for 24 hours before the procedure.
- Withhold medications, as directed, before the procedure.
- Check that informed consent or pre-testing forms are signed, as required by facility policy.
- Check the injection site for bleeding after the procedure.

Thyroid function test

A **thyroid uptake,** also called **radioactive iodine uptake** or **RAIU**, is used to measure the amount of radioactive iodine taken up by the thyroid gland in 24 hours. This measurement evaluates thyroid function.

Nursing actions
- Explain the procedure to the client.
- Instruct the client not to ingest iodine-rich foods for 24 hours before the test.
- Discontinue all thyroid and cough medications 7 to 10 days before the test.

Radiograph of the 'roid

A **thyroid scan** gives visual imaging of radioactivity distribution in the thyroid gland that helps assess size, shape, position, and anatomic function of the thyroid.

Nursing actions
- Explain the procedure to the client.
- If iodine-123 (^{123}I) or ^{131}I is to be used, tell the client to fast after midnight the night before the test. Fasting isn't required if an I.V. injection of ^{99m}Tc pertechnetate is used.
- Withhold any medications that may interfere with the procedure.
- Instruct the client to stop consuming iodized salt, iodinated salt substitutes, and seafood one week before the procedure.
- Imaging follow soral administration (^{123}I or ^{131}I) by 24 hours and I.V. injection (^{99m}Tc pertechnetate) by 20 to 30 minutes.
- Remove dentures, jewelry, and other materials that may interfere with imaging.
- After the procedure, tell the client he may resume medications that were suspended for testing.

Keep abreast of psychological tests

Psychological tests evaluate the client's mood, personality, and mental status. Here's a review of the most common psychological tests.

Pop quiz
The **Mini–Mental Status Examination** measures orientation, registration, recall, calculation, language, and motor skills.

Cognitive capacity
The **Cognitive Capacity Screening Examination** measures orientation, memory, calculation, and language.

General knowledge
The **Cognitive Assessment Scale** measures orientation, general knowledge, mental ability, and psychomotor function.

Measuring what's lost
The **Global Deterioration Scale** assesses and stages primary degenerative dementia, based on orientation, memory, and neurologic function.

Getting by
The **Functional Dementia Scale** measures orientation, affect, and the ability to perform activities of daily living.

Measuring depression
The **Beck Depression Inventory** helps diagnose depression, determine its severity, and monitor the client's response during treatment.

What's on the menu?
The **Eating Attitudes Test** detects patterns that suggest an eating disorder.

Who are you?
The **Minnesota Multiphasic Personality Inventory** helps assess personality traits and ego function in adolescents and adults. Test results include information on coping strategies, defenses, strengths, gender identification, and self-esteem. The test pattern may strongly suggest a diagnostic category, point to a suicide risk, or indicate the potential for violence.

Alcoholism test #1
The **Michigan Alcoholism Screening Test** is a 24-item timed test in which a score of 5 or better classifies the client as an alcoholic.

Alcoholism test #2
The **CAGE Questionnaire** is a four-question tool in which two or three positive responses indicate alcoholism.

Cocaine addiction tests
The **Cocaine Addiction Severity Test** and **Cocaine Assessment Profile** are used when cocaine use is suspected.

Polish up on client care

Various treatment options coexist in psychiatric and mental health care. Nurses may use one specific treatment approach or a combination of approaches to guide client care.

One on one
Individual therapy is the establishment of a structured relationship between nurse and client in an attempt to achieve change in the client. The nurse works with the client to develop an approach to resolve conflict, decrease emotional pain, and develop appropriate ways of meeting the client's needs. This relationship with the client consists of three overlapping phases:
- the orientation phase, in which the nurse builds a connection with the client by establishing rapport and a sense of trust (goals are formulated in this phase)
- the working phase, in which the client becomes increasingly involved in self-exploration (the nurse assists the client as he tries to develop self-understanding and encourages him to take risks in terms of changing dysfunctional behavior)
- the termination phase, in which the client and nurse determine that closure of the relationship is appropriate (both parties agree that the problem that initiated the relationship has been alleviated or has become manageable).

Milling around
During **milieu therapy,** the nurse uses all aspects of the hospital environment in a therapeutic manner. Clients are exposed to rules, expectations, peer pressure, and social interactions. Nurses encourage communication and decision making and provide opportunities for enhancing self-esteem and learning new skills and behaviors. The goal of therapy is to enable the client to live outside the institutional setting.

Treating disease and imbalance
Biological therapies are called for when emotional and behavioral disturbances are thought to be caused by chemical imbalances or by disease-causing organisms.

Some examples of biological therapies are:
- psychoactive drugs
- electroconvulsive therapy
- nonconvulsive electrical stimulation.

Changing ideas
Cognitive behavioral therapy employs strategies to modify the beliefs and attitudes that influence a client's feelings and behaviors.

Some basic cognitive interventions include:
- teaching thought substitution
- identifying problem-solving strategies
- finding ways to modify negative self-talk
- role playing
- modeling coping strategies.

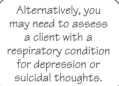

It's a balancing act! While identifying the disordered thought of a schizophrenic client, also assess for physiologic complications.

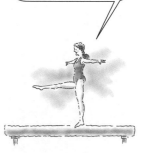

Alternatively, you may need to assess a client with a respiratory condition for depression or suicidal thoughts.

The real world
Reality therapy focuses on assisting the client meet two basic emotional needs:
- loving and being loved
- feeling worthwhile and feeling that others are worthwhile.

The nurse emphasizes personal responsibility for behavior, controlling one's own life, and fulfilling basic needs.

All in the family
During **family therapy,** the entire family is considered the treatment unit. The primary goal of therapy is to improve the functioning of the family. The types of clients that can benefit most from family therapy are those involved in marital issues, intergenerational conflicts, sibling concerns, and family crises, such as death and divorce.

The gang's all here
Group therapy includes an advanced practice nurse–therapist and six to eight people who meet regularly for the purpose of increasing self-awareness, improving interpersonal relationships, and changing maladaptive behavioral problems. Like individual therapy, group therapy goes through the orientation phase, working phase, and termination phase.

Urgent care
Crisis intervention is a systemic approach to short-term therapy in which the nurse works with a client, family, or group that's experiencing a potentially dangerous situation. The nurse initiates actions to decrease the client's sense of personal danger and facilitate the client's ability to control the situation.

Trance time
Hypnosis is used to induce deep relaxation by altering the client's state of consciousness. The result of hypnotic induction is a trancelike state during which clients use memories, mental associations, and concentration to discover experiences that are connected to their current distress. Hypnosis is effective for dealing with anxiety disorders, some types of pain, repressed traumatic events, and addictive disorders.

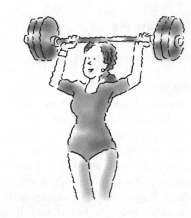

Pump up on practice questions

1. A client tells the nurse that he never disagrees with anyone and that he has loved everyone he's ever known. What would be the nurse's best response to this client?
1. "How do you manage to do that?"
2. "That's hard to believe. Most people couldn't do that."
3. "What do you do with your feelings of dissatisfaction or anger?"
4. "How did you come to adopt such a way of life?"

Answer: 4. Inquiring about the client's way of life allows for further exploration of the message he's trying to convey. Asking him how he's managed to do that has too narrow a focus and doesn't permit maximal exploration of the client's experience. Expressing disbelief is incorrect because the client could misinterpret it as a challenge and become even more defensive. Asking about feelings of dissatisfaction or anger is incorrect because the nurse shouldn't identify the client's feelings for him.

➡ *NCLEX keys*
Client needs category: Psychosocial integrity
Client needs subcategory: None
Cognitive level: Application

2. A nurse is working with a client who has just stimulated her anger by using a condescending tone of voice. Which response by the nurse is most therapeutic?
1. "I feel angry when I hear that tone of voice."
2. "You make me so angry when you talk to me that way."
3. "Are you trying to make me angry?"
4. "Why do you use that condescending tone of voice with me?"

Answer: 1. This response allows the nurse to provide feedback without making the client responsible for the nurse's reaction. Stating that the client makes you angry is accusatory and blocks communication. "Are you trying to make me angry" is a challenging remark that can lead to power struggles, lowers the client's self-esteem, and blocks opportunities for open communication. Avoid "why" questions such as "Why do you use that condescending tone of voice with me" because these questions put the client on the defensive.

➡ *NCLEX keys*
Client needs category: Psychosocial integrity
Client needs subcategory: None
Cognitive level: Application

3. A client on the unit tells the nurse that his wife's nagging really gets on his nerves. He asks the nurse if she'll talk with his wife about her nagging during their family session tomorrow afternoon. Which response is the most therapeutic?
1. "Tell me more specifically about her complaints."
2. "Can you think why she might nag you so much?"
3. "I'll help you think about how to bring this up yourself tomorrow."
4. "Why do you want me to initiate this discussion in tomorrow's session rather than you?"

Answer: 3. The client needs to learn how to communicate directly with his wife about her behavior. The nurse's assistance will enable him to practice a new skill and will communicate the nurse's confidence in his ability to confront this situation directly. Asking about the wife's specific complaints or reasons for nagging inappropriately directs attention away from the client and toward his wife, who isn't present. Asking why you should initiate the discussion implies that there might be a legitimate reason for the nurse to assume responsibility for something that rightfully belongs to the client. Instead of focusing on his problems, he will waste time convincing the nurse why she should do his work.

➡ *NCLEX keys*
Client needs category: Psychosocial integrity
Client needs subcategory: None
Cognitive level: Application

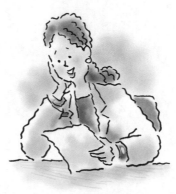

4. A nurse is caring for a client diagnosed with conversion disorder who has developed paralysis of her legs. Diagnostic tests fail to uncover a physiologic cause. During the working phase of the nurse-client relationship, the client says to her nurse, "You think I could walk if I wanted to, don't you?" Which response by the nurse would be best?
1. "Yes, if you really wanted to, you could."
2. "Tell me why you're concerned about what I think."
3. "Do you think you could walk if you wanted to?"
4. "I think you are unable to walk now, whatever the cause."

Answer: 4. This response answers the question honestly and nonjudgmentally and helps to preserve the client's self-esteem. Telling the client that she could walk if she really wanted to is an open and candid response but diminishes the client's self-esteem. Asking the client why she's concerned about what you think doesn't answer the client's question and isn't helpful. Asking her if she thought she could walk if she really wanted to would increase the client's anxiety because her inability to walk is directly related to an unconscious psychological conflict that hasn't yet been resolved.

➡ *NCLEX keys*

Client needs category: Psychosocial integrity
Client needs subcategory: None
Cognitive level: Application

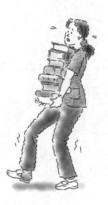

5. A 42-year-old homemaker arrives at the emergency department with uncontrollable crying and anxiety. Her husband of 17 years has recently asked her for a divorce. The client is sitting in a chair, rocking back and forth. Which is the best response for the nurse to make?
1. "You must stop crying so that we can discuss your feelings about the divorce."
2. "Once you find a job, you'll feel much better and more secure."
3. "I can see how upset you are. Let's sit in the office so that we can talk about how you're feeling."
4. "Once you have a lawyer looking out for your interests, you will feel better."

Answer: 3. This response validates the client's distress and provides an opportunity for her to talk about her feelings. Because clients in crises have difficulty making decisions, the nurse must be directive as well as supportive. Telling the client to stop crying doesn't provide the client with adequate support. Telling her that she will feel better after she has a job or a lawyer doesn't acknowledge the client's distress. Moreover, clients in crises can't think beyond the immediate moment, so discussing long-range plans isn't helpful.

➡ *NCLEX keys*

Client needs category: Psychosocial integrity
Client needs subcategory: None
Cognitive level: Application

6. A widower is hospitalized after complaining of difficulty sleeping, extreme apprehension, shortness of breath, and a sense of impending doom. Which response by the nurse would be best?
1. "You have nothing to worry about. You're in a safe place. Try to relax."
2. "Has anything happened recently or in the past that may have triggered these feelings?"
3. "We have given you a medication that will help to decrease these feelings of anxiety."
4. "Take some deep breaths and try to calm down."

Answer: 2. This question provides support, reassurance, and an opportunity to gain insight into the cause of the client's anxiety. Brushing off the client's anxiety by telling him he has nothing to worry about dismisses the client's feelings and offers false reassurance. Simply administering medication or instructing him to calm down doesn't allow the client to discuss his feelings, which he must do to understand and resolve the cause of his anxiety.

➡ *NCLEX keys*

Client needs category: Psychosocial integrity
Client needs subcategory: None
Cognitive level: Application

7. A client is admitted to an inpatient psychiatric hospital after having been picked up by the local police while walking around the neighborhood at night without shoes in the snow. He appears confused and disoriented. Which action should take priority?

1. Assess and stabilize the client's medical needs.
2. Assess and stabilize the client's psychological needs.
3. Attempt to locate the nearest family members to get an accurate history.
4. Arrange a transfer to the nearest medical facility.

Answer: 1. The possibility of frostbite must be evaluated before the other interventions. Attending to the client's psychological needs, locating family members, or arranging for transfer doesn't address the client's immediate medical needs.

➡ *NCLEX keys*

Client needs category: Physiological integrity
Client needs subcategory: Reduction of risk potential
Cognitive level: Analysis

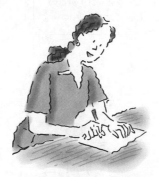

8. What occurs during the working phase of the nurse-client relationship?

1. The nurse assesses the client's needs and develops a care plan.
2. The nurse and client evaluate and modify the goals of the relationship.
3. The nurse and client discuss their feelings about terminating the relationship.
4. The nurse and client explore each other's expectations of the relationship.

Answer: 2. The therapeutic nurse-client relationship consists of three overlapping phases, the orientation, the working, and the termination. During the working phase, the nurse and the client together evaluate and refine goals established during the orientation phase. In addition, major therapeutic work takes place, and insight is integrated into a plan of action. The orientation phase involves assessing the client, formulating a contract, exploring feelings, and establishing expectations about the relationship. During the termination phase, the nurse prepares the client for separation and explores feelings about the end of the relationship.

➡ *NCLEX keys*

Client needs category: Psychosocial integrity
Client needs subcategory: None
Cognitive level: Knowledge

9. When preparing to conduct group therapy, an advanced practice nurse keeps in mind that the optimal number of clients in a group should be:

1. 3 to 5.
2. 6 to 8.
3. 10 to 12.
4. unlimited.

Answer: 2. Clinicians generally consider 6 to 8 people to be the ideal number of clients for a therapeutic group. The size allows opportunities for maximum therapeutic exchange and participation. In groups of 5 or fewer, participation commonly is inhibited by self-consciousness and insecurity. In groups larger than 8, participation and exchange among certain members may be lost.

➡ *NCLEX keys*

Client needs category: Psychosocial integrity
Client needs subcategory: None
Cognitive level: Application

10. A therapeutic nurse-client relationship begins with the nurse's:

1. sincere desire to help others.
2. acceptance of others.
3. self-awareness and understanding.
4. sound knowledge of psychiatric nursing.

Answer: 3. Although all of the options are desirable, knowledge of self is the basis for building a strong, therapeutic nurse-client relationship. Being aware of and understanding personal feelings and behavior is a prerequisite for understanding and helping clients.

➡ *NCLEX keys*

Client needs category: Safe and effective care environment

Client needs subcategory: Management of care

Cognitive level: Knowledge

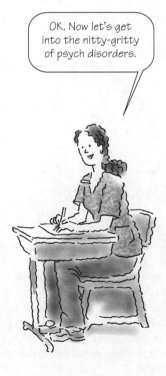

OK. Now let's get into the nitty-gritty of psych disorders.

13 Somatoform & sleep disorders

Brush up on key concepts

The client with a sleep disorder commonly suffers from excessive daytime sleepiness and impaired ability to perform daily tasks safely or properly. The client with a somatoform disorder commonly suffers physical symptoms related to an inability to handle stress. These physical symptoms have no physiologic cause but are overwhelming to the client.

At any time, you can review the major points of each disorder by consulting the *Cheat sheet* on pages 388 and 389.

Somatoform disorders

The *Diagnostic and Statistical Manual of Mental Disorders,* Fourth edition, *Text Revision (DSM-IV-TR)* categorizes somatic symptoms of psychiatric origins as somatoform disorders.

The client with a somatoform disorder complains of physical symptoms and typically travels from physician to physician in search of sympathetic and enthusiastic treatment. Physical examinations and laboratory tests, however, fail to uncover an organic basis for the client's symptoms. Because the client doesn't produce the symptoms intentionally or feel a sense of control over them, he's usually unable to accept that his illness has a psychological cause.

From mind to body
Psychosomatic is a term used to describe conditions in which a psychological state contributes to the development of a physical illness.

An expression of emotional stress
Somatization is the manifestation of physical symptoms that result from psychological distress. Anyone who feels the pain of a sore throat or the ache of flu has a somatic symptom, but it isn't considered somatization unless the physical symptoms are an expression of emotional stress.

All bottled up
Internalization refers to the condition in which a client's anxiety, stress, and frustration are expressed through physical symptoms rather than confronted directly.

Sleep disorders

The client with a primary sleep disorder is unable to initiate or maintain sleep. Primary sleep disorders may be categorized as dyssomnias or parasomnias.

Too much or not enough
Dyssomnias involve excessive sleep or difficulty initiating and maintaining sleep. Examples of dyssomnias include primary insomnia, circadian rhythm sleep disorder, obstructive sleep apnea syndrome, primary hypersomnia, and narcolepsy.

Strange things in the night
Parasomnias are physiologic or behavioral reactions *during* sleep. Examples of parasomnias include nightmare disorder, sleep terror disorder, and sleepwalking disorder.

You're getting sleepy...
Sleep can be broken down into two major phases, **rapid-eye-movement** (REM) sleep and **non–rapid-eye-movement** (NREM) sleep, which alternate throughout the sleep period.

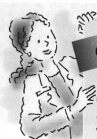

Somatoform & sleep disorders refresher

CONVERSION DISORDER
Key signs and symptoms
• La belle indifference (a lack of concern about the symptoms or limitation on functioning)

Key test results
• The absence of expected diagnostic findings can confirm the disorder.

Key treatments
• Individual therapy
• Hypnosis
• Stress management

Key interventions
• Establish a supportive relationship that communicates acceptance of the client but keeps the focus away from symptoms.
• Review all laboratory and diagnostic study results.

HYPOCHONDRIASIS
Key signs and symptoms
• Abnormal focus on bodily functions and sensations
• Anger, frustration, depression
• Frequent visits to physicians and specialists despite assurance from health care providers that the client is healthy
• Intensified physical symptoms around sympathetic people
• Rejection of the idea that the symptoms are stress related
• Use of symptoms to avoid difficult situations

Key treatments
• Individual therapy
• Cognitive behaviorial therapy
• Tricyclic antidepressants: amitriptyline (Elavil), imipramine (Tofranil), doxepin (Sinequan)
• Selective serotonin reuptake inhibitors: citalopram (Celexa), fluoxetine (Prozac), paroxetine (Paxil), sertraline (Zoloft)

Key interventions
• Assess the client's level of knowledge about how emotional issues can impact physiologic functioning.

> Falling asleep during studying doesn't count as a sleep disorder.

• Encourage emotional expression.
• Respond to the client's symptoms in a matter-of-fact way.

PAIN DISORDER
Key signs and symptoms
• Acute and chronic pain not associated with a psychological cause
• Frequent visits to multiple physicians to seek pain relief

Key test results
• Test results don't support client complaints.

Key treatments
• Individual therapy
• Biofeedback
• Cognitive behavioral threapy
• Tricyclic antidepressants: amitriptyline (Elavil), imipramine (Tofranil), doxepin (Sinequan)

Key interventions
• Acknowledge the client's pain.
• Encourage the client to recognize situations that precipitate pain.

DYSSOMNIAS
Key signs and symptoms
Primary insomnia
• History of light or easily disturbed sleep or difficulty falling asleep
• Insomnia
Circadian rhythm sleep disorder
• Cardiovascular and GI distubances, such as palpitations, peptic ulcer disease, and gastritis
• Fatigue
Breathing-related sleep disorder
• Abnormal breathing events during sleep including apnea, abnormally slow or shallow respirations, and hypoventilation (abnormal blood oxygen and carbon dioxide levels)
• Fatigue
• Snoring while sleeping
Primary hypersomnia
• Confusion upon awakening
• Difficulty awakening
• Poor memory

Somatoform & sleep disorders refresher (continued)

DYSSOMNIAS (CONTINUED)

Narcolepsy
- Cataplexy (bilateral loss of muscle tone triggered by strong emotion)
- Generalized daytime sleepiness
- Hypnagogic hallucination (intense dreamlike images)
- Irresistible attacks of refreshing sleep

Key test results
- Polysomnography is diagnostic for individual sleep disorder.

Key treatments
Primary insomnia or circadian rhythm sleep disorder
- Hypnotics: zolpidem (Ambien), eszopiclone (Lunesta)
- Benzodiazepines: lorazepam (Ativan), alprazolam (Xanax)
Primary hypersomnia or narcolepsy
- Stimulants: caffeine, methylphenidate (Ritalin), dextroamphetamine (Dexedrine); modafinil (Provigil)

Key interventions
Primary insomnia and circadian rhythm disturbance
- Encourage the client to discuss concerns that may be preventing sleep.
- Schedule regular sleep and awakening times.
Breathing-related sleep disorder
- Administer continuous positive nasal airway pressure.
Primary hypersomnia and narcolepsy
- Administer medication as prescribed.

- Develop strategies to manage symptoms and integrate them into their daily routine, such as taking naps during lunchtime or work breaks.

PARASOMNIAS

Key signs and symptoms
Nightmare disorder
- Dream recall
- Mild autonomic arousal upon awakening (sweating, tachycardia, tachypnea)
Sleep terror disorder
- Autonomic signs of intense anxiety (tachycardia, tachypnea, flushing, sweating, increased muscle tone, dilated pupils)
- Screaming or crying
Sleepwalking disorder
- Amnesia of the episode or limited recall
- Sitting up, talking, walking, or engaging in inappropriate behavior during episode

Key test results
- Polysomnography is diagnostic for individual sleep disorder.

Key treatments
- Relaxation techniques
- Individual counseling

Key interventions
- Lock windows and doors if sleepwalking occurs.
- Provide emotional support.

NREM sleep consists of four stages:

☝ Stage 1 NREM sleep is a transition from wakefulness to sleep characterized by low-voltage mixed-frequency EEG and slow eye movement and occupies about 5% of time spent asleep in healthy adults.

✌ Stage 2 NREM sleep, which is characterized by specific EEG waveforms (sleep spindles and K complexes), occupies about 50% of time spent asleep.

🖖 Stages 3 and 4 NREM sleep (also known collectively as *slow-wave sleep* or *delta sleep*) are the deepest levels of sleep and occupy about 10% to 20% of sleep time declining to 0% in the elderly.

🖐 REM sleep, during which the majority of typical storylike dreams occur, occupies about 20% to 25% of total sleep.

Light intensity can affect sleep patterns causing changes in cortisol, melatonin, and core body temperature.

Patterns after dark

Stages of sleep have a characteristic temporal organization. NREM stages 3 and 4 tend to occur in the first one-third to one-half of the night. REM sleep occurs in cycles throughout the night, alternating with NREM sleep about every 80 to 100 minutes. REM sleep periods increase in duration during the last half of the night, toward the morning.

Sparks in the night

Polysomnography is the monitoring of multiple electrophysiologic parameters during sleep and generally includes measurement of EEG activity, electro-oculographic activity (electrographic tracings made by movement

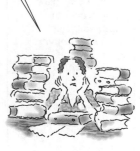

I'm sick of studying! Does that qualify as a somatoform disorder?

of the eye), and electromyographic activity (electrographic tracings made by skeletal muscles at rest).

Additional polysomnographic measures may include oral or nasal airflow, respiratory effort, chest and abdominal wall movement, oxyhemoglobin saturation, or exhaled carbon dioxide concentration. These measures are used to monitor respiration during sleep and to detect the presence and severity of sleep apnea. Measurement of peripheral electromyographic activity may be used to detect abnormal movements during sleep such as those that occur with restless leg syndrome.

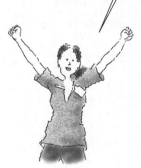

Absence means presence. The absence of expected diagnostic findings can confirm conversion disorder.

You can do it during the daytime, too!

Most polysomnographic studies are performed during the client's usual sleeping hours — that is in a sleep laboratory overnight. However daytime polysomnographic studies are also used to quantify daytime sleepiness.

Polish up on client care

Major somatoform disorders include conversion disorder, hypochondriasis, and pain disorder. Sleep disorders include dyssomnias (primary insomnia, circadian rhythm sleep disorder, breathing-related sleep disorder, primary hypersomnia, and narcolepsy) and parasomnias (nightmare disorder, sleep terror disorder, and sleepwalking disorder).

Conversion disorder

Memory jogger

When thinking of **conversion disorder,** think of the term **convert,** which means "to change from one form or function to another." Clients with conversion disorder convert stress into physical ailments.

The client with conversion disorder exhibits symptoms that suggest a physical disorder, but evaluation and observation can't determine a physiologic cause. The onset of symptoms is preceded by psychological trauma or conflict, and the physical symptoms are a manifestation of the conflict. Resolution of the symptoms usually occurs spontaneously.

CONTRIBUTING FACTORS
- Psychological conflict
- Overwhelming stress
- History of trauma

ASSESSMENT FINDINGS
- Aphonia (inability to produce sound)
- Laryngitis
- Blindness
- Deafness
- Dysphagia
- Impaired balance and impaired coordination
- La belle indifference (a lack of concern about the symptoms or limitation on functioning)
- Loss of touch sensation
- Lump in the throat
- Paralysis
- Seizures or pseudoseizures
- Urinary retention

DIAGNOSTIC TEST RESULTS
- Test results are inconsistent with physical findings.
- The absence of expected diagnostic findings can confirm the disorder.

NURSING DIAGNOSES
- Ineffective coping
- Anxiety
- Chronic low self-esteem

TREATMENT
- Individual therapy
- Hypnosis
- Relaxation training
- Stress management

Drug therapy
- Benzodiazepines: lorazepam (Ativan), alprazolam (Xanax), clonazepam (Klonopin)

INTERVENTIONS AND RATIONALES
- Ensure and maintain a safe environment *to protect the client.*
- Establish a supportive relationship that communicates acceptance of the client but keeps the focus away from symptoms *to help the client learn to recognize and express anxiety.*

- Review all laboratory and diagnostic study results *to ascertain whether any physical problems are present.*
- Encourage the client to identify any emotional conflicts occurring before the onset of physical symptoms *to make the relationship between the conflict and the symptoms clearer.*
- Promote social interaction *to decrease the client's level of self-involvement.*
- Identify constructive coping mechanisms *to encourage the client to use practical coping skills and relinquish the role of being sick.*
- Teach relaxation techniques and effective coping mechanisms and help the client identify areas of stress *to help decrease symptoms.*

Teaching topics
- Explanation of the disorder and treatment plan
- Medication use and possible adverse effects
- Setting limits on the client's sick role behavior while continuing to provide support (for family members)
- Stress-reduction methods

Hypochondriasis

In hypochondriasis, the client is preoccupied by fear of a serious illness, despite medical assurance of good health. The client with hypochondriasis interprets all physical sensations as indications of illness, impairing his ability to function normally.

CONTRIBUTING FACTORS
- Death of a loved one
- Family member with a serious illness
- Previous serious illness
- Marital problems
- Career changes
- History of anxiety and depression

ASSESSMENT FINDINGS
- Abnormal focus on bodily functions and sensations
- Anger, frustration, depression
- Frequent visits to physicians and specialists despite assurance from health care providers that the client is healthy

- Intensified physical symptoms around sympathetic people
- Rejection of the idea that the symptoms are stress related
- Use of symptoms to avoid difficult situations
- Vague physical symptoms

DIAGNOSTIC TEST RESULTS
- Test results are inconsistent with the client's complaints and physical findings.

NURSING DIAGNOSES
- Deficient knowledge (treatment plan)
- Ineffective coping
- Ineffective health maintenance
- Anxiety
- Disturbed sensory perception

TREATMENT
- Individual therapy
- Cognitive behavioral therapy

Drug therapy
- Benzodiazepines: lorazepam (Ativan), alprazolam (Xanax)
- Tricyclic antidepressants: amitriptyline (Elavil), imipramine (Tofranil), doxepin (Sinequan)
- Selective serotonin reuptake inhibitors (SSRIs): paroxetine (Paxil), citalopram (Celexa), fluoxetine (Prozac), sertraline (Zoloft)
- Serotonin–norepinephrine reuptake inhibitor (SNRI): venlafaxine (Effexor)

INTERVENTIONS AND RATIONALES
- Assess the client's level of knowledge about how emotional issues can impact physiologic functioning *to promote understanding of the condition.*
- Encourage emotional expression *to discourage emotional repression, which can have physical consequences.*
- Respond to the client's symptoms in a matter-of-fact way *to reduce secondary gain the client achieves from talking about symptoms.*

Teaching topics
- Explanation of the disorder and treatment plan
- Medication use and possible adverse effects

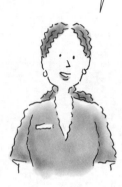

Acknowledging the client's pain helps to discourage him from striving to convince you the pain is real.

- Relaxation and assertiveness techniques
- Initiating conversations that focus on topics other than physical maladies

Pain disorder

In pain disorder, the client experiences pain in which psychological factors play a significant role in the onset, severity, exacerbation, or maintenance of the pain. The pain isn't intentionally produced or feigned by the client. The pain becomes a major focus of life, and the client is often unable to function socially or at work. The client may have a physical ailment but shouldn't be experiencing such intense pain.

CONTRIBUTING FACTORS
- Traumatic, stressful, or humiliating experience

ASSESSMENT FINDINGS
- Acute and chronic pain not associated with a physiologic cause
- Anger, frustration, depression, anxiety
- Drug-seeking behavior in an attempt to relieve pain
- Frequent visits to multiple physicians to seek pain relief
- Insomnia

DIAGNOSTIC TEST RESULTS
- Test results don't support client complaints.
- With psychotherapy, the client may recall a traumatic event.

NURSING DIAGNOSES
- Acute or chronic pain
- Ineffective coping
- Anxiety

TREATMENT
- Individual therapy
- Biofeedback
- Cognitive behavioral therapy

Drug therapy
- Anxiolytics (benzodiazepines): lorazepam (Ativan), alprazolam (Xanax)

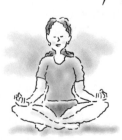

Nursing care in pain disorder may focus on pain management techniques, such as relaxation and meditation.

- Tricyclic antidepressants: amitriptyline (Elavil), imipramine (Tofranil), doxepin (Sinequan)
- SSRIs: paroxetine (Paxil), citalopram (Celexa), fluoxetine (Prozac)
- SNRI: venlafaxine (Effexor)

INTERVENTIONS AND RATIONALES
- Ensure a safe, accepting environment for the client *to promote therapeutic communication.*
- Acknowledge the client's pain *to discourage the client from striving to convince you that pain is real and to reinforce a therapeutic relationship.*
- Encourage the client to recognize situations that precipitate pain *to foster an understanding of the disorder.*

Teaching topics
- Explanation of the disorder and treatment plan
- Medication use and possible adverse effects
- Promoting social interaction
- Establishing constructive coping mechanisms
- Problem-solving techniques
- Nonpharmacologic pain management, such as guided imagery, massage, therapeutic touch, relaxation, heat, and cold

Dyssomnias

Dyssomnias are primary disorders of initiating or maintaining sleep or excessive sleepiness. These disorders are characterized by a disturbance in the amount, quality, or timing of sleep.

Primary insomnia is characterized by a subjective complaint of difficulty initiating or maintaining sleep that lasts for at least 1 month. Alternatively, the client may report that sleep isn't refreshing. A key symptom of primary insomnia is the client's intense focus and anxiety about not getting sleep, resulting in signficant distress or impairment. Commonly, the client reports being a "light sleeper."

In **circadian rhythm sleep disorder,** there's a mismatch between the internal sleep-wake circadian rhythm and timing and the duration of sleep. The client may report insomnia at particular times during the day and excessive sleepiness at other times. Causes can be intrinsic such as delays in the sleep phases or extrinsic as in jet lag or shift work.

Another class of sleep disorder identified by the *DSM-IV-TR* is **breathing-related sleep disorder.** Specific disorders in this class include central sleep apnea syndrome, central alveolar hypoventilation syndrome, and obstructive sleep apnea syndrome. Obstructive sleep apnea syndrome is the most commonly diagnosed breathing-related sleep disorder.

In breathing-related sleep disorder, a disturbance in breathing leads to a disruption in sleep that leads to excessive sleepiness or insomnia. Excessive sleepiness is the most common complaint of clients. Naps usually aren't refreshing and may be accompanied by a dull headache. These clients typically minimize the problem by bragging that they can sleep anywhere and at any time.

In **narcolepsy,** the client develops an overwhelming urge to sleep at any time of the day regardless of the amount of previous sleep. The client may fall asleep two to six times a day during inappropriate times, such as while driving the car or attending class. The client's sleepiness typically decreases after a sleep attack, only to return several hours later. The sleep attacks must occur daily over a period of 3 months to confirm the diagnosis.

In **primary hypersomnia,** the client experiences excessive sleepiness lasting at least 1 month. The client may take daytime naps or sleep extended periods at night. People with primary hypersomnia typically sleep 8 to 12 hours per night. They fall asleep easily and sleep through the night but often have trouble awakening in the morning. Some mornings they awake confused and combative. These clients have great difficulty with morning obligations.

CONTRIBUTING FACTORS
Primary insomnia
- Illness (especially pheochromocytoma or hyperthyroidism)
- Many illegal drugs
- Age older than 65

- Stress
- Life changes
- Use of certain legal drugs (see *Drugs that affect sleep,* page 394)

Circadian rhythm sleep disorder
- Delayed sleep phase
- Jet lag
- Shift work

Breathing-related sleep disorder
- Instability in the respiratory control center, which causes apnea
- Obstruction or collapse of airway, which causes apnea
- Slow or shallow breathing, which causes arterial oxygen desaturation
- Obesity; short, fat neck
- Elongated uvula

Primary hypersomnia
- Autonomic nervous system dysfunction
- Genetic predisposition
- Corticol hypoactivity

Narcolepsy
- Genetic predisposition

ASSESSMENT FINDINGS
Primary insomnia
- Anxiety related to sleep loss
- Fatigue
- Haggard appearance
- Slowed response to stimuli
- Personality changes
- History of light or easily disturbed sleep or difficulty falling asleep
- Insomnia
- Poor concentration
- Tension headache
- Poor memory

Circadian rhythm sleep disorder
- Cardiovascular and GI disturbances, such as palpitations, peptic ulcer disease, and gastritis
- Fatigue
- Haggard appearance
- Poor concentration
- Poor memory

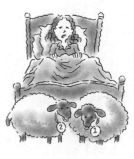

It takes more than counting sheep to cure most sleep disorders.

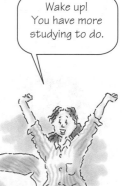

Wake up! You have more studying to do.

Management moments

Drugs that affect sleep

When caring for a client with a sleep disorder, keep in mind that medications and alcohol can affect sleep. Review the client's medication list to see if he's receiving any medications that affect sleep such as those listed here.

INCREASED TOTAL SLEEP TIME
- Barbiturates
- Benzodiazepines
- Alcohol (during the first half of the night)
- Phenothiazines

DECREASED TOTAL SLEEP TIME
- Amphetamines
- Alcohol (during the second half of the night)
- Caffeine

ALTERED DREAMING AND REM SLEEP
- Beta-adrenergic blockers: decreased rapid-eye-movement (REM) sleep, possible nightmares
- Antiparkinsonian: vivid dreams and nightmares
- Amphetamines: decreased REM sleep

- Tricyclic antidepressants and monoamine oxidase inhibitors: decreased REM sleep
- Barbiturates: decreased REM sleep
- Benzodiazepines: decreased REM sleep
- Selective serotonin reuptake inhibitors (SSRIs): decreased REM sleep, vivid dreams

INCREASED WAKING AFTER SLEEP ONSET
- Steroids
- Opioids
- Beta-adrenergic blockers
- Alcohol
- SSRIs

DECREASED WAKING AFTER SLEEP ONSET
- Benzodiazepines
- Barbiturates

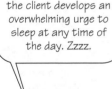

In narcolepsy, the client develops an overwhelming urge to sleep at any time of the day. Zzzz.

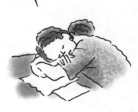

Breathing-related sleep disorder
- Abnormal breathing events during sleep including apnea, abnormally slow or shallow respirations, and hypoventilation (abnormal blood oxygen and carbon dioxide levels)
- Dull headache upon awakening
- Fatigue
- Gastroesophageal reflux
- Mild systemic hypertension with elevated diastolic blood pressure
- Snoring while sleeping

Primary hypersomnia
- Confusion upon awakening
- Difficulty awakening
- Poor memory

Narcolepsy
- Cataplexy (bilateral loss of muscle tone triggered by strong emotion)
- Frequent, intense, and vivid dreams may occur during nocturnal sleep
- Generalized daytime sleepiness

- Hypnagogic hallucination (intense dream-like images)
- Irresistible attacks of refreshing sleep

DIAGNOSTIC TEST RESULTS
Primary insomnia
- Polysomnography shows poor sleep continuity, increased stage 1 sleep, decreased stages 3 and 4 sleep, increased muscle tension, or increased amounts of EEG alpha activity during sleep.
- Psychophysiologic testing may show high arousal (increased muscle tension or excessive physiologic reactivity to stress).

Circadian rhythm sleep disorder
- Polysomnography shows short sleep latency (length of time it takes to fall asleep), reduced sleep duration, and sleep continuity disturbances. (Results may vary depending on the time of day testing is performed.)

Breathing-related sleep disorder

• Polysomnography measures of oral and nasal airflow are abnormal and oxyhemoglobin saturation is reduced.

Primary hypersomnia

• Polysomnography demonstrates a normal to prolonged sleep duration, short sleep latency, normal to increased sleep continuity, and normal distributions of REM and NREM sleep. Some individuals may have increased amounts of slow-wave sleep.

Narcolepsy

• Polysomnography shows sleep latencies of less than 10 minutes and frequent sleep onset REM periods, frequent transient arousals, decreased sleep efficiency, increased stage 1 sleep, increased REM sleep, and increased eye movements within the REM periods. Periodic limb movements and episodes of sleep apnea are also often noted.

NURSING DIAGNOSES

• Disturbed sleep pattern
• Fatigue
• Impaired home maintenance
• Risk for injury

TREATMENT

• Relaxation techniques
• Sleep restrictions (clients are instructed to avoid napping and to stay in bed only when sleeping)
• Regular exercise
• Light therapy

Drug therapy

Primary insomnia or circadian rhythm sleep disorder
• Antidepressant: trazodone
• Benzodiazepines: lorazepam (Ativan), alprazolam (Xanax)
• Diphenhydramine (Benadryl)
• Hypnotics: zolpidem (Ambien), eszopiclone (Lunesta)
• Melatonin
Primary hypersomnia or narcolepsy
• Stimulants: caffeine, methylphenidate (Ritalin), dextroamphetamine (Dexedrine), modafinil (Provigil)

INTERVENTIONS AND RATIONALES

• Assess the client and document symptoms of sleep disturbance *to gain information for care plan development.*

Primary insomnia and circadian rhythm disturbance

• Encourage the client to discuss concerns that may be preventing sleep. *Active listening helps elicit underlying causes of sleep disturbance such as stress.*
• Establish a sleep routine *to promote relaxation and sleep.*
• Schedule regular sleep and awakening times *to help ensure that progress is maintained after the client leaves the hospital.*
• Administer medications, as prescribed, *to induce sleep and to reduce anxiety.*
• Provide warm milk at bedtime. *L-tryptophan, found in milk, is a precursor to serotonin, a neurotransmitter necessary for sleep.*
• Plan activities that require the client to wake at a regular hour and stay out of bed during the day *to reinforce natural circadian rhythms.*
• Encourage regular exercise early in the day.
• Teach relaxation techniques *to decrease symptoms.*

Breathing-related sleep disorder

• Administer continuous positive nasal airway pressure *to treat obstructive sleep disorders.*
• Encourage weight loss, as appropriate, *to decrease incidence of apnea.*
• Suggest sleeping in reclining position *to help maintain a patent airway.*

Primary hypersomnia and narcolepsy

• Administer medications, as prescribed, *to help the client stay awake and maintain client safety.*
• Develop strategies to manage symptoms and integrate them into the client's daily routine, such as taking naps during lunch or work breaks, *to help maintain client safety and promote normal functioning.*

Teaching topics

All types
• Explanation of the disorder and treatment plan

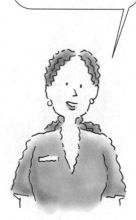

For the client with primary insomnia or circadian rhythm disturbance, plan activities that require him to wake at a regular hour and stay out of bed during the day.

- Medication use and possible adverse effects

Primary insomnia and circadian rhythm disorder

- Relaxation techniques
- Importance of limiting caffeine and alcohol
- Need to avoid exercising within 3 hours before bedtime
- Ways to identify and reduce stressors
- Healthy diet and regular exercise routine

Breathing-related sleeping disorder

- Use of home positive nasal airway pressure device
- Weight loss information

Primary hypersomnia and narcolepsy

- Integrating nap period into daily routine

Parasomnias

Parasomnias are characterized by abnormal, unpleasant motor or verbal arousals and behaviors that occur during sleep. They include nightmare disorder, sleep terror disorder, and sleepwalking disorder. The client is able to perform the behaviors but does not have conscious awareness or responsibility for them.

Nightmare disorder is characterized by the recurrence of frightening dreams that cause the client to awaken from sleep. When the client awakens, he's fully alert and experiences persistent anxiety or fear. Typically, the client can recall details of the dream involving physical danger.

Sleep terror disorder is characterized by episodes of sleep terrors that cause distress or impairment of social or occupational functioning. The client may sit up in bed screaming or crying with a frightened expression and signs of intense anxiety. During such episodes, the client is difficult to awaken and, if he does awaken, he's generally confused or disoriented. The client has no recollection of the dream content.

In **sleepwalking disorder,** the client arises from bed and walks about. The client has limited recall of the event upon awakening.

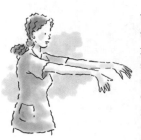

Zzzz... Sleepwalkers may also sit up, talk, or engage in inappropriate behavior with little or no recall of the incident.

CONTRIBUTING FACTORS

- Severe psychosocial stressors
- Genetic predisposition
- Sleep deprivation
- Fever

ASSESSMENT FINDINGS

Nightmare disorder

- Anxiety
- Depression
- Dream recall
- Excessive sleepiness
- Irritability
- Mild autonomic arousal upon awakening (sweating, tachycardia, tachypnea)
- Poor concentration

Sleep terror disorder

- Autonomic signs of intense anxiety (tachycardia, tachypnea, flushing, sweating, increased muscle tone, dilated pupils)
- Inability to recall dream content
- Screaming or crying

Sleepwalking disorder

- Amnesia of the episode or limited recall
- Sitting up, talking, walking, or engaging in inappropriate behavior during episode

DIAGNOSTIC TEST RESULTS

Nightmare disorder

- Polysomnography demonstrates abrupt awakenings from REM sleep that correspond to the individual's report of nightmares. These awakenings usually occur during the second half of the night. Heart rate and respiratory rate may increase or show increased variability before the awakening.

Sleep terror disorder

- Polysomnography reveals that sleep terrors begin during deep NREM sleep characterized by slow-frequency EEG activity.

Sleepwalking disorder

- Polysomnography reveals episodes of sleepwalking that begin within the first few hours of sleep, usually during NREM stage 3 or 4 sleep.

NURSING DIAGNOSES
- Disturbed sleep pattern
- Fatigue
- Ineffective role performance
- Risk for injury

TREATMENT
- Relaxation training
- Guided imagery
- Individual counseling

Drug therapy
- Rarely used

INTERVENTIONS AND RATIONALES
- Assess the client and document the symptoms of sleep disturbance *to aid in formulating a treatment plan.*
- Lock windows and doors if sleepwalking occurs *to maintain client safety.*
- Provide emotional support *to allay the client's anxiety.*
- Establish a sleep routine *to promote relaxation and sleep.*
- Schedule regular sleep and awakening times *so that the client can learn specific planning strategies for managing sleep.*
- Administer medications, as prescribed *to promote sleep.*
- Help the client identify stressors to sleep disturbance *to help reduce incidence.*

Teaching topics
- Safety measures for the client with sleepwalking disorder
- Ways to identify and reduce stressors

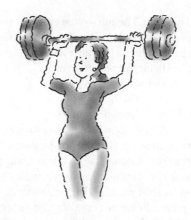

Pump up on practice questions

1. A client complains of experiencing an overwhelming urge to sleep. He states that he's been falling asleep while working at his desk. He reports that these episodes occur about five times daily. This client is most likely experiencing which sleep disorder?
1. Breathing-related sleep disorder
2. Narcolepsy
3. Primary hypersomnia
4. Circadian rhythm disorder

Answer: 2. Narcolepsy is characterized by irresistible attacks of refreshing sleep that occur two to six times per day and last for 5 to 20 minutes. The client with breathing-related sleep disorder suffers interruptions in sleep that leave the client with excess sleepiness. In hypersomnia, the client suffers excess sleepiness and reports prolonged periods of nighttime sleep or daytime napping. With circadian rhythm disorder, the client has periods of insomnia followed by periods of increased sleepiness.

➡ *NCLEX keys*
Client needs category: Psychosocial integrity
Client needs subcategory: None
Cognitive level: Application

2. A nurse is caring for a client who complains of fatigue, inability to concentrate, and palpitations. The client states that she has been experiencing these symptoms for the past 6 months. The nurse suspects that the client is experiencing circadian rhythm sleep disturbance related to which factor?

1. History of recent fever
2. Shift work
3. Hyperthyroidism
4. Pheochromocytoma

Answer: 2. The client is experiencing circadian rhythm sleep disorder (palpitations, GI disturbances, fatigue, haggard appearance, and poor concentration), which is typically caused by shift work, jet lag, or a delayed sleep phase. Fever is a contributing factor in parasomnias. Hyperthyroidism and pheochromocytoma are causative factors for primary insomnia.

➡ *NCLEX keys*

Client needs category: Psychosocial integrity
Client needs subcategory: None
Cognitive level: Analysis

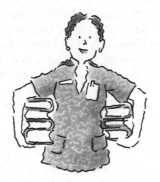

3. A client comes to the clinic complaining of the inability to sleep over the past 2 months. He states that his inability to sleep is ruining his life because "getting sleep" is all he can think about. This client is most likely experiencing which sleep disorder?

1. Circadian rhythm sleep disorder
2. Breathing-related sleep disorder
3. Primary insomnia
4. Primary hypersomnia

Answer: 3. The client with primary insomnia experiences difficulty initiating or maintaining sleep. A key symptom of primary insomnia is the client's intense focus and anxiety about not getting to sleep. The client diagnosed with circadian rhythm sleep disorder reports periods of insomnia at particular times during a 24-hour period and excessive sleepiness

at other times. Excessive sleepiness is the most common complaint of clients affected by breathing-related sleep disorder. The client experiencing primary hypersomnia typically sleeps 8 to 12 hours per night. They fall asleep easily and sleep through the night but commonly have trouble awakening in the morning.

➡ *NCLEX keys*

Client needs category: Psychosocial integrity
Client needs subcategory: None
Cognitive level: Analysis

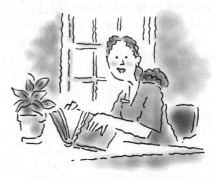

4. A nurse is preparing a teaching plan for a client diagnosed with primary insomnia. Which teaching topic should be included?

1. Eating unlimited spicy foods and limiting caffeine and alcohol
2. Exercising 1 hour before bedtime to promote sleep
3. Importance of sleeping whenever the client tires
4. Drinking warm milk before bed to induce sleep

Answer: 4. Clients diagnosed with primary insomnia should be taught that drinking warm milk before bedtime can help induce sleep. They should also be taught the importance of limiting spicy foods, alcohol, and caffeine; avoiding exercise within 3 hours before bedtime; establishing a routine bedtime; and avoiding napping.

➡ *NCLEX keys*

Client needs category: Psychosocial integrity
Client needs subcategory: None
Cognitive level: Application

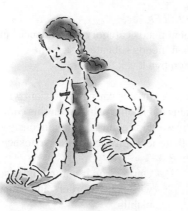

5. A nurse is caring for a client hospitalized on numerous occasions for complaints of chest pain and fainting spells, which she attributes to her deteriorating heart condition. No relatives or friends report ever actually seeing a fainting spell. After undergoing an extensive cardiac, pulmonary, GI, and neurologic work-up, she's told that all test results are completely negative. The client remains persistent in her belief that she has a serious illness. What diagnosis is appropriate for this client?

1. Exhibitionism
2. Somatoform disorder
3. Degenerative dementia
4. Echolalia

Answer: 2. Somatoform disorders are characterized by recurrent and multiple physical symptoms that have no organic or physiologic base. Exhibitionism involves public exposure of genitals. Degenerative dementia is characterized by deterioration of mental capacities. Echolalia is a repetition of words or phrases.

➡ NCLEX keys

Client needs category: Safe and effective care environment
Client needs subcategory: Management of care
Cognitive level: Analysis

6. A client is prescribed sertraline (Zoloft), a selective serotonin reuptake inhibitor. Which adverse effects about this drug should the nurse include when creating a medication teaching plan? Select all that apply.

1. Agitation
2. Agranulocytosis
3. Sleep disturbance
4. Intermittent tachycardia
5. Dry mouth
6. Seizures

Answer: 1, 3, 5. Common adverse effects of sertraline are agitation, sleep disturbance, and dry mouth. Agranulocytosis, intermittent tachycardia, and seizures are adverse effects of clonazepam (Klonopin).

➡ NCLEX keys

Client needs category: Physiological integrity
Client needs subcategory: Pharmacological and parenteral therapies
Cognitive level: Application

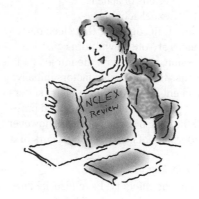

7. A nurse is caring for a client who exhibits signs of somatization. Which statement is most relevant?

1. Clients with somatization are cognitively impaired.
2. Anxiety rarely coexists with somatization.
3. Somatization exists when medical evidence supports the symptoms.
4. Clients with somatization often have lengthy medical records.

Answer: 4. Clients with somatization are prone to "physician shop" and have extensive medical records as a result of their multiple procedures and tests. Clients with somatization aren't usually cognitively impaired.

These clients have coexisting anxiety and depression and no medical evidence to support a clear-cut diagnosis.

➡ *NCLEX keys*
Client needs category: Psychosocial integrity
Client needs subcategory: None
Cognitive level: Analysis

8. A nurse is caring for a client who reveals symptoms of a sleep disorder during the admission assessment. The client also admits that he has "broken down and cried for no apparent reason." Which criterion is most important for the nurse to initially consider to gain insight into the client's patterns of sleep and feelings of depression?
   1. Stressors in the client's life
   2. The client's weight
   3. Periods of apnea
   4. Sexual activity
Answer: 1. Recognizing that sleep disturbances are often symptoms of stress, depression, and anxiety, the nurse is prudent to discuss these possible factors initially. If the client has a weight problem, suffers from sleep apnea, or reports sexual problems, these also can affect sleep; however, consideration of life stressors occurs first.

➡ *NCLEX keys*
Client needs category: Psychosocial integrity
Client needs subcategory: None
Cognitive level: Application

9. A nurse is caring for a client who displays gait disturbances, paralysis, pseudoseizures, and tremors. These symptoms may be manifestations of what psychiatric disorder?
   1. Pain disorder
   2. Adjustment disorder
   3. Delirium
   4. Conversion disorder
Answer: 4. Conversion disorders are most frequently associated with psychologically mediated neurologic deficits, such as gait disturbances, paralysis, pseudo-seizures, and tremors. Pain disorders and adjustment disorders aren't generally expressed in terms of neurologic deficits. Delirium is associated with cognitive impairment.

➡ *NCLEX keys*
Client needs category: Psychosocial integrity
Client needs subcategory: None
Cognitive level: Analysis

10. A nurse is caring for a client who complains of chronic pain. Given this complaint, why would the nurse simultaneously evaluate both general physical and psychosocial problems?
   1. Depression is commonly associated with pain disorders and somatic complaints.
   2. Combining evaluations will save time and allow for quicker delivery of health care.
   3. Most insurance plans won't cover evaluation of both as separate entities.
   4. The physician doesn't have the training to evaluate for psychosocial considerations.
Answer: 1. Psychosocial factors should be suspected when pain persists beyond the normal tissue healing time and physical causes have been investigated. The other choices may or may not be correct but certainly aren't credible in all cases.

➡ *NCLEX keys*
Client needs category: Psychosocial integrity
Client needs subcategory: None
Cognitive level: Analysis

You've finished the chapter on sleep disorders. You may want to nap before the next chapter.

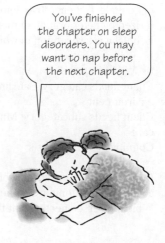

14 Anxiety & mood disorders

Brush up on key concepts

Anxiety disorders are characterized by anxiety and avoidant behavior. Clients are overwhelmed by feelings of impending catastrophe, guilt, shame, and worthlessness. Clients with anxiety cling to maladaptive behaviors in an attempt to alleviate their own distress, but these behaviors only increase their symptoms.

Mood disorders are characterized by depressed or elevated moods that alter the client's ability to cope with reality and to function normally.

At any time, you can review the major points of each disorder by consulting the *Cheat sheet* on pages 402 and 403.

Polish up on client care

Major mood disorders include bipolar disorder and major depression. Major anxiety disorders include generalized anxiety, obsessive-compulsive disorder, panic disorder, phobias, and posttraumatic stress disorder (PTSD).

Bipolar disorder

Bipolar disorder is a severe disturbance in affect, manifested by episodes of extreme sadness alternating with episodes of euphoria. Severity and duration of episodes vary. The exact biological basis of bipolar disorder remains unknown, although it's thought that a combination of genetic factors and stressful events contribute to the development of mania.

Two common patterns of bipolar disorder include:
• bipolar I, in which depressive episodes alternate with full manic episodes (hyperactive behavior, delusional thinking, grandiosity, and often hostility)
• bipolar II, characterized by recurrent depressive episodes and occasional manic episodes.

CONTRIBUTING FACTORS
• Concurrent major illness
• Environment
• Heredity
• History of psychiatric illnesses
• Seasons and circadian rhythms that affect mood
• Sleep deprivation
• Stressful events may produce limbic system dysfunction

ASSESSMENT FINDINGS
During episodes of mania
• Bizarre and eccentric appearance
• Cognitive manifestations, such as difficulty concentrating, flight of ideas, delusions of grandeur, impaired judgment
• Decreased sleep
• Deteriorated physical appearance
• Euphoria and hostility
• Feelings of grandiosity
• Impulsiveness
• Increased energy (feeling of being charged up)
• Increased sexual interest and activity
• Increased social contacts
• Inflated sense of self-worth
• Lack of inhibition
• Rapid, jumbled speech

(Text continues on page 404.)

Cheat sheet

Anxiety & mood disorders refresher

BIPOLAR DISORDER

Key signs and symptoms

During episodes of mania
- Euphoria and hostility
- Feelings of grandiosity
- Substance abuse
- Increased sexual interest and activity
- Inflated sense of self-worth
- Increased energy (feeling of being charged up)

During episodes of depression
- Altered sleep patterns
- Anorexia and weight loss
- Helplessness
- Irritability
- Lack of motivation
- Low self-esteem
- Sadness and crying
- Suicidal ideation or attempts

Key test results
- EEG is abnormal during the depressive episodes of bipolar I disorder and major depression.

Key treatments
- Individual therapy
- Family therapy
- Antimanic agents: lithium carbonate (Eskalith), lithium citrate

Key interventions

During manic phase
- Decrease environmental stimuli by behaving consistently and supplying external controls.
- Ensure a safe environment.
- Define and explain acceptable behavior and then set limits.
- Monitor drug levels, especially lithium and carbamazepine.

During depressive phase
- Assess the level and intensity of the client's depression.
- Ensure a safe environment.
- Assess the risk for suicide and formulate a safety contract with the client, as appropriate.
- Observe the client for medication compliance and adverse effects.
- Encourage the client to identify current stressors and support systems.

GENERALIZED ANXIETY DISORDER

Key signs and symptoms
- Easy startle reflex
- Excessive worry and anxiety
- Diaphoresis
- Fatigue
- Fears of grave misfortune or death
- Muscle tension and aches
- Trembling and tingling of hands and feet

Key test results
- Laboratory tests exclude physiologic causes.

Key treatments
- Relaxation training
- Cognitive behavioral therapy
- Anxiolytics: alprazolam (Xanax), lorazepam (Ativan), clonazepam (Klonopin), buspirone (BuSpar)
- Serotonin norepinephrine reuptake inhibitors (SNRIs): venlafaxine (Effexor), duloxetine (Cymbalta)
- Selective serotonin reuptake inhibitors (SSRIs): fluoxetine (Prozac), paroxetine (Paxil), sertraline (Zoloft), citalopram (Celexa)

Key interventions
- Help the client identify and explore coping mechanisms used in the past.
- Observe for signs of mounting anxiety.

MAJOR DEPRESSION

Key signs and symptoms
- Altered sleep patterns
- Appetite changes resulting in weight loss or gain
- Anorexia and weight loss
- Helplessness
- Irritability
- Lack of motivation
- Low self-esteem
- Sadness and crying
- Suicidal ideation or attempts

Key test results
- Beck Depression Inventory indicates depression.

Key treatments
- SSRIs: paroxetine (Paxil), fluoxetine (Prozac), sertraline (Zoloft), citalopram (Celexa)

> Don't get frazzled if you don't have time to study the whole chapter. Just peek at the Cheat sheet.

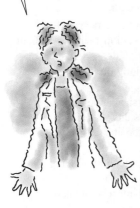

Anxiety & mood disorders refresher *(continued)*

MAJOR DEPRESSION *(CONTINUED)*
- Tricyclic antidepressants (TCAs): imipramine (Tofranil), desipramine (Norpramin), amitriptyline (Elavil)
- SNRIs: venlafaxine (Effexor), duloxetine (Cymbalta)

Key interventions
- Assess the level and intensity of the client's depression.
- Ensure a safe environment for the client.
- Assess the risk of suicide and formulate a safety contract with the client as appropriate.
- Observe the client for medication compliance and adverse effects.

OBSESSIVE-COMPULSIVE DISORDER
Key signs and symptoms
- Compulsive behavior (which may include repetitive touching or counting, doing and undoing small tasks, or any other repetitive activity or hoarding of certain items such as newspapers)
- Obsessive thoughts (which may include thoughts of contamination, repetitive worries about impending tragedy, repeating and counting images or words)

Key test results
- Positron emission tomography shows increased activity in the frontal lobe of the cerebral cortex.

Key treatments
- Cognitive behavioral therapy
- Individual therapy
- Benzodiazepines: alprazolam (Xanax), lorazepam (Ativan), clonazepam (Klonopin)
- SSRIs: fluoxetine (Prozac), paroxetine (Paxil), sertraline (Zoloft), fluvoxamine (Luvox)

Key interventions
- Encourage the client to express his feelings.
- Encourage the client to identify situations that produce anxiety and precipitate obsessive-compulsive behavior.

PANIC DISORDER
Key signs and symptoms
- Diminished ability to focus, even with direction from others
- Edginess, impatience
- Loss of objectivity
- Severely impaired rational thought
- Uneasiness and tension

Key test results
- Medical tests eliminate physiologic cause.

Key treatments
- Cognitive behavioral therapy
- Benzodiazepines: alprazolam (Xanax), lorazepam (Ativan), clonazepam (Klonopin)

Key interventions
During panic attacks
- Distract the client from the attack.
- Approach the client calmly and unemotionally.
- Use short, simple sentences.

PHOBIAS
Key signs and symptoms
- Panic when confronted with the feared object
- Persistent fear of specific things, places, or situations

Key test results
- No specific tests can be used to diagnose phobias.

Key treatments
- Benzodiazepines: alprazolam (Xanax), lorazepam (Ativan), clonazepam (Klonopin)
- Cognitive behavioral therapy
- Family therapy
- Supportive therapy

Key interventions
- Help the client to identify the feared object or situation.
- Assist in desensitizing the client.

POSTTRAUMATIC STRESS DISORDER
Key signs and symptoms
- Anxiety
- Flashbacks of the traumatic experience
- Nightmares about the traumatic experience
- Poor impulse control
- Social isolation
- Survivor guilt

Key test results
- No specific tests identify or confirm posttraumatic stress disorder.

Key treatments
- Cognitive behavioral therapy
- Group therapy
- Systematic desensitization
- Benzodiazepines: alprazolam (Xanax), lorazepam (Ativan), clonazepam (Klonopin)
- TCAs: imipramine (Tofranil), amitriptyline (Elavil)

Key interventions
- Help the client to identify stressors.
- Provide for client safety.
- Encourage the client to explore the traumatic event and the meaning of the event.
- Assist the client with problem solving and resolving guilt.

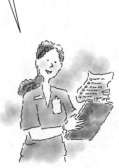

> Bipolar disorder isn't indicated by mood swings alone. It involves extreme behavior during both manic and depressive phases.

- Recklessness and poor judgment
- Substance abuse

During episodes of depression
- Altered sleep patterns
- Amenorrhea
- Anorexia and weight loss
- Confusion and indecisiveness
- Constipation
- Decreased alertness
- Delusions, hallucinations
- Difficulty thinking logically
- Guilt
- Helplessness
- Impotence and lack of interest in sex
- Inability to experience pleasure
- Irritability
- Lack of motivation
- Low self-esteem
- Pessimism
- Poor hygiene
- Poor posture
- Sadness and crying
- Suicide ideation or attempts

DIAGNOSTIC TEST RESULTS
- Abnormal dexamethasone suppression test results indicate bipolar I disorder.
- Cortisol secretion increases during manic episodes of bipolar I disorder.
- EEG is abnormal during the depressive episodes of bipolar I disorder and major depression.

NURSING DIAGNOSES
- Bathing self-care deficit
- Disturbed sleep pattern

TREATMENT
- Electroconvulsive therapy (ECT), if drug therapy fails
- Individual therapy
- Family therapy
- Interpersonal and social rhythm therapy
- Rehabilitation for substance abuse

Drug therapy
- Anticonvulsant agents: carbamazepine (Tegretol), gabapentin (Neurontin), divalproex sodium (Depakote)

- Antimanic agents: lithium carbonate (Eskalith), lithium citrate
- Selective serotonin reuptake inhibitors (SSRIs): paroxetine (Paxil), fluoxetine (Prozac), sertraline (Zoloft), citalopram (Celexa)
- Antipsychotic: aripiprazole (Abilify) for acute agitation

INTERVENTIONS AND RATIONALES
During manic phase
- Decrease environmental stimuli by behaving consistently and supplying external controls *to promote relaxation and enable sleep.*
- Ensure a safe environment *to protect the client from injuring himself.*
- Define and explain acceptable behaviors and then set limits *to begin a process in which the client will eventually define and set his own limits.*
- Monitor drug levels, especially lithium and carbamazepine, *to keep the dosage within the therapeutic range.*
- Monitor for suicidal ideations and innitiate safety measures *to prevent injury.*

During depressive phase
- Assess the level and intensity of the client's depression *because baseline information is essential for effective nursing care.*
- Ensure a safe environment *to protect the client from self-inflicted harm.*
- Assess the risk for suicide and formulate a safety contract with the client, as appropriate, *to ensure well-being and open lines of communication.*
- Observe the client for medication compliance and adverse effects; *without compliance, there's little hope of progress.*
- Encourage the client to identify current stressors and support systems *so that he can begin therapeutic treatment.*
- Promote opportunities for increased involvement in activities through a structured, daily program *to help the client feel comfortable with himself and others.*
- Select activities that ensure success and accomplishment *to increase self-esteem.*
- Help the client to modify negative expectations and think more positively; *positive thinking helps begin a healing process.*
- Spend time with the client *to enhance a therapeutic relationship.*

Teaching topics
- Explanation of the disorder and treatment plan
- Medication and possible adverse effects
- Recognizing signs of relapse
- Strategies to reduce stress
- Contacting the National Depressive and Manic Depressive association for support

Generalized anxiety disorder

A client with generalized anxiety disorder worries excessively and experiences tremendous anxiety almost daily. The worry lasts for longer than 6 months and is usually disproportionate to the situation. Both adults and children can be diagnosed with generalized anxiety disorder, though the content of the worry may differ.

CONTRIBUTING FACTORS
- Family history of anxiety
- Preexisting psychiatric problems, such as social phobia, panic disorder, and major depression

ASSESSMENT FINDINGS
- Autonomic hyperactivity
- Chest pain
- Distractibility
- Diaphoresis
- Easy startle reflex
- Excessive attention to surroundings
- Excessive worry and anxiety
- Fatigue
- Fears of grave misfortune or death
- Headaches
- Motor tension
- Muscle tension and aches
- Pounding heart
- Repetitive thoughts
- Sleep disorder
- Strained expression
- Trembling and tingling of hands and feet
- Vigilance and scanning

DIAGNOSTIC TEST RESULTS
- Laboratory tests exclude physiologic causes.

NURSING DIAGNOSES
- Anxiety
- Ineffective coping
- Deficient knowledge (disorder and treatment plan)

TREATMENT
- Relaxation training
- Cognitive behavioral therapy

Drug therapy
- Serotonin norepinephrine reuptake inhibitors (SNRIs): venlafaxine (Effexor), duloxetine (Cymbalta)
- Anxiolytics: alprazolam (Xanax), lorazepam (Ativan), clonazepam (Klonopin), buspirone (BuSpar)
- Beta-adrenergic blocker: propranolol (Inderal)
- Antihypertensive: clonidine (Catapres)
- Monoamine oxidase inhibitors (MAOIs): phenelzine (Nardil), tranylcypromine (Parnate)
- SSRIs: paroxetine (Paxil), sertraline (Zoloft), fluoxetine (Prozac), citalopram (Celexa)
- Tricyclic antidepressants (TCAs): imipramine (Tofranil), desipramine (Norpramin)

INTERVENTIONS AND RATIONALES
- Help the client identify and explore coping mechanisms used in the past. *Establishing a baseline for the level of current functioning will enable the nurse to build on the client's knowledge.*
- Observe for signs of mounting anxiety *to direct measures to moderate it.*
- Negotiate a contract to work on goals *to give the client control of his own situation.*
- Alter the environment *to reduce anxiety or meet the client's needs.*
- Monitor diet and nutrition; reduce caffeine intake *to reduce anxiety.*

Teaching topics
- Explanation of the disorder and treatment plan
- Medication use and possible adverse effects
- Recognizing signs of anxiety

Finding the most effective drug and dosage for anxiety and mood disorders is often a process of trial and error.

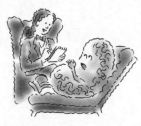

Treatment for depression usually requires collaboration with the client to find an effective program of drug therapy and psychotherapy.

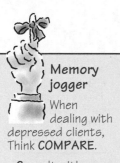

• Altering diet when receiving MAOIs (caffeine can cause arrhythmias; foods containing tyramine, such as fava beans, yeast-containing and fermented foods, and red wine, can cause hypertensive crisis)
• Contact information for counseling and support groups

Major depression

Major depression is a syndrome of persistent sad, dysphoric mood accompanied by disturbances in sleep and appetite from lethargy and an inability to experience pleasure. Depression is confirmed when the client exhibits five or more classic symptoms of depression for at least 2 weeks.

Major depression can profoundly alter social functioning, but the most severe complication of major depression is the potential for suicide.

CONTRIBUTING FACTORS
• Current substance abuse
• Deficiencies in the receptor sites for some neurotransmitters: norepinephrine, serotonin, dopamine, and acetylcholine
• Family history of depressive disorders
• Hormonal imbalances
• Lack of social support
• Nutritional deficiencies
• Prior episode of depression
• Significant medical problems
• Stressful life events

ASSESSMENT FINDINGS
• Altered sleep patterns
• Amenorrhea
• Appetite changes resulting in weight loss or gain
• Confusion and indecisiveness
• Constipation
• Decreased alertness
• Delusions, hallucinations
• Difficulty thinking logically
• Guilt
• Helplessness
• Impotence or lack of interest in sex

• Inability to experience pleasure
• Irritability
• Lack of motivation
• Low self-esteem
• Pessimism
• Poor hygiene
• Poor posture
• Sadness and crying
• Suicidal ideation or attempt

DIAGNOSTIC TEST RESULTS
• Thyroid test is abnormal in major depression.
• Beck Depression Inventory indicates depression.

NURSING DIAGNOSES
• Hopelessness
• Impaired social interaction
• Chronic low self-esteem

TREATMENT
• ECT
• Individual therapy
• Family therapy
• Phototherapy

Drug therapy
• MAOI: phenelzine (Nardil)
• SSRIs: paroxetine (Paxil), fluoxetine (Prozac), sertraline (Zoloft), citalopram (Celexa)
• TCAs: imipramine (Tofranil), desipramine (Norpramin), amitriptyline (Elavil)
• SNRIs: venlofaxine (Effexor), duloxetine (Cymbalta)

INTERVENTIONS AND RATIONALES
• Assess the level and intensity of the client's depression *because baseline information is essential for effective nursing care.*
• Address issues that trigger depression, and assist the client in using effective coping skills *to minimize depressive episodes.*
• Ensure a safe environment for the client *to protect the client from self-inflicted harm.*
• Assess the risk of suicide and formulate a safety contract with the client, as appropriate,

to ensure his well-being and open lines of communication.
- Reorient the client undergoing ECT as needed. *Clients receiving ECT often have temporary memory loss.*
- Observe the client for medication compliance and adverse effects*; without compliance, there's little hope of progress.*
- Encourage the client to identify current stressors and support systems *so that he can begin therapeutic treatment.*
- Promote opportunities for increased involvement in activities through a structured, daily program *to help the client feel comfortable with himself and others.*
- Select activities that ensure success and accomplishment *to increase self-esteem.*
- Help the client to modify negative expectations and think more positively; *positive thinking helps the client begin the healing process.*
- Spend time with the client *to enhance the therapeutic relationship.*

Teaching topics
- Explanation of the disorder and treatment plan
- Medication use and possible adverse effects
- Learning relaxation and sleep methods
- Complying with therapy
- If taking MAOIs, avoiding tyramine-containing foods, such as wine, beer, cheese, fermented fruits, meats, and vegetables

Obsessive-compulsive disorder

Obsessive-compulsive disorder is characterized by recurrent obsessions (intrusive thoughts, images, and impulses) and compulsions (repetitive behaviors in response to an obsession). The obsessions and compulsions may cause intense stress and impair the client's functioning. Some clients have simultaneous symptoms of depression.

CONTRIBUTING FACTORS
- Brain lesions
- Childhood trauma
- Lack of role models to teach coping skills
- Multiple stressors

ASSESSMENT FINDINGS
- Compulsive behavior (which may include repetitive touching or counting, doing and undoing, or any other repetitive activity or hoarding of items such as newspapers)
- Obsessive thoughts (which may include thoughts of contamination, repetitive worries about impending tragedy, repeating and counting images or words)
- Social impairment

DIAGNOSTIC TEST RESULTS
- Positron emission tomography shows increased activity in the frontal lobe of the cerebral cortex and abnormal metabolic rate of basal ganglia.

NURSING DIAGNOSES
- Anxiety
- Ineffective coping
- Chronic low self-esteem

TREATMENT
- Cognitive behavioral therapy
- Individual therapy

Drug therapy
- Benzodiazepines: alprazolam (Xanax), lorazepam (Ativan), clonazepam (Klonopin)
- MAOIs: phenelzine (Nardil), tranylcypromine (Parnate)
- SSRIs: fluoxetine (Prozac), sertraline (Zoloft), paroxetine (Paxil), fluvoxamine (Luvox)
- TCAs: imipramine (Tofranil), desipramine (Norpramin)

INTERVENTIONS AND RATIONALES
- Encourage the client to express his feelings *to decrease the client's level of stress.*

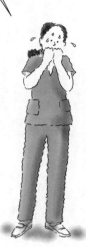

Don't worry. Dreading the exam doesn't mean you've developed panic disorder.

- Help the client assess how his obsessions and compulsive behaviors affect his functioning. The client needs *to realistically evaluate the consequences of his behavior.*
- Encourage the client to identify situations that produce anxiety and precipitate obsessive-compulsive behavior *to help him evaluate and cope with his condition.*
- Work with the client to develop appropriate coping skills *to reduce anxiety.*

Teaching topics
- Explanation of the disorder and treatment plan
- Medication use and possible adverse effects

Panic disorder

Although everyone experiences some level of anxiety, clients with panic disorder experience a nonspecific feeling of terror and dread, accompanied by symptoms of physiologic stress. This level of anxiety makes it difficult, if not impossible, for the client to carry out the normal functions of everyday life.

CONTRIBUTING FACTORS
- Agoraphobia (fear of being alone or in public places)
- Asthma
- Cardiovascular disease
- Familial pattern
- GI disorders
- History of anxiety disorders
- History of depression
- Neurologic abnormalities: abnormal activity on the medial portion of the temporal lobe in the parahippocampal area and significant asymmetrical atrophy of the temporal lobe
- Neurotransmitter involvement
- Stressful lifestyle

ASSESSMENT FINDINGS
- Abdominal discomfort or pain, nausea, heartburn, or diarrhea
- Avoidance (the client's refusal to encounter situations that may cause anxiety)
- Chest pressure, lump in throat, or choking sensation

Memory jogger

Note the differences in how to define fear, anxiety, and panic:

Fear is a response to external stimuli.

Anxiety is a response to internal conflict.

Panic is an extreme level of anxiety.

- Confusion
- Decreased ability to relate to others
- Diminished ability to focus, even with direction from others
- Dizziness or light-headedness
- Edginess, impatience
- Eyelid twitching
- Fidgeting or pacing
- Flushing or pallor
- Generalized weakness, tremors
- Increased or decreased blood pressure
- Insomnia
- Loss of appetite or revulsion toward food
- Loss of objectivity
- Palpitations and tachycardia
- Physical tension
- Potential for dangerous, impulsive actions
- Rapid speech
- Rapid, shallow breathing or shortness of breath
- Severely impaired rational thought
- Startle reaction
- Sudden urge and frequent urination
- Sweating, itching
- Trembling
- Uneasiness and tension

DIAGNOSTIC TEST RESULTS
- Medical tests eliminate physiologic cause.
- Urine and blood tests check for presence of psychoactive agents.

NURSING DIAGNOSES
- Anxiety
- Ineffective coping
- Powerlessness

TREATMENT
- Cognitive behavioral therapy
- Group therapy
- Relaxation training

Drug therapy
- Benzodiazepines: alprazolam (Xanax), lorazepam (Ativan), clonazepam (Klonopin)
- MAOIs: phenelzine (Nardil); in clients with severe panic disorder, tranylcypromine (Parnate)
- SSRI: paroxetine (Paxil)

- TCAs: imipramine (Tofranil), desipramine (Norpramin)

INTERVENTIONS AND RATIONALES
During panic attacks
- Distract the client from the attack *to alleviate the effects of panic.*
- Approach the client calmly and unemotionally *to reduce the risk of further stressing the client.*
- Use short, simple sentences *because the client's ability to focus and to relate to others is diminished.*
- Administer medications, as needed, *to ensure a therapeutic response.*

After panic attacks
- Attempt to identify triggers to panic attacks *to assist with treatment.*
- Discuss other methods of coping with stress *to make the client aware of alternatives.*

Teaching topics
- Explanation of the disorder and treatment plan
- Medication use and possible adverse effects
- Learning decision-making and problem-solving skills
- Learning relaxation techniques

Phobias

A phobia is an intense, irrational fear of something external. It's a fear that persists, even though the client recognizes its irrationality. Phobias are resistant to insight-oriented therapies.

CONTRIBUTING FACTORS
- Biochemical, involving neurotransmitters
- Familial patterns
- Traumatic events

ASSESSMENT FINDINGS
- Displacement (shifting of emotions from their original object) and symbolization
- Disruption in social life or work life
- Panic when confronted with the feared object
- Persistent fear of specific things, places, or situations

DIAGNOSTIC TEST RESULTS
- No specific test is used to diagnose phobias.

NURSING DIAGNOSES
- Anxiety
- Fear
- Powerlessness

TREATMENT
- Cognitive behavioral therapy
- Family therapy
- Social skills training
- Supportive therapy
- Systematic desensitization

Drug therapy
- Beta-adrenergic blocker: propranolol (Inderal) for phobia related to public speaking
- Benzodiazepines: alprazolam (Xanax), lorazepam (Ativan), clonazepam (Klonopin)
- MAOIs: phenelzine (Nardil), tranylcypromine (Parnate)
- SSRI: paroxetine (Paxil)
- TCAs: imipramine (Tofranil), desipramine (Norpramin)

INTERVENTIONS AND RATIONALES
- Help the client to identify the feared object or situation *to develop an effective treatment plan.*
- Assist in desensitizing the client *to diminish his fear.*
- Remind the client about resources and personal strengths *to build self-esteem.*

Teaching topics
- Explanation of the disorder and treatment plan
- Medication use and possible adverse effects
- Learning assertiveness techniques
- Learning relaxation techniques
- Participating in the desensitizing process

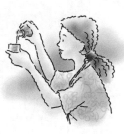

Note that depressed or anxious clients often attempt to self-medicate. Be aware of possible interactions with prescribed treatments.

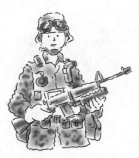

PTSD was originally called "shell shock" because participation in active combat is a common cause of this disorder.

Posttraumatic stress disorder

PTSD is a group of symptoms that develop after a traumatic event. This traumatic event may involve death, injury, or threat to physical integrity. In PTSD, ordinary coping behaviors fail to relieve the anxiety. The client may experience reactions that are acute, chronic, or delayed.

CAUSES
• Personal experience of threatened injury or death
• Witnessing a traumatic event happen to a close friend or family member
• Extreme distress causing a profound sense of fear, terror, or helplessness

CONTRIBUTING FACTORS
• Anxiety
• Low self-esteem
• Preexisting psychopathology

ASSESSMENT FINDINGS
• Anger
• Anxiety
• Apathy
• Avoidance of people involved in the trauma
• Avoidance of places where the trauma occurred
• Chronic tension
• Detachment
• Difficulty concentrating
• Difficulty falling or staying asleep
• Emotional numbness
• Flashbacks of the traumatic experience
• Hyperalertness
• Inability to recall details of the traumatic event
• Labile affect
• Nightmares about the traumatic experience
• Poor impulse control
• Social isolation
• Survivor guilt

DIAGNOSTIC TEST RESULTS
• No specific tests identify or confirm PTSD.

NURSING DIAGNOSES
• Fear
• Posttrauma syndrome
• Powerlessness
• Situational low self-esteem

TREATMENT
• Alcohol and drug rehabilitation, when indicated
• Cognitive behavioral therapy
• Group therapy
• Relaxation training
• Systematic desensitization

Drug therapy
• Benzodiazepines: alprazolam (Xanax), lorazepam (Ativan), clonazepam (Klonopin)
• Beta-adrenergic blocker: propranolol (Inderal)
• MAOIs: phenelzine (Nardil), tranylcypromine (Parnate)
• SSRIs: fluoxetine (Prozac), paroxetine (Paxil), sertraline (Zoloft)
• TCAs: imipramine (Tofranil), amitriptyline (Elavil)

INTERVENTIONS AND RATIONALES
• Help the client to identify stressors *to initiate effective coping.*
• Provide for client safety *because the client's ineffective coping, coupled with the intensity of the reaction and poor impulse control, increases the risk of injury.*
• Encourage the client to explore the traumatic event and the meaning of the event *to promote effective coping.*
• Assist the client with problem solving and resolving guilt *to help him understand that uncontrollable factors were responsible for the trauma and the event was beyond his personal control.*

Teaching topics

• Explanation of the disorder and treatment plan
• Medication use and possible adverse effects
• Learning relaxation techniques
• Promoting social interaction
• Contact information for counseling and support groups

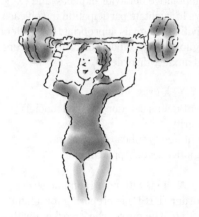

Pump up on practice questions

1. A nurse is caring for a client who is experiencing a panic attack. Which intervention is most appropriate?
1. Tell the client that there's no need to panic.
2. Speak in short, simple sentences.
3. Explain that there's no need to worry.
4. Give the client a detailed explanation of his panic reaction.

Answer: 2. The client experiencing a panic attack is unable to focus and his ability to relate to others is diminished; therefore, short, simple sentences are the most effective means of communication. Telling the client that there's no need to panic or that he's safe, or offering detailed explanations invalidates the client's feelings of anxiety.

➡ *NCLEX keys*
Client needs category: Psychosocial integrity
Client needs subcategory: None
Cognitive level: Analysis

2. A nurse is caring for a client who reports that she feels a choking sensation in her throat, a racing heart, and fearfulness. These symptoms have occurred almost daily for the past 3 months. Suspecting a psychological component the nurse anticipates administering:
1. benzodiazepines.
2. proton pump inhibitors.
3. nitroprusside.
4. lithium carbonate.

Answer: 1. Pharmacologic management would consist of either tricyclic antidepressants or benzodiazepines. Proton pump inhibitors are used for GI disorders. Nitroprusside is a vasodilator used for hypertensive emergencies. Lithium carbonate is an antimanic agent.

➡ *NCLEX keys*
Client needs category: Physiological integrity
Client needs subcategory: Pharmacological and parenteral therapies
Cognitive level: Application

3. A client who experiences panic disorder states that he's frequently overwhelmed by feelings of powerlessness. In working with this client, the nurse should initiate which intervention?
1. Assist the client to recognize unnecessary risk-taking.
2. Explore with the client issues related to identity problems.
3. Teach the client problem-solving and decision-making skills.
4. Have the client discuss the things he desires in a relationship.

Answer: 3. A client with panic disorder commonly has feelings of powerlessness and helplessness, and can easily feel out of control.

Teaching the client problem-solving and decision-making skills can promote the ability to cope and to have a sense of personal control. A client who experiences panic disorder typically doesn't tend to engage in high-risk behaviors or have identity problems. A discussion about relationships is premature for this client.

➡ **NCLEX keys**

Client needs category: Psychosocial integrity
Client needs subcategory: None
Cognitive level: Application

4. A nurse is assessing a client who struggles with social phobia. Which assessment question does the nurse need to ask?
1. "Do you drink alcohol or use illicit drugs?"
2. "Do you use physical outlets to handle anger?"
3. "Do you often struggle to control your impulses?
4. "Do you have a history of being an underachiever?"

Answer: 1. Clients with social phobia are highly likely to consume alcohol or use or abuse other substances to control the fear they experience in specific social situations. Clients with social phobia don't tend to be angry or aggressive, struggle to control their impulses, or have a history of underachievement.

➡ **NCLEX keys**

Client needs category: Psychosocial integrity
Client needs subcategory: None
Cognitive level: Application

5. After a nurse teaches a client with generalized anxiety disorder some strategies for coping with stressors, another goal for the client would be to:
1. recognize the signs associated with an elevation in mood.
2. learn to obtain assistance when his anxiety is increasing.

3. develop guidelines for decreasing manipulative behavior of peers.
4. explore ways to facilitate participation in self-care activities.

Answer: 2. It's important for a client to identify when his anxiety is escalating, when his anxiety may be getting out of control, and when seeking help is necessary. Recognizing the signs associated with an elevation in mood, developing guidelines for decreasing manipulative behavior of peers, and exploring ways to facilitate participation in self-care activities are goals appropriate for a client diagnosed with bipolar disorder, not generalized anxiety disorder.

➡ **NCLEX keys**

Client needs category: Psychosocial integrity
Client needs subcategory: None
Cognitive level: Application

6. A client with posttraumatic stress disorder (PTSD) is preparing for a family meeting. The nurse who's working with the client should encourage him to share which topic with family members?
1. Struggling to stop engaging in people-pleasing behaviors
2. Using medications to help cope with feelings of survivor guilt
3. Difficulty being emotionally attached to people
4. Difficulty handling the hallucinations experienced after a trauma

Answer: 3. Clients who suffer from PTSD tend to avoid emotional attachments as a way to protect themselves from the trauma they've experienced. Clients with PTSD don't tend to engage in people-pleasing behaviors or experience hallucinations after the experience of extreme trauma and loss. Although clients with PTSD may be prescribed medications to assist in symptom reduction, there aren't any drugs used specifically to help clients handle their feelings of survivor guilt.

➡ NCLEX keys

Client needs category: Psychosocial integrity
Client needs subcategory: None
Cognitive level: Application

7. A nurse is observing a client on a medical unit who's pacing the room, shaking his head from side to side, and clasping and unclasping his hands. As the nurse reviews the client's health history, she should be alert for information about which medication that could be linked to the client's behavior?

   1. Anticholinergics
   2. Vasodilators
   3. Antiemetics
   4. Steroids

Answer: 4. Clients who have taken steroids can experience a manic episode. Anticholinergic, vasodilator, and antiemetic drugs don't induce a manic episode.

➡ NCLEX keys

Client needs category: Psychosocial integrity
Client needs subcategory: None
Cognitive level: Application

8. A nurse is caring for a client who has generalized anxiety disorder. Which statement about this client is true?

   1. The client has regular obsessions.
   2. Relaxation techniques are necessary for cure.
   3. Nightmares and flashbacks are common in this client.
   4. His anxiety lasts longer than 6 months.

Answer: 4. Constant patterns of anxiety that affect the client for more than 6 months and interfere with normal activities are characteristic of generalized anxiety disorder. Pharmaceutical therapy with benzodiazepines can help. Clients having regular obsessions are probably suffering from obsessive-compulsive disorder. Nightmares and flashbacks are typical symptoms of posttraumatic stress disorder.

➡ NCLEX keys

Client needs category: Psychosocial integrity
Client needs subcategory: None
Cognitive level: Analysis

9. A client with the nursing diagnosis of *fear related to being embarrassed in the presence of others* exhibits symptoms of social phobia. What should be the goals for this client? Select all that apply.

   1. Manage his fear in group situations.
   2. Develop a plan to avoid situations that may cause stress.
   3. Verbalize feelings that occur in stressful situations.
   4. Develop a plan for responding to stressful situations.
   5. Deny feelings that may contribute to irrational fears.
   6. Use suppression to deal with underlying fears.

Answer: 1, 3, 4. Improving stress management skills, verbalizing feelings, and anticipating and planning for stressful situations should be goals for this client. Avoidance, denial, and suppression are maladaptive defense mechanisms.

➡ NCLEX keys

Client needs category: Psychosocial integrity
Client needs subcategory: None
Cognitive level: Application

10. A nurse is caring for a client who suffers from depression. She tells the client that he must avoid cheese, yogurt, preserved meats, and vegetables. Based on this information, the client is most likely receiving which drug therapy to treat his depression?

   1. Monoamine oxidase inhibitor (MAOI)
   2. Benzodiazepine
   3. Selective serotonin reuptake inhibitor (SSRI)
   4. Tricyclic antidepressant (TCA)

Answer: 1. This client is receiving an MAOI, which requires the client to avoid tyramine-rich foods, such as cheese, beer, wine, yogurt, and preserved fruits, vegetables, and meats. Benzodiazepines, SSRIs, and TCAs don't require dietary restrictions except avoiding alcoholic beverages.

➡ *NCLEX keys*
Client needs category: Psychosocial integrity
Client needs subcategory: None
Cognitive level: Analysis

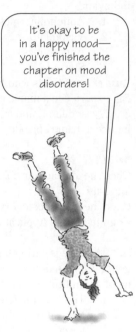

It's okay to be in a happy mood— you've finished the chapter on mood disorders!

Brush up on key concepts

Cognitive disorders result from any condition that alters or destroys brain tissue and, in turn, impairs cerebral functioning. Symptoms of cognitive disorders include cognitive impairment, behavioral dysfunction, and personality changes. The most common cognitive disorders described in the *Diagnostic and Statistical Manual of Mental Disorders*, Fourth edition, *Text Revision* are delirium, dementia, and amnestic disorders.

At any time, you can review the major points of each disorder by consulting the *Cheat sheet* on pages 416 and 417.

Catching up on cognitive disorders

Cognitive disorders are characterized by the disruption of cognitive functioning. Clinically, cognitive disorders are manifested as mental deficits in clients who hadn't previously exhibited such deficits.

Cognitive disorders are difficult to identify and treat. The key to diagnosis lies in the discovery of an organic problem with the brain's tissue.

Cognitive disorders may result from:
* a primary brain disease
* the brain's response to a systemic disturbance such as a medical condition
* the brain tissue's reaction to a toxic substance as in substance abuse.

Brain disruptions

Delirium is commonly caused by the disruption of brain homeostasis. When the source of the disturbance is eliminated, cognitive deficits generally resolve.

Common causes of delirium include postoperative conditions or metabolic disorders, withdrawal from alcohol and drugs, and toxic substances. Toxic substances are especially difficult to deal with because they can have residual effects. Drugs present another problem—a medication may be innocuous by itself but deadly when taken with another medication or food. Elderly clients are especially susceptible to the toxic effects of medication.

Brain defects

Unlike delirium, **dementia** is caused by primary brain pathology. Consequently, reversal of cognitive defects is less likely. Dementia can easily be mistaken for delirium, so the cause needs to be thoroughly investigated.

Polish up on client care

Major cognitive disorders include Alzheimer's-type dementia, amnesic disorder, delirium, and vascular dementia.

Alzheimer's-type dementia

A client with Alzheimer's-type dementia suffers from a global impairment of cognitive functioning, memory, and personality. The dementia occurs gradually but with continuous decline. Damage from Alzheimer's-type dementia is irreversible. Because of the difficulty of obtaining direct pathological evidence of Alzheimer's disease, the diagnosis can be made only when the etiologies for the dementia have been eliminated.

Researchers have developed different scales to measure the progression of symptoms. The Clinical Dementia Rating delineates five stages in the disease. Another, the Global Deterioration Scale, delineates seven.

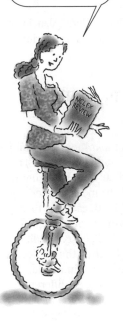

Cheat sheet

Cognitive disorders refresher

ALZHEIMER'S-TYPE DEMENTIA

Key signs and symptoms

Stage 1 (mild symptoms)
• Confusion and memory loss
• Disorientation to time and place
• Difficulty performing routine tasks
• Changes in personality and judgment
• Sleep disturbances

Stage 2 (moderate symptoms)
• Difficulty performing activities of daily living
• Anxiety
• Suspiciousness
• Agitation
• Wandering
• Pacing
• Repetitive behaviors
• Sleep disturbances
• Difficulty recognizing family members

Stage 3 (severe symptoms)
• Loss of speech
• Loss of appetite
• Weight loss
• Loss of bowel and bladder control
• Total dependence on caregiver

Key test results
• Cognitive assessment scale demonstrates cognitive impairment.
• Functional dementia scale shows degree of dementia.
• Magnetic resonance imaging shows apparent structural and neuralgic changes.
• Mini–Mental Status Examination reveals disorientation and cognitive impairment.

Key treatments
• Group therapy
• Anticholinesterase agents: tacrine (Cognex), donepezil (Aricept), rivastigmine (Exelon), galantamine (Razadyne)

Key interventions
• Remove hazardous items or potential obstacles from the client's environment.
• Provide verbal and nonverbal communication that's consistent and structured.
• Increase social interaction.
• Encourage the use of community resources; make appropriate referrals as necessary

AMNESIC DISORDER

Key signs and symptoms
• Confusion, disorientation, and lack of insight
• Inability to learn and retain new information
• Tendency to remember remote past better than more recent events

Key test results
• Mini–Mental Status Examination shows disorientation and lack of recall.

Key treatments
• Correction of the underlying medical cause
• Group therapy

Key interventions
• Ensure the client's safety.
• Encourage exploration of feelings.
• Provide simple, clear medical information.

DELIRIUM

Key signs and symptoms
• Altered psychomotor activity, such as apathy, withdrawal, and agitation
• Bizarre, destructive behavior that worsens at night
• Disorganized thinking
• Distractibility
• Impaired decision making
• Inability to complete tasks
• Insomnia or daytime sleepiness
• Poor impulse control
• Rambling, bizarre, or incoherent speech

Key test results
• Laboratory results indicate delirium is a result of a physiologic condition, intoxication, substance withdrawal, toxic exposure, prescribed medicines, or a combination of these factors.

Key treatments
• Correction of underlying physiologic problem
• Cholinesterase inhibitor: physostigmine (Antilirium)
• Antipsychotic agent: risperidone (Risperdal)

Key interventions
• Determine the degree of cognitive impairment.
• Create a structured and safe environment.
• Keep the client's room lit.

Don't forget about the Cheat sheet.

Cognitive disorders refresher (continued)

VASCULAR DEMENTIA

Key signs and symptoms
- Depression
- Difficulty following instructions
- Emotional lability
- Inappropriate emotional reactions
- Memory loss
- Wandering and getting lost in familiar places

Key test results
- Cognitive Assessment Scale shows deterioration in cognitive ability.
- Global Deterioration Scale signifies degenerative dementia.
- Mini–Mental Status Examination reveals disorientation and recall difficulty.

Key treatments
- Carotid endarterectomy to remove blockages in the carotid artery
- Treatment of underlying condition (hypertension, high cholesterol, or diabetes)
- Aspirin to decrease platelet aggregation and prevent clots

Key interventions
- Orient the client to his surroundings.
- Monitor the environment.
- Encourage the client to express feelings of sadness and loss.

However, most health care providers categorize the disease in only three stages: mild, moderate, and severe. These three stages may overlap, and the appearance and progression of symptoms may vary from one individual to the next.

CONTRIBUTING FACTORS
- Alterations in acetylcholine (a neurotransmitter)
- Altered immune function, with autoantibody production in the brain
- Familial history, such as a first-degree relative with Alzheimer's disease or Down syndrome
- Increased brain atrophy with wider sulci and cerebral ventricles than seen in normal aging
- Neurofibrillary tangles and beta amyloid neuritic plaques, mainly in the cerebral cortex and hippocampus (early) and later in the frontal, parietal, and temporal lobes

ASSESSMENT FINDINGS
Stage 1 (mild symptoms)
- Confusion and memory loss
- Disorientation to time and place
- Difficulty performing routine tasks
- Changes in personality and judgment
- Sleep disturbances

Stage 2 (moderate symptoms)
- Difficulty performing activities of daily living, such as feeding and bathing

- Anxiety
- Suspiciousness
- Agitation
- Wandering
- Pacing
- Repetitive behaviors
- Sleep disturbances
- Difficulty recognizing family members

Stage 3 (severe symptoms)
- Loss of speech
- Loss of appetite
- Weight loss
- Loss of bowel and bladder control
- Total dependence on caregiver

DIAGNOSTIC TEST RESULTS
- Cognitive assessment scale demonstrates cognitive impairment.
- Functional dementia scale shows degree of dementia.
- Magnetic resonance imaging (MRI) shows apparent structural and neurologic changes.
- Mini–Mental Status Examination reveals disorientation and cognitive impairment.
- Spinal fluid contains increased beta amyloid.

NURSING DIAGNOSES
- Bathing self-care deficit
- Impaired memory
- Caregiver role strain

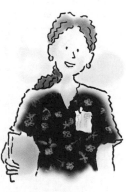

To recall symptoms, it may help to remember that people with Alzheimer's used to be described as "going senile."

TREATMENT
- Group therapy
- Palliative medical treatment
- Diet adequate in folic acid

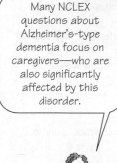

Many NCLEX questions about Alzheimer's-type dementia focus on caregivers—who are also significantly affected by this disorder.

Drug therapy
- Anticholinesterase agents: tacrine (Cognex), donepezil (Aricept), rivastigmine (Exelon), galantamine (Razadyne)
- Antipsychotic agents: haloperidol (Haldol), risperidone (Risperdal) in low doses, olanzapine (Zyprexa)
- Benzodiazepines: alprazolam (Xanax), lorazepam (Ativan), oxazepam
- Vitamin E supplements
- Antidepressants: citalopram (Celexa), fluoxetine (Prozac), paroxetine (Paxil), sertraline (Zoloft)

INTERVENTIONS AND RATIONALES
- Remove any hazardous items or potential obstacles from the client's environment *to maintain a safe environment.*
- Monitor food and fluid intake *to ensure adequate nutrition.*
- Identify triggers to agitation (typically, changes in the client's environment) *to maintain client and caregiver safety.*
- When the client is agitated, redirect the client's focus, *to prevent worsening agitation.*

- Simplify the client's environmental tasks and routines *to prevent agitation.*
- Encourage the consumption of foods containing folic acid, such as green, leafy vegetables, citrus fruits and juices, whole wheat bread, and dry beans *to help decrease symptoms of diagnosis.*
- Encourage the client and his caregiver to initiate health care directives and decisions while the client still has the capacity to do so *to ease the burden on the caregiver as the disease progresses.*
- Provide verbal and nonverbal communication that's consistent and structured *to prevent added confusion.*
- State expectations simply and completely *to orient the client.*
- Increase social interaction *to provide stimuli for the client.*
- Encourage the use of community resources; make appropriate referrals as necessary *to find outside support for caregivers.*
- Promote physical activity and sensory stimulation *to alleviate symptoms of the disorder.*

Teaching topics
- Explanation of the disorder and treatment plan
- Medication use and possible adverse effects

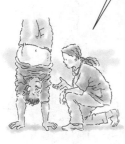

Because clients with Alzheimer's are confused, communication with them should be consistent, direct, and structured.

Management moments

Caring for the caregiver

Caring for a family member or friend with Alzheimer's disease can place considerable strain on the caregiver. Therefore, encourage the caregiver to express his feelings. In many cases, caregivers feel confused, fearful, guilty, and grief stricken when a family member is diagnosed with Alzheimer's disease. Help the caregiver cope by:
- discussing situations that are typically stressful, such as dealing with the client's hostility, anxiety, and suspicion
- discussing resources needed to provide adequate, safe care (caring for a client with

Alzheimer's disease can place financial strain on the family)
- developing a plan for the caregiver to obtain assistance from other family members, neighbors, friends, and community resources
- reinforcing the importance of the caregiver establishing a plan for maintaining personal well-being, including recreation, rest, and exercise (the stress of caring for a client with Alzheimer's disease can leave the caregiver susceptible to illness).

- Finding support and education (for caregivers) (see *Caring for the caregiver*)
- Learning stress-relief techniques (for caregivers)
- Contacting the Alzheimer's Association and local support services

Amnesic disorder

In amnesic disorder, the client experiences a loss of both short-term and long-term memory. He can't recall some or many past events. The client's abstract thinking, judgment, and personality usually remain intact. Symptoms may have a sudden or gradual onset and may be transient or long-lasting.

Amnesic disorder differs from dissociative amnesia in that it results from an identifiable physical cause, rather than psychosocial stressors.

CONTRIBUTING FACTORS
- Adverse effects of certain medications
- Brain surgery
- Cerebrovascular events
- Encephalitis
- Exposure to a toxin
- Poorly controlled type 1 diabetes
- Substance abuse
- Sustained nutritional deficiency
- Traumatic brain injury

ASSESSMENT FINDINGS
- Apathy, emotional blandness
- Confabulation in early stages
- Confusion, disorientation, and lack of insight
- Inability to learn and retain new information
- Tendency to remember remote past better than more recent events

DIAGNOSTIC TEST RESULTS
- Medical tests (electrolyte levels, MRI, and computed tomography [CT] scan) confirm a physical basis.
- Mini–Mental Status Examination shows disorientation and lack of recall.
- Neuropsychological testing demonstrates memory deficits.

NURSING DIAGNOSES
- Dressing self-care deficit
- Impaired memory
- Deficient knowledge (disease process and treatment plan)

TREATMENT
- Correction of the underlying medical cause
- Group therapy

Drug therapy
- Anticholinisterase agents: tacrine (Cognex), donepezil (Aricept), rivastigmine (Exelon)

INTERVENTIONS AND RATIONALES
- Ensure the client's safety *because the client may be unable to maintain a safe environment.*
- Use environmental cues—for example, post the client's name and schedule in his room—*to promote orientation.*
- Spend time with the client and talk about the client's health and self-care needs *to encourage greater self-understanding.*
- Identify realistic short-term goals *so the client doesn't become overwhelmed.*
- Encourage exploration of feelings, *which can spark memory.*
- Provide simple, clear medical information *to help the client understand the condition.*

Teaching topics
- Understanding the underlying illness and its relationship to amnestic disorder

Delirium

Delirium is a disturbance of consciousness accompanied by a change in cognition that can't be attributed to preexisting dementia. Delirium is characterized by an acute onset and may last from several hours to several days. It's potentially reversible but can be life-threatening if not treated.

CONTRIBUTING FACTORS
- Cerebral hypoxia
- Effects of medication
- Fever
- Fluid and electrolyte imbalances

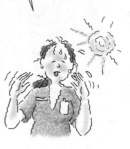

Dehydration is a common cause of delirium, especially in older clients.

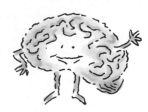

Treatment of delirium focuses on the underlying cause.

Memory jogger

To help remember the difference between delirium and dementia, think DR. DID (delirium reversible; dementia irreversible damage):

Delirium is reversible (though serious if not treated).

Dementia stems from irreversible damage.

- Infection (especially of the urinary tract and upper respiratory system)
- Metabolic disorders
- Neurotransmitter imbalance
- Pain
- Polypharmacy, especially anticholinergics
- Sensory overload or deprivation
- Sleep deprivation
- Stress
- Substance intoxication or withdrawal

ASSESSMENT FINDINGS
- Altered psychomotor activity, such as apathy, withdrawal, and agitation
- Altered respiratory depth or rhythm
- Bizarre, destructive behavior that worsens at night
- Disorganized thinking
- Disorientation (especially to time and place)
- Distractibility
- Impaired decision making
- Inability to complete tasks
- Insomnia or daytime sleepiness
- Picking at bed linen and clothes
- Poor impulse control
- Rambling, bizarre, or incoherent speech
- Tremors, generalized seizures
- Visual and auditory illusions

DIAGNOSTIC TEST RESULTS
- Laboratory test results indicate delirium is a result of a physiologic condition, intoxication, substance withdrawal, toxic exposure, prescribed medicines, or a combination of these factors.

NURSING DIAGNOSES
- Risk for injury
- Impaired memory
- Disturbed sensory perception (visual)

TREATMENT
- Correction of underlying physiologic problem
- Individual therapy

Drug therapy
- Tranquilizer: droperidol (Inapsine)
- Benzodiazepine: low-dose lorazepam (Ativan)

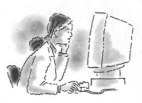

Hmmm... Slurred speech and wandering, along with stroke symptoms? That sounds like vascular dementia.

- Antipsychotic agent: risperidone (Risperdal)
- B vitamins (if related to alcohol)

INTERVENTIONS AND RATIONALES
- Determine the degree of cognitive impairment *to understand and treat the client.*
- Create a structured and safe environment *to prevent the client from harming himself.*
- Institute measures to help the client relax and fall asleep *to comfort him.*
- Keep the client's room lit *to allay his fears and prevent visual hallucinations.*
- Monitor the effects of medications *to prevent exacerbating symptoms.*

Teaching topics
- Explanation of the disorder and treatment plan (to the client's family)
- Medication use and possible adverse effects (to family)
- Contacting community resources
- Managing the client's basic needs

Vascular dementia

Also called *multi-infarct dementia,* vascular dementia impairs the client's cognitive functioning, memory, and personality but doesn't affect the client's level of consciousness. It's caused by an irreversible alteration in brain function that damages or destroys brain tissue.

CONTRIBUTING FACTORS
- Cerebral emboli or thrombosis
- Diabetes
- Heart disease
- High cholesterol level
- Hypertension (leading to stroke)
- Transient ischemic attacks

ASSESSMENT FINDINGS
- Depression
- Difficulty following instructions
- Dizziness
- Emotional lability
- Inappropriate emotional reactions
- Memory loss
- Neurologic symptoms that last only a few days

- Rapid onset of symptoms
- Slurred speech
- Wandering and getting lost in familiar places
- Weakness in an extremity

DIAGNOSTIC TEST RESULTS
- Cognitive Assessment Scale shows deterioration in cognitive ability.
- Global Deterioration Scale signifies degenerative dementia.
- Mini–Mental Status Examination reveals disorientation and recall difficulty.
- Structural and neurologic changes can be seen on MRI or CT scans.

NURSING DIAGNOSES
- Impaired memory
- Risk for injury

TREATMENT
- Carotid endarterectomy to remove blockages in the carotid artery
- Low-fat diet
- Smoking cessation
- Treatment of underlying condition (hypertension, high cholesterol, or diabetes)

Drug therapy
- Aspirin to decrease platelet aggregation and prevent clots

INTERVENTIONS AND RATIONALES
- Orient the client to his surroundings *to alleviate client anxiety.*
- Monitor the environment *to prevent overstimulation.*
- Encourage the client to express feelings of sadness and loss *to foster a healthy therapeutic environment.*

Teaching topics
- Explanation of the disorder and treatment plan (to the client's family)
- Medication use and possible adverse effects (to family)
- Controlling weight and diet
- Exercising to decrease cardiovascular risk factors

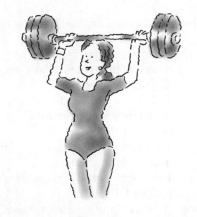

Pump up on practice questions

1. A client is experiencing acute confusion due to poisoning from an accidental exposure to toxic chemicals in the workplace. What type of behavior should the nurse expect this client to demonstrate upon admission to the nursing unit?
1. Inability to eat without experiencing nausea
2. Frequently verbalizing ambivalent feelings
3. Difficulty expressing ideas and needs
4. Despondency in the presence of family members

Answer: 3. A client with delirium has disorganized thinking and has difficulty expressing his ideas and needs to the nurse. A client in a state of confusion can usually eat without experiencing nausea, doesn't tend to verbalize feelings of ambivalence, and doesn't demonstrate irritability in the presence of others.

➡ *NCLEX keys*
Client needs category: Physiological integrity
Client needs subcategory: Reduction of risk potential
Cognitive level: Application

2. A nurse is caring for a 78-year-old client hospitalized with bilateral pneumonia. Shortly after admission, he became extremely belligerent, confused, and hypotensive, and he developed tachypnea. The nurse prepares the client for intubation, administers anti-infectives stat, and requests that the computed tomography (CT) scan of his head be delayed. Why?

1. His change in mental status was related to hypoxia, metabolic encephalopathy, and sepsis.
2. Taking this client to the radiology department would jeopardize his condition.
3. The client exhibited no signs of focal neurologic impairment.
4. His prognosis was poor and didn't justify a CT scan.

Answer: 1. Severe functional abnormalities and confusion are commonly caused by nonneurologic diseases, especially in elderly clients. Encephalopathies such as these are reversible if the underlying cause is treated. An unstable condition, absence of signs of focal neurologic impairment, and poor prognosis aren't appropriate justifications for delaying a diagnostic CT scan.

➡ *NCLEX keys*

Client needs category: Physiological integrity
Client needs subcategory: Reduction of risk potential
Cognitive level: Analysis

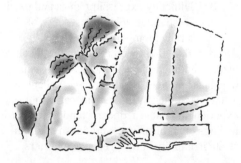

3. A client with dementia suffers from sundown syndrome. Which nursing action should be included in this client's care plan?

1. Integrate the client's cultural preferences into the care provided.
2. Maintain a consistent schedule and sequence of daily activities.
3. Provide opportunities for the client to learn and practice new skills.
4. Serve a warm beverage and snacks in the early evening.

Answer: 2. A client with dementia benefits from a consistent schedule of activities; routine is reassuring and can promote comfort. Cultural preferences don't tend to influence the client's agitation. Providing opportunities to learn and practice new skills could upset the routine and cause additional agitation. Although serving a beverage and snack is a thoughtful strategy to implement, it won't decrease the potential for agitation associated with sundown syndrome.

➡ *NCLEX keys*

Client needs category: Physiological integrity
Client needs subcategory: Reduction of risk potential
Cognitive level: Application

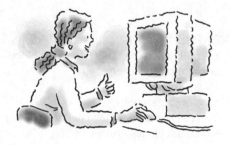

4. A nurse is teaching the wife of a client who has mild symptoms of dementia how to more effectively communicate with her spouse. The teaching would be considered successful if the nurse observed the wife:

1. having a face-to-face conversation with her husband.
2. talking quietly into her husband's ear.
3. discussing only events related to their past.
4. speaking loudly and enunciating each word.

Answer: 1. Speaking face-to-face is the most effective strategy to use when communicating with a cognitively impaired client because it allows the client to pick up visual cues to assist him in understanding his wife. Talking directly into the client's ear prohibits the client from having access to the reinforcement of non-verbal communication. It isn't good practice to assume that all recent memory is gone; it is better to stay current, explain things, and orient as necessary. There's no need to speak loudly and enunciate each word to a client with mild dementia unless he has a hearing impairment.

➡ *NCLEX keys*
Client needs category: Physiological integrity
Client needs subcategory: Reduction of risk potential
Cognitive level: Application

5. A nurse is assessing a client for vascular dementia. Which finding helps confirm the diagnosis?
1. Positive drug screen for toxicology
2. Findings upon autopsy
3. Magnetic resonance imaging (MRI)
4. Response to electroconvulsive therapy

Answer: 3. Vascular dementia is commonly caused by cerebrovascular disease and small infarctions, which can be detected with MRI. A positive drug screen wouldn't be helpful in diagnosing dementia caused by vascular problems. Attempts to diagnosis vascular dementia wouldn't be delayed until autopsy. Electroconvulsive therapy is occasionally used in the treatment for selected psychiatric disorders but isn't a diagnostic tool for dementia.

➡ *NCLEX keys*
Client needs category: Physiological integrity
Client needs subcategory: Reduction of risk potential
Cognitive level: Comprehension

6. A nurse is caring for a client with vascular dementia. When planning activities for this client, the nurse should select which activity?
1. Simple crafts
2. Memory games
3. Playing cards
4. Chair exercising

Answer: 4. A client with vascular dementia can benefit from exercising, even chair exercising. Doing simple crafts, playing memory games, and playing cards are inappropriate because a client with vascular dementia manifests memory loss and has difficulty following directions.

➡ *NCLEX keys*
Client needs category: Physiological integrity
Client needs subcategory: Reduction of risk potential
Cognitive level: Application

7. A nurse is planning care for a client with substance abuse delirium. When the nurse implements care that addresses the client's hygiene needs, which action should be taken?
1. Provide an electric shaver instead of a razor.
2. Administer medication before starting care.
3. Set limits for staff involvement in the client's daily care.
4. Bathe the client, but permit the client's family to dress him.

Answer: 1. For a client with delirium, using an electric shaver is preferable because the client may be predisposed to injury if a standard razor is used. Medication is administered to promote comfort and address illness issues, not to promote the client's participation in self-hygiene. The client requires assistance during the recovery process, not limits for staff involvement. Bathing the client facilitates dependency; the goal is to provide optimal functioning and self-care ability.

➡ *NCLEX keys*
Client needs category: Physiological integrity
Client needs subcategory: Reduction of risk potential
Cognitive level: Application

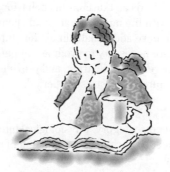

8. A nurse is caring for a client who is diagnosed with delirium. What must the nurse provide for the client?

1. A safe environment
2. An opportunity to release frustration
3. Prescribed medications
4. Medications, as needed, judiciously

Answer: 1. Keeping the client with delirium safe is the most important aspect of care. All other choices are logical and appropriate, but safety issues and meeting the client's basic physiologic needs are of primary importance.

➡ *NCLEX keys*

Client needs category: Safe and effective care environment
Client needs subcategory: Safety and infection control
Cognitive level: Application

9. An elderly male client develops symptoms of delirium after a surgical procedure. To effectively minimize the client's agitation, which action should the nurse take?

1. Discuss the behavior change with the client.
2. Maintain continuous staff-client contact.
3. Introduce appropriate sensory stimulation.
4. Limit unnecessary interactions with the client.

Answer: 2. A client with delirium will benefit from the reassuring presence of familiar staff monitoring his condition and maintaining a consistent environment. A client suffering from delirium can't discuss his behavior change with the nurse. An agitated client must not have additional stimulation. Interactions are necessary to promote calmness, reinforce reality, build trust, and provide support during this stressful period.

➡ *NCLEX keys*

Client needs category: Physiological integrity
Client needs subcategory: Reduction of risk potential
Cognitive level: Application

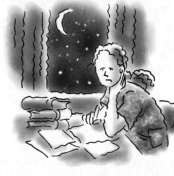

10. A 76-year-old client is admitted to a long-term-care facility with a diagnosis of Alzheimer's-type dementia. The client has been wearing the same dirty clothes for several days and the nurse contacts the family to bring in clean clothing. Which intervention would best prevent further regression in the client's personal hygiene?

1. Encouraging the client to perform as much self-care as possible
2. Making the client assume responsibility for physical care
3. Assigning a staff member to take over the client's physical care
4. Accepting the client's desire to go without bathing

Answer: 1. Clients with Alzheimer's-type dementia tend to fluctuate in their capabilities. Encouraging self-care to the extent possible will help increase the client's orientation and promote a trusting relationship with the nurse. Making the client assume responsibility for physical care is unreasonable. Assigning a staff member to take over restricts the client's independence. Accepting the client's desire to go without bathing promotes bad hygiene.

➡ *NCLEX keys*

Client needs category: Physiological integrity
Client needs subcategory: Reduction of risk potential
Cognitive level: Application

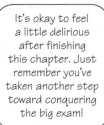

It's okay to feel a little delirious after finishing this chapter. Just remember you've taken another step toward conquering the big exam!

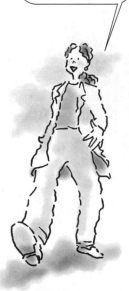

16 Personality disorders

Brush up on key concepts

Personality traits are patterns of behavior that reflect how people perceive and relate to others and themselves. Personality disorders occur when these traits become **rigid** and **maladaptive.** According to the *Diagnostic and Statistical Manual of Mental Disorders*, Fourth edition, *Text Revision,* a personality disorder is a problematic pattern occurring in two of the following four areas: cognition, affectivity, interpersonal functioning, and impulse control. A person with a personality disorder uses maladaptive behavior to relate to others and fulfill basic emotional needs.

At any time, you can review the major points of each disorder by consulting the *Cheat sheet* on pages 426 and 427.

Polish up on client care

Major personality disorders include antisocial personality disorder, borderline personality disorder, dependent personality disorder, and paranoid personality disorder.

Antisocial personality disorder

Antisocial personality disorder leads the client to have a total disregard for the rights of others. Antisocial personality disorder can begin in early childhood and continue into adulthood, but the actual diagnosis requires that the client be at least 18 years old and that the client has displayed some symptoms of the disorder before age 15.

CONTRIBUTING FACTORS
- Childhood trauma
- Genetic predisposition
- Physical abuse
- Sexual abuse
- Social isolation
- Transient friendships
- Unstable or erratic parenting

ASSESSMENT FINDINGS
- Destructive tendencies
- Excessively opinionated nature
- General disregard for the rights and feelings of others
- Impulsive actions
- Inability to learn from past experiences
- Inability to maintain close personal or sexual relationships
- Inflated and arrogant self-appraisal
- Lack of remorse
- Possible concurrent psychiatric disorders
- Power-seeking behavior
- Previous violations of societal norms or rules
- Substance abuse
- Sudden or frequent changes in job, residence, or relationships
- Superficial charm (manipulative)

DIAGNOSTIC TEST RESULTS
- Minnesota Multiphasic Personality Inventory reveals antisocial personality disorder.

NURSING DIAGNOSES
- Social isolation
- Risk for other-directed violence
- Chronic low self-esteem

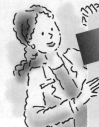

Personality disorders refresher

ANTISOCIAL PERSONALITY DISORDER

Key signs and symptoms
- Destructive tendencies
- General disregard for the rights and feelings of others
- Lack of remorse
- Sudden or frequent changes in job, residence, or relationships

Key test results
- Minnesota Multiphasic Personality Inventory reveals antisocial personality disorder.

Key treatments
- Cognitive behavioral therapy
- Antipsychotic: lithium (Eskalith)
- Anxiolitics: alprazolam (Xanax), lorazepam (Ativan) for severe anxiety, insomnia, or agitation
- Beta-adrenergic blocker: propranolol (Inderal) for controlling aggressive outbursts
- Selective serotonin reuptake inhibitors (SSRIs): paroxetine (Paxil), sertraline (Zoloft)

Key interventions
- Help the client to identify manipulative behaviors.
- Establish a behavioral contract.
- Hold the client responsible for his behavior.

BORDERLINE PERSONALITY DISORDER

Key signs and symptoms
- Destructive behavior
- Impulsive behavior
- Inability to develop a sense of self
- Inability to maintain relationships
- Moodiness
- Self-mutilation

Key test results
- Standard psychological tests reveal a high degree of dissociation.

Key treatments
- Milieu therapy
- Individual therapy
- Antimanic medications: carbamazepine (Tegretol), lithium (Eskalith)
- Anxiolytic: buspirone (BuSpar)
- SSRIs: paroxetine (Paxil), fluoxetine (Prozac), sertraline (Zoloft), citalopram (Celexa)

Key interventions
- Recognize behaviors that the client uses to manipulate others.
- Set appropriate expectations for social interaction, and make sure these expectations are met.

DEPENDENT PERSONALITY DISORDER

Key signs and symptoms
- Clinging, demanding behavior
- Fear and anxiety about losing the people they're dependent upon
- Hypersensitivity to potential rejection and decision making
- Low self-esteem

Key test results
- Laboratory tests rule out an underlying medical condition.

Key treatments
- Behavior modification through assertiveness training
- Individual therapy
- Benzodiazepines: alprazolam (Xanax), lorazepam (Ativan), clonazepam (Klonopin)
- SSRIs: paroxetine (Paxil), citalopram (Celexa)
- Tricyclic antidepressants: imipramine (Tofranil), desipramine (Norpramin)

Key interventions
- Encourage activities that require decision making (balancing a checkbook, planning meals, paying bills).
- Help the client to identify manipulative behaviors, focusing on specific examples.

PARANOID PERSONALITY DISORDER

Key signs and symptoms
- Feelings of being deceived
- Hostility
- Major distortions of reality
- Social isolation
- Suspiciousness, mistrusting friends and relatives

Loosen up. Personality disorders occur when traits become rigid and maladaptive.

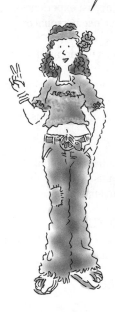

TREATMENT
• Alcohol or drug rehabilitation (if appropriate)
• Cognitive behavioral therapy
• Group therapy
• Individual therapy

Drug therapy
• Antipsychotic agent: lithium (Eskalith)
• Anxiolytics: alprazolam (Xanax), lorazepam (Ativan) for severe anxiety, insomnia, or agitation
• Beta-adrenergic blocker: propranolol (Inderal) for controlling aggressive outbursts
• Selective serotonin reuptake inhibitors (SSRIs): paroxetine (Paxil), sertraline (Zoloft)

INTERVENTIONS AND RATIONALES
• Help the client to identify manipulative behaviors *to help counteract the perception that others are extensions of himself.*
• Establish a behavioral contract *to communicate to the client that other behavior options are available.*
• Avoid confrontations and power struggles *to maintain the opportunity for therapeutic communication.* (See *Dealing with antisocial personality disorder*, page 428.)
• Hold the client responsible for his behavior *to promote development of a collaborative relationship.*
• Help the client to manage anger and observe for physical and verbal signs of agitation *to maintain a healthy therapeutic environment.*

Teaching topics
• Explanation of the disorder and treatment plan
• Medication use and possible adverse effects
• Learning appropriate behaviors
• Continuing treatments after discharge

Borderline personality disorder

Borderline personality disorder results in a pattern of instability in a person's mood, interpersonal relationships, self-esteem, self-identity, behavior, and cognition. Impulsiveness is its most prominent characteristic. Borderline personality disorder appears to originate in early childhood.

CONTRIBUTING FACTORS
• Brain dysfunction in the limbic system or frontal lobe
• Decreased serotonin activity
• Early parental loss or separation
• Increased activity in $alpha_2$-noradrenergic receptors
• Major losses early in life
• Physical abuse
• Sexual abuse
• Substance abuse

ASSESSMENT FINDINGS
• Compulsive behavior
• Destructive behavior
• Dissociation (separating objects from their emotional significance)
• Dysfunctional lifestyle
• Emotional reactions, with few coping skills
• Extreme fear of abandonment
• High self-expectations
• Impulsive behavior
• Inability to develop a healthy sense of self

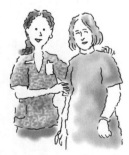

Be prepared for defensiveness. Clients suffering from a personality disorder aren't likely to recognize it in themselves.

Management moments

Dealing with antisocial personality disorder

Aggressive behavior makes caring for the client with antisocial personality disorder a challenge. Clients with this disorder are typically impulsive. They tend to lash out at those who interfere with their need for immediate gratification. Therefore, helping these clients express their anger in a nonviolent manner takes priority. Taking the following precautions may be helpful:
• Maintain a safe environment.
• Encourage the client to verbalize aggressive feelings.
• Talk with the client about appropriate ways to handle anger such as channeling energy into socially acceptable activities.
• Teach the client coping strategies, such as negotiation skills, stress reduction techniques, and ways to communicate anger effectively.

Be careful! Clients receiving drug therapy for borderline personality disorder should take medications only for targeted symptoms and only for a short period.

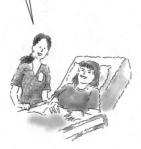

• Inability to maintain relationships
• Moodiness
• Paranoid ideation
• Self-directed anger
• Self-mutilation
• Shame
• Suicidal behavior
• View of others as either extremely good or bad

DIAGNOSTIC TEST RESULTS
• Standard psychological tests reveal a high degree of dissociation.

NURSING DIAGNOSES
• Impaired social interaction
• Risk for self-directed violence
• Chronic low self-esteem

TREATMENT
• Alcohol and drug rehabilitation, as indicated
• Milieu therapy
• Group therapy
• Family therapy
• Individual therapy

Drug therapy
• Antimanic medications: carbamazepine (Tegretol), lithium (Eskalith)
• Anxiolytic: buspirone (BuSpar)
• Monoamine oxidase inhibitor: phenelzine (Nardil)
• Opioid detoxification adjunct agent: naltrexone (ReVia)

• SSRIs: paroxetine (Paxil), fluoxetine (Prozac), sertraline (Zoloft), citalopram (Celexa)

INTERVENTIONS AND RATIONALES
• Recognize behaviors that the client uses to manipulate others *to avoid unconsciously reinforcing these behaviors*.
• Set appropriate expectations for social interaction, and praise the client when these expectations are met *to create a healthy therapeutic environment*.
• Respect the client's sense of personal space *to increase trust*.
• Provide a safe environment. Observe the client frequently *to prevent self-injury*.

Teaching topics
• Explanation of the disorder and treatment plan
• Medication use and possible adverse effects
• Developing problem-solving skills
• Developing therapeutic communication skills
• Implementing relaxation techniques

Dependent personality disorder

The client with dependent personality disorder experiences an extreme need to be taken care of that leads to submissive, clinging behavior and fear of separation. This pattern begins by early adulthood, when behaviors designed to elicit caring from others become predominant. These behaviors arise from the client's perception that he's unable to function adequately without others.

CONTRIBUTING FACTORS

- Childhood traumas
- Closed family system that discourages relationships with others
- Genetic predisposition
- Physical abuse
- Sexual abuse
- Social isolation

ASSESSMENT FINDINGS

- Clinging, demanding behavior
- Exaggerated fear of losing support and approval
- Fear and anxiety about losing the people they're dependent upon
- Hypersensitivity to potential rejection and decision making
- Indirect resistance to occupational and social performance
- Low self-esteem
- Over-reliance on family members
- Tendency to be passive

DIAGNOSTIC TEST RESULTS

- Laboratory tests rule out underlying medical condition.

NURSING DIAGNOSES

- Interrupted family processes
- Ineffective coping
- Chronic low self-esteem

TREATMENT

- Behavior modification through assertiveness training
- Individual therapy
- Group therapy

Drug therapy

- Benzodiazepines: alprazolam (Xanax), lorazepam (Ativan), clonazepam (Klonopin)
- SSRIs: paroxetine (Paxil), citalopram (Celexa)
- Tricyclic antidepressants: imipramine (Tofranil), desipramine (Norpramin)

INTERVENTIONS AND RATIONALES

- Encourage activities that require decision making (balancing a checkbook, planning meals, paying bills) *to promote independence.*
- Help the client establish and work toward goals *to foster a sense of independence.*
- Help the client identify manipulative behaviors, focusing on specific examples, *to decrease the perception that others are an extension of the self.*
- Limit interactions with the client to a few consistent staff members *to increase the client's sense of security.*

Teaching topics

- Explanation of the disorder and treatment plan
- Medication use and possible adverse effects
- Expressing ideas and feelings assertively
- Improving social skills and promoting social interaction

Paranoid personality disorder

Paranoid personality disorder is characterized by extreme distrust of others. Paranoid people avoid relationships in which they aren't in control or have the potential of losing control.

CONTRIBUTING FACTORS

- Genetic predisposition
- Neurochemical alteration
- Parental antagonism

ASSESSMENT FINDINGS

- Bad temper
- Delusional thinking
- Emotional reactions, including nervousness, jealousy, anger, or envy
- Feelings of being deceived
- Hostility
- Hyperactivity
- Hypervigilance
- Irritability
- Lack of humor
- Lack of social support systems
- Major distortions of reality
- Need to be in control
- Refusal to confide in others

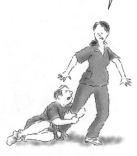

Client stuck on you? Help the client with dependent personality disorder feel secure but maintain appropriate boundaries.

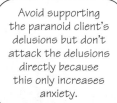

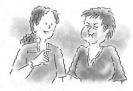

Avoid supporting the paranoid client's delusions but don't attack the delusions directly because this only increases anxiety.

- Self-righteousness
- Social isolation
- Sullen attitude
- Suspiciousness (mistrust of friends and relatives)

DIAGNOSTIC TEST RESULTS
- There are no specific tests for paranoid personality disorder.

NURSING DIAGNOSES
- Ineffective coping
- Chronic low self-esteem
- Social isolation

TREATMENT
- Possible drug-free treatment to reduce the chance of causing increased paranoia
- Individual therapy

Drug therapy
- Antipsychotic agents: olanzapine (Zyprexa), risperidone (Risperdal), chlorpromazine, thioridazine, fluphenazine, haloperidol (Haldol) in low doses
- SSRIs: paroxetine (Paxil), citalopram (Celexa), sertraline (Zoloft)

INTERVENTIONS AND RATIONALES
- Establish a therapeutic relationship by listening and responding to the client *to initiate therapeutic communication.*
- Encourage the client to take part in social interactions *to introduce other people's perceptions and realities to him.*
- Help the client identify negative behaviors that interfere with relationships *so the client can see how his behavior impacts others.*
- Instruct the client in and help him to practice strategies that facilitate the development of social skills *so the client can gain confidence and practice interacting with others.*

Teaching topics
- Explanation of the disorder and treatment plan
- Medication use and possible adverse effects
- Learning coping strategies
- Understanding the disorder (for family and client)

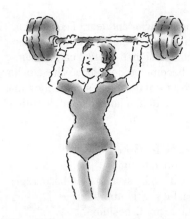

Pump up on practice questions

1. A client with a personality disorder is on a general medical-surgical unit after a recent surgery. The nurse deliberately interacts with this client more than she interacts with another client, who had the same surgery. Both clients are recovering equally well. Why would the nurse do this?
1. Other caregivers commonly minimize contact with such clients.
2. The nurse feels sorry for the client.
3. One client has health insurance; the other client doesn't.
4. The nurse suspects that the first client isn't recovering as well as reported.

Answer: 1. Because clients with personality disorders tend to be demanding and difficult, health care providers with little psychiatric experience commonly try to limit their contact with them. This approch tends to perpetuate behavioral problems, not improve them. This nurse is acting to balance that trend. Sympathy for a client, lack of health insurance, and unfounded suspicions aren't relevant considerations.

➡ *NCLEX keys*
Client needs category: Safe and effective care environment
Client needs subcategory: Management of care
Cognitive level: Application

2. A nurse is caring for a client diagnosed with paranoid personality disorder in an acute care facility. Which intervention should the nurse use to control the client's suspiciousness?

1. Keeping messages clear and consistent, while avoiding deception
2. Providing pharmacologic therapy
3. Providing social interactions with others on the unit
4. Attending to basic daily needs of the client on a consistent basis

Answer: 1. Keeping messages consistent, fostering trust, and avoiding deception will help to decrease suspiciousness. Encouraging social interactions, attending to basic daily needs, and providing pharmacologic therapy are general nursing interventions that are appropriate for any psychiatric disorder.

➡ *NCLEX keys*

Client needs category: Safe and effective care environment
Client needs subcategory: Management of care
Cognitive level: Analysis

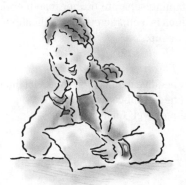

3. A client arrived on the psychiatric unit from the emergency department. His diagnosis is personality disorder, and he exhibits manipulative behavior. As the nurse reviews the unit rules with him, the client asks "Can I go to the snack shop just one time and then I will answer whatever you ask?" What is the nurse's most appropriate response?

1. "Yes, but hurry, because I need to finish your assessment."
2. "Okay but be back in 5 minutes."
3. "No, you can't go."
4. "No, you can't go. The rules here apply to everyone."

Answer: 4. This response sets limits with an appropriate explanation. Allowing the client to go gives in to his manipulative behavior. Simply saying no doesn't explain the purpose of the refusal.

➡ *NCLEX keys*

Client needs category: Psychosocial integrity
Client needs subcategory: None
Cognitive level: Application

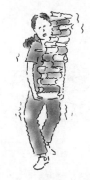

4. During group therapy on the addiction disorder unit, one client says to another client, "That's a stupid thing to be worried about." Which statement by the nurse group facilitator would address the client's unacceptable comment?

1. "It's important to let a person speak about the things that he finds bothersome."
2. "There are alternative social behaviors that you must demonstrate in this group."
3. "Think before you speak or others in the group will act disrespectful to you."
4. "Restate in a positive way what you want to share with your colleague."

Answer: 4. Clients with personality disorders, especially antisocial personality disorder, are typically insensitive to the feelings and rights of others. A nursing response that encourages the client to identify and practice appropriate behavior and provides the opportunity to perform in socially acceptable ways is considered therapeutic care. Telling the client that others should be able to say what they want doesn't address the client's unacceptable behavior. Telling the client that he must demonstrate alternate behaviors helps correct his behavior but doesn't help him correct the situation. Telling the client that others in the group may act disrespectful to him has the potential to come across as threatening or punitive and doesn't assist the client in addressing the issue.

➡ *NCLEX keys*

Client needs category: Physiological integrity
Client needs subcategory: None
Cognitive level: Application

5. A client with a borderline personality has a history of unsuccessful suicidal behavior. After creating a safe environment for this client, the nurse should implement which intervention?
1. Direct the client to make a personal inventory of his resentful situations.
2. Have the client work on addressing the source of his pain and anger.
3. Address with the client how to document problematic conditions as they arise.
4. Tell the client to verbalize disturbing and disorganized thoughts as they occur.

Answer: 2. After securing a safe environment for a client with borderline personality disorder who has a history of incomplete suicide attempts, the nurse should work with the client to discover the origin of his pain and anger. Often, these clients displace their anger and hurt themselves rather than recognize actual painful situations. If the client takes a personal inventory of resentful situations, he won't learn how to work on his hurtful feelings.

Documenting problematic conditions only identifies negative events; it doesn't address how to handle them. Telling the client to verbalize disturbing thoughts as they occur contributes to promoting impulsive and reckless behavior.

➡ *NCLEX keys*

Client needs category: Physiological integrity
Client needs subcategory: None
Cognitive level: Application

6. A nurse is teaching a client about healthy interpersonal relationships. Which characteristic should the nurse include?
1. Minimal self-revelation
2. Willingness to risk self-revelation
3. Ego-dystonic behavior
4. Intimacy and merging of identities

Answer: 2. Willingness to risk self-revelation is a characteristic of a healthy interpersonal relationship. Minimal self-revelation is holding back on the relationship. Ego-dystonic behavior refers to thoughts, impulses, attitudes and behavior that the client feels are distressing, repugnant, or inconsistent with the rest of his personality. Intimacy while maintaining separate (rather than merging) identities is a characteristic of a healthy relationship.

➡ *NCLEX keys*

Client needs category: Psychosocial integrity
Client needs subcategory: None
Cognitive level: Analysis

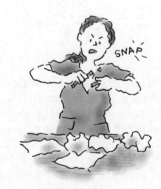

7. A client is court mandated to attend an anger management course. The client uses an aggressive tone to ask the nurse who's teaching the educational session, "Why can't I talk the way I want?" Which is the best therapeutic response from the nurse?

1. "Sometimes our words don't adequately express the point we want to make."
2. "There's often a problem when an attitude of superiority is shown to others."
3. "Tomorrow you may feel differently and you can't change the way you spoke today."
4. "The way a person speaks can be a way of acting out intense feelings."

Answer: 4. The nurse should respond in a way that helps the client recognize that the way a person speaks can escalate anger and arouse anxiety and aggressive responses in others. Although the other responses spoken could be true for some clients, they don't address the client's acting out verbally and attempting to use aggressive words to intimidate others.

➡ *NCLEX keys*

Client needs category: Physiological integrity
Client needs subcategory: None
Cognitive level: Application

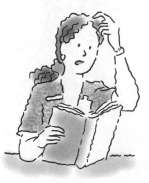

8. The nurse is assisting a client with a dependent personality disorder to work on the goal of developing healthy relationships with family members. Which nursing intervention should the nurse initiate to help the client develop healthy relationships?

1. Determine a structure for each part of the day spent alone.
2. Establish a nurse-client contract based on mutual cooperation.
3. Practice disagreeing with statements verbalized by the nurse.
4. Talk about self while participating in outside activities.

Answer: 3. A client with a dependent personality disorder can become incapacitated by a family member's criticism or disagreement. It is beneficial for the client to practice respectfully refuting or disagreeing with a person (the nurse) who will still remain in the relationship. Determining a structure for time spent alone, establishing a nurse-client contract, and talking about oneself during outside activities won't help a client with dependent personality disorder develop healthy relationships.

➡ *NCLEX keys*

Client needs category: Physiological integrity
Client needs subcategory: None
Cognitive level: Application

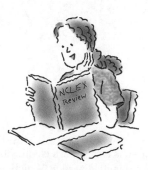

9. A nurse notices that a client with paranoid personality disorder demonstrates some instances of spying behaviors on other clients on the unit. Which nursing intervention should the nurse institute?

1. Address the client's actions that interfere with creating social relationships.
2. Talk with the client about the need to follow the rules established for the unit.

3. Encourage the client to evaluate and change personal thinking patterns.
4. Tell the client that his negative feelings are causing personality changes.

Answer: 1. By addressing the client's actions that interfere with creating social relationships, the nurse can assist the client in becoming aware of the impact of inappropriate behaviors on others and begin to work on how to prevent them. Talking with the client about following unit rules, encouraging him to change thinking patterns, and telling him that his negative feelings are causing personality changes don't address how his spying behavior influences other clients and isolates him from effectively interacting with peers.

➡ *NCLEX keys*
Client needs category: Physiological integrity
Client needs subcategory: None
Cognitive level: Application

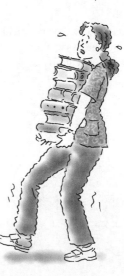

10. A nurse is caring for a client with borderline personality disorder. Which interventions should the nurse perform?
1. Setting limits on manipulative behavior
2. Allowing the client to set limits
3. Using restraints judiciously
4. Encouraging acting out behavior

Answer: 1. Setting limits on manipulative behavior provides the structure that the client needs. Encouraging acting out behavior and allowing the client to set limits would be contraindicated. The need for restraints in a client with borderline personality disorder would be rare, unless coexisting disorders exist.

➡ *NCLEX keys*
Client needs category: Psychosocial integrity
Client needs subcategory: None
Cognitive level: Application

I think I'm getting a borderline anti-NCLEX disorder!

17 Schizophrenic & delusional disorders

Brush up on key concepts

Schizophrenic and delusional disorders fall under the diagnostic umbrella **psychosis.** A psychotic illness is a brain disorder characterized by an impaired perception of reality, commonly coupled with mood disturbances. Psychosis can be either progressive or episodic.

Schizophrenia is characterized by disturbances (for at least 6 months) in thought content and form, perception, affect, sense of self, volition, interpersonal relationships, work and self-care, and psychomotor behavior. Schizophrenia is usually a chronic disorder, equally prevalent in men and women. It begins in young adulthood. It's more common in African and Asian Americans.

Delusional disorders are marked by false beliefs with a plausible basis in reality. Once referred to as *paranoid disorders,* delusional disorders affect less than 1% of the population.

At any time, you can review the major points of each disorder by consulting the *Cheat sheet* on pages 436 and 437.

Positive or negative
Symptoms of schizophrenia may be characterized as positive or negative. **Positive symptoms** focus on a distortion of normal functions; **negative symptoms** focus on a loss of normal functions. Examples of positive symptoms are delusions, hallucinations, disorganized speech, and grossly disorganized or catatonic behavior. Examples of negative symptoms include flat affect, alogia (poverty of speech), avolition (lack of self-initiated behaviors), and anhedonia (minimal enjoyment of activities).

Thought broadcasting
Delusions are false, fixed beliefs that aren't shared by other members of the client's social, cultural, or religious background. Delusions may occur in the form of thought broadcasting, in which the client believes that his personal thoughts are broadcast to the external world. Many times, he believes that his feelings, thoughts, or actions aren't his own.

Look for a theme
Common themes characterize delusions. Delusional themes are described as **persecutory, somatic, erotomanic, jealous,** or **grandiose.** An example of a persecutory delusion is the idea that one is being followed, tricked, tormented, or made the subject of ridicule. The client with erotomanic delusions falsely believes he shares an idealized relationship with another person, usually someone of higher status such as a celebrity. An example of a somatic delusion is a client who believes his body is deteriorating from within. An example of a jealous delusion is the client's feeling that his or her spouse or partner is unfaithful. The client with grandiose delusions has an exaggerated sense of self-importance.

Hearing voices
Most commonly, schizophrenics experience **auditory hallucinations.** When the client hears voices, he perceives these voices as being separate from his own thoughts. The content of the voices is usually threatening and derogatory. Many times, the voices tell the client to commit an act of violence against himself or others.

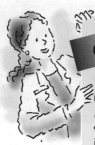

Cheat sheet

Schizophrenic & delusional disorders refresher

CATATONIC SCHIZOPHRENIA

Key signs and symptoms

• Bizarre postures, waxy flexibility (posture held in odd or unusual fixed positions for extended periods), and resistance to being moved
• Excessive motor activity
• Extreme negativism (resistance to instruction or movement)
• Displacement (switching emotions from their original object to a more acceptable substitute)
• Dissociation (separation of things from their emotional significance)
• Echolalia (repetition of another's words)
• Echopraxia (involuntary imitation of another person's movements and gestures)

Key test results

• Magnetic resonance imaging (MRI) shows possible enlargement of lateral ventricles, an enlarged third ventricle, enlarged sulci, cortical atrophy, and decreased cerebral blood flow.
• Clients show impaired performance on neuropsychological and cognitive tests.

Key treatments

• Milieu therapy
• Supportive psychotherapy
• Antipsychotics: chlorpromazine, risperidone (Risperdal), olanzapine (Zyprexa)

Key interventions

• Provide skin care and reposition the client every 2 hours.
• Monitor for adverse effects of antipsychotic drugs, such as akathesia, akinesia, parkinsonism, neuroleptic malignant syndrome, dystonic reactions, and tardive dyskinesia.
• Be aware of the client's personal space; use gestures and touch judiciously.
• Provide appropriate measures to ensure safety and explain to the client why you're doing so.
• Collaborate with the client to identify anxious behavior as well as probable causes.

DISORGANIZED SCHIZOPHRENIA

Key signs and symptoms

• Cognitive impairment
• Fantasy

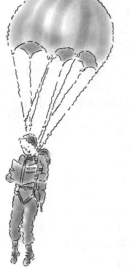

• Hallucinations
• Loose associations
• Word salad
• Disorganized behavior
• Flat or inappropriate affect

Key test results

• Neuropsychological and cognitive tests indicate impaired performance.

Key treatments

• Milieu therapy
• Social skills training
• Supportive psychotherapy
• Antipsychotics (traditional): chlorpromazine, fluphenazine, haloperidol (Haldol), olanzapine (Zyprexa), thioridazine, thiothixene (Navane)
• Antipsychotics (atypical): clozapine (Clozaril), aripiprazole (Abilify), quetiapine (Seroquel), risperidone (Risperdal), ziprasidone (Geodon)

Key interventions

• Help the client meet basic needs for food, comfort, and a sense of safety.
• During an acute psychotic episode, remove potentially hazardous items from the environment.
• If the client experiences hallucinations, don't attempt to reason with him or challenge his perception of the hallucinations. Instead, ensure safety and provide comfort and support.
• Encourage the client with auditory hallucinations to reveal what voices are telling him.
• Encourage the client to participate in one-on-one interactions, and then progress to small groups.
• Provide positive reinforcement for socially acceptable behavior such as efforts to improve hygiene and table manners.
• Encourage the client to express feelings related to experiencing hallucinations.

Schizophrenic & delusional disorders refresher *(continued)*

PARANOID SCHIZOPHRENIA

Key signs and symptoms
• Delusions and auditory hallucinations
• Dissociation
• Inability to trust

Key test results
• MRI shows possible enlargement of ventricles and enlarged sulci. The presence of the enlarged sulci suggests cortical loss, particularly in the frontal lobe.

Key treatments
• Milieu therapy
• Supportive psychotherapy
• Antipsychotics (traditional): chlorpromazine, fluphenazine, haloperidol (Haldol), olanzapine (Zyprexa), thioridazine, thiothixene (Navane)
• Antipsychotics (atypical): clozapine (Clozaril), aripiprazole (Abilify), quetiapine (Seroquel), risperidone (Risperdal), ziprasidone (Geodon)

Key interventions
• Inform the client that you will help him control his behavior.
• Set limits on aggressive behavior and communicate your expectations to the client.
• Use nonphysical techniques, such as redirecting the client's focus and verbal deescalation.
• Maintain a low level of stimuli.
• Provide reality-based diversional activities.
• Provide a safe environment.
• Reorient the client to time and place, as appropriate.

DELUSIONAL DISORDER

Key signs and symptoms
• Hallucinations that are visual, auditory, or tactile
• Inability to trust
• Projection
• Delusions that are erotomanic, grandiose, jealous, persecutory, or somatic

Key test results
• Blood and urine tests eliminate an organic or chemical cause.
• Endocrine function tests rule out hyperadrenalism, pernicious anemia, and thyroid disorders.
• Neurologic evaluations rule out an organic cause.

Key treatments
• Milieu therapy
• Supportive psychotherapy
• Antipsychotics (traditional): chlorpromazine, fluphenazine, haloperidol (Haldol), olanzapine (Zyprexa), thioridazine, thiothixene (Navane)
• Antipsychotics (atypical): clozapine (Clozaril), aripiprazole (Abilify), quetiapine (Seroquel), risperidone (Risperdal), ziprasidone (Geodon)

Key interventions
• Explore events that trigger delusions.
• Don't directly attack the client's delusion.
• When the dynamics of the delusions are understood, discourage repetitious talk about delusions and refocus the conversation on the client's underlying feelings.
• Recognize delusion as the client's perception of the environment.

All over the place

Disorganized thinking or **looseness of associations** is where speech shifts randomly from one topic to another, with only a vague connection between topics. The client may digress to unrelated topics, make up new words (neologisms), repeat words involuntarily (perseveration), or repeat words or phrases similar in sound only (clang association).

Loss of self

The client may demonstrate a blunted, flat, or inappropriate affect manifested by poor eye contact; a distant, unresponsive facial expression; and very limited body language. The sense of self is disturbed, an experience referred to as **loss of ego boundaries.** This loss of a coherent sense of self causes the client to experience difficulty in maintaining an ongoing sense of identity. This may make

it impossible for the client to maintain interpersonal relationships or function at work and in other life roles.

Polish up on client care

Major psychotic disorders include catatonic schizophrenia, disorganized schizophrenia, paranoid schizophrenia, and delusional disorder.

Catatonic schizophrenia

Clients with catatonic schizophrenia show little reaction to their environments. Catatonic

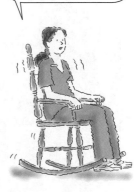

Some catatonic clients may repeat the same motion continuously for hours.

behavior involves remaining completely motionless or continuously repeating one motion. This behavior can last for hours at a time. Catatonic schizophrenia is the least common type of schizophrenia.

CONTRIBUTING FACTORS
- A fragile ego that can't withstand the demands of reality
- Brain abnormalities
- Developmental abnormalities
- Genetic factors
- Hyperactivity of the neurotransmitter dopamine
- An infectious agent or autoimmune response (unproven cause)
- Social or environmental stress, interacting with the person's inherited biological makeup

ASSESSMENT FINDINGS
- Agitation that may be unexpected and dangerous
- Bizarre postures, waxy flexibility (posture held in odd or unusual fixed positions for extended periods), and resistance to being moved
- Excessive motor activity
- Extreme negativism (resistance to instruction or movement)
- Childlike, regressed behavior
- Clang association
- Displacement (switching emotions from their original object to a more acceptable substitute)

- Dissociation (separation of things from their emotional significance)
- Echolalia (repetition of another's words)
- Echopraxia (involuntary imitation of another person's movements and gestures)
- Episodes of impulsiveness
- Fantasy
- Inability to trust
- Little reaction to environment
- Mutism
- Neologism
- Projection
- Purposeless overactivity or underactivity
- Ritualistic mannerisms
- Social isolation
- Speech resembling a word salad (string of words that aren't connected in any way)

DIAGNOSTIC TEST RESULTS
- Magnetic resonance imaging (MRI) shows possible enlargement of lateral ventricles, an enlarged third ventricle, enlarged sulci, cortical atrophy, and decreased cerebral blood flow.
- Clients show impaired performance on neuropsychological and cognitive tests.

NURSING DIAGNOSES
- Risk for impaired skin integrity
- Imbalanced nutrition: Less than body requirements
- Ineffective coping
- Dressing self-care deficit

TREATMENT
- Electroconvulsive therapy (if client isn't responsive to medication)
- Family therapy
- Milieu therapy
- Outpatient group therapy
- Psychoeducational programs
- Social skills training
- Stress management
- Supportive psychotherapy

Drug therapy
- Antiparkinsonian agents: benztropine (Cogentin) for adverse effects of antipsychotics

Here's a major difficulty in treating schizophrenia: After clients' more troubling symptoms recede, they believe they can discontinue therapy and medication.

Yet, when treatment stops, the symptoms inevitably recur in full force.

Understanding antipsychotics

Antipsychotic medications act against the symptoms of schizophrenia and other psychoses and are first-line therapy for schizophrenia. These medications can't "cure" the illness, but they alleviate and eliminate symptoms. In some cases, they can shorten the course of the illness.

TRADITIONAL NEUROLEPTICS

There are several antipsychotic (neuroleptic) medications available. The main differences among the medications is in their potency, their therapeutic effects, and their adverse effects. Physicians consider several factors when prescribing an antipsychotic medication, including:
- degree and type of illness
- client's age
- client's body weight
- client's medical history.

TARDIVE DYSKINESIA

Although maintenance treatment is helpful for many people, a drawback is the possibility of developing long-term adverse effects from long-term treatment with antipsychotics. In particular, a condition called tardive dyskinesia, characterized by involuntary movements (usually of the facial muscles), can occur. The disorder may range from mild to severe and can be irreversible.

ATYPICAL NEUROLEPTICS

In 1990, clozapine (Clozaril), an "atypical neuroleptic," was introduced in the United States. This medication is a more effective tool for treating individuals with treatment-resistant schizophrenia, and the risk of tardive dyskinesia is lower. However, because of the potential adverse effect of a serious blood disorder, agranulocytosis, clients who are on clozapine must have weekly blood tests. The expense involved in this monitoring, together with the cost of the medication, has made maintenance on clozapine difficult for many persons with schizophrenia.

Since clozapine was approved in the United States, other atypical neuroleptics have been introduced. Risperidone (Risperdal) was released in 1994, olanzapine (Zyprexa) in 1996, and quetiapine (Seroquel) in 1997. These agents help relieve positive and negative symptoms of schizophrenia. Although they have some adverse effects, these newer medications are generally better tolerated than clozapine or traditional antipsychotics, such as chlorpromazine (Thorazine), and they don't cause agranulocytosis. Disadvantages of atypical neuroleptics include higher cost and a tendency to cause weight gain. They also show a higher incidence of metabolic syndrome, which includes type 2 diabetes mellitus, hypertension, obesity, hyperlipidemia, and coagulation abnormalities.

- Antipsychotics: chlorpromazine, risperidone (Risperdal), olanzapine (Zyprexa) (see *Understanding antipsychotics*)

INTERVENTIONS AND RATIONALES

- Provide skin care and reposition the client every 2 hours *to prevent skin breakdown.*
- Monitor intake and output. *Body weight may decrease as a result of inadequate intake.*
- Monitor for adverse effects of antipsychotic drugs, such as akathesia, akinesia, parkinsonism, neuroleptic malignant syndrome, dystonic reactions, and tardive dyskinesia. *Early identification of extrapyramidal effects can help diminish or eliminate the client's anxiety about these symptoms.*
- Be aware of the client's personal space; use gestures and touch judiciously. *Invading the client's personal space can increase his anxiety.*
- When discussing care, give short, simple explanations at the client's level of understanding *to increase cooperation.*

- Provide appropriate measures to ensure safety and explain to the client why you're doing so. *Implementing and explaining safety measures can promote trust and decrease anxiety while increasing the client's sense of security.*
- Promote a trusting relationship *to create a safe environment in which the client can prepare for social interaction.*
- Briefly explain procedures, routines, and tests *to allay the client's anxiety.*
- Collaborate with the client to identify anxious behavior as well as probable causes. *Involving the client in examination of behavior can increase his sense of control.*
- Provide opportunities for the client to learn adaptive social skills in a nonthreatening environment. *Learning new social skills can enhance the client's adjustment after discharge.*

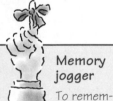

Memory jogger

To remember the major needs of schizophrenic clients, think **SDS**.

Structure — because they tend to have too little in their lives

Diversion — to distract them from disturbing thoughts

Stress reduction — to minimize the severity of the disorder

Teaching topics

- Explanation of the disorder and treatment plan
- Medication use and possible adverse effects
- Importance of continuing medications as prescribed
- Preventing photosensitivity reactions to drugs by avoiding exposure to sunlight

Disorganized schizophrenia

Disorganized schizophrenics have a flat or inappropriate affect and incoherent thoughts. Clients with this disorder exhibit loose associations and disorganized speech and behaviors.

CONTRIBUTING FACTORS

- A fragile ego that can't withstand the demands of external reality
- Brain abnormalities
- Developmental involvement
- Genetic factors
- Neurotransmitter abnormalities
- Social or environmental stress, interacting with the person's inherited biological makeup

ASSESSMENT FINDINGS

- Cognitive impairment
- Disorganized behavior
- Displacement
- Fantasy
- Flat or inappropriate affect
- Grimacing
- Hallucinations
- Lack of coherence
- Loose associations
- Magical thinking (client believes his thoughts can control others)
- Word salad

DIAGNOSTIC TEST RESULTS

- MRI shows possible enlargement of the ventricles and prominent cortical sulci.
- Neuropsychological and cognitive tests indicate impaired performance.

NURSING DIAGNOSES

- Social isolation
- Dressing self-care deficit
- Ineffective role performance

Forming a trusting relationship is a key intervention for schizophrenic clients.

TREATMENT

- Family therapy
- Milieu therapy
- Psychoeducational programs
- Social skills training
- Stress management
- Supportive psychotherapy

Drug therapy

- Antiparkinsonian agents: benztropine (Cogentin) for adverse effects of antipsychotic medications
- Antipsychotics (traditional): chlorpromazine, fluphenazine, haloperidol (Haldol), olanzapine (Zyprexa), thioridazine, thiothixene (Navane)
- Antipsychotics (atypical): clozapine (Clozaril), aripiprazole (Abilify), quetiapine (Seroquel), risperidone (Risperdal), ziprasidone (Geodon)

INTERVENTIONS AND RATIONALES

- Help the client meet basic needs for food, comfort, and a sense of safety *to ensure the client's well-being and to build trust.*
- During an acute psychotic episode, remove potentially hazardous items from the client's environment *to promote safety.*
- Briefly explain procedures, routines, and tests *to decrease the client's anxiety.*
- Protect the client from self-destructive tendencies or aggressive impulses *to ensure safety.*
- Convey sincerity and understanding when communicating *to promote a trusting relationship.*
- Formulate realistic goals with the client. *Including the client in formulating goals can help diminish suspicion while increasing self-esteem and a sense of control.*
- If the client experiences hallucinations, don't attempt to reason with him or challenge his perception of the hallucinations. Instead, ensure the client's safety and provide comfort and support. *Attempts to reason with the client increase anxiety, possibly making hallucinations worse.*
- Encourage the client with auditory hallucinations to reveal what voices are telling him *to help prevent harm to the client and others.*

- Encourage the client to participate in one-on-one interactions, and then progress to small groups *to enable the client to practice newly acquired social skills.*
- Provide positive reinforcement for socially acceptable behavior, such as efforts to improve hygiene and table manners, *to foster improved social relationships and acceptance from others.*
- Encourage the client to express feelings related to experiencing hallucinations *to promote better understanding of the client's experiences and to allow him to vent emotions, thereby reducing anxiety.*

Teaching topics
- Explanation of the disorder and treatment plan
- Medication use and possible adverse effects
- Learning to use distraction techniques

Paranoid schizophrenia

Clients with paranoid schizophrenia have delusions or frequent auditory hallucinations unrelated to reality. They commonly display bizarre behavior, are easily angered, and are at high risk for violence. The prognosis for independent functioning is usually better than for other types of schizophrenia.

CONTRIBUTING FACTORS
- A fragile ego that can't withstand the demands of external reality
- Brain abnormalities
- Developmental involvement
- Genetic factors
- Neurotransmitter abnormalities
- Social or environmental stress, interacting with the person's inherited biological makeup

ASSESSMENT FINDINGS
- Anxiety
- Argumentativeness
- Delusions and auditory hallucinations
- Displacement
- Dissociation
- Easily angered
- Inability to trust
- Potential for violence

- Projection
- Withdrawal or aloofness

DIAGNOSTIC TEST RESULTS
- MRI shows possible enlargement of ventricles and enlarged sulci. The presence of the enlarged sulci suggests cortical loss, particularly in the frontal lobe.
- Neuropsychological and cognitive tests indicate impaired performance.

NURSING DIAGNOSES
- Social isolation
- Ineffective coping
- Risk for other-directed violence
- Anxiety

TREATMENT
- Family therapy
- Group therapy
- Behavior management techniques
- Milieu therapy
- Psychoeducational programs
- Social skills training
- Stress management
- Supportive psychotherapy

Drug therapy
- Antiparkinsonian agents: benztropine (Cogentin) for adverse effects of antipsychotic drugs
- Antipsychotics (traditional): chlorpromazine, fluphenazine, haloperidol (Haldol), olanzapine (Zyprexa), thioridazine, thiothixene (Navane)
- Antipsychotics (atypical): clozapine (Clozaril), aripiprazole (Abilify), quetiapine (Seroquel), risperidone (Risperdal), ziprasidone (Geodon)

INTERVENTIONS AND RATIONALES
- Inform the client that you will help him control his behavior *to promote feelings of safety.*
- Set limits on aggressive behavior and communicate your expectations to the client *to prevent injury to the client and others.*
- Use behavior management techniques *to promote adaptive behavior.*

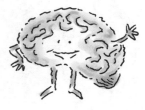

Distraction techniques such as singing along with music can alleviate hallucinations, helping to bring the client back to reality.

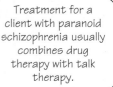

Treatment for a client with paranoid schizophrenia usually combines drug therapy with talk therapy.

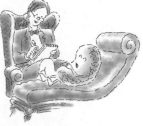

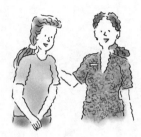

Interventions for schizophrenia promote the client's safety, meet physical needs, and help the client deal with reality.

• Use nonphysical techniques, such as redirecting the client's focus or verbal deescalation *to help the client become calm.*
• Enforce "time-outs" *to prohibit threatening or intimidating behavior.*
• Utilize seclusion and restraints only when nonphysical interventions are ineffective and there's an imminent threat of injury *to protect the client and caregivers from harm.*
• Designate one nurse to communicate with the client and to direct other staff members who care for the client *to foster trust and a stable environment and to minimize opportunities for the client to exhibit hostility.*
• Maintain a low level of stimuli *to minimize the client's anxiety, agitation, and suspiciousness.*
• Provide reality-based diversional activities *to maintain the client's focus and help him stay in touch with reality.*
• Provide a safe environment *to protect the client and others from harm.*
• Reorient the client to time and place as appropriate *to help him cope with his hallucinations and maintain orientation.*
• Be flexible — allow the client to have some control. Approach him in a calm and unhurried manner. Let him talk about anything he wishes, but keep the conversation light and social *to avoid entering into power struggles.*
• Don't take the client's remarks personally. If he tells you to leave him alone, do leave but return soon. *Brief contacts with the client may be most useful at first.*
• Don't make attempts to combat the client's delusions with logic. Instead, respond to feelings, themes, or underlying needs. *Combatting delusions may increase feelings of persecution or hostility.*
• If the client is taking clozapine, stress the importance of returning weekly to the facility or an outpatient setting to have his blood checked *to monitor for adverse effects and prevent toxicity.*
• Teach the client the importance of complying with the medication regimen. Tell him to report adverse reactions instead of discontinuing the drug *to maintain therapeutic drug levels.*

• If the client takes a slow-release formula, make sure that he understands when to return for his next dose *to promote compliance.*

Teaching topics
• Explanation of the disorder and treatment plan
• Medication use and possible adverse effects
• Avoiding exposure to sunlight (to prevent photosensitive reactions to antipsychotics)
• Reporting adverse affects of antipsychotic medications
• Visiting the hospital weekly to monitor blood chemistry

Delusional disorder

Clients with delusional disorder hold firmly to false belief despite contradictory information. They tend to be intelligent and can have a high level of competence but have impaired social and personal relationships. One indication of delusional disorder is an absence of hallucinations.

CONTRIBUTING FACTORS
• Brain abnormalities
• Developmental involvement
• Family history of schizophrenic, avoidant, and paranoid personality disorders
• Lower socioeconomic status
• Neurotransmitter abnormalities
• Social or environmental stress, interacting with the person's inherited biological makeup

ASSESSMENT FINDINGS
• Antagonism
• Brushes with the law
• Delusions that are erotomanic, grandiose, jealous, persecutory, or somatic
• Denial
• Hallucinations that are visual, auditory, or tactile
• Ideas of reference (everything in the environment takes on a personal significance)
• Inability to trust
• Irritable or depressed mood
• Marked anger and violence
• Projection

- Stalking behavior (as in erotomania [the belief that the client is loved by a prominent person])

DIAGNOSTIC TEST RESULTS
- Blood and urine tests eliminate an organic or chemical cause.
- Endocrine function tests rule out hyperadrenalism, pernicious anemia, and thyroid disorders.
- Neurologic evaluations rule out an organic cause.

NURSING DIAGNOSES
- Impaired social interaction
- Ineffective coping
- Risk for other-directed violence

TREATMENT
- Family therapy
- Group therapy
- Milieu therapy
- Psychoeducational programs
- Stress management
- Supportive psychotherapy

Drug therapy
- Antiparkinsonian agent: benztropine (Cogentin) for adverse effects of antipsychotic medications
- Antipsychotics (traditional): chlorpromazine, fluphenazine, haloperidol (Haldol), olanzapine (Zyprexa), thioridazine, thiothixene (Navane)
- Antipsychotics (atypical): clozapine (Clozaril), aripiprazole (Abilify), quetiapine (Seroquel), risperidone (Risperdal), ziprasidone (Geodon)

INTERVENTIONS AND RATIONALES
- Formulate realistic, modest goals with the client. *Including the client when setting goals may help diminish suspicion while increasing the client's self-esteem and sense of control.*
- Establish a therapeutic relationship *to foster trust.*
- Designate one nurse to communicate with the client and to supervise other staff members with regard to the client's care *to build trust and to minimize opportunities for the client to exhibit hostility.*

- Explore events that trigger delusions. Discuss anxiety associated with triggering events. *Exploring triggers will help you understand the dynamics of the client's delusional system.*
- Don't directly attack the client's delusion. *Doing so will increase the client's anxiety.* Instead, be patient in formulating a trusting relationship.
- When the dynamics of the delusions are understood, discourage repetitious talk about delusions and refocus the conversation on the client's underlying feelings. *As the client identifies and explores his feelings, he will decrease reliance on delusional thought.*
- Recognize delusion as the client's perception of the environment. Avoid getting into arguments with the client regarding the content of delusions *to foster trust.*

Teaching topics
- Explanation of the disorder and treatment plan
- Medication use and possible adverse effects
- Learning decision-making, problem-solving, and negotiating skills

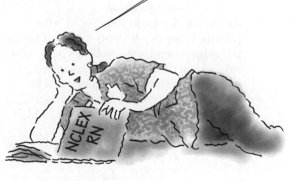

Differentiating delusional disorder from schizophrenia can be tricky. Delusions reflect reality in a somewhat distorted way. Schizophrenia is indicated by scattered and incoherent thoughts unrelated to reality.

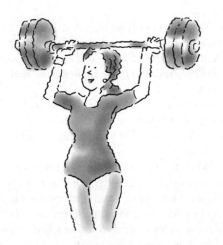

Pump up on practice questions

1. The family of a client with schizoaffective disorder tells the nurse that they haven't been successful in meeting their goal for home management of their son. They report that he's posing a threat to their safety. What primary recommendation should the nurse make based on this information?

　　1. Have the client evaluated for a voluntary admission to a mental health facility.
　　2. Discuss what the family can do to chemically restrain the client at home.
　　3. Tell the family that the client's behavior releases them from the duty of care.
　　4. Arrange for respite care because the family could be aggravating the client's condition.

Answer: 1. A voluntary admission is the preferred approach because it involves having the client recognize the problems being experienced and facilitates the client's involvement in treatment. The client's rights would be violated by the use of chemical restraints because the client has the right to freedom from the use of restraints and seclusion. The duty of care is a legal relationship that applies only to the nurse-client relationship—not to the family relationship. Respite care isn't an appropriate recommendation at this time because the safety issue must be addressed and effective treatment and care instituted. It would be prudent to talk to the family about caregiver burden and the option of using respite care after the safety issue is resolved.

➡ *NCLEX keys*

Client needs category: Safe and effective care environment
Client needs subcategory: Management of care
Cognitive level: Application

2. A nurse is caring for a client who was found huddled in her apartment by the police. The client stares toward one corner of the room and seems to be responding to something not visible to others. She appears hyperalert and scared. How should the nurse assess the situation?

　　1. The client may be hallucinating.
　　2. The client is suicidal.
　　3. Nothing is wrong because the client isn't a threat to society.
　　4. The client is malingering.

Answer: 1. The scenario is typical of a client who's hallucinating. Not enough information is available to suggest that she's a threat to society or to herself. Malingering refers to a medically unproven symptom that's consciously motivated.

➡ *NCLEX keys*

Client needs category: Psychosocial integrity
Client needs subcategory: None
Cognitive level: Analysis

3. A nurse is caring for a client whom she suspects is paranoid. How should the nurse confirm this assessment?
1. Indirect questioning
2. Direct questioning
3. Lead-in sentences
4. Open-ended sentences

Answer: 2. Direct questions (such as "Do you hear voices?" or "Do you feel safe right now?") are the most appropriate technique for eliciting verifiable responses from a psychotic client. The other options may not elicit helpful responses.

➡ *NCLEX keys*
Client needs category: Psychosocial integrity
Client needs subcategory: None
Cognitive level: Application

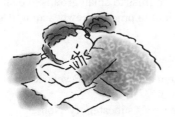

4. A nurse is caring for a client who's experiencing auditory hallucinations. What should be most crucial for the nurse to assess?
1. Possible hearing impairment
2. Family history of psychosis
3. Content of the hallucinations
4. Possible sella turcica tumors

Answer: 3. To prevent the client from harming himself or others, the nurse should encourage him to reveal the content of auditory hallucinations. Assessing for hearing impairment would be inappropriate. Family history, although important because of a possible genetic component, isn't an immediate concern. Olfactory hallucinations, not auditory hallucinations, are associated with sella turcica tumors.

➡ *NCLEX keys*
Client needs category: Safe and effective care environment
Client needs subcategory: Management of care
Cognitive level: Application

5. A client with schizophrenia is being prepared for discharge. He tells the nurse that he has no home or family and has been living on the street. Which response by the nurse is most appropriate?
1. Offer the name and phone numbers of various homeless shelters in the community.
2. Ask him to further explain how he feels living in such desperate conditions.
3. Contact the physician for a referral to social services for further evaluation.
4. Document the client's response and inform the charge nurse of the situation.

Answer: 3. A person who's homeless may have complex underlying needs and issues that need to be further explored by a trained social service worker to provide the most appropriate interventions. Offering the name and number of shelters may be helpful, but the nurse isn't in a position to follow up on the client's care after discharge. Having the client discuss his feelings may be therapeutic, but at this point, there's a need for direct intervention to ensure the client's safety and well-being. Documenting and informing the charge nurse is useful, but doesn't ensure that there will be appropriate intervention.

➡ *NCLEX keys*
Client needs category: Safe and effective care environment
Client needs subcategory: Management of care
Cognitive level: Analysis

6. A nurse is preparing to care for a client diagnosed with catatonic schizophrenia. In anticipation of this client's arrival, what should the nurse do?
1. Notify security.
2. Prepare a magnesium sulfate drip.
3. Place a specialty mattress overlay on the bed.
4. Communicate the client's nothing-by-mouth status to the dietary department.

Answer: 3. The nurse should first focus on meeting the client's immediate physical needs and preventing complications related to the catatonic state. The need for intervention from security personnel is unlikely. A magnesium sulfate drip isn't indicated. Nutritional status should be addressed after the client is fully assessed and admitted.

➡ *NCLEX keys*
Client needs category: Physiological integrity
Client needs subcategory: Basic care and comfort
Cognitive level: Application

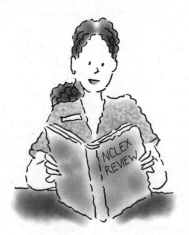

7. A nurse is caring for a client with disorganized schizophrenia. The client is responding well to therapy but has had limited social contact with others. Which of the following interventions is most appropriate?
1. Discourage the client from interacting with others because, if his efforts fail, it will be too traumatic for him.
2. Encourage the client to attend a party thrown for the residents of the facility.
3. Encourage the client to participate in one-on-one interactions.
4. Encourage the client to place a personal advertisement in the local newspaper but not to reveal his mental disability.

Answer: 3. First, encourage the client to participate in one-on-one interactions, and then progress to small groups to enable the client to practice newly acquired social skills.

➡ *NCLEX keys*
Client needs category: Psychosocial integrity
Client needs subcategory: None
Cognitive level: Application

8. A nurse is caring for a schizophrenic client who's well managed on medications. He reveals that he's doing so well, he doesn't think he needs to take medication anymore. What response indicates the nurse best understands the client's diagnosis?
1. "The medications are helping you and if you stop suddenly you could get sick again."
2. "I'll pass this information on to your doctor to see if he feels this might be wise."

3. "You should take the medication for several months after you go home."
4. "You have to take your pills because the doctor has ordered them for you."

Answer: 1. Many schizophrenic clients feel that they can stop taking their medication when their symptoms decrease. The nurse needs to plan client education to reinforce to the client that the medication is what is keeping the symptoms under control. The client will have to take the medication for life, not for a few months after discharge. Telling the client that he has to take the medications doesn't address the client's diagnosis.

➡ *NCLEX keys*
Client needs category: Safe and effective care environment
Client needs subcategory: Management of care
Cognitive level: Analysis

9. A client with schizophrenia is taking the atypical antipsychotic medication clozapine (Clozaril). Which signs and symptoms indicate the presence of adverse effects associated with this medication? Select all that apply.
1. Sore throat
2. Pill-rolling movements
3. Polyuria
4. Fever
5. Flulike symptoms
6. Orthostatic hypotension

Answer: 1, 4, 5. Sore throat, fever, and a sudden onset of other flulike symptoms are signs of agranulocytosis. The condition is caused by a lack of sufficient granulocytes (a type of white blood cell [WBC]), which causes the individual to be susceptible to infection. The client's WBC count should be monitored at least weekly throughout the course of treatment. Pill-rolling movements can occur in those experiencing extrapyramidal adverse effects associated with antipsychotic medication that has been prescribed for much longer than a medication such as clozapine. Polyuria (increased urine) is a common adverse effect of lithium. Orthostatic hypotension is an adverse effect of tricyclic antidepressants.

➡ *NCLEX keys*
Client needs category: Physiological integrity
Client needs subcategory: Pharmacological and parenteral therapies
Cognitive level: Application

10. A nurse is caring for a client who has schizophrenia. What's the first-line treatment for this client?
1. Group therapy
2 Thyroid replacement therapy in selected individuals
3. Milieu therapy
4. Antipsychotics

Answer: 4. Antipsychotics are used as the first-line treatment for schizophrenia. Although thyroid disorders can be a cause of psychotic-like symptoms, they aren't a cause of schizophrenia. Milieu therapy may be helpful but isn't a first-line treatment. Group therapy also wouldn't be a first-line treatment.

➡ *NCLEX keys*
Client needs category: Physiological integrity
Client needs subcategory: Pharmacological and parenteral therapies
Cognitive level: Application

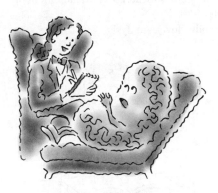

If you can't get enough of psych disorders, you're in luck. There are more coming up in the next chapter.

18 Substance-related disorders

Brush up on key concepts

The relationship between mental illness and substance use and abuse is complex. Alcohol and psychoactive drugs alter a person's perceptions, feelings, and behavior. People may use substances for just that reason. Many people who suffer from emotional disorders or mental illness turn to drugs and alcohol to self-medicate as a way of tolerating feelings. Yet, this method of self-treating doesn't work and commonly makes matters worse.

Nursing care for a substance abuser begins with a thorough assessment to determine which substance is being abused. During the acute phase, care focuses on maintaining the client's vital functions and safety. Rehabilitation involves helping the client to recognize his substance abuse problem and find alternative methods of dealing with stress. The nurse helps the client to achieve recovery and stay drug-free.

At any time, you can review the major points of each disorder by consulting the *Cheat sheet* on page 450.

Social use?
Substance intoxication is the development of a reversible substance-specific syndrome due to ingestion of or exposure to a substance. The clinically significant maladaptive behavior or psychological changes vary from substance to substance.

It's a problem
The essential feature of **substance abuse** is a maladaptive pattern of substance use coupled with recurrent and significant adverse consequences.

The monkey ON the back
Substance dependence is characterized by physical, behavioral, and cognitive changes resulting from persistent substance use. Persistent drug use can result in tolerance and withdrawal.

Just can't get enough
Tolerance is defined as an increased need for a substance or a need for an increased amount of the substance to achieve an effect.

The monkey OFF the back
Withdrawal occurs when the tissue and blood levels of the substance decrease in a person who has engaged in prolonged, heavy use of the substance.

When uncomfortable withdrawal symptoms persist, the person usually takes the drug to relieve the symptoms. Withdrawal symptoms vary from substance to substance.

Classes of controlled substances

Each class of a controlled substance has a different effect on the body and thus produces different reactions. Common classes of controlled substances include:
- cannabis
- depressants
- designer drugs
- hallucinogens
- inhalants
- opiates
- phencyclidine (PCP)
- stimulants.

CANNABIS
Tetrahydrocannabinol, the active ingredient in hashish and marijuana, produces a type

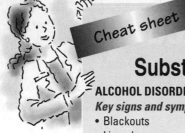

Cheat sheet

Substance-related disorders refresher

ALCOHOL DISORDER

Key signs and symptoms
- Blackouts
- Liver damage
- Pathologic intoxication

Key test results
- CAGE questionnaire indicates alcoholism.
- Michigan Alcoholism Screening test indicates alcoholism.

Key treatments
- Alcoholics Anonymous
- Individual and group therapy
- Medical detoxification and rehabilitation
- Benzodiazepines: chlordiazepoxide (Librium), diazepam (Valium), lorazepam (Ativan)
- Disulfiram (Antabuse) to prevent relapse into alcohol abuse (the client must be alcohol-free for 12 hours before administering this drug)
- Naltrexone (Revia) to prevent relapse into alcohol abuse
- Selective serotonin reuptake inhibitors (SSRIs): fluoxetine (Prozac), paroxetine (Paxil)

Key interventions
- Assess the client's use of denial as a coping mechanism.
- Set limits on denial and rationalization.
- Monitor for signs and symptoms of withdrawal, such as elevated blood pressure, tachycardia, nausea, vomiting, anxiety, agitation, and seizures.
- Have the client formulate goals for maintaining a drug-free lifestyle.

COCAINE-USE DISORDER

Key signs and symptoms
- Elevated energy and mood
- Grandiose thinking
- Impaired judgment

Key test results
- Drug screening is positive for cocaine.

Key treatments
- Detoxification
- Rehabilitation (inpatient or outpatient)

- Narcotics Anonymous
- Individual therapy
- Anxiolytics: lorazepam (Ativan), alprazolam (Xanax)
- Dopamine agent: bromocriptine (Parlodel)
- SSRIs: fluoxetine (Prozac), paroxetine (Paxil)

Key interventions
- Establish a trusting relationship with the client.
- Provide the client with well-balanced meals.
- Set limits on the client's attempts to rationalize behavior.

OTHER SUBSTANCE ABUSE DISORDERS

Key signs and symptoms
- Blaming others for problems
- Development of biological or psychological need for a substance
- Dysfunctional anger
- Feelings of grandiosity
- Impulsiveness
- Use of denial and rationalization to explain consequences of behavior

Key test results
- Drug screening is positive for the abused substance.

Key treatments
- Individual therapy
- Clonidine (Catapres) for opiate withdrawal symptoms
- Methadone maintenance for opiate addiction detoxification
- Levo-alpha-acetylmethadol to treat heroin addiction

Key interventions
- Ensure a safe, quiet environment free from stimuli.
- Monitor for withdrawal symptoms, such as tremors, seizures, anxiety, elevated blood pressure, nausea, and vomiting.
- Help the client understand the consequences of substance abuse.
- Encourage the client to vent fear and anger.

Remember, you can always refer to the *Cheat sheet* for a quick review of a chapter.

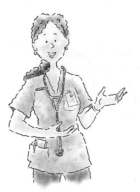

of euphoria, increased appetite, sensory alterations, tachycardia, lack of coordination, and impaired judgment and memory.

DEPRESSANTS

These substances slow down central nervous system (CNS) functioning, causing slurred speech, impaired judgment, and mood swings and can cause respiratory distress when taken in overdose. Common depressants include:
- alcohol
- barbiturates
- benzodiazepines.

DESIGNER DRUGS

These substances are similar to other classes of drugs but they're manufactured with chemical changes that, in some cases, make them more dangerous. The most common designer drugs are:
- adam (ecstasy)
- china white (synthetic type of heroin).

HALLUCINOGENS

These substances produce euphoria, sympathetic and parasympathetic stimulation, and hallucinations, dissociative states, and bizarre, maniclike behavior. They include:
- lysergic acid diethylamide (LSD)
- mushrooms (psilocybin)
- mescaline (from peyote cactus).

INHALANTS

Use of inhalants is called *huffing*. These substances aren't drugs, but some people have found that they can "catch a buzz" from inhaling the fumes. The following products are commonly used:
- glue
- cleaning solutions
- nail polish remover
- aerosols
- petroleum products
- paint thinners.

OPIATES AND RELATED ANALGESICS

These substances, which dull the senses, resulting in sedation and a dreamlike state, can cause respiratory depression and cardiac arrest:
- heroin
- morphine
- codeine

- opium
- methadone
- meperidine (Demerol).

PHENCYCLIDINE

PCP, also known as *angel dust*, heightens CNS function, distorts perception, and causes agitation and aggressive behavior and physiological symptoms, such as hypertension and tachycardia.

STIMULANTS

These substances stimulate the CNS:
- methamphetamines
- cocaine (including crack cocaine)
- caffeine
- nicotine.

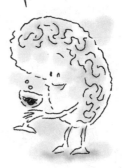

Note that alcohol is a depressant.

Polish up on client care

Almost any controlled substance can potentially become addictive. Although specific circumstances may vary, causes and treatments remain similar for each substance. Common disorders include alcohol disorder, cocaine-use disorder, and other substance abuse disorders.

Alcohol disorder

Although alcohol abuse and dependence are considered substance-related abuse disorders, assessment findings and treatment differ somewhat from that for other substances. Alcohol is a sedative but it creates a feeling of euphoria. Sedation increases with the amount ingested. Respiratory depression and coma can occur with excessive intake.

CAUSES
- Interaction of hereditary, biological, psychological, and environmental factors

CONTRIBUTING FACTORS
- Familial tendency
- Gender (males have increased likelihood of addiction)

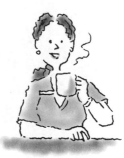

Caffeine and nicotine are classified as stimulants because of the effect they have on the body.

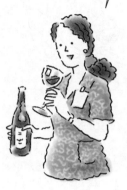

Because alcohol use is widely accepted, therapeutic communication may involve dealing with a client's rationalizations.

- History of abuse, depression, or anxiety
- Influence of nationality and ethnicity
- Personality disorders

ASSESSMENT FINDINGS
- Adrenocortical insufficiency
- Alcoholic cardiomyopathy
- Alcoholic cirrhosis
- Alcoholic hepatitis
- Alcoholic paranoia
- Blackouts
- Erection problems
- Esophageal varices
- Gastritis or gastric ulcers
- Hallucinations
- Korsakoff's syndrome
- Liver damage
- Muscular myopathy
- Pancreatitis
- Pathologic intoxication
- Peripheral neuropathy
- Wernicke's encephalopathy

DIAGNOSTIC TEST RESULTS
- Drug screening is positive for alcohol.
- CAGE questionnaire indicates alcoholism. (See *The CAGE questionnaire*.)
- Michigan Alcoholism Screening test indicates alcoholism.

NURSING DIAGNOSES
- Ineffective denial
- Ineffective coping
- Risk for injury
- Dysfunctional family processes
- Risk for impaired liver function

TREATMENT
- Alcoholics Anonymous
- Individual and group therapy
- Medical detoxification and rehabilitation

Drug therapy
- Antidepressant: bupropion (Wellbutrin)
- Benzodiazepines: chlordiazepoxide (Librium), diazepam (Valium), lorazepam (Ativan) to treat withdrawal symptoms
- Disulfiram (Antabuse) to prevent relapse into alcohol abuse (the client must be alcohol-free for 12 hours before administering this drug)

- Naltrexone (Revia) to prevent relapse into alcohol abuse
- Selective serotonin reuptake inhibitors (SSRIs): fluoxetine (Prozac), paroxetine (Paxil)

INTERVENTIONS AND RATIONALES
- Monitor for signs and symptoms of withdrawal, such as elevated blood pressure, tachycardia, nausea, vomiting, anxiety, agitation, and seizures. The client may also experience hallucinations, tremors, and delirium tremens. *Monitoring these effects helps identify complications and promotes rapid treatment.*
- Assess the client's use of denial as a coping mechanism *to begin a therapeutic relationship.*
- Encourage the verbalization of anger, fear, inadequacy, grief, and guilt *to promote healthy coping behaviors.*
- Set limits on denial and rationalization *to help the client gain control and perspective.*
- Have the client formulate goals for maintaining of a drug-free lifestyle *to help avoid relapses.*

Teaching topics
- Explanation of the disorder and treatment plan
- Medication use and possible adverse effects
- Understanding substance abuse and relapse prevention
- Maintaining good nutrition
- Available rehabilitation and support groups

Cocaine-use disorder

Cocaine-use disorder results from the potent euphoric effects of the drug. Individuals exposed to cocaine develop dependence after a very short period. Maladaptive behavior follows, resulting in social dysfunction. Cocaine use can also cause serious physical complications, such as cardiac arrhythmias, myocardial infarction, seizures, and stroke.

CONTRIBUTING FACTORS
- Genetic predisposition
- History of abuse, depression, or anxiety
- Personality disorder

ASSESSMENT FINDINGS
- Assault or violent behavior
- Elevated energy and mood
- Grandiose thinking
- Impaired judgment
- Impaired social functioning
- Paranoia
- Weight loss

DIAGNOSTIC TEST RESULTS
- Drug screening is positive for cocaine.

NURSING DIAGNOSES
- Ineffective health maintenance
- Imbalanced nutrition: Less than body requirements
- Risk for other-directed violence

TREATMENT
- Detoxification
- Rehabilitation (inpatient or outpatient)
- Narcotics Anonymous
- Individual therapy

Drug therapy
- Anxiolytics: lorazepam (Ativan), alprazolam (Xanax)
- Dopamine agent: bromocriptine (Parlodel)
- SSRIs: fluoxetine (Prozac), paroxetine (Paxil)
- Propranolol (Inderal)
- Modanafil (Provigil)

INTERVENTIONS AND RATIONALES
- Establish a trusting relationship with the client *to alleviate anxiety or paranoia.*
- Provide the client with well-balanced meals *to compensate for nutritional deficits.*
- Provide a safe environment during withdrawal. *The client may pose a risk to himself or others.*
- Set limits on the client's attempts to rationalize behavior *to reduce inappropriate behavior.*

Teaching topics
- Explanation of the disorder and treatment plan
- Medication use and possible adverse effects
- Contacting Narcotics Anonymous
- Coping strategies
- Managing stress

Other substance abuse disorders

Other substance abuse disorders include all patterns of abuse excluding alcohol and cocaine. These disorders have a great deal in common; however, symptoms vary depending upon the abused substance.

CONTRIBUTING FACTORS
- Familial tendency
- Gender (females have increased likelihood of abusing prescription drugs; males have generally increased likelihood of addiction)
- History of abuse, depression, or anxiety
- Influence of nationality and ethnicity
- Personality disorders

ASSESSMENT FINDINGS
- Attempts to avoid anxiety and other emotions
- Attempts to avoid conscious feelings of guilt and anger
- Attempts to meet needs by influencing others
- Blaming others for problems
- Development of biological or psychological need for a substance
- Dysfunctional anger
- Feelings of grandiosity
- Impulsiveness
- Manipulation and deceit
- Need for immediate gratification
- Pattern of negative interactions
- Possible malnutrition
- Symptoms of withdrawal
- Use of denial and rationalization to explain consequences of behavior

DIAGNOSTIC TEST RESULTS
- Drug screening is positive for the abused substance.

NURSING DIAGNOSES
- Ineffective health maintenance
- Imbalanced nutrition: Less than body requirements
- Risk for other-directed violence

The CAGE questionnaire

This questionnaire is a brief, unscored examination meant to provide a standard for assessing alcohol addiction. Any two positive responses to these four yes-or-no questions strongly suggest alcohol dependence.

1. Have you ever felt you should **C**ut down on your drinking?

2. Have people **A**nnoyed you by criticizing your drinking?

3. Have you ever felt bad or **G**uilty about your drinking?

4. Have you ever had an **E**ye-opener first thing in the morning because of a hangover, or just to get the day started?

> During a psychiatric evaluation, always rule out drug or alcohol use; these substances produce symptoms that mimic those of mental illness.

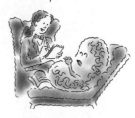

TREATMENT
- Behavior modification
- Employee assistance programs
- Family counseling
- Group therapy
- Halfway houses
- Individual therapy
- Informal social support
- Self-help groups

Drug therapy
- Clonidine (Catapres) for opiate withdrawal symptoms
- Methadone maintenance for opiate addiction detoxification
- Levo-alpha-acetylmethadol to treat heroin addiction
- Buprenorphine (Suleoxone) for opiate withdrawal

INTERVENTIONS AND RATIONALES
- Ensure a safe, quiet environment free from stimuli *to provide a therapeutic setting and to alleviate withdrawal symptoms.*
- Monitor for withdrawal symptoms, such as tremors, seizures, anxiety, elevated blood pressure, nausea, and vomiting *to provide the most comfortable environment possible.*
- Assess the client for polysubstance abuse *to plan appropriate interventions.*
- Help the client understand the consequences of substance abuse *to assist recovery.*
- Provide measures to induce sleep *to help the client manage the discomfort of withdrawal.*
- Encourage the client to vent fear and anger *so that he can begin the healing process.*
- Help the client identify appropriate lifestyle changes *to promote health and prevent complications.*

Teaching topics
- Explanation of the disorder and treatment plan
- Medication use and possible adverse reactions
- Contacting addiction support agencies
- Learning healthy coping mechanisms

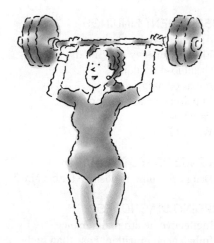

Pump up on practice questions

1. A depressed client states that her daughter uses amphetamines, then asks the nurse, "What will happen when my daughter can't get them and goes into withdrawal from them?" Which response by the nurse would be helpful information for the client?
1. "Your daughter will become very tired and may experience depression."
2. "It's hard to say because she may not have any problems except mild nausea."
3. "Sometimes it can cause people to become agitated and act aggressively toward others."
4. "There's a high risk of seizures and other neurological problems."

Answer: 1. A person withdrawing from amphetamines will become very lethargic and can experience depression or even suicidal tendencies. Telling the client that her daughter may only experience nausea, agitation, or neurological problems wouldn't be providing the client with accurate information about amphetamine withdrawal.

➡ *NCLEX keys*
Client needs category: Physiological integrity
Client needs subcategory: Reduction of risk potential
Cognitive level: Application

2. A nurse is caring for a client who has a history of alcohol abuse. Why would the client act as if he didn't have a problem?

1. The client has never taken the CAGE questionnaire.
2. Denial is a defense mechanism commonly used by alcoholics.
3. Thought processes are distorted.
4. Alcohol is inexpensive.

Answer: 2. Denial is a defense mechanism commonly used by alcoholics. The CAGE questionnaire is a direct method of discovering whether the client is a substance abuser, but the client is likely to deny the problem regardless of whether he's familiar with this assessment tool. Distorted thought processes and the cost of alcohol are less likely to influence the client's use of denial.

➡ *NCLEX keys*
Client needs category: Psychosocial integrity
Client needs subcategory: None
Cognitive level: Analysis

3. A nurse is caring for a client who exhibits pinpoint pupils as well as decreased blood pressure, pulse, respirations, and temperature. These symptoms may be a sign of intoxication with which substance?

1. Opiate
2. Amphetamine
3. Cannabis
4. Alcohol

Answer: 1. Opiates, such as morphine or heroin, cause these changes. Amphetamines dilate pupils. Cannabis intoxication causes tachycardia, dry mouth, and increased appetite. Alcohol intoxication causes unsteady gait, incoordination, nystagmus, and flushed face.

➡ *NCLEX keys*
Client needs category: Physiological integrity
Client needs subcategory: Physiological adaptation
Cognitive level: Application

4. A nurse is caring for a client in a substance abuse clinic. The client tells the nurse he needs more heroin to produce the same effect that he experienced a few weeks ago. How should the nurse describe this condition?

1. Tolerance
2. Dependence
3. Withdrawal delirium
4. Compulsion

Answer: 1. Tolerance occurs when more drug is required to produce the same effect. Dependence is a physiologic dependence on a substance. Withdrawal delirium occurs when cessation of a substance produces physiologic symptoms. Compulsion refers to an unwanted repetitive act.

➡ *NCLEX keys*
Client needs category: Physiological integrity
Client needs subcategory: Physiological adaptation
Cognitive level: Application

5. A nurse is interviewing a client who's currently under the influence of a controlled substance and shows signs of becoming agitated. What should the nurse do?

1. Use confrontation.
2. Express disgust with the client's behavior.
3. Be aware of hospital security.
4. Communicate a scolding attitude to intimidate the client.

Answer: 3. The nurse, for her own protection, should be aware of hospital security and other assisting personnel. The other options may cause a relatively docile client to become belligerent.

➡ *NCLEX keys*
Client needs category: Safe and effective care environment
Client needs subcategory: Management of care
Cognitive level: Application

6. A nurse is assessing a client who's manifesting the long-term effects of using illicit inhalant drugs. Which laboratory finding should alert the nurse to the need for further assessment and diagnostic testing?

1. Blood dyscrasia
2. Renal dysfunction
3. Thyroid abnormality
4. Muscle atrophy

Answer: 2. A client with a history of using illicit inhalant drugs will have laboratory values that indicate renal problems, and these problems should be addressed immediately by additional assessment and diagnostic testing. Blood dyscrasia, thyroid abnormality, and muscle atrophy aren't typical physiological problems that occur in clients who use illicit inhalant drugs.

➡ *NCLEX keys*
Client needs category: Physiological integrity
Client needs subcategory: Reduction of risk potential
Cognitive level: Application

7. A nurse is caring for a client with a history of substance abuse. Depending on the substance abused, what might treatment include?
　1. Antabuse or methadone
　2. Morphine
　3. Demerol
　4. Lithium
Answer: 1. Antabuse assists in recovery from alcoholism; methadone maintenance is used for opiate abusers. Morphine and Demerol are controlled substances and aren't used in substance abuse treatment. Lithium is used to treat bipolar disorder.

➡ *NCLEX keys*
Client needs category: Physiological integrity
Client needs subcategory: Pharmacological and parenteral therapies
Cognitive level: Application

8. A nurse is using the CAGE questionnaire as a screening tool for alcohol problems. What do these initials represent?
　1. Cut down, Annoyed, Guilty, Eye-opener
　2. Consumed, Angry, Gastritis, Esophageal varices
　3. Cancer, Alcoholic liver, Gastric ulcer, Erosive gastritis
　4. Cunning, Anger, Guilt, Excess
Answer: 1. CAGE stands for "Have you felt the need to **C**ut down on your drinking? Have you ever been **A**nnoyed by criticism of your drinking? Have you felt **G**uilty about your drinking? Have you felt the need for an **E**ye-opener in the morning?"

➡ *NCLEX keys*
Client needs category: Psychosocial integrity
Client needs subcategory: None
Cognitive level: Analysis

9. A nurse is administering disulfiram (Antabuse) to a client with a history of alcohol abuse. Before receiving therapy, which of the following is required of the client?
　1. Be committed to attending AA meetings weekly
　2. Admit to himself and another person that he's an alcoholic
　3. Remain alcohol-free for 6 hours
　4. Remain alcohol-free for 12 hours
Answer: 4. The client must be alcohol-free for 12 hours before initiating disulfiram therapy. Attending AA and acknowledging alcoholism aren't necessary before therapy.

➡ *NCLEX keys*
Client needs category: Physiological integrity
Client needs subcategory: Pharmacological and parenteral therapies
Cognitive level: Application

10. A client with a history of alcoholism returns to the hospital 3 hours later than the time specified on his day pass. His breath smells of alcohol and his gait is unsteady. What should the nurse say?
　1. "Why are you 3 hours late?"
　2. "How much did you drink tonight? Drinking is against the rules."
　3. "I'm disappointed that you weren't responsible with your day pass."
　4. "Please go to bed now. We'll talk in the morning."
Answer: 4. The client can best discuss his behavior when he's no longer under the influence of alcohol. Asking why he's late encourages the client to invent excuses. Being judgmental by admonishing the client or expressing disappointment discourages open communication.

➡ *NCLEX keys*
Client needs category: Psychosocial integrity
Client needs subcategory: None
Cognitive level: Analysis

You finished another chapter. Reward yourself—but remember, moderation in all things.

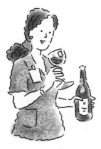

19 Dissociative disorders

Brush up on key concepts

A client with a **dissociative disorder** experiences a disruption in the usual relationship among memory, identity, consciousness, and perceptions. This disturbance may occur suddenly or appear gradually. It's more common in women. Typically, dissociation is a mechanism used to protect the self and gain relief from overwhelming anxiety.

At any time, you can review the major points of each disorder by consulting the *Cheat sheet* on pages 458 and 459.

Polish up on client care

Common dissociative disorders include depersonalization disorder, dissociative amnesia, dissociative fugue, and dissociative identity disorder.

Depersonalization disorder

In depersonalization disorder, the client may feel like a detached observer, passively watching his mental or physical activity as if in a dream. Reality testing remains intact. The onset of depersonalization is sudden and the progression of the disorder may be chronic, characterized by remissions and exacerbations.

CONTRIBUTING FACTORS
- History of physical and emotional abuse
- History of substance abuse
- Neurophysiologic predisposition
- Obsessive-compulsive disorder
- Sensory deprivation
- Severe stress, such as military combat, violent crime, or other traumatic events

ASSESSMENT FINDINGS
- Anxiety symptoms
- Depressive symptoms
- Disturbance in sense of time
- Fear of going insane
- Impaired occupational functioning
- Impaired social functioning
- Low self-esteem
- Persistent or recurring feelings of detachment from mind and body

DIAGNOSTIC TEST RESULTS
- Standard dissociative disorder tests demonstrate a high degree of dissociation. These tests include:
  - diagnostic drawing series
  - dissociative experience scale
  - dissociative interview schedule
  - structured clinical interview for dissociative disorders.

NURSING DIAGNOSES
- Anxiety
- Posttrauma syndrome
- Ineffective role performance
- Ineffective coping

Establishing a support system is a key intervention for depersonalization disorder.

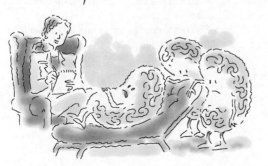

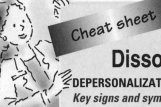

Cheat sheet

Dissociative disorders refresher

DEPERSONALIZATION DISORDER

Key signs and symptoms
- Fear of going insane
- Impaired occupational functioning
- Impaired social functioning
- Persistent or recurring feelings of detachment from mind and body

Key test results
- Standard dissociative disorder tests demonstrate a degree of dissociation. These tests include:
  - dissociative experience scale
  - dissociative interview schedule.

Key treatments
- Individual psychotherapy
- Benzodiazepines: alprazolam (Xanax), lorazepam (Ativan), clonazepam (Klonopin)
- Nonbenzodiazipine: buspirone (Buspar)
- Selective serotonin reuptake inhibitors (SSRIs): fluoxetine (Prozac), citalopram (Celexa), sertraline (Zoloft), paroxetine (Paxil)

Key interventions
- Encourage the client to recognize that depersonalization is a defense mechanism used to deal with anxiety and trauma.
- Assist the client in establishing supportive relationships.

DISSOCIATIVE AMNESIA AND DISSOCIATIVE FUGUE

Key signs and symptoms
Dissociative amnesia
- Altered memory
- Low self-esteem
- No conscious recollection of a traumatic event, yet colors, sounds, sites, or odors of the event may trigger distress or depression
- Sudden onset of amnesia and inability to recall personal information
Dissociative fugue
- Sudden, unplanned travel away from home or place of work
- Confusion about personal identity or taking on a new identity

Key test results
- Standard dissociative disorder tests demonstrate a degree of dissociation. These tests include:
  - diagnostic drawing series
  - dissociative experience scale
  - dissociative interview schedule
  - structured clinical interview for dissociative disorders.

Key treatments
- Individual therapy
- Benzodiazepines: alprazolam (Xanax), lorazepam (Ativan)
- Nonbenzodiazepine: buspirone (BuSpar)
- SSRIs: paroxetine (Paxil), citalopram (Celexa)

Key interventions
- Encourage the client to verbalize feelings of distress.
- Encourage the client to recognize that memory loss is a defense mechanism used to deal with anxiety and trauma.

DISSOCIATIVE IDENTITY DISORDER

Key signs and symptoms
- Guilt and shame
- Lack of recall (beyond ordinary forgetfulness)
- Presence of two or more distinct identities or personality states
- Disturbances not due to direct physiologic effects of a substance

Key test results
- Standard dissociative disorder tests demonstrate a degree of dissociation. These tests include:
  - diagnostic drawing series
  - dissociative experience scale
  - dissociative interview schedule
  - structured clinical interview for dissociative disorders.
- EEG readings may vary markedly among the different identities.

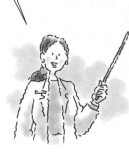

Don't forget to review the highlights of each disorder in the Cheat sheet.

Dissociative disorders refresher *(continued)*

DISSOCIATIVE IDENTITY DISORDER *(CONTINUED)*
Key treatments
• Long-term reconstructive psychotherapy
• Benzodiazepines: alprazolam (Xanax), lorazepam (Ativan), clonazepam (Klonopin)
• Nonbenzodiazepine: buspirone (BuSpar)
• SSRIs: paroxetine (Paxil), escitalopram (Lexapro)
• Tricyclic antidepressants: imipramine (Tofranil), desipramine (Norpramin)

Key interventions
• Assist the client in identifying each personality.
• Encourage the client to identify emotions that occur under duress.
• Monitor risk of self-harm.

TREATMENT
• Individual psychotherapy

Drug therapy
• Benzodiazepines: alprazolam (Xanax), lorazepam (Ativan), clonazepam (Klonopin)
• Nonbenzodiazepine: buspirone (BuSpar)
• Selective serotonin reuptake inhibitors (SSRIs): fluoxetine (Prozac), citalopram (Celexa), sertraline (Zoloft), paroxetine (Paxil)

INTERVENTIONS AND RATIONALES
• Establish a trusting relationship by conveying acceptance and respect *to provide a safe environment for the client to express distressing feelings*.
• Encourage the client to recognize that depersonalization is a defense mechanism used to deal with anxiety and trauma *because the client needs to first recognize how depersonalization works*.
• Assist the client in establishing supportive relationships *because social interaction reduces the tendency toward depersonalization*.

Teaching topics
• Explanation of the disorder and treatment plan
• Medication use and possible adverse effects
• Effective stress management

Dissociative amnesia and dissociative fugue

In dissociative amnesia, acute memory loss is triggered by severe psychological stress. The client may repress disturbing memories or dissociate from anxiety-laden experiences.

The client may not recall important life events in an attempt to avoid traumatic memories. Recovery from dissociative amnesia is common and recurrences are rare.

With dissociative fugue, the client may travel from home or work and become suddenly confused about personal identity. The client may take on a new identity and can't recall the past.

CONTRIBUTING FACTORS
• Emotional abuse
• Low self-esteem
• Past traumatic event
• Physical abuse
• Sexual abuse

ASSESSMENT FINDINGS
Dissociative amnesia
• Altered memory
• Clinically significant distress or impairment in social or occupational functioning
• Depression
• Emotional numbness
• Low self-esteem
• No conscious recollection of a traumatic event, yet colors, sounds, sites, or odors of the event may trigger distress or depression
• Self-mutilation, suicidal or aggressive urges
• Sudden onset of amnesia and inability to recall personal information

Dissociative fugue
• Sudden unplanned travel away from home or place of work
• Confusion about personal identity or taking on a new identity

NURSING DIAGNOSES
• Anxiety
• Impaired memory

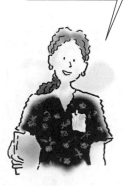

Remember, when working with clients who have dissociative disorders, keep the focus on the client, not on the symptoms.

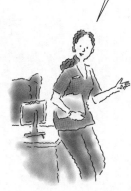

Help psychiatric clients recognize strengths as well as weaknesses to bolster confidence as they begin to cope with trauma.

- Social isolation
- Ineffective coping

DIAGNOSTIC TEST RESULTS
- Standard dissociative disorder tests demonstrate a degree of dissociation. These tests include:
  – diagnostic drawing series
  – dissociative experience scale
  – dissociative interview schedule
  – structured clinical interview for dissociative disorders.

TREATMENT
- Hypnosis
- Individual therapy

Drug therapy
- Benzodiazepines: alprazolam (Xanax), lorazepam (Ativan)
- Nonbenzodiazepine: buspirone (BuSpar)
- SSRIs: paroxetine (Paxil), citalopram (Celexa)
- Tricyclic antidepressants (TCAs): imipramine (Tofranil), desipramine (Norpramin)

INTERVENTIONS AND RATIONALES
- Encourage the client to verbalize feelings of distress *to help him deal with anxiety before it escalates.*
- Encourage the client to recognize that memory loss is a defense mechanism used to deal with anxiety and trauma *to help him understand his condition.*

Teaching topics
- Explanation of the disorder and treatment plan
- Medication use and possible adverse effects
- Promoting positive coping skills
- Utilizing relaxation techniques

Dissociative identity disorder

In dissociative identity disorder, formerly known as *multiple personality disorder,* the client has at least two unique identities. Each identity can have unique behavior patterns and unique memories, though usually one

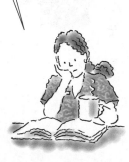

Until recently, dissociative identity disorder was known as *multiple personality disorder.*

primary identity is associated with the client's name. The client may also have traumatic memories that intrude into his awareness. This disorder tends to be chronic and recurrent.

CONTRIBUTING FACTORS
- Emotional, physical, or sexual abuse
- Genetic predisposition
- Lack of nurturing experiences to assist in recovery from abuse
- Low self-esteem
- Traumatic experience before age 15

ASSESSMENT FINDINGS
- Eating disorders
- Guilt and shame
- Hallucinations (auditory and visual)
- Lack of recall (beyond ordinary forgetfulness)
- Low self-esteem
- Posttraumatic symptoms (flashbacks, startle responses, nightmares)
- Presence of two or more distinct identities or personality states
- Recurrent depression
- Sexual dysfunction and difficulty forming intimate relationships
- Sleep disorders
- Somatic pain syndromes
- Substance abuse
- Suicidal tendencies
- Disturbances not due to direct physiological effects of a substance

DIAGNOSTIC TEST RESULTS
- Standard dissociative disorder tests demonstrate a degree of dissociation. These tests include:
  – diagnostic drawing series
  – dissociative experience scale
  – dissociative interview schedule
  – structured clinical interview for dissociative disorders.
- EEG readings may vary markedly among the different identities.

NURSING DIAGNOSES
- Risk for self-mutilation
- Disturbed personal identity
- Chronic low self-esteem
- Ineffective coping

TREATMENT
- Hypnosis to revisit the trauma
- Implementation of suicide precautions, if necessary
- Long-term reconstructive psychotherapy
- Treatment for eating disorders, sleeping disorders, and sexual dysfunction

Drug therapy
- Benzodiazepines: alprazolam (Xanax), lorazepam (Ativan), clonazepam (Klonopin)
- Nonbenzodiazepine: buspirone (BuSpar)
- Monoamine oxidase inhibitors: phenelzine (Nardil), tranylcypromine (Parnate)
- SSRIs: paroxetine (Paxil), escitalopram (Lexapro)
- TCAs: imipramine (Tofranil), desipramine (Norpramin)

INTERVENTIONS AND RATIONALES
- Establish a trusting relationship. *Because of a history of abuse, the client will have trouble developing a trusting relationship.*
- Assist the client in identifying each personality *to work toward integration.*
- Encourage the client to identify emotions that occur under duress *to demonstrate that extreme emotions are a normal result of stress.*
- Monitor risk of self-harm *to help maintain client safety.*

Teaching topics
- Explanation of the disorder and treatment plan
- Medication use and possible adverse effects
- Coping techniques to maintain safety

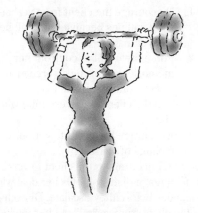

Pump up on practice questions

1. A client who was diagnosed with intermittent explosive disorder is prescribed carbamazepine (Tegretol). What type of blood study would be drawn before discharge as a baseline parameter for determining if the client is experiencing adverse effects of the medication?
　1. Fasting blood glucose
　2. Complete blood count (CBC)
　3. Electrolyte tests
　4. Cholesterol studies

Answer: 2. Because carbamazepine has the potential to cause immunosuppression, the nurse should draw blood for a CBC before discharge. Carbamazepine doesn't alter a client's fasting blood glucose. Neither electrolyte tests nor cholesterol studies would be needed because carbamazepine doesn't alter electrolytes (unless the client experiences an overdose) or affect cholesterol or triglyceride levels.

➡ NCLEX keys
Client needs category: Safe and effective care environment
Client needs subcategory: Management of care
Cognitive level: Analysis

2. A nurse is caring for a client diagnosed with dissociative amnesia. The client recently experienced a divorce. How should the nurse help the client deal with traumatic memories?

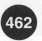

1. Discourage the client from verbalizing feelings because they will be too traumatic.
2. Force the client to confront her memories about the divorce in a direct, confrontational manner.
3. Tell the client that everything will be all right.
4. Encourage the client to verbalize feelings of distress.

Answer: 4. Encouraging the client to verbalize feelings of distress helps her deal with her anxieties before they escalate. Discouraging the client from verbalizing her feelings may cause anxiety to escalate. Forcing the client to confront her memories will increase her anxiety. Telling the client that everything will be all right offers false reassurance.

➡ *NCLEX keys*
Client needs category: Psychosocial integrity
Client needs subcategory: None
Cognitive level: Application

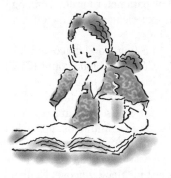

3. A nurse is caring for a client who frequently complains of vague, inconsistent symptoms. Which nursing intervention would be the most appropriate?
1. Screen the client for recent life changes and symptoms of depression, while focusing on physical symptoms.
2. Attempt to minimize physical symptoms, while screening the client for psychological disorders.
3. Exhaust all diagnostic options in ruling out disease before focusing on psychological issues.
4. Refer the client to a psychiatrist.

Answer: 1. It's important not to minimize physical symptoms so that the nurse can demonstrate empathy and establish rapport. The nurse should simultaneously investigate recent life changes and the risk of depression. Although tests and imaging studies may be done in certain cases, review of previous medical records and a physical examination should first be performed to determine the likelihood of physical findings. Referral may be indicated, but not enough information is available.

➡ *NCLEX keys*
Client needs category: Psychosocial integrity
Client needs subcategory: None
Cognitive level: Analysis

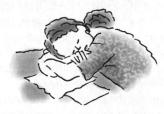

4. A nurse is caring for a client who reports feeling "estranged and separated from himself." How should the nurse describe such symptoms?
1. Intoxication
2. Antimotivational syndrome
3. Existentialism
4. Depersonalization

Answer: 4. Depersonalization is characterized by feelings of separateness from oneself. Intoxication is described as feelings of calm, omnipotence, or euphoria. When a relative lack of motivation occurs within an individual, antimotivational syndrome is present. Existentialism is the philosophy that a person finds meaning in life through experiences.

➡ *NCLEX keys*
Client needs category: Psychosocial integrity
Client needs subcategory: None
Cognitive level: Comprehension

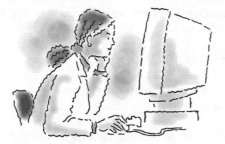

5. A nurse is caring for a client named Susan who has been diagnosed with dissociative identity disorder. Usually, the client arrives to therapy sessions dressed in a tasteful business suit. One day, the client comes to the clinic dressed in a gold lamé mini-dress and insists that her name is Ruby. How should the nurse respond?

1. Ask the client why she's wearing that ridiculous outfit.
2. Refuse to call the client anything but Susan.
3. Ignore the client's behavior.
4. Help client explore the characteristics of this newly emerged personality.

Answer: 4. The nurse should help the client explore the characteristics of this newly emerged personality to work toward integration. Asking the client about her outfit would further decrease the client's self-esteem. Not calling the client by the name she requests would jeopardize the trusting nurse-client relationship. Ignoring the behavior doesn't help the client work toward integration.

➡ *NCLEX keys*
Client needs category: Psychosocial integrity
Client needs subcategory: None
Cognitive level: Application

6. A nurse is caring for a client who has a dissociative identity disorder. Which statement about this client is true?

1. The client's sense of selfhood, which sustains an integrated personality structure, is diminished.
2. The client's sense of selfhood continuously sustains an integrated personality structure.
3. The physician has requested that the client dissociate from her usual medical caregivers and be referred to a psychiatrist.
4. The client is experiencing a gender identity crisis.

Answer: 1. Identity is described as a person's sense of selfhood that sustains an integrated personality structure. In a client with a dissociative identity disorder, this sense is altered. The other choices aren't logical.

➡ *NCLEX keys*
Client needs category: Psychosocial integrity
Client needs subcategory: None
Cognitive level: Comprehension

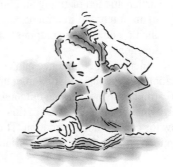

7. A nurse is caring for a client who seems to lack spontaneity, have difficulty distinguishing himself from others, and have difficulty distinguishing between internal and external stimuli. The client describes a vague feeling of estrangement. Which statement would describe this client?

1. He's depressed and should be placed on antidepressants.
2. He may have a depersonalization disorder.
3. He may benefit from electroconvulsive therapy (ECT).
4. He should be placed on suicide precautions.

Answer: 2. The client has characteristics of a depersonalization disorder. He may also suffer from depression, but antidepressants aren't indicated given the available information. ECT wouldn't be appropriate. At this point, the client's behavior doesn't seem suicidal; therefore, such precautions aren't needed.

➡ *NCLEX keys*

Client needs category: Psychosocial integrity
Client needs subcategory: None
Cognitive level: Analysis

8.   A nurse is caring for a client who has a depersonalization disorder. Which clear and explicit outcomes should the nurse work toward?
1. Emphasizing strengths, rather than the pathologic condition
2. Focusing on past accomplishments, rather than the current condition
3. Increasing confidence and active participation in planning and implementation of the treatment
4. Eliciting empathetic responses from the client

Answer: 3. Increasing confidence and active participation in planning and implementation of the treatment are measurable outcomes. The active involvement expected of this client will allow for concise documentation. The other options are vague and inappropriate.

➡ *NCLEX keys*

Client needs category: Psychosocial integrity
Client needs subcategory: None
Cognitive level: Application

9.   A nurse is caring for a client who has a dissociative disorder. What should the nurse do to assist the client in goal achievement?
1. Provide opportunities for the client to experience success.
2. Praise the client frequently, whether warranted or not.
3. Evaluate components of the client's self-concept.
4. Discuss with the client three categories of behavior commonly associated with an altered self-concept.

Answer: 1. Providing opportunities for the client to experience success would assist him in achieving goals. Praise, if offered in unwarranted situations, will inevitably cause the client to question the caregiver's sincerity.

The other two choices are merely academic exercises and won't assist the client in achieving goals.

➡ *NCLEX keys*

Client needs category: Psychosocial integrity
Client needs subcategory: None
Cognitive level: Application

10.   A nurse is caring for a client who has a dissociative disorder and is experiencing amnesia. What could have triggered the amnesia?
1. Severe psychosocial stress
2. Short-acting sedation
3. Conscious sedation
4. Syndrome of inappropriate antidiuretic hormone (SIADH)

Answer: 1. Amnesia in the client with a dissociative disorder can be triggered by severe psychosocial stress. Certain pharmacologic agents given for sedation actually have an amnesic affect, but this doesn't qualify as a dissociative disorder. SIADH isn't associated with amnesia.

➡ *NCLEX keys*

Client needs category: Psychosocial integrity
Client needs subcategory: None
Cognitive level: Analysis

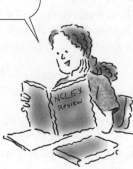

I'm ready to dissociate from this chapter. On to the next one!

20 Sexual disorders

Brush up on key concepts

Sexual disorders described in the *Diagnostic and Statistical Manual of Mental Disorders,* Fourth Edition, Text Revision (*DSM-IV-TR*) include **gender identity disorder, paraphilias,** and **sexual dysfunctions.** Gender identity disorder is characterized by an intense and ongoing cross-gender identification. Paraphilias are characterized by an intense, recurring sexual urge centered on inanimate objects or on human suffering and humiliation. Sexual dysfunctions are characterized by a deficiency or loss of desire for sexual activity or by a disturbance in the sexual response cycle.

At any time, you can review the major points of each disorder by consulting the *Cheat sheet* on page 466.

Polish up on client care

This section discusses care for clients with gender identity disorders, paraphilias, and sexual dysfunctions.

Gender identity disorder

Clients with gender identity disorders want to become or be like the opposite sex and are extremely uncomfortable with their assigned gender roles. This disorder can occur in childhood, adolescence, or adulthood.

CONTRIBUTING FACTORS
• Concurrent paraphilias, especially transvestic fetishism
• Feelings of sexual inadequacy and being in the body of the wrong gender

• Generalized anxiety disorder
• Personality disorders

ASSESSMENT FINDINGS
• Anxiety
• Attempts to mask sex organs
• Requests for surgery to remove primary and secondary sex characteristics
• Cross-dressing
• Depression
• Disturbance in body image
• Dreams of cross-gender identification
• Fear of abandonment by family and friends
• Finding one's own genitals "disgusting"
• Ineffective coping strategies
• Peer ostracism
• Persistent distress about sexual orientation
• Preoccupation with appearance
• Self-hatred
• Self-medication such as hormonal therapy
• Strong attraction to stereotypical activities of the opposite sex
• Suicide attempts
• Impairment of social and occupational function

DIAGNOSTIC TEST RESULTS
• Karyotyping for sex chromosomes (not usually indicated) may reveal an abnormality.
• Psychological testing may reveal cross-gender identification or behavior patterns.
• Sex hormones assay (not usually indicated) may reveal an abnormality.

NURSING DIAGNOSES
• Disturbed body image
• Chronic low self-esteem
• Disturbed personal identity
• Ineffective coping
• Risk for suicide

TREATMENT
• Group and individual psychotherapy
• Hormonal therapy

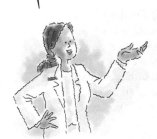

Cheat sheet

Sexual disorders refresher

GENDER IDENTITY DISORDER
Key signs and symptoms
- Dreams of cross-gender identification
- Finding one's own genitals "disgusting"
- Persistent distress about sexual orientation
- Preoccupation with appearance
- Self-hatred

Key test results
- Psychological testing may reveal cross-gender identification or behavior patterns.

Key treatments
- Group and individual psychotherapy
- Hormonal therapy
- Sex-reassignment surgery

Key interventions
- Be careful to demonstrate a nonjudgmental attitude at all times. Don't say anything that would make the client feel ashamed.
- Help the client to identify positive aspects of himself.

PARAPHILIAS
Key signs and symptoms
- Development of a hobby or change in occupation that makes the paraphilia more accessible
- Recurrent paraphilic fantasies
- Social isolation
- Troubled social or sexual relationships

Key treatments
- Individual therapy

Key interventions
- Be careful to demonstrate a nonjudgmental attitude at all times. Don't say anything that would make the client feel ashamed.
- If the client is a threat to others, institute safety precautions per facility protocol.
- Initiate a discussion about how emotional needs for self-esteem, respect, love, and intimacy influence sexual expression.

- Encourage the client to identify feelings, such as pleasure, reduced anxiety, increased control, or shame associated with sexual behavior and fantasies.

SEXUAL DYSFUNCTIONS
Key signs and symptoms
- Anxiety
- Decreased sexual desire (sexual desire disorder)
- Delayed or absent orgasm (orgasmic disorder)
- Depression
- Inability to maintain an erection (sexual arousal disorder)
- Pain with sexual intercourse (sexual pain disorder)
- Premature ejaculation (orgasmic disorder)

Key test results
- Diagnostic tests are used to rule out a physiologic cause for the dysfunction.

Key treatments
- Individual therapy
- Hormone replacement
- Phosphodiesterase inhibitors: sildenafil (Viagra), tadalafil (Cialis), vardenafil (Levitra)

Key interventions
- Encourage the client to discuss feelings and perceptions about his sexual dysfunction.
- Teach the client and his partner alternative ways of expressing sexual intimacy and affection.
- Encourage the client to seek evaluation and therapy from a qualified professional.

Use the Cheat sheet for a quick review of sexual disorders.

• Sex-reassignment surgery

INTERVENTIONS AND RATIONALES

• Be careful to demonstrate a nonjudgmental attitude at all times. Don't say anything that would make the client feel ashamed. *It's the client's needs and feelings, not your opinions, that matter.*
• Provide emotional support and empathy as the client discusses fears and concerns *to help him deal with anxiety.*
• Help the client to identify positive aspects of himself *to alleviate feelings of shame and distress.*
• Encourage the client to participate in support groups *so the client can gain empathy from others and find a safe environment to discuss concerns.*

Teaching topics

• Explanation of the disorder and treatment plan
• Medication use and possible adverse effects
• Available support groups and follow-up care

Paraphilias

A paraphilia is defined as a recurrent, intense sexual urge or fantasy, generally involving nonhuman subjects, children, nonconsenting partners, or the degradation, suffering, and humiliation of the client or partners. The client may report that the fantasy is always present but there are periods when the frequency of the fantasy and intensity of the urge vary. The disorder tends to be chronic and lifelong but, in adults, both the fantasy and behavior commonly diminish with advancing age. Inappropriate sexual behavior may increase in response to psychological stressors, in relation to other mental disorders, or when opportunity to engage in the paraphilia becomes more available.

Common paraphilias include:
• exhibitionism (exposing genitals and occasionally masturbating in public)
• fetishism (use of an object to become sexually aroused)
• frotteurism (rubbing one's genital on another nonconsenting person to become aroused)

• pedophilia (sexual activity with a child)
• sexual masochism (being humiliated or feeling pain to become aroused)
• sexual sadism (causing physical or emotional pain to another to become aroused)
• transvestic fetishism (cross-dressing)
• voyeurism (watching others who are nude or engaging in sex to become aroused).

CONTRIBUTING FACTORS

• Childhood incest
• Concurrent mental disorders
• Emotional trauma
• Gender (more likely in males)
• Personality disorders
• Central nervous system tumors
• Closed head injury
• Neuroendocrine disorders
• Psychosocial stressors
• Lack of knowledge about sex
• Sexual trauma

ASSESSMENT FINDINGS

• Anxiety
• Depression
• Development of a hobby or change in occupation that makes the paraphilia more accessible
• Disturbance in body image
• Guilt or shame
• Ineffective coping
• Multiple paraphilias at the same time
• Obsessive-compulsive tendencies
• Purchase of books, films, or magazines related to the paraphilia
• Recurrent paraphilic fantasies
• Sexual dysfunction
• Social isolation
• Troubled social or sexual relationships

DIAGNOSTIC TEST RESULTS

• Penile plethysmography testing may measure sexual arousal in response to visual imagery; however, the results of this procedure can be unreliable.

NURSING DIAGNOSES

• Ineffective sexuality patterns
• Chronic low self-esteem
• Risk for other-directed violence
• Anxiety
• Impaired social interaction

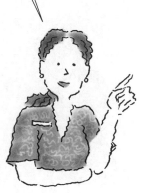

Inappropriate sexual behavior may increase in response to stress.

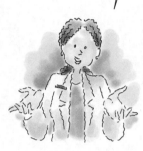

Institute safety precautions if the client with paraphilia is a threat to others.

TREATMENT
- Behavior therapy
- Cognitive therapy
- Individual therapy

INTERVENTIONS AND RATIONALES
- Be careful to demonstrate a nonjudgmental attitude at all times. Don't say anything that would make the client feel ashamed. *It's the client's needs and feelings, not your opinions, that matter.*
- If the client is a threat to others, institute safety precautions per facility protocol *to protect the client and others.*
- Initiate a discussion about how emotional needs for self-esteem, respect, love, and intimacy influence sexual expression *to help the client understand the disorder.*
- Encourage the client to identify feelings, such as pleasure, reduced anxiety, increased control, or shame associated with sexual behavior and fantasies, *to provide insight for developing appropriate interventions.*
- Help the client distinguish practices that are distressing because they don't conform to social norms or personal values from those that may place him or others in serious emotional, medical, or legal jeopardy *to reinforce the need to stop behaviors that could harm the client or others.*

Teaching topics
- Explanation of the disorder and treatment plan
- Contacting Sexaholics Anonymous

Sexual dysfunctions

Sexual dysfunctions are characterized by a disturbance during one or more phases of the sexual response cycle. The most common dysfunctions are:
- orgasmic disorders — The *DSM-IV-TR* lists female orgasmic disorder, male orgasmic disorder, and premature ejaculation. Male and female orgasmic disorders are characterized by a persistent or recurrent delay in or absence of orgasm following a normal sexual excitement phase. Premature ejaculation is marked by persistent and recurrent onset of orgasm and ejaculation with minimal sexual stimulation.
- sexual arousal disorders — These include female sexual arousal disorder and male erectile disorder. With female sexual arousal disorder, the client has a persistent or recurrent inability to attain or maintain adequate lubrication, swelling, and response of sexual excitement until the completion of sexual activity. In male erectile disorder, the client has a persistent or recurrent inability to attain or maintain an adequate erection until completion of sexual activity.
- sexual desire disorders — This category includes hypoactive sexual desire disorder and sexual aversion disorder. The key feature of hypoactive sexual desire disorder is a deficiency or absence of sexual fantasies and the desire for sexual activity. The client usually doesn't initiate sexual activity and may only engage in it reluctantly when it's initiated by the partner. With sexual aversion disorder, the client has an aversion to and active avoidance of genital sexual contact with a sexual partner.
- sexual dysfunction due to a medical condition — Sexual dysfunction may occur as a result of a physiologic problem.
- sexual pain disorders — This category includes dyspareunia and vaginismus. The essential feature of dyspareunia is genital pain associated with sexual intercourse. Most commonly experienced during intercourse, dyspareunia may also occur before or after intercourse. The disorder can occur in males and females. Vaginismus is recurrent or persistent involuntary contraction of the perineal muscles surrounding the outer third of the vagina when vaginal penetration is attempted. In some clients, even the anticipation of vaginal insertion may result in muscle spasm. The contractions may be mild to severe.
- substance-induced sexual dysfunction — This term is used to describe sexual dysfunction resulting from direct physiologic effects of a substance, such as from drug abuse, medication use, or toxin exposure.

CONTRIBUTING FACTORS
- Anger or hostility
- Depression
- Disability

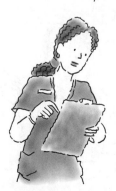

Sexual dysfunction usually accompanies other medical situations, such as surgery, pregnancy, or pharmacologic treatment.

- Drugs or alcohol
- Endocrine disorders
- Genital surgery
- Genital trauma
- Infections
- Lifestyle disruptions
- Medications
- Paraphilia
- Pregnancy
- Religious or cultural taboos that reinforce guilty feelings about sex
- Stress

ASSESSMENT FINDINGS
- Anxiety
- Decreased sexual desire (sexual desire disorder)
- Delayed or absent orgasm (orgasmic disorder)
- Depression
- Disturbance in body image
- Frustration and feelings of being unattractive
- Inability to maintain an erection (sexual arousal disorder)
- Ineffective coping
- Pain with sexual intercourse (sexual pain disorder)
- Poor self-concept
- Premature ejaculation (orgasmic disorder)
- Social isolation

DIAGNOSTIC TEST RESULTS
- Diagnostic tests are used to rule out a physiologic cause for the dysfunction.

NURSING DIAGNOSES
- Impaired social interaction
- Chronic low self-esteem
- Sexual dysfunction

TREATMENT
- Changing medications to decrease symptoms (as appropriate)
- Individual therapy
- Marital or couples therapy
- Penile implant or vacuum pump (for erectile dysfunction)
- Sex therapy
- Treatment of underlying medical condition
- Vaginal dilators
- Vascular surgery for erectile dysfunction

Drug therapy
- Hormone replacement
- Phosphodiesterase inhibitors: sildenafil (Viagra), tadalafil (Cialis), vardenafil (Levitra)
- Alprostadil (Caverject) intracavernously to induce erection

INTERVENTIONS AND RATIONALES
- Establish a therapeutic relationship with the client *to provide a safe and comfortable atmosphere for discussing sexual concerns.*
- Encourage the client to discuss feelings and perceptions about his sexual dysfunction *to help validate his perceptions and reduce emotional distress.*
- Teach the client and his partner alternative ways of expressing sexual intimacy and affection. *Alternative expressions of intimacy may raise the client's self-esteem.*
- Encourage the client to seek evaluation and therapy from a qualified professional *to enable the client to obtain proper diagnosis and treatment.*

Teaching topics
- Explanation of the disorder and treatment plan
- Medication use and possible adverse effects
- Understanding sexual response
- Using alternative sexual positions to promote comfort
- Performing relaxation exercises
- Performing Kegel exercises to improve urethral and vaginal tone
- Contacting self-help groups

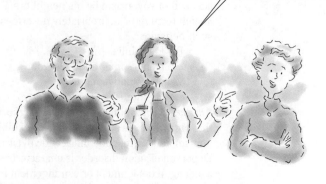

Teach the client and his partner alternative ways of expressing sexual intimacy and affection.

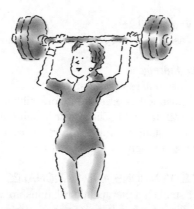

Pump up on practice questions

1. A nurse is caring for a client who's experiencing hypoactive sexual desire. How should the nurse classify this condition?
   1. Sexual arousal disorder
   2. Sexual pain disorder
   3. Sexual desire disorder
   4. Orgasmic disorder

Answer: 3. Sexual desire disorders include sexual aversion and hypoactive sexual desire disorder. Sexual arousal disorders include male erectile and female arousal disorders. Examples of sexual pain disorders include dyspareunia and vaginismus. Orgasmic disorders, such as premature ejaculation, affect males and females.

➡ *NCLEX keys*

Client needs category: Psychosocial integrity
Client needs subcategory: None
Cognitive level: Application

2. A nurse is caring for a client who was accused of voyeurism by his neighbors. Which term most appropriately describes such behavior?
   1. Paraphilia
   2. Depersonalization disorder
   3. Dissociative fugue
   4. Gender identity disorder

Answer: 1. Paraphilia is a general diagnosis that encompasses such disorders as exhibitionism, fetishism, pedophilia, and voyeurism. Depersonalization disorder is characterized by a feeling of detachment or estrangement from one's self. Dissociative fugue is characterized by sudden, unexpected travel away from home, accompanied by an inability to recall one's past. Gender identity disorder is a separate diagnostic category and isn't related to paraphilias.

➡ *NCLEX keys*

Client needs category: Psychosocial integrity
Client needs subcategory: None
Cognitive level: Application

3. A nurse is caring for a female client who's about to begin thrombolytic therapy to treat an acute myocardial infarction (MI). When the physician questions the client about her last menstrual period, she becomes embarrassed and asks him to leave the room. She then tells the nurse that she underwent sex-reassignment surgery. What should be the nurse's most appropriate response?
   1. "I understand your reluctance to tell the physician, but it may have an impact on your treatment."
   2. "Based on client confidentiality, I won't tell the physician if you wish."
   3. "Your sex change and your hormones have nothing to do with your heart attack."
   4. "Tell me about your sexual preference. Are you attracted to men or women?"

Answer: 1. During the history and physical examination of any female client being screened for thrombolytic therapy, the physician must know about the last menstrual period before the MI. Although not an absolute contraindication to thrombolytics, the possibility of pregnancy or menstruation must be documented. According to the ethics of client confidentiality, information may be shared in a professional manner with those who require it for the client's care. Hormones are an important factor in the pathogenesis of MI. Estrogen is cardioprotective, while replacement hormones after sex-reassignment surgery can impact how prone a person is to an MI. The client's sexual preference is of no consequence in this situation.

➡ *NCLEX keys*

Client needs category: Physiological integrity
Client needs subcategory: Reduction of risk potential
Cognitive level: Application

4. A client arrives at her physician's office crying. Her husband of 17 years has asked her for a divorce. She admits that recently she has avoided having sexual intercourse with him. Which response by the nurse would be most appropriate when talking with this client?

1. "Please stop crying so that we can discuss your feelings about the divorce."
2. "Once you have intercourse with him, you'll be able to get your relationship back on track."
3. "I can see how upset you are. Let's sit in the office so that we can talk about how you're feeling."
4. "Find a good lawyer who'll look out for your interests, and then you'll feel better."

Answer: 3. This response validates the client's distress and provides her the opportunity to talk about her feelings. Because a client in crisis has difficulty making decisions, the nurse must be directive as well as supportive. Telling the client to stop crying doesn't provide the client with adequate support. Suggesting that the client have intercourse or hire a lawyer doesn't acknowledge the client's distress. Moreover, the client in crisis can't think beyond the immediate moment, so discussing long-range plans isn't helpful.

➡ *NCLEX keys*
Client needs category: Psychosocial integrity
Client needs subcategory: None
Cognitive level: Application

5. A client explains to the nurse that she has felt distant from her spouse for a long period. Which question would be appropriate for the nurse to ask this client to assess female sexual functioning?

1. "Have you been spending time with friends?"
2. "What problems are you having with sleep?"
3 "Are you experiencing any signs of depression?"
4. "When did your family allow you to be independent?"

Answer: 3. A client who feels distant from her spouse may be experiencing hypoactive sexual desire disorder, and it may be related to negativity or cognitive distortions. It's important for the nurse to explore the client's feelings of depression and factors that may contribute to decreased sexual desire. Asking about time with friends, sleep problems, and independence doesn't address potential factors that contribute to hypoactive sexual desire disorder.

➡ *NCLEX keys*
Client needs category: Psychosocial integrity
Client needs subcategory: Psychosocial adaptation
Cognitive level: Application

6. A male client tells the nurse that he's experiencing problems with sexual arousal, and he asks her if he'll get anything out of attending the educational session on sexual disorders. Which response by the nurse would provide useful information to the client?

1. "I'm not sure if the class is appropriate for you; please ask your doctor what he thinks."
2. "I'll be talking about how certain medications can enhance sexual functioning."
3. "If you have a substance abuse problem, the class won't be helpful."
4. "I think that everyone can benefit from an educational class on sexual functioning."

Answer: 2. A male client with a sexual arousal disorder is typically experiencing an erectile disorder. In the educational session the nurse will speak about such medications as sildenafil (Viagra), tadalafil (Cialis), and vardenafil (Levitra), which are used to enhance male sexual functioning. The other responses don't directly answer the client's question about problems with sexual functioning.

➡ *NCLEX keys*
Client needs category: Psychosocial integrity
Client needs subcategory: Psychosocial adaptation
Cognitive level: Application

7. A client is diagnosed with erectile disorder. Which drug may be beneficial in treating a client with this disorder?

1. Methyldopa (Aldomet)
2. Alprostadil (Caverject)

3. Benazepril (Lotensin)
4. Clonidine (Catapres)

Answer: 2. Alprostadil is indicated for erectile disorder. It can be administered intracavernously before sexual intercourse. Methyldopa, benazepril, and clonidine are antihypertensive agents that can cause erectile disorder.

➡ *NCLEX keys*

Client needs category: Psychosocial integrity
Client needs subcategory: None
Cognitive level: Analysis

8. A nurse is caring for a male client awaiting sex-reassignment surgery. When interacting with this client, it's important that the nurse:

1. discourage the client from undergoing the procedure.
2. demonstrate a nonjudgmental attitude.
3. discuss with the client the option of undergoing hypnosis as an alternative to the surgery.
4. tell the client that his life will be less complicated and more peaceful after the surgery is complete.

Answer: 2. When caring for a client with gender identity disorder, the nurse should demonstrate a nonjudgmental attitude toward the client. It's the client's needs and feelings that matter most, not the nurse's opinions. The nurse shouldn't discourage the client's decision to go ahead with the procedure. Hypnosis isn't a treatment for gender identity disorder, and it isn't appropriate for the nurse to suggest hypnosis to the client. Telling the client his life will be less complicated and more peaceful after surgery offers false reassurance.

➡ *NCLEX keys*

Client needs category: Psychosocial integrity
Client needs subcategory: None
Cognitive level: Analysis

9. A nurse explains exhibitionism, a sexual disorder, to a mother whose 24-year-old son displays the disorder. Which statement by the woman indicates her understanding of the disorder?

1. "The genetic factors make the disorder out of his control."

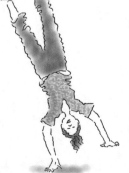

2. "There's no real treatment except for aversion therapy."
3. "Getting caught is the only thing that will stop this behavior."
4. "The pleasure that he got from the behavior reinforced it."

Answer: 4. A client who displays exhibitionism will continue to display this behavior when negative consequences don't occur and the pleasure he obtains continues to be reinforced. There are no genetic factors associated with exhibitionism. Aversion therapy isn't appropriate treatment for exhibitionism. Getting caught doesn't necessarily stop the behavior of this sexual disorder.

➡ *NCLEX keys*

Client needs category: Psychosocial integrity
Client needs subcategory: None
Cognitive level: Application

10. A 14-year old male who prefers to dress in female clothing is brought to the psychiatric crisis room by his mother. The client's mother states, "He is always dressing in female clothing. There must be something wrong with him." Which of the following responses from the nurse is most appropriate?

1. "Your son will be evaluated shortly."
2. "I will explain to your son that his behavior isn't appropriate."
3. "I see you're upset. Would you like to talk?"
4. "You're being judgmental. There's nothing wrong with a boy wearing female clothing."

Answer: 3. Acknowledging the mother's feelings and offering her an opportunity to verbalize her concerns provides a forum for open communication. Telling the boy's mother that he will be evaluated shortly doesn't address the mother's concerns. Telling the client that his behavior is inappropriate isn't therapeutic. The nurse shouldn't offer an opinion regarding whether the client's behavior is acceptable.

➡ *NCLEX keys*

Client needs category: Psychosocial integrity
Client needs subcategory: None
Cognitive level: Application

21 Eating disorders

Brush up on key concepts

Eating disorders are characterized by severe disturbances in eating behaviors. The two most common disorders, anorexia nervosa and bulimia nervosa, put the client at risk for severe cardiovascular and GI complications and can ultimately result in death.

Clients with these disorders exhibit severe disturbances in body image and self-perception. Their behavior may include self-starvation, binge eating, and purging. The causes of eating disorders aren't fully understood. They're more prevalent in females (90%) and can be chronic with periods of remission.

At any time, you can review the major points of each disorder by consulting the *Cheat sheet* on page 474.

Polish up on client care

Here's a review of anorexia nervosa and bulimia nervosa, the two most common eating disorders.

Anorexia nervosa

In anorexia nervosa, the client deliberately starves herself or engages in binge eating and purging. A client with anorexia nervosa wants to become as thin as possible and refuses to maintain an appropriate weight. A key clinical finding is a refusal to sustain weight at or above minimum requirements for the client's age and height and an intense fear of gaining weight or becoming fat. If left untreated, anorexia nervosa can be fatal.

CONTRIBUTING FACTORS
- Age (most prominent in adolescents)
- Distorted body image
- Gender (primarily affects females)
- Genetic predisposition
- Low self-esteem
- Neurochemical changes
- Poor family relations
- Poor self-esteem
- Preoccupation with weight and dieting
- Sexual abuse

ASSESSMENT FINDINGS
- Amenorrhea, fatigue, loss of libido, infertility
- Body image disturbance
- Cognitive distortions, such as overgeneralization, dichotomous thinking, or ideas of reference
- Compulsive behavior
- Decreased blood volume, evidenced by lowered blood pressure and orthostatic hypotension
- Dependency on others for self-worth
- Electrolyte imbalance, evidenced by muscle weakness, seizures, or arrhythmias
- Emaciated appearance
- GI complications, such as constipation or laxative dependence
- Guilt associated with eating
- Impaired decision making
- Need to achieve and please others
- Obsessive rituals concerning food
- Overly compliant attitude
- Perfectionist attitude
- Refusal to eat

DIAGNOSTIC TEST RESULTS
- Eating Attitude Test suggests an eating disorder.
- Electrocardiogram reveals non-specific ST interval, prolonged PR interval, and T-wave changes.

Eating disorders refresher

ANOREXIA NERVOSA

Key signs and symptoms
• Decreased blood volume, evidenced by lowered blood pressure and orthostatic hypotension
• Electrolyte imbalance, evidenced by muscle weakness, seizures, or arrhythmias
• Emaciated appearance
• Need to achieve and please others
• Obsessive rituals concerning food
• Refusal to eat

Key test results
• Eating Attitude Test suggests an eating disorder.
• Electrocardiogram reveals nonspecific ST interval, prolonged PR interval, and T-wave changes.
• Laboratory tests show elevated blood urea nitrogen level and electrolyte imbalances.
• Female clients exhibit low estrogen levels.
• Male clients exhibit low serum testosterone levels.

Key treatments
• Individual and group therapy
• Nutritional counseling
• Antianxiety agents: lorazepam (Ativan), alprazolam (Xanax)
• Antidepressants: amitriptyline (Elavil), imipramine (Tofranil)
• Selective serotonin reuptake inhibitors: paroxetine (Paxil), fluoxetine (Prozac), sertraline (Zoloft), citalopram (Celexa)

Key interventions
• Contract with the client for amount to be eaten.
• Provide one-on-one support before, during, and after meals.
• Prevent the client from using the bathroom for 90 minutes after eating.
• Help the client identify coping mechanisms for dealing with anxiety.
• Weigh the client once or twice per week at the same time of day using the same scale.

• Help the client and her family understand the anorectic cycle.
• Monitor for suicidal ideation, maladaptive substance use, and medical complications.

BULIMIA NERVOSA

Key signs and symptoms
• Alternating episodes of binge eating and purging
• Constant preoccupation with food
• Disruptions in interpersonal relationships
• Eroded tooth enamel
• Extreme need for acceptance and approval
• Irregular menses
• Russell sign (bruised knuckles due to induced vomiting)
• Sporadic, excessive exercise

Key test results
• Beck Depression Inventory may reveal depression.
• Eating Attitude Test suggests an eating disorder.
• Metabolic acidosis may occur from diarrhea caused by enemas and excessive laxative use.
• Metabolic alkalosis may occur from frequent vomiting.

Key interventions
• Explain the purpose of a nutritional contract.
• Avoid power struggles around food.
• Prevent the client from using the bathroom for 90 minutes after eating.
• Provide one-on-one support before, during, and after meals.
• Weigh the client once or twice per week at the same time of day using the same scale.
• Help the client and her family identify the cause of the disorder.
• Point out cognitive distortions.

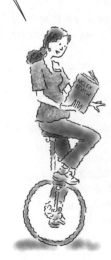

I can use the Cheat sheet to study while I get my exercise.

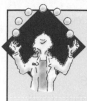

Management moments

Communication counts

Communication strategies play a key role when caring for the client with anorexia nervosa. Many clients with this disorder communicate on a superficial level and have difficulty forming interpersonal relationships. Therefore, you should focus on developing a therapeutic relationship. Use an accepting, nonjudgmental approach, and encourage the client to discuss her feelings, which may include sadness, depression, and loneliness. Teach the client effective communication techniques that focus on assertiveness skills.

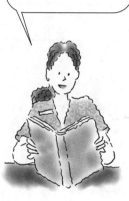

The largest obstacle to treating anorexia is that clients don't want to be treated. Yet quick intervention is essential. Anorexia nervosa can be fatal.

- Laboratory tests show elevated blood urea nitrogen and electrolyte imbalances.
- Female clients exhibit low estrogen levels.
- Leukopenia and mild anemia are apparent.
- Male clients exhibit low serum testosterone levels.
- Thyroid study findings are low.

NURSING DIAGNOSES
- Imbalanced nutrition: Less than body requirements
- Disturbed body image
- Chronic low self-esteem
- Anxiety
- Ineffective coping
- Decreased cardiac output

TREATMENT
- Behavioral modification
- Individual and group therapy
- Nutritional counseling
- Family therapy

Drug therapy
- Antianxiety agents: lorazepam (Ativan), alprazolam (Xanax)
- Antidepressants: amitriptyline (Elavil), imipramine (Tofranil)
- Selective serotonin reuptake inhibitors (SSRIs): paroxetine (Paxil), fluoxetine (Prozac), sertraline (Zoloft), citalopram (Celexa)

INTERVENTIONS AND RATIONALES
- Obtain a complete physical assessment *to identify complications of anorexia nervosa.*
- Contract with the client for amount to be eaten *to avoid conflict between staff members and the client.*

- Provide one-on-one support before, during, and after meals *to foster a strong nurse-client relationship and to ensure that the client is eating.*
- Prevent the client from using the bathroom for 90 minutes after eating *to break the purging cycle.*
- Encourage verbal expression of feelings *to foster open communications about body image.* (See *Communication counts.*)
- Help the client identify coping mechanisms for dealing with anxiety *to promote health-coping techniques.*
- Weigh the client once or twice per week at the same time of day using the same scale *to accurately monitor weight gain.* Be aware of objects in pockets or heavy clothing the client may be wearing in an attempt *to increase her weight.*
- Help the client and her family understand the anorectic cycle *to prevent future anorectic behavior.*
- Discuss the client's perception of her appearance. Explain that she has a right to think of herself as beautiful regardless of how she compares with others *to build self-esteem.*
- Discuss the client's progress with her *to increase awareness of achievements and promote continued effort.*
- Monitor for suicidal ideation, maladaptive substance use, and medical complications *to better understand the client history.*

Teaching topics
- Explanation of the disorder and treatment plan
- Medication use and possible adverse effects
- Need for gradual weight gain
- Nutritional support measures

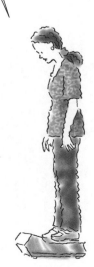

Weigh the client once or twice each week but not more; weighing too often reinforces the focus on weight.

- Treatment options
- Support services and community resources

Bulimia nervosa

Bulimia nervosa is characterized by episodic binge eating, followed by purging in the form of vomiting. The client may also use laxatives, enemas, diuretics, or syrup of ipecac. The client's weight may remain normal or close to normal. The severity of the disorder depends on the frequency of the binge and purge cycle as well as physical complications. The client commonly views food as a source of comfort. The condition can be chronic or intermittent.

Tell the client that she has a right to think of herself as beautiful regardless of how she compares with others.

CONTRIBUTING FACTORS
- Distorted body image
- History of sexual abuse
- Low self-esteem
- Neurochemical changes
- Poor family relations

ASSESSMENT FINDINGS
- Alternating episodes of binge eating and purging
- Anxiety
- Avoidance of conflict
- Cognitive distortions such as with anorexia nervosa
- Constant preoccupation with food
- Eroded tooth enamel
- Disruptions in interpersonal relationships
- Dissatisfaction with body image
- Extreme need for acceptance and approval
- Feelings of helplessness
- Focus on changing a specific body part
- Frequent lies and excuses to explain behavior
- Guilt and self-disgust
- Irregular menses
- Perfectionist attitude
- Parotid and salivary gland swelling
- Pharyngitis
- Physiologic problems as in anorexia nervosa (amenorrhea, fatigue, loss of libido, infertility, electrolyte imbalance, GI complications)
- Possible use of amphetamines or other drugs to control hunger
- Problems caused by frequent vomiting
- Repression of anger and frustration
- Russell sign (bruised knuckles due to induced vomiting)
- Sporadic, excessive exercise

DIAGNOSTIC TEST RESULTS
- Beck Depression Inventory may reveal depression.
- Eating Attitude Test suggests an eating disorder.
- Metabolic acidosis may occur from diarrhea caused by enemas and excessive laxative use.
- Metabolic alkalosis (the most common metabolic complication) may occur from frequent vomiting.

NURSING DIAGNOSES
- Imbalanced nutrition: Less than body requirements
- Anxiety
- Powerlessness
- Fatigue
- Disturbed body image

TREATMENT
- Cognitive therapy to identify triggers for binge eating and purging
- Family therapy

Drug therapy
- SSRIs: paroxetine (Paxil), fluoxetine (Prozac)
- Topiramate (Topamax) to reduce binge eating and preoccupation with food
Note: Drug therapy is most effective when combined with cognitive therapy.

INTERVENTIONS AND RATIONALES
- Perform a complete physical assessment *to identify complications associated with bulimia nervosa*.
- Explain the purpose of a nutritional contract *to encourage a dietary change without initiating arguments or struggles*.
- Avoid power struggles around food *to keep the focus on establishing and maintaining a positive self-image and self-esteem*.
- Prevent the client from using the bathroom for 90 minutes after eating *to help the client avoid purging behavior*.
- Provide one-on-one support before, during, and after meals *to monitor and assist the client with eating*.

• Encourage the client to express her feelings *to facilitate conversation and promote understanding.*

• Weigh the client once or twice per week at the same time of day using the same scale *to monitor weight.*

• Help the client and her family identify the cause of the disorder *to help her gain understanding and work toward wellness.*

• Point out cognitive distortions *to help identify sources of the problem.*

• Discuss the client's perception of her appearance. Explain that she has a right to think of herself as beautiful regardless of how she compares with others *to build self-esteem.*

• Discuss the client's progress with her *to increase awareness of achievements and promote continued effort.*

Teaching topics

• Explanation of the disorder and treatment plan
• Medication use and possible adverse effects
• Need to gain weight gradually
• Treatment options
• Support services and community resources

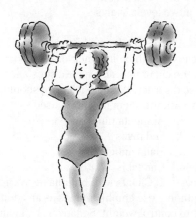

Pump up on practice questions

1. During the health history, a 16-year-old female client is looking for her prescription medication in her purse. The nurse notices a bottle of ipecac among the contents. Which concern should this observation cause the nurse?

1. Does the client frequently self-induce vomiting?
2. Will the client sell this drug to a minor at school?
3. Is the client aware that it's illegal to have this drug?
4. How should the nurse notify the client's parents about the client's possession of this drug?

Answer: 1. The only reason a client would have a bottle of ipecac is to self-induce vomiting. This information strongly indicates the possibility that the client has an eating disorder. Ipecac isn't an illegal drug and it would be unlikely that the client would sell it at school. The nurse isn't mandated to report possession of this drug to the client's parents.

➡ *NCLEX keys*

Client needs category: Physiological integrity
Client needs subcategory: Reduction of risk potential
Cognitive level: Application

2. A nurse is monitoring a client diagnosed with anorexia nervosa. In addition to monitoring the client's eating, the nurse should do which of the following after meals?

1. Encourage the client to go for a walk to get some exercise.
2. Prevent the client from using the bathroom for 90 minutes after eating.
3. Tell the client to lie down for 2 hours after eating.
4. Instruct the client to get plenty of exercise.

Answer: 2. After observing the client while she eats, the nurse should prevent the client from using the bathroom for at least 90 minutes to break the purging cycle. Exercise should be restricted until the client has shown adequate weight gain, and then it should be encouraged in moderation. It isn't necessary for the client to lie down for 90 minutes after eating.

➡ *NCLEX keys*

Client needs category: Physiological integrity
Client needs subcategory: Reduction of risk potential
Cognitive level: Application

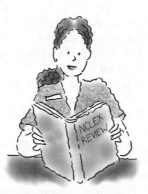

3.   A nurse has taken the health history of a client who admits to binge eating. Which health concern should the nurse assess further during the next meeting with the client?

1.   Adolescent turmoil
2.   Emotional hunger
3.   Disorganized behavior
4.   Extreme restlessness

Answer: 2. A client who engages in binge eating will commonly eat when already feeling full and as a way to cope with emotions that aren't being handled effectively. A history of adolescent turmoil isn't necessarily associated with binge eating. Disorganized behavior and extreme restlessness are associated with bipolar disorder, not binge eating.

➡ *NCLEX keys*

Client needs category: Psychosocial integrity
Client needs subcategory: None
Cognitive level: Analysis

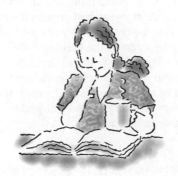

4.   A nurse overhears a female client with bulimia nervosa talk in a disparaging way about herself to another client before the beginning of the group therapy session. Which intervention should the nurse initiate during group therapy?

1.   Help the client realize and admit that she has socialization problems.
2.   Discuss with the client ways to acknowledge and accept her angry feelings.
3.   Encourage the client to recognize and change misperceptions about herself.
4.   Teach the client to identify and tolerate frustrations about her daily life.

Answer: 3. A client who has distorted perceptions about herself would benefit from recognizing and changing these distorted perceptions. The nurse needs to address the issue of negative verbalizations about the self, rather than focus on socialization issues, anger management, or tolerance of frustrations.

➡ *NCLEX keys*

Client needs category: Psychosocial integrity
Client needs subcategory: None
Cognitive level: Analysis

5.   A nurse is taking a history from a woman diagnosed with bulimia nervosa and suspects that the client may also have a substance abuse disorder. Which illicit drug should the nurse ask the client if she has used?

1.   Amphetamines
2.   Sedatives
3.   Hallucinogens
4.   Cannabis

Answer: 1. Clients with bulimia nervosa will commonly use amphetamines as an additional way to control weight. Sedatives, hallucinogens, and cannabis aren't typically used by bulimic clients to control weight.

➡ *NCLEX keys*

Client needs category: Psychosocial integrity
Client needs subcategory: None
Cognitive level: Application

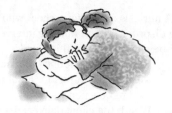

6. A client with bulimia nervosa tells the nurse that she wants to stop her binge eating. Which intervention should the nurse use to meet the client's request for help?
1. Discuss the binge-purge cycle and identify where the cycle could be interrupted.
2. Address the defense mechanism of projection and talk about underlying conflicts.
3. Provide anger management counseling and later involve the client's family in the treatment.
4. Focus on dysfunctional family and peer relationships and teach positive self-talk.

Answer: 1. Educating a client with bulimia nervosa about the binge-purge cycle can assist her to change her eating behavior and regain control over her eating. The defense mechanism commonly seen in a client with an eating disorder is denial, not projection. Anger management and learning positive self-talk wouldn't be the interventions of choice for assisting someone to stop binge eating behavior.

➡ *NCLEX keys*
Client needs category: Physiological integrity
Client needs subcategory: Reduction of risk potential
Cognitive level: Application

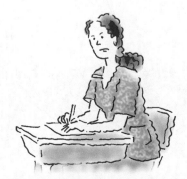

7. A nurse is caring for a client who has bulimia. Which treatment option is most effective?
1. Antidepressants
2. Cognitive-behavioral therapy
3. Antidepressants and cognitive-behavioral therapy
4. Total parenteral nutrition (TPN) and antidepressants

Answer: 3. The combined approach of antidepressants and cognitive-behavioral therapy has been effective, even when clients don't present with depression. TPN isn't indicated.

➡ *NCLEX keys*
Client needs category: Physiological integrity
Client needs subcategory: Pharmacological and parenteral therapies
Cognitive level: Application

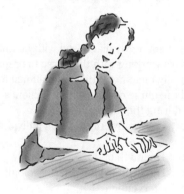

8. A nurse is caring for several clients who have eating disorders. Based on appearance, how would the nurse distinguish bulimic clients from anorectic clients?
1. By their teeth
2. By body size and weight
3. By looking for Mallory-Weiss tears
4. The clients are indistinguishable upon physical examination

Answer: 2. Behaviors of the anorectic client and the bulimic client are commonly similar, especially because both implement rituals to lose weight; however, the bulimic client tends to eat much more, due to binge episodes, and therefore can be near-normal weight. Not all persons with the purge disorder have loss of enamel on teeth, especially if the disorder has developed recently. Mallory-Weiss tears are small tears in the esophageal mucosa caused by forceful vomiting, but they aren't always present in bulimic clients.

➡️ *NCLEX keys*
Client needs category: Physiological integrity
Client needs subcategory: Physiological adaptation
Cognitive level: Application

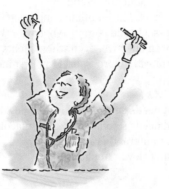

9. A client newly diagnosed with bulimia nervosa is working with the nurse to prepare for a family meeting. Which educational topic should the nurse discuss with the client's family during the meeting?
1. The family emphasis on individualism
2. The myth of the perfect family
3. The need to stop pharmacological intervention
4. The correlation of learning disabilities with disordered eating

Answer: 2. A client with a diagnosis of bulimia nervosa commonly comes from a family in which there's strong parental criticism. The family also places a high value on the idea of being perfect in all aspects of someone's life; the nurse needs to begin dismantling the myth of the perfect family. The emphasis on individualism wouldn't contribute to an eating disorder. Pharmacological intervention is frequently a necessary part of treatment and isn't discontinued in the early phase of treatment. There's no correlation between learning disabilities and eating disorders.

➡️ *NCLEX keys*
Client needs category: Physiological integrity
Client needs subcategory: Reduction of risk potential
Cognitive level: Analysis

10. A nurse is caring for a client who has an eating disorder. Which nursing interventions would be appropriate for this client?
1. Weigh the client once or twice per week, and contract for amount of food to be eaten.
2. Weigh the client daily, and allow the client to use the bathroom ½ hour after eating.
3. Provide one-on-one support before meals.
4. Contract amount of food to be eaten, and weigh the client twice daily.

Answer: 1. Weighing the client more often than once or twice per week reinforces the client's excessive emphasis on weight. The client shouldn't be allowed to use the bathroom any sooner than 90 minutes after eating without supervision. One-on-one support for the client must be undertaken before, during, and after meals — not just before meals.

➡️ *NCLEX keys*
Client needs category: Physiological integrity
Client needs subcategory: Physiological adaptation
Cognitive level: Application

It's been a long, strange trip through the mind, so give your brain a rest. Then move on to the next section.

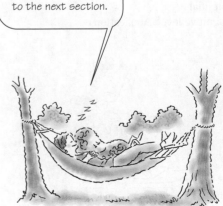

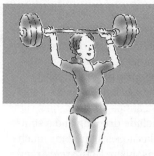

Pump up on more practice questions

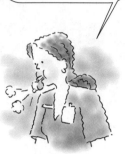

Get set for the exam with 30 psych practice questions. Go for it!

1. A nurse is caring for a client who's sarcastic and critical and commonly expresses feelings that are the opposite of what he's actually feeling. This client is exhibiting which type of behavior?
1. Passive
2. Aggressive
3. Passive-aggressive
4. Assertive

Answer: 3. The passive-aggressive person is commonly sarcastic and critical and expresses feelings that are the opposite of what he actually feels. He defends his rights through resistance. The goal is to dominate through retaliation. Passive behavior is characterized by denying one's own rights to please others. Aggressive behavior is characterized by trying to violate the rights of others, controlling through humiliation. Assertive behavior is characterized by honest, direct assertion of one's rights through effective communication.

➡ *NCLEX keys*
Client needs category: Psychosocial integrity
Client needs subcategory: None
Cognitive level: Application

2. A client is prescribed sertraline (Zoloft), a selective serotonin reuptake inhibitor. Which adverse effect about this drug should the nurse include in medication teaching?
1. Sleep disturbance
2. Agranulocytosis
3. Seizures
4. Pseudoparkinsonism

Answer: 1. A client taking sertraline may experience sleep disturbance. Agranulocytosis and seizures are adverse effects of clozapine (Clozaril). Pseudoparkinsonism is an adverse effect of haloperidol (Haldol).

➡ *NCLEX keys*
Client needs category: Physiological integrity
Client needs subcategory: Reduction of risk potential
Cognitive level: Application

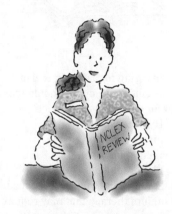

3. A nurse is teaching a client receiving a monoamine oxidase inhibitor (MAOI) about his drug therapy. The client demonstrates understanding by expressing the need to avoid tyramine-containing foods and that even moderate amounts of tyramine must be avoided to prevent hypertensive crisis. The nurse asks the client to list specific tyramine-containing foods. The client would be correct in naming which of the following foods?
1. Swiss cheese
2. Cream cheese
3. Milk
4. Ice cream

Answer: 1. Fermented, aged, or smoked foods tend to be high in tyramine and should be avoided. Cream cheese, milk, and ice cream are unfermented milk products that may be taken with MAOIs without incident.

➡ *NCLEX keys*
Client needs category: Physiological integrity
Client needs subcategory: Pharmacological and parenteral therapies
Cognitive level: Application

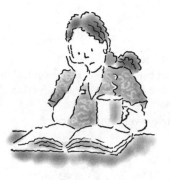

4. When caring for a client receiving lithium (Eskalith), the nurse should monitor the client for which adverse effect?
1. Hypertension
2. Fine hand tremors
3. Weight loss
4. Fluid retention

Answer: 2. Fine hand tremors are an adverse effect of lithium therapy that may require a dosage adjustment. Other adverse effects include hypotension, weight gain, polyuria, and dehydration. Hypertension, weight loss, and fluid retention aren't adverse effects associated with lithium therapy.

➡ *NCLEX keys*
Client needs category: Physiological integrity
Client needs subcategory: Pharmacological and parenteral therapies
Cognitive level: Knowledge

5. A client on antipsychotic drugs begins to exhibit bizarre facial and tongue movements. Based on these findings, the client is most likely exhibiting signs and symptoms of which disorder?
1. Akinesia
2. Pseudoparkinsonism
3. Tardive dyskinesia
4. Oculogyric crisis

Answer: 3. Clients on long-term antipsychotic therapy are at risk for tardive dyskinesia, which causes bizarre facial and tongue movements. Symptoms are potentially irreversible. Pseudoparkinsonism may also occur in clients on antipsychotic drugs; signs and symptoms include drooling and a shuffling gait. Akinesia causes symptoms much like pseudoparkinsonism. Both are extrapyramidal adverse effects. Oculogyric crisis is uncontrolled rolling back of the eyes, which sometimes occurs in epidemic encephalitis or postencephalitic parkinsonism.

➡ *NCLEX keys*
Client needs category: Physiological integrity
Client needs subcategory: Pharmacological and parenteral therapies
Cognitive level: Application

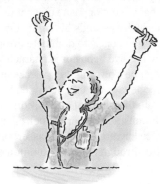

6. The emergency department nurse admits a client who ingested 12 lithium tablets instead of 2 tablets 12 hours ago. Which equipment should the nurse make available to use with this critically ill client?
1. Gastric lavage
2. Balloon tamponade
3. Peritoneal dialysis
4. Insulin pump

Answer: 3. A client suffering from lithium toxicity is a candidate for peritoneal dialysis or hemodialysis. Gastric lavage should only be used within 1 hour of ingestion of the lithium. Balloon tamponade is a modality used for esophageal bleeding, not lithium toxicity. An insulin pump wouldn't be useful to treat lithium toxicity.

Client needs category: Physiological integrity
Client needs subcategory: Pharmacological and parenteral therapies
Cognitive level: Application

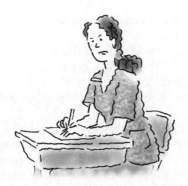

7. The brother of a client admitted to the hospital in an acute manic phase questions the nurse about why the psychiatrist would discuss electroconvulsive therapy (ECT) as a potential treatment modality with the family. Which response best answers the family member's question?

1. "Clients with bipolar disorder are given ECT to prevent the depression side of the bipolar cycle."
2. "Clients who don't tolerate the medications used for bipolar disorder are considered for ECT treatment."
3. "Clients with bipolar disorder and chronic undifferentiated schizophrenia are commonly given ECT."
4. "Clients experiencing disordered eating patterns and difficulty with control of manic symptoms are ECT candidates."

Answer: 2. A client diagnosed with bipolar disorder in the acute manic phase who isn't responding to any type of antimanic medication is a candidate for ECT. ECT is never given to prevent depression in clients with bipolar disorder, to clients with bipolar disorder and chronic undifferentiated schizophrenia disorders, or to clients with eating disorders.

➡ *NCLEX keys*
Client needs category: Physiological integrity
Client needs subcategory: Pharmacological and parenteral therapies
Cognitive level: Application

8. Which nursing diagnosis would be most appropriate for the client who has undergone the full course of electroconvulsive therapy (ECT)?

1. *Deficient knowledge related to memory loss*
2. *Noncompliance related to knowledge deficit*
3. *Disturbed thought processes related to adverse effects of ECT*
4. *Fear related to the unknown*

Answer: 3. Because memory loss is a common adverse effect of ECT, *disturbed thought processes* is the most appropriate nursing diagnosis for this client. Every attempt should be made to educate the client's family so they can adequately care for the client at home. *Noncompliance* isn't an appropriate diagnosis for a client who has undergone a full course of ECT. *Fear* related to the unknown would be an appropriate diagnosis for the client before ECT.

➡ *NCLEX keys*
Client needs category: Psychosocial integrity
Client needs subcategory: None
Cognitive level: Analysis

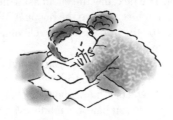

9. Which nursing intervention is most appropriate when planning care for the client with anorexia nervosa?

1. Have the client weigh herself at the same time every day.
2. Have the client record her food intake after she has eaten.
3. Remain with the client during mealtime and observe her for 2 hours after eating.
4. Recommend that the client not eat snacks so that she can eat at mealtime.

Answer: 3. The client with an eating disorder requires supervision during and after meals to ensure that she eats and doesn't try to vomit after eating. The client may record her weight, but the nurse must be present to weigh the client to ensure that the weight is recorded accurately. The nurse should leave snacks for the client so food is always available.

➡ NCLEX keys
Client needs category: Physiological integrity
Client needs subcategory: Reduction of risk potential
Cognitive level: Application

10. A depressed client is voluntarily admitted to the inpatient unit after a suicide attempt. The next day the client asks the nurse when he can leave the hospital. Which response by the nurse gives the client accurate information?
1. "I really can't say; you'll need to talk to your psychiatrist."
2. "Let's talk more about discharge after you have been fully evaluated."
3. "After you've been admitted, you'll have no say without a lawyer."
4. "After 1 week of therapy you'll probably be permitted to leave."

Answer: 2. The client was admitted voluntarily; however, after an evaluation by the health team, the client may be found to be a danger to himself and be required to remain hospitalized. Telling the client that you don't know doesn't accurately provide the client with information about discharge. Telling the client that he'll have no say without a lawyer or that he'll be able to leave after 1 week are inaccurate.

➡ NCLEX keys
Client needs category: Psychosocial integrity
Client needs subcategory: None
Cognitive level: Application

11. Which intervention by the nurse takes top priority when caring for a client with dementia?
1. Providing foods that are easy to eat
2. Providing the opportunity for rest and sleep
3. Keeping the incontinent client clean and dry
4. Creating a safe environment

Answer: 4. Safety takes top priority when caring for the client with dementia. Providing foods that are easy to eat, providing rest and sleep, and keeping the incontinent client clean and dry are all important when caring for the client with dementia, but safety takes top priority.

➡ NCLEX keys
Client needs category: Psychosocial integrity
Client needs subcategory: None
Cognitive level: Application

12. The adult daughter of a client manifesting dementia expresses concern about her elderly father still driving his car. Which response by the nurse will educate the woman about mild dementia?
1. "His inability to concentrate and the tendency to get lost is a problem to address."
2. "The agitation that will occur when you stop him from driving will be severe."
3. "His inability to obtain adequate sleep poses the risk of reckless driving."
4. "The sundowning effect that occurs in people with mild dementia prohibits driving."

Answer: 1. A client with mild dementia can't concentrate and has a tendency to get lost due to memory loss. The symptoms of agitation, disordered sleep, and sundowning occur in the later stage of dementia.

Client needs category: Safe and effective care environment
Client needs subcategory: Safety and infection control
Cognitive level: Application

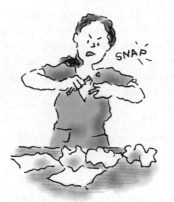

13. A postoperative client who had outpatient surgery for hernia repair begins to experience tremors, irritability, and headache upon discharge. For which information would the nurse check in the history and physical examination section of the client's chart?

1. Panic attacks
2. Substance use
3. Transient disorientation
4. Situational crisis

Answer: 2. A postoperative client experiencing tremors, irritability, and headache upon discharge is most likely going into alcohol withdrawal, which tends to occur 4 to 12 hours after stopping a heavy intake of alcohol. The symptoms that the client is experiencing are not typical symptoms of panic attacks, transient disorientation, or situational crisis.

➡ *NCLEX keys*
Client needs category: Safe and effective care environment
Client needs subcategory: Safety and infection control
Cognitive level: Application

14. A client who has a long history of alcohol abuse is experiencing cardiac problems. The client says to the nurse, "I never had heart problems before, and I don't

understand why I need to stop drinking." Which response by the nurse helps the client understand the relationship between his heart condition and drinking alcohol?

1. "Alcohol can do odd things to the physical functioning of the body."
2. "Alcohol can cause weight gain, and the extra weight can cause heart problems."
3. "Alcohol decreases blood flow to the heart and causes muscle weakness."
4. "Alcohol causes a vitamin D deficiency that over time injures the heart muscle."

Answer: 3. A client with a long history of alcohol abuse will experience cardiac problems because alcohol decreases blood flow to the heart muscle, causing the heart to become weak and deteriorate. Cardiomyopathy is a common condition that results from long-term alcohol abuse. Telling the client that odd things can happen to his body isn't providing him with useful information about his situation. Clients who abuse alcohol can have weight gain or weight loss. A vitamin D deficiency contributes to the development of peripheral neuropathy, not cardiac disease.

➡ *NCLEX keys*
Client needs category: Health promotion and maintenance
Client needs subcategory: None
Cognitive level: Analysis

15. A client who abuses cocaine tells the nurse that he's seeking treatment because he's struggling with withdrawal symptoms. Which assessment question should help the nurse to understand the withdrawal symptoms the client is experiencing?

1. "Have you had the sensation of wanting to yawn?"
2. "Have you experienced discharge from your nose?"
3. "Have you felt cold and had goose bumps?"
4. "Have you been feeling depressed or hopeless?"

Answer: 4. A client withdrawing from cocaine is prone to severe depression (*post coke blues*) and the nurse needs to assess for this health problem. A yawning sensation, discharge from the nose, and feeling cold with goose bumps are all symptoms related to opioid withdrawal.

➡ *NCLEX keys*

Client needs category: Physiological integrity
Client needs subcategory: Reduction of risk potential
Cognitive level: Application

16. A nurse is caring for a client with

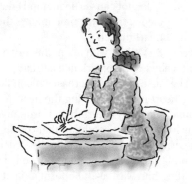

Wernicke's encephalopathy. When developing a teaching plan for the client and his family, the nurse should stress the importance of including which vitamin in his diet?
1. Niacin
2. Riboflavin
3. Ascorbic acid
4. Thiamine

Answer: 4. Wernicke's encephalopathy is a neurologic disorder seen in a client with chronic alcohol abuse that results from thiamine deficiency. The client should be encouraged to eat a diet rich in thiamine. Niacin, riboflavin, and ascorbic acid deficiencies aren't implicated in Wernicke's encephalopathy.

➡ *NCLEX keys*

Client needs category: Physiological integrity
Client needs subcategory: Reduction of risk potential
Cognitive level: Analysis

17. A client with alcohol dependence has completed a rehabilitation program and now attends Alcoholics Anonymous (AA) meetings three times per week. Which statement by the client best reflects an understanding of AA?

1. "I have to attend these meetings until I can control my drinking."
2. "The organization will see that I get therapy if I begin to drink again."
3. "AA will help me remain sober."
4. "AA will help me find shelter and a job."

Answer: 3. AA is a self-help organization that helps attendees maintain sobriety through mutual support. Total abstinence is the only effective treatment for alcohol abuse. Social drinking isn't possible for the alcoholic. AA doesn't provide counseling, shelter, or jobs.

➡ *NCLEX keys*

Client needs category: Psychosocial integrity
Client needs subcategory: None
Cognitive level: Analysis

18. A client tells the nurse that he has been using ecstasy every weekend with his friends. He states, "Using ecstasy isn't dangerous because there are no withdrawal problems." Which response by the nurse is the most appropriate?
1. "There's psychological addiction because people usually become dependent on taking the drug."
2. "It's hard to say if a physical addiction exists, but that shouldn't be an excuse to use the drug."
3. "Sometimes these types of drugs have individual adverse effects that are not well known."
4. "All drugs have withdrawal symptoms and adverse effects, and they can cause health problems."

Answer: 1. The withdrawal effects of hallucinogens are not clearly established because these drugs are not known to be physically addictive. However, there's usually a psychological addiction that occurs because the user feels increasingly dependent on them. The other responses don't provide the client with accurate information about the hallucinogens.

➡ *NCLEX keys*

Client needs category: Physiological integrity
Client needs subcategory: Reduction of risk potential
Cognitive level: Application

19. On the treatment plan for a client diagnosed with schizophrenia, one of the goals is to discuss issues that reinforce reality. Which intervention should the nurse use to assist the client to meet this goal?

1. Tell the client to look for discrepancies between what he thinks and feels.
2. Teach the client how external stressors can cause him to have hallucinations.
3. Limit the number of interpersonal relationships that he has while in treatment.
4. Discourage his use of illegal substances and explain how they can cause him to hallucinate.

Answer: 2. Helping a client to understand that external stressors can provoke hallucinations can assist the client to recognize and avoid these stressors and enhance coping ability. Telling him to look for discrepancies between what he thinks and feels and limiting the number of relationships he has during treatment encourage the client to focus internally on himself and not engage with external reality. Discouraging his use of illegal substances assumes that he abuses substances that can alter his perceptions of reality.

➡ *NCLEX keys*
Client needs category: Psychosocial integrity
Client needs subcategory: Psychosocial adaptation
Cognitive level: Analysis

20. A client tells the nurse that he can't eat because his food has been poisoned. This statement is an indication of:

1. paranoia.
2. delusions of persecution.
3. hallucination.
4. illusion.

Answer: 1. Paranoia is described as extreme suspiciousness of others and their intentions. Delusions of persecution are feelings that others intend harm or persecution. A hallucination is a false sensory perception associated without real external stimuli. Illusions are misperceptions of real external stimuli.

➡ *NCLEX keys*
Client needs category: Psychosocial integrity
Client needs subcategory: None
Cognitive level: Application

21. A client tells the nurse that a voice keeps telling him to crawl on his hands and knees like a dog. Which response by the nurse is the most appropriate for this client?

1. "They're just imaginary voices and they will go away."
2. "If it makes you feel better, do what the voices tell you."
3. "I don't hear them, but I understand that you do."
4. "Even though I don't hear the voices, I understand that you do."

Answer: 4. By telling the client that she doesn't hear the voices, the nurse lets the client know that the voices aren't real to her. The nurse follows with a validation of the client's statement that opens a line of communication and encourages the client to talk about his hallucinations. In the other comments, using the words "they" and "them" in describing the voices reinforces the client's perception that they actually exist, which isn't appropriate.

➡ *NCLEX keys*
Client needs category: Psychosocial integrity
Client needs subcategory: None
Cognitive level: Analysis

22. A nurse is developing a teaching plan for the client receiving clozapine (Clozaril). The nurse should include the importance of which aspect of follow-up care?

  1. A monthly EEG
  2. A cardiology consult
  3. An echocardiogram
  4. Routine complete blood count with differential

Answer: 4. Clozapine can cause a potentially fatal blood dyscrasia characterized by decreased white blood cells and severe neutropenia. Although this adverse effect is rare, it's potentially fatal if not detected early. Clozapine can also cause drowsiness, sedation, excessive salivation, tachycardia, dizziness, and seizures. A monthly EEG, a cardiology consult, and an echocardiogram aren't a necessary part of follow-up care for the client taking clozapine.

➡ *NCLEX keys*
Client needs category: Physiological integrity
Client needs subcategory: Pharmacological and parenteral therapies
Cognitive level: Application

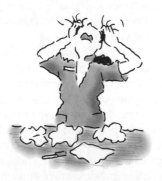

23. A client is admitted to the facility in the manic phase of bipolar disorder. When placing a diet order for the client, which foods are most appropriate?

  1. A bowl of soup, crackers, and a dish of peaches
  2. A cheese sandwich, carrot sticks, fresh grapes, and cookies
  3. Roast chicken, mashed potatoes, and peas
  4. A tuna sandwich, an apple, and a dish of ice cream

Answer: 2. The client may have a difficult time sitting long enough to eat his meal; therefore, finger foods that can be eaten easily are most appropriate. The other foods require the client to sit and eat, a task the client will be unable to achieve at this time.

➡ *NCLEX keys*
Client needs category: Physiological integrity
Client needs subcategory: Basic care and comfort
Cognitive level: Application

24. A client with a history of panic attacks seeks to increase social interaction. Each time the client tries to go to the day room, she begins to perspire and becomes short of breath. Which action by the nurse will help ease the client's feelings of panic?

  1. Have other clients volunteer to accompany the client.
  2. Tell the client she has to overcome her fear.
  3. Allow the client to stay in her room.
  4. Walk with the client and stay with her while she's in the day room.

Answer: 4. The client may find security in the presence of a trusted person. Her fears are very real and she'll need the emotional support of caring professionals, rather than other clients, to overcome them. Telling the client she has to overcome her fears minimizes her feelings. Allowing the client to stay in her room doesn't help the client overcome her feelings of panic.

➡ *NCLEX keys*
Client needs category: Psychosocial integrity
Client needs subcategory: None
Cognitive level: Application

25. During the night, a 50-year-old Vietnam veteran with posttraumatic stress syndrome wakens shaking and tells you that someone is trying to smother him. What's the appropriate response for the nurse in this situation?

  1. "It was a bad dream. You're safe. I'll stay here with you until you go back to sleep."
  2. "We can talk about it tomorrow. Try to see if you can get back to sleep."
  3. "It was only a dream. There's nothing to be frightened about."

4. "I'll call the physician and see whether I can get you medication to help you go back to sleep."

Answer: 1. The important intervention is to assist the client to feel safe. Staying with him until he can sleep again or listening to him if he wants to talk is the most appropriate action for the nurse to take in this situation. Talking about it in the morning won't comfort the client when he's most upset. Stating that it was only a dream trivializes his experience. Calling the physician for a sleeping aid doesn't help the client cope with stress.

➡ *NCLEX keys*
Client needs category: Psychosocial integrity
Client needs subcategory: None
Cognitive level: Application

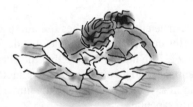

26. A 45-year-old female has constant complaints of dizziness and weakness. The client has been referred to specialists for medical evaluation. All tests have been negative. The physician has concluded that the client has a somatic disorder. How should the nurse deal with this client?
1. Review the test results with the client so she understands there's nothing physically wrong with her.
2. Tell the client that if she develops more outside interests she won't focus on her physical symptoms so much.
3. Accept the fact that the physical complaint is real to the client.
4. Ignore the client's complaints.

Answer: 3. To deny the client's physical complaint is nontherapeutic and prevents the development of a trusting, therapeutic relationship. The nurse should accept the client's problem despite the fact that it isn't organic. Other actions, such as reviewing test results, telling her to develop outside interests, or ignoring the client's complaints, aren't appropriate ways to deal with this client.

➡ *NCLEX keys*
Client needs category: Psychosocial integrity
Client needs subcategory: None
Cognitive level: Application

27. A client is being taught how to manage the adverse effects of the antipsychotic medication that he has been prescribed. Which information does the nurse need to include in the teaching plan?
1. Always keep an over-the-counter (OTC) bottle of loperamide (Imodium) available.
2. Have vision checked by an ophthalmologist to prevent double vision.
3. Use OTC artificial tears as an effective treatment for eye dryness.
4. Drink caffeinated beverages throughout the day to handle the feeling of being sleepy.

Answer: 3. A client taking an antipsychotic medication will commonly experience the adverse effect of dry eyes and should be instructed to use artificial tears. Antipsychotic medications tend to cause constipation, not diarrhea. Antipsychotic medications tend to cause blurred vision, not double vision. Sedation is a less common adverse effect of antipsychotic drugs and it will resolve itself; the client needs to be reminded to stay active.

➡ *NCLEX keys*
Client needs category: Physiological integrity
Client needs subcategory: Basic care and comfort
Cognitive level: Application

28. A client recently prescribed antipsychotic medication comes to the hospital emergency department with a high fever and parkinsonian-type symptoms. The staff suspects the client may have neuroleptic malignant syndrome (NMS). What's the most common progression of symptoms of NMS? Use all the options.
1. Stupor
2. Elevated vital signs
3. Muscle rigidity
4. Deteriorated mental status

Answer:
3. Muscle rigidity
2. Elevated vital signs
4. Deteriorated mental status
1. Stupor

A client with NMS first demonstrates severe parkinsonian muscle rigidity. Next, he experiences an elevation in temperature and pulse and respiratory rates. Last, there's a deterioration in mental status that leads to stupor and coma.

➡ *NCLEX keys*

Client needs category: Safe and effective care environment
Client needs subcategory: Management of care
Cognitive level: Application

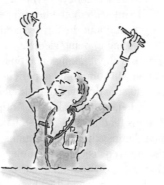

29. A physician starts a client on the antipsychotic medication haloperidol (Haldol). The nurse is aware that this medication has extrapyramidal adverse effects. Which measures should the nurse take during haloperidol administration? Select all that apply.
1. Review subcutaneous injection technique.
2. Closely monitor vital signs, especially temperature.
3. Provide the client with the opportunity to pace.
4. Monitor blood glucose levels.
5. Provide the client with hard candy.
6. Monitor for signs and symptoms of urticaria.

Answer: 2, 3, 5. Neuroleptic malignant syndrome is a life-threatening extrapyramidal adverse effect of antipsychotic medications such as haloperidol. It's associated with a rapid increase in temperature. The most common extrapyramidal adverse effect, akathisia, is a form of psychomotor restlessness that can usually be relieved by pacing. Haloperidol and the anticholinergic medications that are provided to alleviate its extrapyramidal effects can result in dry mouth. Providing the client with hard candy to suck on can help alleviate this problem. Haloperidol isn't given subcutaneously and doesn't affect blood glucose levels. Urticaria isn't usually associated with haloperidol administration.

➡ *NCLEX keys*

Client needs category: Physiological integrity
Client needs subcategory: Pharmacological and parenteral therapies
Cognitive level: Analysis

30. A male client approaches the nurse and says "Hey cutie, can you take me outside for a smoke?" The nurse is aware that the client isn't supposed to go out to smoke for another 15 minutes. Which response by the nurse is most therapeutic?
1. "Sure, I'm not busy right now."
2. "You can ask the technician. I'm busy right now."
3. "You'll be able to smoke in 15 minutes. Calling me cutie is disrespectful."
4. "You know the rules. It isn't time yet for you to go out to smoke."

Answer: 3. The client's behavior indicates that he has difficulty adhering to limits and respecting boundaries. The nurse must place limits on the client's manipulative behavior. Taking the client outside to smoke is inappropriate because the nurse is allowing the client to manipulate her. Referring the client to the technician is incorrect because the nurse isn't addressing the client's manipulative behavior. Offering an abrupt response, such as "You know the rules," may cause the client to act defensively.

➡ *NCLEX keys*

Client needs category: Psychosocial integrity
Client needs subcategory: None
Cognitive level: Application

Part IV   Maternal-neonatal care

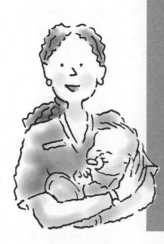

22 Antepartum care

Brush up on key concepts

Antepartum care refers to care of a mother before childbirth. Knowledge of the physiologic changes that accompany pregnancy and fetal development is essential to understanding client care during the antepartum period.

At any time, you can review the major points of this chapter by consulting the *Cheat sheet* on pages 494 to 496.

Normal antepartum period

Nursing care during the normal antepartum period includes taking a thorough maternal history, performing a complete physical examination, and educating the client about antepartum health.

SIGNS AND SYMPTOMS OF PREGNANCY

The client may experience presumptive, probable, or positive signs of pregnancy.

Could be

Presumptive signs of pregnancy include:
• amenorrhea or slight, painless spotting of unknown cause in early gestation
• breast enlargement and tenderness
• fatigue
• increased skin pigmentation
• nausea and vomiting
• quickening (first recognizable movement of fetus)
• urinary frequency and urgency.

Probably is

Probable signs of pregnancy include:
• ballottement (passive fetal movement in response to tapping the lower portion of the uterus or cervix)
• Braxton Hicks contractions (painless uterine contractions that occur throughout pregnancy)
• Chadwick's sign (color of the vaginal walls changes from normal light pink to deep violet)
• Goodell's sign (softening of the cervix)
• Hegar's sign (softening of the lower uterine segment) may be present at 6 to 8 weeks' gestation
• positive pregnancy test results
• abdominal and uterine enlargement
• abdominal strain.

Definitely is

Positive signs of pregnancy include:
• detection of fetal heartbeat (by 17 to 20 weeks' gestation)
• detection of fetal movements (after 16 weeks' gestation)
• ultrasound findings (as early as 6 weeks' gestation).

PHYSIOLOGIC ADAPTATIONS

Here's a review of how body systems adapt to pregnancy.

My ever changin' heart

Cardiovascular system changes include:
• cardiac hypertrophy from increased blood volume and cardiac output
• displacement of the heart upward and to the left from pressure on the diaphragm
• progressive increase in blood volume, peaking in the third trimester at 30% to 50% of levels before pregnancy
• resting pulse rate fluctuations, with increases ranging from 15 to 20 beats/minute at term

(Text continues on page 496.)

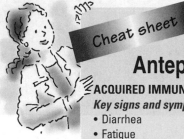

Antepartum care refresher

ACQUIRED IMMUNODEFICIENCY SYNDROME
Key signs and symptoms
- Diarrhea
- Fatigue
- Kaposi's sarcoma
- Mild flulike symptoms
- Opportunistic infections, such as toxoplasmosis, oral and vaginal candidiasis, herpes simplex, *Pneumocystis carinii,* and *Candida* esophagitis
- Anorexia and weight loss

Key test results
- $CD4^+$ T-cell level is less than 200 cells/µl.
- Enzyme-linked immunosorbent assay shows positive human immunodeficiency virus antibody titer.
- Western blot test is positive.

Key treatments
- If the client is newly diagnosed, zidovudine (Retrovir) or didanosine (Videx) treatment initiated at 14 to 34 weeks' gestation

Key interventions
- Assess whether the client can care for her infant after delivery.

ADOLESCENT PREGNANCY
Key signs and symptoms
- Denial of pregnancy, which may deter the adolescent from seeking medical attention early in the pregnancy

Key test results
- Pregnancy test is positive.

Key treatments
- Diet with caloric intake that supports the growing adolescent and her developing fetus

Key interventions
- Monitor the adolescent's weight gain.
- Advise the adolescent of her options, including terminating the pregnancy, continuing the pregnancy and giving up the infant for adoption, or continuing the pregnancy and keeping the infant.

DIABETES MELLITUS
Key signs and symptoms
- Glycosuria
- Ketonuria
- Polyuria

Key test results
- One-hour glucose tolerance test reveals glucose level greater than 140 mg/dl.

Key treatments
- 1,800- to 2,200-calorie diet divided into three meals and three snacks that should also include low fat and cholesterol and high fiber
- Insulin or glyburide (DiaBeta) after the first trimester

Key interventions
- Encourage adherence to dietary regulations.
- Encourage the client to exercise moderately.
- Prepare the client for antepartum fetal surveillance testing, including oxytocin challenge testing, nipple stimulation stress testing, amniotic fluid index, biophysical profile, and nonstress test (NST).

ECTOPIC PREGNANCY
Key signs and symptoms
- Irregular vaginal bleeding; possible amenorrhea followed by bleeding
- Abdominal or pelvic pain; may be sharp or dull
- Rupture of tubes, causing sudden and severe abdominal pain, syncope, and referred shoulder pain as the abdomen fills with blood
- Uterine size smaller than expected for gestational age

Key test results
- Human chorionic gonadotropin (HCG) titers are abnormally low when compared to a normal pregnancy.
- Serum progesterone levels are lower than in a normal pregnancy.

Key treatments
- Laparotomy to ligate the bleeding vessels and remove or repair damaged fallopian tube
- If the tube hasn't ruptured, methotrexate (Trexall) followed by leucovorin to stop trophoblastic cells from growing (therapy continues until negative HCG levels are achieved)

Key interventions
- Monitor for severe abdominal pain, orthostatic hypotension, tachycardia, and dizziness.
- Administer blood products and monitor closely during infusion.
- Administer $Rh_o(D)$ immune globulin (RhoGAM) to clients who are Rh-negative.

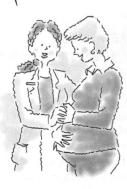

Don't forget, pregnancy itself is NOT a disorder. Effective nursing care usually involves listening to and reassuring healthy mothers.

Antepartum care refresher *(continued)*

HEART DISEASE

Key signs and symptoms
- Tachycardia
- Dyspnea
- Fatigue
- Diastolic murmur at the heart's apex
- Crackles at the base of the lungs

Key test results
- Echocardiography, electrocardiography, and chest X-ray may reveal cardiac abnormalities, impaired cardiac function, and cardiovascular decompensation.

Key treatments
Class III and IV
- Anticoagulant: heparin
- Antiarrhythmics: digoxin (Lanoxin), procainamide, beta-adrenergic blockers
- Thiazide diuretics and furosemide (Lasix) to control heart failure if activity restriction and reduced sodium intake don't prevent it

Key interventions
- Assess cardiovascular and respiratory status.
- Administer oxygen by nasal cannula or face mask during labor.
- Position the client on her left side with her head and shoulders elevated during labor.

HYDATIDIFORM MOLE

Key signs and symptoms
- Intermittent or continuous bright red or brownish vaginal bleeding by 12 weeks' gestation
- Absence of fetal heart sounds

Key test results
- HCG levels are extremely high for early pregnancy
- Ultrasound fails to reveal a fetal skeleton.

Key treatments
- Therapeutic abortion (suction and curettage) if a spontaneous abortion doesn't occur
- Weekly monitoring of HCG levels until they remain normal for 3 consecutive weeks
- Periodic follow-up for 1 to 2 years because of increased risk of neoplasm

Key interventions
- Monitor vaginal bleeding.
- Send contents of uterine evacuation to the laboratory for analysis.

HYPEREMESIS GRAVIDARUM

Key signs and symptoms
- Continuous, severe nausea and vomiting
- Dehydration
- Oliguria

Key test results
- Arterial blood gas analysis reveals metabolic alkalosis.
- Hemoglobin level and hematocrit are elevated.
- Serum potassium level reveals hypokalemia.

Key treatment
- Restoration of fluid and electrolyte balance

Key interventions
- Monitor fundal height and the client's weight.
- Provide small, frequent meals.
- Maintain I.V. fluid replacement and total parenteral nutrition.

HYPERTENSIVE DISORDERS OF PREGNANCY

Key signs and symptoms
Gestational hypertension
- Onset of hypertension without associated proteinuria after 20 weeks' gestation; blood pressure returns to baseline by 12 weeks' postpartum

Preeclampsia
- Hypertension plus proteinuria
- Three categories of preeclampsia
  - Mild preeclampsia: Blood pressure 140/90 mm Hg; 300 mg of proteinuria in 24 hours
  - Severe preeclampsia: Blood pressure 160/110 mm Hg; 5 gm of proteinuria in 24 hours; less than 500 ml of urine in 24 hours
    - Vision disturbances
    - Right upper quadrant tenderness
    - Fetal growth restriction
  - Eclampsia
    - Presence of new-onset grand mal seizures in a client with preeclampsia

Chronic hypertension
- Medically diagnosed hypertension exists before pregnancy
- Gestational hypertension doesn't resolve within 12 weeks of delivery
- Superimposed preeclampsia
- Chronic hypertension plus new-onset proteinuria or other signs and symptoms of preeclampsia

Key test results
- Blood chemistry reveals increased blood urea nitrogen, creatinine, and uric acid levels and elevated liver function studies.

Key treatments
- Bed rest in a left lateral position
- Delivery: with mild preeclampsia, when the fetus is mature and safe induction is possible; with severe preeclampsia regardless of gestational age
- High-protein diet with moderate sodium intake
- Fluid and electrolyte replacement balanced with output

(continued)

Antepartum care refresher *(continued)*

HYPERTENSIVE DISORDERS OF PREGNANCY *(CONTINUED)*

• With severe preeclampsia: antihypertensives, such as hydralazine or labetalol
• Corticosteroid: betamethasone to accelerate fetal lung maturation
• Magnesium sulfate to reduce the amount of acetylcholine produced by motor nerves, thereby preventing seizures

Key interventions
For all clients
• Assess the client for edema and proteinuria.
• Maintain seizure precautions.
• Encourage bed rest in a left lateral recumbent position.
• Monitor blood pressure.
For clients with severe preeclampsia
• Assess maternal blood pressure every 1 to 4 hours or more frequently if unstable.
• Be prepared to obtain a blood sample for typing and cross-matching.
• Keep calcium gluconate (antidote to magnesium sulfate) nearby for administration at first sign of magnesium sulfate toxicity (elevated serum levels, decreased deep tendon reflexes, muscle flaccidity, central nervous system depression, and decreased respiratory rate and renal function).

MULTIFETAL PREGNANCY
Key signs and symptoms
• More than one set of fetal heart sounds
• Uterine size greater than expected for dates

Key test results
• Alpha fetoprotein levels are elevated.
• Ultrasonography is positive for multifetal pregnancy.

Key treatments
• Bed rest if early dilation occurs or at 24 to 28 weeks' gestation
• Biweekly NST to document fetal growth, beginning at 28 weeks' gestation
• Increased intake of calories, iron, folate, and vitamins
• Ultrasound examinations monthly to document fetal growth

Key interventions
• Monitor fetal heart sounds.
• Monitor maternal vital signs and weight.
• Monitor cardiovascular and pulmonary status.

PLACENTA PREVIA
Key signs and symptoms
• Painless, bright red vaginal bleeding, especially during the third trimester

Key test results
• Early ultrasound evaluation reveals the placenta implanted in the lower uterine segment.

Key treatments
• Treatment based on gestational age, when first episode occurs, and amount of bleeding
• If gestational age less than 34 weeks, hospitalizing the client and restricting her to bed rest to avoid preterm labor
• Treatment of choice: surgical intervention (by cesarean deliver) depending on placental placement and maternal and fetal stability

Key interventions
• Don't perform rectal or vaginal examinations unless equipment is available for vaginal and cesarean delivery.

• pulmonic systolic and apical systolic murmurs resulting from decreased blood viscosity and increased blood flow
• increased femoral venous pressure caused by impaired circulation from the lower extremities (resulting from the pressure of the enlarged uterus on the pelvic veins and inferior vena cava)
• decreased cerebrospinal fluid space from enlargement of the vessels surrounding the spinal cord's dura mater
• increased fibrinogen levels (up to 50% at term) from hormonal influences
• increased levels of blood coagulation factors VII, IX, and X, leading to a hypercoagulable state

• increase of about 33% in total red blood cell (RBC) volume, despite hemodilution and decreasing erythrocyte count
• hematocrit (HCT) decrease of about 7%
• increase of 12% to 15% in total hemoglobin (Hb) level; this is less than the overall plasma volume increase, thus reducing Hb concentration and leading to physiologic anemia of pregnancy
• leukocyte production equal to or slightly greater than blood volume increase (average leukocyte count is 10,000 to 11,000/μl; peaks at 25,000/μl during labor, possibly through an estrogen-related mechanism).

Cravings and more

GI system changes include:
• gum swelling from increased estrogen levels; gums may be spongy and bleed easily
• lateral and posterior displacement of the intestines
• superior and lateral displacement of the stomach
• delayed intestinal motility and gastric and gallbladder emptying time from smooth-muscle relaxation caused by high placental progesterone levels, causing heartburn
• nausea and vomiting (usually subside after the first trimester)
• hemorrhoids late in pregnancy from venous pressure
• constipation from increased progesterone levels, resulting in increased water absorption from the colon
• displacement of the appendix from McBurney point (making diagnosis of appendicitis difficult)
• bile saturation with cholesterol, sometimes leading to gallstone formation.

Hormonal changes

Endocrine system changes include:
• increased basal metabolic rate (up 25% at term) caused by demands of the fetus and uterus and by increased oxygen consumption
• increased iodine metabolism from slight hyperplasia of the thyroid caused by increased estrogen levels
• slight hyperparathyroidism from increased requirement for calcium and vitamin D
• elevated plasma parathyroid hormone levels, peaking between 15 and 35 weeks' gestation
• slightly enlarged pituitary gland
• increased production of prolactin by the pituitary gland late in pregnancy
• increased estrogen levels and hypertrophy of the adrenal cortex
• increased cortisol levels to regulate protein and carbohydrate metabolism
• possibly decreased maternal blood glucose levels
• decreased insulin production early in pregnancy
• increased production of estrogen, progesterone, and human chorionic somatomammotropin by the placenta and increased

levels of maternal cortisol, which reduce the mother's ability to use insulin, thus ensuring an adequate glucose supply for the fetus and placenta.

Altered breathing

Respiratory system changes include:
• increased vascularization of the respiratory tract caused by increased estrogen levels
• compression of the lungs caused by the enlarging uterus
• upward displacement of the diaphragm by the uterus
• increased tidal volume, causing slight hyperventilation
• increased chest circumference (by about 2 3/8" [6 cm])
• altered breathing, with abdominal breathing replacing thoracic breathing as pregnancy progresses
• slight increase (2 breaths/minute) in respiratory rate
• lowered threshold for carbon dioxide due to increased levels of progesterone.

Everything increases

Metabolic system changes include:
• increased water retention caused by higher levels of steroidal sex hormones, decreased serum protein levels, and increased intracapillary pressure and permeability
• increased levels of serum lipids, lipoproteins, and cholesterol
• increased iron requirements caused by fetal demands
• increased carbohydrate needs
• increased protein retention from hyperplasia and hypertrophy of maternal tissues
• weight gain of 25 to 35 lb (11.3 to 16 kg). (See *What causes weight gain in pregnancy?*)

Is it getting hot in here?

Integumentary system changes include:
• hyperactive sweat and sebaceous glands
• changing pigmentation from the increase of melanocyte-stimulating hormone caused by increased estrogen and progesterone levels (darkened line from symphysis pubis to umbilicus known as linea nigra)
– darkened nipples, areola, cervix, vagina, and vulva

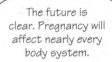

The future is clear. Pregnancy will affect nearly every body system.

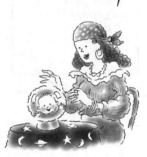

What causes weight gain in pregnancy?

The following factors are responsible for the weight gain that occurs during pregnancy:
• fetus (7.5 lb [3.4 kg])
• placenta and membranes (1.5 lb [0.7 kg])
• amniotic fluid (2 lb [0.9 kg])
• uterus (2.5 lb [1.1 kg])
• breasts (3 lb [1.4 kg])
• blood volume (2 to 4 lb [0.9 to 1.8 kg])
• extravascular fluid and fat reserves (4 to 9 lb [1.8 to 4.1 kg])

– pigmentary changes on nose, cheeks, and forehead known as facial chloasma
• striae gravidarum, commonly known as *stretch marks*, caused by weight gain and enlarged uterus.

Time to go (often)

Changes to the genitourinary system include:

• dilated ureters and renal pelvis caused by progesterone and pressure from the enlarging uterus, increasing the risk of urinary tract infection (UTI)
• increased glomerular filtration rate (GFR) and renal plasma flow (RPF) early in pregnancy; elevated GFR until delivery, but a near-normal RPF by term
• increased clearance of urea and creatinine from increased renal function
• decreased blood urea and nonprotein nitrogen values from increased renal function
• glycosuria from increased glomerular filtration without an increase in tubular reabsorptive capacity
• decreased bladder tone, causing urinary urgency and frequency
• increased sodium retention from hormonal influences
• increased dimensions of uterus
• hypertrophied uterine muscle cells (5 to 10 times normal size)
• increased vascularity, edema, hypertrophy, and hyperplasia of the cervical glands

• increased vaginal secretions with a pH of 3.5 to 6.0
• discontinued ovulation and maturation of new follicles
• thickening of vaginal mucosa, loosening of vaginal connective tissue, and hypertrophy of small-muscle cells. (See *Estimating delivery dates and gestational age*.)

Not just pickles and ice cream

Nutritional needs also change during pregnancy. For example:
• Calorie requirements during pregnancy exceed prepregnancy needs by 300 calories/day (from 2,100 to 2,400 calories/day).
• Protein requirements during pregnancy exceed prepregnancy needs by 30 g/day (from 46 to 76 g/day).
• Intake of all vitamins should increase, and a prenatal vitamin with iron is usually recommended.
• Folic acid intake is particularly important to help prevent fetal anomalies such as neural tube defects. Intake should be increased from 400 to 800 mg/day. Dietary sources of folic acid include green, leafy vegetables and whole-grain breads.
• Intake of all minerals, especially iron, should be increased. (See *Battling discomforts of pregnancy*.)
• Intake of fiber and fluid should be increased.

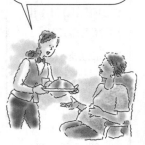

or
toward
9 months
7 days

Estimating delivery dates and gestational age

• Nägele's rule determines the estimated date of delivery by subtracting 3 months from the first day of the last menses and adding 7 days; for example, October 5 − 3 months = July 5 + 7 days = July 12.
• Quickening is described as light fluttering fetal movement felt by the mother and is usually felt between 16 and 22 weeks' gestation.
• Fetal heart sounds can be detected with a Doppler ultrasound at 12 weeks' gestation and can be auscultated with a fetoscope at 16 to 20 weeks' gestation.

• Fetal crown-to-rump measurements, determined by ultrasound, can be used to assess the fetus's age until the head can be defined.
• Biparietal diameter is the widest transverse diameter of the fetal head. Measurements can be made by about 12 to 13 weeks' gestation.
• McDonald's rule uses fundal height in centimeters to determine the duration of pregnancy in weeks. To use this rule, place a tape measure at the symphysis pubis and measure up and over the fundus. Fundal height in centimeters $\times \, ^8/_7 =$ duration of pregnancy in weeks.

Battling discomforts of pregnancy

Education plays an important role in helping the client deal with discomforts.

FIRST-TRIMESTER DISCOMFORTS
Nausea and vomiting
Symptoms may occur at any time during pregnancy but are most prevalent during the first trimester. Teach the client to avoid greasy, highly seasoned foods; to eat small, frequent meals; and to eat dry toast or crackers before arising in the morning. Instruct the client to rise slowly from a lying or sitting position.

Nasal stuffiness, discharge, or obstruction
Advise the client to use a cool-mist vaporizer.

Breast enlargement and tenderness
Tell the client to wear a well-fitting support bra.

Urinary frequency and urgency
Instruct the client to decrease fluid intake in the evening to prevent nocturia, to avoid caffeine-containing fluids, and to respond to the urge to void immediately to prevent bladder distention and urinary stasis. Also teach the client how to perform Kegel exercises, and tell her to promptly report signs of urinary tract infections.

Fatigue
Tell the client to rest periodically throughout the day and to get at least 8 hours of sleep each night.

Increased leukorrhea
Advise the client to bathe daily and wear absorbent cotton underwear.

SECOND- AND THIRD-TRIMESTER DISCOMFORTS
Heartburn
Encourage the client to eat small, frequent meals; avoid fatty or fried foods; remain upright for at least 1 hour after eating; and use antacids that don't contain sodium bicarbonate.

Constipation
Encourage the client to exercise daily, increase fluid and dietary fiber intake, and maintain regular elimination patterns.

Hemorrhoids
Tell the client to avoid constipation, prolonged standing, and constrictive clothing, and advise her to use topical ointments, warm soaks, and anesthetic ointments to relieve symptoms.

Backache
Teach the client how to use proper body mechanics and maintain good posture. Also tell her to avoid wearing high heels.

Leg cramps
Instruct the client to increase calcium, frequently rest with legs elevated, wear warm clothing on the legs and, during a leg cramp, pull the toes up toward the leg while pressing down on the knee.

Shortness of breath
Encourage the client to maintain proper posture, especially when standing, and to sleep in semi-Fowler's position.

Ankle edema
Advise the client to wear loose-fitting garments, elevate the legs during rest periods, and ensure dorsiflexion of the feet if standing or sitting for prolonged periods.

Insomnia
Encourage the client to use relaxation techniques. Tell her to lie on her left side, using pillows to support her legs and abdomen.

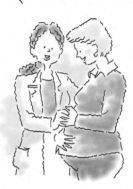

May I suggest you eat small, frequent meals and avoid fatty and fried foods.

Fetal development and structures

Structures unique to the fetus include fetal membranes, the umbilical cord, the placenta, and amniotic fluid.

His and her cells
Intrauterine development begins with **gametogenesis,** the production of specialized sex cells called *gametes.*

- The male gamete (spermatozoon) is produced in the seminiferous tubules of the testes during spermatogenesis.
- The female gamete (ovum) is produced in the graafian follicle of the ovary during oogenesis.
- As gametes mature, the number of chromosomes they contain is halved (through meiosis) from 46 to 23.

The moment of truth
Conception, or fertilization, occurs with the fusion of a spermatozoon and an

ovum (oocyte) in the ampulla of the fallopian tube.
- The fertilized egg is called a **zygote.**
- The diploid number of chromosomes (a pair of each chromosome; 44 autosomes and 2 sex chromosomes) is restored when the zygote is formed.
- A male zygote is formed if the ovum is fertilized by a spermatozoon carrying a Y chromosome.
- A female zygote is formed if the ovum is fertilized by a spermatozoon carrying an X chromosome.

A place to stay
Implantation occurs when the cellular wall of the blastocyst (trophoblast) implants itself in the endometrium of the anterior or posterior fundal region, about 7 to 9 days after fertilization.
- Primary villi appear within weeks after implantation.
- After implantation, the endometrium is called the *decidua.*

The beginning of the placenta
During **placental formation,** chorionic villi invade the decidua and become the fetal portion of the future placenta. By 4 weeks' gestation, a normal fetus begins to show noticeable signs of growth.

Fetal linings
Two fetal membranes are unique to the fetus:
- The **chorion** is the fetal membrane closest to the uterine wall; it gives rise to the placenta.
- The **amnion** is the thin, tough, inner fetal membrane that lines the amniotic sac.

Construction under way
Embryonic germ layers generate these fetal tissues:
- The **ectoderm** generates the epidermis, nervous system, pituitary gland, salivary glands, optic lens, lining of the lower portion of the anal canal, hair, and tooth enamel.

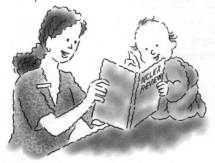

If this is the client's first pregnancy, she'll be referred to as a *primigravida*; otherwise, she's referred to as a *multigravida.*

- The **endoderm** generates the epithelial lining of the larynx, trachea, bladder, urethra, prostate gland, auditory canal, liver, pancreas, and alimentary canal.
- The **mesoderm** generates the connective and supporting tissues; the blood and vascular system; the musculature; teeth (except enamel); mesothelial lining of the pericardial, pleural, and peritoneal cavities; and kidneys and ureters.

The lifeline
The **umbilical cord** serves as the lifeline from the embryo to the placenta. At term, it measures from 20" to 22" (51 to 56 cm) in length and about ¾" (2 cm) in diameter. The umbilical cord contains two arteries, one vein, and Wharton's jelly (which prevents kinking of the cord in utero). Blood flows through the cord at about 400 ml/minute.

Red on the outside, gray on the inside
The **placenta,** weighing about 1 to 1¼ lb (454 to 590 g) and measuring from 6" to 10" (15 to 25 cm) in diameter, contains 15 to 20 subdivisions called cotyledons and is 1" to 1¼" (2.5 to 3 cm) thick at term. Rough in texture, the placenta appears red on the maternal surface and shiny and gray on the fetal surface. The placenta:
- functions as a transport mechanism between the mother and the fetus
- has a life span and function that depends on oxygen consumption and maternal circulation; circulation to the fetus and placenta improves when the mother lies on her left side
- receives maternal oxygen by way of diffusion
- produces hormones, including human chorionic gonadotropin, human placental lactogen, gonadotropin-releasing hormone, thyrotropin-releasing factor, corticotropin, estrogen, and progesterone
- supplies the fetus with carbohydrates, water, fats, protein, minerals, and inorganic salts
- carries end products of fetal metabolism to the maternal circulation for excretion

• transfers passive immunity by way of maternal antibodies.

Fetal protection
The **amniotic fluid** prevents heat loss, preserves constant fetal body temperature, cushions the fetus, and facilitates fetal growth and development. Amniotic fluid is replaced every 3 hours.

At term, the uterus contains 800 to 1,200 ml of amniotic fluid, which is clear and yellowish and has a specific gravity of 1.007 to 1.025 and a pH of 7.0 to 7.25. Maternal serum provides amniotic fluid in early gestation, with increasing amounts derived from fetal urine late in gestation. Amniotic fluid contains:
• albumin
• bilirubin
• creatinine
• enzymes
• fat
• lanugo
• lecithin
• leukocytes
• sphingomyelin
• urea.

Blood movers
Fetal circulation structures include:
• one umbilical vein, which carries oxygenated blood to the fetus from the placenta
• two umbilical arteries, which carry deoxygenated blood from the fetus to the placenta
• the foramen ovale, which serves as the septal opening between the atria of the fetal heart
• the ductus arteriosus, which connects the pulmonary artery to the aorta, allowing blood to shunt around the fetal lungs
• the ductus venosus, which carries oxygenated blood from the umbilical vein to the inferior vena cava, bypassing the liver.

Keep abreast of diagnostic tests

Here's a brief review of tests performed as part of antepartum care.

The routine
These routine laboratory tests can confirm pregnancy and reveal maternal complications:
• **blood type, Rh, and abnormal antibodies** to identify the fetus at risk for erythroblastosis fetalis or hyperbilirubinemia
• **immunologic tests** such as rubella antibodies to detect the presence of rubella, rapid plasma reagin to detect untreated syphilis, hepatitis B surface antigen to detect hepatitis B, and human immunodeficiency virus (HIV) antibodies to detect HIV infection
• **urine tests** to detect UTI and to measure human chorionic gonadotropin (HCG) to confirm pregnancy
• **hematologic studies,** in which blood samples are used to analyze and measure RBCs, white blood cells (WBCs), erythrocyte sedimentation rate, platelets, Hb level, and HCT
• **coagulation studies,** in which a blood sample is used to analyze and measure prothrombin time (PT), partial thromboplastin time (PTT), and International Normalized Ratio (INR)
• **genital cultures,** such as a gonorrhea smear and chlamydia test, to detect sexually transmitted disease (STD)
• **triple screen** between 15 and 20 weeks' gestation to identify if the fetus is at increased risk for Down syndrome and neural tube defects
• **alpha fetoprotein,** which involves using a blood sample to measure alpha fetoprotein levels (high maternal serum levels may suggest fetal neural tube defects, such as spina bifida and anencephaly).

Nursing actions
Before the procedure
• Explain the procedure to the client.
After the procedure
• Check the venipuncture site for bleeding if blood was drawn.
• Label the specimen and send it to the laboratory.

Check your fluid?
Amniocentesis is usually performed after 14 weeks' gestation, when amniotic fluid is

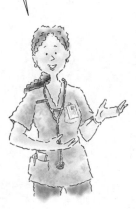

After amniocentesis, monitor the client for hemorrhage, infection, premature labor, and amnionitis.

sufficient and the uterus has moved into the abdominal cavity. This procedure involves transabdominal insertion of a spinal needle into the uterus to aspirate amniotic fluid. This procedure helps determine:
- gestational age by way of a lecithin-sphingomyelin ratio
- fetal lung maturity by analyzing lecithin-sphingomyelin ratio, two key components of surfactant
- creatinine levels.

Amniocentesis is used to diagnose genetic disorders, such as chromosomal aberrations, sex-linked disorders, inborn errors of metabolism, and neural tube defects. It may also be used to diagnose and evaluate isoimmune disorders, including Rh sensitization and ABO blood type incompatibility.

Nursing actions
Before the procedure
- Explain the procedure to the client.
- Make sure informed, written consent is obtained.

After the procedure
- Monitor the fetal heart rate (FHR) and uterine activity with an external fetal or fetal uterine monitor for several hours.
- Monitor for maternal hemorrhage, infection, premature labor, fetal hemorrhage, and amnionitis.
- Administer $Rh_O(D)$ immune globulin (RhoGAM) to Rh-negative mothers to prevent fetal isoimmunization.

Tissue sample
Chorionic villi sampling can be performed as early as 8 weeks' gestation. It involves removal and analysis of a small tissue specimen from the fetal portion of the placenta. This test helps determine the genetic makeup of the fetus, providing earlier diagnosis and allowing earlier and safer abortion if the fetus carries the risk of spontaneous abortion, infection, hematoma, fetal limb defects, and intrauterine death.

Nursing actions
Before the procedure
- Explain the procedure to the client.

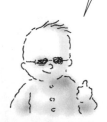

You guessed it...the nonstress test doesn't bother me at all.

After the procedure
- Administer RhoGAM to Rh-negative mothers to prevent Rh sensitization.
- Monitor the FHR and uterine activity with an external fetal monitor for several hours.

Sound picture
Ultrasound, a painless procedure, uses ultrasonic waves reflected by tissues of different densities to visualize deep structures of the body. Reflected signals are then amplified and processed to produce a visual display, providing immediate results without harm to the fetus or mother. It may be performed vaginally, if necessary. Ultrasound can detect fetal death, malformation, or malpresentation; placental abnormalities; multiple gestation; and hydramnios or oligohydramnios. It's used to monitor fetal growth and estimate gestational age.

Nursing actions
Before the procedure
- Explain the procedure to the client.
- Instruct the client to drink a glass of water every 15 minutes, beginning 1½ hours before the procedure.
- Instruct the client not to void until immediately after the procedure.
- If the vaginal approach is necessary, instruct the client to void before the procedure and to avoid fluids.

After the procedure
- Offer a damp cloth to remove the conduction gel used to perform the study.

Stress-free
The **nonstress test** (NST) is used to detect fetal heart accelerations in response to fetal movement. This noninvasive test provides simple, inexpensive, immediate results without contraindications or complications. It may be indicated for a client at risk for uteroplacental insufficiency or for altered fetal movements.

The NST can be given between 32 and 34 weeks' gestation. A nonreactive test result indicates the possibility of fetal hypoxia, fetal sleep cycle, or the effects of drugs. The results may be inconclusive if the client is extremely obese.

Nursing actions
Before the procedure
- Explain the procedure to the client.
- Advise the client to eat a snack before testing.

After the procedure
- Allow the client to resume normal activities.

Contraction action
The **oxytocin challenge test** (OCT) evaluates fetal ability to withstand an oxytocin-induced contraction. This test, given after a nonreactive NST result, requires I.V. administration of oxytocin in increasing doses every 15 to 20 minutes until three high-quality uterine contractions are obtained within 10 minutes.

The OCT is performed on a client at risk for uteroplacental insufficiency or fetal compromise from diabetes, heart disease, hypertension, or renal disease or on a client with a history of stillbirth. The OCT isn't indicated for those with previous classic cesarean delivery or third-trimester bleeding or for those at high risk for preterm labor.

Nursing actions
Before the procedure
- Explain the procedure to the client.

During and after the procedure
- Monitor the FHR and uterine contractions with an external fetal monitor.

Breast test
The **nipple stimulation stress test** induces contractions by activating sensory receptors in the areola, triggering the release of oxytocin by the posterior pituitary gland. The receptors are activated by rolling the nipple manually or by applying a warm washcloth. This test has the same reactive pattern as the reactive NST result.

Nursing actions
Before the procedure
- Explain the procedure to the client.

During and after the procedure
- Monitor the FHR and uterine contractions with an external fetal monitor.

Good vibrations
The **vibroacoustic stimulation** test uses vibration and sound to induce fetal reactivity during an NST. Vibration is produced by an artificial larynx or a fetal acoustic stimulator (over the fetus's head for 1 to 5 seconds). This test is noninvasive, quick, and convenient.

Nursing actions
Before the procedure
- Explain the procedure to the client.

During and after the procedure
- Monitor the FHR with an external fetal monitor.

Six profiles in one
The **biophysical profile** assesses four to six parameters — fetal breathing movements, body movements, muscle tone, amniotic fluid volume, heart rate reactivity, and placental grade — using real-time ultrasound. This test is noninvasive and quick and can detect central nervous system (CNS) depression.

Nursing actions
Before the procedure
- Explain the procedure to the client.

During and after the procedure
- Monitor the FHR with an external fetal monitor.

How does the flow go?
Fetal blood flow studies use umbilical or uterine Doppler velocimetry to evaluate vascular resistance, especially in a client with hypertension, diabetes, isoimmunization, or lupus. These studies are useful when congenital anomalies or cardiac arrhythmias are suspected.

Nursing actions
Before and during the procedure
- Explain the procedure to the client.
- Before the procedure, obtain a baseline FHR.
- During the procedure, continue to monitor the mother and fetus for signs of problems, such as changes in vital signs or FHR or continuation of uterine contractions.

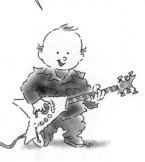

Vibroacoustic stimulation...I dig it!

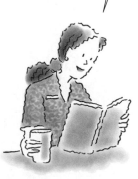

Put it together. Determination and knowledge. That's what you need to pass the exam.

Risky business

Percutaneous umbilical blood sampling (PUBS) is an invasive procedure that involves inserting a spinal needle into the umbilical cord to obtain fetal blood samples or to transfuse blood to the fetus in utero.

Usually performed during the second or third trimester, PUBS is indicated when the fetus is at risk for congenital and chromosomal abnormalities, congenital infection, or anemia. It carries a 1% to 2% risk of fetal loss.

Nursing actions

Before the procedure
- Explain the procedure to the client.
- Obtain a signed informed consent for the procedure.

During and after the procedure
- Monitor fetal and maternal status throughout the procedure.
- Administer RhoGAM to an Rh-negative mother after PUBS to prevent sensitization.

Every kick counts

Fetal movement count identifies the presence and frequency of fetal movement. Normally, fetal movement occurs about 280 times per day. Decreased movement may indicate fetal compromise.

Nursing actions

Before the procedure
- Explain the procedure to the client.
- Teach the client to record fetal movement for 30 minutes three times per day.
- Instruct the client to report fewer than 10 movements in 2 hours.

Polish up on client care

Potential antepartum complications and accompanying conditions include acquired immunodeficiency syndrome (AIDS), adolescent pregnancy, diabetes mellitus, ectopic pregnancy, heart disease, hydatidiform mole, hyperemesis gravidarum, hypertensive disorders of pregnancy, multifetal pregnancy, and placenta previa.

Acquired immunodeficiency syndrome

A female client may be first identified as positive for HIV antibodies during pregnancy or when the neonate's HIV status is identified. Because of the effects of pregnancy on immunosuppression, the progression from HIV infection to full-blown AIDS may be expedited during pregnancy.

CAUSES
- Exposure to HIV through blood transfusions, contaminated needles, or handling of blood
- Exposure to semen or vaginal secretions containing HIV

ASSESSMENT FINDINGS
- Diarrhea
- Fatigue
- HIV-associated dementia
- Kaposi's sarcoma
- Mild flulike symptoms
- Night sweats
- Opportunistic infections, such as toxoplasmosis, oral and vaginal candidiasis, herpes simplex, *Pneumocystis jiroveci* pneumonia, and *Candida* esophagitis
- Anorexia and weight loss

DIAGNOSTIC TEST RESULTS
- Blood chemistry shows increased transaminase, alkaline phosphatase, and gamma globulin level and decreased albumin level.
- $CD4^+$ T-cell level is less than 200 cells/µl.
- Enzyme-linked immunosorbent assay shows positive HIV antibody titer.
- Hematology shows decreased WBC, RBC, and platelet counts.
- Western blot test is positive.

NURSING DIAGNOSES
- Fear
- Fatigue
- Ineffective protection
- Anxiety
- Ineffective coping

TREATMENT

• Care during pregnancy and delivery same as that for any other client with HIV (see "Acquired immunodeficiency syndrome," page 131)
• Fetus monitored closely; serial ultrasounds performed to identify intrauterine growth restrictions; NST performed weekly after 32 weeks' gestation

Drug therapy

• If the client is newly diagnosed, zidovudine (Retrovir) or didanosine (Videx) is typically initiated at 14 to 34 weeks' gestation

INTERVENTIONS AND RATIONALES

• Assess for fever, chest tightness, and shortness of breath *to evaluate for possible recurrent acute pneumonia or pulmonary tuberculosis, which may indicate AIDS.*
• Administer total parenteral nutrition (TPN), if necessary, *to improve and support nutritional status.*
• Provide rest periods *to prevent fatigue.*
• Provide emotional support to the client and her family *to allay her fears.*
• Assess whether the client can care for her infant after delivery *to evaluate the need for additional support services.*

Teaching topics

• Explanation of the disorder and treatment plan
• Medication use and possible adverse effects
• Preventing the spread of infection
• Decreasing the risk of transmission to the fetus by avoiding unsafe sex practices or discontinuing I.V. drug use
• Counseling the client to help her decide whether to terminate the pregnancy

Adolescent pregnancy

A pregnant teenager is at risk for such complications as hypertensive disorders of pregnancy, cephalopelvic disproportion, anemia, and nutritional deficiencies. Teenagers also have a high incidence of STDs, posing a concern for both mother and neonate.

Infants born to teenagers are at risk for such complications as prematurity and low birth weight.

CONTRIBUTING FACTORS

• Peer pressure to be sexually active
• Desire to gain love, adulthood, and independence through pregnancy
• Fear of reporting sexual activity to parents
• High level of adolescent sexual activity
• Lack of appropriate role models
• Limited access to contraceptives
• Low level of education correlated with incorrect use of contraceptives
• Sporadic use of contraceptives
• Naiveté about ability to become pregnant

ASSESSMENT FINDINGS

• Amenorrhea
• Denial of pregnancy, which may deter the adolescent from seeking medical attention early in pregnancy

DIAGNOSTIC TEST RESULTS

• Pregnancy test is positive.
• Ultrasound confirms presence of fetus.

NURSING DIAGNOSES

• Deficient knowledge (pregnancy and care options)
• Imbalanced nutrition: Less than body requirements
• Interrupted family processes
• Fear

TREATMENT

• Diet with caloric intake sufficient to support the growing adolescent and her developing fetus
• Regular prenatal checkups

Drug therapy

• Antibiotics for STDs, if necessary
• Prenatal vitamins with iron

INTERVENTIONS AND RATIONALES

• Monitor the adolescent's weight gain *to assess for nutritional deficiencies.*
• Assess the adolescent's knowledge of her pregnancy *to determine the need for further teaching.*

> Be aware! Teenage mothers are at risk for insufficient or delayed medical care.

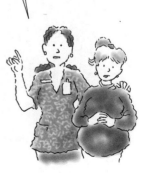

- Collect data about the adolescent's family and available support *to determine the need for referrals.*
- Provide nutritional support and encouragement *to promote the well-being of the mother and fetus.*
- Stress the importance of attending scheduled prenatal appointments *to promote the well-being of mother and fetus.*
- Advise the adolescent of her options, including terminating the pregnancy, continuing the pregnancy and giving up the infant for adoption, or continuing the pregnancy and keeping the infant, *to promote informed decision making.*
- Allow the adolescent to express her feelings about her pregnancy and herself *to promote mental and emotional well-being.*

Teaching topics
- Condition and any identified complications and the treatment plan
- Encouraging attendance at prenatal and birthing classes and infant care classes
- Recognizing the importance of prenatal care

Diabetes mellitus

In gestational diabetes mellitus, the client's pancreas, stressed by the normal adaptations to pregnancy, can't meet the increased demands for insulin.

A client may have preexisting diabetes or may develop gestational diabetes while she's pregnant. Gestational diabetes is associated with an increased risk of congenital anomalies, hydramnios, macrosomia, hypertensive disorders of pregnancy, spontaneous abortion, and fetal death. Additionally, the infant of a client with diabetes is at risk for developing sacral agenesis, a congenital anomaly characterized by incomplete formation of the vertebral column.

The client with gestational diabetes has an increased risk of developing diabetes mellitus at a later time.

RISK FACTORS
- Family history of diabetes
- Gestational diabetes in previous pregnancies
- Maternal age older than 25
- Obesity

ASSESSMENT FINDINGS
- Glycosuria
- Ketonuria
- Polydipsia
- Polyphagia
- Polyuria
- Fatigue
- Acetone breath
- Possible monilial infection (vaginal yeast infection)
- Possible UTI

DIAGNOSTIC TEST RESULTS
- One-hour glucose tolerance test reveals glucose level greater than 140 mg/dl.
- Three-hour glucose tolerance test reveals fasting serum glucose level of 105 mg/dl or greater.
- Three-hour glucose tolerance test reveals 1-hour serum glucose level of 190 mg/dl or greater.
- Three-hour glucose tolerance test reveals 2-hour serum glucose level of 165 mg/dl or greater.
- Three-hour glucose tolerance test reveals 3-hour serum glucose level of 145 mg/dl or greater.

NURSING DIAGNOSES
- Imbalanced nutrition: More than body requirements
- Risk for deficient fluid volume
- Ineffective coping
- Fear
- Anxiety

TREATMENT
- Monitoring of capillary blood sugar
- Exercise
- 1,800- to 2,200-calorie diet, divided into three meals and three snacks that should also include low fat and cholesterol and high fiber

Drug therapy
- Insulin or glyburide (DiaBeta) after the first trimester
- Other oral antidiabetic agents contraindicated because of adverse effects on the fetus

INTERVENTIONS AND RATIONALES
- Encourage adherence to dietary regulations *to maintain euglycemia.*
- Encourage the client to exercise moderately *to reduce blood glucose levels and decrease the need for insulin.*
- Prepare the client for antepartum fetal surveillance testing, including OCT, nipple stimulation stress testing, amniotic fluid index, biophysical profile, and NST, *to assess fetal well-being.*
- Encourage the client to verbalize her feelings *to allay her fears.*
- Provide emotional support *to reduce anxiety.*

Teaching topics
- Explanation of the disorder and treatment plan
- Medication use and possible adverse effects
- Performing capillary glucose monitoring
- Performing fetal "kick counts" to assess fetal well-being during the third trimester

Ectopic pregnancy

Ectopic pregnancy refers to implantation of the fertilized ovum outside the uterine cavity. Most commonly, ectopic pregnancy occurs in a fallopian tube; other sites include the cervix, ovary, and abdominal cavity. It's the second most frequent cause of vaginal bleeding early in pregnancy.

CAUSES
- Hormonal factors
- Malformed fallopian tubes
- Ovulation induction drugs
- Progestin-only hormonal contraceptives
- Tubal atony
- Tubal damage from pelvic inflammatory disease
- Tubal damage from previous pelvic or tubal surgery
- Tubal spasms
- Use of intrauterine devices

ASSESSMENT FINDINGS
- Hypotension
- Irregular vaginal bleeding; possible amenorrhea followed by bleeding
- Abdominal or pelvic pain; may be sharp or dull
- Nausea and vomiting
- Rapid, thready pulse
- Rupture of tubes, causing sudden and severe abdominal pain, syncope, and referred shoulder pain as the abdomen fills with blood
- Shock with profuse hemorrhage
- Uterine size smaller than expected for gestational age

DIAGNOSTIC TEST RESULTS
- HCG titers are abnormally low when compared to a normal pregnancy.
- Ultrasound is positive for ruptured tube and collective pelvic fluid.
- Vaginal examination reveals a palpable tender mass in Douglas' cul-de-sac.
- Serum progesterone levels are lower than in a normal pregnancy.

NURSING DIAGNOSES
- Deficient fluid volume
- Risk for infection
- Acute pain
- Fear

TREATMENT
- Laparotomy to ligate the bleeding vessels and remove or repair damaged fallopian tube
- Transfusion therapy: packed RBCs (if bleeding is uncontrolled)

Drug therapy
- If the tube hasn't ruptured, methotrexate (Trexall) followed by leucovorin to stop trophoblastic cells from growing (therapy continues until negative HCG levels are achieved)

INTERVENTIONS AND RATIONALES
- Monitor vital signs and intake and output *to assess for intense blood loss and shock.*
- Monitor for severe abdominal pain, orthostatic hypotension, tachycardia, and dizziness, *which may indicate rupturing ectopic pregnancy.*
- Administer I.V. fluid *to compensate for blood loss.*
- Administer blood products and monitor closely during infusion *to detect adverse reactions.*

Severe abdominal pain, orthostatic hypotension, tachycardia, and dizziness may indicate a rupturing ectopic pregnancy.

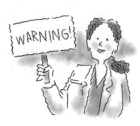

- Administer RhoGAM *to combat isoimmunization in the client who's Rh-negative.*
- Provide routine postoperative care *to promote recovery.*
- Provide emotional support *for parents grieving over the loss of the pregnancy.*

Teaching topics
- Explanation of the disorder and treatment plan
- Medication use and possible adverse effects
- Importance of follow-up medical care

Heart disease

Heart disease occurs in about 1% of pregnant women. Pregnancy may reveal an underlying heart condition that previously produced no symptoms, or it may aggravate a known heart condition. A client with heart disease is at greatest risk when blood volume peaks between 28 and 32 weeks' gestation.

Successful delivery of a healthy baby depends on the type and extent of the disease. Decreased placental perfusion may lead to intrauterine growth retardation, fetal distress, and prematurity.

Pregnant clients with heart disease are graded as class I to IV.

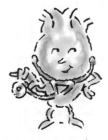

Pregnancy may reveal an underlying heart condition that previously produced no symptoms, or it may aggravate a known heart condition.

CAUSES
- Regurgitation, which permits blood to leak through an incompletely closed valve, thereby increasing the workload on heart chambers on either side of the affected valve
- Valvular stenosis (decreases blood flow through a valve, increasing workload on heart chambers located before the stenotic valve)

ASSESSMENT FINDINGS
- Tachycardia
- Dyspnea
- Fatigue
- Diastolic murmur at the heart's apex
- Crackles at the base of the lungs
- Cough
- Orthopnea
- Pitting edema
- Hemoptysis

DIAGNOSTIC TEST RESULTS
- Echocardiography, electrocardiogram (ECG), and chest X-ray may reveal cardiac abnormalities, impaired cardiac function, and cardiovascular decompensation.
- 12-lead ECG may reveal arrhythmias.

NURSING DIAGNOSES
- Activity intolerance
- Excess fluid volume
- Decreased cardiac output
- Ineffective breathing pattern

TREATMENT
- Low-sodium, low-fat diet with fluid restriction, if applicable
- Rest periods to prevent fatigue
- Oxygen therapy

Drug therapy
Class I and II
- Antibiotics: ampicillin (Omnipen-N), gentamicin to prevent bacterial endocarditis
Class III and IV
- Anticoagulant: heparin
- Antiarrhythmics: digoxin (Lanoxin), procainamide, beta-adrenergic blockers
- Antibiotics: ampicillin, gentamicin to prevent bacterial endocarditis
- Thiazide diuretics and furosemide (Lasix) to control heart failure if activity restriction and reduced sodium intake don't prevent it

INTERVENTIONS AND RATIONALES
- Monitor maternal and fetal vital signs *to assess for maternal and fetal well-being.*
- Assess cardiovascular and respiratory status *to assess for signs of maternal cardiac decompensation (tachycardia, tachypnea, moist crackles, exhaustion).*
- Administer anticoagulants, antiarrhythmics, antibiotics, and diuretics, as prescribed, *to achieve therapeutic regimens.*
- Encourage the client to monitor her intake *to avoid excessive weight gain.*
- Encourage the client to limit her physical activity according to her ability and symptoms *to ensure adequate rest.*
- Encourage the client to get 8 to 10 hours of sleep each night *to ensure adequate rest.*
- Monitor I.V. fluid intake and output *to maintain proper fluid levels.*

Polish up on client care   **509**

- Administer oxygen by nasal cannula or face mask during labor *to maintain fetal oxygenation.*
- Position the client on her left side with her head and shoulders elevated during labor *to prevent supine hypotension syndrome.*
- Continue to monitor the client during the postpartum period *to assess for signs of cardiac decompensation, even if distress is absent during pregnancy and labor.*

Teaching topics
- Explanation of the disorder and treatment plan
- Medication use and possible adverse effects
- Dietary modification
- Avoiding infection
- Recognizing signs and symptoms of heart failure
- Receiving adequate rest

Hydatidiform mole

Also known as *gestational trophoblastic disease,* hydatidiform mole is a developmental anomaly of the placenta that converts the chorionic villi into a mass of clear vesicles (hydatid vesicles). There are two types:
- *complete mole,* in which there's neither an embryo nor an amniotic sac
- *partial mole,* in which there's an embryo (usually with multiple abnormalities) and an amniotic sac.

CAUSES
- Possibly poor maternal nutrition or a defective ovum

ASSESSMENT FINDINGS
- Disproportionate enlargement of the uterus
- Excessive nausea and vomiting
- Intermittent or continuous bright red or brownish vaginal bleeding by 12 weeks' gestation
- Absence of fetal heart sounds
- Passage of clear, fluid-filled vesicles along with vaginal bleeding
- Symptoms of gestational hypertension before 20 weeks' gestation

DIAGNOSTIC TEST RESULTS
- HCG levels are extremely high for early pregnancy.
- Ultrasound fails to reveal a fetal skeleton.

NURSING DIAGNOSES
- Deficient fluid volume
- Complicated grieving
- Acute pain

TREATMENT
- Therapeutic abortion (suction and curettage) if a spontaneous abortion doesn't occur to prevent choriocarcinoma
- Pelvic examinations and chest X-rays at regular intervals
- Weekly monitoring of HCG levels until they remain normal for 3 consecutive weeks
- Periodic follow-up for 1 to 2 years because of increased risk of neoplasm

Drug therapy
- Methotrexate (Trexall) prophylactically (the drug of choice for choriocarcinoma)

INTERVENTIONS AND RATIONALES
- Monitor and record vital signs and intake and output *to assess for changes that may indicate complications.*
- Provide emotional support for the grieving couple *to demonstrate concern and understanding for the client and the family.*
- Monitor vaginal bleeding *to assess for hemorrhage.*
- Send contents of uterine evacuation to the laboratory for analysis *to assess for the presence of hydatid vesicles.*
- Advise the client to avoid pregnancy until HCG levels are normal (may take up to 2 years) *to avoid future complications.*

Teaching topics
- Explanation of the disorder and treatment plan
- Dealing with an uncertain obstetric and medical future
- Information on birth control

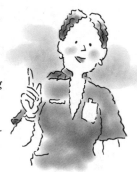

Hydatidiform mole is a chorionic tumor. The chorion is the fetal membrane closest to the uterine wall; it gives rise to the placenta.

Hyperemesis gravidarum

Hyperemesis gravidarum is persistent, uncontrolled vomiting that begins in the first weeks of pregnancy and may continue throughout pregnancy. Unlike "morning sickness," hyperemesis can have serious complications, including severe weight loss, dehydration, and electrolyte imbalance.

CAUSES
- Gonadotropin production
- Psychological factors
- Trophoblastic activity

ASSESSMENT FINDINGS
- Continuous, severe nausea and vomiting
- Dehydration
- Dry skin and mucous membranes
- Electrolyte imbalance
- Jaundice
- Metabolic alkalosis
- Nonelastic skin turgor
- Oliguria
- Significant weight loss

DIAGNOSTIC TEST RESULTS
- Arterial blood gas analysis reveals alkalosis.
- Hb level and HCT are elevated.
- Serum potassium level reveals hypokalemia.
- Urine ketone levels are elevated.
- Urine specific gravity is increased.

NURSING DIAGNOSES
- Imbalanced nutrition: Less than body requirements
- Deficient fluid volume
- Acute pain

TREATMENT
- TPN
- Restoration of fluid and electrolyte balance

Drug therapy
- Antiemetics, as necessary, for vomiting

INTERVENTIONS AND RATIONALES
- Monitor vital signs and fluid intake and output *to assess for fluid volume deficit.*

- Obtain blood samples and urine specimens *for laboratory tests, including Hb level, HCT, urinalysis, and electrolyte levels.*
- Monitor fundal height and the client's weight *to detect complications.*
- Provide small, frequent meals *to maintain adequate nutrition.*
- Maintain I.V. fluid replacement and TPN *to reduce fluid deficits and pH imbalances.*
- Provide emotional support *to help the client cope with her condition.*

Teaching topics
- Explanation of the disorder and treatment plan
- Recognizing triggers of nausea and vomiting
- Using salt on foods to replace sodium lost by vomiting

Hypertensive disorders of pregnancy

Hypertensive disorders of pregnancy include gestational hypertension, preeclampsia, chronichypertension, and superimposed hypertension. The client is at risk for cerebral hemorrhage, circulatory collapse, heart failure, hepatic rupture, and renal failure. If delivery occurs before term, the fetal prognosis is poor because of hypoxia, acidosis, and immaturity.

Maternal mortality from eclampsia is 10% to 15%, usually resulting from intracranial hemorrhage and heart failure.

RISK FACTORS
- Adolescence
- Antiphospholipid antibodies
- Diabetes mellitus
- Familial tendency
- Hydatidiform mole
- Hydramnios
- Hydrops fetalis
- Hypertension
- Malnutrition
- Maternal age older than 35
- Multifetal pregnancy
- Obesity
- Renal disease

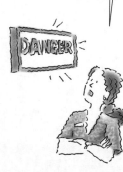

A mother with gestational hypertension is at risk for cerebral hemorrhage, circulatory collapse, heart failure, hepatic rupture, and renal failure.

DANGER

Preeclampsia
HTN + Proteinuria

ASSESSMENT FINDINGS
Gestational hypertension
• Onset of hypertension without associated proteinuria after 20 weeks' gestation
• Blood pressure returning to baseline by 12 weeks' postpartum

Preeclampsia
• Hypertension plus proteinuria
• Three categories of preeclampsia
– Mild preeclampsia
▪ Blood pressure at least 140/90 mm Hg
▪ 300 mg of proteinuria in 24 hours
▪ Mild edema in upper extremities or face
– Severe preeclampsia
▪ Blood pressure 160/110 mm Hg
▪ 5 gm of proteinuria in 24 hours
▪ Less than 500 ml of urine in 24 hours
▪ Vision disturbances
▪ Pulmonary edema
▪ Headaches, hyperreflexia, nausea
▪ Right upper quadrant tenderness
▪ Fetal growth restriction
▪ Thrombocytopenia
– Eclampsia
▪ Presence of new-onset grand mal seizures in a client with preeclampsia

Chronic hypertension
• Medically diagnosed hypertension exists before pregnancy
• Gestational hypertension that doesn't resolve within 12 weeks of delivery
• Superimposed preeclampsia
• Chronic hypertension plus new-onset proteinuria or other signs and symptoms of preeclampsia

DIAGNOSTIC TEST RESULTS
• Blood chemistry reveals increased blood urea nitrogen, creatinine, and uric acid levels and elevated liver function studies.
• Hematology reveals thrombocytopenia (HELLP syndrome).

NURSING DIAGNOSES
• Activity intolerance
• Excess fluid volume
• Risk for injury
• Ineffective breathing pattern
• Decreased cardiac output

TREATMENT
• Bed rest in a left lateral position
• Delivery: with mild preeclampsia, when the fetus is mature and safe induction is possible; with severe preeclampsia, regardless of gestational age
• High-protein diet with moderate sodium intake
• Fluid and electrolyte replacement balanced with output

Drug therapy
• With severe preeclampsia: antihypertensives, such as hydralazine or labetalol
• Corticosteroid: betamethasone to accelerate fetal lung maturation
• Magnesium sulfate to reduce the amount of acetylcholine produced by motor nerves, thereby preventing seizures
• Diuretic: furosemide (Lasix) if pulmonary edema develops

INTERVENTIONS AND RATIONALES
For all clients
• Assess the client for edema and proteinuria, *which may indicate impending eclampsia.*
• Assess neurologic status *to detect early signs of deterioration, which might suggest impending eclampsia.*
• Monitor daily weight *to identify sodium and water retention.*
• Maintain a high-protein diet with moderate sodium restriction *as a measure against gestational hypertension.*
• Maintain seizure precautions *to ensure safety.*
• Encourage bed rest in a left lateral recumbent position *to improve uterine and renal perfusion.*
• Monitor blood pressure *to evaluate the effectiveness of treatment.*
• Monitor the FHR continuously during labor *to assess fetal well-being.*

For clients with severe preeclampsia
• Assess maternal blood pressure every 1 to 4 hours or more frequently if unstable *to assess for abnormalities.*
• If necessary, prepare for amniocentesis *to assess fetal maturity.*

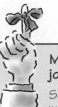

Memory jogger

Some women who develop preeclampsia also develop **HELLP** syndrome, so be alert if you notice the following signs:

Hemolysis

Elevated **L**iver enzyme levels

Low **P**latelet count.

Encourage bed rest in a left lateral recumbent position to improve uterine and renal perfusion.

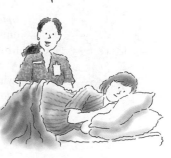

- Maintain I.V. fluids, as prescribed. *I.V. fluids are restricted based on urine output and total fluid intake per hour.*
- Obtain blood samples for complete blood count, platelet count, and liver function studies and to determine serum levels of blood urea nitrogen, creatinine, and fibrin degradation products *to detect signs of complications.*
- Be prepared to obtain a blood sample for typing and crossmatching *because of the risk of placenta previa.*
- Obtain urine specimens to determine urine protein levels and specific gravity, and perform 24-hour urine collection for protein and creatinine, as ordered, *to evaluate renal function.*
- Monitor urine output *to assess fluid status.*
- Keep calcium gluconate (antidote to magnesium sulfate) nearby *to administer at the first sign of magnesium sulfate toxicity* (elevated serum levels, decreased deep tendon reflexes, muscle flaccidity, CNS depression, and decreased respiratory rate and renal function).
- Promote relaxation *to reduce fatigue.*
- Encourage the client to verbalize her feelings *to allay anxiety.*
- Provide a quiet environment *to help prevent complications.*

(handwritten margin notes) calcium gluconate ↑ Mag Sulfate toxicity ↓ deep tendon muscle flaccidity CNS ↓ resp ↓ renal

Teaching topics
- Explanation of the disorder and treatment plan
- Importance of bed rest and adequate nutrition
- Recognizing signs and symptoms of severe preeclampsia and eclampsia

Multifetal pregnancy

A multifetal pregnancy, also known as *multiple gestation,* occurs when two or more embryos or fetuses exist simultaneously. Multifetal pregnancies are formed as follows:
- Single-ovum (monozygotic, identical) twins usually have one chorion, one placenta, two amnions, and two umbilical cords and are of the same sex.

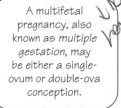

A multifetal pregnancy, also known as *multiple gestation,* may be either a single-ovum or double-ova conception.

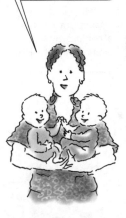

- Double-ova (dizygotic, nonidentical) twins have two chorions, two placentas, two amnions, and two umbilical cords and may be of the same or different sex.
- Multifetal pregnancies of three or more fetuses may be single-ovum conceptions, multiple-ova conceptions, or a combination of both.

CAUSES
- In vitro fertilization
- Family history
- Gamete intrafallopian tube transfer
- Ovulation stimulation with such drugs as clomiphene (Clomid)

ASSESSMENT FINDINGS
- More than one set of fetal heart sounds
- Uterine size greater than expected for dates

DIAGNOSTIC TEST RESULTS
- Alpha fetoprotein levels are elevated.
- Ultrasonography is positive for multifetal pregnancy.

NURSING DIAGNOSES
- Anxiety
- Deficient knowledge (pregnancy)
- Risk for injury
- Fear

TREATMENT
- Activity, as tolerated, with increased rest periods
- Bed rest if early dilation occurs or at 24 to 28 weeks' gestation to improve uterine blood flow and, possibly, increase birth weight of the fetuses
- Biweekly NST to document fetal growth, beginning at 28 weeks' gestation
- Increased intake of calories, iron, folate, and vitamins
- Prenatal visits every 2 weeks, increasing to weekly between 24 and 28 weeks' gestation; cervical examinations performed at each visit to check for premature dilation
- Ultrasound examinations monthly to document fetal growth

INTERVENTIONS AND RATIONALES
- Monitor fetal heart sounds *to evaluate fetal well-being*.
- Monitor maternal vital signs and weight *to assess maternal well-being*.
- Monitor cardiovascular and pulmonary status *to assess for signs of gestational hypertension*.
- Ensure adequate nutrition and increased intake of folate, calories, vitamins, and iron *to ensure adequate weight gain*.
- Encourage frequent rest periods, especially during the third trimester, or to maintain bed rest, if indicated, *to prevent fatigue*.
- Provide emotional support and encouragement *to reduce anxiety*.
- Advise the client to return for ultrasound examination and NST as scheduled *to assess for fetal well-being*.

Teaching topics
- Pregnancy needs and expected course
- Notifying physician immediately if signs of premature labor occur
- Refraining from coitus during the third trimester

Placenta previa   *Painless bleeding*

In placenta previa, the placenta is implanted in the lower uterine segment (low implantation). The placenta can occlude the cervix partially or totally.

RISK FACTORS
- Maternal age older than 35
- Multiple pregnancies
- Placental villi torn from the uterine wall as the lower uterine segment contracts and dilates in the third trimester
- Uterine fibroid tumors
- Uterine scars from surgery
- Uterine sinuses exposed at the placental site and bleeding

ASSESSMENT FINDINGS
- Painless, bright red vaginal bleeding, especially during the third trimester (possibly increasing with each successive incident)

DIAGNOSTIC TEST RESULTS
- Early ultrasound evaluation reveals the placenta implanted in the lower uterine segment.

NURSING DIAGNOSES
- Fear
- Anxiety
- Deficient fluid volume
- Risk for injury

TREATMENT
- Treatment based on gestational age, when first episode occurs, and amount of bleeding
- If gestational age less than 34 weeks, hospitalizing the client and restricting her to bed rest to avoid preterm labor
- Administering supplemental iron if anemia is present
- Restricting maternal activities (for example, no lifting heavy objects, long-distance travel, or sexual intercourse)
- Transfusion of packed RBCs if Hb level and HCT are low
- Treatment of choice: surgical intervention (by cesarean delivery), depending on placental placement and maternal and fetal stability

INTERVENTIONS AND RATIONALES
- Monitor maternal vital signs, including uterine activity, *to assess maternal well-being*.
- Monitor for vaginal bleeding *to estimate blood loss*.
- Monitor for signs of infection; *clients with placenta previa are at increased risk for infection*.
- Monitor the FHR, using electronic fetal monitoring, *to assess for complications*.
- Don't perform rectal or vaginal examinations unless equipment is available for vaginal and cesarean delivery *to avoid stimulating uterine activity*.
- Obtain blood samples for HCT, Hb level, PT, INR, PTT, fibrinogen level, platelet count, and typing and crossmatching *to assess for complications*.
- Provide routine postoperative care if cesarean delivery is performed *to ensure the client's well-being*.
- Monitor for postpartum hemorrhage *because clients with placenta previa are more prone to hemorrhage*.

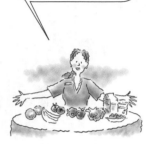

The nutritional needs of a client with a multifetal pregnancy exceed those of other pregnant women. Try some calories, iron, folate, and vitamins.

• Provide emotional support *to reduce anxiety.*
• Administer I.V. fluids, as ordered, *to reduce fluid loss.*
• Be prepared to administer betamethasone *to increase fetal lung maturity if preterm labor can't be halted.*

Teaching topics

• Explanation of the disorder and treatment plan
• Limiting activity
• Reporting increased bleeding immediately
• Understanding possible need for preterm delivery

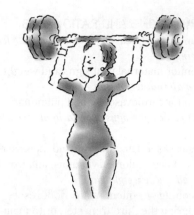

Pump up on practice questions

1. A 15-year-old client is 26 weeks pregnant. She has been admitted to the labor and delivery unit with a complaint of abdominal pain. Her parents want to speak with the nurse in reference to her condition. The nurse's best response to the parents is:

   1 "I'll need a signed consent from your daughter to give you medical information."
   2. "The physician can give you more information without consent."
   3. "She'll be OK. It's just a stomachache."
   4. "She's experiencing Braxton-Hicks contractions and is too young to understand the difference."

Answer: 1. A pregnant minor becomes emancipated to make decisions for herself and her baby. The client's right to confidentiality means that medical information of any kind can't be divulged without a signed consent from her. The physician can't give out information without consent.

➡ *NCLEX keys*
Client needs category: Safe and effective care environment
Client needs subcategory: Management of care
Cognitive level: Analysis

2. A client who's 32 weeks pregnant presents to the emergency department with bright red bleeding and no abdominal pain. Which action should the nurse take *first*?
1. Perform a pelvic examination.
2. Assess the client's blood pressure.
3. Assess the fetal heart rate (FHR).
4. Order a stat hemoglobin and hematocrit.

Answer: 3. The nurse should assess FHR for fetal distress or viability. A pelvic examination shouldn't be attempted because of the possibility of placenta previa, in which symptoms present as bright red bleeding without abdominal pain. The client's blood pressure should be addressed after fetal heart tones are attempted. Ordering a hemoglobin and hematocrit is a physician intervention, not a nursing intervention.

➡ *NCLEX keys*
Client needs category: Safe and effective care environment
Client needs subcategory: Management of care
Cognitive level: Analysis

3. Which finding is considered normal during the antepartum period of pregnancy?
1. Resting pulse rate fluctuations ranging from 15 to 20 beats/minute
2. Slight decrease in respiratory rate
3. Altered breathing pattern with thoracic breathing replacing abdominal breathing
4. Hematocrit (HCT) increase of about 7%

Answer: 1. Cardiovascular system changes associated with pregnancy lead to resting pulse rate fluctuation with increases ranging from 15 to 20 beats/minute at term. Other pregnancy-related changes include a slight increase (2 breaths/minute) in respiratory rate, altered breathing pattern with abdominal breathing replacing thoracic breathing as pregnancy progresses, and a decrease in HCT of about 7%.

➡ *NCLEX keys*
Client needs category: Health promotion and maintenance
Client needs subcategory: None
Cognitive level: Knowledge

4. A client comes to the clinic for her 12-week pregnancy checkup. The client asks the nurse when she should begin to feel her baby move. Which response should the nurse offer?
1. "You should have already felt it move."
2. "Typically women feel their baby move for the first time when they're 20 weeks pregnant."
3. "You'll probably feel your baby move after your 16th week of pregnancy."
4. "Each person experiences the baby's first movement at a different time throughout their pregnancy."

Answer: 3. Although each client does detect fetal movement at a different time, it's typically experienced just after the 16th week. If movement isn't detected around this time, problems with the pregnancy may exist.

➡ *NCLEX keys*
Client needs category: Health promotion and maintenance
Client needs subcategory: None
Cognitive level: Application

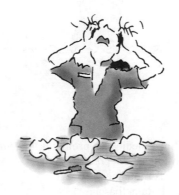

5. A client at a routine prenatal visit mentions to the nurse that she's nervous and afraid to go home. The nurse should respond by:

1. reassuring her that most new parents are nervous and that it's normal to feel this way.
2. contacting the admissions department to extend her stay.
3. asking her if she's unsafe at home.
4. excusing herself and reporting her remarks to the nurse in charge.

Answer: 3. The nurse has a legal responsibility to assess for and report abuse. False reassurance and extending her stay do not pinpoint the client's concern. The charge nurse may need to be notified after the nurse has defined the issue.

➡ *NCLEX keys*
Client needs category: Safe and effective care environment
Client needs subcategory: Management of care
Cognitive level: Application

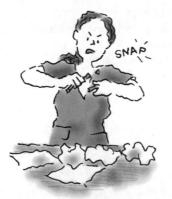

6. Which medication promotes fetal lung maturity in cases of preterm labor?
1. Terbutaline
2. Betamethasone

3. Co-trimoxazole (Bactrim)
4. Clarithromycin (Biaxin)

Answer: 2. Preterm labor raises concerns about the fetus's respiratory potential. Therefore, betamethasone is used to stimulate the development of surfactant in the lungs. Terbutaline is a beta-adrenergic agonist used to treat preterm labor. Co-trimoxazole is a sulfonamide commonly used to treat urinary tract infections, and clarithromycin is an antibiotic used to treat upper respiratory tract infections.

➡ *NCLEX keys*
Client needs category: Physiological integrity
Client needs subcategory: Pharmacological and parenteral therapies
Cognitive level: Application

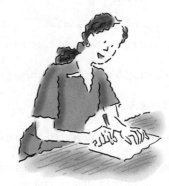

7. A multigravida client at 38 weeks' gestation has come to the emergency department complaining of chest pain. She tells the nurse that she has recently inhaled crack cocaine. The nurse's top priority is to assess the client for:
1. abruptio placentae.
2. placenta accreta.
3. malnutrition.
4. hypotension.

Answer: 1. The use of crack cocaine during pregnancy is associated with abruptio placentae, along with hypertension, stroke, tachycardia, hemorrhage, low birth weight, and preterm neonates. Crack cocaine isn't associated with placenta accreta (unusually deep attachment of the placenta to the uterine myometrium) or hypotension. Although malnutrition may exist, it isn't life-threatening at this point.

➡ *NCLEX keys*
Client needs category: Physiological integrity
Client needs subcategory: Reduction of risk potential
Cognitive level: Analysis

8. A multigravida client at 39 weeks' gestation is diagnosed with gestational hypertension and HELLP syndrome. The nurse's top priority is to assess the client's:
1. white blood count (WBC) count.
2. blood glucose levels.
3. serum iron levels.
4. platelet count.

Answer: 4. Women diagnosed with HELLP syndrome have hemolysis of red blood cells, elevated liver enzyme levels, and a low platelet count, so the nurse should assess the client's platelet count. This syndrome can lead to disseminated intravascular coagulation or hemorrhage. Monitoring WBC count, blood glucose levels, and serum iron levels isn't a priority for clients diagnosed with HELLP syndrome.

➡ *NCLEX keys*
Client needs category: Physiological integrity
Client needs subcategory: Reduction of risk potential
Cognitive level: Analysis

9. A hospitalized client who's 26 weeks pregnant has been diagnosed with gestational diabetes. She is overweight and doesn't understand the diet that has been suggested to her by the physician. The nurse asks the physician to order consults from which health care team member to demonstrate a gestational diabetic diet?
1. Social worker
2. Dietician
3. Psychologist
4. Lactation consultant

Answer: 2. A dietician can create a meal plan that will fit into the client's daily lifestyle and ensure specific calorie needs suggested by the physician. Dietary considerations will take into account the client's culture, food preferences, and activities of daily living. A social worker or psychologist would be consulted if psychological needs needed to be addressed. A lactation consultant could be consulted in the postpartum stage to address the client's and neonate's needs associated with breastfeeding.

➡ *NCLEX keys*
Client needs category: Safe and effective care environment
Client needs subcategory: Management of care
Cognitive level: Application

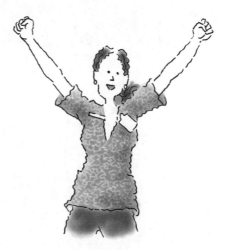

10. A nurse is performing a prenatal assessment on a client who's 32 weeks pregnant. She performs Leopold's maneuvers and determines that the fetus is in the cephalic position. Identify where the nurse should place the Doppler to auscultate fetal heart tones.

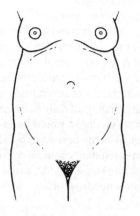

Answer: When the fetus is in the cephalic position (head down), fetal heart tones are best auscultated midway between the symphysis pubis and the umbilicus. When the fetus is in the breech position, fetal heart tones are best heard at or above the level of the umbilicus.

NCLEX keys
Client needs category: Health promotion and maintenance
Client needs subcategory: None
Cognitive level: Analysis

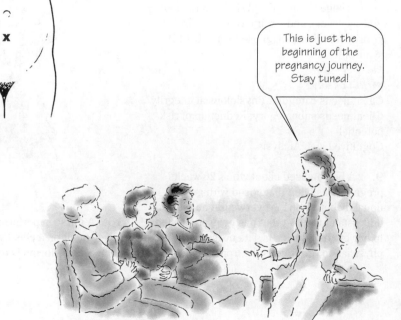

This is just the beginning of the pregnancy journey. Stay tuned!

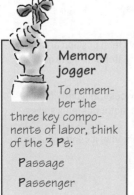

Memory jogger

To remember the three key components of labor, think of the 3 Ps:

Passage

Passenger

Power.

Brush up on key concepts

Intrapartum care refers to care of the client during labor. In this section, you'll find a brief review of the signs and symptoms that indicate the onset of labor, the client's physiologic and psychosocial responses to labor, basic obstetric procedures, and methods of monitoring the client and fetus.

At any time, you can review the major points of this chapter by consulting the *Cheat sheet* on pages 520 to 523.

Components of labor

The three major components of labor are the passage, the passenger, and the power. These components must work together for labor to progress normally.

Long and winding road

Passage refers to the maternal pelvis and soft tissues, the passageway through which the fetus exits the body. This area is affected by the shape of the inlet, the structure of the pelvis, and pelvic diameters.

Coach or first class?

Passenger refers to the fetus and its ability to move through the passage. This ability is affected by such fetal features as:
• the skull
• the lie (relationship of the long axis [spine] of the fetus to the long axis of the mother)
• presentation (portion of the fetus that enters the pelvic passageway first)
• position (relationship of the presenting part of the fetus to the front, back, and sides of the maternal pelvis).

Attitude refers to the relationship of the fetal parts (such as the chest, chin, or arms) to one another during the passage through the birth canal. The fetal head may be in a flexed (chin-to-chest) or extended (head-to-back) position. Pressure exerted by the maternal pelvis and birth canal during labor and delivery causes the sutures of the skull to allow the cranial bones to shift, resulting in molding of the fetal head.

What kind of engine?

Power refers to uterine contractions, which cause complete cervical effacement (thinning) and dilation (expansion).

Along for the ride

Other factors that affect labor are:
• accomplishment of the tasks of pregnancy
• coping mechanisms
• mother's ability to bear down (voluntary use of abdominal muscles to push during the second stage of labor)
• past experiences
• placental positioning
• preparation for childbirth
• psychological readiness
• support systems.

Let's get this show on the road

Preliminary signs that indicate the onset of labor may occur anywhere from 24 hours to 3 weeks before onset of true labor. They include:
• lightening, or fetal descent into the pelvis, which usually occurs 2 to 3 weeks before term in a primiparous client and later or during labor in a multiparous client
• Braxton Hicks contractions, which can occur irregularly and intermittently throughout pregnancy and may become uncomfortable and produce false labor

(Text continues on page 523.)

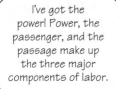

Cheat sheet

Intrapartum care refresher

ABRUPTIO PLACENTAE

Key signs and symptoms
- Acute abdominal pain and rigid abdomen
- Hemorrhage with dark red vaginal bleeding

Key test results
- Ultrasonography locates the placenta and may reveal a clot or hematoma.

Key treatments
- Transfusion: packed red blood cells (RBCs), platelets, and fresh frozen plasma, if necessary
- Cesarean birth

Key interventions
- Avoid pelvic or vaginal examinations and enemas.
- Administer blood products and monitor vital signs.
- Position the client in a left lateral recumbent position.

AMNIOTIC FLUID EMBOLISM

Key signs and symptoms
- Cyanosis and chest pain
- Tachypnea and sudden dyspnea

Key test results
- Electronic fetal monitor reveals fetal distress (during the intrapartum period).
- Arterial blood gas results reveal hypoxemia.

Key treatments
- Oxygen therapy: endotracheal intubation and mechanical ventilation if respiratory arrest occurs
- Cardiopulmonary resuscitation (CPR) if client is apneic and pulseless
- Emergency delivery by cesarean birth

Key interventions
- Assess respiratory and cardiovascular status.
- Assess fetal heart rate (FHR).
- Perform CPR, if necessary.
- Assist with immediate delivery of the neonate.

DISSEMINATED INTRAVASCULAR COAGULATION

Key signs and symptoms
- Abnormal bleeding (petechiae, hematomas, ecchymosis, cutaneous oozing)
- Oliguria

Key test results
- Coagulation studies reveal decreased fibrinogen level, positive D-dimer test specific for disseminated intravascular coagulation, prolonged prothrombin time (PT), and prolonged partial thromboplastin time (PTT).
- Hematology studies reveal decreased platelet count.

Key treatments
- Transfusion therapy: packed RBCs, fresh frozen plasma, platelets, and cryoprecipitate
- Treatment of the underlying condition
- Immediate delivery of the fetus by cesarean birth

Key interventions
- Monitor cardiovascular, respiratory, neurologic, GI, and renal status.
- Monitor vital signs frequently.
- Monitor intake and output.
- Administer blood products and monitor client closely for signs and symptoms of a transfusion reaction.
- Monitor the results of serial blood studies.

DYSTOCIA

Key signs and symptoms
- Arrested descent
- Hypotonic contractions

Key test results
- Ultrasonography shows fetal position or malformation or fetal weight greater than 4,500 g.

Key treatments
- Delivery of the fetus by cesarean birth if labor fails to progress and the mother or fetus shows signs of compromise
- Uterotonic: oxytocin (Pitocin) if contractions are ineffective

I've got the power! Power, the passenger, and the passage make up the three major components of labor.

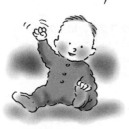

Intrapartum care refresher *(continued)*

DYSTOCIA *(CONTINUED)*
Key interventions
- Monitor maternal vital signs and FHR.
- Assist the patient to a left side-lying position.
- Monitor the effectiveness of oxytocin therapy, and watch for complications.

EMERGENCY BIRTH
Key signs and symptoms
For prolapsed umbilical cord
- Cord visible at the vaginal opening
- Variable decelerations or bradycardia noted on the fetal monitor strip
For uterine rupture
- Abdominal pain and tenderness, especially at the peak of a contraction, or the feeling that "something ripped"
- Excessive external bleeding
- Late decelerations, reduced FHR variability, tachycardia and bradycardia, and cessation of FHR
- Palpation of the fetus outside the uterus
For amniotic fluid embolism
- Chest pain
- Coughing with pink, frothy sputum
- Increasing restlessness and anxiety
- Sudden dyspnea
- Tachypnea

Key test results
For prolapsed umbilical cord
- Ultrasonography confirms that the cord is prolapsed.
For uterine rupture
- Ultrasonography may reveal the absence of the amniotic cavity within the uterus.
For amniotic fluid embolism
- Arterial blood gas analysis reveals hypoxemia.

Key treatments
- Administration of oxygen by nasal cannula or mask (endotracheal intubation and mechanical ventilation may be necessary in the case of amniotic fluid embolism)
- Emergency cesarean delivery

Key interventions
- Monitor maternal vital signs, pulse oximetry, and intake and output as well as FHR.
- Administer maternal oxygen by cannula or mask at 8 to 10 L/minute.
- Maintain I.V. fluid replacement.
- Place the client in a left lateral recumbent position.

- Obtain blood samples to determine hematocrit (HCT), hemoglobin (Hb) level, PT and PTT, fibrinogen level, and platelet count and to type and crossmatch blood.
- Monitor administration of blood products as necessary.
- Prepare the client and her family for the possibility of cesarean delivery.

FETAL DISTRESS
Key signs and symptoms
- Electronic fetal monitor showing bradycardia or FHR greater than 180 beats/minute
- Loss of fetal movement

Key test results
- Fetal scalp blood sampling reveals acidosis.

Key treatments
- Supplemental oxygen by face mask, typically at 6 to 8 L/minute
- I.V. fluid administration
- Emergency fetal delivery by vacuum aspiration, forceps, or cesarean birth

Key interventions
- Monitor FHR, fetal activity, and fetal heart variability.
- Assist the client to a left side-lying position.

INVERTED UTERUS
Key signs and symptoms
- Large, sudden gush of blood from the vagina
- Severe uterine pain

Key test results
- Hematology tests reveal decreased levels of Hb and HCT.

Key treatments
- Fluid resuscitation with I.V. fluids and blood products
- Supplemental oxygen administration
- Immediate manual replacement of the uterus
- Possible emergency hysterectomy
- Tocolytic agent: terbutaline

Key interventions
- Administer supplemental oxygen.
- Monitor vital signs frequently.
- Monitor intake and output.

LACERATION
Key signs and symptoms
- Increased vaginal bleeding after delivery of placenta

Key test results
- Hematology studies may reveal decreased levels of Hb and HCT.

(continued)

Intrapartum care refresher *(continued)*

LACERATION *(CONTINUED)*

Key treatments
- Laceration repair
- Analgesics: ibuprofen (Motrin), acetaminophen and oxycodone (Percocet), acetaminophen (Tylenol)

Key interventions
- Monitor vital signs, including temperature.
- Monitor laceration site for signs of infection and bleeding.
- Insert indwelling urinary catheter, if indicated.

PRECIPITATE LABOR

Key signs and symptoms
- Cervical dilation greater than 5 cm/hour in a nulliparous woman; more than 10 cm/hour in a multiparous woman

Key test results
- There are no diagnostic test findings specific to this complication.

Key treatments
- Controlled delivery to prevent maternal and fetal injury

Key interventions
- Monitor FHR and variability.

PREMATURE RUPTURE OF MEMBRANES

Key signs and symptoms
- Blood-tinged amniotic fluid gushing or leaking from the vagina
- Uterine tenderness

Key test results
- Vaginal probe ultrasonography allows detection of amniotic sac tear or rupture.

Key treatments
- Hospitalization to monitor for maternal fever and leukocytosis and fetal tachycardia if pregnancy is between 28 and 34 weeks. If infection is confirmed, labor must be induced.
- Oxytocic agent: oxytocin (Pitocin) for labor induction if term pregnancy and labor doesn't result within 24 hours after membrane rupture

Key interventions
- Assess for signs of infection or fetal distress.
- Administer antibiotics as prescribed.
- Encourage the client to express her feelings and concerns.

PRETERM LABOR

Key signs and symptoms
- Feeling of pelvic pressure or abdominal tightening
- Increased vaginal discharge

- Intestinal cramping
- Uterine contractions that result in cervical dilation and effacement

Key test results
- Electronic fetal monitoring confirms uterine contractions.
- Vaginal examination confirms cervical effacement and dilation.

Key treatments
- Betamethasone administered I.M. at regular intervals over 48 hours to increase fetal lung maturity in a fetus expected to be delivered preterm
- Tocolytic agents, such as terbutaline and ritodrine (Yutopar), to inhibit uterine contractions
- Magnesium sulfate to maintain uterine relaxation

Key interventions
- Monitor maternal vital signs, contractions, and FHR every 15 minutes during tocolytic therapy (otherwise, provide continuous fetal monitoring).
- Monitor for maternal adverse reactions to terbutaline or ritodrine.
- Monitor for magnesium sulfate toxicity, and make sure calcium gluconate is available.
- Assess the neonate for possible adverse affects of indomethacin (Indocin), such as premature closure of the ductus arteriosus.

PROLAPSED UMBILICAL CORD

Key signs and symptoms
- Cord visible at the vaginal opening
- Variable decelerations or bradycardia noted on the fetal monitor strip

Key test results
- Ultrasonography may reveal the cord as the presenting part.

Key treatments
- Immediate delivery of the fetus

Key interventions
- Place the client in Trendelenburg's position (position the woman's hips higher than her head in a knee-to-chest position).
- Monitor FHR and variability.

UTERINE RUPTURE

Key signs and symptoms
- Abdominal pain and tenderness, especially at the peak of a contraction, or the feeling that "something ripped"
- Late decelerations, reduced FHR variability, tachycardia and bradycardia, and cessation of FHR

Intrapartum care refresher (continued)

UTERINE RUPTURE *(CONTINUED)*
Key test results
• Hematology tests reveal decreased levels of Hb and HCT.

Key treatments
• Fluid resuscitation: I.V. fluids and blood products via rapid infusion

• Surgery to remove the fetus and repair the tear, or hysterectomy, if necessary
• Oxytocic agent: oxytocin (Pitocin) to help contract the uterus

Key interventions
• Monitor vital signs frequently.
• Prepare the client for immediate surgery.

• cervical changes, including softening, effacement, and slight dilation several days before the initiation of labor
• a sudden burst of energy before the onset of labor, commonly demonstrated by housecleaning activities and called the *nesting instinct* (See *True or false?*)
• bloody show as the mucus plug is expelled from the cervix
• increase in clear vaginal secretions
• rupture of membranes, occurring before the onset of labor in about 12% of clients and within 24 hours for about 80% of clients.

Evaluating the mother during true labor

Here's a review of methods and techniques used to monitor the progress of true labor and the mother's condition.

Starting to open
Observe **dilation.** The cervical os should increase from 0 to 10 cm.

The thick and thin of it
Observe **effacement,** cervical thinning and shortening, which is measured from 0% (thick) to 100% (paper thin).

What's the situation?
Using abdominal palpation (Leopold's maneuvers), determine **fetal position and presentation.** The process consists of four maneuvers.

Palpate the fundus to identify the occupying fetal part: the fetus's head is firm and rounded and moves freely; the breech is softer and less regular and moves with the trunk.

Palpate the abdomen to locate the fetus's back: the back should feel firm, smooth, and convex, whereas the front is soft, irregular, and concave.

Determine the level of descent of the head by grasping the lower portion of the abdomen above the symphysis pubis to identify the fetal part presenting over the inlet; an unengaged head can be rocked from side to side.

True or false?
Use the chart below to help distinguish between true and false labor.

True labor	False labor
Regular contractions	Irregular, brief contractions
Back discomfort that spreads to the abdomen	Discomfort that's localized in the abdomen
Progressive cervical effacement and dilation	No cervical change
Gradually shortened intervals between contractions	No change or irregular change in intervals between contractions
Increased intensity of contractions with ambulation	Contractions that may be relieved with ambulation
Contractions that increase in duration and intensity	Usually no change in duration and intensity of contractions
Usually bloody show	Usually no bloody show

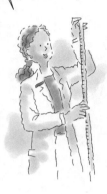

Uterine contractions are measured by duration, frequency, and intensity.

Determine head flexion by moving fingers down both sides of the uterus to assess the descent of the presenting part into the pelvis; greater resistance is met as the fingers move downward on the cephalic prominence (brow) side.

What's the relationship?

Check the **station,** the relationship of the presenting part to the pelvic ischial spines:
- The presenting part is even with the ischial spines at 0 station.
- The presenting part is above the ischial spines at −3, −2, or −1.
- The presenting part is below the ischial spines at +1, +2, or +3.

Thirsty?

Monitor the client for signs of **dehydration,** such as poor skin turgor, decreased urine output, and dry mucous membranes.

I need a little rest

Use an external pressure transducer to monitor the client for **tetanic contractions,** sustained prolonged contractions with little rest in between that reduce oxygen supply to the fetus.

Measuring contractions

Phases of **uterine contractions** include increment (buildup and longest phase), acme (peak of the contraction), and decrement (letting-down phase). Contractions are measured by duration, frequency, and intensity. Here's how to measure each:
- **Duration** is measured from the beginning of the increment of the contraction to the end of the decrement of the contraction and averages 30 seconds early in labor and 60 seconds later in labor.
- **Frequency** is measured from the beginning of one contraction to the beginning of the next and averages 5 to 30 minutes apart early in labor and 2 to 3 minutes apart later in labor.
- **Intensity** is assessed during the acme phase and can be measured with an intrauterine catheter or by palpation; normal resting pressure when using an intrauterine catheter is 5 to 15 mm Hg; pressure increases to 30 to 50 mm Hg during the acme. When assessing intensity by palpation, the contraction is considered mild, moderate, or strong.

All around adaptations

Labor also prompts a series of responses throughout the mother's body, including changes in the cardiovascular, respiratory, and GI systems. (See *Maternal responses to labor.*)

Maternal responses to labor

During labor, the mother undergoes physiologic changes.

CARDIOVASCULAR SYSTEM
- Increased intrathoracic pressure during pushing in the second stage
- Increased peripheral resistance during contractions, which elevates blood pressure and decreases pulse rate
- Increased cardiac output

FLUID AND ELECTROLYTE BALANCE
- Increased water loss from diaphoresis and hyperventilation

- Increased evaporative water volume from increased respiratory rate

RESPIRATORY SYSTEM
- Increased oxygen consumption
- Increased respiratory rate

HEMATOPOIETIC SYSTEM
- Increased plasma fibrinogen level and leukocyte count
- Decreased blood coagulation time and blood glucose levels

GI SYSTEM
- Decreased gastric motility and absorption

- Prolonged gastric emptying time

RENAL SYSTEM
- Forward and upward displacement of the bladder base at engagement
- Possibly proteinuria from muscle breakdown
- Possibly impaired blood and lymph drainage from the bladder base, resulting from edema caused by the presenting fetal part
- Decreased bladder sensation if epidural anesthetic has been administered

Evaluating the fetus during true labor

Evaluation of uterine contractions and fetal heart rate (FHR) during true labor involves external and internal monitoring.

Heart check

FHR can be monitored either intermittently with a handheld device or continuously with an electronic fetal monitor.

Pressure check

Contraction frequency and intensity is monitored externally with a **tocotransducer.** This pressure-sensitive device records uterine motion during contractions. Contractions may also be monitored by palpation.

From the inside out

Internal electronic fetal monitoring can evaluate fetal status during labor more accurately than external methods. A spiral electrode attached to the presenting fetal part provides the baseline FHR and allows evaluation of FHR variability.

Intense info

To determine the true intensity of contractions, a **pressure-sensitive catheter** is inserted into the uterine cavity alongside the fetus.

Stages of labor

The labor process is divided into four stages, ranging from the onset of true labor through delivery of the fetus and placenta to the first hour after delivery.

FIRST STAGE

The first stage is measured from the onset of true labor to complete dilation of the cervix. This period lasts from 6 to 18 hours in a primiparous client and from 2 to 10 hours in a multiparous client. There are three phases of stage one.

This is getting exciting

During the **latent phase,** the cervix is dilated 0 to 3 cm, contractions are irregular, and the client may experience anticipation, excitement, or apprehension. Cervical effacement is almost complete.

This is getting serious

During the **active phase,** the cervix is dilated 4 to 7 cm. Cervical effacement is complete. Contractions are about 5 to 8 minutes apart and last 45 to 60 seconds with moderate to strong intensity. During this phase, the client becomes serious and concerned about the progress of labor; she may ask for pain medication or use breathing techniques. If membranes haven't ruptured spontaneously, amniotomy may be performed.

Whole lotta shakin' going on

During the **transitional phase,** the cervix is dilated 8 to 10 cm. Contractions are about 1 to 2 minutes apart and last 60 to 90 seconds with strong intensity. During this phase, the client may lose control, thrash in bed, groan, or cry out.

SECOND STAGE

The second stage of labor extends from complete dilation to delivery. This stage lasts an average of 40 minutes (20 contractions) for the primiparous client and 20 minutes (10 contractions) for the multiparous client. It may last longer if the client has had epidural anesthesia.

The client may become exhausted and dehydrated as she moves from coping with contractions to actively pushing. During this stage, the fetus is moved along the birth canal by the mechanisms of labor described here.

A brief engagement

The fetus's head is considered to be **engaged** when the biparietal diameter passes the pelvic inlet.

Going down

The movement of the presenting part through the pelvis is called **descent.**

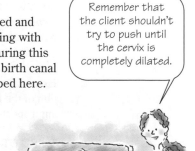

Remember that the client shouldn't try to push until the cervix is completely dilated.

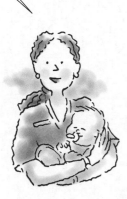

Nursing care during labor and delivery

Nursing actions include interventions that correspond to all stages of labor as well as those that apply only to certain stages.

CARE DURING ALL STAGES OF LABOR
• Monitor and record vital signs, I.V. fluid intake, and urine output.
• Provide emotional support to the client and her coach.
• Assess the need for pain medication, and evaluate the effectiveness of pain-relief measures.
• Maintain sterile technique and standard precautions.
• Maintain the client's comfort by offering mouth care, ice chips, and a change of bed linen.
• Explain the purpose of all nursing actions and medical equipment.

CARE DURING FIRST AND SECOND STAGES
• Monitor the frequency, duration, and intensity of contractions.

• Monitor fetal heart rate during and between contractions, and report changes.
• Observe for rupture of membranes, noting the time, color, odor, amount, and consistency of amniotic fluid.
• Watch for signs of hypotensive supine syndrome; if blood pressure falls, position the client on the left side and report changes immediately.
• During the second stage, observe the perineum for show and bulging.

CARE DURING FIRST, SECOND, AND THIRD STAGES
• Assist with breathing techniques.
• Encourage rest between contractions.

CARE DURING THE FOURTH STAGE
• Assess lochia and the location and consistency of the fundus.
• Encourage bonding.
• Initiate breast-feeding.

Flex that chin
During **flexion,** the head flexes so that the chin moves closer to the chest.

Head rotation I
Internal rotation is the rotation of the head in order to pass through the ischial spines.

Stretch as you go by
Extension is when the head extends as it passes under the symphysis pubis.

Head rotation II
External rotation involves the external rotation of the head as the shoulders rotate to the anteroposterior position in the pelvis.

THIRD STAGE
The third stage of labor extends from delivery of the neonate to expulsion of the placenta and lasts from 5 to 30 minutes.

Pain, then placenta
During this period, the client typically focuses on the neonate's condition. The client may experience discomfort from uterine contractions before expelling the placenta.

FOURTH STAGE
The fourth stage of labor is the 1 to 4 hours after delivery, when the primary activity is the promotion of maternal-neonatal bonding.

For a review of nursing actions during the delivery process, see *Nursing care during labor and delivery.*

Pain relief during labor and delivery

Pain relief is an important element of client care during labor and delivery. Pain relief during labor includes nonpharmacologic methods, analgesics, and general or regional anesthetics.

Just relax
Relaxation techniques may be effective.

Just rub it
Effleurage, a light abdominal stroking with the fingertips in a circular motion, is effective for mild to moderate discomfort.

Hey, look over here
Distraction can divert attention from mild discomfort early in labor. Focal point imaging and music are sometimes effective diversions.

Breathing, breathing, breathing
Three patterns of controlled chest breathing, called **Lamaze breathing,** are used primarily during the active and transitional phases of labor.

Ancient pain relief
The stimulation of key trigger points with needles (**acupuncture**) or finger pressure (**acupressure**) can reduce pain and enhance energy flow.

Pain relief but not without risk
Opioids, such as nalbuphine, can be used to relieve pain. If an opioid is given within 2 hours of delivery, it can cause neonatal respiratory depression, hypotonia, and lethargy.

Less pain but still awake
Lumbar epidural anesthesia requires an injection of medication into the epidural space in the lumbar region, leaving the client awake and cooperative. An epidural provides analgesia for the first and second stages of labor and anesthesia for delivery without adverse fetal effects. Hypotension is uncommon, but its incidence increases if the client doesn't receive a proper fluid load before the procedure. Epidural anesthesia may decrease the woman's urge to push.

Urgent cases
Spinal anesthesia involves an injection of medication into the cerebrospinal fluid in the spinal canal. Because of its rapid onset, spinal anesthesia is useful for urgent cesarean deliveries.

Delivery relief
Local infiltration involves an injection of anesthetic into the perineal nerves. It offers no relief from discomfort during labor but relieves pain during delivery.

Pain blocker I
A **pudendal block** involves blockage of the pudendal nerve. This procedure is used only for delivery.

Pain blocker II
A **paracervical block** involves the blockage of nerves in the peridural space at the sacral hiatus, which provides analgesia for the first and second stages of labor and anesthesia for delivery. This procedure increases the risk of forceps delivery.

Knockout drops
General anesthetics can be administered I.V. or through inhalation, resulting in unconsciousness. General anesthetics should be used only if regional anesthetics are contraindicated or in a rapidly developing emergency.

I.V. anesthetics, which are usually reserved for clients with massive blood loss, include ketamine (Ketalar).

Inhalation anesthetics include nitrous oxide and isoflurane (Forane).

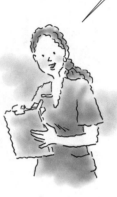

Hypotension after an epidural is uncommon but can occur if the client doesn't receive enough fluids beforehand.

Keep abreast of diagnostic tests

The key diagnostic test in the intrapartum period is fetal blood sampling.

Scratch the scalp
Fetal blood sampling is a method of monitoring fetal blood pH when indefinite or suspicious FHR patterns occur. The blood sample is usually taken from the scalp but may also be taken from the presenting part if the fetus

is in a breech presentation. Fetal blood sampling requires that:
- membranes be ruptured
- the cervix be dilated 2 to 3 cm
- the presenting part be no higher than −2 station.

A pH of 7.25 or higher is normal, 7.20 to 7.24 is preacidotic, and lower than 7.20 constitutes severe acidosis.

Nursing actions
- Explain the procedure to the client.
- After the procedure, observe the FHR and observe the client for vaginal bleeding, which may indicate fetal scalp bleeding.

Polish up on client care

Some potential intrapartum complications are abruptio placentae, amniotic fluid embolism, disseminated intravascular coagulation (DIC), dystocia, fetal distress, inverted uterus, laceration, precipitate labor, premature rupture of membranes (PROM), prolapsed umbilical cord, and uterine rupture.

Abruptio placentae

Abruptio placentae refers to premature separation of the placenta from the uterine wall after 20 to 24 weeks of gestation. It may occur as late as the first or second stage of labor. Placental separation is measured by degree (from grades 0 to 3) to determine the fetal and maternal outcome.

Perinatal mortality depends on the degree of placental separation and fetal level of maturity. Most serious complications stem from hypoxia, prematurity, and anemia. The maternal mortality rate is about 6% and depends on the severity of bleeding, the presence of coagulation defects, hypofibrinogenemia, and the time lapse between placental separation and delivery.

CAUSES
- Abdominal trauma
- Cocaine or "crack" use

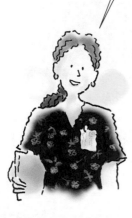

Abruptio placentae can occur anytime from 20 weeks' gestation through the second stage of labor.

- Decreased blood flow to the placenta
- Hydramnios
- Multifetal pregnancy
- Other risk factors (low serum folic acid levels, vascular or renal disease, hypertensive disorders of pregnancy)

ASSESSMENT FINDINGS
- Acute abdominal pain
- Frequent, low-amplitude contractions (noted with an external fetal monitor)
- Hemorrhage, either concealed or apparent, with dark red vaginal bleeding
- Rigid abdomen
- Shock
- Uteroplacental insufficiency

DIAGNOSTIC TEST RESULTS
- Ultrasonography locates the placenta and may reveal a clot or hematoma.
- Coagulation studies may show evidence of DIC — increased partial thromboplastin time (PTT) and prothrombin time (PT), elevated level of fibrinogen degradation products, and decreased fibrinogen level.
- Hematology may reveal decreased platelet count if DIC is present.

NURSING DIAGNOSES
- Anxiety
- Deficient fluid volume
- Risk for decreased cardiac tissue perfusion

TREATMENT
- Transfusion: packed red blood cells (RBCs), platelets, and fresh frozen plasma, if necessary
- Cesarean birth

INTERVENTIONS AND RATIONALES
- Monitor maternal vital signs, FHR, uterine contractions, and vaginal bleeding *to assess maternal and fetal well-being.*
- Assess fluid and electrolyte balance *to assess renal function.*
- Avoid pelvic or vaginal examinations and enemas *to prevent further placental disruption.*
- Administer blood products and monitor vital signs *to detect adverse reactions.*

- Provide oxygen by mask *to minimize fetal hypoxia*.
- Position the client in a left lateral recumbent position *to help relieve pressure on the vena cava from an enlarged uterus, which could further compromise fetal circulation*.
- Provide emotional support *to allay client anxiety*.

Teaching topics
- Explanation of the disorder and treatment plan
- Activity restrictions

Amniotic fluid embolism

In amniotic fluid embolism, amniotic fluid escapes into the maternal circulation because of a defect in the membranes after rupture or partial abruptio placentae. During labor (or in the postpartum period), solid particles, such as skin cells, enter the maternal circulation and reach the lungs as small emboli, forcing a massive pulmonary embolism.

CAUSES
- Oxytocin (Pitocin) administration
- Abruptio placentae
- Polyhydramnios

ASSESSMENT FINDINGS
- Chest pain
- Hypertension
- Coughing with pink, frothy sputum
- Cyanosis
- Hemorrhage
- Increasing restlessness and anxiety
- Shock disproportionate to blood loss
- Sudden dyspnea
- Tachypnea
- Fetal bradycardia

DIAGNOSTIC TEST RESULTS
- Electronic fetal monitor reveals fetal distress (during the intrapartum period).
- Arterial blood gas (ABG) results reveal hypoxemia.
- Coagulation studies may reveal DIC.
- Chest X-ray reveals pulmonary edema.

NURSING DIAGNOSES
- Decreased cardiac output
- Impaired gas exchange
- Ineffective breathing pattern

TREATMENT
- Oxygen therapy: endotracheal intubation and mechanical ventilation if respiratory arrest occurs
- Cardiopulmonary resuscitation (CPR) if client is apneic and pulseless
- Continuous fetal monitoring
- Emergency delivery by cesarean birth
- Blood transfusion, if indicated
- Fluid replacement

Drug therapy
- Anticoagulant: heparin for DIC
- Vasopressor: dopamine
- Uterotonic: oxytocin (Pitocin)
- Activated factor VIIa for severe hemorrhage

INTERVENTIONS AND RATIONALES
- Monitor and record vital signs *to watch for tachycardia and tachypnea, which may indicate hypoxemia*.
- Assess respiratory and cardiovascular status *to detect early signs of compromise*.
- Assess FHR *to detect fetal distress*.
- Administer oxygen, as prescribed, *to improve oxygenation*.
- Assist with endotracheal intubation and mechanical ventilation, if necessary, *to maintain pulmonary function*.
- Perform CPR, if necessary, *to restore breathing and circulation*.
- Monitor and record intake and output *to detect deficient fluid volume*.
- Assist with immediate delivery of the neonate *to prevent fetal compromise*.

Teaching topics
- Explaining the disorder and treatment options to the client and her family

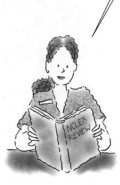

In amniotic fluid embolism, amniotic fluid escapes into the maternal circulation. It's an emergency that can require CPR.

Disseminated intravascular coagulation

DIC refers to increased production of pro-thrombin, platelets, and other coagulation factors, leading to widespread thrombus formation, depletion of clotting factors, and hemorrhage.

CAUSES
• Abruptio placentae
• Amniotic fluid embolism
• Retained fetus after demise

ASSESSMENT FINDINGS
• Abnormal bleeding (petechiae, hema-tomas, ecchymosis, cutaneous oozing)
• Nausea
• Oliguria
• Severe muscle, back, and abdominal pain
• Shock
• Vomiting

DIAGNOSTIC TEST RESULTS
• Coagulation studies reveal decreased fibrinogen level, positive D-dimer test specific for DIC, prolonged PT, and prolonged PTT.
• Hematology studies reveal decreased platelet count.

NURSING DIAGNOSES
• Risk for deficient fluid volume
• Ineffective tissue perfusion: Cardiopulmonary
• Decreased cardiac output

TREATMENT
• Transfusion therapy: packed RBCs, fresh frozen plasma, platelets, and cryoprecipitate
• Oxygen therapy
• Treatment of underlying condition
• Immediate delivery of the fetus by cesarean birth

Drug therapy
• Anticoagulant: heparin

INTERVENTIONS AND RATIONALES
• Monitor cardiovascular, respiratory, neuro-logic, GI, and renal status *to detect early signs of complications.*
• Monitor vital signs frequently *to detect signs of shock (increased tachycardia and hypo-tension).*
• Check all I.V. and venipuncture sites frequently for bleeding. Apply pressure to injection sites for at least 10 minutes. Alert other personnel to the client's tendency to hemorrhage. *These measures help to prevent hemorrhage.*
• Monitor intake and output *to detect signs of hypovolemia.*
• Enforce complete bed rest *to protect the client from injury.*
• Administer blood products and monitor the client closely for signs and symptoms of a transfusion reaction *to detect life-threatening complications.*
• Administer oxygen *to meet the body's increased oxygen demands.*
• Monitor the results of serial blood studies *to help guide the treatment plan.*

Teaching topics
• Explaining the disorder and treatment options to the client and her family
• Bleeding prevention

Dystocia

Dystocia is long, difficult, or abnormal labor. It's estimated that approximately 10% of women experience dystocia during the first stage of labor when the fetus assumes the vertex position.

CAUSES
• Problems with the power:
  – hypertonic uterine patterns
  – hypotonic uterine patterns
• Problems with the passenger:
  – fetal weight of 4500 g or more
  – malposition or malformation of the fetus
• Problems with the passage:
  – inadequate pelvic inlet

Dystocia is long, difficult labor. It's experienced by about 10% of women during the first stage of labor.

ASSESSMENT FINDINGS
- Arrested descent
- Hypertonic contractions
- Hypotonic contractions
- Prolonged active phase
- Prolonged deceleration phase
- Protracted latent phase
- Uncoordinated contractions

DIAGNOSTIC TEST RESULTS
- Ultrasonography shows fetal position or malformation or fetal weight greater than 4,500 g.
- Clinical pelvimetry identifies inadequate size of pelvic inlet.

NURSING DIAGNOSES
- Acute pain
- Deficient fluid volume
- Fear

TREATMENT
- Active management of labor
- I.V. fluid administration
- Delivery of the fetus by cesarean birth if labor fails to progress and the mother or fetus shows signs of compromise

Drug therapy
- Uterotonic: oxytocin (Pitocin) if contractions are ineffective

INTERVENTIONS AND RATIONALES
- Monitor maternal vital signs and FHR *to detect early signs of compromise.*
- Provide emotional support and encouragement *to help alleviate fear and anxiety.*
- Assist the client to a left side-lying position *to increase comfort and to relieve pressure on the vena cava from an enlarged uterus, which could compromise fetal circulation.*
- Encourage the client to void every 2 hours *to keep the bladder empty.*
- Monitor the effectiveness of oxytocin therapy and watch for complications *to ensure prompt intervention if complications occur.*

Teaching topics
- Explanation of the disorder and treatment plan

Fetal distress

Fetal distress refers to fetal compromise that results in a stressful and potentially lethal condition.

CAUSES
- Fetal hypoxia
- Prolapsed umbilical cord
- Unfavorable uterine environment
- Maternal causes: fever, drug use, illness
- Moderate to severe Rh factor isoimmunization

ASSESSMENT FINDINGS
- Meconium-stained fluid
- Electronic fetal monitoring reveals bradycardia or FHR greater than 180 beats/minute
- Maternal signs and symptoms of underlying illness
- Unsatisfactory progress of labor
- Loss of fetal movement

DIAGNOSTIC TEST RESULTS
- Fetal scalp blood sampling reveals acidosis.

NURSING DIAGNOSES
- Anxiety
- Fear
- Risk for decreased cardiac tissue perfusion

TREATMENT
- Supplemental oxygen by face mask, typically at 6 to 8 L/minute
- Amnioinfusion if the fetus exhibits variable deceleration not relieved by oxygen, positioning, or discontinuation of oxytocin (Pitocin) infusion (see *Understanding amnioinfusion*)
- I.V. fluid administration
- Emergency fetal delivery by vacuum aspiration, forceps, or cesarean birth

Drug therapy
- Discontinuing oxytocin infusion

INTERVENTIONS AND RATIONALES
- Monitor FHR, fetal activity, and fetal heart variability *to detect early signs of fetal compromise.*

Understanding amnioinfusion

Amnioinfusion is the replacement of amniotic fluid volume through intrauterine infusion of a saline solution, using a pressure catheter. This procedure is indicated for the treatment of repetitive variable decelerations not alleviated by maternal position change and oxygen administration.

Amnioinfusion relieves umbilical cord compression in such conditions as:
- oligohydramnios associated with post-maturity
- intrauterine growth retardation
- premature rupture of membranes.

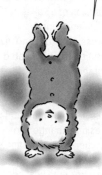

• Monitor maternal vital signs and pulse oximetry *to detect early signs of compromise.*
• Notify the physician immediately of signs of compromise *to ensure prompt treatment.*
• Monitor intake and output *to detect early signs of deficient fluid volume.*
• Assist the client to a left side-lying position *to relieve pressure on the vena cava from an enlarged uterus, which could compromise fetal circulation.*

Teaching topics
• Explanation of the disorder and treatment plan

Inverted uterus

An inverted uterus can occur during delivery of the placenta. The inversion can be partial or total.

CAUSES
• Excessive cord traction
• Excessive fundal pressure

ASSESSMENT FINDINGS
• Large, sudden gush of blood from the vagina
• Signs of blood loss, such as hypotension, tachycardia, dizziness, paleness, and diaphoresis, which can progress to shock if blood loss continues unchecked for more than a few minutes
• Inability to palpate the fundus
• Severe uterine pain
• Uterine mass within the vaginal canal

DIAGNOSTIC TEST RESULTS
• Hematology tests reveal decreased levels of hemoglobin (Hb) and hematocrit (HCT).

NURSING DIAGNOSES
• Acute pain
• Deficient fluid volume
• Risk for decreased cardiac tissue perfusion

TREATMENT
• Fluid resuscitation with I.V. fluids and blood products
• Supplemental oxygen administration

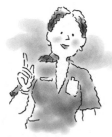

• Immediate manual replacement of the uterus
• Possible emergency hysterectomy

Drug therapy
• Vasodilator: nitroglycerin to relax the uterus
• Tocolytic agent: terbutaline
• Oxytocic agent: oxytocin (Pitocin) after replacing the uterus to aid contraction
• Antibiotics to prevent infection because the uterus was exposed
• Analgesics: meperidine, morphine

INTERVENTIONS AND RATIONALES
• Administer supplemental oxygen *to meet increased oxygen demand.*
• Monitor vital signs frequently *to detect early signs of shock.*
• Monitor intake and output *to detect signs of deficient fluid volume.*
• Initiate CPR, if needed, *to restore circulation and breathing.*
• Assess the uterus for firmness, height, and position during the recovery phase *to detect complications.*
• Provide emotional support to the client and her family *to help allay fears and anxiety.*

Teaching topics
• Explanation of the disorder and treatment plan

Laceration

Laceration refers to tears in the perineum, vagina, or cervix from the stretching of tissues during delivery. Lacerations are classified as first, second, third, or fourth degree.

First-degree laceration involves the vaginal mucosa and the skin of the perineum and fourchette.

Second-degree laceration involves the vagina, perineal skin, fascia, levator ani muscle, and perineal body.

Third-degree laceration involves the entire perineum and the external anal sphincter.

Fourth-degree laceration involves the entire perineum and rectal sphincter and portions of the rectal mucosa.

CAUSES
- Large infant size
- Instruments used to facilitate birth
- Position of the fetus

ASSESSMENT FINDINGS
- Increased vaginal bleeding after delivery of placenta
- Evidence of laceration

DIAGNOSTIC TEST RESULTS
- Hematology studies may reveal decreased levels of Hb and HCT.

NURSING DIAGNOSES
- Acute pain
- Deficient fluid volume
- Fear

TREATMENT
- Laceration repair
- Cold application followed by heat application
- Sitz bath

Drug therapy
- Antibiotics possibly needed in some cases
- Analgesics: ibuprofen (Motrin), acetaminophen and oxycodone (Percocet), acetaminophen (Tylenol)
- Stool softener: docusate sodium (Colace)

INTERVENTIONS AND RATIONALES
- Monitor vital signs, including temperature, *to detect early signs of infection.*
- Monitor the laceration site for signs of infection and bleeding *to ensure prompt treatment interventions.*
- Insert an indwelling urinary catheter, if indicated, *to keep the perineal area clean and promote healing.*
- Provide maternal support and explain procedures *to allay anxiety.*

- Refrain from administering suppositories or enemas to a client with a third- or fourth-degree laceration *to prevent trauma to the repaired laceration site.*
- Apply cold packs to the perineal area for 12 hours, followed by heat packs and sitz baths for the next 12 hours, *to promote comfort and healing.*

Teaching topics
- Explanation of the disorder and treatment plan
- Perineal care
- Medication use and possible adverse effects

Precipitate labor

Precipitate labor occurs when uterine contractions are so strong that the woman delivers with only a few rapidly occurring contractions. It's commonly defined as labor completed within less than 3 hours. Such rapid labor may occur with multiparity. It may also follow induction of labor by oxytocin (Pitocin) or an amniotomy.

CAUSES
- Lack of maternal tissue resistance to the passage of the fetus
- Oxytocin administration
- Amniotomy

ASSESSMENT FINDINGS
- Cervical dilation greater than 5 cm/hour in a nulliparous woman; more than 10 cm/hour in a multiparous woman

DIAGNOSTIC TEST RESULTS
- There are no diagnostic test findings specific to this complication.

NURSING DIAGNOSES
- Anxiety
- Fear
- Risk for injury

TREATMENT
- Nonpharmacologic measures for pain control
- Controlled delivery to prevent maternal and fetal injury

Drug therapy
• Tocolytic agent: terbutaline to reduce the force and frequency of contractions

INTERVENTIONS AND RATIONALES
• Monitor FHR and variability *to detect early signs of fetal distress.*
• Monitor the infusion of a tocolytic drug *to detect early signs of adverse reactions.*
• Institute nonpharmacologic measures *to control pain, such as breathing exercises and distraction.*
• Provide emotional support *to allay anxiety and fear.*

Teaching topics
• Explanation of the disorder and treatment plan

Premature rupture of membranes

PROM is the rupture of membranes beyond 37 weeks' gestation but before the onset of labor. Chorioamnionitis may occur if the time between rupture of membranes and onset of labor is longer than 24 hours.

Preterm PROM is the rupture of membranes before 37 weeks' gestation.

CAUSES AND CONTRIBUTING FACTORS
• Cause unknown (however, malpresentation and a contracted pelvis commonly accompany the rupture)
• Lack of proper prenatal care
• Poor nutrition and hygiene
• Maternal smoking
• Incompetent cervix
• Increased uterine tension from hydramnios or multiple gestation
• Reduced amniotic membrane tensile strength
• Uterine infection

ASSESSMENT FINDINGS
• Fetal tachycardia
• Blood-tinged amniotic fluid gushing or leaking from the vagina
• Foul-smelling amniotic fluid if infection is present

• Maternal fever
• Uterine tenderness

DIAGNOSTIC TEST RESULTS
• Hematology studies may reveal an elevated white blood cell count if infection is present.
• Vaginal probe ultrasonography allows detection of an amniotic sac tear or rupture.
• Amniotic fluid culture and sensitivity identifies the causative organism of infection.

NURSING DIAGNOSES
• Anxiety
• Risk for infection
• Risk for injury

TREATMENT
• Hospitalization to monitor for maternal fever and leukocytosis and fetal tachycardia if the pregnancy is between 28 and 34 weeks (if infection is confirmed, labor must be induced)
• Cesarean birth if labor induction fails

Drug therapy
• Oxytocic agent: oxytocin (Pitocin) for labor induction if term pregnancy and labor doesn't result within 24 hours after membrane rupture
• Antibiotics according to culture and sensitivity results if infection is present

INTERVENTIONS AND RATIONALES
• Monitor for signs of labor and then progression of labor *to assess fetal progression.*
• Assess for signs of infection or fetal distress *to avoid treatment delay.*
• Administer antibiotics as prescribed *to treat infection and prevent complications.*
• Encourage the client to express her feelings and concerns *to allay her anxiety.*
• Monitor intake and output closely *to quickly identify signs of deficient fluid volume.*
• Assess the client for adverse reactions to oxytocin *to prevent complications.*

Teaching topics
• Explanation of the disorder and treatment plan

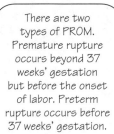

There are two types of PROM. Premature rupture occurs beyond 37 weeks' gestation but before the onset of labor. Preterm rupture occurs before 37 weeks' gestation.

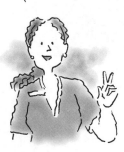

Prolapsed umbilical cord

A prolapsed umbilical cord occurs when the umbilical cord descends into the vagina before the presenting fetal part.

CAUSES
- Premature rupture of membranes
- Fetal presentation other than cephalic
- Placenta previa
- Intrauterine tumors that prevent the presenting part from engaging
- Small fetus
- Cephalopelvic disproportion that presents firm engagement
- Hydramnios
- Multiple gestation

ASSESSMENT FINDINGS
- Cord palpable during vaginal examination
- Cord visible at the vaginal opening
- Variable decelerations or bradycardia noted on the fetal monitor strip

DIAGNOSTIC TEST RESULTS
- Ultrasonography may reveal the cord as the presenting part.

NURSING DIAGNOSES
- Anxiety
- Risk for injury
- Risk for suffocation

TREATMENT
- Supplemental oxygen therapy at 10 L/ minute by face mask
- Maternal positioning on her hands and knees or with her hips elevated
- Immediate delivery of the fetus
- Nurse or physician maintaining a hand in the client's vagina until delivery occurs

Drug therapy
- Tocolytic agent: terbutaline may be used to reduce the force and frequency of contractions

INTERVENTIONS AND RATIONALES
- Place the client in Trendelenburg's position (position the woman's hips higher than her head in a knee-to-chest position) *to relieve pressure on the umbilical cord and restore blood flow to the fetus.*
- Administer supplemental oxygen *to help meet increased oxygen demands of the mother and fetus.*
- Apply warm saline-moistened towels to the protruding cord *to prevent drying and retard cooling of the cord.*
- Monitor FHR and variability *to detect early signs of fetal distress.*
- Assist with immediate delivery of the fetus *to prevent fetal death.*

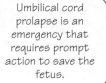

Umbilical cord prolapse is an emergency that requires prompt action to save the fetus.

Uterine rupture

Uterine rupture occurs when the uterus undergoes more strain than it can bear. Without emergency intervention, maternal and fetal death may occur.

CAUSES
- Prolonged labor
- Previous cesarean delivery
- Faulty presentation
- Multiple gestation
- Obstructed labor
- Uterine trauma

ASSESSMENT FINDINGS
- Abdominal pain and tenderness, especially at the peak of a contraction, or the feeling that "something ripped"
- Cessation of uterine contractions
- Chest pain or pain on inspiration
- Excessive external bleeding
- Hypovolemic shock caused by hemorrhage
- Late decelerations, reduced FHR variability, tachycardia and bradycardia, and cessation of FHR
- Palpation of the fetus outside the uterus
- Pathological retraction ring (indentation apparent across the abdomen and over the uterus)

DIAGNOSTIC TEST RESULTS
Diagnostic testing may not be possible in light of the life-threatening situation.
- Hematology tests reveal decreased levels of Hb and HCT.

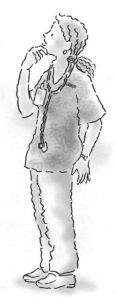

NURSING DIAGNOSES
- Acute pain
- Deficient fluid volume
- Ineffective tissue perfusion: Cardiopulmonary

TREATMENT
- Fluid resuscitation: I.V. fluids and blood products via rapid infusion
- Supplemental oxygen therapy, which may include endotracheal intubation and mechanical ventilation
- Surgery to remove the fetus and repair the tear, or hysterectomy, if necessary

Drug therapy
- Oxytocic agent: oxytocin (Pitocin) to help contract the uterus

INTERVENTIONS AND RATIONALES
- Monitor vital signs frequently *to detect signs of shock.*
- Prepare the client for immediate surgery *to avoid life-threatening treatment delay.*
- Administer supplemental oxygen *to meet increased oxygen demands.*
- Monitor I.V. fluid administration *to detect early signs of infiltration.*
- Monitor intake and output *to detect early signs of deficient fluid volume.*
- Assess cardiovascular, neurologic, and renal status *to detect early signs of compromise.*
- Provide emotional support to the parents *to promote healing in the occurrence of fetal demise or hysterectomy.*

Teaching topics
- Explanation of the disorder and treatment plan
- Postoperative care
- Availability of grief counseling

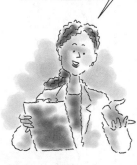

Note the most common complications requiring emergency birth: prolapsed umbilical cord, uterine rupture, and amniotic fluid embolism.

Emergency birth and preterm labor

Emergency birth and preterm labor are two examples of conditions requiring nursing care that may occur during the intrapartum period.

Emergency birth

Emergency delivery of the fetus may become necessary when the well-being of the mother or fetus is in jeopardy. Causes may include a prolapsed umbilical cord, uterine rupture, or amniotic fluid embolism.

CONTRIBUTING FACTORS
Contributing factors vary for each emergency birth situation.

Prolapsed umbilical cord
- Fetus presentation other than cephalic
- Hydramnios (excess of amniotic fluid)
- Multiple gestation
- Placenta previa
- Premature rupture of membranes

Uterine rupture
- Uterine trauma
- Previous uterine surgery
- Multiple gestation

Amniotic fluid embolism
- Abruptio placentae
- Polyhydramnios

ASSESSMENT FINDINGS
Data collection findings vary for each emergency birth situation.

Prolapsed umbilical cord
- Cord palpable during vaginal examination
- Cord visible at the vaginal opening
- Variable decelerations or bradycardia noted on the fetal monitor strip

Uterine rupture
- Abdominal pain and tenderness, especially at the peak of a contraction, or the feeling that "something ripped"
- Cessation of uterine contractions
- Chest pain or pain on inspiration
- Excessive external bleeding
- Hypovolemic shock caused by hemorrhage
- Late decelerations, reduced FHR variability, tachycardia and bradycardia, and cessation of FHR
- Palpation of the fetus outside the uterus

Amniotic fluid embolism
- Chest pain
- Coughing with pink, frothy sputum
- Cyanosis
- Hemorrhage
- Increasing restlessness and anxiety
- Shock disproportionate to blood loss
- Sudden dyspnea
- Tachypnea

DIAGNOSTIC TEST RESULTS
Prolapsed umbilical cord
- Ultrasonography confirms that the cord is prolapsed.

Uterine rupture
- Urinalysis can detect gross hematuria.
- Ultrasonography may reveal the absence of the amniotic cavity within the uterus.

Amniotic fluid embolism
- ABG analysis reveals hypoxemia.
- Hematology reveals thrombocytopenia, decreased fibrinogen level and platelet count, prolonged PT, and a PTT consistent with DIC.

NURSING DIAGNOSES
- Ineffective coping
- Acute pain
- Risk for infection

TREATMENT
- Administration of I.V. fluid
- Administration of oxygen by nasal cannula or mask (endotracheal intubation and mechanical ventilation may be necessary in the case of amniotic fluid embolism)
- Placing the client in left lateral recumbent position (for uterine rupture)
- Emergency hysterectomy (for uterine rupture)
- Emergency cesarean birth (see *Cesarean birth*)
- Possible transfusion of packed RBCs, fresh frozen plasma, or platelets

INTERVENTIONS AND RATIONALES
- Monitor maternal vital signs, pulse oximetry and intake and output as well as FHR *to assess for complications.*
- Administer maternal oxygen by cannula or mask at 8 to 10 L/minute *to maintain uteroplacental oxygenation.*

Management moments

Cesarean birth

Cesarean birth is the planned or emergency removal of the neonate from the uterus through an abdominal incision. A midline and vertical (classic) incision, allowing easy access to the fetus, is usually used in emergency situations. A low-segment, transverse, or Pfannenstiel (bikini) incision is usually chosen in a planned cesarean birth.

NURSING ACTIONS
- Provide emotional support and reassurance to the patient and her family, including reassurance about the well-being of the fetus.
- Assess fetal heart rate and maternal vital signs and intake and output.
- Monitor uterine contractions and labor progress, when appropriate.
- Obtain blood samples for hematocrit, hemoglobin level, prothrombin and partial thromboplastin times, fibrinogen level, platelet count, and typing and crossmatching.
- Maintain I.V. fluid replacement as necessary.
- Prepare the patient for surgery, including shaving of the abdomen and perineal area as necessary.
- Insert an indwelling urinary catheter as ordered.
- Provide preoperative teaching as necessary.
- Administer preoperative sedation as ordered.
- Provide immediate postoperative care.

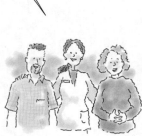

Therapeutic communication is key during emergency birth situations. The client and her family rely on you for support, reassurance, and information.

• Maintain I.V. fluid replacement *to replace volume loss.*
• Place the client in a left lateral recumbent position *to relieve pressure on the vena cava due to an enlarged uterus, which would compromise fetal circulation.*
• Provide emotional support and reassurance to the client *to allay fears and reduce anxiety.*
• Obtain blood samples to determine HCT, Hb level, PT and PTT, fibrinogen level, and platelet count and to type and crossmatch blood *to establish baseline values.*
• Monitor blood product administration, as necessary, *to replace volume loss.*
• Prepare the client and her family for the possibility of cesarean birth *to reduce anxiety.*

Teaching topics
• Reason for emergency birth
• Learning about procedures
• Understanding preoperative instruction
• Using breathing techniques

Preterm labor

Preterm labor, occurs before the end of the 37th week of gestation. Preterm labor can place both the mother and the fetus at high risk.

CAUSES AND CONTRIBUTING FACTORS
Causes of and contributing risk factors to preterm labor can be maternal or fetal.

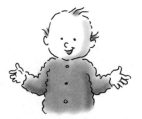

What can I say...sometimes I show up late, sometimes I show up early!

Maternal causes
• Abdominal surgery or trauma
• Cardiovascular and renal disease
• Dehydration
• Diabetes mellitus
• Incompetent cervix
• Infection
• Placental abnormalities
• Gestational hypertension
• PROM
• Smoking

Fetal causes
• Hydramnios
• Infection
• Multifetal pregnancy

ASSESSMENT FINDINGS
• Feeling of pelvic pressure or abdominal tightening
• Increased vaginal discharge
• Intestinal cramping
• Menstrual-like cramps
• Pain or discomfort in the vulva or thighs
• Persistent, low, dull backache
• Uterine contractions that result in cervical dilation and effacement
• Vaginal spotting

DIAGNOSTIC TEST RESULTS
• Electronic fetal monitoring confirms uterine contractions.
• Vaginal examination confirms cervical effacement and dilation.

NURSING DIAGNOSES
• Anxiety
• Deficient knowledge (treatment plan)
• Risk for injury

TREATMENT
• Suppression of preterm labor (if the fetal membranes are intact, there's no evidence of bleeding, the well-being of the fetus and mother isn't in jeopardy, cervical effacement is no more than 50%, and cervical dilation is less than 4 cm)
• Bed rest

Drug therapy
• Antibiotics according to organism sensitivity if urinary tract infection is present
• Betamethasone administered I.M. at regular intervals over 48 hours to increase fetal lung maturity in a fetus expected to be delivered preterm
• Nifedipine (Procardia), a calcium channel blocker, to decrease the production of calcium, a substance associated with the initiation of labor (adverse maternal effects include dizziness, nausea, bradycardia, and flushing)
• Indomethacin (Indocin) to decrease the production of prostaglandins and lipid compounds associated with the initiation of labor (adverse maternal effects include nausea, vomiting, and dyspepsia; premature closure of the fetus's ductus arteriosus can occur if indomethacin is given before 32 weeks' gestation)

• Magnesium sulfate to prevent a reflux of calcium into the myometrial cells, thereby maintaining a relaxed uterus

• Tocolytic agents, such as terbutaline and ritodrine (Yutopar), to inhibit uterine contractions (maternal adverse effects include tachycardia, hypoglycemia, hypokalemia, hypotension, and nervousness)

INTERVENTIONS AND RATIONALES

• Monitor maternal vital signs, contractions, and FHR every 15 minutes during tocolytic therapy (otherwise, provide continuous fetal monitoring) *to assess maternal and fetal well-being.*

• Notify the physician if the maternal pulse rate exceeds 120 beats/minute or the FHR exceeds 180 beats/minute *to expedite medical evaluation of maternal and fetal status.*

• Monitor the mother's respiratory status *to assess for pulmonary edema, an adverse effect associated with tocolytic therapy.*

• Monitor for maternal adverse reactions to terbutaline or ritodrine *to detect possible tachycardia, diarrhea, nervousness, tremors, nausea, vomiting, headache, hyperglycemia, hypoglycemia, hypokalemia, or pulmonary edema.*

• Provide emotional support to the mother *to ease anxiety and establish a therapeutic relationship.*

• Place the client in the lateral position *to increase placental perfusion.*

• Monitor for magnesium sulfate toxicity, which causes central nervous system depression in the mother and fetus, and make sure calcium gluconate is available *to reverse these effects.*

• Assess the neonate for possible adverse effects of indomethacin, such as premature closure of the ductus arteriosus.

Teaching topics

• Explanation of the disorder and treatment plan

• Medication use and possible adverse effects

• Following instructions for ongoing tocolytic therapy, if appropriate

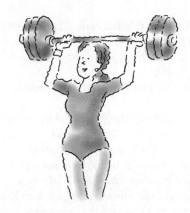

Pump up on practice questions

1. A client in the 28th week of gestation comes to the emergency department because she thinks that she's in labor. To confirm a diagnosis of preterm labor, the nurse would expect the physical examination to reveal:

    1. irregular uterine contractions with no cervical dilation.

    2. painful contractions with no cervical dilation.

    3. regular uterine contractions with cervical dilation.

    4. regular uterine contractions with no cervical dilation.

Answer: 3. Regular uterine contractions (every 10 minutes or more) along with cervical dilation before 36 weeks' gestation or rupture of fluids indicates preterm labor. Uterine contractions without cervical dilation don't indicate preterm labor.

➡ *NCLEX keys*
Client needs category: Physiological integrity
Client needs subcategory: Physiological adaptation
Cognitive level: Application

2. A client in the active phase of labor has a reactive fetal monitor strip and has been encouraged to walk. When she returns to bed for a monitor check, she complains of an urge to push. The nurse notes that the amniotic membranes have ruptured and that she can visualize the umbilical cord. What should the nurse do next?

1. Put the client in a knee-to-chest position.
2. Call the physician or midwife.
3. Push down on the uterine fundus.
4. Arrange for fetal blood sampling to assess for fetal acidosis.

Answer: 1. The knee-to-chest position decreases pressure on the baby and umbilical cord and improves blood flow. Calling the physician or midwife and arranging for blood sampling are important, but they have a lower priority than decreasing pressure on the cord. Pushing down on the fundus would increase the danger by further compromising blood flow.

➡ *NCLEX keys*

Client needs category: Physiological integrity
Client needs subcategory: Reduction of risk potential
Cognitive level: Analysis

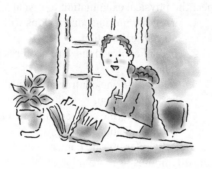

3. A client is attempting to deliver vaginally despite the fact that her previous delivery was by cesarean birth. Her contractions are 2 to 3 minutes apart, lasting from 75 to 100 seconds. Suddenly, the client complains of intense abdominal pain, and the fetal monitor stops picking up contractions. The nurse recognizes that which of the following has occurred?

1. Abruptio placentae
2. Prolapsed cord
3. Partial placenta previa
4. Complete uterine rupture

Answer: 4. In complete uterine rupture, the client would feel a sharp pain in the lower abdomen and contractions would cease. Fetal heart rate would also cease within a few minutes. Uterine irritability would continue to be

indicated by the fetal heart monitor tracing with abruptio placentae. With a prolapsed cord, contractions would continue and there would be no pain from the prolapse itself. There would be vaginal bleeding with a partial placenta previa, but no pain outside of the expected pain of contractions.

➡ *NCLEX keys*

Client needs category: Physiological integrity
Client needs subcategory: Physiological adaptation
Cognitive level: Application

4. A client with gravida 3 para 2 (three pregnancies and two children) at 40 weeks' gestation is admitted with spontaneous contractions. The physician performs an amniotomy to augment her labor. The priority nursing action is to:

1. explain the rationale for the amniotomy to the client.
2. assess fetal heart tones after the amniotomy.
3. ambulate the client to strengthen the contraction pattern.
4. position the client in a lithotomy position to administer perineal care.

Answer: 2. The nurse should assess fetal heart tones after an amniotomy is performed because the umbilical cord may be washed down below the presenting part and cause umbilical cord compression. An explanation of the rationale for amniotomy would be given before the procedure. The nurse would ambulate the client only if the presenting part were engaged. Perineal care can be provided after assessing the fetal response to the amniotomy.

➡ *NCLEX keys*

Client needs category: Physiological integrity
Client needs subcategory: Reduction of risk potential
Cognitive level: Analysis

5. A nurse can consider the fetus's head to be engaged when:

1. the presenting part moves through the pelvis.
2. the fetal head rotates to pass through the ischial spines.

3. the fetal head extends as it passes under the symphysis pubis.
4. the biparietal diameter passes the pelvic inlet.

Answer: 4. The fetus's head is considered engaged when the biparietal diameter passes the pelvic inlet. The presenting part moving through the pelvis is called *descent.* Rotation of the head to pass through the ischial spines is called *internal rotation.* Extension of the head as it passes under the symphysis pubis is called *extension.*

➡ *NCLEX keys*

Client needs category: Health promotion and maintenance
Client needs subcategory: None
Cognitive level: Analysis

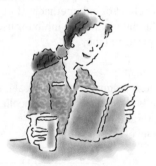

6. A client is dilated to 4 cm. She's asking for an epidural; however, her mother states that because of their culture, she has to "bite the bullet" as she did. What should the nurse do to make sure her client's request is honored?

1. Ask the client in a non-threatening way if it's her wish to have an epidural and then speak with the physician.
2. Honor the client's mother's request for no epidural.
3. Knowing the client's culture, have the family call a meeting to make the decision.
4. Call the anesthesiologist and request that he perform the epidural because the client is uncomfortable.

Answer: 1. It's up to the client to decide if she wants to have an epidural. The nurse is in the role of the advocate for the client. If a client is pregnant (at any age), she becomes emancipated and can make her own decisions. The client's mother or family can't override the client's decision. The nurse can't make the decision to call the physician without the client's consent. The nurse needs to clarify that the client does, in fact, want an epidural before contacting the anesthesiologist.

➡ *NCLEX keys*

Client needs category: Safe and effective care environment
Client needs subcategory: Management of care
Cognitive level: Analysis

7. The nurse receives orders for a client to receive a titrated infusion of oxytocin. Before starting the infusion, the nurse first:

1. initiates I.V. access.
2. checks the label on the infusion bag for proper concentration.
3. sets the infusion pump for the ordered rate.
4. identifies the client.

Answer: 4. The nurse must first identify the client because the infusion must be given to the correct client. Initiating I.V. access, checking the label on the infusion bag, and setting the infusion pump all address proper I.V. medication administration; however, the main concern is providing the infusion to the correct client.

➡ *NCLEX keys*

Client needs category: Safe and effective care environment
Client needs subcategory: Safety and infection control
Cognitive level: Application

8. A client in the second stage of labor experiences rupture of the membranes. The most appropriate intervention by the nurse is to:

1. assess the client's vital signs immediately.
2. observe for a prolapsed cord and monitor fetal heart rate (FHR).
3. administer oxygen through a face mask at 6 to 10 L/minute.
4. position the client on her left side.

Answer: 2. The nurse should immediately check for a prolapsed cord and monitor FHR. When the membranes rupture, the cord may become compressed between the fetus and the maternal cervix or pelvis, thus compromising fetoplacental perfusion. It isn't necessary to monitor maternal vital signs, administer oxygen, or position the client on her left side when the client's membranes rupture.

➡ *NCLEX keys*

Client needs category: Physiological integrity
Client needs subcategory: Reduction of risk potential
Cognitive level: Application

9. On the waveform, identify the area that indicates possible umbilical cord compression.

Answer: Variable decelerations are decreases in fetal heart rate that aren't related to the timing of contractions. Characteristic of umbilical cord compression, variable decelerations generally occur as drops of 10 to 60 beats/minute below the baseline.

➡ *NCLEX keys*

Client needs category: Physiological integrity
Client needs subcategory: Reduction of risk potential
Cognitive level: Analysis

10. A client is receiving magnesium sulfate to help suppress preterm labor. The nurse should watch for which sign of magnesium toxicity?

1. Headache
2. Loss of deep tendon reflexes
3. Palpitations
4. Dyspepsia

Answer: 2. Magnesium toxicity causes signs of central nervous system depression, such as loss of deep tendon reflexes, paralysis, respiratory depression, drowsiness, lethargy, blurred vision, slurred speech, and confusion. Headache may be an adverse effect of calcium channel blockers, which are sometimes used to treat preterm labor. Palpitations are an adverse effect of terbutaline and ritodrine (Yutopar), which are also used to treat preterm labor. Dyspepsia may occur as an adverse effect of indomethacin (Indocin), a prostaglandin synthetase inhibitor used to suppress preterm labor.

➡ *NCLEX keys*

Client needs category: Physiological integrity
Client needs subcategory: Pharmacological and parenteral therapies
Cognitive level: Application

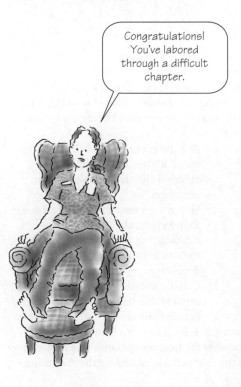

Congratulations! You've labored through a difficult chapter.

24 Postpartum care

Brush up on key concepts

A client undergoes both physiologic and psychological changes after delivery. Understanding these changes is essential to providing safe, effective client care.

At any time, you can review the major points of this chapter by consulting the *Cheat sheet* on page 544.

Physiologic changes after delivery

Here's a brief review of body system changes that occur immediately after delivery.

Circulation gyration

In the **vascular system,** blood volume decreases and hematocrit (HCT) increases after vaginal delivery. Excessive activation of blood-clotting factors also occurs. Blood volume returns to prenatal levels within 3 weeks.

Reproductive regeneration

In the **reproductive system,** uterine involution occurs rapidly immediately after delivery. Progesterone production ceases until the client's first ovulation. Endometrial regeneration begins after 6 weeks. The cervical opening is permanently altered from a circle to a jagged slit.

Hungry for hard work

GI system changes include:
• increased hunger after labor and delivery
• delayed bowel movement from decreased intestinal muscle tone and perineal discomfort
• increased thirst from fluids lost during labor and delivery.

Increasing capacity

Genitourinary system changes include:
• increased urine output during the first 24 to 72 hours after delivery due to an increased glomerular filtration rate and a drop in progesterone levels
• increased bladder capacity
• proteinuria caused by the catalytic process of involution (in 50% of women)
• decreased bladder-filling sensation caused by swollen and bruised tissues
• return of dilated ureters and renal pelvis to prepregnancy size after 6 weeks.

Hormone readjustment

In the **endocrine system,** thyroid function and the production of anterior pituitary gonadotropic hormones is increased. Simultaneously, the production of other hormones, including estrogen, aldosterone, progesterone, human chorionic gonadotropin, corticoids, and ketosteroids, decreases.

Psychological changes after pregnancy

More than 50% of women experience transient mood alterations immediately after pregnancy. This mood change is called **postpartum depression,** or the "baby blues," and signs and symptoms include sadness, crying, fatigue, and low self-esteem. Possible causes include hormonal changes, genetic predisposition, and adjustment to an altered role and self-concept.

Teach the client that mood swings and bouts of depression are normal postpartum responses; they typically occur during the

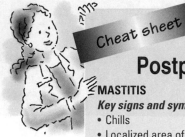

Cheat sheet

Postpartum care refresher

MASTITIS

Key signs and symptoms
- Chills
- Localized area of redness and inflammation on the breast with possible streaks over the breast
- Temperature of 101.1° F (38.4° C) or higher

Key test results
- Culture of purulent discharge may test positive for *Staphylococcus aureus*.

Key treatments
- Incision and drainage if abscess occurs
- Moist heat application to local area
- Pumping breasts to preserve breast-feeding ability if abscess occurs
- Analgesics: acetaminophen (Tylenol), ibuprofen (Advil)
- Antibiotics: cephalexin (Keflex), cefaclor (Raniclor), clindamycin (Cleocin)

Key interventions
- Administer antibiotic therapy.
- Apply moist heat.
- Encourage the client to breast-feed on the affected side before the unaffected side.

POSTPARTUM HEMORRHAGE

Key signs and symptoms
- Blood loss greater than 500 ml within a 24-hour period; may occur up to 6 weeks after delivery
- Signs of shock (tachycardia, hypotension, oliguria)
- Uterine atony

Key test results
- Hematology studies show decreased hemoglobin and hematocrit levels, a low fibrinogen level, and decreased partial thromboplastin time.

Key treatments
- Bimanual compression of the uterus and dilatation and curettage to remove clots
- I.V. replacement of fluids and blood
- Parenteral administration of methylergonovine (Methergine)
- Rapid I.V. infusion of dilute oxytocin (Pitocin)

Key interventions
- Massage the fundus and express clots from the uterus.
- Perform a pad count.
- Monitor the fundus for location.
- Monitor I.V. infusion of dilute oxytocin, as ordered.

PSYCHOLOGICAL MALADAPTATION

Key signs and symptoms
- Inability to stop crying
- Increased anxiety about self and neonate's health
- Overall feeling of sadness
- Unwillingness to be left alone

Key treatments
- Counseling for the client and family at risk
- Psychotherapy for the client
- Antidepressants: imipramine (Tofranil), nortriptyline (Pamelor)

Key interventions
- Obtain a health history during the antepartum period.
- Assess the client's support systems.
- Assess maternal-infant bonding.
- Provide emotional support and encouragement.

PUERPERAL INFECTION

Key signs and symptoms
- Abdominal pain and tenderness
- Purulent, foul-smelling lochia
- Tachycardia

Key test results
- Complete blood count may show an elevated white blood cell count in the upper ranges of normal (more than 30,000/µl) for the postpartum period.
- Cultures of the blood or the endocervical and uterine cavities may reveal the causative organism.

Key treatments
- Broad-spectrum I.V. antibiotic therapy, unless a causative organism is identified

Key interventions
- Monitor vital signs every 4 hours.
- Place the client in Fowler's position.
- Maintain I.V. fluid administration as ordered.
- Administer antibiotics as prescribed.

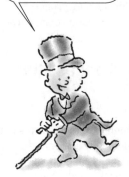

Expecting mothers spend 9 months imagining what I MIGHT be like...it takes them a little while to get used to the real me!

first 3 weeks after delivery and subside within 1 to 10 days.

Maternal behavior after delivery is divided into three phases:
- taking-in phase
- taking-hold phase
- letting-go phase.

What have I gotten myself into?

During the **taking-in phase** (1 to 2 days after delivery), the mother is passive and dependent, directing energy toward herself instead of toward her neonate. She may relive her labor and delivery experience to integrate the process into her life and may have difficulty making decisions.

Getting to know you

During the **taking-hold phase** (about 2 to 7 days after delivery), the mother has more energy and begins to act independently and initiate self-care activities. Although she may express a lack of confidence in her abilities, she accepts responsibility for her neonate and becomes receptive to neonate care and client teaching about self-care activities.

Assuming the role

During the **letting-go phase** (about 7 days after delivery), the mother begins to readjust to family members, assuming the mother role and the responsibility that comes with it. She relinquishes the neonate she has imagined during her pregnancy and accepts her real neonate as an entity separate from herself.

Keep abreast of postpartum assessment

The period immediately after labor and delivery is crucial to good postpartum nursing care. An understanding of normal and abnormal assessment findings is essential.

Monitor, monitor, monitor

The client's respiratory rate should return to normal after delivery. Other findings are listed below.
- The client's temperature may be elevated to 100.4° F (38° C) from dehydration and the exertion of labor.
- Blood pressure is usually normal within 24 hours of delivery.
- Bradycardia of 50 to 70 beats/minute is common during the first 6 to 10 days after delivery because of reductions in cardiac strain, stroke volume, and the vascular bed.

Nursing actions
- Monitor vital signs every 15 minutes for the first 1 to 2 hours, then every 4 hours for the first 24 hours, and then during every shift.

Fundal features

Check the tone and location of the **fundus** (the uppermost portion of the uterus) every 15 minutes for the first 1 to 2 hours after delivery and then during every shift. The involuting uterus should be at the midline. The fundus is usually:
- midway between the umbilicus and symphysis 1 to 2 hours after delivery
- 1 cm above or at the level of the umbilicus 12 hours after delivery
- 3 cm below the umbilicus by the third day after delivery
- firm to the touch.

The fundus will continue to descend about 1 cm/day until it isn't palpable above the symphysis (about 9 days after delivery). The uterus shrinks to its prepregnancy size 5 to 6 weeks after delivery.

A firm uterus helps control postpartum hemorrhage by clamping down on uterine blood vessels. The physician may prescribe oxytocin (Pitocin), ergonovine (Ergotrate), or methylergonovine (Methergine) to maintain uterine firmness. (See *Fundal assessment and massage,* page 546.)

Nursing actions
- Massage a boggy (soft) fundus gently; if the fundus doesn't become firm, use a stronger touch.

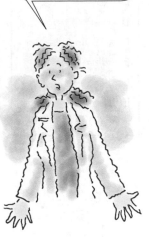

Studying for a big test can also cause mood swings—sometimes you may feel confident, other times anxious. Remind yourself that it's a normal reaction.

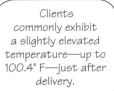

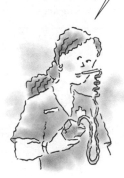

Clients commonly exhibit a slightly elevated temperature—up to 100.4° F—just after delivery.

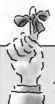

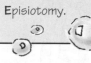

Fundal assessment and massage

WHY YOU DO IT

Fundal assessment is done to evaluate the progress of the uterus after birth, including uterine size, firmness, and descent. Fundal massage helps to maintain or stimulate uterine contractions, which are essential in preventing postpartum hemorrhage.

Assessment and massage should be performed every 15 minutes for the first hour after delivery, every 30 minutes for the next 2 hours, every hour for the next 4 hours, and then every 4 hours for the first postpartum day.

HOW YOU DO IT

• Explain the procedure to the client, and answer any questions. Provide privacy.
• Place the client in the supine position or with her head slightly elevated.
• Expose the abdomen and perineum.
• Gently compress the uterus between your hands to evaluate firmness and position in relation to the umbilicus (in fingerbreadths or centimeters).
• If the fundus seems soft and boggy, massage it gently in a circular motion until it's firm.
• Observe lochia flow during massage.
• Document the client's position, the firmness of the fundus, and the response to massage (if performed).

• Be aware that the uterus may relax if overstimulated by massage or medications.
• Suspect a distended bladder if the uterus isn't firm at the midline. A distended bladder can impede the downward descent of the uterus by pushing it upward and, possibly, to the side.
• Assess maternal-infant bonding by observing how the mother responds to her neonate.
• Assess for excessive vaginal bleeding.

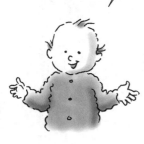

Don't forget to communicate with my mother… she might have questions or might just need a little reassurance.

Discharge diagnosis

Lochia is the discharge from the sloughing of the uterine decidua.
• **Lochia rubra** is the vaginal discharge that occurs for the first 2 to 3 days after delivery; it has a fleshy odor and is bloody with small clots.
• **Lochia serosa** refers to the vaginal discharge that occurs during days 3 through 9; it is pinkish or brown with a serosanguineous consistency and fleshy odor.
• **Lochia alba** is a yellow to white discharge that usually begins about 10 days after delivery; it may last from 2 to 6 weeks.

Some lochia characteristics may indicate the need for further intervention:
• Foul-smelling lochia may indicate an infection.

• Continuous seepage of bright red blood may indicate a cervical or vaginal laceration.
• Lochia that saturates a sanitary pad within 45 minutes usually indicates an abnormally heavy flow.
• Lochia may diminish after a cesarean birth.
• Numerous large clots should be evaluated further; they may interfere with involution.
• Lochia may be scant but should never be absent; absence may indicate postpartum infection.

Nursing actions

• Collect data on the color, amount, odor, and consistency of lochia every shift.

Breast check

Collect data on the size and shape of the client's **breasts** every shift, noting reddened areas, tenderness, and engorgement. Check the nipples for cracking, fissures, and soreness.

Nursing actions

• Advise the client to wear a support bra to maintain breast shape and enhance comfort.
• Tell the non-breast-feeding client that she can relieve discomfort from engorged breasts by wearing a support bra, applying ice packs, and taking prescribed medications.

- If the client is breast-feeding, advise her that she can relieve breast engorgement by feeding the infant frequently, applying warm compresses, and expressing milk manually.
- Explain that nipples should be washed with plain water and allowed to air-dry. Soap and towel drying dries out nipples, causing cracking.

Elimination examination

Assess the client's **elimination** patterns. The client should void within the first 6 to 8 hours after delivery. If she doesn't, assess for a distended bladder, which can interfere with elimination and increase the risk of hemorrhage within the first few hours after delivery.

Nursing actions

- If the client can't urinate, pour warm water over the perineum to help stimulate voiding or insert a urinary catheter.
- Apply required ice packs or analgesic preparations to the client with hemorrhoids.
- Encourage the client to increase her fluid and fiber intake to prevent constipation.
- Administer laxatives, stool softeners, suppositories, or enemas as needed.
- Avoid rectal temperatures and enemas in clients who have a fourth-degree laceration.
- Alleviate maternal anxieties regarding pain from or damage to the episiotomy site.
- Encourage ambulation.

Evaluating episiotomy

The site of **episiotomy** (surgical incision into the perineum and vagina) should be assessed every shift to evaluate healing, noting erythema, intactness of stitches, edema, and any odor or drainage. Twenty-four hours after delivery, the edges of an episiotomy are usually sealed.

Nursing actions

- Administer medications to relieve discomfort from the episiotomy, uterine contractions, incisional pain, or engorged breasts as prescribed. Medications may include analgesics, stool softeners and laxatives, or oxytocic agents.

Teaching topics

- Explanation of the disorder and treatment plan
- Changing perineal pads frequently, removing from front to back
- Reporting lochia with a foul odor, heavy flow, or clots
- Showering daily to relieve discomfort of normal postpartum diaphoresis
- Following instructions on sexual activity and contraception
- Performing Kegel exercises to help strengthen the pubococcygeal muscles
- Sitting with the legs elevated for 30 minutes if lochia increases or lochia rubra returns, either of which may indicate excessive activity (notifying the physician if excessive vaginal discharge persists)
- Increasing protein and caloric intake to restore body tissues (if breast-feeding, increasing daily caloric intake by 200 kcal over the pregnancy requirement of 2,400 kcal)
- Relieving perineal discomfort from an episiotomy by using ice packs (for the first 8 to 12 hours to minimize edema); spray peri bottles; sitz baths; anesthetic sprays, creams, and pads; and prescribed pain medications

> During assessment, position the client with a mediolateral episiotomy on her side to provide better visibility and prevent discomfort.

Polish up on client care

Potential postpartum complications include mastitis, postpartum hemorrhage, psychological maladaptation, and puerperal infection.

Mastitis

Mastitis is an infection of the lactating breast. It most commonly occurs during the second and third weeks after birth but can occur at any time.

CAUSES

- *Staphylococcus aureus* (the most common causative pathogen)

CONTRIBUTING FACTORS
- Altered immune response
- Constriction from a bra that's too tight (may interfere with complete emptying of the breast)
- Engorgement and stasis of milk (usually precede mastitis)
- Injury to the nipple, such as a crack or blister, which may allow causative organism to enter

ASSESSMENT FINDINGS
- Aching muscles
- Chills
- Edema and breast heaviness
- Fatigue
- Headache
- Localized area of redness and inflammation on the breast with possible streaks over the breast
- Malaise
- Purulent drainage
- Temperature of 101.1° F (38.4° C) or higher

DIAGNOSTIC TEST RESULTS
- Culture of the purulent discharge may test positive for the *S. aureus* bacteria.

NURSING DIAGNOSES
- Ineffective coping
- Acute pain
- Situational low self-esteem

TREATMENT
- Incision and drainage if abscess occurs
- Moist heat application to local area
- Pumping breasts to preserve breast-feeding ability if abscess occurs

Drug therapy
- Analgesics: acetaminophen (Tylenol), ibuprofen (Advil)
- Antibiotics: cephalexin (Keflex), cefaclor (Raniclor), clindamycin (Cleocin)

INTERVENTIONS AND RATIONALES
- Monitor vital signs *to assess for complications.*
- Administer antibiotic therapy *to treat infection.*
- Apply moist heat *to increase circulation and reduce inflammation and edema.*

- Encourage the client to breast-feed on the affected side before the unaffected side *to promote complete emptying;* breast-feeding should be stopped and pumping initiated if an abscess occurs *to ensure emptying of the unaffected breast.*

Teaching topics
- Positioning the infant during breast-feeding to avoid trauma to the nipples and milk stasis
- Avoiding bras that are too tight and that may restrict the flow of milk
- Breast-feeding every 2 to 3 hours and completely emptying the breasts
- Changing nipple shields as soon as they become wet to prevent infection
- Using a breast pump and discarding milk if breast abscess has developed

Postpartum hemorrhage

Postpartum hemorrhage is maternal blood loss from the uterus greater than 500 ml within a 24-hour period. It can occur immediately after delivery (within the first 24 hours) or later (during the remaining days of the 6-week puerperium).

CAUSES
- Administration of magnesium sulfate
- Cesarean birth
- Clotting disorders
- Disseminated intravascular coagulation
- Forceps delivery
- General anesthesia
- Low implantation of placenta or placenta previa
- Multiparity
- Overdistention of uterus (multifetal pregnancy, hydramnios, large infant)
- Perineal laceration
- Precipitate labor or delivery
- Previous postpartum hemorrhage
- Previous uterine surgery
- Prolonged labor
- Retained placental fragments
- Soft, boggy uterus, indicating relaxed uterine tone
- Subinvolution of the uterus
- Urinary bladder distention
- Use of tocolytic drugs

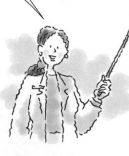

Uterine blood loss greater than 500 ml in a 24-hour period indicates postpartum hemorrhage.

ASSESSMENT FINDINGS

- Blood loss greater than 500 ml within a 24-hour period; may occur up to 6 weeks after delivery
- Perineal lacerations
- Retained placental fragments
- Signs of shock (tachycardia, hypotension, oliguria)
- Uterine atony

DIAGNOSTIC TEST RESULTS

- Hematology studies show decreased hemoglobin and HCT levels, a low fibrinogen level, and decreased partial thromboplastin time.

NURSING DIAGNOSES

- Ineffective peripheral tissue perfusion
- Deficient fluid volume
- Risk for infection

TREATMENT

- Bimanual compression of the uterus and dilatation and curettage to remove clots
- I.V. replacement of fluids and blood
- Abdominal hysterectomy if other interventions fail to control blood loss
- Urinary catheterization to empty the bladder

Drug therapy

- Parenteral administration of methylergonovine (Methergine)
- Rapid I.V. infusion of dilute oxytocin (Pitocin)

INTERVENTIONS AND RATIONALES

- Monitor vital signs *to assess for complications*.
- Massage the fundus and express clots from the uterus *to increase uterine contraction and tone*.
- Perform a pad count *to assess the amount of vaginal bleeding*.
- Monitor lochia, including amount, color, and odor, *to assess for infection*.
- Monitor the fundus for location *to assess for uterine displacement*.
- Monitor I.V. infusion of dilute oxytocin, as ordered, *to increase uterine contraction and tone*.
- Administer methylergonovine, as ordered, *to increase uterine contraction and tone*.
- Administer blood products and I.V. fluids, as prescribed, *to replace volume loss*.

- Provide emotional support *to help alleviate fears and anxiety*.
- Advise the client to request assistance with ambulation *to prevent injury*.

Teaching topics

- Explanation of the disorder and treatment plan
- Learning about surgical procedures, if appropriate
- Reporting changes in vaginal bleeding

Psychological maladaptation

Known as *postpartum depression*, psychological maladaptation is depression of a significant depth and duration after childbirth. Many postpartum clients experience some level of mood swings; psychological maladaptation refers to depression that lasts longer than 2 weeks, indicating a serious problem.

CAUSES AND CONTRIBUTING FACTORS

- Difficult pregnancy, labor, or delivery
- Neonatal complications
- History of depression
- Hormonal shifts as estrogen and progesterone levels decline
- Lack of support from family and friends
- Lack of self-esteem
- Stress in the home or work
- Troubled childhood

ASSESSMENT FINDINGS

- Extreme fatigue
- Inability to make decisions
- Inability to stop crying
- Increased anxiety about self and neonate's health
- Overall feeling of sadness
- Postpartum psychosis (hallucinations, delusions, potential for suicide or homicide)
- Psychosomatic symptoms (nausea, vomiting, diarrhea)
- Unwillingness to be left alone

DIAGNOSTIC TEST RESULTS

- There are no diagnostic test findings specific to this complication (diagnosis is based on signs and symptoms).

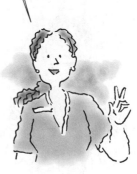

Although many clients experience some depression after childbirth, depression that lasts longer than 2 days should trigger your assessment alarm.

Women who have undergone cesarean delivery are at higher risk for puerperal infection.

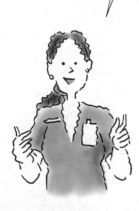

NURSING DIAGNOSES
- Fatigue
- Ineffective coping
- Social isolation

TREATMENT
- Counseling for the client and family at risk
- Group therapy
- Psychotherapy for the client

Drug therapy
- Antidepressants: imipramine (Tofranil), nortriptyline (Pamelor)

INTERVENTIONS AND RATIONALES
- Obtain a health history during the antepartum period *to assess whether the client is at risk for postpartum depression.*
- Assess the client's support systems *to determine the need for additional help.*
- Assess maternal-neonate bonding *to check for signs of depression.*
- Provide emotional support and encouragement *to reduce anxiety.*
- Notify a skilled professional if you observe psychotic symptoms in the client *to obtain necessary treatment.*

Teaching topics
- Explanation of the disorder and treatment plan
- Medication use and possible adverse effects
- Understanding that continued depression may require psychiatric counseling
- Understanding how to meet her own physical and emotional needs

Puerperal infection

Puerperal infection occurs after childbirth in 2% to 5% of all women who have vaginal deliveries and in 15% to 20% of those who have cesarean births. Puerperal infection affects the uterus and structures above it and is one of the leading causes of maternal death.

CAUSES AND CONTRIBUTING FACTORS
- Bladder catheterization
- Cesarean birth
- Colonization of lower genital tract with pathogenic organisms, such as group B streptococci, *Chlamydia trachomatis, Staphylococcus aureus, Escherichia coli,* and *Gardnerella vaginalis*
- Episiotomy
- Forceps delivery
- Excessive number of vaginal examinations
- Intrauterine fetal monitoring
- Laceration
- History of previous infection
- Low socioeconomic status
- Medical conditions such as diabetes mellitus
- Poor general health
- Poor nutrition
- Prolonged labor
- Premature rupture of membranes
- Retained placental fragments
- Trauma

ASSESSMENT FINDINGS
- Abdominal pain and tenderness
- Anorexia
- Chills
- Fever
- Lethargy
- Malaise
- Purulent, foul-smelling lochia
- Subinvolution of the uterus
- Tachycardia
- Uterine cramping

DIAGNOSTIC TEST RESULTS
- Urine specimen may reveal the causative organism.
- Complete blood count may show an elevated white blood cell count in the upper ranges of normal (more than 30,000/µl) for the postpartum period.
- Cultures of the blood or of the endocervical and uterine cavities may reveal the causative organism.

NURSING DIAGNOSES
- Acute pain
- Risk for infection
- Social isolation

TREATMENT
- Administration of I.V. fluids (if hydration is needed)

Drug therapy
- Broad-spectrum I.V. antibiotic therapy, unless a causative organism is identified

Placing the client in Fowler's position helps with the drainage of lochia.

INTERVENTIONS AND RATIONALES
• Monitor vital signs every 4 hours *to assess for complications.*
• Place the client in Fowler's position *to facilitate drainage of lochia.*
• Administer pain medication, as ordered, *to relieve pain and discomfort.*
• Provide emotional support and reassurance *to ease anxiety.*
• Maintain I.V. fluid administration, as ordered, *to replace volume loss.*
• Administer antibiotics, as prescribed, *to fight infection.*

Teaching topics
• Explanation of the disorder and treatment plan
• Medication use and possible adverse effects
• Recognizing signs and symptoms of a worsening condition, such as nausea, vomiting, absent bowel sounds, abdominal distention, and severe abdominal pain

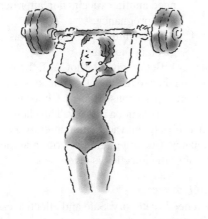

Pump up on practice questions

1. When checking a postpartum client for uterine bleeding, the nurse finds the fundus to be boggy. After fundal massage by the nurse, the physician prescribes 0.2 mg of methylergonovine (Methergine) by mouth. What should the nurse tell the client?

1. "Methergine is commonly used to help the uterus contract so that the bleeding will decrease. You may experience more cramping as your uterus becomes firmer."
2. "You'll probably take this medication until you're discharged from the hospital. Every client usually needs to take this medication."
3. "If your blood pressure is low, you won't be able to take this medication; I'll establish a new I.V. line so I can start Pitocin again."
4. "Most people don't experience additional pain or cramping from taking this medication."

Answer: 1. Methylergonovine, an ergot alkaloid, is commonly given to stimulate sustained uterine contraction. It allows the uterus to remain contracted and firm, thus decreasing postpartum bleeding. Abdominal cramping, which may become painful, is a common adverse effect. Methylergonovine is discontinued when the lochia flow has decreased or the client complains of severe cramping. Clients may need only a few doses of methylergonovine to keep the uterus contracted. Methylergonovine is contraindicated in clients with high—not low—blood pressure.

➡ NCLEX keys
Client needs category: Physiological integrity
Client needs subcategory: Pharmacological and parenteral therapies
Cognitive level: Application

2. A client had a cesarean birth and is postpartum day 1. She's asking for pain medication when the nurse enters the room to do her shift assessment. She states that her pain level is an 8 on a scale of 1 to 10. What should be the nurse's priority of care?

1. Have the client get up to wash so that the bed can be made and the medication orders checked.
2. Start the postpartum assessment.
3. Check the orders for a pain medication and return for the assessment after the medication has relieved her discomfort.
4. Tell the client to relax and the pain will subside.

Answer: 3. Pain management is a priority. Control of pain will enable the client to move, eliminating other potential complications of delivery. In addition, bonding with the infant will be facilitated if the client is without discomfort. The assessment should be initiated after pain management. Relaxation techniques will act as an adjunct therapy but isn't useful by itself for pain management during the postpartum period.

➡ *NCLEX keys*

Client needs category: Safe and effective care environment
Client needs subcategory: Management of care
Cognitive level: Analysis

3. A client delivered a neonate with spina bifida. She had been informed during the pregnancy that this was a potential risk. The nurse giving report states that this woman's decision to continue with the pregnancy was selfish, and now the neonate will suffer. In spite of the nurse's opinion, what ethical position should the nurse take when caring for this client and neonate?
1. Ask the client why she didn't have an abortion.
2. Accept the client's decision and care for the family as with any other patient.
3. Ask for another assignment because she doesn't agree with the decision the client made to continue the pregnancy.
4. Avoid going into the client's room if not necessary.

Answer: 2. It's the nurse's responsibility to care for and support the client and neonate. It isn't within the scope of care to judge a client or avoid responsibility.

➡ *NCLEX keys*

Client needs category: Safe and effective care environment
Client needs subcategory: Management of care
Cognitive level: Analysis

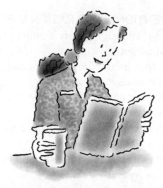

4. This is the client's first pregnancy. Her blood type is A– and her baby's blood type is A+. Before discharge, the client is scheduled to have a Rho(D) immune globulin (RhoGAM) vaccine. What's the most important action the nurse should take before administering the medication?
1. Ensure that the client understands and signs a consent form for the vaccination.
2. Choose a site for the injection that isn't tender.
3. Instruct the client that she won't need another vaccination after her next pregnancy.
4. Document that the injection was given in the chart.

Answer: 1. Before giving RhoGAM, the nurse needs to educate the client and make sure the client signs a consent form. Choosing a nontender site is not a priority. The client will need a subsequent vaccination after every pregnancy. Documentation is written in the chart after the injection is given.

➡ *NCLEX keys*

Client needs category: Safe and effective care environment
Client needs subcategory: Management of care
Cognitive Level: Application

5. During the third postpartum day, which finding is a nurse most likely to find in a client?
1. She's interested in learning more about neonate care.
2. She talks a lot about her birth experience.

3. She sleeps whenever the baby isn't present.
4. She requests help in choosing a name for the baby.

Answer: 1. The second to seventh days of postpartum care are the "taking-hold" phase, in which the new mother strives for independence and is eager for her baby. Talking about the birth experience, sleeping excessively, and asking for help in choosing a baby name describe the "taking-in phase," in which the mother relives her birth experience.

➡ *NCLEX keys*
Client needs category: Health promotion and maintenance
Client needs subcategory: None
Cognitive level: Analysis

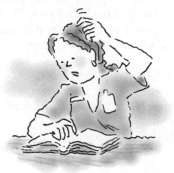

6.   A client is 3 days postpartum. She states that she hasn't had a bowel movement since before delivery and is experiencing discomfort. She has had a fourth-degree laceration. The nurse knows that the best remedy is:
1. a suppository.
2. an enema to alleviate gas pains quickly.
3. stool softeners and fluids.
4. pain medication for the discomfort.

Answer: 3. A client with a fourth-degree laceration is at risk for dehiscence. Stool softeners and fluid will gently promote stool evacuation. Suppositories and an enema would be too harsh, and pain medications would slow down peristalsis of the intestines, slowing evacuation.

➡ *NCLEX keys*
Client needs category: Safe and effective environment
Client needs subcategory: Management of care
Cognitive level: Analysis

7.   A nurse is providing care for a post-partum client. Which condition places this client at greater risk for a postpartum hemorrhage?
1. Hypertension
2. Uterine infection
3. Placenta previa
4. Severe pain

Answer: 3. A client with placenta previa is at greatest risk for postpartum hemorrhage. In placenta previa, the lower uterine segment doesn't contract as well as the fundal part of the uterus; therefore, more bleeding occurs. Hypertension, uterine infection, and severe pain don't place the client at increased risk for postpartum hemorrhage.

➡ *NCLEX keys*
Client needs category: Health promotion and maintenance
Client needs subcategory: None
Cognitive level: Analysis

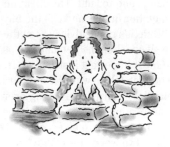

8.   In performing a routine fundal assessment, a nurse finds that a client's fundus is boggy. What should the nurse do first?
1. Call the physician.
2. Massage the fundus.
3. Assess lochia flow.
4. Obtain an order for methylergon-ovine (Methergine).

Answer: 2. The nurse should begin to massage the uterus so that it will be stimulated to contract. Lochia flow can be assessed while the uterus is being massaged. The nurse shouldn't leave the client to call the physician. If the fundus remains boggy and the uterus continues to bleed, the nurse should use the call button to ask another nurse to call the physician. Methylergonovine may be prescribed, if needed.

➡ NCLEX keys

Client needs category: Physiological integrity
Client needs subcategory: Reduction of risk potential
Cognitive level: Application

9. Early discharge from the postpartum unit has safety issues that need to be discussed with the client during discharge education. What's the most important instruction that the nurse should give the new mom?
    1. "Sleep when the neonate sleeps to avoid exhaustion."
    2. "Don't sleep with the neonate in bed with you."
    3. "If you have excessive vaginal bleeding, massage your fundus and call the physician."
    4. "Don't worry; women have been having babies for years without postpartum problems."

Answer: 3. Excessive bleeding can lead to hemorrhage, causing the client to lose fluid balance and to faint. The client needs to massage her fundus and call the physician. While it's good advice to tell the client to sleep when the neonate sleeps, it isn't the most important instruction. Having the neonate sleep with the mother can be a potential hazard when rolling over causes suffocation; however, it isn't the most important instruction to give a client. Telling the client not to worry doesn't give her information about how to prevent a potentially life-threatening problem with postpartum hemorrhage.

➡ NCLEX keys

Client needs category: Safe and effective care environment
Clients needs subcategory: Management of care
Cognitive Level: Application

10. On a client's second postpartum visit, the physician reviews the chart note here regarding the client's lochia. What's the best term for the lochia described?

Flowsheet		
Lochia		
Date	10/12/10	10/13/10
Time	0945	0930
Color	Red	Red
Odor	Normal	Normal
Consistency	Few tiny clots	No clots
Amount	4 pads/ 24 hours	3 pads/ 24 hours

    1. Alba
    2. Thrombis
    3. Rubra
    4. Serosa

Answer: 3. Lochia rubra is a red discharge that occurs 1 to 3 days after birth. It consists almost entirely of blood with only small clots and mucus. Lochia alba is a creamy white or colorless discharge that occurs 10 to 14 days postpartum and may continue for up to 6 weeks. Lochia thrombis isn't a valid term. Lochia serosa is a pink or brownish discharge that occurs 4 to 10 days postpartum.

➡ NCLEX keys

Client needs category: Physiological integrity
Clients needs subcategory: Physiological adaptation
Cognitive level: Application

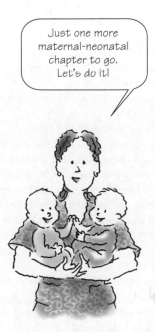

Just one more maternal-neonatal chapter to go. Let's do it!

Brush up on key concepts

A neonate experiences many changes as he adapts to life outside the uterus. Knowledge of these changes and of the normal physiologic characteristics of the neonate provides the basis for normal neonatal care.

At any time, you can review the major points of this chapter by consulting the *Cheat sheet* on pages 556 and 557.

Adaptations to extrauterine life

Here's a review of how the neonate's body systems change.

Heart seals
The **cardiovascular system** changes from the very first breath, which expands the neonate's lungs and decreases pulmonary vascular resistance. Clamping the umbilical cord increases systemic vascular resistance and left atrial pressure, which functionally closes the foramen ovale (fibrosis may take from several weeks to a year).

Every breath you take
The **respiratory system** also begins to change with the first breath. The neonate's breathing is a reflex triggered in response to noise, light, and temperature and pressure changes. Air immediately replaces the fluid that filled the lungs before birth.

A delicate balance
Renal system function doesn't fully mature until between the second and third year of life; as a result, the neonate has a minimal range of chemical balance and safety. The neonate's limited ability to excrete drugs, coupled with excessive neonatal fluid loss, can rapidly lead to acidosis and fluid imbalances.

Digestive difficulties
The **GI system** also isn't fully developed because normal bacteria aren't present in the neonate's GI tract. The lower intestine contains meconium at birth; the first meconium (sterile, greenish black, and viscous) usually passes within 24 hours. Some aspects of GI development include:
• audible bowel sounds 1 hour after birth
• uncoordinated peristaltic activity in the esophagus for the first few days of life
• a limited ability to digest fats because amylase and lipase are absent at birth
• frequent regurgitation because of an immature cardiac sphincter.

Bun from the oven
Changes in neonatal **thermogenesis** depend on environment. In an optimal environment, the neonate can produce sufficient heat, but rapid heat loss may occur in a suboptimal thermal environment.

Disease control
The neonatal **immune system** depends largely on three immunoglobulins: immunoglobulin (Ig) G, IgM, and IgA. IgG (detected in the fetus at the third month of gestation) is a placentally transferred immunoglobulin, providing antibodies to bacterial and viral agents. The infant synthesizes its own IgG during the first 3 months of life, thus compensating for concurrent catabolism of maternal antibodies. By the 20th week of gestation, the fetus synthesizes IgM, which is undetectable at birth because it doesn't cross the placenta.

High levels of IgM in the neonate indicate a nonspecific infection. Secretory IgA (which

(Text continues on page 558.)

Because the renal system hasn't fully matured yet, the neonate can easily develop acidosis and fluid imbalances.

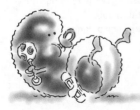

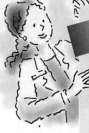

Cheat sheet

Neonatal care refresher

FETAL ALCOHOL SYNDROME

Key signs and symptoms
- Central nervous system dysfunction (decreased I.Q., developmental delays, neurologic abnormalities)
- Facial deformities
- Prenatal and postnatal growth retardation

Key test results
- Chest X-ray may reveal congenital heart defect.

Key treatments
- Swaddling
- I.V. phenobarbital

Key interventions
- Provide a stimulus-free environment for the neonate; darken the room, if necessary.
- Provide gavage feedings, if necessary.

HUMAN IMMUNODEFICIENCY VIRUS (HIV)

Key signs and symptoms
- Produces no symptoms (at birth)

Key test results
- Test interpretation is problematic because most neonates with an HIV-positive mother test positive at birth. Uninfected neonates lose this maternal antibody at 8 to 15 months, and infected neonates remain seropositive. Therefore, testing should be repeated at age 15 months.

Key treatments
- Antimicrobial therapy to treat opportunistic infections
- Zidovudine (Retrovir) recommended during the first 6 weeks of life based on the neonate's lymphocyte count

Key interventions
- Assess cardiovascular and respiratory status.
- Maintain standard precautions.
- Keep the umbilical stump meticulously clean.

HYPOTHERMIA

Key signs and symptoms
- Kicking and crying (a mechanism to increase the metabolic rate to produce body heat)

- Core body temperature lower than 97.7° F (36.5° C)

Key test results
- Arterial blood gas (ABG) analysis shows hypoxemia.
- Blood glucose level reveals hypoglycemia.

Key treatments
- Radiant warmer
- Skin-to-skin warmth (place neonate close to the mother)

Key interventions
- Dry the neonate immediately after delivery.
- Allow the mother to hold the neonate.
- Monitor vital signs every 15 to 30 minutes.
- Provide a knitted cap for the neonate.
- Place the neonate in a radiant warmer.

NEONATAL DRUG DEPENDENCY

Key signs and symptoms
- High-pitched cry
- Irritability
- Jitteriness
- Poor sleeping pattern
- Tremors

Key treatments
- Gavage feedings, if necessary
- Paregoric and phenobarbital to treat withdrawal symptoms; methadone shouldn't be given to neonates because of its addictive nature

Key interventions
- Monitor cardiovascular status.
- Use tight swaddling for comfort.
- Place the neonate in a dark, quiet environment.
- Encourage the use of a pacifier (in cases of heroin withdrawal).
- Be prepared to administer gavage feedings (in cases of methadone withdrawal).
- Maintain fluid and electrolyte balance.

> Time for a change. I experience many bodily changes as I adapt to life outside the uterus.

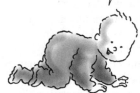

Neonatal care refresher (continued)

NEONATAL INFECTIONS
Key signs and symptoms
- Feeding pattern changes, such as poor sucking or decreased intake
- Sternal retractions
- Subtle, nonspecific behavioral changes, such as lethargy or hypotonia
- Temperature instability

Key test results
- Blood and urine cultures are positive for the causative organism, most commonly gram-positive beta-hemolytic streptococci and the gram-negative *Escherichia coli, Aerobacter, Proteus,* and *Klebsiella.*
- Complete blood count shows an increased white blood cell count.

Key treatments
- I.V. therapy to provide adequate hydration
- Antibiotic therapy: broad-spectrum until the causative organism is identified and then a specific antibiotic

Key interventions
- Assess cardiovascular and respiratory status.
- Administer broad-spectrum antibiotics before culture results are received and specific antibiotic therapy after results are received.

NEONATAL JAUNDICE
Key signs and symptoms
- Jaundice
- Lethargy

Key test results
- Bilirubin levels are elevated, with the rate of rise based on gestational age.

Key treatments
- Phototherapy (preferred treatment)
- Increased fluid intake

Key interventions
- Assess neurologic status.
- Monitor serum bilirubin levels.
- Initiate and maintain phototherapy (provide eye protection while under phototherapy lights and remove eye shields promptly when removed from the phototherapy lights).

RESPIRATORY DISTRESS SYNDROME
Key signs and symptoms
- Expiratory grunting
- Fine crackles and diminished breath sounds
- Seesaw respirations
- Sternal and substernal retractions
- Tachypnea (more than 60 breaths/minute)
- Tachycardia (more than 160 beats/minute)

Key test results
- ABG analysis reveals respiratory acidosis.
- Chest X-rays reveal bilateral diffuse reticulogranular density.

Key treatments
- Oxygen therapy with endotracheal intubation and mechanical ventilation
- Nutrition supplements (total parenteral nutrition [TPN] or enteral feedings, if possible)
- Surfactant replacement by way of endotracheal tube
- Temperature regulation with a radiant warmer

Key interventions
- Assess cardiovascular, respiratory, and neurologic status.
- Monitor vital signs and pulse oximetry readings.
- Initiate and maintain ventilatory support status.
- Administer medications, including endotracheal surfactant, as prescribed.
- Provide adequate nutrition through enteral feedings, if possible, or TPN.

TRACHEOESOPHAGEAL FISTULA
Key signs and symptoms
- Difficulty feeding, such as choking or aspiration; cyanosis during feeding
- Signs of respiratory distress (tachypnea, cyanosis, sternal and substernal retractions)

Key test results
- Abdominal X-ray shows the fistula and a gas-free abdomen.

Key treatments
- Emergency surgical intervention to prevent pneumonia, dehydration, and fluid and electrolyte imbalances
- Maintenance of a patent airway

Key interventions
- Assess cardiovascular, respiratory, and GI status.
- Place the neonate in high Fowler's position.
- Keep a laryngoscope and endotracheal tube at the bedside.
- Provide the neonate with a pacifier.
- Provide gastrostomy tube feedings postoperatively.

limits bacterial growth in the GI tract) is found in colostrum and breast milk.

Poietic license

In the neonatal **hematopoietic system,** blood volume accounts for 80 to 85 ml/kg of body weight. The neonate experiences prolonged coagulation time after birth because maternal stores of vitamin K become depleted and the neonate's immature liver can't produce enough to maintain adequate levels.

Nervous energy

The full-term neonate's **neurologic system** should produce equal strength and symmetry in responses and reflexes. Diminished or absent reflexes may indicate a serious neurologic problem, and asymmetrical responses may indicate trauma during birth, including nerve damage, paralysis, or fracture. Some neonatal reflexes gradually weaken and disappear during the early months.

Liver concerns

Increased serum levels of unconjugated bilirubin from increased red blood cell (RBC) lysis, altered bilirubin conjugation, or increased bilirubin reabsorption from the GI tract may cause jaundice — a major complication for the neonatal hepatic system. Physiologic jaundice appears after the first 24 hours of extrauterine life; pathologic jaundice is evident at birth or within the first 24 hours of extrauterine life; and breast milk jaundice appears after the 1st week of extrauterine life when physiologic jaundice is declining.

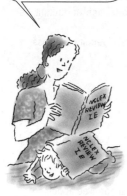

Physiologic jaundice is a mild jaundice that lasts for the first few days after birth.

Keep abreast of neonatal assessment

Neonatal assessment includes initial and ongoing assessments as well as a thorough physical examination.

First things first

Initial neonatal assessment involves detecting abnormalities and keeping accurate records.

Nursing actions

• Ensure a proper airway by suctioning, and administer oxygen as needed.
• Dry the neonate under a warmer while keeping the head lower than the trunk (to promote drainage of secretions).
• Apply a cord clamp, and monitor the neonate for abnormal bleeding from the cord; check the number of cord vessels.
• Observe the neonate for voiding and meconium; document the first void and stools.
• Check the neonate for gross abnormalities and clinical manifestations of suspected abnormalities.
• Continue to assess the neonate by using the Apgar score criteria even after the 5-minute score is received. (See *Apgar scoring.*)
• Obtain clear footprints and fingerprints (the neonate's footprints are kept on a record that includes the mother's fingerprints).
• Apply identification bands with matching numbers to the mother (one band) and neonate (two bands) before they leave the delivery room.
• Promote bonding between the mother and neonate.

Keep on keepin' on

Ongoing neonatal physical assessment includes observing and recording vital signs and administering prescribed medications.

Nursing actions

• Monitor the neonate's vital signs.
• Take the first temperature by the rectal route to determine whether the rectum is patent. Temperatures obtained by this route must be done gently to prevent injury to the rectal mucosa.
• Take the apical pulse for 60 seconds (normal rate is 120 to 160 beats/minute).
• Count respirations with a stethoscope for 60 seconds (normal rate is 30 to 60 breaths/minute).
• Measure and record blood pressure (normal reading ranges from 60/40 mm Hg to 90/45 mm Hg).
• Measure and record the neonate's vital statistics (weight, length, and head and chest circumference).
• Complete a gestational age assessment.

Apgar scoring

The Apgar scoring system provides a way to evaluate the neonate's cardiopulmonary and neuro-logic status. The assessment is performed at 1 and 5 minutes after birth and repeated every 5 minutes until the infant stabilizes. A score of 8 to 10 indicates that the neonate is in no apparent distress; a score below 8 indicates that resuscitative measures may be needed.

Sign	0	1	2
Heart rate	Absent	Less than 100 beats/minute	Greater than 100 beats/minute
Respiratory effort	Absent	Slow, irregular	Good crying
Muscle tone	Flaccid	Some flexion of extremities	Active motion
Reflex irritability	None	Grimace	Vigorous cry
Color	Pale, blue	Body pink, blue extremities	Completely pink

• Administer prescribed medications such as vitamin K, which is a prophylactic against transient deficiency of coagulation factors II, VII, IX, and X.
• Administer erythromycin ointment, the drug of choice for neonatal eye prophylaxis, to prevent damage and blindness from conjunctivitis caused by *Neisseria gonorrhoeae* and *Chlamydia;* treatment is required by law.
• Administer the first hepatitis B vaccine within 12 hours after birth after obtaining parental consent.
• Perform laboratory tests.
• Monitor glucose levels and hematocrit (test results help assess for hypoglycemia and anemia).

Neonatal physical examination

The neonate should receive a thorough visual and physical examination of each body part. The following is a brief review of normal and abnormal neonatal physiology.

Heads up

The neonate's head is about one-fourth of its body size. The term **molding** refers to the shaping of the fetal head as it adapts to the shape of the birth canal. This is a normal occurrence with most births. The heads of most neonates return to their normal shape within 3 days after delivery.

Cranial complications that can occur include:
• cephalohematoma — blood collects between the skull and the periosteum; may occur on one or both sides of the head but doesn't cross the suture lines
• caput succedaneum — swelling in the soft tissues of the scalp, which can extend across the suture lines.

Closing time

The neonatal skull has two **fontanels:** a diamond-shaped anterior fontanel and a triangular-shaped posterior fontanel. The anterior fontanel is located at the juncture of the frontal and parietal bones, measures 1⅛" to 1⅝" (3 to 4 cm) long and ¾" to 1⅛" (2 to 3 cm) wide, and closes in about 18 months. The posterior fontanel is located at the juncture of the occipital and parietal bones,

The heads of most neonates return to their normal shape within 3 days after delivery.

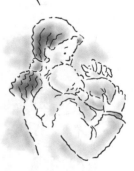

measures about ¾" across, and closes in 12 to 16 weeks. The fontanels:

- should feel soft to the touch
- shouldn't be depressed—a depressed fontanel may indicate dehydration
- shouldn't bulge—bulging fontanels require immediate attention because they may indicate increased intracranial pressure.

Jeepers peepers

- The neonate's eyes are usually blue or gray because of scleral thinness. Permanent eye color is established within 3 to 12 months.
- Lacrimal glands are immature at birth, resulting in tearless crying for up to 2 months.
- The neonate may demonstrate transient strabismus.
- Doll's eye reflex (when the head is rotated laterally, the eyes deviate in the opposite direction) may persist for about 10 days.
- Subconjunctival hemorrhages may appear from vascular tension changes during birth.

Nose only

Because infants are obligatory nose breathers for the first few months of life, nasal passages must be kept clear to ensure adequate respiration. Neonates instinctively sneeze to remove obstruction.

Dry mouth

The neonate's mouth usually has scant saliva and pink lips. Epstein's pearls (pearly, white, pinpoint papules) may be found on the gums or hard palate, and precocious teeth may also be apparent.

Sound check

The neonate's ears are characterized by incurving of the pinna and cartilage deposition. The top of the ear should be above or parallel to an imaginary line from the inner to the outer canthus of the eye. Low-set ears are associated with several syndromes, including chromosomal abnormalities.

The neonate should respond to sudden sounds by increasing his heart and respiratory rates.

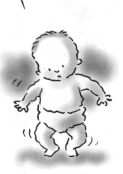

All neonates are bowlegged and have flat feet. Not to worry—most of us outgrow it.

For the neck of it

The neonate's neck is typically short and weak with deep folds of skin.

Flexi-chest

The neonatal chest is characterized by a cylindrical thorax and flexible ribs. Breast engorgement from maternal hormones may be apparent, and supernumerary nipples may be located below and medially to the true nipples.

Nice abs

The neonatal abdomen is usually cylindrical with some protrusion. A scaphoid appearance indicates diaphragmatic hernia. The umbilical cord is white and gelatinous with two arteries and one vein and begins to dry within 1 to 2 hours after delivery.

Teeny, tiny genitalia

Characteristics of a male neonate's genitalia include rugae on the scrotum and testes descended into the scrotum. The urinary meatus is located in one of three places:

- at the penile tip (normal)
- on the dorsal surface (epispadias)
- on the ventral surface (hypospadias).

In the female neonate, the labia majora cover the labia minora and clitoris, vaginal discharge from maternal hormones appears, and the hymenal tag is present.

Extreme measures

All neonates are bowlegged and have flat feet. Some neonates may have abnormal extremities. They may be polydactyl (more than five digits on an extremity) or syndactyl (two or more digits fused together).

Soldier straight

The neonatal spine should be straight and flat, and the anus should be patent without any fissure. Dimpling at the base of the spine is commonly associated with spina bifida.

Baby-smooth skin

The skin of a neonate can indicate many conditions—some quite normal and others requiring more serious attention. Assessment findings include:

- acrocyanosis (cyanosis of the hands and feet), which results from high levels of hemoglobin and vasomotor instability during the first week of life
- milia (clogged sebaceous glands) on the nose or chin
- lanugo (fine, downy hair) appearing after 20 weeks of gestation on the entire body except the palms and soles
- vernix caseosa (a white, cheesy protective coating composed of desquamated epithelial cells and sebum)
- erythema toxicum neonatorum (a transient, maculopapular rash)
- telangiectasia (flat, reddened vascular areas) appearing on the neck, upper eyelid, or upper lip
- port-wine stain (nevus flammeus), a capillary angioma located below the dermis and commonly found on the face
- strawberry hemangioma (nevus vasculosus), a capillary angioma located in the dermal and subdermal skin layers indicated by a rough, raised, sharply demarcated birthmark
- Mongolian spot, an area of bluish skin discoloration sometimes found in Blacks, Native Americans, and neonates of Mediterranean descent.

Reflections on reflexes

Normal neonates display a number of reflexes, which include:

- sucking: sucking motion begins when a nipple is placed in the neonate's mouth
- Moro's: when lifted above the crib and suddenly lowered, the arms and legs symmetrically extend and then abduct while the fingers spread to form a "C"
- rooting: when the cheek is stroked, the neonate turns his head in the direction of the stroke
- tonic neck (fencing position): when the neonate's head is turned while the neonate is lying supine, the extremities on the same side straighten while those on the opposite side flex
- Babinski's: when the sole on the side of the small toe is stroked, the neonate's toes fan upward
- palmar grasp: when a finger is placed in each of the neonate's hands, the neonate's

fingers grasp tightly enough to be pulled to a sitting position

- dancing or stepping: when held upright with the feet touching a flat surface, the neonate exhibits dancing or stepping movements
- startle: a loud noise, such as a hand clap, elicits neonatal arm abduction and elbow flexion; the neonate's hands stay clenched
- trunk incurvature: when a finger is run laterally down the neonate's spine, the trunk flexes and the pelvis swings toward the stimulated side.

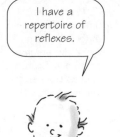

I have a repertoire of reflexes.

Polish up on client care

Potential neonatal complications and disorders include fetal alcohol syndrome (FAS), human immunodeficiency virus (HIV), hypothermia, drug dependency, infections, jaundice, respiratory distress syndrome, and tracheoesophageal fistula.

Fetal alcohol syndrome

FAS results from a mother's chronic or periodic intake of alcohol during pregnancy. The degree of alcohol consumption necessary to cause the syndrome varies. Because alcohol crosses the placenta in the same concentration as is present in the maternal bloodstream, alcohol consumption (particularly binge drinking) is especially dangerous during critical periods of organogenesis. The fetal liver isn't mature enough to detoxify alcohol.

CAUSES

- Risk of teratogenic effects increases proportionally with daily alcohol intake; FAS has been detected in neonates of even moderate drinkers (1 to 2 oz of alcohol daily)

ASSESSMENT FINDINGS

- Central nervous system dysfunction (decreased I.Q., developmental delays, neurologic abnormalities)

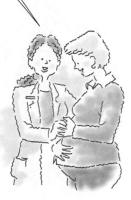

Warn mothers-to-be that binge drinking is even more detrimental than moderate daily alcohol consumption.

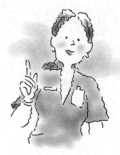

Prevention point: Administering zidovudine to an HIV-positive pregnant woman significantly reduces the risk of transmission to the neonate.

- Facial anomalies (microcephaly, microophthalmia, maxillary hypoplasia, short palpebral fissures)
- Prenatal and postnatal growth retardation
- Sleep disturbances (either always awake or always asleep, depending on the mother's alcohol level close to birth)
- Weak sucking reflex

DIAGNOSTIC TEST RESULTS

- Chest X-ray may reveal congenital heart defect.

NURSING DIAGNOSES

- Imbalanced nutrition: Less than body requirements
- Delayed growth and development
- Risk for impaired parenting

TREATMENT

- Swaddling

Drug therapy

- I.V. phenobarbital (to control hyperactivity and irritability)

INTERVENTIONS AND RATIONALES

- Provide a stimulus-free environment for the neonate; darken the room, if necessary, *to minimize stimuli.*
- Provide gavage feedings, as necessary, *to ensure adequate nutrition for the infant.*
- Refer the mother to an alcohol treatment center *for ongoing support and rehabilitation.*

Teaching topics

- Explanation of the disorder and treatment plan
- Expectations for the neonate's behavior
- Alcohol rehabilitation program

Human immunodeficiency virus

A mother can transmit HIV to her fetus transplacentally at various gestational ages — perinatally through maternal blood and bodily fluids and postnatally through breast milk. Administration of zidovudine to HIV-positive pregnant women significantly reduces the risk of transmission to the fetus.

CAUSES

- Transmission of the virus to the fetus or neonate from an HIV-positive mother

ASSESSMENT FINDINGS

- Produces no symptoms (at birth)
- Opportunistic infections (may appear by ages 3 to 6 months)

DIAGNOSTIC TEST RESULTS

- Test interpretation is problematic because most neonates with an HIV-positive mother test positive at birth. Uninfected neonates lose this maternal antibody at 8 to 15 months, and infected neonates remain seropositive. Therefore, testing should be repeated at age 15 months.
- HIV-deoxyribonucleic acid polymerase chain reaction or viral cultures for HIV should be performed at birth and again between ages 1 and 2 months.

NURSING DIAGNOSES

- Imbalanced nutrition: Less than body requirements
- Ineffective protection
- Risk for infection

TREATMENT

- I.V. fluid administration
- Nutritional supplements to prevent weight loss

Drug therapies

- Antimicrobial therapy to treat opportunistic infections
- Routine immunizations with killed viruses, except the varicella vaccines
- Zidovudine (Retrovir): recommended during the first 6 weeks of life based on the neonate's lymphocyte count to prevent perinatal transmission.
- Combination therapy: recommended when HIV infection is confirmed; therapy should include zidovudine combined with lamivudine (Epivir) or didanosine (Videx); or lamivudine combined with didanosine

INTERVENTIONS AND RATIONALES
- Assess the neonate's cardiovascular and respiratory status *for complications*.
- Monitor vital signs and fluid intake and output *to assess for dehydration*.
- Monitor fluid and electrolyte status *to guide fluid and electrolyte replacement therapy*.
- Keep the umbilical stump meticulously clean *to prevent opportunistic infection*.
- Maintain standard precautions *to prevent the spread of infection*.
- Administer medications, as indicated, *to treat infection and improve immune function*.
- Provide emotional support to the family *to allay anxiety*
- Monitor the neonate for signs of opportunistic infection *to prevent treatment delay*.

Teaching topics
- Explanation of the disorder and treatment plan
- Medication use and possible adverse effects
- Avoiding infection
- Importance of nutrition
- Providing the child with all necessary immunizations

Hypothermia

A neonate's temperature is about 99° F (37.2° C) at birth. Inside the womb, the fetus was confined in an environment where the temperature was constant. At birth, this temperature can fall rapidly.

CAUSES
- Cold temperature in delivery environment
- Heat loss due to evaporation, conduction, radiation, or convection
- Immature temperature-regulating system
- Inability to conserve heat because of little subcutaneous fat (brown fat store)

ASSESSMENT FINDINGS
- Kicking and crying (a mechanism to increase the metabolic rate to produce body heat)
- Core body temperature lower than 97.7° F (36.5° C)
- Lethargy with extreme hypothermia

DIAGNOSTIC TEST RESULTS
- Arterial blood gas (ABG) analysis shows hypoxemia.
- Blood glucose level reveals hypoglycemia.

NURSING DIAGNOSES
- Hypothermia
- Ineffective thermoregulation
- Risk for impaired parenting

TREATMENT
- Radiant warmer
- Skin-to-skin warmth (place the neonate close to the mother)

INTERVENTIONS AND RATIONALES
- Dry the neonate immediately after delivery *to prevent heat loss*.
- Wrap the neonate in a warm blanket *to help stabilize body temperature*.
- Allow the mother to hold the neonate *to provide warmth*.
- Monitor vital signs every 15 to 30 minutes *to assess temperature fluctuations and complications*.
- Provide a knitted cap for the neonate *to prevent heat loss through the head*.
- Place the neonate in a radiant warmer *to maintain thermoregulation*.

Teaching topics
- Preventing hypothermia
- Stressing infant-parent bonding (see *Teaching neonatal care to parents,* page 564)

Neonatal drug dependency

Neonates born to drug-addicted mothers are at risk for preterm birth, aspiration pneumonia, meconium-stained fluid, and meconium aspiration. Drug-dependent neonates also may experience withdrawal from such substances as heroin and cocaine.

CAUSES
- Drug addiction in the mother

ASSESSMENT FINDINGS
- Diarrhea
- Frequent sneezing and yawning

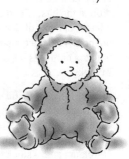

Brrr... In the womb, the temperature was constant. At birth, my temperature may fall rapidly.

Teaching neonatal care to parents

Here are some topics to include when teaching parents about caring for their neonate.

CORD CARE

With every diaper change, wipe the umbilical cord with water, especially around the base. Report any odor, discharge, or signs of skin irritation around the cord. Fold the diaper below the cord until the cord falls off, usually in 1 to 2 weeks.

CIRCUMCISION CARE

Gently clean the circumcised penis with water, and apply fresh petroleum gauze with each diaper change. Loosen the petroleum gauze stuck to the penis by pouring warm water over the area. Don't remove yellow discharge that covers the glans after circumcision; this is part of normal healing. Report any foul-smelling, purulent discharge promptly. Apply diapers loosely until the circumcision heals after about 5 days.

If the plastibell method of circumcision was used, leave the plastic ring in place until it falls off on its own, typically in 5 to 8 days. No special dressing is applied, and bathing and diapering are performed normally.

UNCIRCUMCISED CARE

Don't retract the foreskin when washing the uncircumcised penis because the foreskin is adhered to the glans.

POTTY PATTERNS

Become familiar with the neonate's voiding and elimination patterns:

- The neonate's first stools are called *meconium;* they are odorless, dark green, and thick.
- Transitional stools occur about 2 to 3 days after the ingestion of milk; they're greenish brown and thinner than meconium.
- The stools change to pasty yellow and pungent (bottle-fed neonate) or loose yellow and sweet-smelling (breast-fed neonate) by the fourth day.
- Change diapers before and after every feeding; expose the neonate's buttocks to the air and light several times a day for about 20 minutes to treat diaper rash.

BATH TIME

Give the neonate sponge baths until the cord falls off; then wash the neonate in a tub containing 3" to 4" (7.5 to 10 cm) of warm water.

MEALTIME AT THE BREAST

Initiate breast-feeding as soon as possible after delivery, and then feed the neonate on demand. Follow these guidelines:

- Position the neonate's mouth slightly differently at each feeding to reduce irritation at one site.
- Burp the neonate before switching to the other breast.
- Insert the little finger into a corner of the neonate's mouth to separate the neonate from the nipple.
- Experiment with various breast-feeding positions.
- Perform thorough breast care to promote cleanliness and comfort.

- Follow a diet that ensures adequate nutrition for the mother and neonate (drink at least four 8-oz glasses of fluid daily, increase caloric intake by 200 kcal over the pregnancy requirement of 2,400 kcal, avoid foods that cause irritability, gas, or diarrhea).
- Consult the physician before taking any medication.
- Know that ingested substances (caffeine, alcohol, and medications) can pass into breast milk.

MEALTIME WITH THE BOTTLE

Follow the pediatrician's instructions for preparing and feeding with formula. Follow these guidelines:

- Feed the neonate in an upright position, and keep the nipple full of formula to minimize air swallowing.
- Burp the neonate after each ounce of formula or more frequently if the neonate spits up.

SAFETY SEATS

Make sure parents understand the importance of using child safety seats. Instruct them to place the neonate in the back seat facing to the rear until the neonate is over 20 lb (9 kg) and older than 1 year. Stress the proper use of car seats by following the manufacturer's recommendations for placement and weight.

- High-pitched cry
- Hyperactive reflexes
- Increased tendon reflexes
- Irritability
- Jitteriness
- Poor feeding habits

- Poor sleeping pattern
- Tremors
- Inability to be consoled
- Vigorous sucking on hands
- Withdrawal symptoms (depend on the length of maternal addiction, the drug

ingested, and the time of last ingestion before delivery; usually appear within 24 hours of delivery)

DIAGNOSTIC TEST RESULTS
• Drug screen reveals agent abused by the mother.

NURSING DIAGNOSES
• Imbalanced nutrition: Less than body requirements.
• Risk for imbalanced fluid volume
• Risk for injury

TREATMENT
• Gavage feedings, if necessary
• I.V. therapy to maintain hydration

Drug therapy
• Paregoric and phenobarbital to treat withdrawal symptoms (methadone shouldn't be given to neonates because of its addictive nature)

INTERVENTIONS AND RATIONALES
• Monitor cardiovascular status *to detect cardiovascular compromise.*
• Monitor vital signs and fluid intake and output *to assess for complications.*
• Encourage the mother to hold the neonate *to promote maternal-infant bonding.*
• Use tight swaddling *for comfort.*
• Place the neonate in a dark, quiet room *to provide a stimulus-free environment.*
• Encourage the use of a pacifier *to meet sucking needs* (in cases of heroin withdrawal).
• Be prepared to administer gavage feedings *because of the neonate's poor sucking reflex* (in cases of methadone withdrawal).
• Maintain fluid and electrolyte balance *to replace fluid loss.*
• Monitor bilirubin levels and assess for jaundice (in cases of methadone withdrawal) *to assess for liver damage.*

Teaching topics
• Explanation of the disorder and treatment plan
• Expectations for the neonate's behavior
• Importance of nutrition
• Avoiding breast-feeding

Neonatal infections

A neonate may contract an infection before, during, or after delivery. Maternal IgM doesn't cross the placenta, and IgA requires time to reach optimum levels after birth, limiting the neonate's immune response. Dysmaturity caused by intrauterine growth retardation, preterm birth, or postterm birth can further compromise the neonate's immune system and predispose him to infection.

Sepsis is one of the most significant causes of neonatal morbidity and mortality. Toxoplasmosis, syphilis, rubella, cytomegalovirus, and herpes are common perinatal infections known to affect neonates. Beta-hemolytic streptococci infection may occur as a result of contact with the maternal genital tract during labor and delivery.

CAUSES
• Chorioamnionitis
• Low birth weight or premature birth
• Maternal substance abuse
• Maternal urinary tract infections
• Meconium aspiration
• Nosocomial infection
• Premature labor
• Prolonged maternal rupture of membranes

ASSESSMENT FINDINGS
• Abdominal distention
• Apnea
• Feeding pattern changes, such as poor sucking or decreased intake
• Hyperbilirubinemia
• Pallor
• Petechiae
• Poor weight gain
• Sternal retractions
• Subtle, nonspecific behavioral changes, such as lethargy or hypotonia
• Tachycardia
• Temperature instability
• Vomiting
• Diarrhea

There's a lot to know about neonatal care... how did we get ourselves into this, anyway?

What do you mean "we"? I'm not taking the NCLEX!

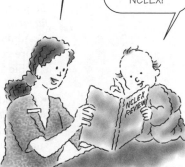

DIAGNOSTIC TEST RESULTS

• Blood and urine cultures are positive for the causative organism, most commonly gram-positive beta-hemolytic streptococci and the gram-negative *Escherichia coli, Aerobacter, Proteus,* and *Klebsiella.*
• Blood chemistry shows increased direct bilirubin levels.
• Complete blood count shows an increased white blood cell count.
• Lumbar puncture is positive for causative organisms.

NURSING DIAGNOSES

• Imbalanced nutrition: Less than body requirements
• Hypothermia
• Risk for imbalanced fluid volume

TREATMENT

• Gastric aspiration
• I.V. therapy to provide adequate hydration

Drug therapy

• Antibiotic therapy: broad-spectrum until the causative organism is identified and then a specific antibiotic

INTERVENTIONS AND RATIONALES

• Assess cardiovascular and respiratory status *for complications.*
• Monitor vital signs *to assess for complications.*
• Monitor fluid and electrolyte status *to assess the need for fluid replacement.*
• Initiate and maintain respiratory support, as needed, *to maintain respiratory filtration.*
• Administer broad-spectrum antibiotics before culture results are received, and specific antibiotic therapy after results are received, *to treat infection.*
• Provide the family with reassurance and support *to reduce anxiety.*
• Provide the neonate with physiologic supportive care *to maintain a neutral thermal environment.*
• Maintain I.V. therapy, as ordered, *to replace fluid loss.*
• Obtain blood samples and urine specimens *to assess antibiotic therapy efficacy.*

Teaching topics

• Explanation of the disorder and treatment plan
• Knowing the importance of continuing drug therapy for the duration prescribed
• Preventing infection

Neonatal jaundice

Also called *hyperbilirubinemia,* neonatal jaundice is characterized by a bilirubin level that:
• exceeds 6 mg/dl within the first 24 hours after delivery
• remains elevated beyond 7 days (in a full-term neonate)
• remains elevated for 10 days (in a premature neonate).

The neonate's bilirubin levels rise as bilirubin production exceeds the liver's capacity to metabolize it. Unbound, unconjugated bilirubin can easily cross the blood-brain barrier, leading to kernicterus (an encephalopathy).

CAUSES

• Absence of intestinal flora needed for bilirubin passage in the bowel
• Enclosed hemorrhage
• Erythroblastosis fetalis (hemolytic disease of the neonate)
• Hypoglycemia
• Hypothermia
• Impaired hepatic functioning
• Neonatal asphyxia (respiratory failure in the neonate)
• Polycythemia
• Prematurity
• Reduced bowel motility and delayed meconium passage
• Sepsis

ASSESSMENT FINDINGS

• Jaundice
• Lethargy
• Decreased reflexes
• High-pitched crying
• Opisthotonos
• Seizures

DIAGNOSTIC TEST RESULTS

- Bilirubin levels are elevated, with the rate of rise based on gestational age.
- Conjugated (direct) bilirubin levels exceed 2 mg/dl.
- Bilirubin levels rise by more than 5 mg/day.

NURSING DIAGNOSES

- Impaired parenting
- Deficient fluid volume
- Risk for injury

TREATMENT

- Phototherapy (preferred treatment)
- Exchange transfusion to remove maternal antibodies and sensitized RBCs if phototherapy fails
- Increased fluid intake
- Treatment for anemia if jaundice is caused by hemolytic disease

INTERVENTIONS AND RATIONALES

- Assess neurologic status *for signs of encephalopathy, which indicates the potential for permanent damage.*
- Maintain a neutral thermal environment *to prevent hypothermia.*
- Monitor serum bilirubin levels *to assess for increased or decreased levels of bilirubin.*
- Initiate and maintain phototherapy (provide eye protection while the neonate is under phototherapy lights, and remove eye shields promptly when he's removed from the phototherapy lights) *to prevent complications.*
- Allow time for maternal-neonate bonding and interaction during phototherapy *to promote bonding.*
- Keep the neonate's anal area clean and dry. *Frequent, greenish stools result from bilirubin excretion and can lead to skin irritations.*
- Provide the parents with support, reassurance, and encouragement *to reduce anxiety.*

Teaching topics

- Explanation of the disorder and treatment plan
- Encouraging frequent feedings to maintain adequate caloric intake and hydration and to facilitate excretion of waste

Respiratory distress syndrome

Respiratory distress syndrome occurs most commonly in preterm neonates of diabetic mothers and neonates delivered by cesarean births. In respiratory distress syndrome, a hyaline-like membrane lines the terminal bronchioles, alveolar ducts, and alveoli, preventing exchange of oxygen and carbon dioxide.

CAUSES

- Inability to maintain alveolar stability
- Low level or absence of surfactant

ASSESSMENT FINDINGS

- Cyanosis
- Expiratory grunting
- Fine crackles and diminished breath sounds
- Hypothermia
- Nasal flaring
- Respiratory acidosis
- Seesaw respirations
- Sternal and substernal retractions
- Tachypnea (more than 60 breaths/minute)
- Tachycardia (more than 160 beats/minute)

DIAGNOSTIC TEST RESULTS

- ABG analysis reveals respiratory acidosis.
- Chest X-rays reveal bilateral diffuse reticulogranular density.

NURSING DIAGNOSES

- Imbalanced nutrition: Less than body requirements
- Ineffective tissue perfusion: Cardiopulmonary
- Impaired gas exchange

TREATMENT

- Acid-base balance maintenance
- Oxygen therapy with endotracheal intubation and mechanical ventilation
- Nutrition supplements (total parenteral nutrition [TPN] or enteral feedings, if possible)
- Surfactant replacement by way of endotracheal tube
- Temperature regulation with a radiant warmer

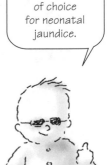

Phototherapy is the treatment of choice for neonatal jaundice.

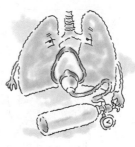

Respiratory distress syndrome occurs most commonly in preterm neonates of diabetic mothers and neonates delivered by cesarean births.

Drug therapy
- Indomethacin (Indocin) to promote closure of the ductus arteriosus (a fetal blood vessel connecting the left pulmonary artery to the descending aorta)

INTERVENTIONS AND RATIONALES
- Assess cardiovascular, respiratory, and neurologic status *for respiratory distress.*
- Monitor vital signs and pulse oximetry readings *to observe for changes.*
- Initiate and maintain ventilatory support status *to maintain air supply.*
- Administer medications, including endotracheal surfactant, as prescribed *to improve respiratory function.*
- Assess hydration status *to assess fluid loss.*
- Maintain I.V. therapy *to maintain fluid levels.*
- Provide adequate nutrition through enteral feedings, if possible, or TPN *to provide adequate nutrition.*
- Maintain thermoregulation *to reduce cold stress.*
- Obtain blood samples, as necessary, *to assess for complications.*

Teaching topics
- Explanation of the disorder and treatment plan
- Promoting maternal-neonatal bonding

Tracheoesophageal fistula

Tracheoesophageal fistula is a congenital anomaly in which the esophagus and trachea don't separate normally. Most commonly, the esophagus ends in a blind pouch, with the trachea communicating by a fistula with the lower esophagus and stomach.

CAUSES
- Abnormal development of the trachea and esophagus during the embryonic period

ASSESSMENT FINDINGS
- Difficulty feeding, such as choking or aspiration; cyanosis during feeding
- Difficulty passing a nasogastric tube
- Excessive mucus secretions
- Maternal polyhydramnios (because fetus can't swallow amniotic fluid)

- Signs of respiratory distress (tachypnea, cyanosis, sternal and substernal retractions)

DIAGNOSTIC TEST RESULTS
- Abdominal X-ray shows the fistula and a gas-free abdomen.
- Bronchoscopy shows a blind pouch.

NURSING DIAGNOSES
- Imbalanced nutrition: Less than body requirements
- Impaired gas exchange
- Risk for aspiration

TREATMENT
- Emergency surgical intervention to prevent pneumonia, dehydration, and fluid and electrolyte imbalances
- Gastrostomy tube placement
- Maintenance of a patent airway

Drug therapy
- Antibiotics (as prophylaxis for aspiration pneumonia)

INTERVENTIONS AND RATIONALES
- Assess cardiovascular, respiratory, and GI status *for complications.*
- Monitor vital signs, fluid intake and output, and transcutaneous blood oxygen tension *to assess fluid replacement needs.*
- Place the neonate in high Fowler's position *to prevent aspiration of gastric contents.*
- Keep a laryngoscope and endotracheal tube at the bedside *in case extreme edema causes obstruction.*
- Provide frequent shallow suctioning for very short periods *to maintain airway patency.*
- Provide the neonate with a pacifier *to meet sucking needs.*
- Provide gastrostomy tube feedings postoperatively *to maintain nutrition.*
- Maintain I.V. fluid therapy *to replace fluid volume.*

Teaching topics
- Explanation of the disorder and treatment plan
- Promoting maternal-neonatal bonding
- Neonatal nutritional needs

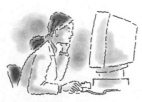

A neonate exhibits difficulty feeding and respiratory distress? That might mean tracheoesophageal fistula.

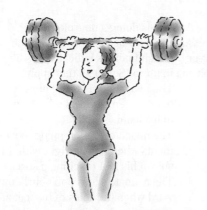

Pump up on practice questions

1. A neonate weighing 1,503 g is born at 32 weeks' gestation. During assessment 12 hours after birth, the nurse notices these signs and symptoms: hyperactivity, persistent shrill cry, frequent yawning and sneezing, and jitteriness. These symptoms indicate:

1. sepsis.
2. hepatitis.
3. drug dependence.
4. hypoglycemia.

Answer: 3. These classic symptoms of drug dependency usually appear within the first 24 hours after birth. Sepsis is indicated by temperature instability and tachycardia. Hepatitis will manifest itself as jaundice. Hypothermia, muscle twitching, diaphoresis, and respiratory distress may be signs of hypoglycemia.

➡ *NCLEX keys*
Client needs category: Physiological integrity
Client needs subcategory: Physiological adaptation
Cognitive level: Analysis

2. A neonate was delivered 1 hour ago. He's pink with acrocyanosis and exhibits occasional shivering movements of his upper extremities. Which nursing action should take priority?

1. Obtain vital signs.
2. Provide warmth with swaddling.
3. Perform a neurologic assessment.
4. Evaluate blood glucose.

Answer: 4. A neonate doesn't shiver to increase body temperature; these are jittery movements that indicate hypoglycemia. The blood glucose should be evaluated and addressed with feeding or I.V. glucose. Obtaining vital signs should have been done before this time; if they're due to be repeated, it shouldn't take priority because this will pose a delay in treatment and resolution of low blood glucose. Swaddling may mask the symptoms and doesn't address the underlying issue. Jittery movements don't indicate seizure activity, but unresolved low blood glucose could lead to seizures.

➡ *NCLEX keys*
Client needs category: Safe and effective care environment
Client needs subcategory: Management of care
Cognitive level: Analysis

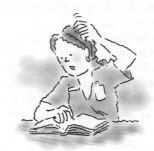

3. A nurse is assessing a 4-hour-old neonate. Which finding should be a cause of concern?

1. Anterior fontanel is ¾" (1.9 cm) wide, head is molded, and sutures are overriding.
2. Hands and feet are cyanotic, abdomen is rounded, and the neonate hasn't voided or passed meconium.
3. Color is dusky, axillary temperature is 97° F (36.1° C), and the neonate is spitting up excessive mucus.
4. The neonate exhibits irregular abdominal respirations and intermittent tremors in the extremities.

Answer: 3. Skin color is expected to be pink-tinged or ruddy, saliva should be scant, and the normal axillary temperature ranges from

97.7° to 98.6° F (36.5° to 37° C). Overriding sutures and molding, when present, may persist for a few days. Acrocyanosis may be present for 2 to 6 hours. The neonate would be expected to pass meconium and to void within 24 hours. Neonatal tremors are common in a full-term neonate; however, they must be evaluated to differentiate them from seizures.

➡ *NCLEX keys*

Client needs category: Health promotion and maintenance
Client needs subcategory: None
Cognitive level: Application

4. Which neonate is at greatest risk for developing respiratory distress syndrome?
    1. A neonate with a history of intrauterine growth retardation
    2. A neonate born at less than 35 weeks' gestation
    3. A neonate whose mother experienced prolonged rupture of membranes
    4. A neonate born at 38 weeks' gestation

Answer: 2. Respiratory distress syndrome is predominantly seen in premature neonates; the more premature the neonate, the more severe the disease. Intrauterine growth retardation and prolonged rupture of membranes are unlikely to be associated with the development of respiratory distress syndrome. A 38-week-gestation neonate usually has mature lungs and isn't at risk for respiratory distress syndrome.

➡ *NCLEX keys*

Client needs category: Physiological integrity
Client needs subcategory: Reduction of risk potential
Cognitive level: Knowledge

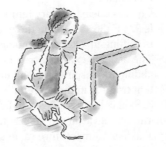

5. A nurse is doing a neurologic assessment on a 1-day-old neonate in the nursery. Which findings indicate possible asphyxia in utero? Select all that apply.
    1. The neonate grasps the nurse's finger when she puts it in the palm of his hand.
    2. The neonate does stepping movements when help upright with the sole of his foot touching a surface.
    3. The neonate's toes don't curl downward when the soles of his feet are stroked.
    4. The neonate doesn't respond when the nurse claps her hands above him.
    5. The neonate turns toward the nurse's finger when she touches his cheek.
    6. The neonate displays weak, ineffective sucking.

Answer: 3, 4, 6. If the neonate's toes don't curl downward when the soles of his feet are stroked and he doesn't respond to a loud sound, it may be evidence that neurologic damage from asphyxia has occurred. A normal neurologic response would be the toes curling downward with stroking and the extension of his arms and legs with a loud noise. Weak, ineffective sucking is another sign of neurologic damage. A neonate should grasp a person's finger when it's placed in the palm of his hand, do stepping movements when help upright with the sole of a foot touching a surface, and turn toward the nurse's finger when she touches his cheek.

➡ *NCLEX keys*

Client needs category: Health promotion and maintenance
Client needs subcategory: None
Cognitive level: Application

6. A nurse assesses a neonate's respiratory rate at 46 breaths/minute 6 hours after birth. Respirations are shallow, with periods of apnea lasting up to 5 seconds. Which action should the nurse take next?
    1. Attach an apnea monitor.
    2. Continue routine monitoring.
    3. Follow respiratory arrest protocol.
    4. Call the pediatrician immediately to report findings.

Answer: 2. The normal respiratory rate is 30 to 60 breaths/minute. Attaching the apnea monitor, following respiratory arrest protocol, and notifying the pediatrician of findings aren't necessary because the listed findings are normal respiratory patterns in neonates.

➡ *NCLEX keys*

Client needs category: Health promotion and maintenance
Client needs subcategory: None
Cognitive level: Application

7. Which statement is true?
1. Binge drinking is less detrimental to the fetus than low-level chronic drinking.
2. The mother's blood alcohol level is greater than that of the fetus.
3. The fetus can stay inebriated for many days.
4. Fetal blood alcohol levels drop off quickly.

Answer: 3. The fetal liver isn't mature enough to detoxify the alcohol. Binge drinking is more detrimental to the fetus than chronic low-level drinking for this reason as well. Alcohol goes directly from mother to fetus at the same level of concentration. High fetal blood alcohol levels stay that way for a long time.

➡ *NCLEX keys*

Client needs category: Physiological integrity
Client needs subcategory: Reduction of risk potential
Cognitive level: Analysis

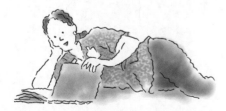

8. The best way to prevent fetal alcohol syndrome (FAS) is for a pregnant woman to:
1. only drink on social occasions.
2. stop drinking when she becomes pregnant.
3. decrease alcohol intake while attempting to become pregnant.
4. abstain from drinking before becoming pregnant and during the entire pregnancy.

Answer: 4. The best prevention is to abstain from alcohol before and during pregnancy. Social drinking can have adverse effects on an unborn child. Because the fetus can be damaged before the mother realizes that she's pregnant, stopping drinking after the pregnancy becomes known may not prevent FAS. Decreasing alcohol intake may not prevent intrauterine growth retardation.

➡ *NCLEX keys*

Client needs category: Health promotion and maintenance
Client needs subcategory: None
Cognitive level: Analysis

9. A baby girl delivered at 38 weeks' gestation weighs 2,325 g (5 lb, 2 oz) and is having difficulty maintaining body temperature. Which nursing action would best prevent cold stress?
1. Immediately after birth, dry the neonate and place her under a radiant warmer for 2 hours.
2. Administer oxygen for the first 30 minutes after birth.
3. Decrease integumentary stimulation after birth.
4. Maintain the environmental temperature at a constant level.

Answer: 1. Drying the neonate and placing her in a radiant warmer helps prevent loss of body heat. Administering oxygen and decreasing integumentary circulation would have no effect in preventing cold stress. Maintaining environmental temperature wouldn't prevent loss of heat via conduction, evaporation, or convection.

➡ *NCLEX keys*
Client needs category: Physiological integrity
Client needs subcategory: Physiological adaptation
Cognitive level: Application

10. A nurse is caring for a drug-dependent neonate. Which intervention should the nurse perform?

1. Limit sensory stimulation of the neonate.
2. Cluster activities.
3. Wrap the neonate loosely in blankets.
4. Increase environmental stimuli.

Answer: 1. Limiting sensory stimulation allows for extensive rest periods. The nurse may want to modulate sensory input as tolerated by the neonate. The neonate needs to be swaddled tightly in a flexed position. Increasing environmental stimuli may exacerbate irritability and restlessness.

➡ *NCLEX keys*
Client needs category: Physiological integrity
Client needs subcategory: Physiological adaptation
Cognitive level: Application

Beautiful. You finished another chapter. Way to goo goo!

Pump up on more practice questions

Get ready to rock these 30 maternal-neonatal practice questions. Pump it up!

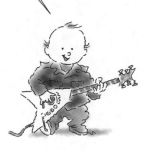

1. A nurse is assessing a neonate with tracheoesophageal fistula. Which finding should the nurse expect to encounter?
1. Increase in saliva
2. Gastric tube easily passed
3. Feeding without difficulty
4. Normal chest X-ray

Answer: 1. The neonate's inability to swallow saliva leads to an increase in saliva. The other options aren't likely findings in tracheoesoph-ageal fistula. The neonate is unable to pass a gastric tube. During feedings, the neonate is at risk for choking and cyanosis. Pulmonary infiltrates, lobar collapse, and atelectasis frequently appear on the chest X-ray.

➡ *NCLEX keys*
Client needs category: Physiological integrity
Client needs subcategory: Physiological adaptation
Cognitive level: Knowledge

2. A client is scheduled for amniocentesis. When preparing her for the procedure, the nurse should:
1. ask her to void.
2. instruct her to drink 1 qt (1 L) of fluid.
3. prepare her for I.V. anesthesia.
4. place her on her left side.

Answer: 1. To prepare a client for amniocentesis, the nurse should ask the client to empty her bladder to reduce the risk of bladder perforation. The nurse may instruct the client to drink 1 qt of fluid to fill the bladder before transabdominal ultrasound (unless ultrasound is done before amniocentesis to locate the placenta). I.V. anesthesia isn't given for amniocentesis. The client should be supine during the procedure; afterward, she should be placed on her left side to avoid supine hypotension, promote venous return, and ensure adequate cardiac output.

➡ *NCLEX keys*
Client needs category: Physiological integrity
Client needs subcategory: Reduction of risk potential
Cognitive level: Application

3. A client is human immunodeficiency virus (HIV)-positive. She states that besides her significant other, her family doesn't know about her health status. Which action should the nurse take to keep the client's health status confidential?
1. Ask the client's family (except for her significant other) to wait outside when educating the client.
2. Discuss the case with the client's mother because she's an immediate family member.
3. Discuss the case at lunch to educate the other staff members on your team.
4. Keep a log of all HIV-infected patients on the floor for statistics used in research.

Answer: 1. To protect client confidentiality, speak only to the client and any other person designated by the client. The nurse should never discuss any client with anyone who doesn't have direct care with that client. Any family member not designated by the client shouldn't be given information about the client's condition. A log of all HIV-infected patients isn't acceptable practice.

➡ *NCLEX keys*
Client needs category: Safe and effective care environment
Client needs subcategory: Management of care
Cognitive level: Application

4. A nurse is the charge nurse of a labor delivery recovery postpartum unit. The census today consists of five mother-neonate couplets, a client in triage with vaginal bleeding, a client in active labor, a client who's scheduled for induction, and a 14-week antepartum client who's being treated for urinary tract infection. There are a limited number of registered nurses (RNs) and licensed practice nurses (LPNs) scheduled for the shift and a call has been placed for additional staff. The available LPNs at the start of the shift should be assigned to which clients?

1. The client in active labor and the client in triage
2. The client scheduled for induction and the antepartum client
3. The mother-neonate couplets and the antepartum client
4. The mother-neonate couplets and the client in active labor

Answer: 3. According to scope of licensure, mother-neonate couplets are usually assigned to LPNs in the maternity setting. An antepartum client who is at 14 weeks' gestation would usually be considered stable enough for the LPN to care for because the risk of preterm labor wouldn't result in the delivery of a viable age neonate. RNs should be assigned to care for clients in active labor and to triage clients with vaginal bleeding. The client scheduled for induction would require the services of an RN.

➡ *NCLEX keys*

Client needs category: Safe and effective care environment
Client needs subcategory: Management of care
Cognitive level: Application

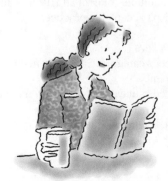

5. Which nursing intervention has priority when feeding a neonate with a cleft lip or palate?

1. Directing the flow of milk in the center of the mouth
2. Providing frequent, small feedings
3. Avoiding breast-feeding
4. Infrequent burping

Answer: 2. Frequent, small feedings help to prevent fatigue and frustration in the neonate. The flow of milk should be directed to the side of the mouth. Breast-feeding may be possible. These neonates need frequent burping because of the large amount of air swallowed while feeding.

➡ *NCLEX keys*

Client needs category: Physiological integrity
Client needs subcategory: Physiological adaptation
Cognitive level: Analysis

6. During a physical examination, a client in her 32nd week of pregnancy becomes pale, dizzy, and light-headed while supine. Which intervention takes priority?

1. Turning the client onto her left side
2. Asking the client to breathe deeply
3. Listening to fetal heart tones
4. Measuring the client's blood pressure

Answer: 1. As the uterus enlarges, pressure on the inferior vena cava increases, compromising venous return and causing blood pressure to drop. This may lead to syncope and other symptoms when the client is supine. Turning the client onto her left side relieves pressure on the vena cava, restoring normal venous return and blood pressure. Deep breathing wouldn't relieve this client's symptoms. Listening to fetal heart tones and measuring the client's blood pressure don't provide relevant information.

➡ *NCLEX keys*

Client needs category: Safe and effective care environment
Client needs subcategory: Safety and infection control
Cognitive level: Comprehension

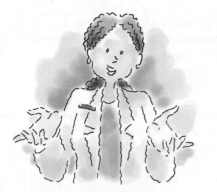

7. A client has meconium-stained amniotic fluid. The fetal monitoring strip shows fetal bradycardia. Fetal blood sampling indicates a pH of 7.12. Based on these findings, which nursing intervention is called for?
   1. Administer oxygen as prescribed.
   2. Prepare for cesarean birth.
   3. Reposition the client.
   4. Start I.V. oxytocin infusion as prescribed.

Answer: 2. Fetal blood pH of 7.19 or lower signals severe fetal acidosis; meconium-stained amniotic fluid and bradycardia are additional signs of fetal distress that warrant cesarean delivery. Oxygen administration and client repositioning may improve utero-placental perfusion but are only temporary measures. Oxytocin administration increases contractions, exacerbating fetal stress.

➡ *NCLEX keys*
Client needs category: Physiological integrity
Client needs subcategory: Reduction of risk potential
Cognitive level: Comprehension

8. A female neonate who was born to a suspected heroin user is now 2 days old and exhibiting signs of drug withdrawal. Which nursing measure is indicated?
   1. Isolate the neonate from the mother until her symptoms subside.
   2. Model behaviors and teach the mother how to reduce stimulation and provide comfort measures.
   3. Order phenobarbital from the pharmacy.
   4. Provide information on contraception to the mother.

Answer: 2. Parents are included in the care of the neonate experiencing withdrawal; these neonates pose a challenge to the limited coping skills of a substance-abusing parent. However, the nurse can't assume that the neonate won't remain in the care or contact of the mother. The nurse should teach the mother how to reduce stimulation and provide comfort measures. Isolation doesn't address the psychosocial needs of the mother or neonate. Ordering medication is the role of the physician, not the nurse. Contraceptive information should be offered, but doesn't address the current needs of the neonate.

➡ *NCLEX keys*
Client needs category: Psychosocial integrity
Client needs subcategory: None
Cognitive level: Application

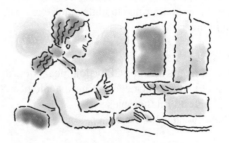

9. Which diagnostic procedure will best determine whether a client in labor has spontaneous rupture of amniotic membranes?
   1. Complete blood count (CBC)
   2. Fern test
   3. Urinalysis
   4. Vaginal examination

Answer: 2. A fern test indicates spontaneous rupture of amniotic membranes. The name of this test refers to the microscopic fern-like pattern produced by sodium chloride crystallization in dried amniotic fluid, which indicates the presence of ruptured amniotic membranes. A CBC might indicate infection (if white blood cells are increased), but it won't indicate whether the amniotic sac has ruptured. Urinalysis doesn't test for the presence of amniotic fluid. A vaginal examination may determine whether the membranes have ruptured but isn't conclusive.

Client needs category: Safe and effective care environment
Client needs subcategory: Safety and infection control
Cognitive level: Analysis

10. A client is admitted to the hospital in preterm labor. To halt her uterine contractions, the nurse expects to administer:
   1. magnesium sulfate.
   2. dinoprostone (Cervidil).
   3. ergonovine (Ergotrate).
   4. terbutaline.

Answer: 4. Terbutaline, a beta$_2$-adrenergic agonist, is used to inhibit preterm uterine contractions. Magnesium sulfate is used to treat gestational hypertension. Dinoprostone is used to induce fetal expulsion and promote cervical dilation and softening. Ergonovine is used to stop uterine blood flow, for example, in hemorrhage.

Client needs category: Physiological integrity
Client needs subcategory: Pharmacological and parenteral therapies
Cognitive level: Comprehension

11. A nurse reviews the history of a postpartum client. Which factor most strongly indicates that this client is at risk for experiencing afterpains?
   1. The client delivered at 39 weeks' gestation.
   2. The client smokes cigarettes.
   3. The client has decided to bottle-feed her neonate.
   4. The client is a gravida 6, para 5.

Answer: 4. In a multiparous client, decreased uterine muscle tone leads to alternating relaxation and contraction during uterine involution; this, in turn, causes afterpains. A gestation of 39 weeks and a history of cigarette smoking don't contribute directly to afterpains. A bottle-feeding client may experience afterpains from lack of oxytocin release, which stimulates the uterus to contract and thus enhances involution. The mere decision to bottle-feed doesn't cause afterpains.

Client needs category: Health promotion and maintenance
Client needs subcategory: None
Cognitive level: Analysis

12. A nurse is assessing a client who's 1 day postpartum. Where should the nurse expect to find the top of the client's fundus?
   1. One fingerbreadth above the umbilicus
   2. One fingerbreadth below the umbilicus
   3. At the level of the umbilicus
   4. Below the symphysis pubis

Answer: 2. After a client gives birth, the height of her fundus should decrease about one fingerbreadth (about 1 cm) each day. So by the end of the first postpartum day, the fundus should be one fingerbreadth below the umbilicus. Immediately after birth, it should be at the level of the umbilicus; 10 days after birth, it should be below the symphysis pubis.

Client needs category: Physiological integrity
Client needs subcategory: Physiological adaptation
Cognitive level: Application

13. High-risk neonates may benefit from the use of positioning aids. Which position is appropriate for a preterm neonate?
   1. Hyperabduction and extension of the arms with external rotation of the hips
   2. Neck extension and back arching with flattened shoulders
   3. Adduction and flexion of the extremities with gently rounded shoulders
   4. Abduction and flexion of the arms with flattened shoulders

Answer: 3. The goal of neonatal positioning is to have the neonate's shoulders gently rounded and elbows flexed and to avoid abduction of the shoulders and hips. This positioning enhances physiologic stability and developmental progress. Hyperabduction and external rotation aren't good for preterm neonates; they may result in contractures.

Neck extension, back arching, and flattened shoulders should be avoided. Abduction and flattened shoulders aren't appropriate positions for preterm neonates because they don't allow neonates to assume a natural position.

➡ *NCLEX keys*

Client needs category: Physiological integrity
Client needs subcategory: Basic care and comfort
Cognitive level: Application

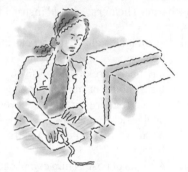

14. A neonate is admitted to the nursery with a maternal history of drug abuse. The neonate's vital signs are axillary temperature, 97° F; heart rate, 168 beats/minute; and respiratory rate, 38 breaths/minute. The neonate's behavior is quiet and drowsy. What's the nurse's priority intervention?

1. Monitor the neonate while obtaining more data about the mother's history.
2. Administer naloxone to reverse the maternal opioids received by the neonate.
3. Place the neonate on seizure precautions because seizures are likely to occur.
4. Obtain permission from the neonate's father to draw blood for toxicology studies.

Answer: 1. The neonate's vital signs and behavior are normal. It would be helpful to identify the types of substances that have been used by the mother to anticipate the neonate's needs. Naloxone shouldn't be administered to a neonate whose mother abused opioids because it could result in withdrawal symptoms in the neonate. There's no indication that the neonate is likely to

have seizures. Obtaining permission from the father to draw a toxicology screen isn't appropriate at this time.

➡ *NCLEX keys*

Client needs category: Psychosocial integrity
Client needs subcategory: None
Cognitive level: Analysis

15. A client has been in labor for 6 hours, and her contractions are occurring every 2 minutes and lasting 80 seconds. She's diaphoretic, restless, and irritable and tells the nurse that she "can't take it anymore." In which stage or phase of labor is the client?

1. Transitional phase
2. Latent phase
3. Second stage
4. Third stage

Answer: 1. During the transitional phase, cervical dilation is between 8 and 10 cm and contractions occur every 1 to 2 minutes, last 60 to 90 seconds, and are strongly intense. Also during this phase, the client may feel overwhelmed and unable to continue with labor, become irritable and restless, groan or cry out, and experience diaphoresis and, possibly, nausea and vomiting. In the latent phase of the first stage, contractions are mild to moderate and irregular. The second stage of labor begins with full cervical dilation and ends with the delivery of the neonate. The third stage begins immediately after delivery.

➡ *NCLEX keys*

Client needs category: Health promotion and maintenance
Client needs subcategory: None
Cognitive level: Application

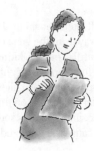

16. A nurse is assessing a pregnant client who states that she smokes one pack of cigarettes per day. What's the priority intervention of the nurse?

1. Ask the client to cut down to one-half a pack daily.
2. Inform the client of the risks to the fetus, and ask if she would like a referral to a stop smoking support group.
3. Insist that the client stop smoking immediately for the health of her fetus.
4. Do nothing; smoking is a personal decision.

Answer: 2. Smoking can be detrimental to the development of the fetus and cause low birth weight or preterm deliveries. Informing the client of the risk factors and offering to help with a referral to a support group provides encouragement and respect for the client to make the decision. Reducing the amount of cigarettes won't reduce the risks; insisting that the client stop smoking may result in a communication breakdown of established trust. Not taking action results in not providing adequate health care information that would affect the mother and fetus.

➡ *NCLEX keys*
Client needs category: Safe and effective care and environment
Client needs subcategory: Management of care
Cognitive level: Application

17. A nurse should advise a pregnant client to use which body position to enhance cardiac output and renal function?

1. Right lateral
2. Left lateral
3. Supine
4. Semi-Fowler's

Answer: 2. The left lateral position shifts the enlarged uterus away from the vena cava and aorta, enhancing cardiac output, kidney perfusion, and kidney function. The right lateral and semi-Fowler's positions don't alleviate pressure of the enlarged uterus on the vena cava. The supine position reduces sodium and water excretion because the enlarged uterus compresses the vena cava and aorta; this decreases cardiac output, leading to decreased renal blood flow, which in turn impairs kidney function.

➡ *NCLEX keys*
Client needs category: Physiological integrity
Client needs subcategory: Reduction of risk potential
Cognitive level: Application

18. A nurse is preparing a postpartum client for discharge. The nurse should instruct her to report:

1. scant lochia alba 2 to 3 weeks after delivery.
2. a temperature of 99.7° F (37.6° C) for 24 hours or more.
3. breast tenderness that's relieved by analgesics.
4. a red, warm, painful area in the breast.

Answer: 4. Signs of postpartum complications include a red, warm, painful area in either breast; heavy vaginal bleeding or passage of clots or tissue fragments; and a temperature of 100.2° F (37.9° C) or higher for 24 hours or longer. Scant lochia alba 2 to 3 weeks after delivery, a temperature of 99.7° F for 24 hours or longer, and breast tenderness that's relieved by analgesics are normal postpartum findings.

➡ *NCLEX keys*
Client needs category: Physiological integrity
Client needs subcategory: Reduction of risk potential
Cognitive level: Application

19. Lower back pain is a common complaint of pregnant clients. Comfort measures are useful to alleviate discomfort. Which comfort measure is inappropriate for the nurse to include in the teaching plan?

1. Wearing high-heel shoes
2. Using a desk seat that's ergonomically correct for the client
3. Tilting the pelvis forward to accommodate the weight of pregnancy
4. Bending at the knees, not from the waist

Answer: 1. Wearing high-heel shoes will promote imbalance and falls. Standing with the neck and shoulders straight and pelvis tilted will alleviate the stress from excess uterine weight. Bending and lifting from the knees will alleviate strain on the lower back muscles.

➡ *NCLEX keys*
Client needs category: Safe and effective care environment
Client needs subcategory: Safety and infection control
Cognitive level: Application

20. At 6 cm dilation, a client in labor receives a lumbar epidural for pain control. Which nursing diagnosis is most appropriate?
1. *Risk for injury related to rapid delivery*
2. *Ineffective breastfeeding after delivery*
3. *Hyperthermia related to effects of anesthesia*
4. *Risk for decreased cardiac tissue perfusion related to effects of anesthesia*

Answer: 4. A disadvantage of a lumbar epidural is the risk of hypotension, which can lead to decreased cardiac perfusion. Epidurals are associated with a longer labor and hypothermia. Epidurals don't affect a client's ability to breast-feed after delivery.

➡ *NCLEX keys*
Client needs category: Physiological integrity
Clients needs subcategory: Pharmacological and parenteral therapies
Cognitive level: Application

21. A neonate is born at 32 weeks' gestation to a mother who has admitted to using heroin. Which neonatal assessment takes priority?
1. Auscultation of breath sounds for signs of pulmonary problems
2. Careful observation of respiratory effort because of the neonate's prematurity
3. Evaluation for signs of drug withdrawal
4. Observation for jaundice

Answer: 3. After delivery, a neonate born to a substance abuser may exhibit signs of drug withdrawal, such as irritability, poor feeding, and continual crying. Auscultating breath sounds, observing respiratory effort, and observing for jaundice are appropriate assessments for *any* neonate, not just the neonate of a substance abuser.

➡ *NCLEX keys*
Client needs category: Safe and effective care environment
Client needs subcategory: Safety and infection control
Cognitive level: Analysis

22. A nurse is assisting with developing a teaching plan for a client who's about to be discharged after delivering a hydatidiform molar pregnancy. Which expected outcome takes highest priority?
1. Client states that she may attempt another pregnancy after 3 months of follow-up care.
2. Client schedules her first follow-up Papanicolaou (Pap) test and gynecologic examination for 6 months after discharge.
3. Client states that she won't attempt another pregnancy until her human chorionic gonadotropin (HCG) level rises.
4. Client uses a reliable contraceptive method until her follow-up care is complete in 1 year and her HCG level is negative.

Answer: 4. After a hydatidiform molar pregnancy, the client should receive follow-up care, including regular HCG testing, for 1 year because of the risk of developing chorionic carcinoma. After removal of a hydatidiform mole, the HCG level gradually falls to a negative reading unless chorionic carcinoma is developing, in which case the HCG level rises. A Pap test isn't an effective indicator of a hydatidiform molar pregnancy. A follow-up examination would be scheduled within weeks of the client's discharge. The client must not become pregnant during follow-up care because pregnancy causes the HCG level to rise, making it indistinguishable from this early sign of chorionic carcinoma.

23. A client expresses concern that her 3-hour-old neonate is difficult to awaken. The nurse explains that this behavior indicates:
1. a physiologic abnormality.
2. probable hypoglycemia.
3. normal progression into the sleep cycle.
4. normal progression into a period of neonatal reactivity.

Answer: 3. Three hours after birth, the neonate is typically difficult to awaken. This finding suggests normal progression into the sleep cycle. During this period, the neonate shows minimal response to external stimuli. Hypoglycemia is characterized by irregular respirations, apnea, and tremors. Periods of neonatal reactivity are characterized by alertness and attentiveness.

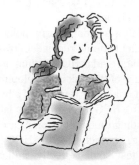

24. A nurse has just finished teaching a postpartum client about breast-feeding her neonate. Which statement is the best indicator that the client knows how to avoid breast engorgement?

1. "I'll apply warm, moist compresses to my breasts."
2. "I'll breast-feed every 1$^1/_2$ to 3 hours."
3. "I'll use an electric breast pump."
4. "I'll wear a bra 24 hours a day."

Answer: 2. Because frequent breast-feeding keeps the breasts relatively empty and increases circulation, it helps remove fluid that may lead to engorgement. Applying warm compresses to the breasts increases circulation and decreases inflammation and edema; it's used to treat, not prevent, breast engorgement. An electric breast pump usually isn't used if the neonate can breast-feed frequently. Although a bra supports the breasts, it can't prevent engorgement.

25. A client expresses concern that her 2-day-old breast-feeding neonate isn't getting enough to eat. The nurse should teach the client that breast-feeding is effective if:
1. the neonate voids once or twice every 24 hours.
2. the neonate breast-feeds four times in 24 hours.
3. the neonate loses 10% to 15% of birth weight within the first 2 days after birth.
4. the neonate latches onto the areola and swallows audibly.

Answer: 4. Breast-feeding is effective if the infant latches onto the mother's areola properly and if swallowing is audible. A breast-feeding neonate should void at least six to eight times per day and should breast-feed every 2 to 3 hours. Over the first few days after birth, an acceptable weight loss is 5% to 10% of the birth weight.

26. At age 5 minutes, a neonate is pink with acrocyanosis, has his knees flexed and fists clenched, has a whimpering cry, has a heart rate of 128 beats/minute, and withdraws his foot when slapped on the sole. What 5-minute Apgar score should the nurse record for this neonate?

Flowsheet

Sign	Apgar score		
	0	*1*	*2*
Heart rate	Absent	Less than 100 beats/minute (slow)	More than 100 beats/minute
Respiratory effort	Absent	Slow, irregular	Good crying
Muscle tone	Flaccid	Some flexion and resistance to extension of extremities	Active motion
Reflex irritability	No response	Grimace or weak cry	Vigorous cry
Color	Pallor, cyanosis	Pink body, blue extremities	Completely pink

1. 4
2. 6
3. 8
4. 10

Answer: 3. Apgar consists of a 0- to 2-point scoring system for a neonate immediately following birth and at age 5 minutes. The nurse evaluates the neonate for heart rate, respiratory effort, muscle tone, reflex irritability, and color. This neonate has a heart rate above 100 beats/minute, which equals 2; has a pink color with acrocyanosis, which equals 1; is well-flexed, which equals 2; has a weak cry, which equals 1; and has a good response to slapping the soles of the feet, which equals 2. Therefore, the nurse should record a total Apgar score of 8.

➡ NCLEX keys
Client needs category: Health promotion and maintenance
Clients needs subcategory: None
Cognitive level: Analysis

27. When assessing a neonate 1 hour after delivery, the nurse measures an axillary temperature of 95.8° F (35.4° C), an apical pulse of 110 beats/minute, and a respiratory rate of 64 breaths/minute. Which nursing diagnosis takes highest priority?

1. *Hypothermia related to heat loss*
2. *Impaired parenting related to the addition of a new family member*
3. *Risk for deficient fluid volume related to insensible fluid losses*
4. *Risk for infection related to transition to the extrauterine environment*

Answer: 1. The neonate's temperature should range from 96° to 97.7° F (35.6° to 36.5° C), and the respiratory rate should be less than 60 breaths/minute. (The respiratory rate increases as hypothermia develops.) Because this neonate's temperature is below normal and because cold stress can lead to respiratory distress and hypoglycemia, hypothermia related to heat loss takes highest priority. The other options may be appropriate but don't take precedence over hypothermia, a potentially life-threatening condition.

➡ NCLEX keys
Client needs category: Physiological integrity
Client needs subcategory: Physiological adaptation
Cognitive level: Analysis

28. A neonate must receive an eye preparation to prevent ophthalmia neonatorum. How should the nurse administer this preparation?

1. By avoiding holding the eyelid open during medication instillation
2. By letting the medication drip onto the surface of the eye
3. By positioning the neonate so that his head remains still
4. By holding the neonate in the football position

Answer: 3. After positioning the neonate securely so that the head remains still, the nurse should hold the eyelid open and instill the medication into the conjunctival sac. Holding the neonate in the football position doesn't secure the head.

➡ NCLEX keys
Client needs category: Safe and effective care environment
Client needs subcategory: Safety and infection control
Cognitive level: Application

29. A nurse is evaluating an external fetal monitoring strip. Identify the area on this strip that causes her to be concerned about uteroplacental insufficiency.

Answer: This fetal monitoring strip illustrates a late deceleration. The decrease in fetal heart rate begins at the end of the contraction and doesn't return to baseline until the contraction is over. Late decelerations are associated with uteroplacental insufficiency, shock, and fetal metabolic acidosis.

➡ *NCLEX keys*
Client needs category: Physiological integrity
Clients needs subcategory: Reduction of risk potential
Cognitive level: Analysis

30. A nurse assesses a 1-day-old neonate. Which finding indicates that the neonate's oxygen needs aren't being adequately met?
1. Respiratory rate of 54 breaths/ minute
2. Abdominal breathing
3. Nasal flaring
4. Acrocyanosis

Answer: 3. Signs of respiratory distress include nasal flaring, a respiratory rate above 60 breaths/minute, labored respirations, grunting, generalized cyanosis, and retractions. Abdominal breathing is a normal finding in neonates. Acrocyanosis (a bluish tinge to the hands and feet) is normal on the first day after birth.

➡ *NCLEX keys*
Client needs category: Health promotion and maintenance
Client needs subcategory: None
Cognitive level: Analysis

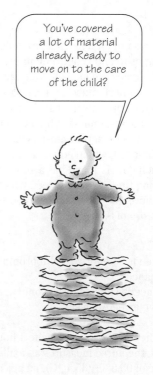

Part V   Care of the child

Brush up on key concepts

Growth and development are fundamental concepts in pediatric nursing. Each developmental stage presents unique client care challenges in such areas as nutrition, language, safety education, medication administration, and pain management.

You can review the major points of this chapter by consulting the *Cheat sheet* on page 586.

An infant's developmental milestones

A child is considered an infant from the time he's born until age 1. During this time, development is marked by five major periods:
- the neonatal period (up to 28 days)
- 1 to 4 months
- 5 to 6 months
- 7 to 9 months
- 10 to 12 months.

NEONATAL PERIOD
The neonatal period covers the time from birth to age 28 days.

Ha, ha. That's a good one. At 4 months, I laugh in response to the environment.

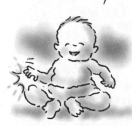

Reflexes reign
During this period, you'll note these findings:
- Head and chest circumferences are approximately equal.
- Behavior is under reflex control.
- Extremities are flexed.
- Vision is poor (the neonate fixates momentarily on light).
- Hearing and touch are well developed.
- When prone, the neonate can lift the head slightly off the bed.

Rapid pulse and respiration
- Normal pulse rate ranges from 110 to 160 beats/minute.
- Normal respiratory rate is 32 to 60 breaths/minute.
- Respirations are irregular and use the diaphragm and abdominal muscles.
- The neonate is an obligate nose breather.

Hot and cold
- Normal blood pressure is 82/46 mm Hg.
- Temperature regulation is poor.

1 TO 4 MONTHS
At age 3 months, the most primitive reflexes begin to disappear, except for the protective and postural reflexes (blink, parachute, cough, swallow, and gag reflexes), which remain for life. The infant reaches out voluntarily but is uncoordinated.

Heads up
The posterior fontanel closes by 2 to 3 months of age. In addition, the infant:
- begins to hold up his head
- begins to put hand to mouth
- develops binocular vision
- cries to express needs
- smiles (the instinctual smile appears at 2 months and the social smile at 3 months)
- laughs in response to the environment (at 4 months).

5 TO 6 MONTHS
At 5 to 6 months, birth weight doubles. In addition, the infant:
- rolls over from stomach to back
- cries when the parent leaves
- attempts to crawl when prone
- voluntarily grasps and releases objects.

7 TO 9 MONTHS
At 7 to 9 months, the infant can self-feed crackers and a bottle. When physically and

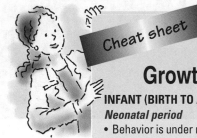

Growth and development refresher

INFANT (BIRTH TO AGE 1)

Neonatal period
- Behavior is under reflex control.
- Extremities are flexed.
- Normal pulse rate ranges from 110 to 160 beats/minute.
- Normal respiratory rate is 32 to 60 breaths/minute. Respirations are irregular and use the diaphragm and abdominal muscles; the neonate is an obligate nose breather.
- Normal blood pressure is 82/46 mm Hg.
- Temperature regulation is poor.

1 to 4 months
- The posterior fontanel closes.
- The infant begins to hold up his head.
- The infant cries to express needs.

5 to 6 months
- The infant rolls over from stomach to back.
- The infant cries when the parent leaves.

7 to 9 months
- The infant sits alone with assistance.
- The infant creeps on the hands and knees the with belly off the floor.
- The infant verbalizes all vowels and most consonants but speaks no intelligible words.
- Fear of strangers appears to peak during the 8th month.

10 to 12 months
- The infant holds onto furniture while walking (cruising) at age 10 months, walks with support at age 11 months, and stands alone and takes first steps at age 12 months.
- The infant says "mama" and "dada" and responds to own name at age 10 months; he can say about five words but understands many more.

TODDLER (AGES 1 TO 3)
- Normal pulse rate is 100 beats/minute.
- Normal respiratory rate is 26 breaths/minute.
- Normal blood pressure is 99/64 mm Hg.
- Separation anxiety arises.
- The child is toilet-trained; day dryness is achieved between ages 18 months and 3 years and night dryness between ages 2 and 5.

PRESCHOOL CHILD (AGES 3 TO 5)
- Normal pulse rate ranges from 90 to 100 beats/minute.
- Normal respiratory rate is 25 breaths/minute.
- Normal blood pressure ranges from 85/60 to 90/70 mm Hg.
- The child may express fear of mutilation or intrusion of his body, animal noises, new experiences, and the dark.

SCHOOL-AGE CHILD (AGES 5 TO 12)
- Normal pulse rate ranges from 75 to 115 beats/minute.
- Normal blood pressure ranges from 106/69 to 117/76 mm Hg.
- Normal respiratory rate ranges from 20 to 25 breaths/minute.
- The child plays with peers, initially prefers friends of the same sex, develops a first true friendship, and develops a sense of belonging, cooperation, and compromise.
- The child learns to read and spell.
- Accidents are a major cause of death and disability during this period.

ADOLESCENT (AGES 12 TO 18)
- The adolescent experiences puberty-related changes in body structure and psychosocial adjustment.
- Peers influence behavior and values.
- Vital signs approach adult levels.

emotionally ready, the infant can be weaned. The infant understands the word "no." Efforts to enforce discipline are appropriate at this time. Fear of strangers appears to peak during the 8th month. Attempts to assess breath and heart sounds should be made while the mother holds the infant.

Sit, creep, and prespeak
In addition, the infant:
- sits alone with assistance

Infants and nutrition

Here's a rundown of primary nutrition guidelines for a child's first year of life:
• Begin with formula (containing iron) or breast milk; give no more than 30 oz (887 ml) of formula each day.
• Iron supplements may be necessary after 4 months.
• No solid foods should be given for the first 6 months.
• Provide rice cereal as the first solid food; follow with other cereals (except wheat-based products).
• Yellow and green vegetables may be given at 8 to 9 months.
• Provide noncitrus fruits at 6½ to 8 months, followed by citrus fruits late in the first year.
• Give junior foods or soft table foods after 9 months.

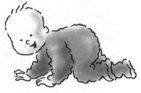

Goo goo. Ga ga. (Translation: I verbalize all vowels and most consonants but don't articulate intelligible words.)

• creeps on the hands and knees with the belly off the floor
• verbalizes all vowels and most consonants but doesn't articulate intelligible words.

10 TO 12 MONTHS
At 10 to 12 months, birth weight triples and birth length increases about 50%. The anterior fontanel normally closes between ages 9 and 18 months. In addition, the infant:
• may walk while holding onto furniture (cruising) at age 10 months
• walks with support at age 11 months, and stands alone and takes first steps at age 12 months
• says "mama" and "dada" and responds to own name at age 10 months
• can say about five words but understands many more
• is ready to be weaned from the bottle and breast. (See *Infants and nutrition*.)

Toddler developmental milestones

The toddler period includes ages 1 to 3. This is a slow growth period with a weight gain of 4 to 9 lb (2 to 4 kg) over 2 years.

Vital measurements
• Normal pulse rate is 100 beats/minute.
• Normal respiratory rate is 26 breaths/minute.
• Normal blood pressure is 99/64 mm Hg.

Me, myself, and I
The toddler exhibits the following behavioral and psychological characteristics:
• egocentricity
• frequent temper tantrums, especially when confronted with the conflict of achieving autonomy and relinquishing dependence on others
• follows the parent wherever he or she goes
• experiences separation anxiety
• lacks the concept of sharing
• prefers solitary play and has little interaction with others; this progresses to parallel play (toddler plays alongside but not with another child).

Look, Ma
The toddler:
• plants his feet wide apart and walks by age 15 months
• climbs stairs at 21 months, runs and jumps by age 2, and rides a tricycle by age 3
• uses at least 400 words as well as two- to three-word phrases and comprehends many more (by age 2)
• uses about 11,000 words (by age 3)
• undergoes toilet training; day dryness should be achieved between ages 18 months and 3 years and night dryness between ages 2 and 5.

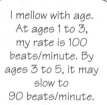

I mellow with age. At ages 1 to 3, my rate is 100 beats/minute. By ages 3 to 5, it may slow to 90 beats/minute.

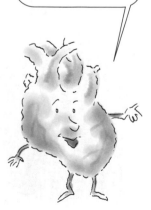

Preschool developmental milestones

The preschool period encompasses ages 3 to 5. Slow growth continues during this period. Birth length doubles by age 4.

Vital measurements
- Normal pulse rate ranges from 90 to 100 beats/minute.
- Normal respiratory rate is 25 breaths/minute.
- Normal blood pressure ranges from 85/60 to 90/70 mm Hg.

Facing fear
The child may begin to express fear. Anticipate the child's fear of mutilation or intrusion of his body, animal noises, new experiences, and the dark. Provide adhesive bandages for cuts because the child may fear losing blood. Using dolls for role-playing may reduce the preschool child's anxiety.

Playtime progress
The child:
- exhibits parallel play, associative play, and group play in activities with few or no rules and independent play accompanied by sharing or talking
- develops a body image
- may count but not understand what numbers mean
- may recognize some letters of the alphabet
- dresses without help but may be unable to tie shoes
- speaks in grammatically correct, complete sentences
- gets along without parents for short periods.

School-age developmental milestones

The school-age years are defined as ages 5 to 12.

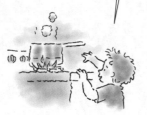

Look out. Accidents are the major cause of school-age disability.

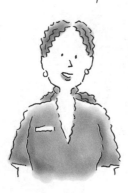

As the child moves into adolescence, nutritional needs increase significantly — remember, most eating disorders emerge during adolescence.

Beat, blood, breath
- Normal pulse rate ranges from 75 to 115 beats/minute.
- Normal blood pressure ranges from 106/69 to 117/76 mm Hg.
- Normal respiratory rate ranges from 20 to 25 breaths/minute.

Watch out
- Accidents are a major cause of death and disability during this period.
- Height increases about 2" (5 cm) a year, and weight doubles between ages 6 and 12.
- The first primary tooth is displaced by a permanent tooth at age 6, and permanent teeth erupt by age 12 except for final molars.
- Vision matures by age 6.

Best friends forever
The child:
- engages in cooperative play
- plays with peers, initially prefers friends of the same sex, develops a first true friendship, and develops a sense of belonging, cooperation, and compromise
- develops concepts of time and place, cause and effect, reversibility, conversation, and numbers
- learns to read and spell
- engages in fantasy play and daydreaming.

Adolescent developmental milestones

Ages 12 to 18 encompass the adolescent period. Adolescence is a period of rapid growth characterized by puberty-related changes in body structure and psychosocial adjustment.

What's happening to me?
During adolescence, these changes are noted:
- Vital signs approach adult levels.
- Peers influence behavior and values.
- Nutritional needs increase significantly.

Ch..ch..changes

Other milestones in adolescent development include:

• increased ability to engage in abstract thinking and to analyze, synthesize, and use logic

• increased attraction to the opposite sex (or same sex)

• breast development in females (the first sign of puberty; begins at about age 9 with the bud stage; may be asymmetrical)

• the onset of menses in females (between ages 8 and 16; possibly irregular initially)

• testicular enlargement in males (the first sign of puberty).

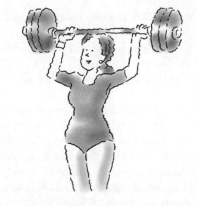

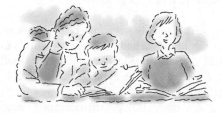

Pump up on practice questions

1. A parent brings a 19-month-old toddler to the clinic for a well-child checkup. When palpating the toddler's fontanels, the nurse should expect to find:

    1. closed anterior fontanel and open posterior fontanel.

    2. open anterior fontanel and closed posterior fontanel.

    3. closed anterior and posterior fontanels.

    4. open anterior and posterior fontanels.

Answer: 3. By age 18 months, the anterior and posterior fontanels should be closed. The diamond-shaped anterior fontanel normally closes between ages 9 and 18 months. The triangular posterior fontanel normally closes between ages 2 and 3 months.

➡ *NCLEX keys*

Client needs category: Health promotion and maintenance
Client needs subcategory: None
Cognitive level: Knowledge

2. A nurse is instructing a mother about the nutritional needs of her full-term, breast-feeding infant age 2 months. Which response shows that the mother understands the infant's dietary needs?

    1. "We won't start any new foods now."

    2. "We'll start the baby on skim milk."

3. "We'll introduce cereal into the diet now."
4. "We should add new fruits to the diet one at a time."

Answer: 1. Because breast milk provides all the nutrients that a full-term infant needs for the first 6 months, the parents shouldn't introduce new foods into the infant's diet at this point. They shouldn't provide skim milk because it doesn't have sufficient fat for infant growth. The parents also shouldn't provide solid foods, such as cereal and fruit, before age 6 months because the infant's GI tract doesn't tolerate them well.

➡ *NCLEX keys*

Client needs category: Health promotion and maintenance
Client needs subcategory: None
Cognitive level: Application

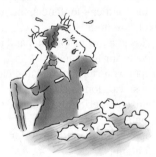

3.   A nurse is teaching the parents of a 6-month-old infant about usual growth and development. Which statements about infant development are true? Select all that apply.
1. A 6-month-old infant has difficulty holding objects.
2. A 6-month-old infant can usually roll from prone to supine and supine to prone positions.
3. A teething ring is appropriate for a 6-month-old infant.
4. Stranger anxiety usually peaks at age 12 to 18 months.
5. Head lag is commonly noted in infants at age 6 months.
6. Lack of visual coordination usually resolves by age 6 months.

Answer: 2, 3, 6. Gross motor skills of the 6-month old infant include rolling from front to back and back to front. Teething usually begins around age 6 months and, therefore, a teething ring is appropriate. Visual coordination is usually resolved by age 6 months. At age 6 months, fine motor skills include purposeful grasps. Stranger anxiety normally peaks at age 8 months. A 6-month-old infant should have good head control and no longer display head lag when pulled up to a sitting position.

➡ *NCLEX keys*

Client needs category: Health promotion and maintenance
Client needs subcategory: None
Cognitive level: Application

4.   A preschooler is admitted to the hospital the day before scheduled surgery. This is the child's first hospitalization. Which action will best help reduce the child's anxiety about the upcoming surgery?
1. Begin preoperative teaching immediately.
2. Describe preoperative and postoperative procedures in detail.
3. Give the child dolls and medical equipment to play out the experience.
4. Explain that the child will be put to sleep during surgery and won't feel anything.

Answer: 3. By playing with medical equipment and acting out the experience with dolls, the preschooler can begin to reduce anxiety. The nurse should schedule teaching shortly before surgery because preschoolers have little concept of time and because a delay between teaching and surgery may increase anxiety by giving the child time to worry. Detailed explanations are inappropriate for this developmental stage and may promote anxiety. The nurse should avoid such phrases as "put to sleep" because they might have a negative meaning to the child.

➡ *NCLEX keys*

Client needs category: Psychosocial integrity
Client needs subcategory: None
Cognitive level: Application

5. Before a well checkup in the pediatrician's office, an 8-month-old infant is sitting contentedly on the mother's lap, chewing a toy. When preparing to examine this infant, which step should the nurse do first?
   1. Obtain body weight.
   2. Auscultate heart and breath sounds.
   3. Check pupillary response.
   4. Measure the head circumference.

Answer: 2. Heart and lung auscultation shouldn't distress the infant, so it should be done early in the assessment. Placing a tape measure on the infant's head, shining a light in the eyes, or undressing the infant before weighing may cause distress, making the rest of the examination more difficult.

➡ *NCLEX keys*
Client needs category: Health promotion and maintenance
Client needs subcategory: None
Cognitive level: Application

6. A nurse is teaching a mother who plans to discontinue breast-feeding after 5 months. The nurse should advise her to include which food in her infant's diet?
   1. Iron-rich formula and baby food
   2. Whole milk and baby food
   3. Skim milk and baby food
   4. Iron-rich formula only

Answer: 4. The American Academy of Pediatrics recommends that infants at age 5 months should receive iron-rich formula and that they shouldn't receive solid food — even baby food— until age 6 months. The Academy doesn't recommend whole milk until age 12 months or skim milk until after age 2 years.

➡ *NCLEX keys*
Client needs category: Health promotion and maintenance
Client needs subcategory: None
Cognitive level: Application

7. A mother tells the nurse that her 22-month-old child says "no" to everything. When scolded, the toddler becomes angry and starts crying loudly, but then immediately wants to be held. What should the nurse tell the mother?

   1. "The toddler isn't effectively coping with stress."
   2. "The toddler's need for affection isn't being met."
   3. "This is normal behavior for a 2-year-old child."
   4. "This behavior suggests the need for counseling."

Answer: 3. Because toddlers are confronted with the conflict of achieving autonomy yet relinquishing the much-enjoyed dependence on the affection of others, their negativism is a necessary assertion of self-control. Therefore, this behavior is a normal part of the child's growth and development. Nothing about the behavior indicates that the child is under stress, isn't receiving sufficient affection, or requires counseling.

➡ *NCLEX keys*
Client needs category: Health promotion and maintenance
Client needs subcategory: None
Cognitive level: Application

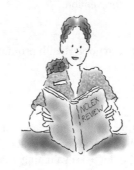

8. A mother asks the nurse how she will know when her son is entering puberty. The nurse tells the mother to watch for which sign?
   1. Appearance of pubic hair
   2. Appearance of axillary hair
   3. Testicular enlargement
   4. Nocturnal emissions

Answer: 3. Testicular enlargement signifies the onset of puberty in the male adolescent. Then sexual development progresses, causing the appearance of pubic hair and axillary hair and the onset of nocturnal emissions.

➡ *NCLEX keys*

Client needs category: Health promotion and maintenance
Client needs subcategory: None
Cognitive level: Application

9.   A nurse is teaching the parents of a school-age child. Which teaching topic should take priority?

1. Accident prevention
2. Keeping a night light on to allay fears
3. Normalcy of fears about body integrity
4. Encouraging the child to dress without help

Answer: 1. Accidents are the major cause of death and disability during the school-age years. Therefore accident prevention should take priority when teaching parents of school-age children. Preschool children are afraid of the dark, have fears concerning body integrity, and should be encouraged to dress without help (with the exception of tying shoes), but none of these should take priority over accident prevention.

➡ *NCLEX keys*

Client needs category: Health promotion and maintenance
Client needs subcategory: None
Cognitive level: Analysis

10.   A mother brings her infant to the pediatrician's office for his 2-week-old checkup. The nurse is evaluating whether the mother has understood teaching points discussed during a previous visit. Which statement indicates that further teaching is needed?

1. "I don't understand why my baby doesn't look at me."
2. "I know I should keep my baby's nasal passages clear."
3. "I should limit my baby's exposure during bath time."
4. "I should cover my baby's head when he's wet or cold."

Answer: 1. Further teaching is indicated if the mother states that she doesn't understand why her 2-week-old infant doesn't look at her. The infant at this period of development has poor vision, is only able to fixate on light momentarily, and can't distinguish objects. The 2-week-old infant should have his nasal passages kept clear because he's an obligate nose breather, he should have limited exposure at bath time, and he should have his head covered when he's wet or cold.

➡ *NCLEX keys*

Client needs category: Health promotion and maintenance
Client needs subcategory: None
Cognitive level: Analysis

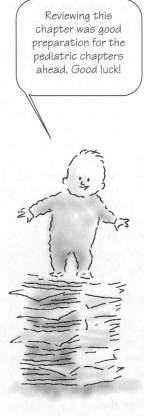

Reviewing this chapter was good preparation for the pediatric chapters ahead. Good luck!

27 Cardiovascular system

Brush up on key concepts

The cardiovascular system consists of the heart and central and peripheral blood vessels. A child's cardiovascular system closely resembles that of an adult. The system's main functions are to pump and circulate blood throughout the body.

At any time, you can review the major points of this chapter by consulting the *Cheat sheet* on pages 594 and 595.

Communication breakdown

A child may have congenital heart defects that impair the movement of blood between the heart's chambers. For example, some congenital heart defects cause a **left-to-right shunt,** in which increased pressure on the left side of the heart forces blood back to the right side. This can lead to tissue hypertrophy on the right side and increased blood flow to the lungs.

Not closed

The blood vessels surrounding the heart may also suffer congenital defects. Soon after birth, the ductus arteriosus (located between the aorta and the pulmonary artery) normally closes. If it doesn't, the infant may experience **patent ductus arteriosus,** in which blood shunts from the aorta to the pulmonary artery. If a large patent ductus arteriosus remains uncorrected, pressure within the pulmonary arteries may increase dramatically and cause blood to flow from the right side of the heart to the left, eventually leading to heart failure.

Keep abreast of diagnostic tests

The most important tests used to diagnose cardiovascular disorders include cardiac catheterization and echocardiography.

Cardiac cath

In **cardiac catheterization,** a catheter is inserted into an artery or vein (in the arm or leg) and advanced to the heart. This procedure is used to:
* evaluate ventricular function
* measure heart pressures
* measure the blood's oxygen saturation level.

Nursing actions
Before the procedure
* Explain the procedure to the child and parents.
* Describe the sensations the child will experience.
* Weigh the child.
* Check the child's color, pulse rate, blood pressure, and temperature of extremities.
* Check the child's activity level.
* Prepare the child based on his developmental level. Show where the catheter is inserted. Make a security object (for example, a teddy bear or toy) available.
After the procedure
* Keep the affected extremity immobile after catheterization to prevent hemorrhage.
* Keep the catheter site clean and dry, and monitor for hematoma formation.
* Monitor peripheral pulses, temperature, and the color of the affected extremity.
* Compare postcatheterization assessment data to precatheterization baseline data, comparing all four extremities.

Cheat sheet

Cardiovascular system refresher

ACYANOTIC HEART DEFECTS

Key signs and symptoms
- Congested cough
- Diaphoresis
- Fatigue
- Machinelike heart murmur (in patent ductus arteriosus)
- Mild cyanosis (if the condition leads to right-sided heart failure)
- Respiratory distress
- Tachycardia
- Tachypnea
- Poor oral intake

Key test results
- Echocardiography and cardiac catheterization confirm the type of defect.

Key treatments
- Cardiac glycoside: digoxin (Lanoxin)
- Diuretic: furosemide (Lasix)
- Surgical repair

Key interventions
- Monitor vital signs, pulse oximetry, and intake and output.
- Assess cardiovascular and respiratory status.
- Take the apical pulse for 1 minute before giving digoxin, and withhold the drug if the heart rate is below 100 beats/minute.
- Monitor fluid status, enforcing fluid restrictions as appropriate.

CYANOTIC HEART DEFECTS

Key signs and symptoms
- Clubbing
- Cyanosis
- History of poor feeding
- Poor weight gain
- Failure to thrive
- Irritability
- Tachycardia
- Tachypnea

Key test results
- Arterial blood gas shows diminished arterial oxygen saturation.

Key treatments
- For transposition of the great vessels or arteries: corrective surgery (called *arterial switch*) performed in the first few days of life
- For tetralogy of Fallot: complete repair or palliative treatment with Blalock-Taussig anastomosis; client's age at repair depends on the degree of pulmonic stenosis
- For hypoplastic left-heart syndrome: surgical repair in three stages (Norwood procedure I, II, and III)
- For truncus arteriosis: Norwood procedure I, II, and III

Key interventions
- Assess cardiovascular and respiratory status.
- Monitor vital signs and pulse oximetry
- Monitor intake and output.
- Administer prophylactic antibiotics.

HEART FAILURE

Key signs and symptoms
- Fussiness
- Lethargy
- Poor feeding
- Poor weight gain

Key test results
- Chest X-ray shows fluid in lungs and possible consolidation.
- Echocardiogram may show decreased or increased cardiac output and poor filling.
- Exercise stress test (in children older than 4) indicates poor activity tolerance.

Key treatments
- Diuretics: furosemide (Lasix), metolazone (Zaroxolyn)
- Cardiac glycoside: digoxin (Lanoxin)
- Inotropic agents: dopamine, dobutamine
- Surgery, if caused by congenital defect
- Extracorporeal membrane oxygenation, in severe cases

Key interventions
- Assess cardiovascular status, including vital signs and hemodynamic variables.
- Assess respiratory status and oxygenation.

A child's cardiovascular system closely resembles that of an adult.

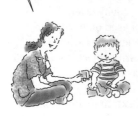

Cardiovascular system refresher *(continued)*

HEART FAILURE *(CONTINUED)*
- Keep the child in semi-Fowler's position.
- Administer oxygen.
- Weigh the child daily.

HYPERTROPHIC CARDIOMYOPATHY
Key signs and symptoms
- Heart failure, in infants
- Murmur, third heart sounds
- Sudden cardiac death
- Syncope, with exertion

Key test results
- Electrocardiogram (ECG) shows left ventricular hypertrophy and nonspecific changes.

Key treatments
- Dual chamber pacing
- Beta-adrenergic blockers: propranolol (Inderal), nadolol (Corgard), metoprolol (Lopressor)
- Calcium channel blockers: verapamil (Calan), diltiazem (Cardizem)
- Diuretics: furosemide (Lasix), spirolactone

Key interventions
- Monitor ECG.
- Assess cardiovascular status, vital signs, and hemodynamic variables.

- Administer oxygen and medications, as prescribed.

RHEUMATIC FEVER
Key signs and symptoms
Major rheumatic fever
- Carditis
- Chorea
- Erythema marginatum (temporary, disk-shaped, nonpruritic, reddened macules that fade in the center, leaving raised margins)
- Polyarthritis
- Subcutaneous nodules

Key test results
- Erythrocyte sedimentation rate is increased.
- Electrocardiogram shows prolonged PR interval.

Key treatments
- Bed rest during fever and until sedimentation rate returns to normal
- Antibiotic: penicillin to prevent additional damage from future attacks

Key interventions
- Monitor vital signs and intake and output.

- Ensure adequate intake (I.V. and oral) to compensate for blood loss during the procedure, nothing-by-mouth status, and diuretic action of some dyes used.

Heart mapping
Echocardiography is a noninvasive test used to evaluate the size, shape, and motion of cardiac structures by recording the echoes of ultrasonic waves of those structures.

Nursing actions
- Explain the procedure to the child and parents.
- Explain to the child and parents that the child may have to lie on his left side, inhale and exhale slowly, or hold his breath at intervals during the test.

Polish up on client care

Major pediatric cardiovascular disorders include acyanotic heart defects, cyanotic heart defects, heart failure, hypertrophic cardiomyopathy, and rheumatic fever. (See *From high to low,* page 596.)

Acyanotic heart defects

In an acyanotic defect, blood is usually shunted from the left (oxygenated) side to the right (unoxygenated) side of the heart. Acyanotic defects include:
- **aortic stenosis** — a narrowing or fusion of the aortic valves, interfering with left ventricular outflow

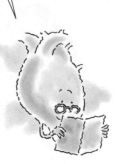

Well, I'll be. Mild cyanosis can occur in an acyanotic heart defect.

From high to low

When cardiac anomalies involve communication — movement of blood through a common opening — between chambers, blood flows from areas of high pressure to areas of low pressure. For example, a left-to-right shunt may result when increased pressure on the left side of the heart causes increased blood flow to the right.

DEFECTS THAT DON'T INVOLVE CHAMBERS

In defects that don't involve the cardiac chambers, blood can also flow from high-pressure to low-pressure areas. In patent ductus arteriosus, for instance, the ductus arteriosus (located between the aorta and pulmonary artery) remains open after birth. This opening causes blood to shunt from the aorta to the pulmonary artery.

- **atrial septal defect** — a defect stemming from a patent foramen ovale or the failure of a septum to develop completely between the atria
- **coarctation of the aorta** — a narrowing of the aortic arch, usually distal to the ductus arteriosus beyond the left subclavian artery
- **patent ductus arteriosus** — a defect resulting from the failure of the ductus to close, causing shunting of blood to the pulmonary artery
- **pulmonary artery stenosis** — a narrowing or fusing of valve leaflets at the entrance of the pulmonary artery, interfering with right ventricular outflow
- **ventricular septal defect** — a defect occurring when the ventricular septum fails to complete its formation between the ventricles, resulting in a left-to-right shunt.

CAUSES
- Defects between structures that inhibit blood flow to the system or alter pulmonary resistance
- Defects in the septa that lead to a left-to-right shunt

ASSESSMENT FINDINGS
- Congested cough
- Diaphoresis
- Fatigue
- Frequent respiratory infections
- Hepatomegaly
- Machinelike heart murmur (in patent ductus arteriosus)
- Mild cyanosis (if the condition leads to right-sided heart failure)

- Poor growth and development as a result of increased energy expenditure for breathing
- Poor oral intake
- Respiratory distress
- Tachycardia
- Tachypnea

DIAGNOSTIC TEST RESULTS
Echocardiography and cardiac catheterization confirm the type of defect.
- In **aortic stenosis,** echocardiography shows left ventricular hypertrophy and prominent pulmonary vasculature. Cardiac catheterization helps determine the degree of shunting and the extent of pulmonary vascular disease.
- In **atrial septal defect,** echocardiography shows enlargement of the right atrium and ventricle and prominent pulmonary vasculature. Cardiac catheterization shows right atrial blood that's more oxygenated than superior vena cava blood. It also helps determine the degree of shunting and the extent of pulmonary vascular disease.
- In **coarctation of the aorta,** echocardiography shows left ventricular hypertrophy, wide ascending and descending aorta, and prominent collateral circulation. Cardiac catheterization shows affected collateral circulation and pressures in the right and left ventricles.
- In **patent ductus arteriosus,** echocardiography shows prominent pulmonary vasculature and enlargement of the left ventricle and aorta. Cardiac catheterization helps determine the extent of pulmonary vascular disease and shows an oxygen content higher in the pulmonary artery than in the right ventricle.

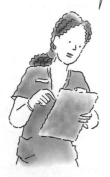

Echocardiography and cardiac catheterization distinguish the various acyanotic heart defects.

- In **pulmonary artery stenosis,** echocardiography shows right ventricular hypertrophy. Cardiac catheterization provides evidence of the degree of shunting.
- In **ventricular septal defect,** echocardiography may be normal for small defects or show cardiomegaly with a large left atrium and ventricle. In a large defect, echocardiography may show prominent pulmonary vasculature. Cardiac catheterization helps determine the size and exact location of ventricular septal defect and the degree of shunting.

NURSING DIAGNOSES
- Anxiety
- Decreased cardiac output
- Impaired gas exchange
- Delayed growth and development

TREATMENT
- **Aortic stenosis:** surgery (valvulotomy or commissurotomy)
- **Atrial septal defect:** surgery to patch the hole (mild defects may close spontaneously) or balloon umbrella device inserted in an opening in the cardiac catheterization laboratory.
- **Coarctation of the aorta:** inoperable if the coarctation is proximal to the ductus arteriosus—a stent is placed in cardiac catheterization laboratory; closed heart resection if the coarctation is distal to the ductus arteriosus
- **Patent ductus arteriosus:** ligation of the patent ductus arteriosus in a closed-heart operation
- **Pulmonary artery stenosis:** open-heart surgery to separate the pulmonary valve leaflets
- **Ventricular septal defect:** as a last resort, permanent correction with a patch later when the heart is larger (spontaneous closure of the ventricular septal defect may occur in some children by age 3) or pulmonary artery banding to prevent heart failure

Drug therapy
- Cardiac glycoside: digoxin (Lanoxin)
- Diuretic: furosemide (Lasix)
- Anti-inflammatory agent: indomethacin (Indocin) to achieve pharmacologic closure

(in patent ductus arteriosus) during the neonatal period only
- Prophylactic antibiotics to prevent endocarditis

INTERVENTIONS AND RATIONALES
- Explain the heart defect and answer any questions *to prepare the child for cardiac catheterization or surgery.*
- Monitor vital signs, pulse oximetry, and intake and output *to assess renal function and detect change.*
- Assess cardiovascular and respiratory status *to detect early signs of decompensation.*
- Take the apical pulse for 1 minute before giving digoxin and hold the drug if the heart rate is below 100 beats/minute *to prevent toxicity.*
- Monitor fluid status, enforcing fluid restrictions as appropriate *to prevent fluid overload.*
- Weigh the child daily *to determine fluid overload or deficit.*
- Organize physical care and anticipate the child's needs *to reduce the child's oxygen demands.*
- Give an infant high-calorie formula. Give a child high-calorie, easy-to-chew, and easy-to-digest foods *to maintain adequate nutrition and decrease oxygen demands.*
- Maintain normal body temperature *to prevent cold stress.*
- Raise the head of the bed or place the infant in an infant car seat *to ease breathing.*

Teaching topics
- Preparing the child and parents for the sights and sounds of the intensive care unit
- Explanation of the disorder and treatment plan
- Medication use and possible adverse effects

Cyanotic heart defects

Cyanotic heart defects result in unoxygenated blood or a mixture of oxygenated and unoxygenated blood being shunted through the cardiovascular system. This shunting can lead to left-sided heart failure, decreased oxygen supply to the body, and the development of

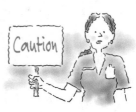

Remember to take an apical pulse for 1 minute before giving digoxin. You're checking for bradycardia, which is a rate below 100 beats/minute for infants.

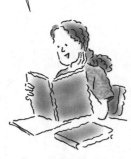

If I keep studying, there won't be anything "defective" about my knowledge of cardiovascular defects.

collateral circulation. Cyanotic heart defects include:
- **transposition of the great vessels or arteries** — a defect in which the aorta arises from the right ventricle, the pulmonary artery arises from the left ventricle, and the position of the coronary arteries is also reversed
- **tetralogy of Fallot** — a defect consisting of pulmonary artery stenosis, ventricular septal defect, hypertrophy of the right ventricle, and an overriding aorta
- **hypoplastic left-heart syndrome** — a defect consisting of aortic valve atresia, mitral atresia or stenosis, diminutive or absent left ventricle, and severe hypoplasia of the ascending aorta and aortic arch
- **truncus arteriosis** — a defect in which there's incomplete division of the common great vessel.

CAUSES
- Any condition that increases pulmonary vascular resistance
- Structural defects

ASSESSMENT FINDINGS
- Clubbing
- Cyanosis
- History of poor feeding
- Poor weight gain
- Diaphoresis when feeding (infants)
- Failure to thrive
- Increasing dyspnea, cyanosis, and tachypnea during the first few days after birth; without treatment, heart failure after closure of the ductus (in hypoplastic left-heart syndrome)
- Irritability
- Tachycardia
- Tachypnea

DIAGNOSTIC TEST RESULTS
- Arterial blood gas analysis shows diminished arterial oxygen saturation.
- Cardiac catheterization results confirm the diagnosis through visualization of defects and measurement of oxygen saturation level.

NURSING DIAGNOSES
- Impaired gas exchange
- Anxiety
- Decreased cardiac output

TREATMENT
For transposition of the great vessels or arteries, several therapies are possible, including:
- corrective surgery (called *arterial switch*) to redirect blood flow by switching the position of the major blood vessels; performed in the first few days of life
- palliative surgery to provide communication between the chambers.

For tetralogy of Fallot, the physician can use:
- complete repair or palliative treatment to increase blood flow to the lungs by bypassing pulmonic stenosis (Blalock-Taussig anastomosis of the right pulmonary artery to the right subclavian artery); age at repair depends on the degree of pulmonic stenosis
- oxygen therapy
- repair of ventricular septal defect and stenosis (may be done in stages).

For hypoplastic left-heart syndrome, surgical repair is done in three stages (Norwood procedure I, II, and III).

For truncus arteriosis, several options include:
- medical management of heart failure
- surgical re-creation of the pulmonary trunk
- corrective surgery to repair ventricular septal defect
- Norwood procedure I, II, and III. (Without surgery, death occurs in early infancy.)

Drug therapy
- Opioid analgesic: morphine during tet spell
- Beta-adrenergic blocker: propranolol (Inderal)
- Prostaglandin E to keep the ductus arteriosus patent

INTERVENTIONS AND RATIONALES
- Assess cardiovascular and respiratory status *to detect early signs of compromise*.
- Monitor vital signs and pulse oximetry *to detect hypoxia*.
- Monitor intake and output *to assess renal status*.
- Provide oxygen, when necessary, *to compensate for impaired oxygen exchange*.

Memory jogger

When a child has a cyanotic heart defect, check for the 4 *C's*:

Cyanosis, especially increasing with crying

Crabbiness or irritability

Clubbing of digits

Crouching, or squatting, which increases systemic venous return, shunts blood from the extremities to the head and trunk, and decreases cyanosis.

- Provide the infant with high-calorie formula *to meet nutritional needs.*
- Anticipate needs and prevent distress *to decrease oxygen demands on the child.*
- Use a preemie nipple *to decrease the energy needed for sucking.*
- Provide adequate hydration *to prevent sequelae of polycythemia.*
- Administer prophylactic antibiotics *to prevent endocarditis.*
- Provide thorough skin care *to prevent skin breakdown.*
- Prepare the child for cardiac catheterization *to decrease anxiety.*

Teaching topics
- Explanation of the disorder and treatment plan
- Preparing the child and parents for the sights and sounds of the intensive care unit
- Explaining the difference between palliative and corrective procedures

Heart failure

Heart failure occurs when the heart can't pump enough blood to meet the body's metabolic needs.

CAUSES
- Congenital defect, such as atrial septal defect, ventricular septal defect, or tetralogy of Fallot
- Infection, causing myocarditis
- Anemia
- Viral infection
- Medications such as chemotherapeutic agents

ASSESSMENT FINDINGS
- Fussiness
- Lethargy
- Diaphoresis
- Poor feeding
- Poor weight gain

DIAGNOSTIC TEST RESULTS
- Chest X-ray shows fluid in lungs and possible consolidation.
- Echocardiogram may show decreased or increased cardiac output and poor filling.
- Exercise stress test (in children older than 4) indicates poor activity tolerance.

NURSING DIAGNOSES
- Decreased cardiac output
- Excess fluid volume
- Impaired gas exchange

TREATMENT
- Oxygen therapy, possibly requiring intubation and mechanical ventilation
- Surgery, if caused by congenital defect
- Left ventricular assist device
- Extracorporeal membrane oxygenation, in severe cases

Drug therapy
- Diuretics: furosemide (Lasix), metolazone (Zaroxolyn)
- Cardiac glycoside: digoxin (Lanoxin)
- Inotropic agents: dopamine, dobutamine

INTERVENTIONS AND RATIONALES
- Assess cardiovascular status, vital signs, and hemodynamic variables *to detect signs of reduced cardiac output.*
- Assess respiratory status and oxygenation *to detect increasing fluid in the lungs and respiratory failure.*
- Keep the child in semi-Fowler's position *to increase chest expansion and improve ventilation.*
- Administer medications, as prescribed, *to enhance cardiac performance and reduce excess fluids.*
- Administer oxygen *to enhance arterial oxygenation.*
- Measure and record intake and output; *intake greater than output may indicate fluid retention.*
- Monitor laboratory studies *to detect electrolyte imbalances, renal failure, and impaired cardiac circulation.*
- Provide suctioning, if necessary, and assist with turning, coughing, and deep breathing *to prevent pulmonary complications.*
- Restrict oral fluids because *excess fluids can worsen heart failure.*
- Weigh the child daily.

Teaching topics
- Explanation of the disorder and treatment plan
- Medications and possible adverse effects
- Limiting sodium intake
- Increasing caloric need to meet metabolic requirements
- Recognizing signs and symptoms of fluid overload

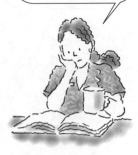

Infants with cyanotic defects have less energy for sucking; use a preemie nipple.

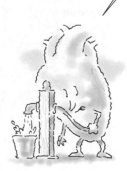

Argh! Sometimes I just can't pump enough to meet demand!

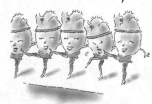

C'mon ladies... you don't want your myocardium to get flabby! And a one, and a two...

Hypertrophic cardiomyopathy

In cardiomyopathy, the myocardium (middle muscular layer) around the left ventricle becomes flabby, altering cardiac function and resulting in decreased cardiac output. Increased heart rate and increased muscle mass compensate in early stages; however, in later stages, heart failure develops.

There are three types of cardiomyopathy: dilated, obstructive, and hypertrophic; hypertrophic is the most common type seen in children. In hypertrophic cardiomyopathy, the hypertrophied left ventricle can't relax and fill properly.

CAUSES
- Congenital
- Genetic link under consideration

ASSESSMENT FINDINGS
- Heart failure, in infants
- Palpitations
- Murmur, third heart sounds
- Syncope, with exertion
- Sudden cardiac death

DIAGNOSTIC TEST RESULTS
- Chest X-ray shows cardiomegaly and pulmonary congestion.
- Electrocardiogram (ECG) shows left ventricular hypertrophy and nonspecific changes.
- Echocardiogram shows decreased myocardial function.

NURSING DIAGNOSES
- Decreased cardiac output
- Impaired gas exchange
- Activity intolerance

TREATMENT
- Dual chamber pacing
- Septal alcohol ablation
- Surgery (when medication fails): heart transplant or ventricular myotomy

Drug therapy
- Antiarrhythmics
- Anticoagulant: warfarin (Coumadin)
- Beta-adrenergic blockers: propranolol (Inderal), nadolol (Corgard), metoprolol (Lopressor)

- Calcium channel blockers: verapamil (Calan), diltiazem (Cardizem)
- Diuretics: furosemide (Lasix), spirolactone

INTERVENTIONS AND RATIONALES
- Monitor ECG *to detect arrhythmias and ischemia.*
- Assess cardiovascular status, vital signs, and hemodynamic variables *to detect heart failure.*
- Monitor respiratory status *to detect evidence of heart failure, such as dyspnea and crackles.*
- Administer oxygen and medications, as prescribed, *to improve oxygenation and cardiac output.*
- Monitor and record intake and output *to detect fluid volume overload.*
- Keep the child in semi-Fowler's position *to enhance gas exchange.*
- Maintain bed rest *to reduce oxygen demands on the heart.*
- Monitor laboratory results *to detect abnormalities, such as hypokalemia, from the use of diuretics.*

Teaching topics
- Explanation of the disorder and treatment plan
- Medications and possible adverse effects
- Early signs and symptoms of heart failure
- Monitoring pulses and blood pressure
- Avoiding straining during bowel movements
- Contacting the Children's Cardiomyopathy Foundation

Rheumatic fever

Rheumatic fever is an inflammatory disease of childhood. It first occurs 1 to 3 weeks after a group A beta-hemolytic streptococcal infection and may recur. Rheumatic fever results in antigen-antibody complexes that ultimately destroy heart tissue.

Rheumatic heart disease refers to the cardiac effects of rheumatic fever and includes pancarditis (inflammation of the heart muscle, heart lining, and sac around the heart) during the early acute phase and chronic heart valve disease later.

In rheumatic fever, antibodies manufactured to combat streptococci react and produce lesions at specific tissue sites, especially in the heart and joints.

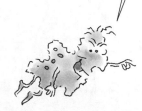

CAUSES
• Production of antibodies against group A beta-hemolytic *Streptococcus*
• Untreated or improperly treated group A beta-hemolytic *Streptococcus* infection (1% to 5% of children infected with *Streptococcus* develop rheumatic fever)

ASSESSMENT FINDINGS
The Jones criteria for assessing major rheumatic fever include:
• carditis
• chorea
• erythema marginatum (temporary, disk-shaped, nonpruritic, reddened macules that fade in the center, leaving raised margins)
• polyarthritis
• subcutaneous nodules.
   The Jones criteria for assessing minor rheumatic fever include:
• arthralgia
• evidence of a *Streptococcus* infection
• fever
• history of rheumatic fever
• new-onset murmur.

DIAGNOSTIC TEST RESULTS
• Antistreptolysin-O titer is elevated.
• Erythrocyte sedimentation rate is increased.
• ECG shows a prolonged PR interval.

NURSING DIAGNOSES
• Decreased cardiac output
• Impaired gas exchange
• Imbalanced nutrition: Less than body requirements

TREATMENT
• Bed rest during fever and until sedimentation rate returns to normal

Drug therapy
• Analgesic: aspirin for arthritis pain
• Antibiotic: penicillin to prevent additional damage from future attacks (taken until age 20 or for 5 years after the attack, whichever is longer)

INTERVENTIONS AND RATIONALES
• Monitor vital signs and intake and output *to detect fluid volume overload or deficit.*
• Institute safety measures for chorea; maintain a calm environment, reduce stimulation, avoid the use of forks or glass, and assist in walking *to prevent injury.*
• Provide appropriate passive stimulation *to maintain growth and development.*
• Provide emotional support for long-term convalescence *to help relieve anxiety.*
• Use sterile technique in dressing changes and standard precautions *to prevent reinfection.*

Teaching topics
• Explanation of the disorder and treatment plan
• Medication use and possible adverse effects
• Understanding the need to inform health care providers of existing medical conditions
• Signs and symptoms of aspirin toxicity (tinnitus, bruising, bleeding gums)

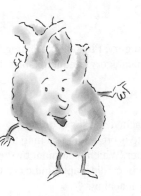

Effective treatment eliminates strep infection, relieves symptoms, and prevents recurrence, reducing the chance I'll suffer permanent damage.

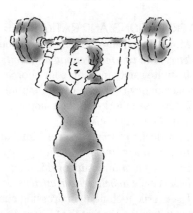

Pump up on practice questions

1.   A child returns to his room after a cardiac catheterization. Which nursing intervention is most appropriate?
1. Maintain the child on bed rest with no further activity restrictions.
2. Maintain the child on bed rest with the affected extremity immobilized.
3. Allow the child to get out of bed to go to the bathroom, if necessary.
4. Allow the child to sit in a chair with the affected extremity immobilized.

Answer: 2. The child should be maintained on bed rest with the affected extremity immobilized after cardiac catheterization to prevent hemorrhage. Allowing the child to move the affected extremity while on bed rest, allowing the child bathroom privileges, or allowing the child to sit in a chair with the affected extremity immobilized places the child at risk for hemorrhage.

➡ *NCLEX keys*
Client needs category: Physiological integrity
Client needs subcategory: Reduction of risk potential
Cognitive level: Application

2.   A child is scheduled for echocardiography. The nurse is providing teaching to the child's mother. Which statement by the mother about echocardiography indicates the need for further teaching?

1. "I'm glad my child won't have an I.V. catheter inserted for this procedure."
2. "I'm glad my child won't need to have dye injected into him before the procedure."
3. "How am I going to explain to my son that he can't have anything to eat before the test?"
4. "I know my child may need to lie on his left side and breathe in and out slowly during the procedure."

Answer: 3. Echocardiography is a noninvasive procedure used to evaluate the size, shape, and motion of various cardiac structures. Therefore, it isn't necessary for the client to have an I.V. catheter inserted, dye injected, or nothing by mouth, as would be the case with a cardiac catheterization. The child may need to lie on his left side and inhale and exhale slowly during the procedure.

➡ *NCLEX keys*
Client needs category: Physiological integrity
Client needs subcategory: Reduction of risk potential
Cognitive level: Analysis

3.   An infant with a ventricular septal defect is receiving digoxin (Lanoxin). Which intervention by the nurse is most appropriate before digoxin administration?
1. Take the infant's blood pressure.
2. Check the infant's respiratory rate for 1 minute.
3. Check the infant's radial pulse for 1 minute.
4. Check the infant's apical pulse for 1 minute.

Answer: 4. Before administering digoxin, the nurse should check the infant's apical pulse for 1 minute. Checking the radial pulse may be inaccurate. Checking the blood pressure and respiratory rate isn't necessary before digoxin administration because the medication doesn't affect these parameters.

➡ *NCLEX keys*
Client needs category: Physiological integrity
Client needs subcategory: Pharmacological and parenteral therapies
Cognitive level: Application

4. A nurse checks an infant's apical pulse before digoxin (Lanoxin) administration and finds that the pulse rate is 90 beats/minute. Which action is most appropriate for the nurse?
1. Withhold the digoxin and notify the physician.
2. Administer the digoxin and notify the physician.
3. Administer the digoxin and document the infant's pulse rate.
4. Withhold the digoxin and document the infant's pulse rate.

Answer: 1. The nurse should withhold the digoxin and notify the physician because an apical pulse below 100 beats/minute in an infant is considered bradycardic. The nurse should also document her findings and interventions in the medical record. Administering the drug to a bradycardic infant could further decrease his heart rate and compromise his status. Withholding the drug and not notifying the physician could compromise the existing treatment plan.

➡ *NCLEX keys*
Client needs category: Physiological integrity
Client needs subcategory: Pharmacological and parenteral therapies
Cognitive level: Application

5. A child has been diagnosed with rheumatic fever. Which statement by the mother indicates an understanding of rheumatic fever?
1. "I should avoid giving my child aspirin for the arthritic pain."
2. "It's very upsetting that my child must take penicillin until he's 20 years old."
3. "I need to wear a gown, gloves, and mask to stay in my child's room."
4. "I don't know how I'll be able to keep my child away from his sister when he gets home."

Answer: 2. Rheumatic fever is an acquired autoimmune-complex disorder that occurs 1 to 3 weeks after an infection of group A beta-hemolytic streptococci, in many cases as a result of strep throat that hasn't been treated with antibiotics. To prevent additional heart damage from future attacks, the child must take penicillin or another antibiotic until the age of 20 or for 5 years after the attack, whichever is longer. Children shouldn't be given aspirin because it may result in Reye's syndrome. Rheumatic fever isn't contagious, so isolation precautions aren't necessary.

➡ *NCLEX keys*
Client needs category: Physiological integrity
Client needs subcategory: Reduction of risk potential
Cognitive level: Analysis

6. A nurse is caring for a child with a cyanotic heart defect. Which signs should the nurse expect to observe?
1. Cyanosis, hypertension, clubbing, and lethargy
2. Cyanosis, hypotension, crouching, and lethargy
3. Cyanosis, irritability, clubbing, and crouching
4. Cyanosis, confusion, clonus, and crouching

Answer: 3. The child with a cyanotic heart defect has cyanosis along with crabiness (irritability), clubbing of the digits, and crouching or squatting. The child with cyanotic heart defect doesn't typically have hypertension, lethargy, confusion, or clonus.

➡ *NCLEX keys*
Client needs category: Physiological integrity
Client needs subcategory: Physiological adaptation
Cognitive level: Comprehension

7. A nurse is caring for an infant with tetralogy of Fallot. Which drug should the nurse anticipate administering during a tet spell?
1. Propranolol (Inderal)
2. Morphine
3. Meperidine (Demerol)
4. Furosemide (Lasix)

Answer: 2. The nurse should anticipate administering morphine during a tet spell to decrease the associated infundibular spasm. Propranolol may be administered as a preventive measure in an infant with tetralogy of Fallot but isn't administered during a tet spell. Furosemide and meperidine aren't appropriate agents for an infant experiencing a tet spell.

➡ **NCLEX keys**
Client needs category: Physiological integrity
Client needs subcategory: Pharmacological and parenteral therapies
Cognitive level: Analysis

8.   An infant is diagnosed with patent ductus arteriosus. Which drug should the nurse anticipate administering to attempt to close the defect?
1. Digoxin (Lanoxin)
2. Prednisone
3. Furosemide (Lasix)
4. Indomethacin (Indocin)

Answer: 4. Indomethacin is administered to an infant with patent ductus arteriosus in the hope of closing the defect. Digoxin and furosemide may be used to treat the symptoms associated with patent ductus arteriosus, but they don't achieve closure. Prednisone isn't used to treat the condition.

➡ **NCLEX keys**
Client needs category: Physiological integrity
Client needs subcategory: Pharmacological and parenteral therapies
Cognitive level: Application

9.   An infant age 2 months has a tentative diagnosis of congenital heart defect. During physical assessment, the nurse notes that the infant has a pulse rate of 168 beats/minute and a respiratory rate of 72 breaths/minute. In which position should the nurse place the infant?
1. Upright in an infant seat
2. Lying on the back
3. Lying on the abdomen
4. Sitting in high Fowler's position

Answer: 1. Because these signs suggest development of respiratory distress, the nurse should position the infant with the head elevated at a 45-degree angle to promote maximum chest expansion. This can be accomplished by placing the infant in an infant seat. Placing an infant flat on the back or abdomen or in high Fowler's position could increase respiratory distress by preventing maximum chest expansion.

➡ **NCLEX keys**
Client needs category: Physiological integrity
Client needs subcategory: Physiological adaptation
Cognitive level: Application

10.   An infant with a congenital cyanotic heart defect has a complete blood count drawn, revealing an elevated red blood cell (RBC) count. Which condition do these findings indicate?
1. Anemia
2. Dehydration
3. Jaundice
4. Hypoxia compensation

Answer: 4. A congenital cyanotic heart defect alters blood flow through the heart and lungs, which produces hypoxia. To compensate for this, the body increases the oxygen-carrying capacity by increasing RBC production, which causes the hemoglobin level and hematocrit to increase. The hemoglobin level and hematocrit are typically decreased in anemia. Altered electrolyte levels and other laboratory values provide better evidence of dehydration. An elevated hemoglobin level and hematocrit aren't associated with jaundice.

➡ **NCLEX keys**
Client needs category: Physiological integrity
Client needs subcategory: Physiological adaptation
Cognitive level: Analysis

28 Respiratory system

Brush up on key concepts

The primary function of the respiratory system is to distribute air to the alveoli in the lungs, where gas exchange takes place. Gas exchange includes:
- the addition of oxygen (O_2) to pulmonary capillary blood
- the removal of carbon dioxide (CO_2) from pulmonary capillary blood.

At any time, you can review the major points of this chapter by consulting the *Cheat sheet* on pages 606 and 607.

Upper and lower
The parts of the respiratory system include the **upper airway** and the **lower airway.**

The upper airway includes the:
- epiglottis
- nasopharynx
- oropharynx
- larynx.

The lower airway includes the:
- trachea
- bronchi
- bronchioles
- alveoli.

Take a deep breath
Breathing delivers inspired gas to the lower respiratory tract and alveoli. Contraction and relaxation of the respiratory muscles move air into and out of the lungs. Here are some important aspects of the breathing process:
- **Ventilation** begins with the contraction of the inspiratory muscles: The diaphragm (the major muscle of respiration) descends while the external intercostal muscles move the rib cage upward and outward.
- Air then enters the lungs in response to the pressure gradient between the atmosphere and the lungs.
- The lungs adhere to the chest wall and diaphragm because of the vacuum created by negative pleural pressure.
- As the thorax expands, the lungs also expand, causing a decrease in pressure in the lungs.
- The accessory muscles of inspiration, which include the scalene and sternocleido-mastoid muscles, raise the clavicles, upper ribs, and sternum.
- To reach the capillary lumen, O_2 diffuses across the alveolocapillary membrane into the blood.
- Normal expiration is passive; the inspiratory muscles cease to contract, and the elastic recoil of the lungs causes the lungs to contract.
- These actions increase the pressure in the lungs above atmospheric pressure, moving air from the lungs to the atmosphere.

Air system under construction
A **child's respiratory tract** differs anatomically from an adult's in ways that predispose the child to many respiratory problems. A child's respiratory tract differs from an adult's in the following ways:
- Lungs aren't fully developed at birth.
- Alveoli continue to grow and increase in size through age 8.
- A child's respiratory tract has a narrower lumen than an adult's until age 5; the narrow airway makes the young child prone to airway obstruction and respiratory distress from inflammation, mucus secretion, or a foreign body.
- Elastic connective tissue becomes more abundant with age in the peripheral part of the lung.
- A child's respiratory rate decreases as body size increases.

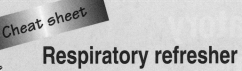

Respiratory refresher

ACUTE RESPIRATORY FAILURE

Key signs and symptoms
- Decreased respiratory excursion, accessory muscle use, retractions
- Difficulty breathing, shortness of breath, dyspnea, tachypnea, orthopnea
- Fatigue
- Fussiness
- Grunting

Key test results
- Arterial blood gas (ABG) levels show hypoxia, acidosis, alkalosis, and hypercapnia.

Key treatments
- Oxygen (O_2) therapy, intubation, and mechanical ventilation
- Analgesic: morphine
- Bronchodilators: terbutaline, aminophylline, theophylline; via nebulizer: albuterol, ipratropium
- Steroids: hydrocortisone, methylprednisolone

Key interventions
- Assess respiratory status.
- Administer O_2.
- Provide suctioning; assist with turning, coughing, and deep breathing; perform chest physiotherapy and postural drainage.
- Maintain bed rest.

ASTHMA

Key signs and symptoms
- Diaphoresis
- Dyspnea
- Prolonged expiration with an expiratory wheeze; in severe distress, possible inspiratory wheeze
- Unequal or decreased breath sounds
- Use of accessory muscles

Key test results
- O_2 saturation via pulse oximetry may show decreased O_2 saturation.
- ABG measurement may show increased partial pressure of arterial carbon dioxide from respiratory acidosis.

Key treatments
- Short-acting bronchodilators (inhaled beta$_2$-adrenergic agonists): albuterol (Proventil-HFA, Ventolin), levalbuterol (Xopenex)

Key interventions
- Assess respiratory and cardiovascular status.
- Monitor vital signs.

During an acute attack
- Allow the child to sit upright; provide moist O_2, if necessary.
- Monitor vital signs.

BRONCHOPULMONARY DYSPLASIA

Key signs and symptoms
- Atelectasis
- Crackles, rhonchi, wheezes
- Dyspnea
- Sternal retractions

Key test results
- Chest X-ray reveals pulmonary changes (bronchiolar metaplasia and interstitial fibrosis).

Key treatments
- Chest physiotherapy
- Ventilatory support and oxygen

Key interventions
- Assess respiratory and cardiovascular status.
- Monitor vital signs, pulse oximetry, and intake and output.

CROUP

Key signs and symptoms
- Barking, brassy cough or hoarseness sometimes described as a "seal bark" cough
- Inspiratory stridor with varying degrees of respiratory distress

Key test results
- Laryngoscopy may reveal inflammation and obstruction in epiglottal and laryngeal areas.
- Neck X-ray shows areas of upper airway narrowing and edema in subglottic folds.

Key treatments
- Cool humidification during sleep with a cool mist tent or room humidifier
- Inhaled racemic epinephrine and corticosteroids such as methylprednisolone sodium succinate
- Tracheostomy, O_2 administration

Key interventions
- Monitor vital signs and pulse oximetry readings.
- Administer O_2 therapy and maintain the child in a cool mist tent, if needed.

Respiratory refresher *(continued)*

CYSTIC FIBROSIS
Key signs and symptoms
• History of a chronic, productive cough and recurrent respiratory infections
• Parents' report of a salty taste on the child's skin

Key test results
• Sweat test using pilocarpine iontophoresis is greater than 60 mEq/L.

Key treatments
• Oral pancreatic enzyme replacement with pancrelipase (Pancrease)

Key interventions
• Assess respiratory and cardiovascular status.
• Administer pancreatic enzymes with meals and snacks.
• Encourage breathing exercises and perform chest physiotherapy two to four times per day.

EPIGLOTTIDITIS
Key signs and symptoms
• Difficult and painful swallowing
• Increased drooling
• Restlessness
• Stridor

Key test results
• Lateral neck X-ray shows an enlarged epiglottis.

Key treatments
• Possible emergency endotracheal intubation or a tracheotomy
• Oxygen therapy or cool mist tent
• Parenteral antibiotics: 10-day course according to the causative organism

Key interventions
• Monitor vital signs and pulse oximetry.
• Assess respiratory and cardiovascular status.
• Don't inspect the oropharynx if epiglottiditis is suspected.

RESPIRATORY SYNCYTIAL VIRUS
Key signs and symptoms
• Sternal retractions, nasal flaring
• Tachypnea
• Increased mucus production

Key test results
• Bronchial mucus culture shows respiratory syncytial virus (RSV).

Key treatments
• Humidified O_2
• I.V. fluids (with severe infection)

Key interventions
• Monitor vital signs and pulse oximetry.
• Assess respiratory and cardiovascular status.
• Administer humidified O_2 therapy.
• Monitor for signs and symptoms of dehydration. Administer and maintain I.V. therapy.

SUDDEN INFANT DEATH SYNDROME
Key signs and symptoms
• Death occurring during sleep without noise or struggle

Key test results
• Autopsy is the only way to diagnose sudden infant death syndrome (SIDS).

Key treatments
• If the child can be resuscitated (near-SIDS): monitoring

Key interventions
• Let the parents touch, hold, and rock the infant, and allow them to say good-bye to the infant.

Keep abreast of diagnostic tests

Here are the most important tests used to diagnose respiratory disorders, along with common nursing interventions associated with each test.

Check the gas
Arterial blood gas (ABG) analysis is used to assess gas exchange:
• Decreased partial pressure of arterial oxygen (PaO_2) may indicate hypoventilation, ventilation-perfusion mismatch, or shunting of blood away from gas exchange sites.
• Increased partial pressure of arterial carbon dioxide ($PaCO_2$) reflects hypoventilation or marked ventilation-perfusion mismatch.
• Decreased $PaCO_2$ reflects increased alveolar ventilation.
• Changes in pH may reflect metabolic or respiratory dysfunction.

Nursing actions
Before the procedure
• Explain the procedure to the parents and child.

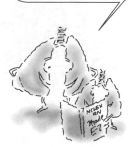

It says here that a decreased PaO_2, along with an increased $PaCO_2$, may indicate hypoventilation or ventilation-perfusion mismatch.

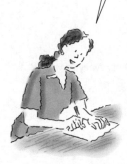

Hmmm. ABG analysis helps to assess gas exchange: pH, $Paco_2$, and Pao_2. Pulse oximetry is used to measure O_2 saturation only.

• Check arterial circulation before making the arterial puncture.

After the procedure
• After the sample is obtained, apply firm pressure to the arterial site.
• Keep the sample on ice, and transport it immediately to the laboratory.
• Assess the puncture site for bleeding or hematoma formation.

Oxygen observation
Pulse oximetry is a painless alternative to ABG analysis for measuring O_2 saturation only. This test may be less effective in jaundiced children or those with dark skin.

Nursing actions
• Explain the procedure to the parents and child.
• Place the oximeter on a site with adequate circulation, such as the finger, toe, or nose.
• Periodically rotate sites to prevent skin breakdown and pressure ulcers.
• Ensure that pulse readings from the site used for oximetry correlate with the child's heart rate before performing oximetry.

Lung function
Pulmonary function tests are used to measure lung volume, flow rates, and compliance. Pulmonary function test results may not be accurate if the young child has difficulty following directions.

Nursing actions
• Explain the procedure to the child and his parents.
• Instruct the child and his parents that he should have only a light meal before the test.
• Tell the parents to withhold bronchodilators and intermittent positive-pressure breathing therapy.
• Just before the test, tell the child to void and loosen tight clothing.

Chest check
Chest X-rays show such conditions as atelectasis, pleural effusion, infiltrates, pneumothorax, lesions, mediastinal shifts, and pulmonary edema.

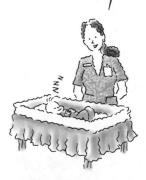

Sleeping like a baby? Not so for neonates and infants who breathe through their nose and develop nasal congestion. In this age-group, it can cause respiratory distress.

Nursing actions
• Explain the procedure to the parents and child.
• Ensure adequate protection by covering the child's gonads and thyroid gland with a lead apron.

Polish up on client care

Major pediatric respiratory disorders include acute respiratory failure, asthma, bronchopulmonary dysplasia, croup, cystic fibrosis, epiglottiditis, respiratory syncytial cirus (RSV) and sudden infant death syndrome (SIDS).

For information about special respiratory treatments for pediatric patients, see *Respiratory assistance for children*.

Acute respiratory failure

In acute respiratory failure, the respiratory system can't adequately supply the body with the O_2 it needs or adequately remove CO_2. The frequency of acute respiratory failure is higher in infants and young children than in adults. This is due to several situations:
• Neonates and infants breathe through the nose until age 6 months because of the proximity of the epiglottis to the nasopharynx. Nasal congestion can lead to significant respiratory distress in this age-group.
• The small size of the airway allows for less room for edema or swelling.
• Infants and young children have a large tongue that fills a small oropharynx.
• The epiglottis is larger and more horizontal to the pharyngeal wall in children than in adults.
• Infants and young children have a narrow subglottic area. A small amount of subglottic edema can lead to clinically significant narrowing, increased airway resistance, and increased work of breathing.
• In slightly older children, adenoidal and tonsillar lymphoid tissue is prominent and can contribute to airway obstruction.

Management moments

Respiratory assistance for children

The oxygen tent, the cool mist tent, the nasal cannula, and chest physiotherapy are specialized treatments for pediatric respiratory disorders. Here are the nursing actions associated with each treatment.

OXYGEN TENT
• Keep the plastic sides down and tucked in; because oxygen is heavier than air, oxygen loss is greater at the bottom of the tent.
• Keep the plastic away from the child's face.
• Prevent the use of toys that produce sparks or friction.
• Frequently assess oxygen concentration.
• To return the child to a tent, put the tent sides down, turn on the oxygen, wait until the oxygen is at the prescribed concentration, and then place the child in the tent.

COOL MIST TENT (CROUP TENT)
• Explain that the cool mist thins mucus, facilitating expectoration.
• Provide the same care as with an oxygen tent.
• Expect the child to be fearful if the mist obscures vision.
• Encourage the use of transitional objects in the tent, except for stuffed toys, which may become damp and promote bacterial growth.
• Keep the child dry by changing bed linens and pajamas frequently.

• Maintain a steady body temperature.
• Teach the parents about cool mist vaporizers for home use; tell them to clean the vaporizers frequently to prevent organisms from being sprayed into the air.

NASAL CANNULA
• Remove nasal secretions from the end of tubing frequently.
• Administer saline nose drops or nasal spray to moisten passages.
• Remove cannula and moisten nares every 8 hours to prevent skin breakdown.

CHEST PHYSIOTHERAPY
• Perform at least 30 minutes before meals.
• Use a cupped hand over a covered rib cage for 2 to 5 minutes on the five major positions (upper anterior lobes, upper posterior lobes, lower posterior lobes, and right and left sides) for a maximum of 30 minutes; for infants, preformed rubber percussors are available.
• Avoid physiotherapy during acute bronchoconstriction (for example, asthma) or airway edema (for example, croup) to prevent mucus plugs from loosening and causing airway obstruction.
• Administer aerosol-nebulized medications immediately before percussion and postural drainage.

CAUSES
• RSV
• Infection
• Atelectasis
• Acute respiratory distress syndrome
• Abdominal or thoracic surgery
• Anesthesia
• Bronchopulmonary dysplasia
• Congential heart defect
• Meningitis
• Muscular dystrophy
• Encephalitis
• Pneumonia
• Ingestion of toxic substance

ASSESSMENT FINDINGS
• Decreased respiratory excursion, accessory muscle use, retractions
• Difficulty breathing, shortness of breath, dyspnea, tachypnea, orthopnea

• Nasal flaring
• Fatigue
• Fussiness
• Grunting
• Adventitious breath sounds (crackles, rhonchi, wheezing)
• Cough, sputum production
• Cyanosis
• Change in mentation
• Tachycardia

DIAGNOSTIC TEST RESULTS
• ABG levels show hypoxia, acidosis, alkalosis, and hypercapnia.
• Chest X-ray shows pulmonary infiltrates, interstitial edema, and atelectasis.
• Lung scan shows ventilation-perfusion ratio mismatch.

NURSING DIAGNOSES
• Activity intolerance

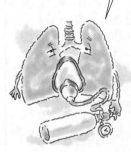

Oxygen can help reduce hypoxemia and relieve respiratory distress!

- Impaired gas exchange
- Ineffective peripheral tissue perfusion
- Ineffective airway clearance
- Anxiety
- Ineffective breathing pattern

TREATMENT
- Chest physiotherapy, postural drainage, incentive spirometry
- Humidity to liquefy secretions
- Inhaled nitric oxide
- O_2 therapy, intubation, and mechanical ventilation

Drug therapy
- Analgesic: morphine
- Bronchodilators: terbutaline, aminophylline, theophylline; via nebulizer: albuterol, ipratropium
- Steroids: hydrocortisone, methylprednisolone
- Exogenous surfactant: calfactant (Infasurf)
- Histamine-2 blockers: famotidine (Pepcid), ranitidine (Zantac), nizatidine (Axid)
- Antibiotics: according to sensitivity of causative organism

INTERVENTIONS AND RATIONALES
- Assess respiratory status *to detect early signs of compromise and hypoxemia.*
- Monitor and record intake and output *to detect fluid volume excess, which may lead to pulmonary edema.*
- Track laboratory values. Report deteriorating ABG levels, such as a fall in PaO_2 levels and rise in $PaCO_2$ levels. *Low hemoglobin and hematocrit levels reduce oxygen-carrying capacity of the blood.*
- Monitor pulse oximetry *to detect a drop in arterial O_2 saturation.*
- Monitor and record vital signs. *Tachycardia and tachypnea may indicate hypoxemia.*
- During steroid therapy, monitor blood glucose level every 6 to 12 hours using a blood glucose meter *to detect hyperglycemia caused by steroid use.*
- Administer O_2 *to reduce hypoxemia and relieve respiratory distress.*
- Monitor mechanical ventilation *to prevent complications and optimize PaO_2.*
- Provide suctioning; assist with turning, coughing, and deep breathing; and perform chest physiotherapy and postural drainage.

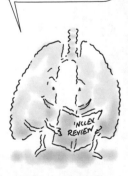

Asthma typically causes prolonged expiration with an expiratory wheeze. However, during severe distress, you may hear an inspiratory wheeze.

- Maintain bed rest.
- Keep the child in semi-Fowler's or high Fowler's position *to promote chest expansion and ventilation.*
- Administer medications as prescribed *to treat infection, dilate airways, and reduce inflammation.*

Teaching topics
- Explanation of the disorder and treatment plan
- Recognizing the early signs and symptoms of respiratory difficulty
- Performing deep-breathing and coughing exercises and incentive spirometry
- Drug therapy

Asthma

Asthma is a reversible, chronic, diffuse, inflammatory disease that produces the following effects:
- increased resistance to airflow
- decreased expiratory flow rates
- smooth-muscle bronchospasm
- increased mucus secretion leading to airway obstruction and air trapping.

CAUSES
- Hyperresponsiveness of the lower airway (may be idiopathic or intrinsic; may be caused by a hyperresponsive reaction to an allergen, exercise, or environmental change)

ASSESSMENT FINDINGS
During an attack
- Increased anteroposterior diameter of chest
- Altered cerebral function (with severe attack)
- Pulsus paradoxus (with moderate to severe attack)
- Diaphoresis
- Tachypnea
- Dyspnea
- Chest tightness
- Tachycardia
- Exercise intolerance
- Fatigue and apprehension
- Agitation
- Prolonged expiration with an expiratory wheeze; in severe distress, possible inspiratory wheeze
- Coarse crackles

- Unequal or decreased breath sounds
- Use of accessory muscles
- Talking in words, not sentences

DIAGNOSTIC TEST RESULTS
- Oxygen saturation via pulse oximetry may show decreased O_2 saturation.
- ABG measurement may show increased $Paco_2$ from respiratory acidosis.
- Skin test identifies the source of the allergy.
- Sputum analysis rules out respiratory infection.
- Exercise challenge (for children younger than age 6) identifies respiratory-induced symptoms and reversibility with aerosolized bronchodilators.

NURSING DIAGNOSES
- Anxiety
- Fear
- Impaired gas exchange
- Ineffective airway clearance

TREATMENT
- Chest physiotherapy (after edema has abated)
- Parenteral fluids to thin mucus secretions
- Oxygen therapy

Status asthmaticus
- Oxygen therapy with possible endotracheal intubation and mechanical ventilation

Drug therapy
Quick relief
- Short-acting bronchodilators (inhaled beta$_2$-adrenergic agonists): albuterol (Proventil-HFA, Ventolin), levalbuterol (Xopenex)

Long-term control
- Inhaled corticosteroid: beclomethasone
- Oral corticosteroid: prednisone
- Long-acting bronchodilator: salmeterol (Serevent)
- Methylxanthene: theophylline
- Mast cell stabilizer: cromolyn (Intal)
- Leukotriene modifier: montelukast (Singulair)

Status asthmaticus
- Corticosteroid: methylprednisolone

INTERVENTIONS AND RATIONALES
- Assess respiratory and cardiovascular status. *Tachycardia, tachypnea, and decreased breath sounds signal worsening respiratory status.*
- Monitor vital signs *to detect changes and prevent complications.*
- Assess the nature of the child's cough (hacking, unproductive progressing to productive), especially at night in the absence of infection. *Early detection and treatment may prevent complications.*
- Modify the environment to avoid an allergic reaction; remove the offending allergen. *Allergens can trigger an asthma attack.*
- Rinse the child's mouth after he inhales medication *to promote comfort and prevent irritation to the oral mucosa.*
- For exercise-induced asthma, give prophylactic treatments of beta-adrenergic blockers or cromolyn 10 to 15 minutes before the child exercises. *Premedication before exercise may prevent an asthma attack.* (See *Living with asthma.*)

> Assess the nature of the child's cough, especially at night. Early detection and treatment can prevent complications.

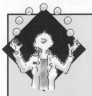

Management moments

Living with asthma

Encourage the parents of a child with asthma to help the child lead as normal a life as possible. Stress the importance of not restricting activities. Encourage participation in exercise and sports. Explain that aerobic activities, such as swimming, running, and brisk walking, increase the efficiency of the body's oxygen use. Prophylactic use of medication typically allows participation in almost any activity, even those that typically precipitate an attack.

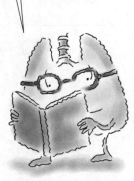

During an acute attack, allow the child to sit upright to ease breathing. Also provide moist oxygen, if necessary.

• For status asthmaticus or severe asthma attack, provide appropriate respiratory support *to prevent complications.*

During an acute attack
• Allow the child to sit upright *to promote chest expansion and ease breathing;* provide moist oxygen, if necessary. *Moist oxygen promotes mobilization of secretions.*
• Monitor vital signs *to detect signs of impending respiratory failure and cardiac decompensation.*
• Monitor the urine for glucose if the child is receiving corticosteroids *to detect early signs of hyperglycemia.*
• Administer inhaled medications through a metered-dose inhaler, and monitor peak flow rates. *Peak flow rates indicate the degree of lung impairment.*
• Maintain a calm environment; provide emotional support and reassurance *to decrease anxiety and decrease oxygen demands.*
• Monitor the effectiveness of drug therapy. *Failure to respond to drugs during an acute attack can result in status asthmaticus.*

Teaching topics
• Explanation of the disorder and treatment plan
• Medication use and possible adverse effects
• Breathing exercises to increase ventilatory capacity
• Proper use of inhalers
• Avoiding smoking areas
• Identifying and avoiding triggers

Bronchopulmonary dysplasia

Bronchopulmonary dysplasia is a chronic lung disease that begins in infancy. It occurs in neonates who require ventilatory support with high positive airway pressure and oxygen in the first 2 weeks of life. Infants at risk may be born prematurely or may have a respiratory disorder.

In this disorder, an acute insult to the neonate's lungs, such as respiratory distress syndrome, pneumonia, or meconium aspiration, requires positive-pressure ventilation

and a high concentration of oxygen over time. These therapies result in tissue and cellular injury to the immature lung.

CONTRIBUTING FACTORS
• Damage to the bronchiolar epithelium (from hyperoxia and positive pressure)
• Difficulty clearing mucus from the lungs
• Illness, such as respiratory distress syndrome, pneumonia, or meconium aspiration
• Oxygen toxicity from administration of a high concentration of oxygen and long-term assisted ventilation
• Possible genetic factors
• Prematurity

ASSESSMENT FINDINGS
• Atelectasis
• Crackles, rhonchi, wheezes
• Delayed development
• Dyspnea
• Hypoxia without ventilator assistance
• Fatigue
• Delayed muscle growth
• Pallor
• Circumoral cyanosis
• Prolonged capillary filling time
• Respiratory distress
• Right-sided heart failure
• Sternal retractions
• Weight loss or difficulty feeding

DIAGNOSTIC TEST RESULTS
• ABG analysis reveals hypoxemia.
• Chest X-ray reveals pulmonary changes (bronchiolar metaplasia and interstitial fibrosis).

NURSING DIAGNOSES
• Delayed growth and development
• Imbalanced nutrition: Less than body requirements
• Impaired gas exchange

TREATMENT
• Chest physiotherapy
• Ventilatory support and oxygen
• Enteral or total parenteral nutrition
• Supportive measures to enhance respiratory function

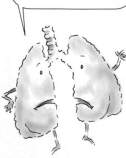

Oxygen may cause injury to the immature lung.

Drug therapy
- Bronchodilator: albuterol (Proventil-HFA) to counter increased airway resistance
- Corticosteroid: dexamethasone therapy to reduce inflammation
- Diuretic: furosemide (Lasix)

INTERVENTIONS AND RATIONALES
- Assess respiratory and cardiovascular status. *Monitoring is essential because children with bronchopulmonary dysplasia are susceptible to lower respiratory tract infections, hypertension, and respiratory failure.*
- Monitor vital signs, pulse oximetry, and intake and output *to assess and maintain adequate hydration, which is necessary to liquefy secretions and detect early signs of respiratory compromise.*
- Provide adequate time for rest *to decrease oxygen demands.*
- Provide chest physiotherapy *to mobilize secretions that interfere with oxygenation.*
- Administer medications as ordered *to improve pulmonary function and improve oxygenation.*
- Provide a quiet environment. *Unnecessary noise or activity may increase the child's anxiety and cause respiratory distress.*

Teaching topics
- Explanation of the disorder and treatment plan
- Medication use and possible adverse effects
- Visiting and becoming involved in the child's care, especially if the child requires lengthy hospitalization

Croup

Croup is a group of related upper airway respiratory syndromes that commonly affect toddlers. It includes acute spasmodic laryngitis, acute obstructive laryngitis, and acute laryngotracheobronchitis.

CAUSES
- Adenoviruses
- Bacteria (pertussis and diphtheria)
- Influenza viruses
- Measles virus
- Parainfluenza viruses
- RSV

ASSESSMENT FINDINGS
- Barking, brassy cough or hoarseness, sometimes described as a "seal bark" cough
- Condition usually begins at night and during cold weather and frequently recurs
- Crackles and decreased breath sounds (indicate that the condition has progressed to the bronchi)
- Increased dyspnea and lower accessory muscle use
- Inspiratory stridor with varying degrees of respiratory distress
- Onset sudden or gradual

DIAGNOSTIC TEST RESULTS
- If bacterial infection is the cause, throat cultures may identify the organisms and their sensitivity to antibiotics as well as rule out diphtheria.
- Laryngoscopy may reveal inflammation and obstruction in epiglottal and laryngeal areas.
- Computed tomography scan of the neck helps differentiate among croup, epiglottiditis, and noninfection.
- Neck X-ray shows areas of upper airway narrowing and edema in subglottic folds and rules out the possibility of foreign body obstruction as well as masses and cysts.

NURSING DIAGNOSES
- Anxiety
- Fear
- Hyperthermia
- Ineffective airway clearance
- Ineffective breathing pattern
- Risk for imbalanced fluid volume

TREATMENT
- Clear liquid diet to keep mucus thin
- Cool humidification during sleep with a cool mist tent or room humidifier
- Rest from activity
- Tracheostomy, O_2 administration

Drug therapy
- Antipyretic: acetaminophen (Tylenol)
- Antibiotics if the cause is bacterial

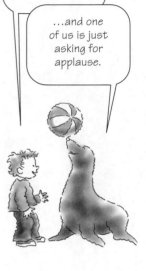

We may sound alike, but one of us has croup...

...and one of us is just asking for applause.

• Inhaled racemic epinephrine and cortico-steroids such as methylprednisolone sodium succinate to alleviate severe respiratory distress

INTERVENTIONS AND RATIONALES
• Assess respiratory and cardiovascular status *to detect any indications that the obstruction is worsening.*
• Monitor vital signs and pulse oximetry readings *to detect early signs of respiratory compromise.*
• Administer O_2 therapy and maintain the child in a cool mist tent, if needed. *Cool mist helps liquefy secretions.*
• Administer medications, as ordered, and note their effectiveness *to maintain or improve the child's condition.*
• Prop the infant in a car seat or with a pillow; position an older child in Fowler's position *to ease respiratory effort.*
• Provide emotional support for the parents *to decrease anxiety.*
• Provide age-appropriate activities for the child confined to the mist tent *to ease anxiety.*
• Monitor for rebound obstruction when administering racemic epinephrine; *the drug's effects are short term and may result in rebound obstruction.*

Teaching topics
• Explanation of the disorder and treatment plan
• Medication use and possible adverse effects
• Humidification method
• Importance of hydration
• Signs and symptoms of complications
• Keeping the child calm to ease respiratory effort and conserve energy

Cystic fibrosis

Cystic fibrosis is a generalized dysfunction of the exocrine glands that affects multiple organ systems. This disorder is characterized by:
• airway obstruction caused by the increased production of thick, tenacious mucus

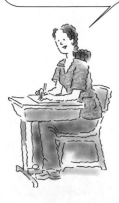

Parents may report a salty taste on the child's skin. In cystic fibrosis, the child's sweat contains two to five times the normal levels of sodium and chloride.

• little or no release of pancreatic enzymes (lipase, amylase, and trypsin).

Transmitted as an autosomal recessive trait, cystic fibrosis is one of the most common inherited diseases in children. The disease occurs equally in both sexes. With improvements in treatment over the past decade, the average life expectancy has risen dramatically. The clinical effects may become apparent soon after birth or take years to develop.

CAUSES
• Autosomal recessive mutation of gene on chromosome 7

ASSESSMENT FINDINGS
• Bulky, greasy, foul-smelling stools that contain undigested food
• Distended abdomen and thin arms and legs from steatorrhea
• Failure to thrive from malabsorption
• History of a chronic, productive cough and recurrent respiratory infections
• Meconium ileus in the neonate from a lack of pancreatic enzymes
• Parents' report of a salty taste on the child's skin
• Voracious appetite from undigested food lost in stools

DIAGNOSTIC TEST RESULTS
• Chest X-ray indicates early signs of obstructive lung disease.
• Sweat test using pilocarpine iontophoresis is greater than 60 mEq/L.
• Stool specimen analysis indicates the absence of trypsin.
• Deoxyribonucleic acid testing shows presence of the delta F 508 cystic fibrosis gene.
• Serum albumin is decreased.

NURSING DIAGNOSES
• Imbalanced nutrition: Less than body requirements
• Impaired gas exchange
• Risk for infection
• Ineffective airway clearance
• Delayed growth and development

TREATMENT
- Chest physiotherapy
- Nebulization and breathing exercises several times a day
- Postural drainage
- Heart-lung transplant
- High-protein formula, if needed

Drug therapy
- Mucolytic (dornase alfa [Pulmozyme]), bronchodilator, or antibiotic nebulizer inhalation treatment before chest physiotherapy
- I.V. antibiotics for a *Pseudomonas* infection when the infection interferes with daily functioning
- Oral pancreatic enzyme replacement with pancrelipase (Pancrease)
- Multivitamins twice per day, especially fat-soluble vitamins A, D, E, and K

INTERVENTIONS AND RATIONALES
- Assess respiratory and cardiovascular status *for early detection of hypoxia.*
- Monitor vital signs and intake and output *to detect dehydration, which may worsen respiratory status.*
- Monitor pulse oximetry readings *to detect early signs of hypoxia.*
- Administer pancreatic enzymes with meals and snacks *to aid digestion and absorption of nutrients.*
- Provide high-calorie, high-protein foods with added salt *to replace sodium loss and promote normal growth.*
- Encourage breathing exercises and perform chest physiotherapy two to four times per day *to mobilize secretions, maintain lung capacity, and increase oxygenation.*
- Encourage physical activity *to promote normal development.*

Teaching topics
- Explanation of the disorder and treatment plan
- Medication use and possible adverse effects
- Chest physiotherapy
- Signs and symptoms of infection or complications

- Avoiding cough suppressants and antihistamines because the child must be able to cough and expectorate
- Genetic counseling for the family

Epiglottiditis

Epiglottiditis, a potentially life-threatening infection, causes inflammation and edema of the epiglottis, a lidlike cartilaginous structure overhanging the entrance to the larynx and serving to prevent food from entering the larynx and trachea while swallowing. Epiglottiditis is most common among preschoolers.

CAUSES
- Bacterial *Haemophilus influenzae* (most common causative organism)
- Pneumococci and group A beta-hemolytic streptococci

ASSESSMENT FINDINGS
- Cough
- Difficult and painful swallowing
- Extending the neck in a sniffing position
- Fever
- Increased drooling
- Irritability
- Lower rib retractions
- Pallor
- Rapid pulse rate
- Rapid respirations
- Refusal to drink
- Restlessness
- Sore throat
- Stridor
- Tripod sitting position
- Use of accessory muscles

DIAGNOSTIC TEST RESULTS
- Lateral neck X-ray shows an enlarged epiglottis.
- Direct laryngoscopy shows a swollen, beefy epiglottis.

NURSING DIAGNOSES
- Fear
- Deficient fluid volume
- Anxiety

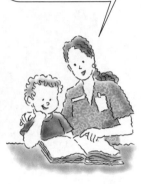

Key assessment findings for epiglottiditis: difficulty swallowing, increased drooling, restlessness, and stridor.

- Ineffective airway clearance
- Ineffective breathing pattern

TREATMENT
- Possible emergency endotracheal intubation or a tracheotomy
- Oxygen therapy or a cool mist tent
- I.V. fluid to prevent dehydration

Drug therapy
- Parenteral antibiotics: 10-day course according to the causative organism

INTERVENTIONS AND RATIONALES
- Monitor vital signs and pulse oximetry *to detect changes in oxygenation.*
- Assess respiratory and cardiovascular status *to determine the severity of the child's condition and prevent respiratory failure or arrest.*
- Don't inspect the oropharynx if epiglottiditis is suspected *because of the risk of occluding the airway.*
- Allow the child to sit on a parent's lap; *sitting on a parent's lap makes breathing easier and decreases anxiety.*
- Have equipment ready for a tracheotomy or intubation. *Emergency intubation and tracheotomy equipment should be on hand in case complete obstruction occurs.*
- Provide humidified oxygen therapy and a cool mist tent. *Humidified oxygen prevents secretions from thickening.*
- Administer medications as ordered *to treat infection and improve respiratory function.*
- Provide emotional support for the child and family *to decrease anxiety.*

Teaching topics
- Explanation of the disorder and treatment plan
- Medication use and possible adverse effects
- Importance of beginning *H. influenzae* immunization at age 2 months

Respiratory syncytial virus

RSV is a lower respiratory infection that's spread by respiratory secretions rather than droplets. It's the leading cause of lower respiratory infections in infants and young children and typically affects infants younger than age 6 months in the winter and spring. Mortality in this age-group is 1% to 6%.

CAUSES
- RSV

ASSESSMENT FINDINGS
- Sternal retractions, nasal flaring
- Tachypnea
- Thick mucus
- Nasal congestion
- Increased mucus production
- Watery drainage from the eyes
- Coughing
- Malaise
- Fever
- Dyspnea
- Sore throat
- Wheezes, rhonchi, crackles

DIAGNOSTIC TEST RESULTS
- Bronchial mucus culture shows RSV.
- Serum RSV antibody titers are elevated.

NURSING DIAGNOSES
- Impaired gas exchange
- Ineffective airway clearance
- Ineffective breathing pattern
- Fear
- Activity intolerance

TREATMENT
- Oral hydration, if possible
- Cool mist tent
- Humidified oxygen
- I.V. fluids (with severe infection)
- Rest periods when fatigued

Drug therapy
- Antiviral agent: ribavirin (Virazole)
- Antiviral immunoglobulin: palivizumab (Synagis) administered prophylactically to high-risk patients to prevent RSV infection

INTERVENTIONS AND RATIONALES
- Monitor vital signs and pulse oximetry *to determine oxygenation needs and to detect deterioration or improvement in the child's condition.*

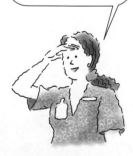

Key findings in RSV: sternal retractions and tachypnea.

- Assess respiratory and cardiovascular status. *Tachycardia may result from hypoxia or the effects of bronchodilator use.*
- Use gloves, gowns, and aseptic hand washing as secretion precautions *to prevent the spread of infection.*
- Administer chest physiotherapy after edema has abated. *Chest physiotherapy helps loosen mucus that may be blocking small airways.*
- Administer humidified oxygen therapy *to liquefy secretions and reduce bronchial edema.*
- Monitor for signs and symptoms of dehydration. Administer and maintain I.V. therapy *to promote hydration and replace electrolytes.*

Teaching topics
- Explanation of the disorder and treatment plan
- Review of medications, dosages, and adverse reactions
- Providing adequate nutrition and hydration
- Importance of humidified environment
- Avoiding people with cold symptoms
- Preventing the spread of infection

Sudden infant death syndrome

SIDS is the sudden death of an infant in which a postmortem examination fails to confirm the cause of death. The peak age is 3 months; 90% of cases occur before age 6 months, especially during the winter and early spring months.

Children who are diagnosed with SIDS are typically described as healthy with no previous medical problems. They're usually found dead sometime after being put down to sleep.

CAUSES
- Possibly viral
- Hypoxia theory
- Apnea theory
- Possible clostridium botulism toxin
- Possibly associated with diphtheria, tetanus, and pertussis vaccines

- Higher incidence with parents who smoke

ASSESSMENT FINDINGS
- History of low birth weight
- History of siblings with SIDS
- Previous near-SIDS event
- Death occurring during sleep without noise or struggle

DIAGNOSTIC TEST RESULTS
- Autopsy is the only way to diagnose SIDS. Autopsy findings indicate pulmonary edema, intrathoracic petechiae, and other minor changes suggesting chronic hypoxia and rules out suffocation and aspiration as a cause of death.

NURSING DIAGNOSES
- Impaired gas exchange
- Impaired spontaneous ventilation

TREATMENT
- None
- If the child can be resuscitated, it's called an *acute life-threatening event* (near-SIDS) and monitoring of the child is initiated.

Drug therapy
- If resuscitation is attempted, drugs are administered according to Pediatric Advanced Life Support protocols; drug therapy may include epinephrine, atropine and, after ABG analysis, sodium bicarbonate, if appropriate.

INTERVENTIONS AND RATIONALES
- Because the infant can't be resuscitated, focus your interventions on providing emotional support for the family. Keep in mind that grief may be coupled with guilt. Allow them to express their feelings. *Parents need to express feelings to prevent dysfunctional grieving.*
- Let the parents touch, hold, and rock the infant, if desired, and allow them to say goodbye to the infant *to facilitate the grieving process.*
- Contact appropriate spiritual support *to help the parents cope with grief.*

Research indicates a decreased incidence of SIDS in infants maintained in a supine position.

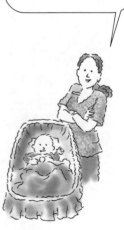

• Provide literature on SIDS and support groups; suggest psychological support for the surviving children *to help prevent maladaptive emotional responses to loss, to promote a realistic perspective on the tragedy, and to promote coping.*
• Act as an advocate for the parents if a police investigation is performed *to provide support.*

Teaching topics
• Explanation of the disorder as a reason for infant death
• Preparing the family for how the infant will look and feel if members touch and hold him
• Providing information on end-of-life procedures

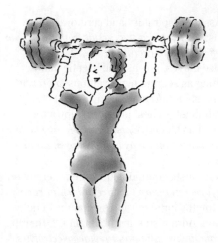

Pump up on practice questions

1. A parent brings her child to the pediatrician's office because of difficulty breathing and a "barking" cough. These signs are associated with which of the following conditions?
   1. Cystic fibrosis
   2. Asthma
   3. Epiglottiditis
   4. Croup
Answer: 4. A "seal bark" cough and difficulty breathing indicate croup. Cystic fibrosis produces a chronic productive cough and recurrent respiratory infections. Asthma may cause prolonged expiration with an expiratory wheeze on auscultation, dyspnea, and accessory muscle use. Epiglottiditis results in increased drooling, difficulty swallowing, tachypnea, and stridor.

➡ *NCLEX keys*
Client needs category: Physiological integrity
Client needs subcategory: Physiological adaptation
Cognitive level: Analysis

2. A woman with a child who awakes at night with a "barking" cough asks the nurse for advice. The nurse should instruct the mother to:
   1. take the child in the bathroom, turn on the shower, and let the room fill with steam.

2. bring the child to the emergency department immediately.
3. notify the pediatrician immediately.
4. call emergency medical services to transport the child to the hospital for an emergency tracheotomy.

Answer: 1. The nurse should instruct the mother to take her child into the bathroom, close the door, turn on the shower's hot-water spigot full-force, and sit with the child as the room fills with steam; this should decrease laryngeal spasm. Epiglottiditis is a potentially life-threatening infection that causes inflammation and edema of the epiglottis. If a child demonstrates symptoms associated with epiglottiditis, not croup (increased drooling, stridor, tachypnea), the mother should notify the pediatrician immediately and call the emergency medical services to transport the child to the hospital; emergency tracheotomy may be necessary. Taking the child to the hospital by herself could jeopardize the child's condition if that condition deteriorates en route.

➡ *NCLEX keys*
Client needs category: Physiological integrity
Client needs subcategory: Reduction of risk potential
Cognitive level: Application

3. A child with croup is placed in a cool mist tent. Which statement should the nurse include when teaching the mother about this type of therapy?
1. "You won't be able to touch your child while he's in the cool mist tent."
2. "The cool mist is necessary because it will thin the child's mucus, making it easier to expectorate."
3. "You can bring in your child's favorite stuffed animal to comfort him while he's in the cool mist tent."
4. "You can bring in any of your child's favorite toys so he can play while he's in the cool mist tent."

Answer: 2. The mother should be taught the purpose of the cool mist tent, which is to thin mucus and facilitate expectoration. The mother is able to touch her child while he's in the cool mist tent. She should be encouraged to bring in toys for the child to play with but to avoid stuffed toys, which may become damp and promote bacterial growth, and toys that produce sparks or friction.

➡ *NCLEX keys*
Client needs category: Physiological integrity
Client needs subcategory: Reduction of risk potential
Cognitive level: Application

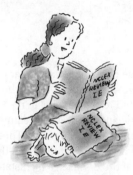

4. A physician orders chest physiotherapy for a child. The nurse shouldn't perform chest physiotherapy when the child is experiencing:
1. a productive cough.
2. retained secretions.
3. acute bronchoconstriction.
4. hypoxia.

Answer: 3. The nurse shouldn't administer chest physiotherapy during episodes of acute bronchoconstriction or airway edema (loosening mucus plugs could cause airway obstruction). Chest physiotherapy aids the elimination of secretions and reexpansion of lung tissue. Successful treatment with chest physiotherapy produces improved breath sounds, improved oxygenation, and increased sputum production and airflow. Therefore, it should be performed when a productive cough, retained secretions, or hypoxia is present.

➡ **NCLEX keys**

Client needs category: Physiological integrity
Client needs subcategory: Reduction of risk
potential
Cognitive level: Application

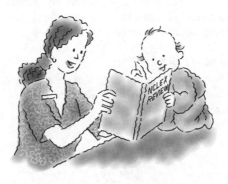

5. A nurse is caring for a 17-year-old
female client with cystic fibrosis who has
been admitted to the hospital to receive
I.V. antibiotic and respiratory treatment for
exacerbation of a lung infection. The client
has questions about her future and the consequences of the disease. Which statements
about the course of cystic fibrosis are true?
Select all that apply.
1. Breast development is commonly
delayed.
2. The client is at risk for developing
diabetes.
3. Pregnancy and child-bearing aren't
affected.
4. Normal sexual relationships can be
expected.
5. Only males carry the gene for the
disease.
6. By age 20, the client can probably decrease the frequency of
respiratory treatment.
Answer: 1, 2, 4. Cystic fibrosis delays growth
and the onset of puberty. Children with cystic
fibrosis tend to be smaller than average
size and develop secondary sex characteristics later in life. In addition, clients with
cystic fibrosis are at risk for developing

diabetes mellitus because the pancreatic duct
becomes obstructed as pancreatic tissues are
destroyed. Clients with cystic fibrosis can
expect to have normal sexual relationships,
but fertility becomes difficult because thick
secretions obstruct the cervix and block
sperm entry. Males and females carry the
gene for cystic fibrosis. Pulmonary disease
commonly progresses as the client ages,
requiring additional (not fewer) respiratory
treatments.

➡ **NCLEX keys**

Client needs category: Physiological integrity
Client needs subcategory: Physiological
adaptation
Cognitive level: Analysis

6. Which test result is a key finding in the
child with cystic fibrosis?
1. Chest X-ray that reveals interstitial
fibrosis
2. Neck X-ray showing areas of upper
airway narrowing
3. Lateral neck X-ray revealing an
enlarged epiglottis
4. Positive pilocarpine iontophoresis
sweat test
Answer: 4. A child with cystic fibrosis has a
positive pilocarpine iontophoresis sweat test.
The child sweats normally, but this sweat
contains two to five times the normal levels
of sodium and chloride. Chest X-ray findings
that reveal bronchiolar metaplasia and interstitial fibrosis are associated with bronchopulmonary dysplasia. A neck X-ray that reveals
upper airway narrowing and edema in the
subglottic folds indicates croup. A lateral neck
X-ray that reveals an enlarged epiglottis indicates epiglottiditis.

➡ **NCLEX keys**

Client needs category: Physiological integrity
Client needs subcategory: Reduction of risk
potential
Cognitive level: Knowledge

7. When communicating with the grieving family after a death from sudden infant death syndrome (SIDS), the nurse should:

  1. instruct the parents to place other infants on their backs to sleep.
  2. stress that the death isn't the parents' fault.
  3. stress that an autopsy must be done to confirm diagnosis.
  4. stress that the parents are still young and can have more children.

Answer: 2. It's most important for the nurse to stress that death from SIDS isn't predictable or preventable and that it isn't the parents' fault. Although it's important to inform the parents that an autopsy is necessary, that's secondary. Instructing the parents to place other infants on their backs to sleep implies that the parents did something wrong to cause the infant's death. Stressing that the parents are still young and can have other children minimizes their grief.

➡ *NCLEX keys*

Client needs category: Psychosocial integrity
Client needs subcategory: None
Cognitive level: Application

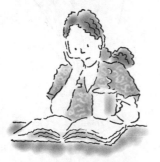

8. A 12-year-old with asthma suddenly becomes short of breath. How should a nurse position the child?

  1. Dorsal recumbent position
  2. Lithotomy position
  3. Semi-Fowler's position
  4. Sims' position

Answer: 3. The nurse should position the child in semi-Fowler's position (or sitting at about 45 degrees) because it facilitates lung expansion. The dorsal recumbent position doesn't ease the work of breathing.

The lithotomy position is normally used for gynecologic examinations. Sims' position is a lateral position with the top leg flexed toward the chest; this position inhibits lung expansion.

➡ *NCLEX keys*

Client needs category: Physiological integrity
Client needs subcategory: Basic care and comfort
Cognitive level: Application

9. A nurse is teaching the parents of a child with cystic fibrosis. The nurse should teach the parents to:

  1. discourage their child from being physically active.
  2. administer pancreatic enzymes after meals and snacks.
  3. avoid administering cough suppressants.
  4. have their child avoid salt intake.

Answer: 3. The parents of a child with cystic fibrosis should be taught to avoid administering cough suppressants and antihistamines to their child. Administration of these drugs interferes with the child's ability to cough and expectorate. The parents should encourage the child to be physically active. Pancreatic enzymes should be administered with meals and snacks, not after meals. Salt shouldn't be avoided; the child with cystic fibrosis has an increased salt loss.

➡ *NCLEX keys*

Client needs category: Physiological integrity
Client needs subcategory: Reduction of risk potential
Cognitive level: Application

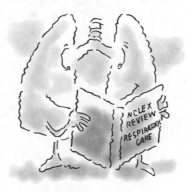

10. Which is the most appropriate nursing diagnosis for the child with epiglottiditis?
1. *Anxiety related to separation from the parent*
2. *Decreased cardiac output related to bradycardia*
3. *Ineffective airway clearance related to laryngospasm*
4. *Impaired gas exchange related to noncompliant lungs*

Answer: 3. Epiglottiditis is a life-threatening emergency that results from laryngospasm and edema. Therefore, ineffective airway clearance is the most appropriate diagnosis for this child. Anxiety related to separation shouldn't apply because the child doesn't need to be separated from the parent. The child will most likely be tachycardic, not bradycardic, unless respiratory failure ensues. The child has impaired gas exchange from impeded airflow, not from a noncompliant lung.

➟ *NCLEX keys*
Client needs category: Physiological integrity
Client needs subcategory: Physiological adaptation
Cognitive level: Analysis

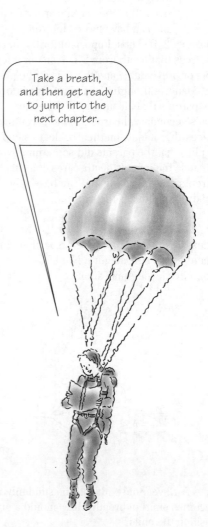

Take a breath, and then get ready to jump into the next chapter.

29 Hematologic & immune systems

Brush up on key concepts

The hematologic and immune systems consist of blood and blood-forming tissues and structures, such as the lymph nodes, thymus, spleen, and tonsils. Reviewing the functions of these systems and the development of a child's immune response lays the groundwork for effective care.

At any time, you can review the major points of this chapter by consulting the *Cheat sheet* on pages 624 and 625.

What blood does
The functions of blood include:
• regulating body temperature by transferring heat from deep within the body to small vessels near the skin
• providing cell nutrition by carrying nutrients from the GI tract to the tissues and removing waste products by transporting them to the lungs, kidneys, liver, and skin for excretion
• defending against foreign antigens by transporting leukocytes and antibodies to the sites of infection, injury, and inflammation
• transporting hormones from endocrine glands to various parts of the body
• maintaining acid-base balance
• carrying oxygen to tissues and removing carbon dioxide.

Each little component does its part
Blood is composed of several components. These include:
• **erythrocytes** (red blood cells [RBCs]), which carry oxygen to the tissues and remove carbon dioxide
• **leukocytes** (white blood cells [WBCs]), which include lymphocytes, monocytes, and granulocytes; these participate in the immune response
• **thrombocytes** (platelets), which contribute to clotting
• **plasma** (the fluid part of blood), which carries antibodies and nutrients to tissues and carries wastes away.

It's common
Communicable diseases and **infections** are commonly seen during the time a child's immune system develops. Over time, a child receives protection from communicable diseases either naturally or artificially.

It's natural
• **Natural (innate) immunity** is present at birth. Examples of natural immunity include barriers against disease, such as skin and mucous membranes, and bacteriocidal substances of body fluids, such as intestinal flora and gastric acidity.
• In **naturally acquired active immunity,** the immune system makes antibodies after exposure to disease. It requires contact with the disease.
• In **naturally acquired passive immunity,** no active immune process is involved. The antibodies are passively received through placental transfer by immunoglobulin G (the smallest immunoglobulin) and breast-feeding (colostrum).

It's artificial
Artificially acquired immunity can be active or passive. In **artificially acquired active immunity,** medically engineered substances are ingested or injected to stimulate the immune response against a specific disease. Immunizations are an example of this kind of immunity.

In **artificially acquired passive immunity,** antibodies are injected without

(Text continues on page 626.)

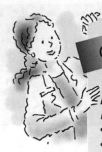

Cheat sheet

Hematologic & immune refresher

ACQUIRED IMMUNODEFICIENCY SYNDROME

Key signs and symptoms
- Failure to thrive
- Mononucleosis-like prodromal symptoms
- Night sweats
- Recurring diarrhea
- Weight loss

Key test results
- $CD4^+$ T-cell count measures the severity of immunosuppression.
- Enzyme-linked immunosorbent assay and Western blot are positive for human immunodeficiency virus (HIV) antibody.
- Polymerase chain reaction detects HIV deoxyribonucleic acid.

Key treatments
- Antibiotic therapy according to sensitivity of infecting organisms
- Antiviral agent: zidovudine (Retrovir)
- Monthly gamma globulin administration

Key interventions
- Monitor vital signs and intake and output
- Monitor developmental progress at regular intervals.
- Assess respiratory and neurologic status.
- Maintain standard precautions.

HEMOPHILIA

Key signs and symptoms
- Multiple bruises without petechiae
- Prolonged bleeding after circumcision, immunizations, or minor injuries

Key test results
- Partial thromboplastin time (PTT) is prolonged (for both types).

Hemophilia A
- Factor VIII assay is 25% of normal or less.

Hemophilia B
- Factor IX assay is deficient.
- Baseline coagulation results are similar to those of hemophilia A but with normal factor VIII.

Key treatments
- Avoiding I.M. injections

Hemophilia A
- Cryoprecipitated antihemophilic factor (AHF), lyophilized AHF, or both
- Desmopressin (Stimate)

Hemophilia B
- Factor IX concentrate

Key interventions
- Monitor vital signs and intake and output.
- When bleeding occurs:
  - elevate the affected extremity above the heart
  - immobilize the site to prevent clots from dislodging
  - apply pressure to the site for 10 to 15 minutes to stop bleeding
  - decrease anxiety to lower the child's heart rate.

IRON DEFICIENCY ANEMIA

Key signs and symptoms
- Fatigue, listlessness
- Increased susceptibility to infection
- Pallor
- Tachycardia
- Numbness and tingling of the extremities
- Vasomotor disturbances

Key test results
- Hemoglobin, hematocrit, and serum ferritin levels are low.
- Serum iron levels are low, with high binding capacity.

Key treatments
- Oral preparation of iron (Fer-In-Sol) or a combination of iron and ascorbic acid (which enhances iron absorption)

Key interventions
- Administer iron before meals with citrus juice. (Iron is best absorbed in an acidic environment.)
- Give liquid iron through a straw to prevent staining the child's skin and teeth; for infants, administer by oral syringe toward the back of the mouth.
- Don't give iron with milk products because these products may interfere with absorption.

Hematologic & immune refresher *(continued)*

LEUKEMIA
Key signs and symptoms
- Fatigue
- Sudden onset of high fever
- Lymphadenopathy
- Pallor
- Petechiae and ecchymosis
- Liver or spleen enlargement

Key test results
- Blast cells appear in the peripheral blood.
- Blast cells may be as high as 95% in the bone marrow.
- Initial white blood cell count may be less than 10,000/µl at the time of diagnosis in a child with acute lymphocytic leukemia between ages 3 and 7.

Key treatments
- Stem cell transplantation
- Chemotherapy: vincristine, high-dose cytarabine (Cytosaru), and daunorubicin (Cerubidine); intrathecal chemotherapy usually with methotrexate
- Radiation therapy

Key interventions
- Provide pain relief, as ordered, and document its effectiveness and adverse effects.
- Monitor vital signs and intake and output.
- Inspect the skin frequently.
- Provide nursing measures to ease adverse effects of radiation and chemotherapy.

REYE SYNDROME
Key signs and symptoms
- Stage 5: seizures, loss of deep tendon reflexes, flaccidity, respiratory arrest (death is usually a result of cerebral edema or cardiac arrest)

Key test results
- Blood test results show elevated serum ammonia levels; serum fatty acid and lactate levels are also elevated.
- Coagulation studies reveal prolonged prothrombin time and PTT.
- Liver biopsy shows fatty droplets distributed through cells.
- Liver function studies show aspartate aminotransferase and alanine aminotransferase are elevated to twice normal levels.

Key treatments
- Endotracheal intubation and mechanical ventilation
- Osmotic diuretic: mannitol

Key interventions
- Monitor vital signs and pulse oximetry.
- Assess cardiac, respiratory, and neurologic status.
- Monitor fluid intake and output.
- Monitor blood glucose levels.

- Maintain seizure precautions.
- Keep the head of the bed at a 30-degree angle.
- Assess pulmonary artery catheter pressure.
- Administer blood products as necessary.
- Administer medications, as ordered, and monitor for adverse effects.
- Maintain a hypothermia blanket as needed, and monitor temperature every 15 to 30 minutes while in use.
- Check for loss of reflexes and signs of flaccidity.

SICKLE CELL ANEMIA
Key signs and symptoms
- In infants and toddlers, colic and splenomegaly
- In preschoolers, hypovolemia, shock, and pain at the site of vaso-occlusive crisis
- In school-age children and adolescents, enuresis, extreme pain at the site of crisis, and priapism

Key test results
- More than 50% hemoglobin S indicates sickle cell disease; a lower level of hemoglobin S indicates sickle cell trait.

Key treatments
- Hydration with I.V. fluid administration
- Transfusion therapy as necessary
- Treatment for acidosis as necessary
- Analgesic: morphine

Key interventions
- Monitor vital signs and intake and output.
- Administer pain medications and note their effectiveness.

THALASSEMIA
Key signs and symptoms
- Jaundice
- Anemia, commonly severe
- Bone abnormalities
- Failure to thrive

Key test results
- Complete blood count shows lowered red blood cell (RBC) and hemoglobin levels, microcytosis, and elevated reticulocyte count.
- Folate level will be decreased.

Key treatments
- Mostly supportive
- Transfusion to raise hemoglobin level; care must be used not to cause iron overload

Key interventions
- Monitor for signs and symptoms of transfusion reaction after RBC transfusions.
- Encourage genetic counseling for the child's parents.

stimulating the immune response. Examples include tetanus antitoxin, hepatitis B immune globulin, and varicella zoster immune globulin.

Keep abreast of diagnostic tests

Here are the most important tests used to diagnose hematologic and immunologic disorders, along with common nursing interventions associated with each test.

Not my type?
Blood typing is used to determine the antigens present in a patient's RBCs. A reaction with standardized sera indicates the presence of specific antigens.

Nursing actions
• Explain the procedure to the child and family.
• Handle the sample gently to prevent hemolysis.
• Apply pressure to the venipuncture site to prevent hematoma or bleeding.

Tuning into the immune system
Laboratory studies, such as **CD4⁺ T-cell count** and **enzyme-linked immunosorbent assay (ELISA),** are used to assess immunosuppression.

Nursing actions
• Explain the procedure to the child and family.
• Handle the sample gently to prevent hemolysis.
• Apply pressure to the venipuncture site to prevent hematoma or bleeding.

Clot measure
A **coagulation study** tests a blood sample to analyze platelet function, platelet count, prothrombin time (PT), International Normalized Ratio, partial thromboplastin time (PTT), coagulation time, and bleeding time.

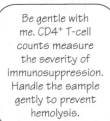

Be gentle with me. CD4⁺ T-cell counts measure the severity of immunosuppression. Handle the sample gently to prevent hemolysis.

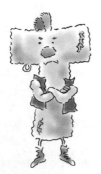

Nursing actions
• Explain the procedure to the child and family.
• Note the child's current drug therapy before procedure.
• Check the venipuncture site for bleeding after the procedure.

A look at the liver
Liver function studies measure levels of hepatic enzymes, such as aspartate aminotransferase (AST) and alanine aminotransferase (ALT).

Nursing actions
• Explain the procedure to the child and family.
• After the test, check the venipuncture site for bleeding.

Polish up on client care

Major pediatric hematologic and immune disorders include acquired immunodeficiency syndrome (AIDS), hemophilia, iron deficiency anemia, leukemia, Reye syndrome, sickle cell anemia, and thalassemia.

Acquired immunodeficiency syndrome

In AIDS, the human immunodeficiency virus (HIV) attacks helper T cells. AIDS may be spread through sexual contact or percutaneous or mucous membrane exposure to needles or other sharp instruments contaminated with blood or bloody body fluid (for example, in I.V. drug abuse). Transmission may also occur between mother and infant during pregnancy or as a result of breast-feeding.

HIV has a much shorter incubation period in children than in adults. In adults, the incubation period may last 10 years or more. By contrast, children who receive the virus by placental transmission are usually HIV-positive by age 6 months and develop clinical signs by age 3.

Because of passive antibody transmission, all infants born to HIV-infected mothers test positive for antibodies to the HIV virus up to about age 18 months. Confirmation of diagnosis during this time requires detection of the HIV antigen.

CAUSES
- Contact with contaminated blood or bloody body fluid
- Infected parent via the birth process or breast-feeding

CONTRIBUTING FACTORS
- Drug use
- Sexual activity

ASSESSMENT FINDINGS
- Failure to thrive
- Lymphadenopathy
- Mononucleosis-like prodromal symptoms
- Neurologic impairment, such as loss of motor milestones and behavioral changes
- Night sweats
- Recurrent opportunistic infections
- Recurring diarrhea
- Weight loss

DIAGNOSTIC TEST RESULTS
- $CD4^+$ T-cell count measures the severity of immunosuppression.
- Culture and sensitivity tests reveal infection with opportunistic organisms.
- ELISA and Western blot are positive for HIV antibody.
- Polymerase chain reaction (PCR) test detects HIV deoxyribonucleic acid (preferred test for children younger than age 18 months).

NURSING DIAGNOSES
- Risk for infection
- Anxiety
- Fear
- Interrupted family processes
- Ineffective protection
- Imbalanced nutrition: Less than body requirements
- Deficient fluid volume

TREATMENT
- Blood administration, if necessary
- Follow-up laboratory studies
- High-calorie diet provided in small, frequent meals
- I.V. fluids to maintain hydration
- Nutrition supplements, if necessary
- Parenteral nutrition, if necessary

Drug therapy
- Antibiotic therapy according to sensitivity of the infecting organisms
- Antiviral agent: zidovudine (Retrovir)
- Monthly gamma globulin administration
- Prophylactic antibiotic therapy with co-trimoxazole (Bactrim) to prevent *Pneumocystis carinii* pneumonia
- Routine immunizations (however, "live" vaccines, such as measles-mumps-rubella, varicella, and the nasal flu vaccine [FluMist] aren't recommended for HIV-infected children)

INTERVENTIONS AND RATIONALES
- Monitor vital signs and intake and output *to detect tachycardia, dyspnea, hypertension, or decreased urine output, which may indicate fluid volume deficit or electrolyte imbalance.*
- Monitor developmental progress at regular intervals *to detect changes in level of functioning and, as appropriate, adapt activity program.*
- Provide appropriate play activities *to promote development.*
- Encourage fluid intake *to prevent dehydration.*
- Assess respiratory and neurologic status *to detect early signs of compromise.*
- Maintain standard precautions *to prevent the spread of infection.*
- Administer medications as ordered *to help boost immune response and prevent opportunistic infections.*
- Provide psychosocial support. *An AIDS diagnosis is devastating for the child and his family.*
- Assess the child's support system and provide referrals. *The child may have no one to care for him.*

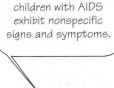

As with adults, children with AIDS exhibit nonspecific signs and symptoms.

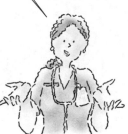

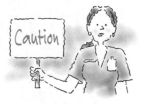

Children with HIV or AIDS and their families must maintain strict personal hygiene.

Caution

Teaching topics
- Explanation of the disorder and treatment plan
- Medication use and possible adverse effects
- Controlling infection in the home using sanitary measures
- Avoiding the consumption of raw or under-cooked meats
- Avoiding swimming in a lake or river
- Avoiding contact with young farm animals
- Understanding risk factors from pets (especially cats)
- Recognizing the signs and symptoms of infection and getting immediate treatment
- Practicing safer sex, if appropriate

Hemophilia

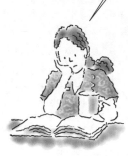

A classic sign of hemophilia: prolonged bleeding after minor injuries.

Hemophilia results from a deficiency in one of the coagulation factors.

The types of hemophilia are:
- hemophilia A (also called *factor VIII deficiency* or *classic hemophilia*), the most common type (75% of all cases)
- hemophilia B (also called *factor IX deficiency* or *Christmas disease*)

Hemophilia is an X-linked recessive disorder. The inheritance pattern is described here:
- If the father has the disorder and the mother doesn't, all daughters will be carriers but sons won't have the disease.
- If the mother is a carrier and the father doesn't have hemophilia, each son has a 50% chance of getting hemophilia and each daughter has a 50% chance of being a carrier.
- If the mother is a carrier and the father has hemophilia, the daughter will inherit the disease, but this situation is extremely rare.

CAUSES
- Genetic inheritance

ASSESSMENT FINDINGS
- Bleeding into the throat, mouth, and thorax
- Hemarthrosis; refusal to move affected joint
- Multiple bruises without petechiae
- Peripheral neuropathies from bleeding near peripheral nerves
- Prolonged bleeding after circumcision, immunizations, or minor injuries

DIAGNOSTIC TEST RESULTS
- PTT is prolonged (for both types).

Hemophilia A
- Factor VIII assay is 25% of normal or less.

Hemophilia B
- Factor IX assay is deficient.
- Baseline coagulation results are similar to those of hemophilia A but with normal factor VIII.

NURSING DIAGNOSES
- Acute pain
- Ineffective protection
- Risk for deficient fluid volume
- Risk for injury

TREATMENT
- Blood transfusion, if necessary
- Avoiding I.M. injections
- Promoting vasoconstriction during bleeding episodes by applying ice, pressure, and hemostatic agents

Drug therapy
- Aminocaproic acid (Amicar)

Hemophilia A
- Cryoprecipitated antihemophilic factor (AHF), lyophilized AHF, or both
- Desmopressin (Stimate)

Hemophilia B
- Factor IX concentrate

INTERVENTIONS AND RATIONALES
- Monitor vital signs and intake and output *to assess renal status and monitor for fluid overload or dehydration.*
- Assess cardiovascular status and check for signs of bleeding; *fever, tachycardia, or hypotension may indicate hypovolemia.*
- Measure the joint's circumference and compare it to that of an unaffected joint *to assess for bleeding into the joint, which may lead to hypovolemia.*
- Note swelling, pain, or limited joint mobility. *Changes may indicate progressive decline in function.*

- Assess for joint degeneration from repeated hemarthroses *to detect extent of damage.*
- Pad toys and other objects in the child's environment *to promote child safety and prevent bleeding.*
- Recommend protective headgear, soft foam Toothettes, soft toothbrush, and stool softeners as appropriate *to prevent bleeding.*
- Discourage abnormal weight gain, *which increases the load on joints.*

When bleeding occurs
- Elevate the affected extremity above the heart *to decrease circulation to the affected area and promote venous return.*
- Immobilize the site *to prevent clots from dislodging.*
- Apply pressure to the site for 10 to 15 minutes *to stop bleeding.*
- Decrease anxiety *to lower the child's heart rate.*
- Apply ice to the site *to promote vasoconstriction.*

To treat hemarthrosis
- Immobilize the affected extremity; elevate it in a slightly flexed position *to prevent further injury.*
- Decrease pain and anxiety *to lower the child's heart rate and minimize blood loss.*
- Avoid excessive handling or weight bearing for 48 hours *to prevent bleeding and to rest the site.*
- Begin mild range-of-motion exercises after 48 hours *to facilitate absorption and prevent contractures.*

Teaching topics
- Explanation of the disorder and treatment plan
- Meticulous dental care
- Medication use and possible adverse effects
- Genetic counseling for the parents
- Encouraging non-contact sports

Iron deficiency anemia

The most common nutritional anemia during childhood, iron deficiency anemia is characterized by poor RBC production. Insufficient body stores of iron lead to:
- depleted RBC mass
- decreased hemoglobin concentration (hypochromia)
- decreased oxygen-carrying capacity of blood.

Most commonly, iron deficiency anemia occurs when the child experiences rapid physical growth, low iron intake, inadequate iron absorption, or loss of blood. Peak incidence is at 12 to 18 months.

CAUSES
- Blood loss secondary to drug-induced GI bleeding (from anticoagulants, aspirin, steroids) or due to heavy menses, hemorrhage from trauma, GI ulcers, or cancer
- Inadequate dietary intake of iron (less than 1 to 2 mg/day), which may occur following prolonged unsupplemented breast-feeding or during periods when the body is stressed, such as rapid growth in children and adolescents; may also occur from excessive consumption of cow's milk rather than iron-fortified foods.
- Iron malabsorption, as in chronic diarrhea, partial or total gastrectomy, and malabsorption syndromes, such as celiac disease and pernicious anemia
- Intravascular hemolysis-induced hemoglobinuria or paroxysmal nocturnal hemoglobinuria
- Mechanical erythrocyte trauma caused by a prosthetic heart valve or vena cava filters

ASSESSMENT FINDINGS
Anemia progresses gradually, and many children are initially asymptomatic, except for symptoms of an underlying condition. Children with advanced anemia display the following symptoms:
- dyspnea on exertion
- fatigue
- headache
- inability to concentrate
- irritability
- listlessness
- pallor
- increased susceptibility to infection
- tachycardia.

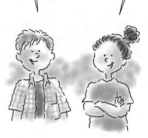

Anemia can follow periods of stress, such as times of rapid growth.

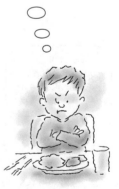

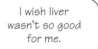

I wish liver wasn't so good for me.

In cases of chronic iron deficiency anemia, children display the following symptoms:
- cracks in corners of the mouth
- dysphagia
- neuralgic pain
- numbness and tingling of the extremities
- smooth tongue
- spoon-shaped, brittle nails
- vasomotor disturbances.

DIAGNOSTIC TEST RESULTS
- Bone marrow studies reveal depleted or absent iron stores and normoblastic hyperplasia.
- Hemoglobin, hematocrit, and serum ferritin levels are low.
- Mean corpuscular hemoglobin is decreased in severe anemia.
- RBC count is low, with microcytic and hypochromic cells. (In early stages, RBC count may be normal, except in infants and children.)
- Serum iron levels are low, with high binding capacity.

NURSING DIAGNOSES
- Activity intolerance
- Imbalanced nutrition: Less than body requirements
- Fatigue
- Impaired gas exchange
- Constipation

TREATMENT
- Increased iron intake (for children and adolescents) by adding foods rich in iron to the diet, or (for infants) adding iron supplements

Drug therapy
- Oral preparation of iron (Fer-In-Sol) or a combination of iron and ascorbic acid (which enhances iron absorption)
- Vitamin supplement: cyanocobalamin (vitamin B_{12}) if intrinsic factor is lacking
- Iron supplement: iron dextran (INFeD) if additional therapy is needed

INTERVENTIONS AND RATIONALES
- Carefully assess a child's drug history. *Certain drugs, such as pancreatic enzymes and vitamin E, may interfere with iron metabolism and absorption.*
- Provide passive stimulation; allow frequent rest; give small, frequent feedings; and elevate the head of the bed *to decrease oxygen demands.*
- Implement proper hand washing *to decrease the risk of infection.*
- Provide foods high in iron (liver, dark leafy vegetables, and whole grains) *to replenish iron stores.*
- Administer iron before meals with citrus juice. *Iron is best absorbed in an acidic environment.*
- Give liquid iron through a straw *to prevent staining the child's skin and teeth.* For infants, administer by oral syringe toward the back of the mouth.
- Don't give iron with milk products. *Milk products may interfere with iron absorption.*
- Monitor bowel patterns *to detect constipation.*
- Be supportive of the family and keep them informed of the child's status *to decrease anxiety.*

Teaching topics
- Explanation of the disorder and treatment plan
- Medication use and possible adverse effects
- Keeping iron supplements safely stored out of the child's reach at home
- Brushing teeth after iron administration
- Reporting reactions to iron supplementation, such as nausea, vomiting, diarrhea, constipation, fever, or severe stomach pain (may require a dosage adjustment)
- Understanding that iron supplements can affect bowel patterns and turn stools tarry black in color

Leukemia

Leukemia is the abnormal, uncontrolled proliferation of WBCs. In leukemia, WBCs are produced so rapidly that immature cells (blast cells) are released into the circulation. These blast cells are nonfunctional, can't fight infection, and are formed continuously without

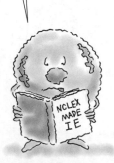

Blast it. In leukemia, I can't get the nutrition I need!

respect to the body's needs. This proliferation robs healthy cells of sufficient nutrition.

In children, the most common type of leukemia is acute lymphocytic leukemia (ALL). This type of leukemia is marked by extreme proliferation of immature lymphocytes (blast cells). In adolescents, acute myelogenous leukemia is more common and is believed to result from a malignant transformation of a single stem cell.

CAUSES AND CONTRIBUTING FACTORS
- Chemical exposure and viruses
- Chromosomal disorders
- Down syndrome
- Ionizing radiation

ASSESSMENT FINDINGS
Clinical findings for leukemia may appear with surprising abruptness in children with few, if any, warning signs. The following are common assessment findings of leukemia:
- blood in urine, stool, or emesis
- bone and joint pain
- decrease in all blood cells when bone marrow undergoes atrophy (leads to anemia, bleeding disorders, and immunosuppression)
- fatigue
- history of infections
- lassitude
- sudden onset of high fever
- lymphadenopathy
- pallor
- pathologic fractures when bone marrow undergoes hypertrophy
- petechiae and ecchymosis
- poor wound healing and oral lesions
- liver or spleen enlargement.

DIAGNOSTIC TEST RESULTS
- Blast cells appear in the peripheral blood (where they normally don't appear).
- Blast cells may be as high as 95% in the bone marrow (they're normally less than 5%) as measured by marrow aspiration in the posterior iliac crest (the sternum can't be used in children).
- Initial WBC count may be less than 10,000/µl at the time of diagnosis in a child with ALL between ages 3 and 7. (This child has the best prognosis.)

- Lumbar puncture indicates whether leukemic cells have crossed the blood-brain barrier.

NURSING DIAGNOSES
- Ineffective protection
- Acute or chronic pain
- Risk for infection
- Anxiety
- Fear
- Interrupted family processes

TREATMENT
- Hematopoietic stem cell transplant: stem cells are harvested and then returned to the recipient; stem cells can also be obtained from a sibling or a donor pool
- High-protein, high-calorie, bland diet
- I.V. fluids as necessary
- Oxygen therapy, if needed
- Radiation therapy
- Transfusion therapy as needed

Drug therapy
- Analgesics
- Antiemetic: ondansetron (Zofran)
- Chemotherapy: vincristine, high-dose cytarabine (Cytosaru), and daunorubicin (Cerubidine); intrathecal chemotherapy, usually with methotrexate
- Corticosteroid: prednisone (Deltasone)

INTERVENTIONS AND RATIONALES
- Monitor vital signs and intake and output *to determine fluid volume deficit and renal status.*
- Monitor for signs of infection. *Children with leukemia are highly susceptible to infection.*
- Give special attention to mouth care *to prevent infection and bleeding.*
- Inspect the skin frequently *to assess for skin breakdown.*

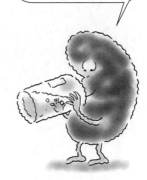

Increased fluid intake helps to flush chemotherapeutic drugs through the kidneys.

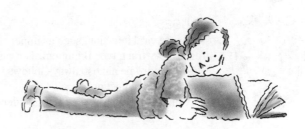

Stem cells may be transfused from a twin or another HLA-identical donor.

- Give increased fluids *to flush chemotherapeutic drugs through the kidneys.*
- Provide a "neutropenic diet" — a high-protein, high-calorie, bland diet with no raw fruits or vegetables. *Eliminating raw fruits and vegetables helps prevent infection. A diet meeting the child's caloric requirements helps ensure that the child's maintenance and growth needs are met.*
- Discourage keeping any live plants in the room *to prevent introduction of bacteria.*
- Provide pain relief, as ordered, and document its effectiveness and adverse effects. *Analgesics depress the central nervous system (CNS), thereby reducing pain.*
- Monitor the CNS *to assess for changes such as confusion that may result from cerebral damage.*
- Provide nursing measures to ease the adverse effects of radiation and chemotherapy *to promote comfort and encourage adequate nutritional intake.*

Teaching topics
- Explanation of the disorder and treatment plan
- Avoiding crowds, people with infection or illness, pets, and raw fruits and vegetables
- Medication use and possible adverse effects
- Adjusting to changes in body image
- Contacting support groups
- Recognizing the signs and symptoms of infection and the need to seek immediate medical attention

Reye syndrome

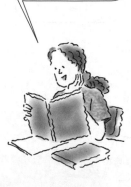

Acute infection plus aspirin use equals risk of Reye syndrome.

Reye syndrome is an acute illness that causes fatty infiltration of the liver, kidneys, brain, and myocardium. It can lead to hyperammonemia, encephalopathy, and increased intracranial pressure (ICP).

CAUSES
- Acute viral infection, such as upper respiratory tract, type B influenza, or varicella (Reye syndrome almost always follows within 1 to 3 days of infection)
- Concurrent aspirin use (high incidence)

ASSESSMENT FINDINGS
Reye syndrome develops in five stages. The severity of signs and symptoms varies with the degree of encephalopathy and cerebral edema:
- Stage 1: vomiting, lethargy, hepatic dysfunction
- Stage 2: hyperventilation, delirium, hyperactive reflexes, hepatic dysfunction
- Stage 3: coma, hyperventilation, decorticate rigidity, hepatic dysfunction
- Stage 4: deepening coma, decerebrate rigidity, large fixed pupils, minimal hepatic dysfunction
- Stage 5: seizures, loss of deep tendon reflexes, flaccidity, respiratory arrest (death is usually a result of cerebral edema or cardiac arrest)

DIAGNOSTIC TEST RESULTS
- Blood test results show elevated serum ammonia levels; serum fatty acid and lactate levels are also increased.
- Cerebrospinal fluid (CSF) analysis shows WBC less than 10/μl; with coma, there's increased CSF pressure.
- Coagulation studies reveal prolonged PT and PTT.
- Liver biopsy shows fatty droplets uniformly distributed throughout cells.
- Liver function studies show AST and ALT elevated to twice normal levels.

NURSING DIAGNOSES
- Decreased intracranial adaptive capacity
- Ineffective thermoregulation
- Risk for imbalanced fluid volume
- Risk for injury

TREATMENT
- Craniotomy
- Endotracheal intubation and mechanical ventilation to control partial pressure of arterial carbon dioxide levels
- Enteral or parenteral nutrition as needed
- Exchange transfusion
- Induced hypothermia
- Transfusion of fresh frozen plasma
- I.V. fluids

Drug therapy
- Osmotic diuretic: mannitol
- Vitamin: phytonadione
- Ammonia detoxicants: sodium phenylacetate and sodium benzoate (Ammonul)

INTERVENTIONS AND RATIONALES
- Monitor ICP with a subarachnoid screw or other invasive device *to closely assess for increased ICP.*
- Monitor vital signs and pulse oximetry *to determine oxygenation status.*
- Assess cardiac, respiratory, and neurologic status *to evaluate the effectiveness of interventions and monitor for complications such as seizures.*
- Monitor fluid intake and output *to prevent fluid overload.*
- Monitor blood glucose levels *to detect hyperglycemia or hypoglycemia and prevent complications.*
- Maintain seizure precautions *to prevent injury.*
- Keep the head of the bed at a 30-degree angle *to decrease ICP and promote venous return.*
- Assess pulmonary artery catheter pressures *to assess cardiopulmonary status.*
- Maintain oxygen therapy, which may include intubation and mechanical ventilation, *to promote oxygenation and maintain thermoregulation.*
- Administer blood products as necessary *to increase oxygen-carrying capacity of the blood and prevent hypovolemia.*
- Administer medications, as ordered, and monitor for adverse effects *to detect complications.*
- Maintain a hypothermia blanket as needed and monitor temperature every 15 to 30 minutes while in use *to prevent injury and maintain thermoregulation.*
- Check for loss of reflexes and signs of flaccidity *to determine the degree of neurologic involvement.*
- Provide good skin and mouth care and range-of-motion exercises *to prevent alteration in skin integrity and promote joint motility.*
- Provide postoperative craniotomy care, if necessary, *to promote wound healing and prevent complications.*

- Be supportive of the family and keep them informed of the child's status *to decrease anxiety.*

Teaching topics
- Explanation of the disorder and treatment plan
- Medication use and possible adverse effects
- Avoiding aspirin products
- Explaining all procedures and nursing care measures to family
- Referring family to support groups as indicated

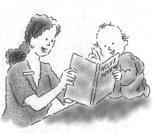

To prevent Reye syndrome, use nonsalicylate analgesics and antipyretics.

Sickle cell anemia

In sickle cell anemia, a defect in the hemoglobin molecule changes the oxygen-carrying capacity and shape of RBCs. The altered hemoglobin molecule is referred to as *hemoglobin S.* In this disorder, RBCs acquire a sickle shape.

The child may experience periodic, painful attacks called *sickle cell crises.* A sickle cell crisis may be triggered or intensified by:
- dehydration
- deoxygenation
- acidosis.

CAUSES
- Genetic inheritance (sickle cell anemia is an autosomal recessive trait; the child inherits the gene that produces hemoglobin S from two healthy parents who carry the defective gene)

ASSESSMENT FINDINGS
Assessment findings vary with the age of the child. Before age 4 months, symptoms are rare (because fetal hemoglobin prevents excessive sickling).

In infants and toddlers
- Colic from pain caused by an abdominal infarction
- Dactylitis or pain in the hands and feet caused by sickling and resulting in decreased blood flow to the hands and feet
- Splenomegaly from sequestered RBCs

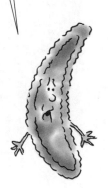

Red blood cells become sickle-shaped. Oh my.

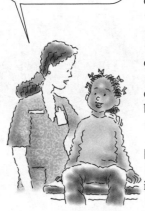

Findings for sickle cell anemia vary with age. For example, the spleen is enlarged in a young child. As the child grows, the spleen atrophies.

In preschoolers
- Hypovolemia and shock from sequestration of large amounts of blood in the spleen
- Pain at the site of vaso-occlusive crisis

In school-age children and adolescents
- Delayed growth and development and delayed sexual maturity
- Enuresis
- Extreme pain at the site of crisis
- History of pneumococcal pneumonia and other infections due to atrophied spleen
- Poor healing of leg wounds from inadequate peripheral circulation of oxygenated blood
- Priapism

DIAGNOSTIC TEST RESULTS
- Laboratory studies show hemoglobin level is 6 to 9 g/dl (in a toddler).
- More than 50% hemoglobin S indicates sickle cell disease; a lower level of hemoglobin S indicates sickle cell trait.
- RBCs are crescent-shaped and prone to agglutination.

NURSING DIAGNOSES
- Ineffective peripheral tissue perfusion
- Impaired gas exchange
- Acute pain

TREATMENT
- Bed rest
- Hydration with I.V. fluid administration (may be increased to 3 L/day during crisis)
- Short-term oxygen therapy (long-term oxygen decreases bone marrow activity, further aggravating anemia)
- Transfusion therapy as necessary
- Treatment for acidosis as necessary

Drug therapy
- Analgesic: morphine
- Antineoplastic: hydroxyurea (Droxia)
- Antibiotics: prophylaxis until age 6 to prevent bacterial septicemia
- Vaccine: pneumococcal vaccine

INTERVENTIONS AND RATIONALES
- Administer pain medication and note their effectiveness *to promote comfort.*
- Assess cardiovascular, respiratory, and neurologic status. *Tachycardia, dyspnea, or hypotension may indicate fluid volume deficit or electrolyte imbalance. Change in level of consciousness may signal neurologic involvement.*
- Assess for symptoms of acute chest syndrome from sickling of cells in the lung *to identify early complications.*
- Assess vision *to monitor for retinal complications.*
- Encourage the child to receive the pneumococcal vaccine *to prevent infection.*
- Give large amounts of oral or I.V. fluids *to prevent fluid volume deficit and prevent complications.*
- Teach the child relaxation techniques *to decrease the child's stress level.*
- Maintain the child's normal body temperature *to prevent stress and maintain adequate metabolic state.*
- Monitor vital signs and intake and output *to assess renal function and hydration status.*
- Provide proper skin care *to prevent skin breakdown.*
- Reduce the child's energy expenditure *to improve oxygenation.*
- Remove tight clothing *to prevent inadequate circulation.*
- Suggest family screening and initiate genetic counseling *to identify possible carriers of the disease.*

Teaching topics
- Explanation of the disorder and treatment plan
- Medication use and possible adverse effects
- Avoiding activities that promote a crisis, such as excessive exercise, mountain climbing, or deep sea diving
- Avoiding high altitudes
- Seeking early treatment of illness to prevent dehydration
- Avoiding aspirin use, which enhances acidosis and promotes sickling

Thalassemia

Thalassemia is characterized by a defective synthesis in the polypeptide chains necessary for hemoglobin production. RBC synthesis is also impaired.

β-thalassemia is the most common form of this disorder. It results from defective beta polypeptide chain synthesis and occurs in three clinical forms: major, intermedia, and minor.

The resulting anemia's severity depends on whether the patient is homozygous or heterozygous for the thalassemic trait. *Thalassemia major* and *thalassemia intermedia* result from homozygous inheritance or the partially dominant autosomal gene responsible for the trait. *Thalassemia minor* results from heterozygous inheritance of the same gene. Thalassemia is most common in people with Mediterranean ancestry, but also occurs in blacks and people from southern China, southeast Asia, and India.

Children with thalassemia major seldom survive to adulthood; children with thalassemia intermedia develop normally into adulthood, although puberty is usually delayed. Those with thalassemia minor can expect a normal life span.

CAUSES
- Genetic

ASSESSMENT FINDINGS
All types
- Jaundice
- Hepatomegaly
- Frequent infections
- Anemia, often severe
- Anorexia
- Bleeding tendencies
- Splenomegaly
- Bone abnormalities
- Failure to thrive

Thalassemia major
- Large head
- Mongoloid features
- Small body

DIAGNOSTIC TEST RESULTS
- Complete blood count shows lowered RBC and hemoglobin levels, microcytosis, and elevated reticulocyte count.
- Folate level is decreased.

- Peripheral blood smear shows target cells, microcytes, pale RBCs, and marked anisocytosis.
- X-ray may show osteoporosis.

NURSING DIAGNOSES
- Risk for injury
- Activity intolerance
- Ineffective protection

TREATMENT
- Mostly supportive
- Transfusion to raise hemoglobin level; care must be used not to cause iron overload
- Bone marrow transplant: showing early success

Drug therapy
- No iron supplements (they're contraindicated)
- Antibiotics: to treat infections
- Folic acid supplements

INTERVENTIONS AND RATIONALES
- Monitor for signs and symptoms after RBC transfusions *to help detect possible transfusion reaction.*
- Administer medications, as prescribed, *to help support the child.*
- Encourage genetic counseling for the parents *because thalassemia is a genetic condition.*

Teaching topics
- Explanation of the disorder and treatment plan
- Medication use and possible adverse effects
- Avoiding products that contain iron
- Recognizing signs and symptoms of hepatitis and iron overload
- Encouraging non-contact sports

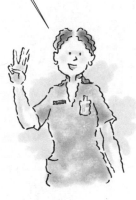

There are three types of β-thalassemia: major, intermedia, and minor.

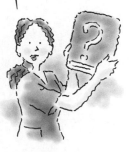

What does an X-ray show with thalassemia? Sometimes, it reveals osteoporosis.

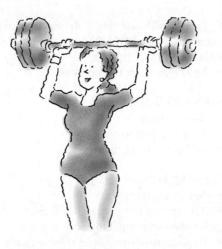

Pump up on practice questions

1. A nurse is taking a history from the mother of a child suspected of having Reye syndrome. The history reveals the use of several medications. Which medication might be implicated in the development of Reye syndrome?

1. Phenytoin (Dilantin)
2. Furosemide (Lasix)
3. Phytonadione
4. Aspirin

Answer: 4. Aspirin use has been implicated in the development of Reye syndrome in children with a history of recent acute viral infection. Phenytoin, furosemide, and phytonadione aren't associated with the development of Reye syndrome.

➡ NCLEX keys

Client needs category: Physiological integrity
Client needs subcategory: Reduction of risk potential
Cognitive level: Application

2. A 3-year-old child has been hospitalized in a vaso-occlusive crisis. To manage the pain associated with this crisis, the nurse should perform which intervention?

1. Apply moist heat and administer analgesics based on pain assessment.
2. Apply ice compresses to the affected areas and initiate range-of-motion exercises.
3. Elevate the affected areas and administer analgesics.
4. Provide a cooling blanket and administer acetaminophen (Tylenol).

Answer: 1. The major clinical feature of sickle cell anemia is pain from a vaso-occlusive crisis. Moist heat is applied to promote tissue oxygenation. Cold should be avoided because it promotes vasoconstriction and sickling. Analgesics should be administered based on the child's pain level, and aren't limited to acetaminophen.

➡ NCLEX keys

Client needs category: Physiological integrity
Client needs subcategory: Basic care and comfort
Cognitive level: Application

3. A nurse is teaching the mother of a child with sickle cell anemia. Which statement by the mother indicates a need for further teaching?

1. "My child can't possibly have sickle cell anemia. He's 4 months old, and he has never been sick before."
2. "I know my child should receive a pneumococcal vaccine when the doctor suggests."
3. "I know I should call the pediatrician immediately if my child begins to vomit."

4. "I know I should try to keep my child's body temperature normal by keeping him away from fluctuations in temperature."

Answer: 1. Further teaching is indicated if the mother states that her child can't have sickle cell anemia because he's 4 months old and has never been sick before. Symptoms of sickle cell anemia rarely appear before age 4 months because the predominance of fetal hemoglobin prevents excessive sickling. The child should receive a pneumococcal vaccine when appropriate. The mother should notify the physician if the child vomits so that treatment can be initiated to prevent dehydration, which can precipitate crisis. Changes in body temperature may also trigger crisis and should be avoided.

➡ *NCLEX keys*
Client needs category: Physiological integrity
Client needs subcategory: Reduction of risk potential
Cognitive level: Analysis

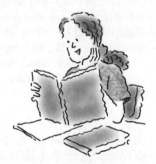

4. A nurse is teaching a mother about the benefits of breast-feeding her infant. Which type of immunity is passed on to the infant during breast-feeding?
1. Natural immunity
2. Naturally acquired active immunity
3. Naturally acquired passive immunity
4. Artificially acquired active immunity

Answer: 3. Naturally acquired passive immunity is received through placental transfer and breast-feeding. Natural immunity is present at birth. Naturally acquired active immunity occurs when the immune system makes antibodies after exposure to disease. Artificially acquired immunity occurs when medically engineered substances are ingested or injected to stimulate the immune response against a specific disease (immunizations).

➡ *NCLEX keys*
Client needs category: Health promotion and maintenance
Client needs subcategory: Safety and infection control
Cognitive level: Application

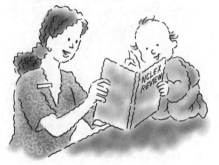

5. Which nursing interventions should a nurse anticipate when caring for a child in acute sickle cell crisis? Select all that apply.
1. Maintaining adequate hydration
2. Providing adequate pain control
3. Assessing family education needs
4. Encouraging healthy eating habits
5. Monitoring vital signs frequently
6. Attending to the child's play needs

Answer: 1, 2, 5. Because the child is in acute crisis, maintaining adequate hydration, providing pain control, and monitoring vital signs frequently are priority points of care. After the child's condition is stabilized, the nurse can then evaluate family learning needs, encourage healthy eating habits, and attend to the child's play needs.

➡ *NCLEX keys*

Client needs category: Physiological integrity
Client needs subcategory: Basic care and comfort
Cognitive level: Application

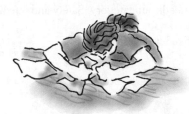

6. A nurse is providing dietary teaching for the mother of a child with iron deficiency anemia. Which iron-rich foods should the nurse instruct the mother to include in her child's diet?
1. Liver, dark leafy vegetables, and whole grains
2. Dark leafy vegetables, chicken, and whole grains
3. Whole grains, citrus fruit, and yogurt
4. Citrus fruit, liver, and whole grains

Answer: 1. The mother should be instructed to give her child iron-rich foods, such as liver, dark leafy vegetables, and whole grains. Chicken is a good source of protein, but it isn't high in iron. Citrus fruits aid iron absorption but aren't high in iron. Yogurt is a good source of calcium but isn't high in iron.

➡ *NCLEX keys*

Client needs category: Physiological integrity
Client needs subcategory: Basic care and comfort
Cognitive level: Application

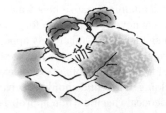

7. A nurse is teaching a child with sickle cell anemia and the child's mother about activities that may promote a vaso-occlusive crisis. Which activity is acceptable for this child?
1. Skiing
2. Mountain climbing
3. Deep sea diving
4. Bowling

Answer: 4. A child with sickle cell anemia should be instructed to avoid activities that promote a crisis, such as excessive exercise, mountain climbing, or deep sea diving. Extremes in temperature can also promote a crisis, so skiing should be avoided. Mountain climbing and deep sea diving may expose the child to altered atmospheric pressures and a deoxygenated state. These conditions can lead to a sickle cell crisis.

➡ *NCLEX keys*

Client needs category: Physiological integrity
Client needs subcategory: Reduction of risk potential
Cognitive level: Application

8. A neonate experiences prolonged bleeding after his circumcision and has multiple bruises without petechiae. These assessment findings suggest which condition?
1. Iron deficiency anemia
2. Hemophilia
3. Sickle cell anemia
4. Leukemia

Answer: 2. Signs of hemophilia include prolonged bleeding after circumcision, immunizations, or minor injuries; multiple bruises without petechiae; peripheral neuropathies from bleeding near peripheral nerves; bleeding into the throat, mouth, and thorax; and hemarthrosis. Some of the signs associated with iron deficiency anemia include dyspnea on exertion, fatigue, and listlessness. Signs and symptoms associated with sickle cell anemia include pain at the site of occlusion, poor healing of leg wounds, priapism, enuresis, and delayed growth and sexual maturity. Signs and symptoms associated with leukemia include history of infections, lymphadenopathy, hematuria, hematemesis, blood in stools, petechiae, and ecchymosis.

➡ *NCLEX keys*
Client needs category: Physiological integrity
Client needs subcategory: Reduction of risk potential
Cognitive level: Application

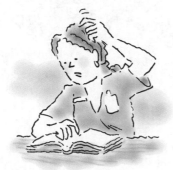

9. A child is admitted to the pediatric floor with hemophilia. The nurse encourages fantasy play and participation in his care. This developmental approach is most appropriate for which pediatric age-group?
1. The school-age child (ages 5 to 12)
2. The preschool child (ages 3 to 5)
3. The toddler (ages 1 to 3)
4. The adolescent (ages 12 to 18)

Answer: 1. School-age children engage in fantasy play and daydreaming. Therefore, it's appropriate for the nurse to encourage this type of play for the hospitalized child. The school-age child is also able to participate in his care. Doll play is helpful for the preschool hospitalized child. The toddler enjoys push-pull toys and games of peek-a-boo. The adolescent can engage in role playing in various situations.

➡ *NCLEX keys*
Client needs category: Health promotion and maintenance
Client needs subcategory: None
Cognitive level: Application

10. A nurse is providing instructions to the parents of an infant recovering from a sickle cell crisis. Which instruction should the nurse include in her teaching?
1. "Discontinue administration of all antibiotics."
2. "Keep the child isolated from all family members."
3. "Restrict the child's nighttime fluids."
4. "Make sure you hold the thermometer tightly under the arm."

Answer: 4. Infants with sickle cell anemia have altered immune function and are highly susceptible to bacterial sepsis. A fever in a child with sickle cell anemia is a medical emergency that requires prompt evaluation. The child should receive antibiotics until he is at least 5 years old. The infant should be isolated from persons with a known illness, but there's no reason to isolate him from all family members. Hydration is necessary for hemodilution and the prevention of sickling.

➡ *NCLEX keys*
Client needs category: Physiological integrity
Client needs subcategory: Reduction of risk potential
Cognitive level: Analysis

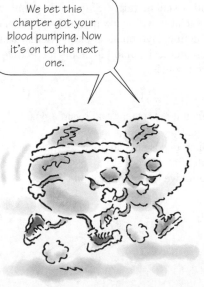

We bet this chapter got your blood pumping. Now it's on to the next one.

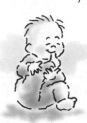

In time, my earliest, reflex-driven responses are replaced by motor responses that are under conscious control.

Brush up on key concepts

The **central nervous system** (CNS) is the body's communication network. It receives sensory stimuli through the five senses and either perceives, integrates, interprets, or retains the stimulus in memory. In an infant, early responses are primarily reflexive; the infant learns to discriminate stimuli and bring motor responses under conscious control. Language helps the older child improve and increase perception. In pediatric patients, flaccid muscles usually indicate a CNS disorder.

At any time, you can review the major points of this chapter by consulting the *Cheat sheet* on pages 642 to 644.

Upward, then downward
In children younger than age 3, the **ear canal** is directed upward. In older children, the ear canal is directed downward and forward. A child's **hearing** develops as follows:
• Sound discrimination is present at birth.
• By ages 5 to 6 months, the infant can localize sounds presented on a horizontal plane and begins to imitate selected sounds.
• By ages 7 to 12 months, the infant can localize sounds in any plane.
• By age 18 months, the child can hear and follow a simple command without visual cues.

Children who have difficulty with language development by age 18 months should have their hearing evaluated.

First, just alert
At birth, **visual function** is limited to alertness to visual stimuli 8" to 12" (20.5 to 30.5 cm) from the eyes. Normal newborns already have a blink reflex. After that, these findings are noted:

• Tear glands begin to secrete within the first 2 weeks of life.
• Transient strabismus (deviation of the eye) is a normal finding in the first few months.
• An infant can fixate on an object and follow a bright light or toy by ages 5 to 6 weeks.
• An infant can reach for objects at varying distances at ages 3 to 4 months.
• Vision reaches 20/20 when the child is about 4 years old.

Keep abreast of diagnostic tests

Here are the most important tests used to diagnose pediatric neurosensory disorders, along with common nursing interventions associated with each test.

Head check
A **basic assessment of cerebral function** includes:
• level of consciousness
• communication
• mental status.

3-D pics
Computed tomography (CT) scanning is a test process that produces three-dimensional images. It can be invasive (if contrast medium is used) or noninvasive.

Nursing actions
• Explain the purpose of the test to the parents and child.
• Make sure that the child holds still during the test.
• Make sure that written, informed consent has been obtained.

(Text continues on page 644.)

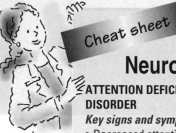

Cheat sheet

Neurosensory refresher

ATTENTION DEFICIT HYPERACTIVITY DISORDER

Key signs and symptoms
- Decreased attention span
- Difficulty organizing tasks and activities
- Easily distracted

Key test results
- Complete psychological, medical, and neurologic evaluations rule out other problems.

Key treatments
- Behavioral modification and psychological therapy
- Amphetamines: methylphenidate (Ritalin), dextroamphetamine (Dexedrine), amphetamine with dextroamphetamine (Adderall), lisdexamfetamine dimesylate (Vyvanse)

Key interventions
- Give one simple instruction at a time.
- Formulate a schedule for the child.
- Reduce environmental stimuli.

CEREBRAL PALSY

Key signs and symptoms
- Abnormal muscle tone and coordination (the most common associated problem)
- Other symptoms specific to cerebral palsy type

Key test results
- Neuroimaging studies determine the site of brain impairment.
- Cytogenic studies (genetic evaluation of the child and other family members) rule out other potential causes.
- Metabolic studies rule out other causes.

Examination findings
- Infant has difficulty sucking or keeping the nipple or food in his mouth.
- Infant seldom moves voluntarily or has arm or leg tremors with voluntary movement.
- Infant crosses legs when lifted from behind rather than pulling them up or "bicycling" like a normal infant.

Key treatments
- Braces or splints and special appliances, such as adapted eating utensils and a low toilet seat with arms, to help child perform activities independently
- Range-of-motion (ROM) exercises to minimize contractures
- Muscle relaxants or neurosurgery to decrease spasticity, if appropriate

Key interventions
- Assist with locomotion, communication, and educational opportunities.
- Divide tasks into small steps.
- Perform ROM exercises if the child is spastic.

DOWN SYNDROME

Key signs and symptoms
- Mild to moderate retardation
- Short stature with pudgy hands
- Simian crease
- Small head with slow brain growth
- Upward slanting eyes

Key test results
- Amniocentesis allows prenatal diagnosis.

Key treatments
- Treatment for coexisting conditions — congenital heart problems, vision defects, or hypothyroidism

Key interventions
- Provide activities and toys appropriate for the child.
- Set realistic, reachable, short-term goals; break tasks into small steps.
- Provide stimulation and communicate at a level appropriate to the child's mental age rather than chronological age.

HYDROCEPHALUS

Key signs and symptoms
- High-pitched cry
- Rapid increase in head circumference and full, tense, bulging fontanels (before cranial sutures close); bulging forehead

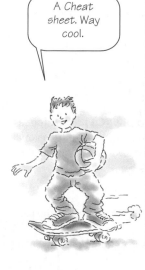

A *Cheat sheet.* Way cool.

Neurosensory refresher (continued)

HYDROCEPHALUS (CONTINUED)
Key test results
• Skull X-rays show thinning of the skull with separation of the sutures and widening of the fontanels.

Key treatments
• Ventriculoperitoneal shunt insertion: to allow cerebrospinal fluid (CSF) to drain from the lateral ventricle in the brain to the peritoneal cavity
• Antiepileptics for seizures: carbamazepine (Tegretol), pheno-barbital (Luminal), diazepam (Valium), phenytoin (Dilantin)

Key interventions
• Monitor vital signs and intake and output.
• Assess neurologic status.
• After the shunt is inserted, position the child on the side of the body opposite from where the shunt is located.
• Lay the child flat.
• If the caudal end of the shunt must be externalized because of infection, keep the bag at ear level.

MENINGITIS
Key signs and symptoms
• Nuchal rigidity that may progress to opisthotonos
• Positive Brudzinski's sign (the child flexes the knees and hips in response to passive neck flexion)
• Positive Kernig's sign (inability to extend the leg when the hip and knee are flexed)

Key test results
• Lumbar puncture shows increased CSF pressure, cloudy color, increased white blood cell count and protein level, and decreased glucose level if meningitis is caused by bacteria.
• Culture and sensitivity of CSF identifies the causative organism.
• Xpert EV test helps distinguish between viral and bacterial meningitis.

Key treatments
• Analgesics to treat the pain of meningeal irritation
• Corticosteroid: dexamethasone (Decadron)
• Droplet precautions (should be maintained until at least 24 hours of effective antibiotic therapy have elapsed; continued isolation recommended for meningitis caused by *Haemophilus influenzae* or *Neisseria meningitidis*)
• Antibiotics (based on results of CSF culture and sensitiv-ity): ceftazidime (Fortaz), ceftriaxone (Rocephin)
• Seizure precautions

Key interventions
• Monitor vital signs and intake and output.
• Assess the child's neurologic status frequently.

• Examine the young infant for bulging fontanels, and measure head circumference.

OTITIS MEDIA
Key signs and symptoms
Acute suppurative otitis media
• Fever (mild to very high)
• Pain that suddenly stops (occurs if the tympanic membrane ruptures)
• Severe, deep, throbbing pain (from pressure behind the tympanic membrane)
• Signs of upper respiratory tract infection (sneezing, coughing)
Acute secretory otitis media
• Popping, crackling, or clicking sounds on swallowing or with jaw movement
• Sensation of fullness in the ear
Chronic otitis media
• Cholesteatoma (cystlike mass in the middle ear)
• Decreased or absent tympanic membrane mobility
• Painless, purulent discharge in chronic suppurative otitis media

Key test results
Acute suppurative otitis media
• Otoscopy reveals obscured or distorted bony landmarks of the tympanic membrane.
Acute secretory otitis media
• Otoscopy reveals clear or amber fluid behind the tympanic membrane and tympanic membrane retraction, which causes the bony landmarks to appear more prominent. If hemorrhage into the middle ear has occurred, as in barotrauma, the tympanic membrane appears blue-black.
Chronic otitis media
• Otoscopy shows thickening, decreased mobility of the tympanic membrane and, sometimes, scarring.

Key treatments
Acute suppurative otitis media
• Myringotomy for children with severe, painful bulging of the tympanic membrane
• Antibiotic therapy, usually amoxicillin (Amoxil)
Acute secretory otitis media
• Inflation of the eustachian tube by performing Valsalva's maneuver several times per day, which may be the only treatment required
• Nasopharyngeal decongestant therapy
Chronic otitis media
• Elimination of eustachian tube obstruction

(continued)

Neurosensory refresher *(continued)*

OTITIS MEDIA *(CONTINUED)*
- Excision for cholesteatoma
- Mastoidectomy
- Broad-spectrum antibiotics: amoxicillin-clavulanate potassium (Augmentin) or cefuroxime (Ceftin) (in selected situations)

Key interventions
- After myringotomy, maintain drainage flow. Place sterile cotton loosely in the external ear. Change the cotton frequently.
- Watch for and report headache, fever, severe pain, or disorientation.
- After tympanoplasty, reinforce dressings and observe for excessive bleeding from the ear canal.
- Instruct the parents not to feed their infant in a supine position or put him to bed with a bottle.

SEIZURE DISORDERS
Key signs and symptoms
- May experience an aura just before the seizure's onset (reports unusual tastes, feelings, or odors)
- Eyes deviating to a particular side or blinking
- Usually unresponsive during tonic-clonic muscular contractions; may experience incontinence
- Irregular breathing with spasms

Key test results
- EEG results help differentiate epileptic from nonepileptic seizures. Each seizure has a characteristic EEG tracing.

Key treatments
- Antiepileptics: I.V. diazepam (Valium) or lorazepam (Ativan), phenobarbital (Luminal) or fosphenytoin (Cerebyx), phenytoin (Dilantin), valproic acid (Depakote), carbamazepine (Tegretol)
- Rectal diazepam (Diastat) for home management of intractable or prolonged seizures

Key interventions
- Assess neurologic status.
- Stay with the child during a seizure.
- Move the child to a flat surface.

- Place the child on his side.
- Don't try to interrupt the seizure.

SPINA BIFIDA
Key signs and symptoms
Spina bifida occulta
- Dimple or tuft of hair on the skin over the spinal defect
- No neurologic dysfunction (usually), except occasional foot weakness or bowel and bladder disturbances
Meningocele
- No neurologic dysfunction (usually)
- Saclike structure protruding over the spine
Myelomeningocele
- Hydrocephalus
- Permanent neurologic dysfunction (paralysis, bowel and bladder incontinence)

Key test results
- Elevated alpha-fetoprotein levels in the mother's blood may indicate the presence of a neural tube defect.
- Amniocentesis reveals neural tube defect.
- Acetylcholinesterase measurement can be used to confirm the diagnosis.

Key treatments
- Surgery (in meningocele and myelomeningocele)

Key interventions
Before surgery
- Assess for signs of hydrocephalus. Measure head circumference daily. Be sure to mark the spot where the measurement was made.
- Assess for signs of meningeal irritation, such as fever or nuchal rigidity.
After surgery
- Assess for hydrocephalus, which commonly follows surgery. Measure the infant's head circumference as ordered.
- Monitor vital signs often.

More detail
Magnetic resonance imaging (MRI) shows the CNS in greater detail than CT scanning. A noniodinated contrast medium may be used to enhance lesions. Advances in MRI allow visualization of cerebral arteries and venous sinuses without administration of a contrast medium.

Nursing actions
- Explain the procedure to the parents and child.
- If the child has any surgically implanted metal objects (such as pins and clips), notify the radiology department because these may interfere with the picture.
- Make sure the child holds still during the test.

Electric pics

Electroencephalogram (EEG) shows abnormal electrical activity in the brain (such as from a seizure, metabolic disorder, or drug overdose).

Nursing actions

• Explain the purpose of the test to the parents and child.
• Make sure the child holds still during the test.

Wavy reflections

Ultrasonography reveals carotid lesions or changes in carotid blood flow and velocity. High-frequency sound waves reflect the velocity of blood flow, which is then reported as a graphic recording of a waveform.

Nursing actions

• Explain the purpose of the test to the parents and child.
• Make sure the child holds still during the test.

Fluid check

A **lumbar puncture** is the insertion of a needle into the subarachnoid space of the spinal cord, usually between L3 and L4 (or L4 and L5) to allow aspiration of cerebrospinal fluid (CSF) for analysis and measurement of CSF pressure.

Nursing actions

Before the procedure
• Explain the procedure to the parents and child.
• Make sure that written, informed consent has been obtained.
• Keep the child in a side-lying, knee-chest position during the procedure.
After the procedure
• Make sure the child rests for 1 hour or as ordered.

Vessel visualization

In **cerebral arteriography,** also known as *angiography*, a catheter is inserted into an artery — usually the femoral artery — and is indirectly threaded up to the carotid artery.

Then a radiopaque dye is injected, allowing X-ray visualization of the cerebral vasculature.

Nursing actions

Before the procedure
• Explain the procedure to the parents and child.
• Make sure that written, informed consent has been obtained.
• Identify allergies before the test.
• Make sure the child holds still during the test, and monitor him for allergic reaction.
After the procedure
• Immobilize the site after the test, and monitor it for pulses and evidence of bleeding.

Pressure check

Intracranial pressure (ICP) monitoring is a direct, invasive method of identifying trends in ICP. A subarachnoid screw and an intra-ventricular catheter convert CSF pressure readings into waveforms that are digitally displayed on an oscilloscope monitor. Another option is to insert a fiber-optic catheter in the ventricle, subarachnoid space, subdural space, or the brain parenchyma. Pressure changes are reported digitally or in waveform.

Nursing actions

Before the procedure
• Explain the procedure to the parents and child.
• Make sure that written, informed consent has been obtained.
After the procedure
• Maintain patency of the catheter, and monitor the waveforms. Alert the physician to changes in trends.
• Maintain sterile technique during care of the catheter and monitoring equipment.
• Monitor the site for signs of infection.

Nerve times

Electromyography detects lower motor neuron disorders, neuromuscular disorders, and nerve damage. A needle inserted into selected muscles at rest and during voluntary contraction picks up nerve impulses and measures nerve conduction time.

> A complete neurologic assessment may require a close look at the eyes, ears, internal structures, fluid pressures, and neural function.

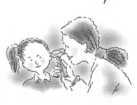

Nursing actions
Before the procedure
• Explain the procedure to the parents and child.
• Check the child's medications for those that may interfere with the test (cholinergics, anticholinergics, skeletal muscle relaxants).
• Make sure that written, informed consent has been obtained.
• Make sure the child holds still during the procedure.
After the procedure
• Monitor the site for infection or bleeding after the procedure.

Ear check
Otoscopic examination allows visualization of the canal and inner structures of the ear.

Nursing actions
• Explain the procedure to the parents and child.
• Use the largest speculum that fits into the ear canal.
• To straighten the ear canal, pull the pinna down and back or out in infants and children younger than age 3. For children older than age 3, the pinna is pulled up and back.

Eye check
Ophthalmoscopic examination helps visualize interior eye structures.

Nursing actions
• Explain the procedure to the parents and child.
• Ensure cooperation during tests by allowing the child to hold a favorite toy, which may decrease anxiety.

Polish up on client care

Major neurologic disorders in pediatric patients are attention deficit hyperactivity disorder (ADHD), cerebral palsy, Down syndrome, hydrocephalus, meningitis, otitis media, seizure disorders, and spina bifida.

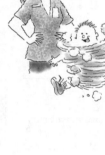

ADHD manifests itself through long-term behaviors that include hyperactivity, impulsiveness, and inattention.

Memory jogger

Here's a tip for remembering diagnostic criteria for ADHD: think of a child who can't **SIT** still.

Seven (age by which symptoms appear)

Impaired social or academic function

Two or more settings

Attention deficit hyperactivity disorder

ADHD, previously called *attention deficit disorder*, includes the following long-term behaviors:
• hyperactivity
• impulsiveness
• inattention.
These manifestations occur in all facets of the child's life and commonly worsen when sustained attention is required such as during school. To qualify as ADHD, behaviors must be present in two or more settings, must be present before age 7, and must result in a significant impairment of social or academic functioning, and the symptoms aren't a result of another mental disorder. Three types of ADHD have been identified based on *Diagnostic and Statistical Manual of Mental Disorders,* Fourth Edition, Text Revision (*DSM-IV-TR*) criteria:
• predominantly inattentive type
• predominantly hyperactive-impulsive type
• combined type.

CAUSES
• Deficit in neurotransmitters (possibly)

ASSESSMENT FINDINGS
• Excessive climbing, running, or talking
• Decreased attention span
• Difficulty organizing tasks and activities
• Difficulty waiting for turns
• Easily distracted
• Failure to give close attention to school work or activity
• Failure to listen when spoken to directly
• Fidgets or squirms in seat
• Frequent forgetfulness; frequently loses things needed for tasks
• Impulsive behavior
• Inability to follow directions

DIAGNOSTIC TEST RESULTS
• Complete psychological, medical, and neurologic evaluations rule out other problems.
• *DSM-IV-TR* criteria is met: Six or more symptoms of inattention, hyperactivity, or impulsiveness have been present for at least

6 months or more and are disruptive or inappropriate for developmental level.

NURSING DIAGNOSES
- Imbalanced nutrition: Less than body requirements
- Risk for impaired parenting
- Risk for injury

TREATMENT
- Behavioral modification and psychological therapy
- Interdisciplinary interventions: pathologic assessment and diagnosis of specific learning needs

Drug therapy
- Amphetamines: methylphenidate (Ritalin), dextroamphetamine (Dexedrine), amphetamine with dextroamphetamine (Adderall), lisdexamfetamine dimesylate (Vyvanse)
- Other medications: imipramine (Tofranil), clonidine (Catapres)

INTERVENTIONS AND RATIONALES
- Monitor growth. *If the child is receiving methylphenidate, growth may be slowed.*
- Give one simple instruction at a time *so the child can successfully complete the task, which promotes self-esteem.*
- Give medications in the morning and at lunch *to avoid interfering with sleep.*
- Ensure adequate nutrition; *medications and hyperactivity may cause increased nutrient needs.*
- Reduce environmental stimuli *to decrease distraction.*
- Formulate a schedule for the child *to provide consistency and routine.*

Teaching topics
- Explanation of the disorder and treatment plan
- Medication use and possible adverse effects
- Allowing the child to expend energy after being in a restrictive environment such as school
- Structuring learning to minimize distractions
- Taking breaks from caregiving to avoid strain

- Teaching important material in the morning (when medication levels peak)

Cerebral palsy

Cerebral palsy is a neuromuscular disorder resulting from damage to or a defect in the part of the brain that controls motor function.

The disorder is most commonly seen in children born prematurely. Cerebral palsy can't be cured; treatment includes interventions that encourage optimum development. Defects are common, including musculoskeletal, neurologic, GI, and nutritional defects as well as other systemic complications (abnormal reflexes, fatigue, growth failure, genitourinary complaints, respiratory infections).

Classifications of cerebral palsy include:
- ataxia type — the least common type; essentially a lack of coordination caused by disturbances in movement and balance
- athetoid type — characterized by involuntary, incoordinate motion with varying degrees of muscle tension (Children with this type of cerebral palsy experience writhing muscle contractions whenever they attempt voluntary movement. Facial grimacing, poor swallowing, and tongue movements cause drooling and poor speech articulation. Despite their abnormal appearance, these children commonly have average or above-average intelligence.)
- spastic type — the most common type; featuring hyperactive stretch in associated muscle groups, hyperactive deep tendon reflexes, rapid involuntary muscle contraction and relaxation, contractions affecting extensor muscles, and scissoring (The child's legs are crossed and the toes are pointed down, so the child stands on his toes.)
- rigidity type — an uncommon type of cerebral palsy characterized by rigid postures and lack of active movement
- mixed type — more than one type of cerebral palsy. (These children are usually severely disabled.)

CAUSES
- Anoxia before, during, or after birth
- Infection
- Trauma (hemorrhage)

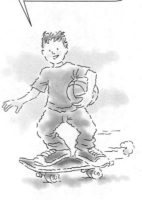

For ADHD, first reduce stimuli during learning times. Then allow the child to expend energy.

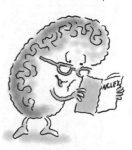

Cerebral palsy arises from a malfunction of motor centers and neural pathways in the brain. Well, I'll be.

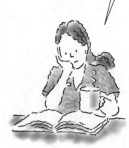

Abnormal muscle tone and coordination characterize all forms of cerebral palsy.

RISK FACTORS
- Low birth weight
- Low Apgar scores at 5 minutes
- Metabolic disturbances
- Seizures

ASSESSMENT FINDINGS
All types
- Abnormal muscle tone and coordination (the most common associated problem)
- Dental anomalies
- Mental retardation of varying degrees in 18% to 50% of cases (most children with cerebral palsy have at least a normal IQ but can't demonstrate it on standardized tests)
- Seizures
- Speech, vision, or hearing disturbances

Ataxic cerebral palsy
- Poor balance and muscle coordination
- Unsteady, wide-based gait

Athetoid cerebral palsy
- Slow state of writhing muscle contractions whenever voluntary movement is attempted
- Facial grimacing
- Poor swallowing
- Drooling
- Poor speech articulation

Rigid cerebral palsy
- Rigid posture
- Lack of active movement

Spastic cerebral palsy
- Hyperactive stretch reflex in associated muscle groups
- Hyperactive deep tendon reflexes
- Rapid involuntary muscle contraction and relaxation
- Contractures affecting the extensor muscles
- Scissoring

Mixed cerebral palsy
- Signs of more than one type of cerebral palsy
- Severely disabled

DIAGNOSTIC TEST RESULTS
- Neuroimaging studies determine the site of brain impairment.

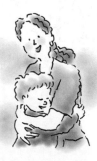

Although cerebral palsy can't be cured, treatment encourages the child to reach his full potential.

- Cytogenic studies (genetic evaluation of the child and other family members) rule out other potential causes.
- Metabolic studies rule out other causes.

Examination findings
- Infant has difficulty sucking or keeping the nipple or food in his mouth.
- Infant seldom moves voluntarily or has arm or leg tremors with voluntary movement.
- Infant crosses his legs when lifted from behind rather than pulling them up or "bicycling" like a normal infant.
- Infant's legs are difficult to separate, making diaper changing difficult.
- Infant persistently uses only one hand or, as he gets older, uses hands — but not legs — well.

NURSING DIAGNOSES
- Impaired physical mobility
- Delayed growth and development
- Impaired verbal communication

TREATMENT
- High-calorie diet, if appropriate
- Artificial urinary sphincter for the incontinent child who can use hand controls
- Braces or splints and special appliances, such as adapted eating utensils and a low toilet seat with arms, to help the child perform activities independently
- Neurosurgery to decrease spasticity, if appropriate
- Orthopedic surgery to correct contractures
- Range-of-motion (ROM) exercises to minimize contractures

Drug therapy
- Muscle relaxants to decrease spasticity, if appropriate
- Anticonvulsants: phenytoin (Dilantin), phenobarbital (Luminal) to control seizures

INTERVENTIONS AND RATIONALES
- Assist with locomotion, communication, and educational opportunities *to enable the child to attain optimal developmental level.*

- Increase caloric intake for the child with increased motor function *to keep up with increased metabolic needs.*
- Promote age-appropriate mental activities and incentives for motor development *to promote growth and development.*
- Provide rest periods *to promote rest and reduce metabolic needs.*
- Perform ROM exercises if the child is spastic *to maintain proper body alignment and mobility of joints.*
- Provide a safe environment, for example, by using protective headgear or bed pads, *to prevent injury.*
- Divide tasks into small steps *to promote self-care and activity and increase self-esteem.*
- Refer the child for speech, nutrition, and physical therapy *to maintain or improve functioning.*
- Use assistive communication devices if the child can't speak *to promote a positive self-concept.*

Teaching topics
- Explanation of the disorder and treatment plan
- Medication use and possible adverse effects
- Contacting appropriate social service agencies, child development specialist, mental health services, and home care assistance
- Understanding the child's condition and prognosis

Down syndrome

The first disorder researchers attributed to a chromosomal aberration, Down syndrome is characterized by:
- mental retardation
- dysmorphic facial features
- other distinctive physical abnormalities.
(Sixty percent of patients have congenital heart defects, respiratory infections, chronic myelogenous leukemia, and a weak immune response to infection.)

CAUSES
- Genetic nondisjunction, with three chromosomes on the 21st pair (total of 47 chromosomes)

CONTRIBUTING FACTORS
- Maternal age (the older the mother, the greater the risk of genetic nondisjunction)

ASSESSMENT FINDINGS
- Brushfield's spots (marbling and speckling of the iris)
- Flat, broad forehead
- Flat nose and low-set ears
- Hypotonia
- Mild to moderate retardation
- Protruding tongue (because of a small oral cavity)
- Short stature with pudgy hands
- Simian crease (a single crease across the palm)
- Small head with slow brain growth
- Upward slanting eyes

DIAGNOSTIC TEST RESULTS
- Amniocentesis allows prenatal diagnosis. It's recommended for women older than age 34, regardless of a negative family history, or a woman of any age if she or the father carries a translocated chromosome.
- Karyotype shows the specific chromosomal abnormality.

NURSING DIAGNOSES
- Delayed growth and development
- Risk for injury
- Risk for aspiration

TREATMENT
- Treatment for coexisting conditions — congenital heart problems, vision defects, or hypothyroidism
- Skeletal, immunologic, metabolic, biochemical, and oncologic problems treated as per specific problem

Drug therapy
- Megavitamin therapy (controversial) to promote growth and development potential

INTERVENTIONS AND RATIONALES
- Provide activities and toys appropriate for the child *to support optimal development.*
- Set realistic, reachable, short-term goals; break tasks into small steps *to make them easier to accomplish.*

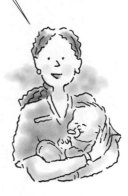

Provide a safe environment for the child with cerebral palsy.

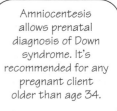

Amniocentesis allows prenatal diagnosis of Down syndrome. It's recommended for any pregnant client older than age 34.

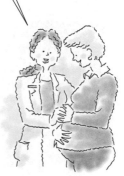

- Use behavior modification, if applicable, *to promote safety and prevent injury to the child and others.*
- Provide stimulation and communicate at a level appropriate to the child's mental age rather than chronological age *to promote a healthy emotional environment.*
- Provide a safe environment *to prevent injury.*
- Mainstream daily routines *to promote normalcy.*

Teaching topics
- Explanation of the disorder and treatment plan
- Contacting early intervention programs
- Contacting support groups for caregivers
- Establishing self-care skills to promote independence

Hydrocephalus

In hydrocephalus, an increase in the amount of CSF occurs in the ventricles and subarachnoid spaces of the brain. The ventricles become dilated because of an imbalance in the rate of production and rate of absorption of CSF. This condition may be congenital or acquired.

In noncommunicating hydrocephalus, an obstruction occurs in the free circulation of CSF, causing increased pressure on the brain or spinal cord. In most cases, congenital hydrocephalus is noncommunicating.

Communicating hydrocephalus involves the free flow of CSF between the ventricles and the spinal theca. Increased pressure on the spinal cord is caused by defective absorption of CSF.

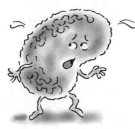

Yikes! In hydrocephalus, an excessive amount of CSF accumulates in the ventricular spaces of the brain.

CAUSES
- Arnold-Chiari malformation (downward displacement of cerebellar components through the foramen magnum into the cervical spinal canal); common in hydrocephalus with spina bifida
- Overproduction of CSF by the choroid plexus
- Scarring, congenital anomalies, or hemorrhage; causes CSF to be absorbed abnormally after it reaches the subarachnoid space (in communicating hydrocephalus)
- Tumors, hemorrhage, or structural abnormalities; block CSF flow, causing fluid to accumulate in the ventricles (in noncommunicating hydrocephalus)

ASSESSMENT FINDINGS
- "Cracked pot" sound when the skull is percussed
- Distended scalp veins
- High-pitched cry
- Inability to support the head when upright
- Irritability or lethargy
- Decreased attention span
- Rapid increase in head circumference and full, tense, bulging fontanels (before cranial sutures close); bulging forehead
- Sunset sign (sclera visible above the iris)
- Widening suture lines
- Vomiting (not related to food intake)

DIAGNOSTIC TEST RESULTS
- Angiography, computed tomography scan, and magnetic resonance imaging differentiate hydrocephalus from intracranial lesions and may demonstrate Arnold-Chiari malformation.
- Light reflects off the opposite side of the skull with skull transillumination.
- Skull X-rays show thinning of the skull with separation of the sutures and widening of the fontanels.

NURSING DIAGNOSES
- Risk for injury
- Delayed growth and development
- Decreased intracranial adaptive capacity

TREATMENT
- Ventriculoperitoneal shunt insertion to allow CSF to drain from the lateral ventricle in the brain to the peritoneal cavity

Drug therapy
- Antiepileptics for seizures: carbamazepine (Tegretol), phenobarbital (Luminal), diazepam (Valium), phenytoin (Dilantin)

INTERVENTIONS AND RATIONALES
• Measure head circumference *to aid in diagnosis of hydrocephalus.*
• Monitor vital signs and intake and output *to assess for fluid volume excess, which can further elevate ICP.*
• Assess neurologic status *to identify changes indicative of increased ICP.*
• After the shunt is inserted, position the child on the side of his body opposite from where it's located *to promote CSF drainage and prevent shunt occlusion.*
• Lay the child flat *to avoid rapid decompression.*
• Observe for signs and symptoms of increased ICP *to prevent complications.*
• Observe for signs of infection. *Signs of shunt infection usually occur within the first month after shunt insertion.*
• If the caudal end of the shunt must be externalized because of infection, keep the bag at ear level *to promote CSF drainage.*
• Support the head when the child is upright *to prevent injury and promote CSF drainage.*
• Provide proper skin care to the head; turn the patient's head frequently *to avoid skin breakdown.*

Teaching topics
• Explanation of the disorder and treatment plan
• Medication use and possible adverse effects
• Recognizing the signs of increasing ICP
• Understanding care required after shunt insertion

Meningitis

Meningitis is an inflammation of the brain and spinal cord meninges. It's most common in infants and toddlers but can occur in other age groups as well. The incidence of meningitis is greatly reduced with routine *Haemophilus influenzae* type B vaccine.

CAUSES
• Viral or bacterial agents, transmitted by the spread of droplets (organisms enter the blood from the nasopharynx or middle ear)

ASSESSMENT FINDINGS
• Nuchal rigidity that may progress to opisthotonos (arching of the back)
• Headache
• Fever
• High-pitched cry
• Irritability
• Delirium
• Coma
• Petechial or purpuric lesions possibly present in bacterial meningitis
• Positive Brudzinski's sign (the child flexes the knees and hips in response to passive neck flexion)
• Positive Kernig's sign (inability to extend the leg when the hip and knee are flexed)
• Projectile vomiting
• Seizures (may occur)

DIAGNOSTIC TEST RESULTS
• Lumbar puncture shows increased CSF pressure, cloudy color, increased white blood cell count and protein level, and decreased glucose level if the meningitis is caused by bacteria.
• Culture and sensitivity of CSF identifies the causative organism.
• Xpert EV test helps distinguish between viral and bacterial meningitis.

NURSING DIAGNOSES
• Decreased intracranial adaptive capacity
• Ineffective breathing pattern
• Risk for injury

TREATMENT
• Droplet precautions (should be maintained until at least 24 hours of effective antibiotic therapy have elapsed; continued precautions recommended for meningitis caused by *H. influenzae* or *Neisseria meningitidis*)
• Hypothermia blanket
• Oxygen therapy may require intubation and mechanical ventilation to induce hyperventilation to decrease ICP
• Seizure precautions
• Treatment for coexisting conditions
• Burr holes to evacuate subdural effusion, if present

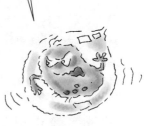
Meningitis is transmitted by the spread of droplets.

Drug therapy

- Analgesics to treat the pain of meningeal irritation
- Corticosteroid: dexamethasone (Decadron)
- Antibiotics (based on results of CSF culture and sensitivity): ceftazidime (Fortaz), ceftriaxone (Rocephin)

INTERVENTIONS AND RATIONALES

- Monitor vital signs and intake and output *to assess for excess fluid volume.*
- Assess the child's neurologic status frequently *to monitor for signs of increased ICP.*
- Provide a dark and quiet environment. *Environmental stimuli can increase ICP or stimulate seizure activity.*
- Maintain seizure precautions *to prevent injury.*
- Administer medications as ordered *to combat infection and decrease ICP.*
- Move the child gently *to prevent a rise in ICP.*
- Maintain isolation precautions as ordered *to prevent the spread of infection.*
- Provide emotional support for the family *to decrease anxiety.*
- Examine the young infant for bulging fontanels, and measure head circumference; *hydrocephalus is a complication that can result from meningitis.*

Teaching topics

- Explanation of the disorder and treatment plan
- Medication use and possible adverse effects
- Understanding the importance of isolation and sanitation

Otitis media

Otitis media is inflammation of the middle ear that may be accompanied by infection. The fluid presses on the tympanic membrane, causing pain and leading to possible rupture or perforation. This condition may be chronic or acute and suppurative or secretory.

Acute otitis media is common in children. Its incidence increases during the winter months, paralleling the seasonal increase in nonbacterial respiratory tract infections. With prompt treatment, the prognosis for acute otitis media is excellent; however, prolonged accumulation of fluid in the middle ear cavity causes chronic otitis media and, possibly, perforation of the tympanic membrane.

CAUSES
All types

- Obstructed eustachian tube
- Wider, shorter, more horizontal eustachian tubes and increased lymphoid tissue in children as well as other anatomic anomalies

Suppurative otitis media

- Bacterial infection with pneumococci, *H. influenzae* (the most common cause in children younger than age 6), *Moraxella (Branhamella) catarrhalis*, group A beta-hemolytic streptococci, staphylococci (most common cause in children age 6 or older), or gram-negative bacteria
- Respiratory tract infection, allergic reaction, nasotracheal intubation, or position changes that allow nasopharyngeal flora to reflux through the eustachian tube and colonize the middle ear

Chronic suppurative otitis media

- Recurrent acute otitis episodes
- Infection by resistant strains of bacteria
- Tuberculosis (rarely)

Secretory otitis media

- Barotrauma (pressure injury caused by an inability to equalize pressure between the environment and the middle ear), as occurs during rapid aircraft descent in a person with upper respiratory tract infection or during rapid underwater ascent in scuba diving (barotitis media)
- Obstruction of the eustachian tube secondary to eustachian tube dysfunction from viral infection or allergy, which causes a buildup of negative pressure in the middle ear that promotes transudation of sterile serous fluid from blood vessels in the membrane of the middle ear

Chronic secretory otitis media

- Persistent eustachian tube dysfunction from mechanical obstruction (adenoidal

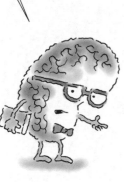

My, oh my... meningitis management mandates meticulous monitoring: Monitor vital signs, intake and output, and neurologic status.

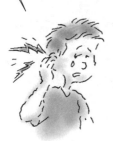

Key clinical fact about acute suppurative otitis media: It HURTS!

tissue overgrowth or tumors), edema (allergic rhinitis or chronic sinus infection), or inadequate treatment of acute suppurative otitis media

ASSESSMENT FINDINGS
Acute suppurative otitis media
• Bulging and erythema of the tympanic membrane
• Dizziness
• Fever (mild to very high)
• Hearing loss (usually mild and conductive)
• Nausea and vomiting (possibly)
• Pain pattern (pulling the pinna doesn't exacerbate pain)
• Pain that suddenly stops (occurs if the tympanic membrane ruptures)
• Purulent drainage in the ear canal from tympanic membrane rupture
• Severe, deep, throbbing pain (from pressure behind the tympanic membrane)
• Signs of upper respiratory tract infection (sneezing and coughing)
• Tinnitus (ringing in the ears)

Acute secretory otitis media
• Echo heard by the patient when speaking; vague feeling of top-heaviness (caused by accumulation of fluid)
• Popping, crackling, or clicking sounds on swallowing or with jaw movement
• Sensation of fullness in the ear
• Severe conductive hearing loss

Chronic otitis media
• Cholesteatoma (cystlike mass in the middle ear)
• Decreased or absent tympanic membrane mobility
• Painless, purulent discharge in chronic suppurative otitis media
• Thickening and scarring of the tympanic membrane

DIAGNOSTIC TEST RESULTS
Acute suppurative otitis media
• Culture of the ear drainage identifies the causative organism.
• Otoscopy reveals obscured or distorted bony landmarks of the tympanic membrane.
• Pneumatoscopy (pneumatic otoscope) may show decreased tympanic membrane

mobility, but this procedure is painful with an obviously bulging, erythematous tympanic membrane.

Acute secretory otitis media
• Otoscopy reveals clear or amber fluid behind the tympanic membrane and tympanic membrane retraction, which causes the bony landmarks to appear more prominent. If hemorrhage into the middle ear has occurred, as in barotrauma, the tympanic membrane appears blue-black.

Chronic otitis media
• Otoscopy shows thickening, decreased mobility of the tympanic membrane and, sometimes, scarring.
• Pneumatoscopy shows decreased or absent tympanic membrane movement.

NURSING DIAGNOSES
• Acute pain
• Disturbed sensory perception (auditory)
• Hyperthermia

TREATMENT
Acute suppurative otitis media
• Myringotomy for children with severe, painful bulging of the tympanic membrane

Drug therapy
• Antibiotic therapy, usually amoxicillin (Amoxil) (antibiotics must be used with discretion to prevent development of resistant strains of bacteria in children with recurring otitis media)
• Antibiotic: amoxicillin-clavulanate potassium (Augmentin) in areas with a high incidence of beta-lactamase–producing *H. influenzae* and in patients who aren't responding to amoxicillin
• Antibiotic: cefaclor (Ceclor) or co-trimoxazole (Bactrim) for patients allergic to penicillin derivatives
• Prevention: broad-spectrum antibiotics, such as amoxicillin-clavulanate potassium (Augmentin) or cefuroxime (Ceftin) in high-risk clients

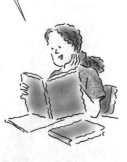

In acute suppurative otitis media, pulling the auricle doesn't worsen the pain.

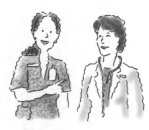

In myringotomy, the physician cuts into the eardrum and gently suctions fluid to relieve pressure.

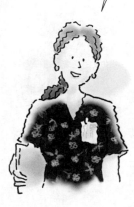

Mastoidectomy is removal of the mastoid process or mastoid cells of the temporal bone.

Acute secretory otitis media
- Concomitant treatment of the underlying cause, such as elimination of allergens, or adenoidectomy for hypertrophied adenoids
- Inflation of the eustachian tube by performing Valsalva's maneuver several times a day, which may be the only treatment required
- Myringotomy and aspiration of middle ear fluid if decongestant therapy fails, followed by insertion of a polyethylene tube into the tympanic membrane for immediate and prolonged equalization of pressure (tube falls out spontaneously after 9 to 12 months)

Drug therapy
- Nasopharyngeal decongestant therapy for at least 2 weeks; sometimes used indefinitely, with periodic evaluation

Chronic otitis media
- Elimination of eustachian tube obstruction
- Excision for cholesteatoma
- Mastoidectomy
- Treatment of otitis externa; myringoplasty and tympanoplasty to reconstruct middle ear structures when thickening and scarring are present

Drug therapy
- Broad-spectrum antibiotic: amoxicillin-clavulanate potassium (Augmentin) or cefuroxime (Ceftin) for exacerbations of otitis media (in selected situations)

INTERVENTIONS AND RATIONALES
- Monitor vital signs *to determine baseline and detect early signs of worsening infection.*
- Watch for and report headache, fever, severe pain, or disorientation *to detect early signs of complications.*
- Administer analgesics, as needed, or recommend applying heat to the ear *to relieve pain.*
- Identify and treat allergies *to prevent recurrences of otitis media.*
- Encourage the child to complete the prescribed course of antibiotic treatment *to prevent reinfection.*
- For children with acute secretory otitis media, watch for and immediately report pain and fever *to detect early signs of secondary infection.*

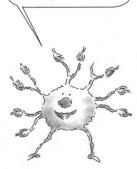

If I become hyperexcitable, it may lead to a seizure.

- Tell the parents to avoid feeding the infant in a supine position or putting him to bed with a bottle *to prevent reflux of nasopharyngeal flora.*
- Encourage the child to perform Valsalva's maneuver several times daily *to promote eustachian tube patency.*
- After myringotomy, maintain drainage flow; place sterile cotton loosely in the external ear *to absorb drainage.* Change the cotton frequently *to prevent infection.*
- After tympanoplasty, reinforce dressings and observe for excessive bleeding from the ear canal *to assess for fluid volume deficit.*

Teaching topics
- Explanation of the disorder and treatment plan
- Medication use and possible adverse effects
- Avoiding blowing the nose or getting the ear wet when bathing
- Instilling nasopharyngeal decongestants properly, if prescribed
- Recognizing upper respiratory tract infections and seeking early treatment
- Returning for follow-up examination after completion of antibiotic therapy

Seizure disorders

A seizure is a sudden, episodic, involuntary alteration in consciousness, motor activity, behavior, sensation, or autonomic function. (See *Classifying seizures.*) Epilepsy is a common, recurrent seizure disorder.

CAUSES
- Excessive neuronal discharges (epilepsy)
- Hyperexcitable nerve cells that surpass the seizure threshold
- Neurons overfiring without regard to stimuli or need

ASSESSMENT FINDINGS
- May experience an aura just before the seizure's onset (the child reports unusual tastes, feelings, or odors)
- Eyes deviating to a particular side or blinking
- Irregular breathing with spasms

Classifying seizures

Seizures can take various forms depending on their origin and whether they're localized to one area of the brain, as occurs in partial seizures, or occur in both hemispheres, as happens in generalized seizures. This chart describes each type of seizure and lists common signs and symptoms.

Type	Description	Signs and symptoms
Partial		
Simple partial	Symptoms confined to one hemisphere	May have motor (change in posture), sensory (hallucinations), or autonomic (flushing, tachycardia) symptoms; no loss of consciousness
Complex partial	Begins in one focal area but spreads to both hemispheres (more common in adults)	Loss of consciousness; aura of visual disturbances; postictal symptoms
Generalized		
Absence (formerly called *petit mal*)	Sudden onset; lasts 5 to 10 seconds; can have 100 daily; precipitated by stress, hyperventilation, hypoglycemia, fatigue; differentiated from daydreaming	Loss of responsiveness but continued ability to maintain posture control and not fall; twitching eyelids; lip smacking; no postictal symptoms
Myoclonic	Movement disorder (not a seizure); seen as the child awakens or falls asleep; may be precipitated by touch or visual stimuli; focal or generalized; symmetrical or asymmetrical	No loss of consciousness; sudden, brief, shocklike involuntary contraction of one muscle group
Clonic	Opposing muscles contract and relax alternately in a rhythmic pattern; may occur in one limb more than others	Mucus production
Tonic	Muscles are maintained in a continuous contracted state (rigid posture)	Variable loss of consciousness; pupils dilate; eyes roll up; glottis closes; possible incontinence; may experience excessive salivation
Tonic-clonic (formerly called *grand mal, major motor*)	Violent total body seizure	Aura; tonic first (20 to 40 seconds); clonic next; postictal symptoms
Atonic	Drop and fall attack; needs to wear protective helmet	Loss of posture tone
Akinetic	Sudden brief loss of muscle tone or posture	Temporary loss of consciousness

(continued)

Classifying seizures *(continued)*

Type	Description	Signs and symptoms
Unclassified		
Febrile	Seizure threshold lowered by elevated temperature; only one seizure per fever; occurs in 4% of population younger than age 5; occurs when temperature is rapidly rising	Lasts less than 5 minutes; generalized, transient, and nonprogressive; doesn't generally result in brain damage; EEG is normal after 2 weeks
Idiopathic	Cause unknown; most common type of pediatric seizures; genetic factors may influence neuronal discharge	Widely variable
Status epilepticus	Prolonged or frequent repetition of seizures without return to baseline; may result in anoxia and cardiac and respiratory arrest.	Consciousness not regained between seizures; lasts more than 30 minutes

- Usually unresponsive during tonic-clonic muscular contractions; may experience incontinence
- May be disoriented to time and place, drowsy, and uncoordinated immediately after seizure

DIAGNOSTIC TEST RESULTS
- EEG results help differentiate epileptic from nonepileptic seizures. Each seizure has a characteristic EEG tracing.

NURSING DIAGNOSES
- Risk for injury
- Ineffective airway clearance
- Disturbed sensory perception (tactile)

TREATMENT
- Drug therapy; if not responsive, ablative therapy
- Supportive until the seizure ends (maintaining airway, protecting from injury)

Drug therapy
- Antiepileptics: I.V. diazepam (Valium) or lorazepam (Ativan), phenobarbital (Luminal) or fosphenytoin (Cerebyx), phenytoin (Dilantin), valproic acid (Depakote), carbamazepine (Tegretol)

- Rectal diazepam (Diastat) for home management of intractable or prolonged seizures

INTERVENTIONS AND RATIONALES
- Monitor vital signs *to determine baseline and detect any changes.*
- Assess neurologic status *to monitor for change in neurologic status.*
- Stay with the child during a seizure *to prevent injury.*
- Move the child to a flat surface *to prevent falling.*
- Place the child on his side *to let saliva drain out, ensuring a patent airway.*
- Don't try to interrupt the seizure *to promote safety.*
- Gently support the head and keep the child's hands from inflicting self-harm, but don't restrain *to prevent injury.*
- Don't use tongue blades; *use of tongue blades during seizure activity may cause trauma to the mouth and result in airway obstruction from an aspirated tooth or laryngospasm.*
- Reduce external stimuli. *External stimuli could worsen seizure activity.*
- Loosen tight clothing *to promote comfort.*
- Record seizure activity. *Description of seizure activity helps to diagnose the type, which will aid in developing a treatment plan.*

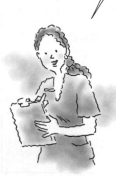

When a seizure occurs, assess neurologic status, move the child to a flat surface, place him on his side, and stay with him.

- Pad the crib or bed *to prevent injury.*
- Monitor serum levels of anticonvulsant medications, such as phenytoin, *to ensure therapeutic levels and prevent toxicity or subtherapeutic levels.*

Teaching topics
- Explanation of the disorder and treatment plan
- Medication use and possible adverse effects
- Importance of follow-up care
- Instituting safety measures during seizure activity

Spina bifida

Spina bifida is exposure of the spinal cord resulting from a defect of the back bone and spinal cord. It has two main forms. Spina bifida occulta, the more common and less severe form, is characterized by incomplete closure of one or more vertebrae without protrusion of the spinal cord or meninges (membranes covering the spinal cord). Spina bifida cystica, the more severe form, is distinguished by incomplete closure of one or more vertebrae that causes protrusion of the spinal contents in an external sac or cystic lesion.

Spina bifida cystica has two classifications:

myelomeningocele: an external sac that contains meninges, CSF, and a portion of the spinal cord or nerve roots

meningocele: an external sac that contains meninges and CSF.

CAUSES
- Combination of genetic and environmental factors
- Exposure to a teratogen
- Part of a multiple malformation syndrome (for example, chromosomal abnormalities such as trisomy 18 or 13 syndrome)
- Low intake of folic acid by the mother during pregnancy

ASSESSMENT FINDINGS
Spina bifida occulta
- Dimple or tuft of hair on the skin over the spinal defect

- No neurologic dysfunction (usually), except occasional foot weakness or bowel and bladder disturbances
- Port wine nevi (commonly found on the skin over the spinal defect)
- Soft fatty deposits (commonly found on the skin over the spinal defect)
- Trophic skin disturbances (ulcerations, cyanosis)

Meningocele
- No neurologic dysfunction (usually)
- Saclike structure protruding over the spine

Myelomeningocele
- Saclike structure protruding over the spine
- Hydrocephalus
- Permanent neurologic dysfunction (paralysis, bowel and bladder incontinence)
- Possible mental retardation
- Knee contractures
- Clubfoot
- Arnold-Chiari syndrome
- Curvature of the spine

DIAGNOSTIC TEST RESULTS
- Elevated alpha-fetoprotein levels in the mother's blood may indicate the presence of a neural tube defect.
- Amniocentesis reveals neural tube defect.
- Acetylcholinesterase measurement can be used to confirm the diagnosis.
- After birth, spinal X-ray can show the bone defect.
- Fetal karyotype should be done in addition to the biochemical tests because of the association of neural tube defects with chromosomal abnormalities.
- Myelography can differentiate spina bifida from other spinal abnormalities, especially spinal cord tumors.
- Ultrasound may identify the open neural tube or ventral wall defect.

NURSING DIAGNOSES
- Delayed growth and development
- Impaired physical mobility
- Impaired adjustment

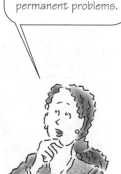

Hmmm. Spina bifida occulta and meningocele rarely cause neurologic dysfunction. However, myelomeningocele may cause permanent problems.

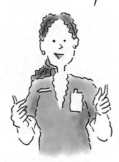

Remember, spina bifida occulta usually requires no treatment. Meningocele and myelomeningocele require surgery.

TREATMENT
- Meningocele: surgical closure of the protruding sac and continual assessment of growth and development
- Myelomeningocele: repair of the sac (doesn't reverse neurologic deficits) and supportive measures to promote independence and prevent further complications
- Spina bifida occulta: usually no treatment

INTERVENTIONS AND RATIONALES
Before surgery
- Hold and cuddle the infant on your lap and position him on his abdomen; handle the infant carefully, and don't apply pressure to the defect *to prevent injury at the site of the defect*.
- Clean the defect, inspect it often, and cover it with sterile dressings moistened with sterile saline solution *to prevent infection*.
- Place the infant in an infant Isolette *to prevent hypothermia*.
- Assess for signs of hydrocephalus. Measure head circumference daily. Be sure to mark the spot where the measurement was made *to ensure accurate readings*.
- Assess for signs of meningeal irritation, such as fever and nuchal rigidity, *to detect signs of meningitis*.
- Provide passive ROM exercises and casting. *To prevent hip dislocation, moderately abduct the hips with a pad between the knees or with sandbags and ankle rolls to prevent hip dislocation.*
- Monitor intake and output. Watch for decreased skin turgor and dryness *to detect dehydration*.

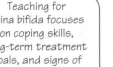

Teaching for spina bifida focuses on coping skills, long-term treatment goals, and signs of complications.

- Provide a diet high in calories and protein *to ensure adequate nutrition.*

After surgery
- Assess for hydrocephalus, which commonly follows surgery. Measure the infant's head circumference as ordered *to detect signs of hydrocephalus and prevent associated complications.*
- Monitor vital signs often *to detect early signs of shock, infection, and increased ICP.*
- Provide wound care and report any signs of drainage, wound rupture, and infection *to promote early treatment and prevent complications.*
- Place the infant in the prone position *to protect and assess the site.*
- If leg casts have been applied to treat deformities, regularly check distal pulses *to ensure adequate circulation.*
- When spina bifida is diagnosed prenatally, refer the prospective parents to a genetic counselor, *who can provide information and support the couple's decisions on how to manage the pregnancy.*

Teaching topics
- Explanation of the disorder and treatment plan
- Handling the infant without applying pressure to the defect
- Coping with the infant's physical problems
- Recognizing early signs of complications, such as hydrocephalus, pressure ulcers, and urinary tract infections
- Maintaining a positive attitude and working through feelings of guilt, anger, and helplessness
- Conducting intermittent catheterization and conduit hygiene
- Bowel training when the child is older
- Recognizing developmental lags (a possible result of hydrocephalus)
- Planning activities appropriate to their child's age and abilities

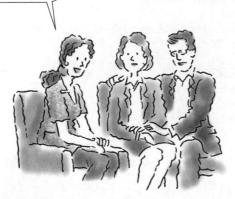

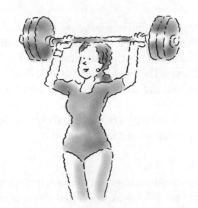

Pump up on practice questions

1. The nurse is assessing a child who may have meningitis. For which of the following assessment findings should the nurse watch?
1. Flat fontanel
2. Irritability, fever, and vomiting
3. Jaundice, drowsiness, and refusal to eat
4. Negative Kernig's sign

Answer: 2. Assessment findings associated with acute bacterial meningitis include irritability, fever, and vomiting along with seizure activity. Fontanels would be bulging as intracranial pressure rises, and Kernig's sign would be present because of meningeal irritation. Jaundice, drowsiness, and refusal to eat may indicate GI disturbance rather than meningitis.

➡ *NCLEX keys*
Client needs category: Physiological integrity
Client needs subcategory: Physiological adaptation
Cognitive level: Application

2. A nurse is assessing a child who may have a seizure disorder. Which option is a description of an absence seizure?
1. Sudden, momentary loss of muscle tone
2. Minimal or no alteration in muscle tone, with a brief loss of consciousness

3. Muscle tone maintained and child frozen into position
4. Brief, sudden contracture of a muscle or muscle group

Answer: 2. Absence seizures are characterized by a brief loss of responsiveness with minimal or no alteration in muscle tone. They may go unrecognized because the child's behavior changes very little. A sudden loss of muscle tone describes atonic seizures. "Frozen positions" describe akinetic seizures. A brief, sudden contraction of muscles describes a myoclonic seizure.

➡ *NCLEX keys*
Client needs category: Physiological integrity
Client needs subcategory: Physiological adaptation
Cognitive level: Knowledge

3. A nurse is caring for a child who's experiencing a seizure. Which nursing intervention takes highest priority when caring for this child?
1. Protect the child from injury.
2. Use a padded tongue blade to protect the airway.
3. Shout at the child to end the seizure.
4. Allow seizure activity to end without interference.

Answer: 1. The nurse should identify the seizure type and protect the child from injury. A padded tongue blade should never be used because it can cause damage to the mouth and airway. Shouting will only agitate or confuse the child. Interfering with seizure activity may cause injury to the child. Allowing the seizure activity to end without interference may cause the child injury. The nurse should position the child on his side to ensure a patent airway and place the child on the ground if he's likely to fall and sustain injury.

➡ *NCLEX keys*
Client needs category: Physiological integrity
Client needs subcategory: Reduction of risk potential
Cognitive level: Analysis

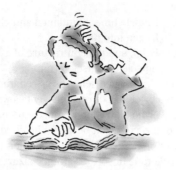

4.   A nurse is caring for a 3-year-old child with viral meningitis. Which signs and symptoms should the nurse expect to find during the initial assessment? Select all that apply.
1.   Bulging anterior fontanel
2.   Fever
3.   Nuchal rigidity
4.   Petechiae
5.   Irritability
6.   Photophobia

Answer: 2, 3, 5, 6. Common signs and symptoms of viral meningitis include fever, nuchal rigidity, irritability, and photophobia. A bulging anterior fontanel is a sign of hydrocephalus, which isn't likely to occur in a toddler because the anterior fontanel typically closes by age 24 months. A petechial, purpuric rash may be seen with bacterial meningitis.

➡ *NCLEX keys*

Client needs category: Physiological integrity
Client needs subcategory: Physiological adaptation
Cognitive level: Application

5.   A nurse is caring for an infant with spina bifida. Which assessment findings suggest hydrocephalus?
1.   Depressed fontanels and suture lines
2.   Deep-set eyes, which appear to look upward only
3.   Rapid increase in head size and irritability
4.   Motor and sensory dysfunction in the foot and leg

Answer: 3. Hydrocephalus is an increase in the amount of cerebrospinal fluid in the ventricles and subarachnoid spaces of the brain.

Assessment findings associated with hydrocephalus include a rapid increase in head size, irritability, suture line separation, and bulging fontanels. The eyes appear to look downward only, with the cornea prominent over the iris (sunset sign). A loss of sensory and motor function is related to the spinal cord defect spina bifida — not hydrocephalus.

➡ *NCLEX keys*

Client needs category: Physiological integrity
Client needs subcategory: Reduction of risk potential
Cognitive level: Application

6.   A nurse is teaching a father whose infant has had several episodes of otitis media. Which statement made by the father indicates that he needs further teaching?
1.   "Children who live in homes where family members smoke have fewer infections."
2.   "The eustachian tube in infants is shorter and less angled than in older children."
3.   "Breast-feeding is one way to help decrease the number of infections."
4.   "I wrap him up and always put a hat on him when we go out."

Answer: 1. Children who live in households where smoking occurs have a greater number of respiratory infections that lead to otitis media, not fewer. The other statements about otitis media are correct.

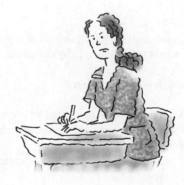

➡ *NCLEX keys*
Client needs category: Health promotion and maintenance
Client needs subcategory: None
Cognitive level: Application

7. A school nurse is monitoring several children with attention deficit hyperactivity disorder who are taking methylphenidate (Ritalin). The nurse should conduct monthly follow-up examinations to monitor:

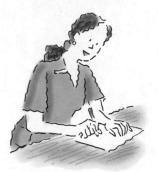

1. whether the child is experiencing dry mouth.
2. whether the child is growing in height.
3. the parent's coping abilities from the child's perspective.
4. when the child is taking the medication.

Answer: 2. Common adverse reactions to methylphenidate include slowed growth in height, sleeplessness, decreased appetite, and crying. Dry mouth is a common adverse reaction to tricyclic antidepressants. Knowing how the parents are coping from the child's perspective may be helpful information but isn't the priority. Knowing when the child takes the medication would be important if the child has problems with sleeplessness.

➡ *NCLEX keys*
Client needs category: Physiological integrity
Client needs subcategory: Pharmacological and parenteral therapies
Cognitive level: Application

8. A nurse is teaching the mother of a child with attention deficit hyperactivity disorder (ADHD) how to manage the child. Which statement by the mother indicates that she needs further teaching?

1. "I give him only one direction at a time."
2. "I encourage my child to ride his bike after school."
3. "My child enjoys rollerblading with friends."
4. "I have my child do homework right after school."

Answer: 4. Children with ADHD need time to expend their energy after being in a restrictive environment such as school. They need time to participate in activities that they enjoy, such as running, bike riding, or inline skating. Homework should be done later in the evening, not right after school. The other statements indicate effective teaching.

➡ *NCLEX keys*
Client needs category: Psychosocial integrity
Client needs subcategory: None
Cognitive level: Application

9. A nurse is caring for an infant with spina bifida. Which technique should the nurse anticipate that the physician will use to diagnose hydrocephalus?

1. Measurement of head circumference
2. Skull X-ray showing a thinning skull
3. Angiography revealing hydrocephalus
4. Magnetic resonance imaging (MRI) revealing hydrocephalus

Answer: 1. Measuring head circumference is the most important assessment technique for diagnosing hydrocephalus and is a key part of the routine infant screening. Skull X-rays, angiography, and MRI may be used to confirm the diagnosis.

➡ *NCLEX keys*
Client needs category: Health promotion and maintenance
Client needs subcategory: None
Cognitive level: Application

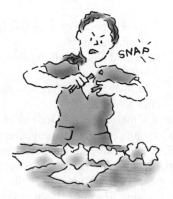

10. A nurse is caring for a child after shunt insertion to relieve hydrocephalus. Which intervention should the nurse perform?
   1. Place the child in an upright position.
   2. Avoid lying the child on the side where the shunt is located.
   3. Place the child in the semi-Fowler position.
   4. Place the child in a prone position.
Answer: 2. After the shunt is inserted, the nurse shouldn't lie the child on the side of the body where the shunt is located. The child should lie supine to avoid rapid decompression. The child shouldn't be in an upright, semi-Fowler, or prone position.

➡ *NCLEX keys*
Client needs category: Physiological integrity
Client needs subcategory: Reduction of risk potential
Cognitive level: Application

Congratulations! Finishing this chapter shows you have a lot of nerve!

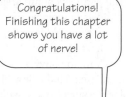

31 Musculoskeletal system

In this chapter, you'll review:

📖 the pediatric musculoskeletal system

📖 tests used to diagnose musculoskeletal disorders

📖 common pediatric musculoskeletal disorders.

Brush up on key concepts

The musculoskeletal system is a complex system of **bones, muscles, ligaments, tendons,** and other **connective tissues.** The functions of the musculoskeletal system include:
- giving the body form and shape
- protecting vital organs
- making movement possible
- storing calcium and other minerals
- providing the site for hematopoiesis (blood cell formation).

At any point, you can review the major points of this chapter by consulting the *Cheat sheet* on pages 664 and 665.

Growing pains

Here are a few facts about the **pediatric musculoskeletal system:**
- Bones and muscles grow and develop throughout childhood.
- Bone lengthening occurs in the epiphyseal plates at the ends of bones; when the epiphyses close, growth stops.
- Bone healing occurs much faster in the child than in the adult because the child's bones are still growing.
- The younger the child, the faster the bone heals.
- Bone healing takes approximately 1 week for every year of life up to age 10.

Fractured logic

The most common fractures in the child are **clavicular fractures** and **greenstick fractures:**
- Clavicular fractures may occur during vaginal birth because the shoulders are the widest part of the body.

- Greenstick fractures of the long bones are related to the increased flexibility of the young child's bones. (The compressed side of the bone bends while the side under tension fractures.)

Keep abreast of diagnostic tests

Here are the most important tests used to diagnose musculoskeletal disorders, along with common nursing interventions associated with each test.

Using physical examination to assess the child's musculoskeletal function and ability is also an important element in diagnosis. (See *Assessing musculoskeletal function and ability*, page 666.)

Look inside the joint

Arthroscopy is the visual examination of the interior of a joint with a fiber-optic endoscope.

Nursing actions
- Explain the procedure to the parents and child.
- Make sure that written, informed consent has been obtained.
- Tell the child and his parents that he may need to fast after midnight before the procedure.
- Note allergies because local anesthesia is used.
- Tell the child that he may feel a thumping sensation as the cannula is inserted in the joint capsule.

Soft-tissue sighting

A **computed tomography scan** is used to identify injuries to the soft tissue, ligaments, tendons, and muscles.

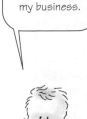

Growing is my business.

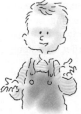

(Text continues on page 666.)

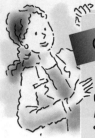

Musculoskeletal refresher

CLUBFOOT

Key signs and symptoms
• Inability to manually correct the deformity (distinguishes true clubfoot from apparent clubfoot)

Key test results
• X-rays show superimposition of the talus and calcaneus and a ladderlike appearance of the metatarsals.

Key treatments
• Correction of the deformity with a series of casts or surgical correction
• Maintenance of correction until the foot gains normal muscle balance
• Close observation of the foot for several years to prevent the deformity from recurring

Key interventions
• Ensure that shoes fit correctly.
• Prepare for surgery, if necessary.

DEVELOPMENTAL HIP DYSPLASIA

Key signs and symptoms
• Increased number of folds on the posterior thigh on the affected side when the child is supine with knees bent
• Appearance of a shortened limb on the affected side
• Restricted abduction of the hips

Key test results
• Barlow's sign: A click is felt when the infant is placed in a supine position with the hips flexed 90 degrees and when the knees are fully flexed and the hip is brought into midabduction.
• Ortolani's click: It can be felt by the fingers at the hip area as the femur head snaps out of and back into the acetabulum. It's also palpable during examination with the child's legs flexed and abducted.
• Positive Trendelenburg's test: When the child stands on the affected leg, the opposite pelvis dips to maintain erect posture.

Key treatments
• Hip-spica cast or corrective surgery (for older children)
• Bryant's traction, if the acetabulum doesn't deepen
• Pavlik harness or casting to keep the neonate's hips and knees flexed and the hips abducted for at least 3 months

Key interventions
• Provide reassurance that early, prompt treatment commonly results in complete correction.
• Reassure the parents that the child will adjust to restricted movement and return to normal sleeping, eating and playing behavior in a few days.

DUCHENNE'S MUSCULAR DYSTROPHY

Key signs and symptoms
• Begins with pelvic girdle weakness, indicated by waddling gait and falling
• Eventual muscle weakness and wasting
• Gowers' sign (use of hands to push self up from floor)

Key test results
• Electromyography typically demonstrates short, weak bursts of electrical activity in the affected muscles.
• Muscle biopsy shows variation in the size of muscle fibers and, in later stages, shows fat and connective tissue deposits, with no dystrophin.

Key treatments
• Physical therapy
• Surgery to correct contractures
• Use of devices, such as splints, braces, trapeze bars, overhead slings, and a wheelchair, to help preserve mobility

Key interventions
• Perform range-of-motion exercises.
• Encourage coughing, deep-breathing exercises, and diaphragmatic breathing.
• Encourage adequate fluid intake, increase dietary fiber, and obtain an order for a stool softener.

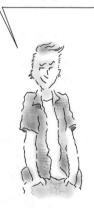

Don't worry. If you use the *Cheat sheet*, I promise I won't tell.

Musculoskeletal refresher *(continued)*

FRACTURES
Key signs and symptoms
- Pain or tenderness
- Skeletal deformity
- Swelling
- Loss of motor function
- Muscle spasm

Key test results
- X-rays confirm the location and type of fracture.

Key treatments
- Reduction and immobilization of the fracture
- Casting
- Surgery: open reduction and external fixation of the fracture

Key interventions
- Keep the affected extremity in proper body alignment.
- Provide support above and below the fracture site when moving the child.
- Elevate the fracture above the level of the heart.
- Apply ice to the fracture to promote vasoconstriction.
- Monitor pulses distal to the fracture every 2 to 4 hours.
- Assess color, temperature, and capillary refill of the affected extremity.

JUVENILE RHEUMATOID ARTHRITIS
Key signs and symptoms
- Inflammation around joints
- Stiffness, pain, and guarding of affected joints

Key test results
- Hematology reveals an elevated erythrocyte sedimentation rate, a positive antinuclear antibody test, and the presence of rheumatoid factor.

Key treatments
- Heat therapy: warm compresses, baths
- Splint application

Key interventions
- Monitor the joints for deformity.

LEGG-CALVE-PERTHES DISEASE
Key signs and symptoms
- Mild hip, thigh, or knee pain
- Persistent thigh or leg pain
- Shortening of affected leg

Key test results
- Hip X-ray confirms the diagnosis, with the findings based on the stage of the disease.

Key treatments
- Bed rest
- Reduced weight-bearing therapy
- Analgesics: acetaminophen (Tylenol), ibuprofen (Motrin)

Key interventions
- Maintain the child on bed rest.
- Provide stimulation for the child on bed rest.
- Monitor for circulatory or neurologic changes in the leg.

OSGOOD-SCHLATTER DISEASE
Key signs and symptoms
- Aching and pain over tibial tubercle
- Swelling
- Tenderness

Key test results
- X-rays show epiphyseal separation and soft tissue swelling in first 6 months after onset; eventually show bone fragmentation.

Key treatments
- Conservative treatment: designed to decrease stress to affected knee
- Avoiding strenuous exercise for the affected knee
- Analgesics: acetaminophen (Tylenol), ibuprofen (Motrin)

Key interventions
- Monitor the child for circulatory or neurologic changes in the leg.

SCOLIOSIS
Key signs and symptoms
- One shoulder higher than the other
- Uneven waist
- Forward bend test with asymmetry of the trunk or abnormal spinal curve

Key test results
- Spinal X-rays identify the degree of deformity.
- Scoliometer measures the amount of curvature.

Key treatments
- Observation for curves 25 to 40 degrees for a child with completed growth
- Bracing for curves above 25 to 30 degrees in a growing child
- Surgery for curves 40 degrees or greater

Key interventions
- Assess brace fit.
After spinal fusion and insertion of rods
- Turn the child by logrolling only.
- Maintain the child in correct body alignment.
- Maintain the bed in a flat position.

Management moments

Assessing musculoskeletal function and ability

To assess a child's musculoskeletal function and ability, perform the following nursing actions:
• Determine the range of motion.
• Note the amount of weight the child can bear.
• Assess gross and fine motor abilities.
• Note whether both arms and legs are used.
• Note whether muscle response is brisk and strong.
• Assess for pain; note whether the child is guarding a body part.
• Determine the relationship of the child's body size or weight to the defect.
• Note whether the child has an adequate and even spread of adipose tissue.
• Note the child's autonomy and independence in terms of mobility and skills.

Nursing actions
• Explain the procedure to the parents and child.
• Make sure written, informed consent has been obtained.
• Tell the child to hold still during the procedure.
• Tell the child that he'll be placed in a tube-like circle for the study and that pictures will be taken of the extremity.

Cross-section check
Magnetic resonance imaging (MRI) allows cross-sectional imaging of bones and joints. MRI, which uses a strong magnetic field and radio waves, has largely replaced arthrography for assessing joint anatomy.

No ionizing radiation is used. MRI studies are also used to assess certain muscle and soft-tissue injuries.

Nursing actions
• Explain the procedure to the parents and child.
• Make sure written, informed consent has been obtained.
• Instruct the child to hold still during the procedure.
• Note whether the child has any metal implants, which may interfere with the study.

Spinal vision
Myelography is an invasive procedure used to evaluate abnormalities of the spinal canal

and cord. It entails injection of a radiopaque contrast medium into the subarachnoid space of the spine. Serial X-rays are then used to visualize the progress of the contrast medium as it passes through the subarachnoid space.

Nursing actions
• Explain the procedure to the parents and child.
• Make sure that written, informed consent has been obtained.
• Before the test, check for allergies to the contrast medium.
• If metrizamide (Amipaque) is used as the contrast medium, discontinue phenothiazines 48 hours before the test.
• When the contrast medium is injected, tell the child that he may experience a burning sensation, warmth, headache, salty taste, nausea, and vomiting.
• After the test, have the child sit in his room or lie in bed with his head elevated 60 degrees. He must not lie flat for at least 8 hours.
• Encourage the child to drink extra fluids.
• Check that the child voids within 8 hours after returning to his room.

Hard tissue check
X-rays are probably the most useful diagnostic tool to evaluate musculoskeletal diseases. They can help to identify joint disruption, calcifications, and bone deformities,

> X-rays are excellent! They're a great tool for identifying calcifications, bone deformities, and fractures as well as bone density.

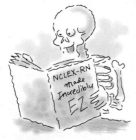

fractures, and destruction as well as measure bone density.

Nursing actions
- Explain the test to the parents and child.
- Tell the child that he must hold still during the X-ray. Cover the genital area with a lead apron.

Polish up on client care

Musculoskeletal disorders in children include clubfoot (talipes), developmental hip dysplasia (dislocated hip), Duchenne's muscular dystrophy, fractures, juvenile rheumatoid arthritis (JRA), Legg-Calve-Perthes disease, Osgood-Schlatter disease, and scoliosis.

Clubfoot

Clubfoot, also known as *talipes,* is a congenital disorder in which the foot and ankle are twisted and can't be manipulated into correct position.

Clubfoot occurs in these five forms:
- equinovarus: combination of positions
- talipes calcaneus: dorsiflexion, as if walking on one's heels
- talipes equinus: plantar flexion, as if pointing one's toes
- talipes valgus: eversion of the ankles, with the feet turning out
- talipes varus: inversion of the ankles, with the soles of the feet facing each other.

CAUSES
- Arrested development during the 9th and 10th weeks of embryonic life, when the feet are formed
- Deformed talus and shortened Achilles tendon
- Possible genetic predisposition
- Intrauterine positioning

ASSESSMENT FINDINGS
- Deformity usually obvious at birth
- Inability to manually correct the deformity (distinguishes true clubfoot from apparent clubfoot)

DIAGNOSTIC TEST RESULTS
- X-rays show superimposition of the talus and calcaneus and a ladderlike appearance of the metatarsals.

NURSING DIAGNOSES
- Delayed growth and development
- Impaired physical mobility
- Risk for peripheral neurovascular dysfunction

TREATMENT
Treatment is administered in three stages:

correcting the deformity either with a series of casts to gradually stretch and realign the angle of the foot and, after cast removal, application of a Denis Browne splint at night until age 1 or surgical correction

maintaining the correction until the foot gains normal muscle balance

observing the foot closely for several years to prevent the deformity from recurring.

INTERVENTIONS AND RATIONALES
- Assess neurovascular status *to ensure circulation to the foot with the cast in place.*
- Ensure that shoes fit correctly *to promote comfort and prevent skin breakdown.*
- Prepare for surgery, if necessary, *to maintain or promote the healing process and decrease anxiety.*

Teaching topics
- Explanation of the disorder and treatment plan
- Using a blow-dryer on the cool setting to provide relief from itching
- Importance of placing nothing inside the cast
- Keeping corrective devices on as much as possible
- Walking as exercise after surgical repair

Developmental hip dysplasia

Developmental hip dysplasia (dislocated hip) results from an abnormal development of the hip socket. It occurs when the head of the

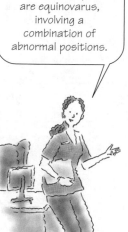

Combos are common. Nearly all cases of talipes are equinovarus, involving a combination of abnormal positions.

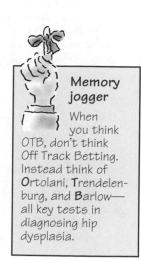

Memory jogger

When you think OTB, don't think Off Track Betting. Instead think of Ortolani, Trendelenburg, and Barlow—all key tests in diagnosing hip dysplasia.

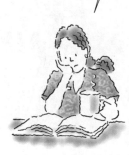

What's the common goal of treatment for developmental hip dysplasia? Enlarging and deepening the socket (acetabulum) through pressure.

femur is still cartilaginous and the acetabulum (socket) is shallow; as a result, the head of the femur comes out of the hip socket. It can affect one or both hips and occurs in varying degrees of dislocation, from partial (subluxation) to complete.

CAUSES
- Breech delivery
- Fetal position in utero
- Genetic predisposition
- Laxity of the ligaments

ASSESSMENT FINDINGS
- Increased number of folds on the posterior thigh on the affected side when the child is supine with knees bent
- Appearance of a shortened limb on the affected side
- Restricted abduction of the hips

DIAGNOSTIC TEST RESULTS
- Barlow's sign is present: A click is felt when the infant is placed supine with hips flexed 90 degrees, knees fully flexed, and the hip brought into midabduction.
- Ortolani's click is present. It can be felt by the fingers at the hip area as the femur head snaps out of and back into the acetabulum. It's also palpable during examination with the child's legs flexed and abducted.
- Sonography and MRI may be used to assess reduction.
- Trendelenburg's test is positive. When the child stands on the affected leg, the opposite pelvis dips to maintain erect posture.
- Ultrasonography shows the involved cartilage and acetabulum.
- X-rays show the location of the femur head and a shallow acetabulum; X-rays can also be used to monitor progression of the disorder.

NURSING DIAGNOSES
- Delayed growth and development
- Impaired physical mobility
- Risk for impaired skin integrity

TREATMENT
- Hip-spica cast or corrective surgery (for older children)
- Bryant's traction, if the acetabulum doesn't deepen

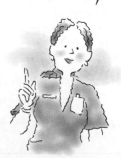

Here's a hint for early assessment: Duchenne's muscular dystrophy begins with a waddling gait and falling. This indicates pelvic girdle weakness.

- Pavlik harness or casting to keep the neonate's hips and knees flexed and the hips abducted for at least 3 months

INTERVENTIONS AND RATIONALES
- Assess circulation before application of a cast or traction; after application, have the child wiggle his toes *to detect signs of impaired circulation.* One finger should fit between the child's skin and the cast.
- Provide skin care *to prevent skin breakdown.*
- Provide reassurance that early, prompt treatment commonly results in complete correction *to decrease anxiety.*
- Reassure the parents that the child will adjust to restricted movement and return to normal sleeping, eating, and play in a few days *to ease anxiety.*
- Inspect the skin, especially around bony prominences, *to detect cast complications and skin breakdown.*

Teaching topics
- Explanation of the disorder and treatment plan
- Correctly splinting or bracing the hips
- Receiving frequent checkups
- Coping with restricted movement
- Removing braces and splints while bathing the child and replacing them immediately afterward
- Stressing good hygiene

Duchenne's muscular dystrophy

A genetic disorder (defect on the X chromosome) that occurs only in males, Duchenne's muscular dystrophy (also called *pseudohypertrophic dystrophy*) is marked by muscular deterioration due to a lack of production of dystrophin that progresses throughout childhood. The absence of dystrophin results in breakdown of muscle fibers. Muscle fibers are replaced with fatty deposits and collagen in muscles. There's no known cure. It generally results in death from cardiac or respiratory failure in the late teens or early 20s.

CAUSES
• Sex-linked recessive trait

ASSESSMENT FINDINGS
• Begins with pelvic girdle weakness, indicated by waddling gait and falling
• Cardiac or pulmonary failure
• Decreased ability to perform self-care activities
• Delayed motor development
• Eventual contractures and muscle hypertrophy
• Eventual muscle weakness and wasting
• Gowers' sign (use of hands to push self up from floor)
• Toe-walking

DIAGNOSTIC TEST RESULTS
• Electromyography typically demonstrates short, weak bursts of electrical activity in affected muscles.
• Muscle biopsy shows variations in the size of muscle fibers and, in later stages, shows fat and connective tissue deposits, with no dystrophin.

NURSING DIAGNOSES
• Impaired physical mobility
• Activity intolerance
• Impaired gas exchange

TREATMENT
• High-fiber, high-protein, low-calorie diet
• Physical therapy
• Surgery to correct contractures
• Use of devices, such as splints, braces, trapeze bars, overhead slings, and a wheelchair, to help preserve mobility
• Gene therapy (under investigation to prevent muscle degeneration)

INTERVENTIONS AND RATIONALES
• Perform range-of-motion (ROM) exercises *to promote joint mobility.*
• Provide emotional support to the child and parents *to decrease anxiety and promote coping mechanisms.*
• Initiate genetic counseling *to inform the child and family about passing the disorder on to future children.*
• Encourage coughing, deep-breathing exercises, and diaphragmatic breathing *to maintain a patent airway and mobilize secretions to prevent complications associated with retained secretions.*
• Encourage the use of a footboard or high-topped sneakers and a foot cradle *to increase comfort and prevent footdrop.*
• Encourage adequate fluid intake, increase dietary fiber, and obtain an order for a stool softener *to prevent constipation associated with inactivity.*

Teaching topics
• Explanation of the disorder and treatment plan
• Recognizing early signs of respiratory complications
• Planning a low-calorie, high-protein, high-fiber diet
• Promoting physical activity within limitations of the disorder
• Promoting peer interaction and preventing social isolation

Fractures

A fracture is a break in the bone's integrity. A complete fracture breaks entirely across, resulting in a break in the continuity of the bone. An incomplete fracture extends only partially through the bone, and the bone remains continuous. In a closed or simple fracture, the break doesn't puncture the skin surface, whereas an open or compound fracture punctures through the skin surface.

Common sites of fractures include the long bones of the arms and legs, clavicle, and knee. The outcome usually depends on the severity of the fracture and the treatment provided. Potential complications include the development of fat emboli, improper bone growth, compartment syndrome, and infection.

CAUSES
• Childhood accidents, such as falls and motor vehicle crashes (most common cause)
• Child abuse
• Pathologic conditions

ASSESSMENT FINDINGS
• Pain or tenderness
• Skeletal deformity

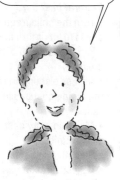

With Duchenne's muscular dystrophy, the goal is to help the child remain as active and independent as possible.

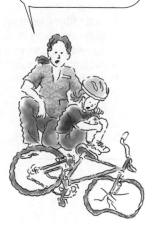

Accidents are the number one cause of fractures in childhood.

Common orthopedic treatments

The use of casts, traction, and braces are common orthopedic treatments.

CASTS

A cast is a hard mold that encases a body part, usually an extremity, to provide immobilization without discomfort.

General cast care

• Turn the child frequently to dry all sides of the cast; use the palms to lift or turn a wet cast to prevent indentations.
• Expose as much of the cast to air as possible to promote drying.
• Assess discomfort in the child because chemical changes in the drying cast cause temperature extremes against the child's skin.
• Maintain a dry cast; wetting the cast softens it and may cause skin irritation.
• Smooth out the cast's rough edges, and petal the edges.
• Assess circulation:
  – Note the capillary refill, color, temperature, and edema of digits.
  – Note the child's ability to wiggle the extremities without tingling or numbness.
• Assess any drainage or foul odor from the cast.
• Prevent small objects or food from falling into the cast.
• Avoid using powder on the skin near the cast; it becomes a medium for bacteria when it absorbs perspiration.

Hip-spica cast care

A hip-spica cast is a body cast extending from the midchest to the legs. The legs are abducted with a bar between them.
• Perform cast care as listed above but with additional measures.
• Line the back edges of the cast with plastic or other water-proof material.
• Keep the cast level but on a slant, with the head of the bed raised (a Bradford frame can be used for this purpose):
  – The body and cast should stay at 180 degrees.
  – The head of the bed is raised on shock blocks or the mattress is raised using a wedge pillow so that the child is on a slant with the head up.
  – Urine and stools drain downward away from the cast.
• Use a mattress firm enough to support the cast; use pillows to support parts of the cast, if needed.
• Reposition frequently to avoid pressure on the skin and the bony prominences; check for pressure as the child grows.

TRACTION

Traction decreases muscle spasms and realigns and positions bone ends by pulling on the distal ends of bones.
• Skin traction pulls indirectly on the skeleton by pulling on the skin with adhesive, moleskin, or elastic bandage.
• Skeletal traction pulls directly on the skeleton with surgically placed pins or tongs.

Traction-related care

• Check that the weights hang free from the bed.
• Monitor for skin irritation, infection at pin sites, and neurovascular response of the extremity.
• Encourage fluids and fiber to prevent constipation.
• Promote pulmonary hygiene using blowing games.
• Provide pain relief through positioning and analgesics.
• Provide stimulation appropriate for the child's age.

Bryant's traction

This skin traction is designed specifically for the lower extremities of the child younger than age 2; the child's body weight provides countertraction. Traction may be followed by application of a hip-spica cast.
• Keep the legs straight and extended 90 degrees toward the ceiling from the trunk (both legs are suspended even if only one is affected).
• Keep the buttocks slightly off the bed to ensure sufficient and continuous traction on the legs.

BRACES

A brace is a plastic shell or metal-hinged appliance that aids mobility and posture.

Brace-related care

• Provide good skin care, especially at the bony prominences.
• Check to ensure accurate fit as the child grows.

Milwaukee brace

This type of brace attempts to slow the progression of spinal curvature of less than 40 degrees until bone growth stops. It can be used until the child reaches skeletal maturity.
• Monitor the use of the brace. It must be worn 20 to 23 hours a day; it may be removed for bathing.

Boston brace

This type of brace functions the same as a Milwaukee brace.
• Make sure the brace extends from the axillary area to the iliac crest.
• Remove the brace for bathing.

- Swelling
- Bony crepitus
- Bruising
- Impaired sensation
- Loss of motor function
- Muscle spasm
- Paralysis
- Paresthesia

DIAGNOSTIC TEST RESULTS

- X-rays confirm the location and type of fracture.

NURSING DIAGNOSES

- Ineffective peripheral tissue perfusion
- Acute pain
- Risk for impaired skin integrity
- Impaired physical mobility

TREATMENT

- Reduction and immobilization of the fracture
- Casting
- Surgery: open reduction and external fixation of the fracture
- Traction, depending on the site of the fracture (see *Common orthopedic treatments*)

Drug therapy

Nonsteroidal anti-inflammatory drug (NSAID): ibuprofen (Motrin)

INTERVENTIONS AND RATIONALES

- Keep the affected extremity in proper body alignment *to promote bone healing and prevent tissue damage.*
- Provide support above and below the fracture site when moving the child *to promote comfort.*
- Monitor pressure areas affected by traction or the child's cast *to prevent impaired tissue perfusion.*
- Elevate the fracture above the level of the heart *to promote venous return and decrease edema.*
- Apply ice to the fracture to promote vasoconstriction, *which inhibits edema and pain.*
- Monitor pulses distal to the fracture every 2 to 4 hours *to assess blood flow to the distal extremity.*
- Assess color, temperature, and capillary refill *to determine whether the affected extremity is adequately perfused.*

- Assess sensation *to determine whether perfusion to the nerves is intact.*
- Assess pain level utilizing pediatric assessment tools and administer analgesia *to provide comfort.*
- Turn and reposition the child every 2 hours *to help relieve skin pressure and prevent skin breakdown.*
- Protect the cast from moisture and petal the edges *to promote healing of the fracture and prevent skin breakdown.*

Teaching topics

- Explanation of the injury and treatment plan
- Caring for a child in cast or traction
- Preventing injury
- Reporting signs of infection or complications

Juvenile rheumatoid arthritis

JRA is an autoimmune disease of the connective tissue. It's characterized by chronic inflammation of the synovia and possible joint destruction. Episodes recur with remissions and exacerbations.

The three main forms of JRA are:
- pauciarticular JRA — asymmetrical involvement of less than five joints, usually affecting large joints such as the knees, ankles, and elbows.
- polyarticular JRA — symmetrical involvement of five or more joints, especially the hands and weight-bearing joints, such as the hips, knees, and feet. Involvement of the temporomandibular joint may cause earache; involvement of the sternoclavicular joint may cause chest pain.
- systemic disease with polyarthritis — involves the lining of the heart and lungs, blood cells, and abdominal organs. Exacerbations may last for months. Fever, rash, and lymphadenopathy may occur.

CAUSES

- Autoimmune response
- Genetic predisposition

ASSESSMENT FINDINGS

- Inflammation around the joints
- Stiffness, pain, and guarding of the affected joints

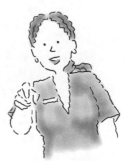

JRA typically involves the joints but can also affect the heart, lungs, liver, and spleen.

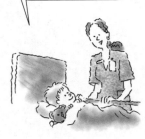

Oh brother! Legg-Calve-Perthes disease occurs most commonly in boys and is seen in families.

DIAGNOSTIC TEST RESULTS
• Hematology reveals an elevated erythrocyte sedimentation rate, a positive antinuclear antibody test, and the presence of rheumatoid factor.
• Slit-lamp evaluation may show iridocyclitis (inflammation of the iris and the ciliary body).

NURSING DIAGNOSES
• Impaired physical mobility
• Chronic pain
• Disturbed body image

TREATMENT
• Heat therapy: warm compresses, baths
• Splint application

Drug therapy
• Low-dose corticosteroids
• Low-dose methotrexate (Trexall) (used as a second-line medication)
• NSAIDs: naproxen (Naprosyn), ibuprofen (Motrin)

INTERVENTIONS AND RATIONALES
• Monitor the joints for deformity *to assess for early changes as a complication of this disease process.*
• Administer medications as prescribed and note the effectiveness *to relieve pain and prevent further joint damage.*
• Assist with exercise and ROM activities *to maintain joint mobility.*
• Apply warm compresses or encourage the child to take a warm bath in the morning *to promote comfort and increase mobility.*
• Apply splints *to maintain position of function and prevent contractures.*
• Provide assistive devices, if necessary, *to encourage the normal performance of daily activities.*

Teaching topics
• Explanation of the disorder and treatment plan
• Medication use and possible adverse effects
• Understanding how stress and climate can influence exacerbations
• ROM exercises

Legg-Calve-Perthes disease

Legg-Calve-Perthes disease is ischemic necrosis that leads to eventual flattening of the head of the femur caused by vascular interruption. Legg-Calve-Perthes disease occurs most commonly in boys ages 4 to 10 and tends to occur in families.

The disease occurs in five stages:
• Growth arrest: avascular phase; may last 6 to 12 months. Early changes include inflammation and synovitis of the hip and ischemic changes in the ossific nucleus of the femoral head.
• Subchondral fracture: Radiographic visualization of the fracture varies with the age of the child at clinical onset and the extent of epiphyseal involvement; may last 3 to 8 months.
• Reabsorption, also called *fragmentation* or *necrosis:* The necrotic bone beneath the subchondral fracture is gradually and irregularly reabsorbed; lasts 6 to 12 months.
• Reossification or healing stage: Ossification of the primary bone begins irregularly in the subchondral area and progresses centrally; takes 6 to 24 months.
• Healed stage, also called *residual stage:* Complete ossification of the epiphysis of the femoral head, with or without residual deformity.

CAUSES
• Unknown
• Theories include trauma, vascular irregularities, increased blood viscosity leading to statis, decreased blood flow

ASSESSMENT FINDINGS
• Mild hip, thigh, or knee pain
• Shortening of affected leg
• Muscle spasm
• Persistent thigh or leg pain
• Muscle atrophy in upper thigh
• Severely restricted abduction and internal rotation of hip

DIAGNOSTIC TEST RESULTS
• Hip X-ray confirms the diagnosis, with the findings based on the stage of the disease.
• MRI helps enhance early diagnosis of necrosis.

NURSING DIAGNOSES

- Impaired physical mobility
- Disturbed body image
- Chronic pain
- Delayed growth and development

TREATMENT

- Bed rest
- Therapy with reduced weight bearing
- Splint, cast, or brace to hold leg in abduction (brace may remain for as long as 18 months)
- Physical therapy after cast removal
- Osteotomy and subtrochanteric derotation: to allow femoral head to return to normal shape (in early stages)

Drug therapy

- Analgesics: acetaminophen (Tylenol), ibuprofen (Motrin)

INTERVENTIONS AND RATIONALES

- Maintain the child on bed rest *to protect the femoral head from further stress and damage.*
- Administer medications, as prescribed, *to reduce the child's pain.*
- Provide stimulation for the child on bed rest *to help promote growth and development.*
- Monitor and record the patient's intake and output and dietary intake. *This helps ensure the child has a diet sufficient for growth without causing excessive weight gain.*
- If the child is in a cast, provide cast care *to help maintain skin integrity.*
- Reposition the child every 2 to 3 hours *to help prevent skin breakdown.*
- Monitor the child for circulatory or neurologic changes in the leg, *which could indicate neurovascular compromise.*
- Provide emotional support to the child and his family.

Teaching topics

- Explanation of the disorder and treatment plan
- Medication use and possible adverse effects
- Following up with physician and therapy appointments
- Importance of socialization

Osgood-Schlatter disease

Osgood-Schlatter disease, also called *osteochondrosis,* is a painful, incomplete separation of the epiphysis of the tibial tubercle from the tibial shaft. This is a common cause of knee pain in adolescents. It's most common in active adolescent boys, but may also be seen in girls ages 10 to 11.

CAUSES

- Trauma before complete fusion of the epiphysis to the main bone
- Locally decreased blood supply
- Genetic factors

ASSESSMENT FINDINGS

- Aching and pain over tibial tubercle
- Swelling
- Tenderness

DIAGNOSTIC TEST RESULTS

- X-rays show epiphyseal separation and soft tissue swelling in first 6 months after onset; eventually show bone fragmentation.
- Bone scan may show increased uptake in area of tibial tuberosity.

NURSING DIAGNOSES

- Impaired physical mobility
- Chronic pain
- Delayed growth and development

TREATMENT

- Conservative: designed to decrease stress to affected knee
- Avoiding strenuous exercise for the affected knee
- Ice application after exercise
- Rest and quadriceps strengthening and hamstring and quadriceps stretching exercises
- Surgery to reposition epiphysis (if conservative methods fail)

Drug therapy

- Analgesics: acetaminophen (Tylenol), ibuprofen (Motrin)

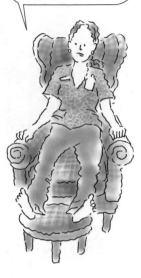

My knees ache from a long day of nursing. Adolescent knee pain could be caused by Osgood-Schlatter disease.

INTERVENTIONS AND RATIONALES

- Monitor the child for circulatory or neurologic changes in the leg, *which could indicate neurovascular compromise.*
- Assess the child for limitations in movement and reposition as needed *to maintain skin integrity.*
- Provide emotional support to the child and family.

Teaching topics

- Explanation of the disorder and treatment plan
- Medication use and possible adverse effects
- Following up with physician and therapy appointments
- Importance of socialization

Scoliosis

Scoliosis is a lateral curvature of the spine. It's commonly identified at puberty and throughout adolescence.

CAUSES

- Congenital: abnormal formation of vertebrae or fused ribs that occurs during prenatal development
- Neuromuscular: scoliosis that occurs as a result of poor muscle control or weakness secondary to another condition, such as cerebral palsy or muscular dystrophy
- Idiopathic: unknown reason for curvature in a previously straight spine

ASSESSMENT FINDINGS

- One shoulder higher than the other
- Tilted pelvis
- Uneven waist
- Backache or lower back pain, especially after prolonged sitting or standing
- Fatigue
- Forward bend test with asymmetry of the trunk or abnormal spinal curve

DIAGNOSTIC TEST RESULTS

- Spinal X-rays identify the degree of deformity.
- Scoliometer measures the amount of curvature.

- MRI may identify additional neurologic changes.

NURSING DIAGNOSES

- Delayed growth and development
- Disturbed body image
- Impaired physical mobility

TREATMENT

- Observation for curves 25 to 40 degrees for a child with completed growth
- Bracing for curves above 25 to 30 degrees in a growing child
- Surgery for curves 40 degrees or greater to insert rods or perform spinal fusion

INTERVENTIONS AND RATIONALES

- Provide emotional support *to help the child develop a positive self image.*
- Assess brace fit *to identify pressure areas and skin irritation and to prevent skin breakdown.*

After spinal fusion and insertion of rods

- Monitor vital signs and intake and output *to prevent fluid volume deficit.*
- Turn the child only by logrolling *to prevent injury.*
- Maintain correct body alignment *to promote joint mobility and prevent injury.*
- Maintain the bed in a flat position *to prevent injury and complications.*
- Help the child adjust to altered self-perception *to promote self-esteem and decrease anxiety.*

Teaching topics

- Explanation of the disorder and treatment plan
- Types of braces needed
- Helping the child maintain self-esteem

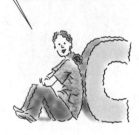

Congenital scoliosis is spinal curvature that occurs before birth.

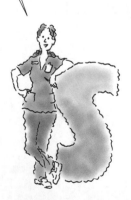

Neuromuscular scoliosis is caused by another condition such as cerebral palsy.

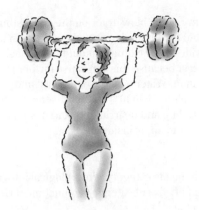

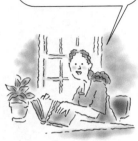

Pump up on practice questions

1. A nurse is caring for a child in traction after a fall. Which action is appropriate when the child is in balanced suspension traction?
1. Increase the weights daily, as ordered.
2. Position the child with his feet against the footboard.
3. Ensure that the weights hang freely.
4. Remove the traction at least three times per day.

Answer: 3. Traction weights must hang freely so that traction and countertraction are properly maintained. The weights aren't increased each day; as the client's muscles relax, the weights may be reduced. To maintain countertraction, position the client in bed so that his feet don't rest against the foot of the bed or against a footboard. Keep the weights in place at all times; neither traction nor the weights are removed until treatment is completed.

➡️ *NCLEX keys*
Client needs category: Physiological integrity
Client needs subcategory: Reduction of risk potential
Cognitive level: Application

2. A child must undergo arthroscopy. Teaching about the procedure is effective when the mother states:
1. "I'm glad he won't feel anything during the procedure."
2. "I'm glad he doesn't have to fast before the procedure."
3. "I need to tell the doctor that he's allergic to lidocaine."
4. "I don't need to sign a consent for the procedure."

Answer: 3. Because a local anesthetic is used before the procedure, teaching is effective when the mother states she must make sure that the physician is aware of her child's allergy to lidocaine. The child may feel a thumping sensation as the cannula is inserted in the joint capsule. The child may need to fast after midnight before the procedure. A parent will need to sign a consent form before the procedure.

➡️ *NCLEX keys*
Client needs category: Safe and effective care environment
Client needs subcategory: Management of care
Cognitive level: Application

3. A nurse is assessing the hand of a child with a long arm cast. The nail bed blanches white with pressure, and the color doesn't return for 5 seconds. The nurse interprets this finding as indicating:
1. fluid accumulation in the fingers.
2. decreased arterial blood supply.
3. a normal response.
4. venous stasis.

Answer: 2. Blanching with slow return to color (capillary refill) is an indication of decreased arterial blood supply. Normally, the color would return to the client's nail bed in less than 3 seconds. Venous stasis and fluid accumulation don't cause blanching.

➡️ *NCLEX keys*
Client needs category: Physiological integrity
Client needs subcategory: Physiological adaptation
Cognitive level: Analysis

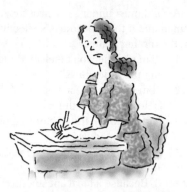

Answer: 3. A blow-dryer on the cool setting should be directed toward the itchy area to provide relief. Nothing should be put inside the cast because this can cause further skin irritation. Water would wet the cast and wouldn't be helpful. Hydrocortisone cream can ball up and be irritating, and it would be difficult to apply inside the cast.

➡ *NCLEX keys*
Client needs category: Physiological integrity
Client needs subcategory: Reduction of risk potential
Cognitive level: Application

4. An adolescent with scoliosis is fitted for a Milwaukee brace. Which statement made by the client indicates successful teaching?
    1. "I'll only have to wear the brace for a few months."
    2. "I can take the brace off only for special occasions like the prom."
    3. "I can take the brace off for 1 hour per day while I bathe."
    4. "The brace will correct the curve if I wear it all the time."

Answer: 3. A Milwaukee brace is used to correct mild scoliosis and needs to be worn approximately 23 hours every day for several months. The brace doesn't correct the curve but prevents the curve from increasing.

➡ *NCLEX keys*
Client needs category: Physiological integrity
Client needs subcategory: Basic care and comfort
Cognitive level: Analysis

5. A child's clubfoot has been placed in a cast. The child develops itching under the cast and asks the nurse for help. The nurse should:
    1. use sterile applicators to relieve the itch.
    2. apply water under the cast.
    3. apply cool air under the cast with a blow-dryer.
    4. apply hydrocortisone cream.

6. A child has undergone repair of a club-foot and is allowed full activity. The nurse is teaching the child's parents about activities for the child. Which activity would benefit the child most?
    1. Walking
    2. Playing catch
    3. Standing
    4. Swimming

Answer: 1. Walking stimulates all of the involved muscles and helps with strengthening. All of the options are good exercises for clubfoot, but walking is the best choice.

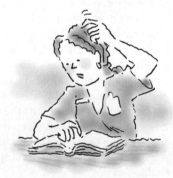

➡ *NCLEX keys*
Client needs category: Physiological integrity
Client needs subcategory: Physiological adaptation
Cognitive level: Application

7. A nurse is doing discharge teaching with a child who has juvenile rheumatoid arthritis (JRA). Which statement indicates that the child and his family understand about exacerbations of JRA?
1. "I should manage stress carefully and stay in a moderate climate."
2. "I should avoid dehydration and exposure to cold."
3. "I should avoid exposure to cold."
4. "I need to limit my exercise."

Answer: 1. Exacerbations of JRA can be precipitated by exposure to stress and climate. Dehydration and exposure to cold can precipitate vaso-occlusive crisis in the client with sickle cell anemia. Exposure to cold can precipitate an exacerbation of Raynaud's disease. Exercise should be encouraged in the child with JRA.

➡ *NCLEX keys*
Client needs category: Physiological integrity
Client needs subcategory: Reduction of risk potential
Cognitive level: Application

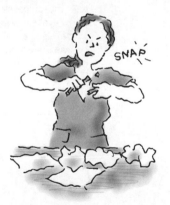

8. A child is admitted with an undiagnosed musculoskeletal condition. Which diagnostic tool is most useful in evaluating a musculoskeletal disorder?
1. Myelography
2. Magnetic resonance imaging (MRI)
3. Computed tomography (CT) scan
4. X-rays

Answer: 4. X-rays are the most useful diagnostic tool to evaluate musculoskeletal diseases and can be used to help identify joint disruption, bone deformities, calcifications, and bone destruction and fractures as well as to measure bone density. Myelography is an invasive procedure used to evaluate abnormalities of the spinal canal and cord. MRI, a form of cross-sectional imaging using a strong magnetic field and radio waves, has largely replaced arthrography for assessing joint anatomy. A CT scan can be used to identify injuries of soft tissue, ligaments, tendons, and muscles.

➡ *NCLEX keys*
Client needs category: Physiological integrity
Client needs subcategory: Reduction of risk potential
Cognitive level: Comprehension

9. A nurse is developing a dietary teaching plan for a child with Duchenne's muscular dystrophy. Which elements are most important for the nurse to include in the child's diet?
1. Lean chicken and brown rice
2. Chicken breast and refined pasta
3. Fried chicken and restricted fluids
4. Chicken breast, brown rice, and supplemental calorie drinks

Answer: 1. A child with muscular dystrophy is prone to constipation and obesity, so dietary intake should include a diet low in calories, high in protein, and high in fiber. Adequate fluid intake should also be encouraged.

➡ *NCLEX keys*
Client needs category: Physiological integrity
Client needs subcategory: Basic care and comfort
Cognitive level: Analysis

10. A nurse is teaching the mother of a child with scoliosis. The nurse knows that teaching has been successful when the mother makes which statement?

1. "I'm glad my daughter will outgrow this deformity."
2. "I'm afraid that my daughter will feel unattractive because she must wear a brace."
3. "I'll make sure that my daughter doesn't do any stretching exercises that could worsen her spine."
4. "I'm glad my daughter will need to wear a brace for only a short time."

Answer: 2. Teaching is successful when the mother shows concern about her daughter's feelings toward wearing a brace for scoliosis treatment. The brace is uncomfortable and unattractive and may make the child self-conscious about her appearance. The child won't outgrow the deformity. Stretching exercises won't worsen the condition. Brace use is determined on an individual basis, so the duration of treatment will vary.

➡ *NCLEX keys*

Client needs category: Physiological integrity
Client needs subcategory: Reduction of risk potential
Cognitive level: Analysis

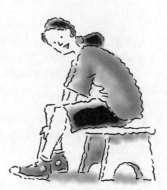

Boning up on the pediatric musculoskeletal system before taking the big exam was smart. Now get ready to muscle your way through the next chapter.

32 Gastrointestinal system

Brush up on key concepts

The GI tract, also known as the **alimentary canal,** consists of a long, hollow, muscular tube that includes several glands and accessory organs. It performs the crucial task of supplying essential nutrients to fuel the other organs and body systems. Because the GI system is so crucial to the rest of the body systems, a problem in this system can quickly affect the overall health, growth, and development of the child.

At any time, you can review the major points of this chapter by consulting the *Cheat sheet* on pages 680 to 682.

GI junior

Characteristics of the pediatric GI system include the following:
• Peristalsis occurs within 2½ to 3 hours of eating in the neonate and extends to 3 to 6 hours in older infants and children.
• Gastric stomach capacity of the neonate is 30 to 60 ml, which gradually increases to 200 to 350 ml by age 12 months and to 1,500 ml as an adolescent.
• The neonatal abdomen is larger than the chest up to ages 4 to 8 weeks, and the musculature is poorly developed.
• The extrusion reflex persists to ages 3 to 4 months (extrusion reflex protects infant from food substances that its system is too immature to digest).
• At age 4 months, saliva production begins and aids in the process of digestion.
• The sucking reflex begins to diminish at age 6 months.
• The neonate has immature muscle tone of the lower esophageal sphincter and low volume capacity of the stomach, which cause the neonate to "spit up" frequently.

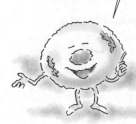

Thanks to the GI tract, I can get a good meal.

• Increased myelination of nerves to the anal sphincter allows for physiologic control of bowel function, usually around age 2.
• The liver's slow development of glycogen storage capacity makes the infant prone to hypoglycemia.
• From ages 1 to 3, composition of intestinal flora becomes more adultlike and stomach acidity increases, reducing the number of GI infections.

Nutrient breakdown

The GI tract breaks down food (carbohydrates, fats, and proteins) into molecules small enough to permeate cell membranes, thus providing cells with the necessary energy to function properly. The GI tract prepares food for cellular absorption by altering its physical and chemical composition. (See *Digestive organs and glands,* page 683.)

Malfunction junction

A malfunction along the GI tract can produce far-reaching metabolic effects, eventually threatening life itself. A common indication of GI problems is referred pain, which makes diagnosis especially difficult.

Keep abreast of diagnostic tests

Here are important tests used to diagnose GI system disorders, along with common nursing interventions associated with each test.

Swallow this

Barium swallow is primarily used to examine the esophagus.

Gastrografin is now used instead of barium for certain patients. Like barium, Gastrografin facilitates imaging through X-rays.

(Text continues on page 682.)

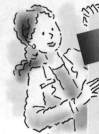

Cheat sheet

Gastrointestinal refresher

ACETAMINOPHEN TOXICITY
Key signs and symptoms
- Diaphoresis
- Nausea and vomiting

Key test results
- Serum aspartate aminotransferase and serum alanine aminotransferase levels become elevated soon after ingestion.

Key treatments
- Gastric lavage or emesis induction with ipecac syrup

Key interventions
- Monitor vital signs and intake and output.
- Assess cardiovascular and GI status.

CELIAC DISEASE
Key signs and symptoms
- Generalized malnutrition and failure to thrive due to malabsorption of protein and carbohydrates
- Steatorrhea and chronic diarrhea due to fat malabsorption
- Weight and height below normal for age-group

Key test results
- Immunoglobulin (Ig) A and IgG anti-tissue transglutaminase antibody test is positive.

Key treatments
- Diet: gluten-free but includes corn and rice products, soy and potato flour, breast milk or soy-based formula, and all fresh fruits

Key interventions
- Monitor growth and development.
- Provide small, frequent, gluten-free meals.

CLEFT LIP AND PALATE
Key signs and symptoms
- Cleft lip: can range from a simple notch on the upper lip to a complete cleft from the lip edge to the floor of the nostril, on either side of the midline but rarely along the midline itself
- Cleft palate without cleft lip: may not be detected until mouth examination or development of feeding difficulties

Key test results
- Prenatal ultrasound may indicate severe defects.

Key treatments
- Cheiloplasty performed between birth and age 3 months to unite the lip and gum edges in anticipation of teeth eruption, providing a route for adequate nutrition and sucking
- Cleft palate repair surgery (staphylorrhaphy); scheduled at about age 18 months to allow for growth of the palate and to be done before the infant develops speech patterns (the infant must be free from ear and respiratory infections)

Key interventions
- Be alert for respiratory distress when feeding.
Before cleft lip repair surgery
- Hold the infant while feeding, and promote sucking between meals.
After cleft lip repair surgery
- Observe for cyanosis as the infant begins to breathe through the nose.
- Keep the infant's hands away from the mouth by using restraints or pinning the sleeves to the shirt; adhesive strips are used to hold the suture line in place.
- Anticipate the infant's needs.
- Place the infant on the right side to prevent aspiration; clean the suture line after each feeding by dabbing it with half-strength hydrogen peroxide or saline solution.
After cleft palate repair surgery
- Position the toddler on the abdomen or side.
- Anticipate edema and a decreased airway from palate closure; this may make the toddler appear temporarily dyspneic; assess for signs of decreased oxygenation.
- Keep hard or pointed objects (utensils, straws, frozen dessert sticks) away from the mouth.

ESOPHAGEAL ATRESIA AND TRACHEO-ESOPHAGEAL FISTULA
Key signs and symptoms
- Sonorous seal bark cough in the delivery room
- Excessive oral secretions and drooling
- Choking when feeding

Gastrointestinal refresher (continued)

ESOPHAGEAL ATRESIA AND TRACHEOESOPHAGEAL FISTULA (CONTINUED)
Key test results
- X-ray confirms esophageal atresia and transesophageal fistula.

Key treatments
- Esophageal atresia repair or tracheoesophageal fistula repair (may be performed immediately or after 2 to 4 months)

Key interventions
- Assess respiratory status.
- Administer I.V. fluids and antibiotics before surgery.
- Keep the neonate warm in an incubator or overhead warmer.
- Maintain continuous suction.

FAILURE TO THRIVE
Key signs and symptoms
- History of feeding problems
- Wasting
- Height, weight, and head circumference less than expected for age

Key test results
- Negative nitrogen balance indicates inadequate intake of protein or calories.

Key treatments
- High-calorie diet
- Parent and child counseling
- Vitamin and mineral supplements

Key interventions
- Properly feed and interact with the child.
- Provide the child with visual and auditory stimulation.
- Provide information on parenting skills.

GASTROENTERITIS
Key signs and symptoms
- Abdominal discomfort
- Diarrhea
- Nausea and vomiting

Key test results
- Stool culture identifies causative bacteria, parasite, or amoebae.

Key treatments
- Increased fluid intake
- I.V. fluid and electrolyte replacement
- Antiemetic: prochlorperazine

Key interventions
- Early intervention with fluid and electrolyte replacement is key.
- Stress hand washing to the child and his family.
- Administer I.V. fluids and medications.

GASTROESOPHAGEAL REFLUX DISEASE
Key signs and symptoms
- Choking or gagging with feeding
- Frequent crying and fussiness
- Frequent or persistent cough
- Frequent or recurrent vomiting

Key test results
- Gastric emptying study shows prolonged emptying time.
- Barium swallow fluoroscopy indicates reflux.
- Esophageal pH probe reveals a low pH, which indicates reflux.

Key treatments
- Positional therapy to help relieve symptoms by decreasing intra-abdominal pressure
- Histamine-2 (H_2) receptor antagonists: ranitidine (Zantac), famotidine (Pepcid)
- Proton-pump inhibitor: esomeprazole (Nexium)

Key interventions
- Encourage the child to eat several small meals during the day to help decrease the pressure on the lower esophageal sphincter.
- Have the parent hold the infant for at least 30 minutes after feeding to reduce intra-abdominal pressure.

INTESTINAL OBSTRUCTION
Key signs and symptoms
- Complete small-bowel obstruction: bowel contents propelled toward mouth (instead of rectum) by vigorous peristaltic waves, along with persistent epigastric or periumbilical pain
- Partial large-bowel obstruction: leakage of liquid stool around the obstruction (common)

Key test results
- With large-bowel obstruction, barium enema reveals a distended, air-filled colon or, in sigmoid volvulus, a closed loop of sigmoid with extreme distention.
- X-rays confirm the diagnosis. Abdominal films show the presence and location of intestinal gas or fluid.

Key treatments
- I.V. therapy to correct fluid and electrolyte imbalances

Key interventions
- Monitor vital signs frequently.
- Assess cardiovascular status; observe the child closely for signs of shock (pallor, rapid pulse, and hypotension).
- Monitor for signs and symptoms of metabolic alkalosis (changes in sensorium; slow, shallow respirations; hypertonic muscles; tetany) or acidosis (dyspnea on exertion, disorientation and, later, deep, rapid breathing, weakness, and malaise).
- Observe for signs and symptoms of secondary infection, such as fever and chills.

(continued)

Gastrointestinal refresher (continued)

LEAD TOXICITY

Key signs and symptoms
• Anorexia, vomiting
• Weight loss

Key test results
• X-rays reveal lead lines near the epiphyseal lines (areas of increased density) of long bones. The thickness of the line shows the length of time the lead ingestion has been occurring.

Key treatments
• Chelating agents: succimer (Chemet) or dimercaprol (BAL In Oil) for a blood lead level greater than 45 mcg/dl.

Key interventions
• Monitor vital signs, intake and output, hydration status, and kidney function.
• Monitor calcium levels (chelating agents also bind with calcium).

PYLORIC STENOSIS

Key signs and symptoms
• Projectile emesis during or soon after feedings, preceded by reverse peristaltic waves (going left to right) but not by nausea (child resumes eating after vomiting)

Key test results
• Ultrasound shows pyloric muscle thickness greater than 4 mm.

Key treatments
• Surgical intervention: pyloromyotomy performed by laparoscopy

Key interventions
• Provide small, frequent, thickened feedings with the head of the bed elevated; burp the child frequently.
• Position the child on his right side.

SALICYLATE TOXICITY

Key signs and symptoms
• High fever
• Petechiae and bleeding tendency

Key test results
• Serum salicylate levels are elevated beyond therapeutic range.

Key treatments
• Gastric lavage
• I.V. fluids
• Alkalinizing agent: sodium bicarbonate

Key interventions
• Administer I.V. fluids.
• Monitor urine pH.
• Assess cardiovascular and GI status.

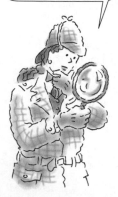

It's alimentary. Barium—or Gastrografin—is swallowed to help visualize the GI tract.

Unlike barium, however, if Gastrografin escapes from the GI tract, it's absorbed by the surrounding tissue. Escaped barium isn't absorbed and can cause complications.

Nursing actions
• Explain the procedure to the child and parents.
• Maintain nothing-by-mouth (NPO) status for 6 to 8 hours before the test.
• Tell the child he must hold still during the X-ray.
• After the test, monitor bowel movements for excretion of barium. Also monitor GI function.

Upper GI imaging

In an **upper GI series,** swallowed barium sulfate proceeds into the esophagus, stomach, and duodenum to reveal abnormalities. The barium outlines stomach walls and delineates ulcer craters and filling defects.

A **small-bowel series,** an extension of the upper GI series, visualizes barium flowing through the small intestine to the ileocecal valve.

Nursing actions
• Explain the procedure to the child and parents.
• Tell the child that he must hold still during the X-ray.
• Make sure the lead apron is properly placed around the genital area.
• After the test, monitor bowel movements for excretion of barium. Also monitor GI function.

Lower GI look

A **barium enema (lower GI series)** allows X-ray visualization of the colon.

Nursing actions
• Explain the procedure to the child and parents.

Digestive organs and glands

Here is a quick rundown of the major organs and glands that facilitate digestion.

SALIVARY GLANDS
The salivary glands provide saliva to moisten the mouth, lubricate food to ease swallowing, and begin food breakdown using the enzyme ptyalin. After food is swallowed, it enters the esophagus and is transported to the stomach.

STOMACH
The stomach is a muscular, saclike organ located between the esophagus and small intestine. Food and fluids enter the stomach and are mixed with stomach secretions. Contractions called *peristalsis* push the food gradually into the small intestine through the pyloric opening at the lower end of the stomach.

INTESTINE
The intestine extends from the pyloric opening to the anus. It's made up of the small and large intestines.
• The small intestine is made up of the duodenum, jejunum, and ileum and is about 20′ (6 m) long. Most digestion takes place in the small intestine; digested food is absorbed through the walls of the small intestine and into the blood for distribution throughout the body.
• The large intestine is about 5′ (1.5 m) long and includes the cecum (and appendix), colon, and rectum. Indigestible food passes into the large intestine, where it's formed into solid feces and eliminated through the rectum.

LIVER
The liver stores and filters blood; secretes bile; processes sugars, fats, proteins, and vitamins; and detoxifies drugs, alcohol, and other substances.

GALLBLADDER
The gallbladder is located beneath the liver and serves as a storage place for bile. Bile is a clear, yellowish fluid that enters the small intestine through bile ducts and aids digestion of fats.

PANCREAS
The pancreas is a large gland located behind the stomach. It secretes digestive enzymes that neutralize stomach acids and break down proteins, carbohydrates, and fats.

• Usually, the child will follow a liquid diet for 24 hours before the test. Bowel preparations are administered before the examination.
• Tell the child that X-rays will be taken on a test table and that he must hold still.
• Cover the genital area with a lead apron during X-ray.

Stool search
A **stool specimen** can be examined for suspected GI bleeding, infection, or malabsorption. Certain tests require several specimens, such as the **guaiac test** for occult blood, a microscopic stool examination for ova and parasites, and tests for fat.

Nursing actions
• Explain the procedure to the child and parents.
• Obtain the specimen in the correct container (the container may need to be sterile or contain preservative).
• Be aware that the specimen may need to be transported to the laboratory immediately or placed in the refrigerator.

Fiber-optic findings
In **esophagogastroduodenoscopy,** insertion of a fiber-optic scope allows direct visual inspection of the esophagus, stomach and, sometimes, duodenum. **Proctosigmoidoscopy** permits inspection of the rectum and

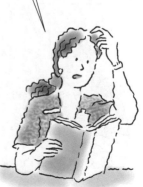

Esophago-
gastro-
duo-
deno-
scopy ...
No problem!

distal sigmoid colon. **Colonoscopy** allows inspection of the descending, transverse, and ascending colon.

Nursing actions
• Explain the procedure to the child and parents.
• Make sure that written, informed consent has been obtained.
• A mild sedative may be administered before the examination.
• The child may be on NPO status before the procedure (upper GI series).
• The child may be placed on a liquid diet for 24 hours before the examination or require enemas or laxatives until clear (lower GI examinations).

Fluoroscopic findings
Endoscopic retrograde cholangiopancreatography is the radiographic examination of the pancreatic ducts and hepatobiliary tree following the injection of contrast media into the duodenal papilla. It's performed on children with suspected pancreatic disease or obstructive jaundice.

Nursing actions
Before the procedure
• Explain the procedure to the child and parents.
• Make sure that written, informed consent has been obtained.
• Check the child's history for allergies to cholinergics and iodine.
• Administer a sedative, and monitor the child for the drug's effect.
After the procedure
• Monitor the child's gag reflex (the child is kept on NPO status until his gag reflex returns).
• Protect the child from aspiration of mucus by positioning the child on his side.
• Monitor the child for urine retention.

Tube topics
Certain GI disorders require insertion of a **gastric tube** for the following purposes:
• to empty the stomach and intestine
• to aid diagnosis and treatment
• to decompress obstructed areas
• to detect and treat GI bleeding
• to administer medications or feedings.

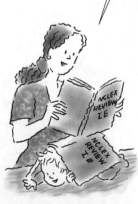

Children who are intubated require diligent oral and nasal care, close monitoring, and emotional support to minimize fear.

Tubes usually inserted through the nose include short nasogastric (NG) tubes (Levin and Salem Sump) and long intestinal tubes (Cantor and Miller-Abbott). The larger Ewald tube is usually inserted orally and is used to empty the stomach.

Nursing actions
• Explain the procedure to the child and parents.
• Maintain accurate intake and output records. Measure gastric drainage every 8 hours; record amount, color, odor, and consistency. When irrigating the tube, note the amount of saline solution instilled and aspirated.
• Monitor for fluid and electrolyte imbalances.
• Provide oral and nasal care. Make sure the tube is secure but isn't causing pressure on the nostrils.
• Anchor the tube to the child's clothing to prevent dislodgment.
• Provide emotional support because many children panic at the sight of a tube. Maintaining a calm, reassuring manner can help minimize the child's fear.

Polish up on client care

Pediatric GI disorders discussed in this chapter include acetaminophen toxicity, celiac disease, cleft lip and palate, esophageal atresia and tracheoesophageal fistula, failure to thrive, gastroenteritis, gastroesophageal reflux disease (GERD), intestinal obstruction, lead toxicity, pyloric stenosis, and salicylate toxicity.

Acetaminophen toxicity

Acetaminophen is an analgesic antipyretic agent that achieves its effect without inhibiting platelet aggregation. Because acetaminophen is an over-the-counter medication commonly found in the home, it's a common cause of poisoning in children.

With acetaminophen toxicity, hepatotoxicity occurs at plasma levels greater than 200 mg/ml at 4 hours after ingestion and greater than 50 mg/ml by 12 hours after ingestion.

CAUSES
- Acetaminophen ingestion beyond the recommended dosage

ASSESSMENT FINDINGS
- Anorexia
- Diaphoresis
- Hypothermia
- Severe hypoglycemia
- Shock
- Oliguria
- Nausea and vomiting
- Pallor
- Right upper quadrant tenderness usually occurring 24 to 48 hours after ingestion; jaundice evident 72 to 96 hours after ingestion
- Hepatic failure, death, or resolution of symptoms occurring 7 to 8 days after ingestion

DIAGNOSTIC TEST RESULTS
- Blood glucose levels are decreased.
- Serum aspartate aminotransferase and serum alanine aminotransferase levels become elevated soon after ingestion.
- Prothrombin time is prolonged.

NURSING DIAGNOSES
- Imbalanced nutrition: Less than body requirements
- Risk for imbalanced fluid volume
- Hypothermia
- Risk for impaired liver function

TREATMENT
- Gastric lavage or emesis induction with ipecac syrup
- Hyperthermia blanket
- I.V. fluid
- Oxygen therapy (intubation and mechanical ventilation may be required)

Drug therapy
- Emetic: ipecac syrup to induce vomiting
- Antidote: acetylcysteine

INTERVENTIONS AND RATIONALES
- Monitor liver function studies *to detect signs of liver damage and to monitor effectiveness of treatment.*
- Monitor vital signs and intake and output. *Tachycardia and decreased urine output may signify dehydration.*

- Assess cardiovascular and GI status *to monitor the effectiveness of treatment.*
- Administer hyperthermia therapy by using a warming blanket, limiting exposure during routine nursing care, and covering the child with warm blankets *to help the child become normothermic.*
- Administer acetylcysteine as ordered *to reduce acetaminophen levels.*

Teaching topics
- Explanation of the disorder and treatment plan
- Storing medication safely and other steps to prevent overdose
- Reading labels carefully (cough and cold preparations may also contain acetominophen)

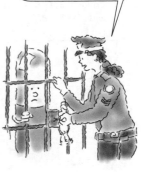

Put it away. Locked medicine storage helps prevent acetaminophen toxicity.

Celiac disease

Celiac disease is an intolerance to gliadin — a gluten protein found in grains, such as wheat, rye, oats, and barley, that causes poor food absorption.

In celiac disease, a decrease in the amount and activity of enzymes in the intestinal mucosal cells causes the villi of the proximal small intestine to atrophy, decreasing intestinal absorption. Celiac disease usually becomes apparent between ages 6 and 18 months.

CAUSES
- Genetic disease that may be triggered by surgery, pregnancy, childbirth, viral infection, or severe emotional stress

ASSESSMENT FINDINGS
- Abdominal distention
- Anorexia
- Generalized malnutrition and failure to thrive due to malabsorption of protein and carbohydrates
- Fatigue
- Bone or joint pain
- Aphthous ulcers
- Itchy rash (dermatitis herpetiform)
- Irritability
- Steatorrhea and chronic diarrhea due to fat malabsorption

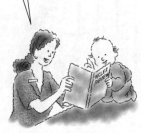

If a child demonstrates malnutrition, steatorrhea, and chronic diarrhea 2 to 4 months after solid foods are introduced, suspect celiac disease.

• Weight and height below normal for age-group

DIAGNOSTIC TEST RESULTS
• Blood chemistry tests reveal hypocalcemia and hypoalbuminemia.
• Hematology reveals decreased hemoglobin level and hypothrombinemia.
• Immunoglobulin (Ig) A and IgG anti-tissue transglutaminase antibody test is positive (not reliable in children younger than age 2).
• IgA and IgG anti-gliadin antibodies are present.
• Intestinal biopsy confirms the diagnosis.
• Stool specimen reveals high fat content.

NURSING DIAGNOSES
• Imbalanced nutrition: Less than body requirements
• Delayed growth and development
• Deficient fluid volume
• Diarrhea

TREATMENT
• Diet: gluten-free but includes corn and rice products, soy and potato flour, breast milk or soy-based formula, and all fresh fruits
• Folate
• Iron (Feosol) supplements
• Vitamins A and D in water-soluble forms

INTERVENTIONS AND RATIONALES
• Provide small, frequent, gluten-free meals *to reduce fatigue and improve nutritional intake.*
• Record the consistency, appearance, and number of stools. *The disappearance of steatorrhea is a good indicator that the child's ability to absorb nutrients is improving.*
• Monitor growth and development *to assess for growth delay and to detect changes in level of functioning* and, as appropriate, plan an activity program for the child.

Teaching topics
• Explanation of the disorder and treatment plan
• Specific foods and formula the child can eat (breads made from rice, corn, soybean, potato, tapioca, sago or gluten-free wheat; dry cereals made with only rice or corn; cornmeal or hominy)

Cleft lip and palate

In cleft lip and palate, the bone and tissue of the upper jaw and palate fail to fuse completely at the midline. The defects may be partial or complete, unilateral or bilateral, and may involve the lip, the palate, or both.

Cleft lip and palate also increase the risk of:
• aspiration because increased open space in the mouth may cause formula or breast milk to enter the respiratory tract
• upper respiratory infection and otitis media, because the increased open space decreases natural defenses against bacterial invasion.

CAUSES
• Congenital defects (in some cases, inheritance plays a role)
• Part of another chromosomal or mendelian abnormality
• Prenatal exposure to teratogens

ASSESSMENT FINDINGS
• Abdominal distention from swallowed air
• Cleft lip: can range from a simple notch on the upper lip to a complete cleft from the lip edge to the floor of the nostril, on either side of the midline but rarely along the midline itself
• Cleft palate: may be partial or complete
• Difficulty swallowing

Note that cleft lip with or without cleft palate is obvious at birth; cleft palate without cleft lip may not be detected until a mouth examination is done or until feeding difficulties develop.

DIAGNOSTIC TEST RESULTS
• Prenatal ultrasonography may indicate severe defects.

NURSING DIAGNOSES
• Imbalanced nutrition: Less than body requirements
• Impaired swallowing
• Risk for aspiration
• Ineffective airway clearance
• Risk for impaired parenting

TREATMENT

- Cheiloplasty performed between birth and age 3 months to unite the lip and gum edges in anticipation of teeth eruption, providing a route for adequate nutrition and sucking
- Cleft palate repair surgery (staphylorrhaphy); scheduled at about age 18 months to allow for growth of the palate and to be done before the infant develops speech patterns (the infant must be free from ear and respiratory infections)
- Long-term, team-oriented care to address speech defects, dental and orthodontic problems, nasal defects, and possible alterations in hearing
- If cleft lip is detected on sonogram while the infant is in utero, possible fetal repair

INTERVENTIONS AND RATIONALES

- Monitor vital signs and intake and output *to determine fluid volume status.*
- Assess respiratory status *to detect signs of aspiration.*
- Assess the quality of the child's suck by determining whether the infant can form an airtight seal around a finger or nipple placed in the infant's mouth *to determine an effective feeding method.*
- Be alert for respiratory distress when feeding *to avoid aspiration.*
- Provide emotional support to the child and parents *to decrease anxiety.*

Preoperative interventions for cleft lip repair

- Feed the infant slowly and in an upright position *to decrease the risk of aspiration.*
- Burp the infant frequently during feeding *to eliminate swallowed air and decrease the risk of emesis.*
- Use gavage feedings *if oral feedings are unsuccessful.*
- Administer a small amount of water after feedings *to prevent formula from accumulating in the cleft and becoming a medium for bacterial growth.*
- Give small, frequent feedings *to promote adequate nutrition and prevent tiring the infant.*
- Hold the infant while feeding and promote sucking between meals. *Sucking is important to speech development.*

Postoperative interventions for cleft lip repair

- Observe for cyanosis as the infant begins to breathe through the nose *to detect signs of respiratory compromise.*
- Keep the infant's hands away from the mouth by using restraints or pinning the sleeves to the shirt; adhesive strips are used to hold the suture line in place *to prevent tension and to maintain an intact suture line.*
- Anticipate the infant's needs *to prevent crying.*
- Use a syringe with tubing to administer foods at the side of the mouth *to prevent trauma to the suture line.*
- Place the infant on the right side *to prevent aspiration;* clean the suture line after each feeding by dabbing it with half-strength hydrogen peroxide or saline solution *to prevent crusts and scarring.*
- Monitor for pain and administer pain medication as prescribed; note the effectiveness of pain medication *to promote comfort.*

Preoperative interventions for cleft palate repair

- Feed the infant with a cleft palate nipple or a Teflon implant *to enhance nutritional intake.*
- Wean the infant from the bottle or breast before cleft palate surgery; *the toddler must be able to drink from a cup.*

Postoperative interventions for cleft palate repair

- Position the toddler on the abdomen or side *to promote a patent airway.*
- Anticipate edema and a decreased airway from palate closure; this may make the toddler appear temporarily dyspneic; assess for signs of decreased oxygenation *to identify airway complications.*
- Keep hard or pointed objects (utensils, straws, frozen dessert sticks) away from the mouth *to prevent trauma to the suture line.*
- Use a cup to feed; don't use a nipple or pacifier *to prevent injury to the suture line.*
- Use elbow restraints *to keep the toddler's hands out of the mouth.*
- Provide soft toys *to prevent injury.*
- Start the toddler on clear liquids and progress to a soft diet; rinse the suture line by giving the toddler a sip of water after each feeding *to prevent infection.*

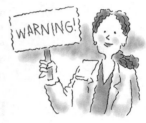

Cleft lip and palate increase the risk of aspiration during feeding as well as the risk of respiratory infection and otitis media.

WARNING!

- Distract or hold the toddler *to try to keep the tongue away from the roof of the mouth.*

Teaching topics
- Explanation of the disorder and treatment options
- Importance of parental involvement (because it results in facial disfigurement, the condition may cause shock, guilt, and grief for the parents and may block parental bonding with the child)
- Need for follow-up speech therapy
- Understanding the child's susceptibility to pathogens and otitis media from the altered position of the eustachian tubes

Esophageal atresia and tracheoesophageal fistula

Esophageal atresia occurs when the proximal end of the esophagus ends in a blind pouch; food can't enter the stomach through the esophagus.

Tracheoesophageal fistula occurs when a connection exists between the esophagus and the trachea. It may result in the reflux of gastric juice after feeding; this can allow acidic stomach contents to cross the fistula, irritating the trachea.

Esophageal atresia and tracheoesophageal fistula occur in many combinations and may be associated with other defects. Esophageal atresia with tracheoesophageal fistula is the most common of these conditions. Esophageal atresia alone is the second most common of these conditions.

Esophageal atresia with tracheoesophageal fistula occurs when either:
- the distal end of the esophagus ends in a blind pouch and the proximal end of the esophagus is linked to the trachea via a fistula
- the proximal end of the esophagus ends in a blind pouch and the distal portion of the esophagus is connected to the trachea via a fistula.

Other birth defects may coexist and should be assessed at birth.

CAUSES
- Unknown

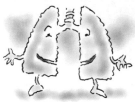

Remember me? Preventing respiratory complications is key to postoperative care in esophageal atresia and tracheoesophageal fistula repair.

ASSESSMENT FINDINGS
- Sonorous seal bark cough in the delivery room
- Excessive oral secretions and drooling
- Choking when feeding
- Regurgitation of undigested formula immediately after feeding; possible respiratory distress and cyanosis if secretions are aspirated
- Abdominal distention (with tracheoesophageal fistula)

DIAGNOSTIC TEST RESULTS
- NG tube doesn't pass because of obstruction 4" to 5" (10 to 12.5 cm) from the neonate's nostrils.
- X-ray confirms esophageal atresia and transesophageal fistula.

NURSING DIAGNOSES
- Imbalanced nutrition: Less than body requirements
- Risk for infection
- Risk for impaired parenting
- Ineffective breathing pattern

TREATMENT
- Gastrostomy tube (PEG tube) insertion and feedings
- Esophageal atresia repair or tracheoesophageal fistula repair (may be performed immediately or after 2 to 4 months)

INTERVENTIONS AND RATIONALES
- Monitor vital signs to detect tachycardia and tachypnea, *which could indicate hypoxemia.*
- Assess respiratory status. *Poor respiratory status may result in hypoxemia.*
- Administer I.V. fluids and antibiotics before surgery *to promote stability.*
- Position the infant with his head elevated to 30 degrees *to decrease reflux at the distal esophagus.*
- Keep the neonate warm in an incubator or overhead warmer *to maintain temperature.*
- Maintain continuous suction *to remove secretions.*
- Suction as needed *to stimulate cough and clear airways.*

After gastrostomy

- Keep the PEG tube open and suspended above the child *for release of gas.*
- If feeding the child through a gastrostomy tube after surgery, anticipate abdominal distention from air; keep the child upright during and after feedings *to reduce the chance of refluxed stomach contents and aspiration pneumonia,* and keep the tube open and elevated before and after feedings.
- Administer gastrostomy feedings only by gravity flow — not a feeding pump — *to help meet nutritional and metabolic requirements.*

Postoperative care

- Maintain chest tube and respiratory support *to prevent respiratory compromise.*
- Suction as needed *to remove secretions and prevent aspiration.*
- Make sure the NG tube is secure and handle with extreme caution *to avoid displacement.*
- Administer antibiotics as prescribed *to prevent infection.*
- Administer total parenteral nutrition or feedings *to maintain nutritional support.*

Teaching topics

- Explanation of the disorder and treatment plan
- Understanding proper care of the child at home, such as feeding and bathing techniques

Failure to thrive

Failure to thrive is a chronic, potentially life-threatening condition characterized by failure to maintain weight and height above the 5th percentile on age-appropriate growth charts. Most children are diagnosed before age 2. It can result from physical, emotional, or psychological causes.

CONTRIBUTING FACTORS

- May be a combination of organic and non-organic factors

Organic

- Prenatal: chromosomal abnormalities; maternal exposure to toxins, such as tobacco, alcohol, or drugs; maternal illness, such as hypertension, preeclampsia, or diabetes mellitus
- Postnatal: inadequate intake due to conditions associated with inability to suck or swallow, lack of appetite resulting from infection, or vomiting associated with GI obstruction; poor absorption of nutrients due to endocrine disorders, GI disorders (such as celiac disease), or renal failure; increased metabolic demand caused by chronic disease (such as inflammatory bowel disease) or malignancy

Nonorganic

- Poor parenting, failure to bond
- Poor feeding skills
- Family dysfunction
- Child neglect
- Difficult child
- Eating disorder

ASSESSMENT FINDINGS

- History of feeding problems
- History of a medical problem or an illness
- History of dysfunctional family or inadequate parenting
- Listlessness
- Noninteractive behavior
- Wasting
- Height, weight, and head circumference less than expected for age
- Rash or skin changes
- Hepatomegaly

DIAGNOSTIC TEST RESULTS

- Negative nitrogen balance indicates inadequate intake of protein or calories.
- Associated physiologic causes may be detected.
- Reduced creatinine-height index reflects muscle mass and estimates muscle protein depletion.

NURSING DIAGNOSES

- Delayed growth and development
- Impaired parenting
- Imbalanced nutrition: Less than body requirements

TREATMENT

- Treatment of underlying medical cause
- High-calorie diet
- Parent and child counseling

Drug therapy

- Vitamin and mineral supplements

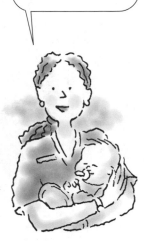

Adequate stimulation helps to prevent failure to thrive.

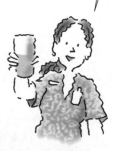

I dig visual and auditory stimulation.

INTERVENTIONS AND RATIONALES
• Weigh the child on admission *to determine baseline weight.*
• Assess growth and development using an appropriate tool, such as the Denver Developmental Screening test, *to determine the child's developmental level.*
• Properly feed and interact with the child *to promote nutrition and growth and development.*
• Establish specific times for feeding, bathing, and sleeping *to establish and maintain a structured routine.*
• Provide the child with visual and auditory stimulation *to promote normal sensory development.*
• Assess interaction of the parent with the child *to determine parent-child relationship and parenting skills.*
• Provide information on parenting skills *to assist parents with proper child care.*

Teaching topics
• Explanation of the disorder and treatment plan
• Understanding healthy parenting skills
• Normal growth and development
• Stimulation techniques
• Obtaining counseling for the parents and child, if necessary
• Understanding dietary needs

Gastroenteritis

A self-limiting disorder, gastroenteritis is characterized by diarrhea, nausea, vomiting, and acute or chronic abdominal cramping. It occurs in children of all ages, and ranks as the fifth leading cause of death in young children. Gastroenteritis can quickly become a major illness in children, especially infants and young children, because of the risk of dehydration.

Drink that water! Increased fluid intake is crucial to combat gastroenteritis.

CAUSES
• Bacteria (responsible for acute food poisoning): *Staphylococcus aureus,* Salmonella, Shigella, *Clostridium botulinum, Eschericheria coli, Clostridium perfringens*
• Viruses: adenovirus, echovirus, coxsackievirus, rotavirus
• Food allergens
• Amoebae, especially *Entamoeba histolytica*
• Drug reactions
• Ingestion of toxins

ASSESSMENT FINDINGS
• Diarrhea
• Nausea and vomiting
• Abdominal discomfort

DIAGNOSTIC TEST RESULTS
• Stool culture identifies causative bacteria, parasite, or amoebae.
• Blood culture identifies causative organism.

NURSING DIAGNOSES
• Diarrhea
• Risk for impaired fluid volume
• Acute pain

TREATMENT
• Increased fluid intake
• I.V. fluid and electrolyte replacement
• Nutritional support

Drug therapy
• Antibiotic therapy according to the sensitivity of the causative organism
• Antidiarrheals: diphenoxylate with atropine, loperamide
• Antiemetic: prochlorperazine

INTERVENTIONS AND RATIONALES
• Early intervention with fluid and electrolyte replacement is key *because of the risk of dehydration in young children.*
• Administer I.V. fluids and medications.
• Encourage clear liquids and electrolyte replacement *to prevent dehydration.*
• Instruct the parents to avoid giving the child milk or milk products, *which may exacerbate the condition.*
• Monitor intake and output. Watch for signs of dehydration, such as sunken fontanels, lack of tears, and lethargy.
• Stress hand washing to the child and his family.

Teaching topics
• Explanation of the disorder and treatment plan

- Increased fluid intake
- Importance of good hand hygiene
- Recognizing signs of dehydration and seeking prompt treatment

Gastroesophageal reflux disease

GERD is the backflow of gastric or duodenal contents, or both, into the esophagus and past the lower esophageal sphincter (LES) without associated belching or vomiting. Until recently, GERD has been underdiagnosed in children. However, many infants diagnosed with GERD outgrow the disorder by age 1.

CAUSES
- Pressure within the stomach that exceeds LES pressure

ASSESSMENT FINDINGS
- Frequent or recurrent vomiting
- Regurgitation and re-swallowing
- Frequent crying and fussiness
- Choking or gagging with feeding
- Frequent or persistent cough

DIAGNOSTIC TEST RESULTS
- Barium swallow fluoroscopy indicates reflux.
- Esophageal pH probe reveals a low pH, which indicates reflux.
- Esophagoscopy shows reflux.
- Gastric emptying study shows prolonged emptying time.

NURSING DIAGNOSES
- Risk for aspiration
- Imbalanced nutrition: Less than body requirements

TREATMENT
- Positional therapy to help relieve symptoms by decreasing intra-abdominal pressure
- Low-fat, high-fiber diet
- Oxygen therapy

Drug therapy
- Histamine-2 receptor antagonists: ranitidine (Zantac), famotidine (Pepcid)

- Proton-pump inhibitor: esomeprazole (Nexium)
- Anti-gas agent: Mylicon

INTERVENTIONS AND RATIONALES
- Have the parent hold the infant for at least 30 minutes after feeding *to reduce intra-abdominal pressure.*
- Offer reassurance and emotional support to the parents *to help them cope with their child's illness.*
- Encourage the child to eat several small meals during the day *to help decrease the pressure on the LES.*

Teaching topics
- Explanation of the disorder and treatment plan
- Medication use and possible adverse effects
- Positional therapy
- Dietary modifications

Intestinal obstruction

Intestinal obstruction is the partial or complete blockage of the lumen in the small or large bowel. Small-bowel obstruction is far more common and usually more serious. Complete obstruction in any part of the bowel, if untreated, can cause death within hours from shock and vascular collapse.

Intestinal obstruction can occur in three forms:

☝ simple: blockage prevents intestinal contents from passing, with no other complications

✌ strangulated: blood supply to part or all of the obstructed section is cut off, in addition to blockage of the lumen

🖐 close-looped: both ends of a bowel section are occluded, isolating it from the rest of the intestine.

CAUSES
Mechanical
- Adhesions and strangulated hernias (most common causes of small-bowel obstruction)

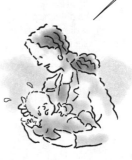

A cranky baby could be a sign of GERD. Check for crying, fussiness, gagging, coughing, and vomiting.

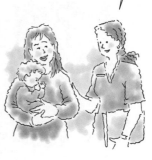

Support parents of a child with GERD. Instruct them to hold their baby for at least 30 minutes after meals to reduce intra-abdominal pressure.

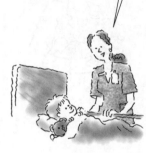

> When the obstruction is high in the intestine, vomiting is marked and abdominal distention is limited. When the obstruction is low, the child has marked distention but little vomiting.

- Carcinomas (most common cause of large-bowel obstruction)
- Compression of the bowel wall due to stenosis, intussusception, volvulus of the sigmoid or cecum, tumors, or atresia
- Congenital bowel deformities
- Ingestion of foreign bodies (such as fruit pits or worms)
- Obstruction after abdominal surgery

Other
- Paralytic ileus
- Electrolyte imbalances
- Toxicity (uremia, generalized infection)
- Neurogenic abnormalities (spinal cord lesions)
- Thrombosis or embolism of mesenteric vessels

ASSESSMENT FINDINGS
Partial small-bowel obstruction
- Abdominal distention
- Colicky pain
- Constipation
- Drowsiness
- Dry oral mucous membranes and tongue
- Intense thirst
- Malaise
- Nausea
- Vomiting (the higher the obstruction, the earlier and more severe the vomiting)

Complete small-bowel obstruction
- Persistent epigastric or periumbilical pain
- Bowel contents propelled toward mouth (instead of rectum) by vigorous peristaltic waves

Partial large-bowel obstruction
- Dramatic abdominal distention
- Colicky abdominal pain; may appear suddenly, producing spasms that last less than 1 minute and recur every few minutes
- Constipation (may be only clinical effect for days)
- Continuous hypogastric pain and nausea; vomiting usually absent at first
- Leakage of liquid stools around the obstruction (common)
- Loops of large bowel becoming visible on the abdomen

Complete large-bowel obstruction
- Continuous abdominal pain
- Vomiting of fecal matter
- Localized peritonitis

DIAGNOSTIC TEST RESULTS
- X-rays confirm the diagnosis. Abdominal films show the presence and location of intestinal gas or fluid.
- With large-bowel obstruction, barium enema reveals a distended, air-filled colon or, in sigmoid volvulus, a closed loop of sigmoid with extreme distention.
- Arterial blood gas (ABG) analysis reveals metabolic alkalosis from dehydration and loss of gastric hydrochloric acid, characteristic of obstruction in the upper intestine.
- ABG analysis reveals metabolic acidosis caused by slower dehydration and loss of intestinal alkaline fluids, characteristic of lower-bowel obstruction.

NURSING DIAGNOSES
- Imbalanced nutrition: Less than body requirements
- Acute pain
- Risk for ineffective gastrointestinal perfusion
- Disturbed body image

TREATMENT
- I.V. therapy to correct fluid and electrolyte imbalances
- NG tube to decompress the bowel to relieve vomiting and distention
- Surgical resection with anastomosis, colostomy, or ileostomy
- Total parenteral nutrition for protein deficit from chronic obstruction, paralytic ileus, infection, or prolonged postoperative recovery time that requires NPO status

Drug therapy
- Analgesics (usually nonopioid to avoid reduced intestinal motility commonly caused by opioid analgesics)
- Antibiotics for peritonitis

INTERVENTIONS AND RATIONALES
- Monitor vital signs frequently. *A drop in blood pressure may indicate reduced circulating blood volume due to blood loss from*

a strangulated hernia. As much as 10 L of fluid can collect in the small bowel, drastically reducing plasma volume.
- Assess cardiovascular status *to observe for signs of shock, such as pallor, rapid pulse, and hypotension.*
- Monitor for signs and symptoms of metabolic alkalosis (changes in sensorium; slow, shallow respirations; hypertonic muscles; tetany) or acidosis (dyspnea on exertion, disorientation and, later, deep, rapid breathing, weakness, and malaise). *This allows for early detection of complications.*
- Observe for signs and symptoms of secondary infection, such as fever and chills. *Sustained temperature elevations after surgery may signal onset of pulmonary complications or wound infection.*
- Monitor intake and output carefully *to assess renal function, circulating blood volume, and possible urine retention caused by bladder compression by the distended intestine.*
- Provide oral and nasal care *to prevent mucosal breakdown.*
- Place the child in Fowler's position as much as possible *to promote pulmonary ventilation and ease respiratory distress from abdominal distention.*
- Assess GI status. Listen for bowel sounds, and watch for signs of returning peristalsis (passage of flatus and mucus through the rectum) *to promote nutritional status.*
- Arrange for an enterostomal therapist to visit the child who has had an ostomy *to provide education and information and relieve anxiety.*

Teaching topics
- Explanation of the disorder and treatment plan
- Signs and symptoms of complications
- Wound care or ostomy care, if appropriate

Lead toxicity

Lead toxicity occurs most commonly in toddlers. Lead is poorly absorbed by the body and slowly excreted, replacing calcium in the bones and increasing the permeability of central nervous system membranes.

CAUSES
- Ingestion of lead from dust, soil, paint chips, folk remedies, or use of old ceramic cookware

ASSESSMENT FINDINGS
- Abdominal pain
- Pallor
- Hyperactivity
- Constipation
- Increased intracranial pressure, cortical atrophy, behavioral changes, altered cognition and motor skills, and seizures
- Peripheral neuritis from calcium release into the blood
- Anorexia, vomiting
- Weight loss

DIAGNOSTIC TEST RESULTS
- Blood lead level (BLL) greater than 10 mcg/dl.
- Hematologic studies reveal anemia and increased erythrocyte protoporphyrin.
- Urinalysis reveals proteinuria, ketonuria, and glycosuria.
- X-rays reveal lead lines near the epiphyseal lines (areas of increased density) of long bones. The thickness of the line shows the length of time the lead ingestion has been occurring.

NURSING DIAGNOSES
- Risk for ineffective cerebral tissue perfusion
- Risk for deficient fluid volume
- Risk for poisoning
- Deficient knowledge (lead toxin)

TREATMENT
- BLL less than 10 mcg/dl: no treatment
- BLL 10 to 14 mcg/dl: repeat test in 1 month and again in 3 months if level isn't lower
- BLL 15 to 19 mcg/dl: repeat test in 1 month and again in 2 months if level isn't lower
- BLL 20 to 44 mcg/dl: repeat test in 1 week; if level remains elevated, environmental evaluation by local health department
- BLL 45 to 69 mcg/dl: repeat test in 2 days; if level confirmed, chelating agents

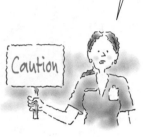

Chelating agents used to treat lead toxicity also bind with calcium, leading to decreased calcium levels. So monitor calcium carefully.

Caution

• BLL over 70 mcg/dl: hospitalization; repeat test, chelating agents
• Oral or I.V. fluid administration to lower BLL and prevent lead encephalopathy
• Low-fat diet with adequate supplies of calcium, magnesium, zinc, iron, and copper; prevents any more lead from being bound and stored in the body's fat tissues

Drug therapy
• Chelating agents: succimer (Chemet) or dimercaprol (BAL In Oil) for BLL greater than 45 mcg/dl
• Benzodiazepines (if seizures occur)

INTERVENTIONS AND RATIONALES
• Monitor calcium levels (chelating agents also bind with calcium) *to prevent tetany and seizures, which may result from hypocalcemia.*
• Monitor vital signs, intake and output, hydration status, and kidney function *to ensure that kidney function is adequate to handle the lead being excreted. If kidney function isn't adequate, EDTA may cause kidney damage.*
• Assess cardiovascular and neurologic status. *Increased levels of lead can cause severe encephalopathy with seizures and permanent neurologic damage.*
• Initiate seizure precautions, if appropriate, *to ensure patient safety.*

Teaching topics
• Explanation of the disorder and treatment plan
• Identifying sources of lead and adjusting the environment appropriately
• Stressing the importance of a well-balanced diet to ensure that the child receives adequate amounts of calcium, magnesium, zinc, iron, and copper
• Signs and symptoms of complications

Pyloric stenosis

With pyloric stenosis, also known as *infantile hypertrophic pyloric stenosis,* hyperplasia and hypertrophy of the circular muscle at the pylorus narrow the pyloric canal, thereby preventing the stomach from emptying normally. The defect is most commonly diagnosed at ages 3 to 12 weeks and occurs four times more often in males.

CAUSES
• Exact cause unknown

ASSESSMENT FINDINGS
• Olive-size bulge palpated below the right costal margin
• Poor weight gain
• Jaundice
• Symptoms of malnutrition and dehydration despite the child's apparent adequate intake of food
• Projectile emesis during or soon after feedings, preceded by reverse peristaltic waves (going left to right) but not by nausea (the child resumes eating after vomiting)
• Tetany

DIAGNOSTIC TEST RESULTS
• ABG analysis reveals metabolic alkalosis.
• Blood chemistry tests may reveal hypocalcemia, hypokalemia, and hypochloremia.
• Hematest reveals emesis containing blood.
• Ultrasound shows pyloric muscle thickness greater than 4 mm.
• Endoscopy reveals a hypertrophied sphincter.

NURSING DIAGNOSES
• Imbalanced nutrition: Less than body requirements
• Risk for imbalanced fluid volume
• Risk for infection
• Delayed growth and development

TREATMENT
• Diet: NPO status before surgery
• I.V. therapy to correct fluid and electrolyte imbalances
• Possible insertion of NG tube, kept open and elevated for gastric decompression
• Surgical intervention: pyloromyotomy performed by laparoscopy

Drug therapy
• Potassium supplements
• Calcium supplement: I.V. calcium
• Atropine sulfate for 21 days (may cause regression of pyloric hypertrophy)

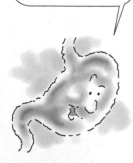

The pylorus is the outlet from the stomach to the duodenum.

INTERVENTIONS AND RATIONALES
- Weigh the child daily *to assess growth.*
- Monitor vital signs and intake and output *to assess renal function and check for signs of dehydration.*
- Assess for metabolic alkalosis and dehydration from frequent emesis *to detect early complications.*
- Assess GI and cardiovascular status *to detect early signs of compromise.*
- Provide small, frequent, thickened feedings with the head of the bed elevated; burp the child frequently (preoperatively) *to promote nutrition and prevent aspiration.*
- Position the child on his right side *to prevent the aspiration of vomitus.*

Postoperative care
- After surgery, feed the infant small amounts of oral electrolyte solution at first; then increase the amount and concentration of food until normal feeding is achieved *to meet nutritional needs and prevent vomiting.*
- Provide a pacifier *to meet nonnutritive sucking needs and maintain comfort.*
- Provide routine postoperative care *to maintain and improve the child's condition and to detect early complications.* Position the child on his side *so if vomiting occurs there's little chance of aspiration. Laying the child on the right side possibly aids the flow of fluid through the pyloric valve by gravity.*

Teaching topics
- Explanation of the disorder and treatment plan
- Feeding the infant, including specific formula, volume, and technique
- Signs and symptoms of complications

Salicylate toxicity

Salicylate (aspirin) is an analgesic, antipyretic, and anti-inflammatory agent that inhibits platelet aggregation. Toxicity may result from an overdose of salicylate. Symptoms begin when children ingest 150 to 200 mg of aspirin per kilogram of body weight. The peak blood level is reached within 2 to 3 hours of ingestion. The

prognosis of the child with salicylate toxicity depends on the amount of salicylate ingested and how quickly treatment begins.

CAUSES
- Ingestion of salicylate beyond the recommended dosage

ASSESSMENT FINDINGS
- Nausea, vomiting
- Tinnitus
- Tachypnea and hyperpnea
- Vertigo
- Restlessness
- Lethargy, which may progress to disorientation, seizures, and coma
- High fever
- Petechiae and bleeding tendency

DIAGNOSTIC TEST RESULTS
- Ferric chloride test reveals the presence of salicylates in urine.
- ABG levels may reveal metabolic acidosis.
- Serum salicylate levels are elevated beyond therapeutic range.

NURSING DIAGNOSES
- Imbalanced nutrition: Less than body requirements
- Hyperthermia
- Risk for imbalanced fluid volume
- Risk for injury
- Ineffective breathing pattern

TREATMENT
- I.V. fluids
- Gastric lavage
- Whole-bowel irrigation with polyethylene glycol
- Hemodialysis (for serum salicylate level over 100 mg/dl)
- Hypothermia blanket
- Intubation and mechanical ventilation if respiratory failure occurs

Drug therapy
- Oral activated charcoal (Liqui-Char)
- Calcium and potassium supplements, if indicated
- Alkalinizing agent: sodium bicarbonate

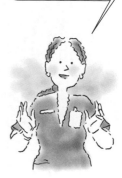

Because aspirin inhibits platelet aggregation, look for petechiae and bleeding in salicylate toxicity.

INTERVENTIONS AND RATIONALES

- Assess respiratory status *to identify respiratory failure.*
- Assess neurologic status *to recognize altered mental staus and level of consciousness and provide appropriate protective measures.*
- Administer I.V. fluids *to dilute the toxin and prevent dehydration.*
- Monitor vital signs and intake and output *to detect dehydration and early signs of compromise.*
- Assess cardiovascular and GI status *to identify signs of metabolic acidosis and GI bleeding.*
- Maintain mechanical ventilation, if required, *to ensure adequate oxygenation.*
- Ensure adequate hydration *to flush the aspirin through the kidneys.*
- Monitor urine pH; *pH over 8 aids salicylate excretion.*
- Dress the child lightly and sponge with tepid water or use a cooling blanket *to reduce high temperature.*
- Monitor body temperature every 15 to 30 minutes according to facility policy while a hypothermia blanket is in use *to evaluate its effectiveness and prevent injury.*
- Monitor ABG values *to assess acid-base balance.*
- Monitor salicylate levels *to assess the effectiveness of treatment.*

Teaching topics

- Explanation of the disorder and treatment plan
- Storing medication and taking steps to prevent aspirin overdose
- Monitoring the child's temperature and encouraging a high fluid intake

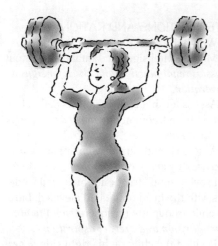

Pump up on practice questions

1. A 3-week-old infant diagnosed with pyloric stenosis is admitted to the hospital during a vomiting episode. Which action by the nurse is most appropriate?

1. Placing the infant on his back to sleep
2. Weighing the infant every 12 hours
3. Positioning the infant on his right side
4. Taking vital signs every 8 hours

Answer: 3. The nurse should position the infant on his right side to prevent aspiration. The infant should be weighed daily, not every 12 hours. Vital signs should be monitored every 4 hours, not every 8 hours.

➡ *NCLEX keys*

Client needs category: Physiological integrity
Client needs subcategory: Reduction of risk potential
Cognitive level: Application

2. A nurse teaches a mother to position an infant with a tracheoesophageal fistula with his head elevated to 30 degrees. The nurse should recognize that teaching was effective when the mother makes which statement?

1. "Positioning him with his head elevated to 30 degrees helps his breathing."
2. "Positioning him with his head elevated to 30 degrees helps with eating."
3. "Positioning him with his head elevated to 30 degrees keeps gastric juices from backing up."
4. "Positioning him with his head elevated to 30 degrees makes him comfortable."

Answer: 3. Placing the infant with his head elevated to 30 degrees helps decrease gastric reflux into the trachea. The child won't be taking food by mouth until after the fistula is surgically repaired. The infant will also breathe easier and be more comfortable with his head elevated, but they aren't the primary reasons for elevating the infant's head to 30 degrees.

➡ *NCLEX keys*
Client needs category: Physiological integrity
Client needs subcategory: Reduction of risk potential
Cognitive level: Application

3. A child with a nasogastric (NG) tube in place complains of nausea. Which action by the nurse is most appropriate?

1. Administer an antiemetic.
2. Irrigate the NG tube.
3. Notify the physician about the nausea.
4. Reposition the NG tube.

Answer: 2. The nurse should first check NG tube placement and then irrigate the tube to check for patency. If nausea continues, the NG tube may be repositioned, depending on the child's condition. If the child continues to complain of nausea after these measures, the physician should be notified and an antiemetic given as ordered.

➡ *NCLEX keys*
Client needs category: Physiological integrity
Client needs subcategory: Reduction of risk potential
Cognitive level: Application

4. The mother of a child diagnosed with celiac disease asks the nurse which foods should be eliminated from her child's diet. The nurse should advise the mother to eliminate:

1. malted milk, wheat bread, and spaghetti.
2. rice cereals, milk, and corn bread.
3. tapioca, potato bread, and peanut butter.
4. corn cereals, milk, and honey.

Answer: 1. The mother should provide her child with celiac disease with a gluten-free diet, eliminating such foods as malted milk, wheat bread, and spaghetti. Rice and corn cereals, milk, corn and potato breads, tapioca, peanut butter, and honey are all appropriate for a gluten-free diet.

➡ *NCLEX keys*
Client needs category: Physiological integrity
Client needs subcategory: Basic care and comfort
Cognitive level: Application

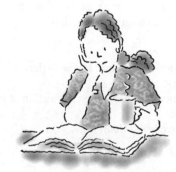

5. A nurse is caring for a toddler after surgical repair of a cleft palate. The nurse should position the child:
   1. on his back.
   2. on his stomach.
   3. on his back with his head slightly elevated.
   4. for comfort.

Answer: 2. After surgical repair of a cleft palate, the child should be positioned on his stomach to prevent pooling of secretions in the oropharynx. The child shouldn't be positioned on his back. The nurse shouldn't choose a position based on comfort.

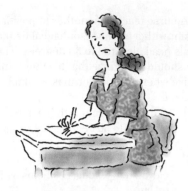

➡ *NCLEX keys*

Client needs category: Physiological integrity
Client needs subcategory: Reduction of risk potential
Cognitive level: Application

6. A nurse is caring for a child with a complete intestinal obstruction. Which is a key finding in this client?
   1. Vomiting
   2. Intense thirst
   3. Visible peristaltic waves
   4. Nausea

Answer: 3. Visible peristaltic waves propel bowel contents toward the mouth instead of the rectum. Vomiting, intense thirst, and nausea are symptoms of a small-bowel obstruction and aren't the key findings in complete intestinal obstruction.

➡ *NCLEX keys*

Client needs category: Physiological integrity
Client needs subcategory: Reduction of risk potential
Cognitive level: Comprehension

7. A nurse is caring for an infant with a cleft lip and palate. This condition places the infant at increased risk for:
   1. upper respiratory infections and otitis media.
   2. otitis media and diarrhea.
   3. upper respiratory infections and diarrhea.
   4. diarrhea and vomiting.

Answer: 1. The infant with a cleft lip and palate is at increased risk for upper respiratory infections and otitis media because the increased open space decreases natural defenses against bacteria. It doesn't increase the risk of vomiting and diarrhea.

➡ *NCLEX keys*

Client needs category: Physiological integrity
Client needs subcategory: Reduction of risk potential
Cognitive level: Application

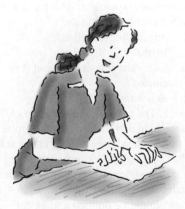

8. A nurse is caring for a toddler with salicylate toxicity. Besides salicylate levels, which values should the nurse be monitoring?

  1. Arterial blood pH
  2. Acetaminophen levels
  3. Calcium levels
  4. Phosphorus levels

Answer: 1. Salicylate toxicity results in metabolic acidosis. Monitoring arterial blood pH helps the nurse evaluate the effectiveness of treatment. Acetaminophen levels should be monitored with acetaminophen toxicity. Calcium and phosphorus levels can be obtained, but they aren't primarily affected by salicylate toxicity.

➡ *NCLEX keys*
Client needs category: Physiological integrity
Client needs subcategory: Reduction of risk potential
Cognitive level: Analysis

9. A 4-week-old infant is brought to the pediatrician's office. The infant has been experiencing projectile vomiting shortly after feedings. The infant most likely has:

  1. an intestinal obstruction.
  2. intussusception.
  3. a tracheoesophageal fistula.
  4. pyloric stenosis.

Answer: 4. Symptoms of pyloric stenosis generally develop between ages 4 and 6 weeks. They include a palpable bulge below the right costal margin, projectile vomiting during or shortly after feeding, resuming feeding after vomiting, poor weight gain, malnutrition, and dehydration. Intestinal obstruction presents with constipation, colicky abdominal pain, nausea, and dramatic abdominal distention. Intussusception causes sudden onset of severe abdominal pain; the infant is usually inconsolable. Tracheo-esophageal fistula causes coughing, choking, and intermittent cyanosis during feeding, and abdominal distention.

➡ *NCLEX keys*
Client needs category: Physiological integrity
Client needs subcategory: Reduction of risk potential
Cognitive level: Application

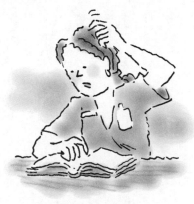

10. Which findings are common in neonates born with esophageal atresia? Select all that apply.

  1. Decreased saliva production
  2. Cyanosis
  3. Coughing
  4. Inadequate swallowing
  5. Choking
  6. Inability to cough

Answer: 2, 3, 5. Cyanosis, coughing, and choking occur when fluid from the blind pouch is aspirated into the trachea. Saliva production doesn't decrease in neonates born with esophageal atresia. The ability to swallow isn't affected by this disorder.

➡ *NCLEX keys*
Client needs category: Physiological integrity
Client needs subcategory: Physiological adaptation
Cognitive level: Analysis

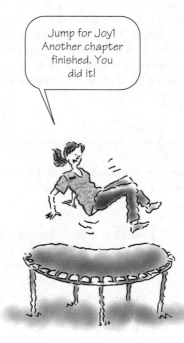

Brush up on key concepts

Together with the nervous system, the endocrine system regulates and integrates the body's metabolic activities. Disorders of the endocrine system involve hyposecretion or hypersecretion of hormones, which affect the body's metabolic processes and function.

At any time, you can review the major points of this chapter by consulting the *Cheat sheet* on page 702.

Endocrine junior

Here are key points about **endocrine functioning in childhood:**
• The pituitary gland controls the release of nine different hormones and is the master gland for all age-groups.
• The adrenal cortex begins secreting glucocorticoids and mineralocorticoids early in embryonic life.
• The thyroid gland, many times larger in children than in adults, is functional at age 2 weeks. It's thought to play a role in immune function.

Ch..ch..changes

The pituitary is stimulated at puberty to produce androgen steroids responsible for **secondary sex characteristics.**

Female secondary sexual development during puberty involves increase in the size of the ovaries, uterus, vagina, labia, and breasts. The first visible sign of sexual maturity is the appearance of breast buds. Body hair appears in the pubic area and under the arms and menarche begins. The ovaries, present at birth, remain inactive until puberty.

Male secondary sexual development consists of genital growth and the appearance of pubic and body hair.

A place to integrate

The endocrine system meets the nervous system at the **hypothalamus.** The hypothalamus, the main integrative center for the endocrine and autonomic nervous systems, controls the function of endocrine organs by neural and hormonal pathways.

Neural pathways connect the hypothalamus to the posterior pituitary, or neurohypophysis. Neural stimulation to the posterior pituitary provokes the secretion of hormones (chemical transmitters released from specialized cells into the bloodstream). Hormones are then carried to specialized organ-receptor cells that respond to them.

Negative feedback

In addition to hormonal and neural controls, a **negative feedback system** regulates the endocrine system. The mechanism of feedback may be either simple or complex:
• **Simple feedback** occurs when the level of one substance regulates secretion of a hormone. For example, low serum calcium levels stimulate parathyroid hormone secretion; high serum calcium levels inhibit it.
• **Complex feedback** occurs through an axis established between the hypothalamus, pituitary gland, and target organ. For example, secretion of the hypothalamic corticotropin-releasing hormone stimulates release of pituitary corticotropin which, in turn, stimulates cortisol secretion by the adrenal gland (the target organ). A rise in serum cortisol levels inhibits corticotropin secretion by decreasing corticotropin-releasing hormone.

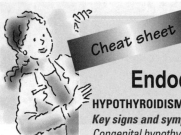

Endocrine refresher

HYPOTHYROIDISM

Key signs and symptoms
Congenital hypothyroidism
- Poor feeding
- Low temperature
- Hoarse crying
- Prolonged jaundice

Acquired hypothyroidism
- Lethargy, decreased energy
- Cold intolerance
- Heat intolerance
- Weight loss

Untreated hypothyroidism in older children
- Bone and muscle dystrophy
- Cognitive impairment
- Stunted growth (cretinism)

Key test results
- Radioimmunoassay confirms hypothyroidism with low triiodothyronine and thyroxine levels.

Key treatments
- Oral thyroid hormone: levothyroxine (Synthroid)

Key interventions
- During early management of infantile hypothyroidism, monitor blood pressure and pulse rate and report hypertension and tachycardia immediately (normal infant heart rate is approximately 120 beats/minute).
- Check rectal temperature every 2 to 4 hours. Keep the infant warm and his skin moist.
- If the infant's tongue is unusually large, position him on his side and observe him frequently.

TYPE 1 DIABETES MELLITUS

Key signs and symptoms
- Polydipsia
- Polyphagia
- Polyuria
- Weight loss and hunger

Key test results
- Two fasting plasma glucose levels (no caloric intake for at least 8 hours) are greater than or equal to 126 mg/dl.
- Glycosylated hemoglobin level is greater than 7%.
- Plasma glucose value in the 2-hour sample of the oral glucose tolerance test is greater than or equal to 200 mg/dl. This test should be performed after a loading dose of 75 g of anhydrous glucose.
- A random plasma glucose value (obtained without regard to the time of the child's last food intake) greater than or equal to 200 mg/dl accompanied by symptoms of diabetes indicates diabetes mellitus.

Key treatments
- Exercise
- Insulin replacement
- Strict diet planned to meet nutritional needs, control blood glucose levels, and reach and maintain appropriate body weight

Key interventions
- Monitor vital signs and intake and output.
- Use age-appropriate teaching materials when teaching about diabetes and the therapeutic regimen.

Keep abreast of diagnostic tests

Here are some important tests used to diagnose endocrine disorders, along with common nursing interventions associated with each test.

Function studies

An **endocrine function study** focuses on measuring the level or effect of a hormone such as the effect of insulin on blood glucose levels.

Sophisticated techniques of hormone measurement have improved diagnosis of endocrine disorders. For example, the human growth hormone stimulation test measures human growth hormone levels after I.V. administration of arginine, an amino acid that, under normal circumstances, stimulates human growth hormone. This test is used to diagnose growth hormone deficiency.

Nursing actions

- Explain the test to the child and his parents.
- Check with the laboratory and consult facility protocol to determine specific actions before the test (nothing-by-mouth for blood glucose test).

Minute measurements

A **radioimmunoassay** is used to measure minute quantities of hormones.

Nursing actions

- Explain the test to the child and his parents.

Polish up on client care

Two major pediatric endocrine disorders are hypothyroidism and type 1 diabetes mellitus.

Hypothyroidism

Hypothyroidism occurs when the body doesn't produce enough thyroid gland hormones, the hormones necessary for normal growth and development. (See *Thyroid gland hormones.*)

Two types of hypothyroidism exist. Congenital hypothyroidism is present at birth. Acquired hypothyroidism is commonly due to thyroiditis, an inflammation of the thyroid gland that results in injury or damage to thyroid tissue. Hypothyroidism is two times more common in girls than in boys.

Early diagnosis and treatment offer the best hope. Infants treated before age 3 months usually grow and develop normally. Children who remain untreated beyond age 3 months and children with acquired hypothyroidism who remain untreated beyond age 2 suffer irreversible cognitive impairment. Skeletal abnormalities may also occur; however, these may be reversible with treatment.

CAUSES

- Antithyroid drugs taken during pregnancy (in infants)
- Chromosomal abnormalities
- Chronic autoimmune thyroiditis (in children older than age 2)
- Defective embryonic development that causes congenital absence or underdevelopment of the thyroid gland (most common cause in infants)
- Inherited enzymatic defect in the synthesis of thyroxine (T_4) caused by an autosomal recessive gene (in infants)
- Irradiation of the thyroid gland

CONTRIBUTING FACTORS

- Prolonged gestation
- High birth weight

ASSESSMENT FINDINGS
General findings

- Delayed dentition
- Enlarged tongue
- Hypotonia
- Legs shorter in relation to trunk size
- Cognitive impairment (develops as the disorder progresses)
- Short stature with the persistence of infant proportions
- Short, thick neck; goiter
- Brittle nails

Congenital hypothyroidism

- Delayed stools at birth
- Prolonged jaundice
- Poor feeding
- Low temperature
- Decreased activity level
- Hoarse crying
- Galactorrhea
- Large fontanels
- Umbilical hernia

Acquired hypothyroidism

- Dry, scaly skin
- Lethargy, decreased energy
- Sleep disturbance
- Cold intolerance
- Constipation
- Heat intolerance
- Weight loss
- Sexual pseudoprecocity

Balance is better. Too many hormones or not enough hormones can cause an endocrine disorder.

Thyroid gland hormones

- The thyroid gland secretes the iodinated hormones thyroxine and triiodothyronine.
- Thyroid hormones, necessary for normal growth and development, act on many tissues to increase metabolic activity and protein synthesis.
- Deficiency of thyroid hormone causes varying degrees of hypothyroidism, from a mild, clinically insignificant form to life-threatening myxedema coma.

Timing is everything. If hypothyroidism is treated before the child is age 3 months, the prognosis is excellent — left untreated, it leads to cognitive impairment and skeletal abnormalities.

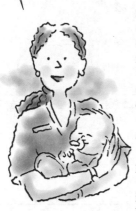

Key test for detecting hypothyroidism: Radioimmunoassay results show low T_3 and T_4 hormone levels.

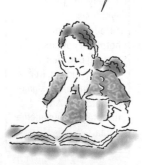

Untreated hypothyroidism in older children
- Bone and muscle dystrophy
- Cognitive impairment
- Stunted growth (cretinism)

DIAGNOSTIC TEST RESULTS
- Electrocardiogram shows bradycardia and flat or inverted T waves in untreated infants.
- Hip, knee, and thigh X-rays reveal absence of the femoral or tibial epiphyseal line and delayed skeletal development that's markedly inappropriate for the child's chronological age.
- In myxedema coma, laboratory tests may also show low serum sodium levels, decreased pH, and increased partial pressure of arterial carbon dioxide, indicating respiratory acidosis.
- Increased gonadotropin levels accompany sexual precocity in older children and may coexist with hypothyroidism.
- Serum cholesterol, alkaline phosphatase, and triglyceride levels are elevated.
- Normocytic normochromic anemia is present.
- Radioimmunoassay confirms hypothyroidism with low triiodothyronine (T_3) and T_4 levels.
- Thyroid scan and ^{131}I uptake tests show decreased uptake levels and confirm the absence of thyroid tissue in athyroid children.
- Thyroid-stimulating hormone (TSH) level is decreased when hypothyroidism results from hypothalamic or pituitary insufficiency.
- TSH level is increased when hypothyroidism results from thyroid insufficiency.

NURSING DIAGNOSES
- Delayed growth and development
- Interrupted family processes
- Deficient knowledge (treatment regimen)
- Imbalanced nutrition: Less than body requirements
- Activity intolerance
- Risk for imbalanced body temperature

TREATMENT
- Routine monitoring of T_4 and TSH levels
- Periodic evaluation of growth to ensure thyroid replacement is adequate
- Surgery to remove massive goiter (rare)

Drug therapy
- Oral thyroid hormone: levothyroxine (Synthroid)

INTERVENTIONS AND RATIONALES
- During early management of infantile hypothyroidism, monitor blood pressure and pulse rate; report hypertension and tachycardia immediately (normal infant heart rate is approximately 120 beats/minute). *These signs of hyperthyroidism indicate that the dose of thyroid replacement medication is too high.*
- Check rectal temperature every 2 to 4 hours. Keep the infant warm and his skin moist *to promote normothermia and reduce metabolic demands.*
- If the infant's tongue is unusually large, position him on his side and observe him frequently *to prevent airway obstruction.*
- Provide parents with support, referrals, and counseling as necessary *to help parents cope with the possibility of caring for a physically and cognitively impaired child.*
- Adolescent girls require future-oriented counseling that stresses the importance of adequate thyroid replacement during pregnancy. *Ideally, women should have excellent control before conception.*

Teaching topics
- Explanation of the disorder and treatment plan
- Medication use and possible adverse effects
- Recognizing signs of overdose of supplemental thyroid hormone (rapid pulse rate, irritability, insomnia, fever, sweating, weight loss)
- Understanding that the child requires life-long treatment with thyroid supplements
- Complying with the treatment regimen to prevent further mental impairment
- Adopting a positive but realistic attitude and focusing on the child's strengths rather than his weaknesses
- Providing stimulating activities to help the child reach maximum potential (referring

parents to appropriate community resources for support)
• Preventing infantile hypothyroidism (emphasize the importance of adequate nutrition during pregnancy, including iodine-rich foods and the use of iodized salt or, in cases of sodium restriction, iodine supplements)

Type 1 diabetes mellitus

Type 1 diabetes mellitus (formerly referred to as juvenile diabetes or insulin-dependent diabetes) is a chronic metabolic disease characterized by absolute insulin insufficiency. Children with this type of diabetes must inject insulin to process carbohydrates, fat, and protein. Type 1 diabetes is most commonly diagnosed during childhood or adolescence but can occur at any time from infancy to about age 30. (See *Understanding type 1 diabetes,* page 706.)

CAUSES
• Genetic predisposition
• Viral infection
• Autoimmune response
• Congenital absence of pancreas or islet cells
• Pancreatic damage secondary to another disorder, such as cystic fibrosis or pancreatitis
• Chromosomal disorders such as Down syndrome

ASSESSMENT FINDINGS
• Polydipsia
• Polyphagia
• Polyuria
• Weight loss and hunger

Hyperglycemia
• Abdominal cramping
• Dry, flushed skin
• Fatigue
• Fruity breath odor
• Headache
• Mental status changes
• Nausea
• Thin appearance and possible malnourishment

• Vomiting
• Weakness

Hypoglycemia in conjunction with diabetes
• Behavior changes (belligerence, confusion, slurred speech)
• Diaphoresis
• Palpitations
• Tachycardia
• Tremors

DIAGNOSTIC TEST RESULTS
• Two fasting plasma glucose levels (no caloric intake for at least 8 hours) are greater than or equal to 126 mg/dl.
• Glycosylated hemoglobin level is greater than 7%.
• Plasma glucose value in the 2-hour sample of the oral glucose tolerance test is greater than or equal to 200 mg/dl. This test should be performed after a loading dose of 75 g of anhydrous glucose.
• A random plasma glucose value (obtained without regard to the time of the child's last food intake) greater than or equal to 200 mg/dl that's accompanied by symptoms of diabetes indicates diabetes mellitus.

NURSING DIAGNOSES
• Disturbed body image
• Risk for imbalanced nutrition: Less than body requirements
• Risk for imbalanced fluid volume
• Deficient knowledge (treatment regimen)

TREATMENT
• Exercise
• Strict diet planned to meet nutritional needs, control blood glucose levels, and reach and maintain appropriate body weight

Drug therapy
• Insulin replacement

INTERVENTIONS AND RATIONALES
• Monitor vital signs and fluid intake and output *to detect signs of hyperglycemia or hypoglycemia.*
• Monitor blood glucose levels and electrolytes *to detect early signs of electrolyte imbalance.*

> Remember that regular study habits do more good than cramming. Plan a realistic, regular schedule and stick to it.

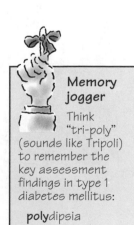

Memory jogger

Think "tri-poly" (sounds like Tripoli) to remember the key assessment findings in type 1 diabetes mellitus:

polydipsia

polyphagia

polyuria.

Understanding type 1 diabetes

Here are important points for understanding how type 1 diabetes develops.

THE KEY PLAYERS
- The endocrine part of the pancreas produces glucagon from the alpha cells and insulin from the beta cells.
- Glucagon, the hormone of the fasting state, releases stored glucose to raise the blood glucose level.
- Insulin, the hormone of the nourished state, facilitates glucose transport, promotes glucose storage, stimulates protein synthesis, and enhances free fatty acid uptake and storage.

WHAT HAPPENS
Absolute or relative insulin deficiency causes diabetes mellitus. Here's what happens:
- Pancreatic beta cells are destroyed, no insulin is produced, and the cells can't utilize glucose.
- Excess glucose in the blood spills into the urine.
- The increased level of blood glucose can act as an osmotic diuretic, resulting in dehydration, hypotension, and renal shutdown.
- The body attempts to compensate for lost energy by breaking down fatty acids to form ketones with resulting metabolic acidosis.

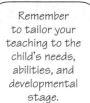

Remember to tailor your teaching to the child's needs, abilities, and developmental stage.

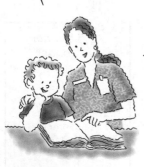

- Observe neurologic status *to detect signs of hyperglycemia or hypoglycemia.*
- Evaluate the child's or adolescent's understanding of type 1 diabetes and his attitude about the need to manage it *to help plan teaching.*
- Use age-appropriate teaching materials when teaching about diabetes and the therapeutic regimen *to increase the child or adolescent's knowledge of his condition and instill confidence in his ability to manage it.*
- Provide an opportunity for the child or adolescent to interact with peers who have experienced diabetes *to decrease his feelings of isolation and being different from others.*

Hyperglycemia
- Administer regular insulin for fast action *to promote euglycemic state and prevent complications.*
- Administer I.V. fluids without dextrose *to flush out acetone and maintain hydration.*
- Monitor electrolyte and arterial blood gas levels *to detect imbalances or acidosis.*
- Monitor blood glucose level *to detect early changes and prevent complications such as diabetic ketoacidosis.*

Hypoglycemia
- Give a fast-acting carbohydrate, such as honey, orange juice, or sugar cubes, followed later by a protein source *to increase glucose levels thereby preventing complications of hypoglycemia.*
- If the child is stuporous or unconscious, administer glucagon (subcutaneously, I.V., or I.M.) or dextrose 50% I.V. *to prevent complications of hypoglycemia.*

Teaching topics
- Explanation of the disorder and treatment plan
- Medication use and possible adverse effects
- Dietary adjustments
- Complying with the prescribed treatment program (see *Teaching about insulin administration*)
- Monitoring blood glucose levels
- Understanding the importance of good hygiene
- Preventing, recognizing, and treating hypoglycemia and hyperglycemia
- Understanding the effect of blood glucose control on long-term health
- Managing diabetes during a minor illness, such as a cold, the flu, or an upset stomach
- Providing the child or adolescent with written materials that cover the teaching topics
- Providing the child and his family with information about the Juvenile Diabetes Foundation

Management moments

Teaching about insulin administration

Teaching about insulin administration is an important part of care management for the child with type 1 diabetes and his parents. Here are some important elements to teach the child and his parents about insulin administration:
• When giving both types of insulin, draw up clear insulin first to prevent contamination.
• To prevent air bubbles, don't shake the vial; intermediate forms are suspensions and should be gently rotated.
• Rotate injection sites to prevent lipodystrophy.
• Make sure the child eats when the insulin peaks, such as midafternoon and bedtime.
• Insulin requirements may be altered with illness, stress, growth, food intake, and exercise; blood glucose measurements are the best way to determine insulin adjustments.

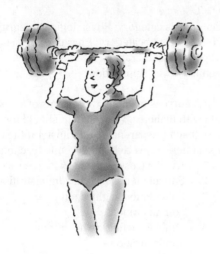

Pump up on practice questions

1. A nurse is teaching the mother of a child diagnosed with type 1 diabetes. The mother asks why her child must inject insulin and can't take pills as her uncle does. Which reply is most appropriate?
1. "Because a child's pancreas is less developed than an adult's, antidiabetic pills aren't recommended for children."
2. "Pills only affect fat and protein metabolism, not sugar."
3. "The only way to replace insulin is by injection."
4. "Your child may be able to take pills when he's older."

Answer: 3. In type 1 diabetes, the pancreas doesn't produce insulin, so the child must receive insulin replacement by injection. Oral antidiabetic agents stimulate the pancreas to produce more insulin and are only effective in treating type 2 diabetes. Because the pancreas in the child with type 1 diabetes doesn't produce insulin, the child will never be a candidate for oral antidiabetic agents.

➡ *NCLEX keys*
Client needs category: Physiological integrity
Client needs subcategory: Pharmacological and parenteral therapies
Cognitive level: Application

2. A nurse is teaching the mother of a child how to recognize the signs and symptoms of hypoglycemia. Which signs and symptoms should the nurse discuss?
1. Behavioral changes, increased heart rate, sweating, and tremors
2. Nausea, fruity breath odor, headache, and fatigue
3. Polydipsia, polyuria, polyphagia, and weight loss
4. Enlarged tongue, hypotonia, easy weight gain, and cool skin temperature

Answer: 1. The nurse should instruct the mother of a child with diabetes to recognize such signs and symptoms of hypoglycemia as behavioral changes, increased heart rate, sweating, and tremors. Nausea, fruity breath odor, headache, and fatigue are present with hyperglycemia. Polydipsia, polyuria, polyphagia, and weight loss are classic signs of diabetes. Enlarged tongue, hypotonia, easy weight gain, and cool skin temperature are associated with hypothyroidism.

➡ *NCLEX keys*

Client needs category: Physiological integrity
Client needs subcategory: Reduction of risk potential
Cognitive level: Comprehension

3. A nurse is assessing a child who might have diabetes. Which laboratory value helps confirm a diagnosis of type 1 diabetes?
   1. A fasting plasma glucose level of 110 mg/dl obtained once
   2. A fasting plasma glucose level of 126 mg/dl obtained at two different times
   3. A random plasma glucose level of 180 mg/dl obtained once
   4. A 2-hour glucose tolerance test of 140 mg/dl obtained at two different times

Answer: 2. According to the American Diabetes Association, diabetes occurs when any of the following conditions exist: symptoms of diabetes plus a random plasma glucose level greater than or equal to 200 mg/dl, two fasting plasma glucose levels greater than or equal to 126 mg/dl, or a 2-hour oral glucose tolerance test greater than or equal to 200 mg/dl.

➡ *NCLEX keys*

Client needs category: Health promotion and maintenance
Client needs subcategory: None
Cognitive level: Application

4. A nurse is caring for a child with type 1 diabetes. The nurse enters the child's room and finds him diaphoretic and unresponsive. The nurse should anticipate which of the following emergency interventions?
   1. Administering honey followed by a protein source
   2. Administering orange juice followed by a protein source
   3. Administering dextrose 50% I.V.
   4. Administering insulin

Answer: 3. The child is unconscious and experiencing a hypoglycemic reaction; therefore, the nurse should be prepared to administer 50% dextrose I.V. The child experiencing a hypoglycemic episode who's conscious should be given a fast-acting carbohydrate, such as honey, orange juice or sugar cubes, followed by a protein source. Insulin administration would further worsen the child's condition.

➡ *NCLEX keys*

Client needs category: Physiological integrity
Client needs subcategory: Pharmacological and parenteral therapies
Cognitive level: Application

5. A nurse is teaching the parents of a child with diabetes. Which agent should the nurse teach the parents to administer if their child suffers a severe hypoglycemic reaction?
   1. I.V. dextrose
   2. Subcutaneous insulin administration
   3. Subcutaneous glucagon administration
   4. Oral fast-acting carbohydrate administration

Answer: 3. The nurse should instruct the parents of a child with diabetes about proper administration of subcutaneous glucagon if their child suffers a severe hypoglycemic episode. Administering insulin subcutaneously would further worsen the child's condition. I.V. dextrose is reserved for health care professionals specially trained in I.V. drug administration. Oral administration of fast-acting carbohydrates is reserved for the conscious child who isn't suffering from a severe hypoglycemic reaction.

➡ *NCLEX keys*

Client needs category: Physiological integrity
Client needs subcategory: Reduction of risk potential
Cognitive level: Application

6. A nurse is teaching an adolescent with diabetes about situations that can alter insulin requirements. Which situation should be emphasized?

1. Illness, stress, growth, food intake, and exercise
2. Water intake, illness, stress, and exercise
3. Exposure to ultraviolet light, illness, stress, and exercise
4. Sodium intake, exercise, stress, and illness

Answer: 1. Illness, stress, growth, food intake, and exercise can alter insulin requirements. Water intake, ultraviolet light exposure, and sodium intake don't alter insulin requirements.

➡ *NCLEX keys*

Client needs category: Physiological integrity
Client needs subcategory: Reduction of risk potential
Cognitive level: Application

7. The nurse is teaching an adolescent with diabetes about his disease. Which statement by the adolescent indicates that teaching was effective?

1. "If I want to eat ice cream, I'll just give myself more insulin."
2. "I'm so busy, I'm glad I can still skip meals if I need to."
3. "I will remember to take my regular dose of insulin even if I'm sick."
4. "I will monitor my blood glucose level to determine how much insulin I need."

Answer: 4. Diabetic teaching is effective when the adolescent verbalizes the importance of monitoring his blood glucose level to determine his insulin needs. Teaching should stress the importance of maintaining a diabetic diet and not skipping meals. It should also address the need for adjusting insulin doses during times of illness.

➡ *NCLEX keys*

Client needs category: Physiological integrity
Client needs subcategory: Reduction of risk potential
Cognitive level: Analysis

8. A 10-year-old boy with type 1 diabetes comes to the pediatrician's office. Which technique best ensures responsible insulin administration?

1. The child observes his parents as they administer his injections.
2. The child learns to administer his insulin with supervision.
3. The child manages his insulin administration independently.
4. The child learns to draw up his own insulin and his parents inject it.

Answer: 2. School-age children should be encouraged to administer their own insulin with adult supervision to ensure correct procedure is followed and the correct dosage is administered. Having the child observe the parents or drawing up his insulin and not injecting it doesn't allow the child to take sufficient responsibility for his care. Allowing the child to administer his insulin without adult supervision gives him too much responsibility.

➡ *NCLEX keys*

Client needs category: Physiological integrity
Client needs subcategory: Reduction of risk potential
Cognitive level: Application

9. A 9-year-old boy with type 1 diabetes takes a mixture of regular and NPH insulin. He's scheduled to go on a camping trip and his mother asks the nurse whether it's safe for him to participate in this activity. What's the most appropriate response?

1. "He needs to understand the physical limitations placed on a client with diabetes."
2. "He should have a light snack before doing any hiking."
3. "He shouldn't go on this trip because it's potentially dangerous."
4. "Have him increase his morning NPH insulin to compensate for higher metabolism while hiking."

Answer: 2. A light meal before rigorous exercise gives the child adequate blood glucose levels during the peak action of his morning NPH insulin. Restricting the child's physical activity discourages a normal lifestyle. The child's diagnosis alone shouldn't be used to evaluate the danger of the trip. Increasing the child's insulin would increase the likelihood of a hypoglycemic reaction.

➡ *NCLEX keys*

Client needs category: Physiological integrity
Client needs subcategory: Reduction of risk potential
Cognitive level: Application

10. A nurse administers oral thyroid hormone to an infant with hypothyroidism. For which signs of overdose should the nurse observe the infant?

1. Tachycardia, fever, irritability, and sweating
2. Bradycardia, cool skin temperature, and dry scaly skin
3. Bradycardia, fever, hypotension, and irritability
4. Tachycardia, cool skin temperature, and irritability

Answer: 1. The infant experiencing an overdose of thyroid replacement hormone exhibits tachycardia, fever, irritability, and sweating. Bradycardia, cool skin temperature, and dry scaly skin are signs of hypothyroidism.

➡ *NCLEX keys*

Client needs category: Physiological integrity
Client needs subcategory: Pharmacological and parenteral therapies
Cognitive level: Application

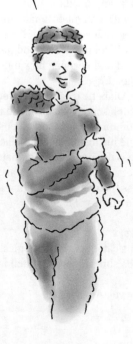

Treat yourself right while studying for the exam. Don't skip meals, miss sleep, or neglect exercise. Stay healthy and, in the long run, you'll stay ahead.

Brush up on key concepts

The genitourinary (GU) system includes the genitalia and urinary structures. This chapter focuses on the kidneys, ureters, and bladder, which are involved in renal and urinary function. The chapter also discusses two sexually transmitted diseases (STDs) that affect children.

You can review the major points of this chapter by consulting the *Cheat sheet* on pages 712 and 713.

High turnover

Water, which is controlled by the GU system, is the body's primary fluid. An infant has a much greater percentage of total body water in extracellular fluid (42% to 45%) than an adult does (20%). Because of the increased percentage of water in a child's extracellular fluid, a child's **water turnover rate** is two to three times greater than an adult's. Every day, 50% of an infant's extracellular fluid is exchanged, compared with only 20% of an adult's; a child is therefore more susceptible than an adult to dehydration.

Sweating it out

A neonate also has a greater ratio of body-surface area to body weight than an adult; this ratio results in greater **fluid loss through the skin.**

Less efficient during stress

A child's kidneys attain the adult number of **nephrons** (about a million in each kidney) shortly after birth. The nephrons, which form urine, continue to mature throughout early childhood.

An infant's renal system can maintain a healthy fluid and electrolyte status. However, it doesn't function as efficiently as an adult's during periods of stress. For example, if a child doesn't receive enough fluid to meet his needs, his kidneys can't adequately concentrate urine to prevent dehydration. Conversely, if a child receives too much fluid, he may be unable to dilute urine appropriately to get rid of the increased volume.

Concentration change

An infant's kidneys don't concentrate urine at an adult level (average **specific gravity** is less than 1.010 for an infant, compared with 1.010 to 1.030 for an adult).

Although the number of daily voidings decreases with increasing age (because of increased urine concentration), the total amount of urine produced daily may not vary significantly.

An infant usually voids 5 to 10 ml/hour, a 10-year-old child usually voids 10 to 25 ml/hour, and an adult usually voids 35 ml/hour.

Short path to the bladder

A child also has a short urethra; therefore, organisms can be easily transmitted into the bladder, increasing the risk of bladder infection.

Keep abreast of diagnostic tests

Here are the most important tests used to diagnose GU disorders, along with common nursing interventions associated with each test.

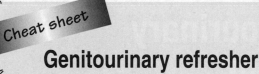

Cheat sheet

Genitourinary refresher

CHLAMYDIA

Key signs and symptoms
With conjunctivitis
- Fiery red conjunctivae with a thick pus
- Edematous eyelids

With pneumonia
- Nasal congestion
- Sharp cough that gradually worsens
- Failure to gain weight
- Tachypnea
- Crackles

Key test results
- Tissue cell cultures from infected sites reveal *Chlamydia trachomatis*.

Key treatments
- Irrigation of eyes with sterile saline solution to clear copious discharge
- Chest physiotherapy to mobilize secretions in a child with pneumonia
- Erythromycin
- Humidified oxygen to ease labored breathing and prevent hypoxemia in a child with pneumonia

Key interventions
- Check the neonate of an infected mother for signs of chlamydial infection.
- Administer medication as prescribed and monitor its effectiveness.
- Auscultate breath sounds and monitor oxygenation.
- Monitor for continued infection.

HYPOSPADIAS

Key signs and symptoms
- Altered angle of urination
- Meatus terminating at some point along lateral fusion line, ranging from the perineum to the distal penile shaft

Key test results
- Examination confirms aberrant placement of the opening.

Key treatments
- Avoiding circumcision (the foreskin may be needed later for surgical repair)

- Tubularized incised plate procedure (for distal and midshaft hypospadias); most commonly used repair for primary tubularization of the urethral plate
- Urethroplasty (surgical procedure in which the urethra is extended into a normal position with a meatus at the top of the penis); may initially be performed to restore normal urinary function
- Orthoplasty when the child is age 12 to 18 months, to release the adherent chordee (fibrous band that causes the penis to curve downward); if extensive repair is needed, delay until age 4
- Indwelling urinary catheter or suprapubic urinary catheter (postoperatively)
- Analgesics: meperidine (Demerol), acetaminophen (Tylenol) for postoperative pain relief
- Antispasmodic agent: propantheline prescribed postoperatively to treat bladder spasms

Key interventions
- Perform diligent perineal care.
- Provide emotional support to parents. Provide accurate information and answer questions thoroughly.

Postoperative care
- After the procedure, apply a pressure dressing.
- Check the tip of the penis frequently.
- Leave the dressing in place for several days.
- Avoid pressure on the child's catheter, and avoid kinking of the catheter.

NEPHRITIS

Key signs and symptoms
- Anorexia
- Burning during urination
- Flank pain
- Urinary frequency
- Shaking chills
- Temperature of 102° F (38.9° C) or higher
- Urinary urgency

> Uh-oh! My renal system doesn't function as well as an adult's when it undergoes stress.

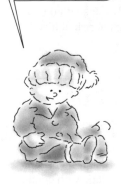

Genitourinary refresher (continued)

NEPHRITIS (CONTINUED)
Key test results
• Pyuria is present (with pyclonephritis). Urine sediment reveals the presence of leukocytes singly, in clumps, and in casts and, possibly, a few red blood cells.
• Urine culture identifies specific bacteria.

Key treatments
• Antibiotics: targeted to specific infecting organism

Key interventions
• Encourage fluid intake to achieve urine output of more than 2 L/day. However, discourage intake greater than 3 L/day.

NEPHROBLASTOMA
Key signs and symptoms
• Nontender mass, usually midline near the liver, that's commonly detected by the parent while bathing or dressing the child
• Associated congenital anomalies, such as microcephaly, mental retardation, genitourinary tract problems

Key test results
• Computed tomography scan or sonography reveals tumor, lymph node involvement, and metastasis.

Key treatments
• Nephrectomy to remove affected kidney and evaluate remaining kidney; may be preceded by chemotherapy to shrink the tumor if it has extended to the vena cava or if there's bilateral involvement
• Radiation therapy (after surgery)
• Chemotherapy (after surgery): dactinomycin (Cosmegen), doxorubicin (Doxil), vincristine

Key interventions
• Monitor vital signs and intake and output.

• Don't palpate the abdomen, and prevent others from doing so.
• Prepare the child and family members for a nephrectomy.
After nephrectomy
• Monitor urine output and report output less than 30 ml/hour.
• Assist with turning, coughing, and deep breathing.
• Encourage early ambulation.
• Provide pain medications as necessary and evaluate their effect.
• Monitor postoperative dressings for signs of bleeding.
• Provide wound care as directed.

URINARY TRACT INFECTION
Key signs and symptoms
• Frequent urges to void with pain or burning on urination
• Lethargy
• Low-grade fever
• Urine that's cloudy and foul-smelling

Key test results
• Clean catch urine culture yields large amounts of bacteria.
• Urine culture identifies specific bacteria.

Key treatments
• Increased fluid intake
• Antibiotics: gentamicin (Garamycin), cefotaxime (Claforan)

Key interventions
• Monitor intake and output.
• Assess toileting habits for proper front-to-back wiping and proper hand washing.
• Encourage increased intake of fluids.
• Assist the child when necessary to ensure that the perineal area is clean after elimination.

Blood analysis
Blood tests are used to analyze serum levels of chemical substances, such as uric acid, creatinine, and blood urea nitrogen.

Nursing actions
• Explain the procedure to the parents and child.
• Allow the child to hold a comfort object, such as a stuffed animal or blanket, to help diminish his anxiety.

Urine tests #1 and #2
Urinalysis is analysis of a urine specimen to determine characteristics, such as:
• presence of red blood cells (RBCs)
• presence of white blood cells
• presence of casts or bacteria
• specific gravity and pH
• physical properties, such as clarity, color, and odor.

Urine culture and sensitivity identifies the type of bacteria present in the urine. Results of this test help direct antibiotic therapy.

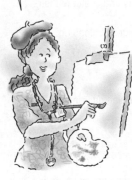

Picture this. Several tests help visualize the renal system: KUB radiography, excretory urography, and voiding cystourethrography.

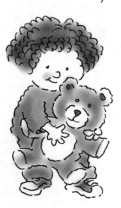

Holding a comfort object such as a stuffed animal may help decrease my anxiety.

Nursing actions

• Explain the procedure to the parents and child.

• Before specimen collection, explain the importance of cleaning the meatal area thoroughly.

• Explain that the culture specimen should be caught midstream, in a sterile container, preferably at the first voiding of the day.

• A urine specimen for culture for an infant should be obtained using a sterile straight catheter.

Urine test #3

A 24-hour urine specimen involves collecting urine over 24 hours to assess urine output or to measure the excretion of certain substances into urine over a 24-hour period.

Nursing actions

• Explain the procedure to the parents and child.

• Begin a 24-hour specimen collection after discarding the first voiding. Specimens typically necessitate special handling or preservatives and should be kept on ice or in the refrigerator until they're ready to be sent to the laboratory.

• When obtaining a urine specimen from a catheterized child, remember to avoid taking the specimen from the collection bag; instead, aspirate a specimen through the collection port in the catheter, with a sterile syringe.

Kidney pictures

Kidney-ureter-bladder (KUB) radiography is an X-ray used to assess the size, shape, position, and possible areas of calcification of the renal organs.

Nursing actions

• Explain the procedure to the parents and child.

• Tell the child that the X-ray only takes a few minutes and remind him to hold still.

• Shield the genitals of a male child to prevent irradiation of the testes.

Crisscrossing the belly

Computed tomography (CT) scan of the abdomen is an X-ray that obtains cross-sectional pictures of abdominal structures.

Nursing actions

• Explain the procedure to the parents and child.

• Complete paperwork required by the facility, including an informed consent if contrast dye is to be used.

• Tell the parents and child that he may be asked to drink barium sulfate 60 to 90 minutes before the test.

• Tell the parents and child that the CT scan should take about 30 minutes and that he'll need to remain still for the test.

• After the test, encourage the child to drink plenty of fluids for 24 to 48 hours.

I.V. action

Excretory urography is an X-ray that aids in checking renal pelvic structures (kidneys, ureters, and bladder). Contrast media is injected into the vein, allowing visualization of the collecting system and ureters.

Nursing actions

• Explain the procedure to the parents and child.

• Check the child's history for allergies.

• Tell the parents and child that the procedure may take up to 1 hour to complete and that the child will need to remain still after the dye is injected.

• Inform the child that a compression device may be placed on the abdomen to keep the contrast dye in the kidneys. The child may feel some pressure.

• Maintain the child on nothing-by-mouth status for 8 hours before the test.

• Make sure that written, informed consent has been obtained.

• Increase hydration after the procedure.

While the water is running

A **voiding cystourethrogram** is an X-ray that views the bladder and related structures during urination.

Nursing actions

• Explain the procedure to the child and parents.

• Check the child's history for allergies.

• Monitor the child's intake and output.

• Make sure that written, informed consent has been obtained.

- Tell the child that a small catheter will be placed in the bladder and that contrast dye will be injected through it.
- Inform the child that he'll be asked to urinate after the catheter is removed and that X-rays will be taken at the same time.
- After the procedure, encourage the child to drink lots of fluids to reduce burning on urination and to flush out residual dye.

Polish up on client care

Common pediatric GU disorders include chlamydia, hypospadias, nephritis, nephroblastoma (Wilms' tumor), and urinary tract infections (UTIs).

Chlamydia

Chlamydial infection is one of the most common STDs in the United States. In infants, the infecting organism is passed from the infected mother to the fetus during passage through the birth canal.

Chlamydia is the most common cause of ophthalmia neonatorum (eye infection at birth or during the first month) and a major cause of pneumonia in infants in the first 3 months of life. With antibiotic therapy, the prognosis is good.

CAUSES
- *Chlamydia trachomatis* exposure

ASSESSMENT FINDINGS
With conjunctivitis (occur within first 10 days of life)
- Fiery red conjunctivae with a thick puslike discharge
- Edematous eyelids

With pneumonia (occur within 3 to 6 weeks of birth)
- Nasal congestion
- Sharp cough that gradually worsens
- Failure to gain weight
- Tachypnea
- Crackles

DIAGNOSTIC TEST RESULTS
- Tissue cell cultures from infected sites reveal *C. trachomatis*.
- Blood studies show elevated levels of immunoglobulin (Ig) G and IgM antibodies.

NURSING DIAGNOSES
- Ineffective airway clearance
- Interrupted family processes
- Acute pain

TREATMENT
- Irrigation of eyes with sterile saline solution to clear copious discharge
- Humidified oxygen to ease labored breathing and prevent hypoxemia in a child with pneumonia
- Chest physiotherapy to mobilize secretions in a child with pneumonia

Drug therapy
- Erythromycin

INTERVENTIONS AND RATIONALES
- Check the neonate of an infected mother for signs of chlamydial infection *to identify infection early and initiate treatment*.
- Obtain appropriate specimens for diagnostic testing *to aid in diagnosis of infection*.
- Administer medication as prescribed and monitor its effectiveness *to improve the infant's condition*.
- Provide eye care for the neonate *to prevent complications*.
- Monitor for continued infection *to evaluate treatment*.
- Auscultate breath sounds and monitor oxygenation *to determine oxygen status and respiratory function*.
- Suction as needed *to provide airway clearance*.
- Assess for signs and symptoms of pain (increased respirations, tachycardia, increased or inconsolable crying, and frequent awakening from sleep).

Teaching topics
- Explanation of the disorder and treatment plan
- Medication use and possible adverse effects
- Completing the entire course of drug therapy

Children born of mothers who have chlamydial infection may contract conjunctivitis or pneumonia during passage through the birth canal.

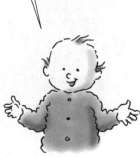

- Eye care
- Signs and symptoms of complications or continued infection
- Information on safe sex practices and prevention of STDs

Hypospadias

Hypospadias is a congenital anomaly of the penis. In this condition, the urethral opening may be anywhere along the ventral side of the penis. The condition shortens the distance to the bladder, offering easier access for bacteria.

CAUSES
- Genetic factors (most likely)
- Idiopathic

ASSESSMENT FINDINGS
- Altered angle of urination
- Meatus terminating at some point along lateral fusion line, ranging from the perineum to the distal penile shaft
- Marked downward curvature of the penis

DIAGNOSTIC TEST RESULTS
- Examination confirms aberrant placement of the opening.

NURSING DIAGNOSES
- Disturbed body image
- Deficient knowledge (disease process and treatment regimen)
- Anxiety

TREATMENT
- Avoiding circumcision (the foreskin may be needed later for surgical repair)

Surgery
- Tubularized incised plate procedure (for distal and midshaft hypospadias); most commonly used repair for primary tubularization of the uretheral plate
- Urethroplasty (procedure in which the urethra is extended into a normal position with a meatus at the tip of the penis); may initially be performed to restore normal urinary function

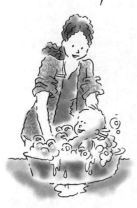

The key intervention in hypospadias is scrupulous cleaning to deter bacteria.

- Orthoplasty when the child is age 12 to 18 months, to release the adherent chordee (fibrous band that causes the penis to curve downward); if extensive repair is needed, delay until age 4
- Indwelling urinary catheter or suprapubic urinary catheter (postoperatively)

Drug therapy
- Analgesics: meperidine (Demerol), acetaminophen (Tylenol) for postoperative pain relief
- Antispasmodic agent: propantheline prescribed postoperatively to treat bladder spasms

INTERVENTIONS AND RATIONALES
- Monitor urine output *to ensure that the infant maintains a normal urine output of 5 to 10 ml/hr.*
- Perform diligent perineal care *to prevent bacteria invasion and infection.*
- Provide emotional support to the parents. Provide accurate information and answer questions thoroughly. Encourage verbalization of feelings. *Encouraging open discussion may help ease the parents' anxiety.*

Postoperative care
- After the procedure, apply a pressure dressing *to reduce bleeding and tissue swelling.*
- Check the tip of the penis frequently *to make sure that it's pink and viable.*
- Leave the dressing in place for several days *to encourage healing of the grafted skin flap.*
- Avoid pressure on the child's catheter *to prevent trauma to the incision site* and avoid kinking of the catheter *to ensure urine flow.*
- Encourage early ambulation *to prevent complications of immobility.*

Teaching topics
- Explanation of the disorder and treatment plan
- Wound care
- Hygiene of uncircumcised penis
- Understanding signs and symptoms of complications
- Follow-up care

Nephritis

Nephritis is a sudden inflammation that primarily affects the interstitial area and the renal pelvis or, less commonly, the renal tubules. Types of nephritis include acute tubulointerstitial nephritis (TIN), pyelonephritis, and glomerulonephritis. One of the most common renal diseases, nephritis is more common in females, probably because of a shorter urethra and the proximity of the urinary meatus to the vagina and the rectum.

With treatment and continued follow-up care, the prognosis is good and extensive permanent damage is rare.

CAUSES
- Bacterial infection of the kidneys (the most common cause); infecting bacteria usually are normal intestinal and fecal flora that grow readily in urine (the most common causative organism is *Escherichia coli,* but *Proteus, Pseudomonas, Staphylococcus aureus,* and *Enterococcus faecalis* [formerly *Streptococcus faecalis*] may also cause such infections)
- Hematogenic infection (as in septicemia or endocarditis)
- Lymphatic infection
- Transplant rejection
- Ureter obstruction
- Allergy or toxic response to a drug (TIN)

ASSESSMENT FINDINGS
- Anorexia
- Burning during urination
- Dysuria
- Flank pain
- Urinary frequency
- General fatigue
- Hematuria (usually microscopic but may be gross)
- Nocturia
- Rash (TIN)
- Shaking chills
- Temperature of 102° F (38.9° C) or higher
- Urinary urgency
- Urine that's cloudy and has an ammonia-like or fishy odor

DIAGNOSTIC TEST RESULTS
- Excretory urography may show asymmetrical or enlarged kidneys.

- Pyuria is present (with pyelonephritis). Urine sediment reveals the presence of leukocytes singly, in clumps, and in casts and, possibly, a few RBCs.
- Urine culture identifies specific bacteria.
- Urine specific gravity and osmolality are low, resulting from a temporarily decreased ability to concentrate urine.
- Urine pH is slightly alkaline.
- Blood chemistry reveals elevated potassium level (TIN).
- KUB radiography may reveal calculi, tumors, or cysts in the kidneys and the urinary tract.
- Kidney biopsy confirms the extent of kidney damage.

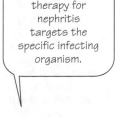

Antibiotic therapy for nephritis targets the specific infecting organism.

NURSING DIAGNOSES
- Impaired urinary elimination
- Hyperthermia
- Fatigue
- Deficient knowledge (disease process; treatment regimen)
- Acute pain

TREATMENT
- Follow-up treatment for antibiotic therapy: reculturing urine 1 week after drug therapy stops and periodically for 1 year after to detect residual or recurring infection
- Dialysis if acute renal failure occurs
- Surgery to relieve obstruction or correct the anomaly responsible for obstruction or vesicoureteral reflux
- Discontinuation of causative drug (TIN)

Drug therapy
- Antibiotics: targeted to specific infecting organism
- Corticosteroid: prednisone (Deltasone) (TIN)
- Antipyretic: acetaminophen (Tylenol)

INTERVENTIONS AND RATIONALES
- Monitor vital signs *to detect fever and hypertension.*
- Monitor intake and output and laboratory studies *to evaluate kidney function.*
- Assess renal status *to determine baseline renal function and detect changes from baseline.*
- Administer antipyretics *to reduce fever.*

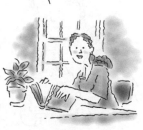

How to survive the big exam? Set goals, have an organized plan of action, and maintain a strong belief in yourself. Stick with it when the going gets tough.

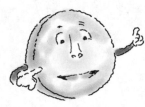

It ain't over till the pill bottle is empty. Emphasize the need to complete the prescribed antibiotic therapy, even after symptoms subside.

• Encourage fluid intake *to achieve urine output of more than 2 L/day.* However, discourage intake greater than 3 L/day. *Excessive fluid intake may decrease the effectiveness of antibiotics.*
• Provide a diet that contains adequate calcium (500 mg for children up to age 3, 800 mg for school-age children, and 1,300 mg for adolescents), moderately restricts sodium intake and protein, and avoids high doses of vitamin C. *These measures help to prevent renal calculi formation.*

Teaching topics

• Explanation of the disorder and treatment plan
• Medication use and possible adverse effects
• Completing prescribed antibiotic therapy, even after symptoms subside
• Understanding long-term follow-up care for high-risk children

Nephroblastoma

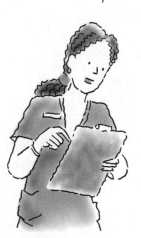

Key assessment finding in nephroblastoma: a nontender mass in the midline area.

Nephroblastoma, also known as *Wilms' tumor,* is an embryonal cancer of the kidney. It's the most common childhood abdominal malignancy. The average age at diagnosis is 2 to 4 years. The prognosis is excellent if metastasis hasn't occurred.

Nephroblastoma is measured in five stages:
• In stage I, the tumor is limited to the kidney.
• In stage II, the tumor extends beyond the kidney but can be completely excised.
• In stage III, the tumor spreads but is confined to the abdomen and lymph nodes.
• In stage IV, the tumor metastasizes to the lung, liver, bone, brain, or lymph nodes outside the abdomenopelvic region.
• In stage V, bilateral renal involvement occurs.

CAUSES

• Genetic predisposition

ASSESSMENT FINDINGS

• Abdominal pain
• Fever
• Constipation
• Hematuria
• Hypertension
• Nontender mass, usually midline near the liver, that's commonly detected by the parent while bathing or dressing the child
• Associated congenital anomalies, such as microcephaly, mental retardation, and GU tract problems

DIAGNOSTIC TEST RESULTS

• CT scan or sonography reveals tumor, lymph node involvement, and metastasis.
• Abdominal ultrasonography identifies a renal mass and possible renal vein or inferior vena cava thrombosis.
• Serum blood studies show anemia.
• Histologic studies at time of nephreotomy confirm diagnosis.

NURSING DIAGNOSES

• Fear
• Chronic pain
• Anxiety

TREATMENT

• Nephrectomy to remove affected kidney and evaluate remaining kidney; may be preceded by chemotherapy to shrink the tumor if it has extended to the vena cava or if there's bilateral involvement
• Radiation therapy (after surgery): for stages III and IV

Drug therapy

• Analgesics (postoperatively)
• Chemotherapy (after surgery): dactinomycin (Cosmegen), doxorubicin (Doxil), vincristine

INTERVENTIONS AND RATIONALES

• Monitor vital signs and intake and output *to determine fluid volume status.*
• Don't palpate the abdomen, and prevent others from doing so; *palpating the abdomen may cause tumor rupture.*
• Prepare the child and family members for a nephrectomy. *Surgery must be performed quickly after diagnosis to prevent metastasis.*
• After surgery, provide routine care for a nephrectomy client:
   – monitor urine output and report output less than 30 ml/hour

– assist with turning, coughing, and deep breathing

– encourage early ambulation

– provide pain medications as necessary and evaluate their effect

– monitor postoperative dressings for signs of bleeding

– provide wound care as directed.

These measures help to prevent postoperative complications, such as pneumonia, wound infection, and kidney failure.

• Evaluate for adverse effects to chemotherapy and radiation therapy *to provide appropriate interventions.*

Teaching topics

• Explanation of the disorder and treatment plan

• Medication use and possible adverse effects

• Providing adequate nutrition and hydration

• Dealing with adverse reactions to chemotherapy

• Signs and symptoms of metastasis or recurrence

• Signs and symptoms of kidney failure

• Follow-up care

• Contacting support groups

Urinary tract infection

A UTI is a microbial invasion of the kidneys, ureters, bladder, or urethra.

The risk of UTIs varies depending on the child's age and the presence of obstructive uropathy or voiding dysfunction. In the neonatal period, UTIs occur most commonly in males, possibly because of the higher incidence of congenital abnormalities in male neonates. By age 4 months, UTIs are much more common in girls than in boys. The increased incidence in girls continues throughout childhood.

After infancy, nearly all UTIs occur when bacteria enter the urethra and ascend the urinary tract. Females are especially at risk for infection because the female urethra is much shorter than the male urethra. The female urethra is more subject to direct contamination because of its proximity to the anal opening. *Escherichia coli* causes approximately 75% to 90% of all UTIs in females.

When evaluating an infant for a UTI, a lumbar puncture may first be performed to rule out meningitis. Urine specimens for culture should be obtained by sterile straight catheterization.

CAUSES

• Incomplete bladder emptying

• Frequent bubble baths

• Poor hygiene

• Reflux

ASSESSMENT FINDINGS

• Abdominal pain

• Flank tenderness

• Enuresis

• Frequent urges to void with pain or burning on urination

• Hematuria

• Lethargy

• Low-grade fever

• Poor feeding patterns

• Urine that's cloudy and foul-smelling

DIAGNOSTIC TEST RESULTS

• Clean-catch urine culture yields large amounts of bacteria.

• Urine culture identifies specific bacteria.

• Urine pH is increased.

NURSING DIAGNOSES

• Impaired urinary elimination

• Acute pain

• Hyperthermia

TREATMENT

• Increased fluid intake

Drug therapy

• Antibiotics: gentamicin (Garamycin), cefotaxime (Claforan)

• Analgesic: acetaminophen (Tylenol)

INTERVENTIONS AND RATIONALES

• Monitor intake and output *to determine if fluid replacement therapy is adequate.*

• Monitor vital signs to detect fever and increased stress on kidneys as evidenced by elevated blood pressure *to identify complications.*

• Assess toileting habits for proper front-to-back wiping and proper hand washing *to prevent recurrent infection.*

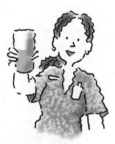

Encourage the client with a UTI to drink fluids. They improve hydration and promote kidney function.

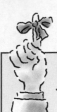

• Encourage increased intake of fluids *to keep the child hydrated and promote kidney function.*
• Assist the child when necessary to ensure that the perineal area is clean after elimination. *Cleaning the perineal area by wiping from the area of least contamination (urinary meatus) to the area of greatest contamination (anus) helps prevent UTIs.*

Teaching topics

• Explanation of the disorder and treatment plan
• Medication use and possible adverse effects
• Avoiding bubble baths
• Encouraging the child to use the toilet every 2 hours
• Performing toilet hygiene; including wiping from front to back

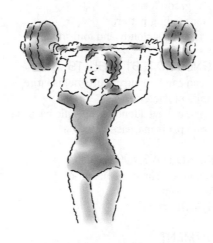

Pump up on practice questions

1. A school-age child is diagnosed with acute glomerulonephritis (nephritis). Which nursing action takes priority when caring for this child?
1. Monitoring blood pressure every 4 hours
2. Checking urine specific gravity every 8 hours
3. Offering the child fluids every hour
4. Providing the child with a regular diet and snacks

Answer: 1. Hypertension is a major complication that can occur during the acute phase of glomerulonephritis; therefore, blood pressure should be monitored at least once every 4 hours. Specific gravity may also be monitored, but it doesn't take priority over blood pressure monitoring. Fluids may be limited and a low-sodium diet initiated if the child is hypertensive.

➡ NCLEX keys

Client needs category: Physiological integrity
Client needs subcategory: Reduction of risk potential
Cognitive level: Application

2. A nurse is assessing a young female child who may have a urinary tract infection (UTI). A female child is more susceptible to UTIs than a male because she has:
1. no pubic hair.
2. a shorter urethra.
3. a smaller bladder.
4. smaller kidneys.

Answer: 2. The female child is more susceptible to UTIs than the male because the female has a shorter urethra, making it easier for organisms to be transmitted into the bladder. The absence of pubic hair is normal in young children; pubic hair growth signals the onset of puberty. A small child voids more frequently because of a small bladder, but this doesn't make the child prone to UTI. The infant's smaller, immature kidneys cause a low glomerular filtration rate but don't make the infant prone to UTI.

➡ NCLEX keys

Client needs category: Health promotion and maintenance
Client needs subcategory: None
Cognitive level: Application

3. An infant is admitted to the pediatric unit for surgical repair of hypospadias. The infant's urine output is 7 ml/hr. Which nursing action is most appropriate?
1. Notify the physician immediately.
2. Prepare to administer I.V. fluids.
3. Offer the infant formula every hour.
4. Continue to monitor urine output.

Answer: 4. The normal urine output for an infant is 5 to 10 ml/hour. The urine output of this infant falls within the normal range;

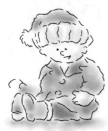

Keep your cool. There's only one more pediatric chapter to go!

therefore, the nurse should continue to monitor urine output. It isn't necessary to notify the physician, administer I.V. fluids, or increase the infant's intake.

➡ NCLEX keys
Client needs category: Physiological integrity
Client needs subcategory: Reduction of risk potential
Cognitive level: Application

4. A nurse must obtain a urine specimen for culture from an infant. The nurse can best obtain a specimen by:
　　1.　inserting a sterile straight catheter for specimen.
　　2.　placing the infant on a pediatric bedpan.
　　3.　inserting an indwelling urinary catheter.
　　4.　wringing out a cloth diaper after the infant voids.
Answer: 1. A sterile straight catheterization is quick and the most accurate way to obtain a sterile urine specimen from an infant. Placing the infant on a pediatric bedpan, inserting an indwelling urinary catheter, or wringing out a urine-filled cloth diaper aren't appropriate methods of collecting urine specimens for culture in infants.

➡ NCLEX keys
Client needs category: Safe and effective care environment
Client needs subcategory: Safety and infection control
Cognitive level: Application

5. A nurse is creating a teaching plan for a school-age child with a urinary tract infection (UTI). Which factor should the nurse assess first?
　　1.　Dietary intake
　　2.　Toileting habits
　　3.　Calcium intake
　　4.　Activity level
Answer: 2. The nurse should assess toileting habits before creating a teaching plan for the school-age child with a UTI. Based on her findings, the nurse should instruct the child in proper front-to-back wiping, hand washing, and toilet use every 2 hours. It isn't necessary to ask about the child's dietary intake, calcium intake, or activity level at this time.

➡ NCLEX keys
Client needs category: Physiological integrity
Client needs subcategory: Reduction of risk potential
Cognitive level: Application

6. A child is admitted to the pediatric unit with a temperature of 102.5° F (39.2° C), shaking chills, and flank pain. From these assessment findings, the nurse should most likely suspect:
　　1.　urinary tract infection (UTI).
　　2.　pyelonephritis.
　　3.　nephroblastoma.
　　4.　urolithiasis.
Answer: 2. With pyelonephritis, the child exhibits such assessment findings as temperature of 102° F (38.9° C) or higher, shaking chills, flank pain, urgency, frequency, and burning during urination. The child experiencing a UTI may exhibit low-grade fever, dysuria, frequency, urgency, lethargy, and urine that's cloudy and foul-smelling. The child with a nephroblastoma typically presents with a nontender mass, usually midline near the liver; abdominal pain; hypertension; hematuria; and constipation. The child with urolithiasis presents with colicky flank pain, nausea, vomiting, hematuria, and dysuria.

➡ NCLEX keys
Client needs category: Physiological integrity
Client needs subcategory: Reduction of risk potential
Cognitive level: Analysis

7. A preschooler is scheduled to have a Wilms' tumor removed. Identify the area of the urinary system where a Wilms' tumor is located.

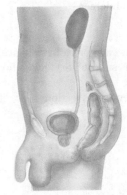

Answer: Wilms' tumor, also known as a *nephroblastoma*, is a tumor located on the kidney. It's most common in children ages 2 to 4.

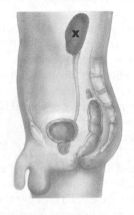

➡ *NCLEX keys*

Client needs category: Physiological integrity
Client needs subcategory: Physiological adaptation
Cognitive level: Application

8. A toddler is admitted to the pediatric unit with a diagnosis of nephroblastoma. When providing routine care for this toddler, the nurse should avoid:
1. palpating the toddler's abdomen.
2. positioning the toddler on the side.
3. bathing the toddler.
4. loosening the toddler's clothing.

Answer: 1. The nurse shouldn't palpate the toddler's abdomen and should prevent others from doing so because it may disseminate cancer cells to other sites. The toddler may be carefully positioned on his side. The toddler may be bathed but must be handled carefully. The toddler's clothes should be loosened around the abdomen.

➡ *NCLEX keys*

Client needs category: Physiological integrity
Client needs subcategory: Reduction of risk potential
Cognitive level: Application

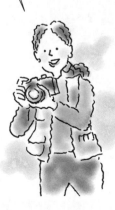

I know you think I'm goofing off, but taking a break and having some fun is also part of preparing for the exam.

9. A parent reports finding a mass in her child's abdomen. After the diagnosis of nephroblastoma is confirmed, the nurse should prepare the child and family for:
1. immediate chemotherapy.
2. immediate radiation therapy.
3. nephrectomy.
4. discharge to home with hospice care.

Answer: 3. The nurse should prepare the child and family for a nephrectomy, which is usually performed within 24 to 48 hours of diagnosis. Chemotherapy and radiation therapy are typically used as follow-up treatment once the nephrectomy is completed. The prognosis is excellent if there's no metastasis, and the tumor usually remains encapsulated for a long time.

➡ *NCLEX keys*

Client needs category: Physiological integrity
Client needs subcategory: Reduction of risk potential
Cognitive level: Knowledge

10. The nurse is doing discharge teaching with the parents of a neonate with hypospadias. Which statement by the parents indicates a need for further teaching?
1. "We'll use disposable diapers."
2. "We'll position him on his back to sleep."
3. "We'll make sure we bathe him in an infant bathtub."
4. "We'll have him circumcised by the pediatrician."

Answer: 4. The parents should be instructed to avoid having the neonate circumcised because the foreskin may be needed for surgical repair. The parents would be permitted to use disposable diapers for their neonate. The parents should be instructed to place the neonate on his back to sleep to decrease the risk of sudden infant death syndrome. It's acceptable for the parents to bathe the neonate in an infant bathtub.

➡ *NCLEX keys*

Client needs category: Physiological integrity
Client needs subcategory: Reduction of risk potential
Cognitive level: Application

35 Integumentary system

Brush up on key concepts

The skin, the primary component of the integumentary system, forms a protective barrier between internal structures and the external environment. Tough and resilient, the skin is virtually impermeable to aqueous solutions, bacteria, or toxic compounds.

At any time, you can review the major points of this chapter by consulting the *Cheat sheet* on pages 724 and 725.

Immature at birth
Like most body systems, the integumentary system isn't mature at birth. Therefore, it provides a less effective barrier to physical elements or microorganisms during birth and infancy than during childhood. This factor helps to explain why infants and young children are more prone to infection.

Untouched
The **skin** of infants and young children appears smoother than that of adults. A child's skin has less terminal hair and hasn't been subjected to long-term exposure to environmental elements.

I'm chilly
Infants have poorly developed **subcutaneous fat,** predisposing them to hypothermia. Eccrine sweat glands don't begin to function until the first month of life, which also inhibits the infant's ability to control body temperature.

Adolescent woes
With the onset of adolescence, **apocrine** glands enlarge and become active. This activity leads to axillary sweating and characteristic body odor. The sebaceous glands begin to produce sebum in response to hormone activity, which predisposes the adolescent to acne. Along with the skin glands becoming active, coarse terminal hair grows in the axillae and pubic areas of both sexes and on the faces of males.

Here's the skinny
Skin performs many vital functions. These functions include:
- protecting against trauma
- regulating body temperature
- serving as an organ of excretion and sensation
- synthesizing vitamin D in the presence of ultraviolet light.

Wearing layers
Skin has three primary layers:

☝ The **epidermis** (the outermost layer) produces keratin as its primary function. It contains two sublayers: the stratum corneum, an outer, horny layer of keratin that protects the body against harmful environmental substances and restricts water loss, and the cellular stratum, where keratin cells are synthesized. It also contains melanocytes, which produce the melanin that gives skin its color, and Langerhans cells, which are involved in various immunologic reactions.

✌ The **dermis** (the middle layer) contains collagen, which strengthens the skin to prevent it from tearing, and elastin to give it resilience.

🖐 The **subcutaneous tissue** (the innermost layer) consists mainly of fat (containing mostly triglycerides), which provides heat, insulation, shock absorption, and a reserve of calories.

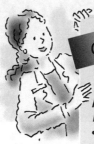

Cheat sheet

Integumentary refresher

ACNE VULGARIS
Key signs and symptoms
- Closed comedo, or whitehead (acne plug not protruding from the follicle and covered by the epidermis)
- Open comedo, or blackhead (acne plug protruding and not covered by the epidermis)
- Inflammation and characteristic acne pustules, papules or, in severe forms, acne cysts or abscesses (caused by rupture or leakage of an enlarged plug into the dermis)

Key treatments
- Phototherapy with blue and red light
- Oral retinoid: isotretinoin (Accutane) limited to those with nodulocystic or recalcitrant acne who don't respond to conventional therapy; contraindicated during pregnancy
- Systemic therapy: usually tetracycline to decrease bacterial growth; alternatively, erythromycin (tetracycline contraindicated during pregnancy and childhood because it discolors developing teeth)
- Topical medications: benzoyl peroxide (Benzac), clindamycin (Cleocin), or erythromycin (Benzamycin) antibacterial agents, alone or in combination with external retinoids such as tretinoin (Accutane, Retin-A), or a keratolytic

Key interventions
- Try to identify predisposing factors.
- Instruct the adolescent receiving tretinoin to apply it at least 30 minutes after washing the face and at least 1 hour before bedtime. Warn against using it around the eyes or lips. After treatments, the skin should look pink and dry.
- Advise the adolescent to avoid exposure to sunlight or to use a sunblock. If the prescribed regimen includes tretinoin and benzoyl peroxide, tell the adolescent to use one preparation in the morning and the other at night.
- Instruct the adolescent to take tetracycline on an empty stomach and not to take it with antacids or milk.
- Tell the adolescent who's taking isotretinoin to avoid vitamin A supplements. Also discuss how

to deal with the dry skin and mucous membranes that usually occur during treatment. Warn the female adolescent about the severe risk of teratogenesis. Monitor liver function and lipid levels.
- Offer emotional support.

BURNS
Key signs and symptoms
Partial-thickness
- Dry, painful skin with edema
- Sunburn appearance
Deep, partial-thickness
- Moist, weeping blisters with edema
- Extreme pain
Full-thickness
- Avascular site without blanching or pain
- Dry, pale, leathery skin

Key test results
- The Lund and Browder chart, a body surface area chart that's corrected for age to determine the extent of injury, estimates extent of the burn.

Key treatments
- I.V. fluids to prevent and treat shock; urine output at 1 to 2 ml/kg
- Protective isolation, depending on burn severity

Key interventions
- Stop the burning in an emergency situation.
- Maintain a patent airway in the immediate postburn phase.
- Monitor vital signs, intake, and output.
- Prevent heat loss.

CONTACT DERMATITIS (DIAPER RASH)
Key signs and symptoms
- Characteristic bright red, maculopapular rash in the diaper area

Key treatments
- Cleaning affected area with mild soap and water
- Leaving affected area open to air
- Zinc oxide or vitamin A ointment

Key interventions
- Keep the diaper area clean and dry.

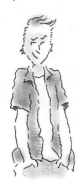

You can read the whole chapter, or you can just go skin deep and study the *Cheat sheet*.

Integumentary refresher (continued)

HEAD LICE

Key signs and symptoms
- Pruritus of the scalp
- Presence of lice eggs, which look like white flecks, firmly attached near the base of hair shafts.

Key treatments
- Pyrethrins (RID) or permethrin (Elimite) shampoos or lindane in resistant cases

Key interventions
- Carefully follow the manufacturer's directions when applying medicated shampoo.

IMPETIGO

Key signs and symptoms
- Red, macular rash progressing to a papular and vesicular rash, which oozes and forms a moist, honey-colored crust

Key treatments
- Washing area with soap and water

Key interventions
- Apply antibiotic ointment.
- Wash the area three times daily with soap and water.

RASHES

Key signs and symptoms
- Papular rash: raised solid lesions with color changes in circumscribed areas
- Pustular rash: vesicles and bullae that fill with purulent exudate
- Vesicular rash: small, raised, circumscribed lesions filled with clear fluid

Key test results
- Aspirate from lesions may reveal cause.
- Patch test may identify cause.

Key treatments
- Antibacterial (bacitracin, neomycin [Cortisporin]), antifungal (clotrimazole [Lotrimin], ketaconazole [Nizoral]), or antiviral agent (acyclovir [Zovirax], penciclovir [Denavir]) if infection is cause
- Antihistamine (diphenhydramine [Benadryl]) if the rash is from an allergy

Key interventions
- Maintain contact precautions.
- Keep draining lesions covered.

SCABIES

Key signs and symptoms
- Minute, linear black burrows between fingers and toes and in palms, axillae, and groin

Key test results
- Drop of mineral oil placed over the burrow, followed by superficial scraping and examination of expressed material under a microscope may reveal ova or mite feces.

Key treatments
- Topical application of permethrin 8% cream (Elimite)

Key interventions
- Apply medication as prescribed.
- Teach the child and parents to apply permethrin from the neck down covering the entire body, wait 15 minutes before dressing, and avoid bathing for 8 to 12 hours.

Thinner, more sensitive

A child's skin differs from an adult's in two important ways:
- The child has thinner and more sensitive skin than the adult.
- Irritation in the neonate's skin can result from the sensitivity of the neonate's skin or clogged pores.

Keep abreast of diagnostic tests

Here are the most important tests used to diagnose skin disorders, along with common nursing interventions associated with each test.

Slide show

In **diascopy,** a lesion is covered with a glass slide or piece of clear plastic and pressure is applied. The area is observed to identify purpura (the lesion remains red) or erythema (the lesion blanches).

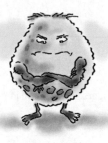

Because a child's skin is thinner and more sensitive than an adult's, it's more prone to infection.

Nursing actions
• Explain the procedure to the child and parents.

Light up and down
Sidelighting shows minor elevations or depressions in lesions; it also helps determine the configuration and degree of eruption.

  Subdued lighting, another test, highlights the difference between normal skin and circumscribed lesions that are hypopigmented or hyperpigmented.

Nursing actions
• Explain the procedure to the child and parents.

Spotlight on disease
Microscopic immunofluorescence identifies immunoglobulins and elastic tissue in detecting skin manifestations of immunologically mediated disease.

Nursing actions
• Explain the procedure to the child and parents.

Organism info
Gram stains and exudate cultures help identify organisms responsible for underlying infections.

Nursing actions
• Explain the procedure to the child and parents.
• Obtain cultures as directed by institutional policy.

Patching it together
Patch tests identify contact sensitivity (usually with dermatitis).

Nursing actions
• Explain the procedure to the child and parents.
• Tell the child that the skin area tested will be evaluated 24 to 48 hours after the patch is applied.

Important nursing actions following skin biopsy include preventing infection, injury, and irritation.

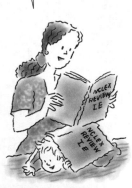

Tissue test
A **skin biopsy** is used to determine the histology of cells. It can be used to diagnose or confirm a disorder.

Nursing actions
Before the procedure
• Explain the procedure to the child and parents.
• Make sure that written, informed consent has been obtained.
After the procedure
• Tell the parents that the child should avoid wool or rough clothing.
• Prevent secondary infections by cutting the child's nails and applying mittens and elbow restraints.
• Suggest the child wear light, loose, nonirritating clothing.

Polish up on client care

Major pediatric skin disorders include acne vulgaris, burns, contact dermatitis (diaper rash), head lice, impetigo, rashes, and scabies.

Acne vulgaris

An inflammatory disease of the sebaceous follicles, acne vulgaris primarily affects adolescents, although lesions can appear as early as age 8. Although acne is more common and more severe in boys, it usually occurs in girls at an earlier age and tends to last longer, sometimes into adulthood. The prognosis is good with treatment.

CAUSES
• Androgen-stimulated sebum production
• Follicular occlusion
• *Propionibacterium acnes,* a normal skin flora

CONTRIBUTING FACTORS
• Androgen stimulation
• Certain drugs, including corticosteroids, corticotropin, androgens, iodides, bromides,

trimethadione (Tridione), phenytoin (Dilantin), isoniazid, lithium (Eskalith), and halothane; cobalt irradiation; or total parenteral nutrition
- Cosmetics
- Exposure to heavy oils, greases, or tars
- Heredity
- Hormonal contraceptives (many females experience acne flare-ups during their first few menses after starting or discontinuing hormonal contraceptives)
- Trauma or rubbing from tight clothing
- Unfavorable climate
- Deficient personal hygiene

ASSESSMENT FINDINGS
- Closed comedo, or whitehead (acne plug not protruding from the follicle and covered by the epidermis)
- Open comedo, or blackhead (acne plug protruding and not covered by the epidermis)
- Inflammation and characteristic acne pustules, papules or, in severe forms, acne cysts or abscesses (caused by rupture or leakage of an enlarged plug into the dermis)
- Acne scars from chronic, recurring lesions

DIAGNOSTIC TEST RESULTS
- Diagnostic testing isn't necessary. The appearance of characteristic acne lesions, especially in an adolescent client, confirms the presence of acne vulgaris.

NURSING DIAGNOSES
- Impaired skin integrity
- Disturbed body image
- Risk for infection

TREATMENT
- Phototherapy with blue and red light
- Exfoliation (mechanical or chemical)

Drug therapy
- Intralesional corticosteroid injection
- Oral retinoid: isotretinoin (Accutane) — limited to those with nodulocystic or recalcitrant acne who don't respond to conventional therapy; contraindicated during pregnancy
- Systemic therapy: usually tetracycline to decrease bacterial growth; alternatively, erythromycin (tetracycline contraindicated

during pregnancy and childhood because it discolors developing teeth)
- Topical medications: benzoyl peroxide (Benzac), clindamycin (Cleocin), or erythromycin (Benzamycin) antibacterial agents; alone or in combination with external retinoids such as tretinoin (Accutane, Retin-A), or a keratolytic
- Antiandrogenic agents: estrogens or spironolactone (Aldactazide)

INTERVENTIONS AND RATIONALES
- Review the adolescent's drug history *because some medications, such as hormonal contraceptives, may cause acne flare-ups.*
- Try to identify predisposing factors *to determine those that can be eliminated or modified.*
- Explain the causes of acne to the adolescent and family. Provide written instructions regarding treatment *to provide education.*
- Instruct the adolescent receiving tretinoin to apply it at least 30 minutes after washing the face and at least 1 hour before bedtime. Warn against using it around the eyes or lips *to prevent damage.* After treatments, the skin should look pink and dry. *If it appears red or starts to peel, the preparation may have to be weakened or applied less often.*
- Advise the adolescent to avoid exposure to sunlight or to use a sunscreen *to prevent a photosensitivity reaction.* If the prescribed regimen includes tretinoin and benzoyl peroxide, tell the adolescent to use one preparation in the morning and the other at night *to avoid skin irritation.*
- Instruct the adolescent to take tetracycline on an empty stomach and not to take it with antacids or milk *because it interacts with their metallic ions and is then poorly absorbed.*
- Tell the adolescent who's taking isotretinoin to avoid vitamin A supplements, *which can worsen adverse effects.* Also discuss how to deal with the dry skin and mucous membranes that usually occur during treatment. Warn the female adolescent about the severe risk of teratogenesis. Monitor liver function and lipid levels *to avoid toxicity.*
- Inform the adolescent that acne takes a long time to clear — possibly even years for complete resolution. Encourage continued local skin care even after acne clears. Explain

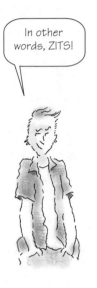

In other words, ZITS!

the adverse effects of all drugs *to promote compliance.*
• Offer emotional support *to help the adolescent cope with the effects of his skin condition.*
• Advise the female adolescent that taking oral antibiotics with hormonal contraceptives may make the contraceptive ineffective.

Teaching topics
• Explanation of the disorder and treatment plan
• Medication use and possible adverse effects
• Avoiding prolonged exposure to sunlight
• Identifying and eliminating predisposing factors, such as cosmetic use and emotional stress

Burns

A burn is tissue damage caused by heat, chemicals, electricity, sunlight, or nuclear radiation. Most pediatric burns occur to children younger than age 5. Overall, burns are the third leading cause of accidental death in children (after motor vehicle accidents and drowning). Burns are classified based on the depth of skin and tissue damage: superficial partial-thickness (first-degree), deep, partial-thickness (second-degree) or full-thickness (third-degree).

> Remember that the Rule of Nines, generally used to determine the extent of a burn, is inaccurate for children. Use the Lund and Browder chart instead.

CAUSES
• Thermal burn: residential fire, motor vehicle accident, playing with matches, improperly stored gasoline, space heater, household accident (such as a child climbing on top of a stove or grabbing a hot iron), excessive exposure to sunlight (sunburn)
• Chemical burn: contact, ingestion, inhalation, or injection of acids, alkalis, or resicants
• Electrical burn: contact with faulty electrical wiring or high-voltage power line, chewing on electric cord

ASSESSMENT FINDINGS
Partial-thickness (first-degree)
• Dry, painful skin with edema
• Sunburn appearance
• Damage limited to the epidermis

Deep, partial-thickness (second-degree)
• Moist, weeping blisters with edema
• Extreme pain
• Damage to the epidermis and part of the dermis

Full-thickness (third-degree)
• Avascular without blanching or pain
• Dry, pale, leathery skin
• Fluid shift from intravascular to interstitial compartments
• Damage to the epidermis and dermis
• Hypovolemia and symptoms of shock from fluid shift, including renal function
• Infection due to altered skin integrity

Fourth-degree burn
• Damage through deeply charred subcutaneous tissue to muscle and bone

DIAGNOSTIC TEST RESULTS
• The Lund and Browder chart, a body surface area chart that's corrected for age to determine the extent of injury, estimates extent of the burn. (The Rule of Nines is inaccurate for children because the head can account for 13% to 19% of body surface area; the legs account for 10% to 16%, depending on the child's age and size.)

NURSING DIAGNOSES
• Deficient fluid volume
• Ineffective airway clearance
• Risk for infection
• Acute pain
• Interrupted family processes
• Disturbed body image

TREATMENT
• Oxygen therapy (may require intubation)
• I.V. fluids to prevent and treat shock; urine output at 1 to 2 ml/kg
• Protective isolation, depending on burn severity
• Total parenteral nutrition
• Debridement
• Escharotomy
• Diet: adequate nutritional support to avoid negative nitrogen balance and prevent overfeeding
• Skin grafting
• Physical and occupational therapy

Drug therapy
- Analgesics: morphine (Arinza), meperidine (Demerol)
- Topical antibiotics: silver sulfadiazine (Silvadene), mafenide acetate (Sulfamylon) to limit infection at the site

INTERVENTIONS AND RATIONALES
- Stop the burning in an emergency situation *to prevent further injury.*
- Maintain a patent airway in the immediate postburn phase; *inhalation of smoke may cause airway edema.*
- Monitor vital signs, intake, and output *to assess for signs of complications.*
- Assess cardiovascular, renal, respiratory, and neurologic status *to assess for signs of shock.*
- Administer I.V. fluids according to recommended rates based on extent of burn damage *to maintain fluid balance.*
- Administer I.V. analgesics *to relieve pain;* don't administer I.M. injections.
- Assist with debridement *to promote healing.*
- Elevate the burned body part *to promote venous drainage and decrease edema.*
- Spread a thin layer of topical medication, such as mafenide acetate, over the burn *to prevent infection.*
- Prevent heat loss *to reduce metabolic demands.*
- Explain treatments, pain management, and the need for the child's active participation in the treatment and offer the child choices, where appropriate, *to help the child feel less afraid and anxious.*
- Encourage family and friends to participate in the child's care when appropriate *to create a loving and supportive atmosphere.*
- Allow the child to participate in everyday activities, such as playing and school activities, *to normalize his situation.*
- Give the child the opportunity to maintain the developmental tasks already achieved, such as eating in a high chair, not using diapers if the child has been toilet-trained, and allowing self-feeding if the child is able, *to prevent regression.*
- Promote a comfortable and loving atmosphere for the child. *This encourages him to talk and act out feelings of depression and hostility and express anxieties.*

Teaching topics
- Explanation of the disorder and treatment plan
- Medication use and possible adverse effects
- Using coping strategies to deal with long-term care
- Understanding burn prevention

Contact dermatitis

Contact dermatitis, also known as *diaper rash*, is a local skin reaction in the areas normally covered by a diaper.

CAUSES
- Irritation caused by acidic urine and fecal enzymes
- Moist, warm environment contained by a plastic diaper lining
- Clothing dyes or the soaps used to wash diapers
- Body soaps, bubble baths, tight clothes, and wool or rough clothing

ASSESSMENT FINDINGS
- Characteristic bright red, maculopapular rash in the diaper area
- Irritability because the rash is painful and warm

DIAGNOSTIC TEST RESULTS
- Diagnostic testing isn't necessary. Diagnosis is based on inspection.

NURSING DIAGNOSES
- Acute pain
- Impaired skin integrity
- Risk for infection

TREATMENT
- Cleaning the affected area with mild soap and water
- Leaving the affected area open to air

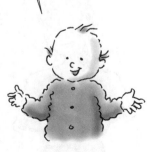

Because contact dermatitis is commonly caused by a moist, warm environment, it makes sense that an important intervention is keeping the area clean, dry, and open to the air.

Drug therapy
• Zinc oxide or vitamin A ointment to help the skin heal
• Antibiotics based on infecting organism if secondary infection occurs: levofloxacin (Levaquin)

INTERVENTIONS AND RATIONALES
• Keep the diaper area clean and dry *to maintain skin integrity.*
• Change the diaper immediately after the child voids or defecates *to prevent skin breakdown.*
• Wash the area with mild soap and water *to promote healing.*
• Keep the area open to the air without plastic bed linings, if possible, *to promote circulation and comfort.*
• Avoid using commercially prepared diaper wipes on broken skin; *the chemicals and alcohol in commercially prepared wipes may be irritating.*

Teaching topics
• Explanation of the disorder and treatment plan
• Medication use and possible adverse effects
• Preventing diaper rash

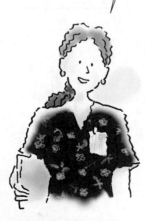

When applying insecticidal treatments, carefully follow the manufacturer's directions to avoid neurotoxicity.

Head lice

Head lice (pediculosis capitis) are a contagious infestation of lice eggs that are firmly attached near the base of hair shafts. The cause of this disorder isn't related to the hygiene of a child or family members; however, head lice are easily transmitted among children and family members.

CAUSES
• Exposure to lice by sharing clothing, hats, or combs or close physical contact with peers

ASSESSMENT FINDINGS
• Pruritus of the scalp
• Presence of lice eggs, which look like white flecks, firmly attached near the base of hair shafts

DIAGNOSTIC TEST RESULTS
• Diagnostic testing isn't necessary.

NURSING DIAGNOSES
• Disturbed body image
• Impaired skin integrity
• Social isolation

TREATMENT
• Removal of lice and eggs using fine-toothed comb

Drug therapy
• Pyrethrins (RID) or permethrin (Elimite) shampoos; lindane in resistant cases
• Preventive drug therapy for other family members and classmates

INTERVENTIONS AND RATIONALES
• Carefully follow the manufacturer's directions when applying medicated shampoo *to avoid neurotoxicity.*
• Repeat treatment in 7 to 12 days *to ensure that all the eggs have been killed.*

Teaching topics
• Explanation of disorder and treatment plan
• Medication use and possible adverse effects
• Washing bed linens, hats, combs, brushes, and anything else that came in contact with the hair to prevent reinfestation
• Assessing for reinfestation
• Refraining from exchanging combs, brushes, headgear, or clothing with other children

Impetigo

Impetigo is a highly contagious superficial infection of the skin, marked by patches of tiny blisters that erupt. It's common in children ages 2 to 5. Infection is spread by direct contact; incubation period is 2 to 10 days after contact.

CAUSE
• Staphylococci

ASSESSMENT FINDINGS
- Red, macular rash that progresses to a papular and vesicular rash, which oozes and forms a moist, honey-colored crust
- Commonly seen on the face and extremities but may spread to other parts of the body by scratching
- Pruritus

DIAGNOSTIC TEST RESULTS
- Diagnostic testing isn't necessary. Diagnosis is based on inspection of skin.

NURSING DIAGNOSES
- Impaired skin integrity
- Risk for infection
- Bathing or hygiene self-care deficit

TREATMENT
- Washing area with soap and water

Drug therapy
- Topical antibiotic ointment
- Systemic antibiotics (in severe cases)

INTERVENTIONS AND RATIONALES
- Apply antibiotic ointment *to eradicate the infection*.
- Wash the area three times daily with soap and water *to promote skin healing*.
- Cover the child's hands, if necessary, *to prevent secondary infection;* cut the child's nails.
- Cover the lesions *to prevent their spread*.

Teaching topics
- Explanation of the disorder and treatment plan
- Medication use and possible adverse effects
- Preventing recurrence

Rashes

A rash is a temporary skin eruption. Three types of rashes — papular, pustular, and vesicular — are described below.

A *papular rash* may erupt anywhere on the body in various configurations and may be acute or chronic. Papular rashes characterize many cutaneous disorders; they may also result from allergy or infectious, neoplastic, or systemic disorders. Common causes of papular rashes in children are infectious diseases, such as molluscum and scarlet fever; scabies; insect bites; allergies or drug reactions; and miliaria.

A *pustular rash* is made up of crops of pustules that fill with purulent exudate. These lesions vary greatly in size and shape and can be generalized or localized to the hair follicles or sweat glands. Pustules appear in skin and systemic disorders, with use of certain drugs, and with exposure to skin irritants. Disorders that produce pustular rash in children include erythema toxicum neonatorum and impetigo. Pustules typify the inflammatory lesions of acne vulgaris, common in adolescents.

A *vesicular rash* is a scattered or linear distribution of vesicles. A vesicular rash may be mild or severe and temporary or permanent. It may result from infection, inflammation, or allergic reactions. Vesicular rashes in children are caused by staphylococcal infections, varicella, hand-foot-mouth disease, and miliaria.

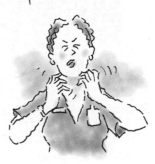

Insidious infectious itch! Impetigo rash may be spread to other parts of the body by scratching.

CAUSES
- Allergic reactions
- Environmental causes
- Viral, fungal, or bacterial infestations

ASSESSMENT FINDINGS
- Papular rash: raised solid lesions with color changes in circumscribed areas
- Pustular rash: vesicles and bullae that fill with purulent exudate
- Vesicular rash: small, raised, circumscribed lesions filled with clear fluid

DIAGNOSTIC TEST RESULTS
- Aspirate from lesions may reveal cause.
- Patch test may identify cause.

NURSING DIAGNOSES
- Impaired skin integrity
- Risk for infection
- Disturbed body image

TREATMENT
- Antibacterial (bacitracin, neomycin [Cortisporin]), antifungal (clotrimazole [Lotrimin], ketoconazole [Nizoral]) or antiviral agent (acyclovir [Zovirax], penciclovir [Denavir]) if infection is cause

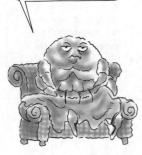

I like to make myself at home. Scabies mites can live their entire lives in human skin, causing chronic infection.

• Antihistamine (diphenhydramine [Benadryl]) if the rash is from an allergy and to decrease pruritis

INTERVENTIONS AND RATIONALES
• Keep the area cool. *Heat aggravates most skin rashes and increases pruritus; coolness decreases pruritus.*
• Keep the affected area clean and pat it dry *to promote healing.*
• Don't apply powder or cornstarch *because these agents encourage bacterial growth.*
• Maintain contact precautions *to prevent the spread of infection.*
• Keep draining lesions covered *to prevent transmission.*

Teaching topics
• Explanation of the disorder and treatment plan
• Medication use and possible adverse effects
• Understanding sanitary techniques
• Avoiding sharing combs or hats
• Avoiding scratching
• Avoiding puncturing vesicles or pustules with needles or hands

Scabies

Scabies is a parasitic skin disorder that causes severe itching. Scabies develops when microscopic itch mites enter a child's skin and provoke a sensitivity reaction. Mites can live their entire lives inside human skin, causing chronic infection. The female mite burrows into the skin to lay her eggs, from which larvae emerge to copulate and then reburrow under the skin. Scabies is transmitted through the skin or through sexual contact.

CAUSES
• Female mite that burrows into the skin and deposits eggs in areas that are thin and moist

ASSESSMENT FINDINGS
• Minute, linear black burrows between fingers and toes and in palms, axillae, and groin
• Severe itching

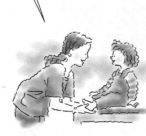

Severe itching marks scabies infestation. Linear black mite burrows may be visible between the fingers and toes or on the palms, axillae, and groin.

DIAGNOSTIC TEST RESULTS
• Drop of mineral oil placed over the burrow, followed by superficial scraping and examination of expressed material under a microscope may reveal ova or mite feces.

NURSING DIAGNOSES
• Disturbed body image
• Impaired skin integrity
• Social isolation

TREATMENT
• Treatment for all members of the family (as well as close contacts of the child)

Drug therapy
• Topical application of permethrin (Elimite) 8% cream

INTERVENTIONS AND RATIONALES
• Apply medication as prescribed *to promote healing.*
• Wash the area thoroughly with soap and water *to promote healing.*
• Teach the child and parents to apply permethrin from the neck down covering the entire body, wait 15 minutes before dressing, and avoid bathing for 8 to 12 hours *to ensure effectiveness of therapy.*
• Explain to the child and parents that if skin irritation or an allergic reaction develops, they should notify the physician immediately, stop using the cream, and wash it off thoroughly *to avoid risk of an anaphylactic reaction.*

Teaching topics
• Explanation of the disorder and treatment plan
• Medication use and possible adverse effects
• Understanding that pruritus may persist for several weeks after treatment
• Practicing proper hygiene measures
• Changing bed linens, towels, and clothing after bathing and lotion application
• Understanding the need to treat family members and close contacts because the parasite is transmitted by close personal contact and through clothes and linens
• Understanding that the length of time between infestation and physical symptoms may be 30 to 60 days

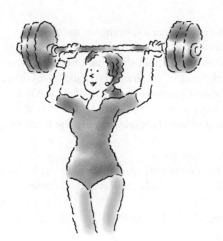

Pump up on practice questions

1. The clothes of a 16-year-old girl catch fire while she's lighting the grill for a family picnic. The girl's mother, a nurse, tells her to drop and roll to extinguish the flames. Which action should the nurse take next?
   1. Move her daughter away from the grill.
   2. Remove her daughter's clothing.
   3. Use the garden hose to wet her daughter down.
   4. Call the fire department.

Answer: 3. In emergency burn care, the priority is to stop the burning. The client shouldn't be moved because flames may intensify. Once the fire is extinguished, the client's clothes should be removed to prevent further injury. Emergency medical personnel should be summoned after the flames are extinguished.

➡ *NCLEX keys*
Client needs category: Physiological integrity
Client needs subcategory: Reduction of risk potential
Cognitive level: Application

2. A child has full-thickness burns of the hands, face, and chest. Which nursing diagnosis takes priority?

   1. *Ineffective airway clearance related to edema*
   2. *Disturbed body image related to physical appearance*
   3. *Impaired urinary elimination related to fluid loss*
   4. *Infection related to epidermal disruption*

Answer: 1. Initially, when a client is admitted to the hospital for burns, the primary focus is on assessing and managing an effective airway. Body image disturbance, impaired urinary elimination, and infection are all integral parts of burn management but aren't the first priority.

➡ *NCLEX keys*
Client needs category: Physiological integrity
Client needs subcategory: Physiological adaptation
Cognitive level: Analysis

3. A nurse is caring for a child with deep, partial-thickness and full-thickness burns. Which analgesic would most effectively manage the client's severe pain?
   1. Acetaminophen administered by suppository
   2. Meperidine administered I.M.
   3. Codeine administered by mouth
   4. Morphine administered I.V.

Answer: 4. A client with severe burns requires strong analgesia. The most effective method of administering analgesics is the I.V. route. Deep partial-thickness burns are commonly too painful to be relieved by acetaminophen. I.M. medication may not be absorbed when the client is physiologically unstable. Codeine may not provide sufficient analgesia, and oral administration usually isn't the best route for severe burn victims.

➡ *NCLEX keys*
Client needs category: Physiological integrity
Client needs subcategory: Pharmacological and parenteral therapies
Cognitive level: Application

To keep up your motivation for studying, remember the big picture. Conquering the exam is one of the keys to fulfilling life goals you have chosen for yourself.

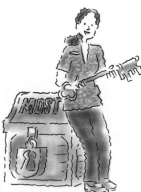

4. A 14-month-old infant is in a private room for treatment of burns. Which intervention can best meet the child's developmental needs?

1. Ask the mother to room with the child.
2. Have nursing personnel visit the child regularly throughout the day.
3. Set the television to the child's favorite cartoon shows.
4. Attach a brightly colored balloon to the child's crib.

Answer: 1. The mother can best provide for the child's developmental needs by being present all of the time. At this age, the child is most susceptible to separation anxiety. A child of this age is likely to be apprehensive toward unfamiliar adults, so regular visits by nursing personnel wouldn't help. Television is a poor substitute for human contact. A balloon is dangerous for a child this age.

➡ *NCLEX keys*
Client needs category: Health promotion and maintenance
Client needs subcategory: None
Cognitive level: Application

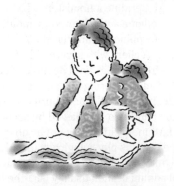

5. A 13-year-old adolescent has received third-degree burns over 20% of his body. When performing an assessment 72 hours after the burn, which finding should the nurse expect?

1. Increasing urine output
2. Severe peripheral edema
3. Respiratory distress
4. Absent bowel sounds

Answer: 1. During the resuscitative-emergent phase of a burn, fluid shifts back into the interstitial space resulting in the onset of diuresis. Edema resolves during the emergent phase, when fluid shifts back to the intravascular space. Respiratory rate increases during the first hours as a result of edema. When edema resolves, respirations return to normal. Absent bowel sounds occur in the initial stage.

➡ *NCLEX keys*
Client needs category: Physiological integrity
Client needs subcategory: Physiological adaptation
Cognitive level: Analysis

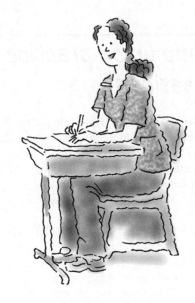

6. A child comes into the emergency department with a rash that's raised and has color changes in circumscribed areas. What type of rash should the nurse document?

1. Macular rash
2. Papular rash
3. Petechial rash
4. Vesicular rash

Answer: 2. A papular rash contains raised solid lesions with color changes in circumscribed areas. A macular rash is flat with color changes in circumscribed areas. Petechiae are pinpoint purple or red spots on the skin caused by minute hemorrhages. A vesicular rash contains small, raised circumscribed lesions filled with clear fluid.

⇒ *NCLEX keys*

Client needs category: Physiological integrity
Client needs subcategory: Reduction of risk potential
Cognitive level: Comprehension

7.   The nurse is developing a teaching plan for the mother of a neonate. The nurse should instruct the mother to prevent diaper rash by:

1. using disposable diapers so she doesn't have to change the infant often.
2. bathing the infant in a tub with bubble bath.
3. not washing the infant with soap.
4. keeping the infant's diaper area clean and dry.

Answer: 4. The mother should be instructed to keep the infant's diaper area clean and dry; to change the diaper immediately after the infant voids or defecates; to avoid bubble bath; and to wash the diaper area with mild soap and water with every diaper change.

⇒ *NCLEX keys*

Client needs category: Health promotion and maintenance
Client needs subcategory: None
Cognitive level: Application

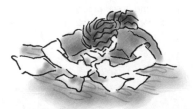

8.   A mother calls the pediatrician's office because there's an outbreak of scabies at her child's day-care center. The nurse should instruct the mother to check her child for which findings associated with scabies infestation?

1. Pruritic papules, pustules, and linear burrows of the fingers and toe webs
2. Oval white dots adhered to the hair shafts
3. Diffuse pruritic wheals
4. Pain, erythema, and edema at the site of the bite

Answer: 1. The mother should be instructed to check her child for pruritic papules, vesicles, and linear burrows. Oval flecks on the hair shaft indicate head lice. Diffuse pruritic wheals can indicate an allergic reaction. The specific site of the bite reveals no trace of the insect bite.

⇒ *NCLEX keys*

Client needs category: Health promotion and maintenance
Client needs subcategory: None
Cognitive level: Application

9.   A 16-month-old infant is being treated with permethrin (Elimite) for scabies. The infant's mother is concerned that the drug hasn't been effective because her child continues to scratch. Which response by the nurse is most appropriate?

1. Stop treatment because the drug isn't safe for children younger than age 2.
2. Tell the mother that pruritus can be present for weeks after treatment.
3. Apply the drug every day until the rash disappears.
4. Tell the mother that pruritus is common in children younger than age 5 treated with permethrin.

Answer: 2. Pruritus may be present for weeks in the child treated with permethrin for scabies. The drug is safe for use in infants as young as age 2 months. Treatment with permethrin can safely be repeated in 2 weeks. Pruritus is caused by secondary reactions of mites.

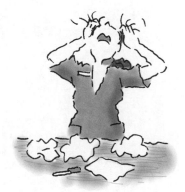

➡ *NCLEX keys*
Client needs category: Physiological integrity
Client needs subcategory: Pharmacological and parenteral therapies
Cognitive level: Application

10. A child is diagnosed with head lice and the mother asks how she should get the nits out of her child's hair. The nurse should tell the mother that:

1. the treatment should be repeated in 7 to 12 days.
2. combing the hair after shampooing is necessary.
3. treatment should be repeated every day for 7 days.
4. all children that had contact with the child should be prophylactically treated.

Answer: 1. Treatment should be repeated in 7 to 12 days to ensure that all of the eggs have been killed. Combing the hair thoroughly isn't necessary to remove lice eggs. People exposed should be observed for infestation before being treated.

➡ *NCLEX keys*
Client needs category: Physiological integrity
Client needs subcategory: Reduction of risk potential
Cognitive level: Application

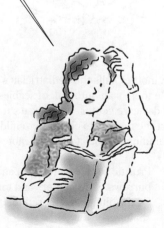

I'm just itching to answer more practice questions. In addition to the questions that follow, don't forget to pump up on practice questions available for free on the Web site.

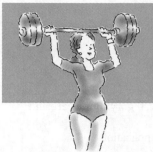

Pump up on more practice questions

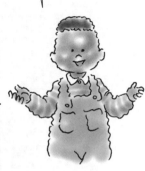

Practice makes perfect. So do these 30 pediatric practice questions.

1. A nurse is teaching the mother of an infant with tetralogy of Fallot. The mother asks what to do when her infant becomes very blue and has trouble breathing after crying. The nurse should tell the mother:

1. "Leave the infant alone until the crying stops."
2. "Put the infant in the knee-chest position."
3. "Offer the infant a bottle of formula."
4. "Take the infant for a ride in the car."

Answer: 2. The infant is having a "tet" or blue spell, which is an acute spell of hypoxia and cyanosis. This occurs when the infant's oxygen requirements are greater than what's supplied in the blood. Treatment involves placing the infant in the knee-chest position to reduce venous return from the extremities because that blood is desaturated. It also increases systemic vascular resistance, which causes more blood to be shunted to the pulmonary artery. Leaving the infant alone until he stops crying causes an increase in cyanosis. An infant who's crying and having trouble breathing shouldn't be offered a bottle because of the danger of aspiration. Taking the infant for a ride in the car may be an alternative if the mother can't quiet the infant.

➡ NCLEX keys
Client needs category: Physiological integrity
Client needs subcategory: Basic care and comfort
Cognitive level: Application

2. A nurse is providing care to a child who had a cardiac catheterization. Which intervention should the nurse perform first?

1. Offer the child liquids immediately on awakening.
2. Allow the child to sleep as much as possible.
3. Assess peripheral pulses for symmetry.
4. Change the dressing over the catheter site.

Answer: 3. The most important nursing intervention after cardiac catheterization is to assess peripheral pulses, especially those distal to the catheter site. The pulse may be weaker initially but typically becomes stronger in a short period. The dressing should be assessed, and the child may want liquids after the procedure. Allowing the child to sleep as much as possible may be appropriate but isn't the most important intervention.

➡ NCLEX keys
Client needs category: Physiological integrity
Client needs subcategory: Basic care and comfort
Cognitive level: Application

3. A nurse notices that the dressing over a child's cardiac catheterization site has a large amount of sanguinous drainage. What should the nurse do first?

1. Notify the on-call physician.
2. Apply pressure 1" (2.5 cm) above the skin site.
3. Check the child's vital signs, including temperature.
4. Assess the peripheral pulse distal to the site.

Answer: 2. When bleeding occurs, it's important to apply direct continuous pressure above the percutaneous skin site to localize pressure over the vessel punctured. All of the other actions are important, but applying pressure is the priority.

Client needs category: Physiological integrity
Client needs subcategory: Basic care and comfort
Cognitive level: Application

4. A nurse is teaching the mother of a toddler with iron deficiency anemia about dietary modifications. Which statement by the mother indicates that she understands?
1. "I can let my child have four glasses of milk every day."
2. "I will feed my child fortified cereal and lots of vegetables."
3. "I plan to offer my child juices and cereal for snacks."
4. "I think my child will drink milk and juices easily."

Answer: 2. For the child with iron deficiency anemia, such iron-rich foods as fortified cereal, green leafy vegetables, and red meat need to be offered in large amounts. Foods that contain less iron — such as milk, juices, yellow vegetables, and nonfortified cereals —should be offered in smaller amounts.

Client needs category: Physiological integrity
Client needs subcategory: Basic care and comfort
Cognitive level: Analysis

5. A 10-year-old child is admitted to the pediatric unit in sickle cell crisis. What should the nurse do first?
1. Assess vital signs.
2. Assess the degree of pain using a pain scale.
3. Determine the rate of I.V. fluids.
4. Obtain pertinent history information from the parents.

Answer: 1. All of the options are important, but the nurse should assess vital signs first to determine the client's baseline. Children with sickle cell disease are prone to developing infections as a result of necrosis of body areas where vaso-occlusive crisis occurs; this crisis is also associated with localized pain at the infection site. It's important for the child to receive adequate fluids to help prevent dehydration and increase blood volume.

History will help determine other coexisting conditions.

Client needs category: Physiological integrity
Client needs subcategory: Basic care and comfort
Cognitive level: Application

6. A nurse is caring for a child with leukemia who has an absolute granulocyte count of 400 μl. Which intervention should the nurse implement?
1. Place the child in strict isolation.
2. Notify the physician immediately.
3. Restrict visitors with active infections.
4. Begin antibiotics per protocol.

Answer: 3. When the absolute granulocyte count is low, a child has difficulty fighting an infection. Visitors with active infections should be restricted to prevent the child from developing an infection. The child should be placed in protective isolation, not strict isolation. Antibiotics shouldn't be started without a septic workup first. The physician must also be notified of the client's condition so that appropriate medical management is initiated.

Client needs category: Safe and effective care environment
Client needs subcategory: Safety and infection control
Cognitive level: Application

7. A client is receiving cyclophosphamide (Cytoxan) as part of a chemotherapy regimen. Which adverse reaction should the nurse teach the family to report right away?
1. Stomatitis
2. Flulike syndrome
3. Ototoxicity
4. Hematuria

Answer: 4. Hematuria is an indication of hemorrhagic cystitis and is an adverse effect of cyclophosphamide. Stomatitis is a rare complication with this medication. Flulike syndrome occurs with decarbazine. Ototoxicity occurs more commonly with cisplatin (Platinol).

➡ *NCLEX keys*
Client needs category: Physiological integrity
Client needs subcategory: Pharmacological
and parenteral therapies
Cognitive level: Comprehension

8. A 15-month-old infant has been admitted to the pediatric unit with a diagnosis of croup. The nurse makes the following assessment: respiratory rate, 36 breaths/minute; heart rate, 120 beats/minute; temperature, 100.7° F (38.2° C); pulse oximetry, 93%; and restlessness. From these findings, the nurse should infer that the:
1. toddler is in respiratory failure.
2. toddler's condition is improving.
3. mother should stay at the bedside.
4. parents can calm the toddler.

Answer: 1. Recognizing more subtle signs of respiratory failure is an extremely important skill for nurses to develop. Subtle signs include restlessness, increase in respiratory effort, tachypnea, tachycardia, and inability of the family to calm the child.

➡ *NCLEX keys*
Client needs category: Physiological integrity
Client needs subcategory: Reduction of risk potential
Cognitive level: Application

9. A 6-year-old child with a history of asthma is brought to the clinic in respiratory distress. The nurse notes the following: respiratory rate, 36 breaths/minute; heart rate, 150 beats/minute; and an anxious child. The nurse should be most concerned about:
1. child's loose cough.
2. prolonged expiratory phase.
3. absence of wheezing.
4. whistling sound on inspiration.

Answer: 3. The most likely explanation for the respiratory distress is an acute asthma attack. These episodes usually begin with a cough, expiratory wheezing, and a prolonged expiratory phase and may progress to more obvious symptoms, such as wheezing on inspiration, shortness of breath, and tight cough. The absence of wheezing during an attack indicates that the child is probably hypoxic and needs immediate medical attention.

➡ *NCLEX keys*
Client needs category: Physiological integrity
Client needs subcategory: Reduction of risk potential
Cognitive level: Application

10. An adolescent with cystic fibrosis has a follow-up appointment after discharge from the hospital for pneumonia. Which assessment question should the nurse ask?
1. "How has your appetite been this past week?"
2. "How many doses of antibiotics have you missed?"
3. "Have you been sleeping well?"
4. "Have you gone back to school yet?"

Answer: 1. An important indication of how clients with cystic fibrosis are doing is their appetite. Poor appetite and weight loss are indications that an infectious process may be occurring. Asking how many doses of antibiotics the client has missed assumes that the client isn't trustworthy, which doesn't help establish a therapeutic relationship. Asking about sleep may give some helpful information about the client's overall health, but it isn't the most important question. When the client returns to school is also an indication of the client's general state.

➡ *NCLEX keys*
Client needs category: Physiological integrity
Client needs subcategory: Reduction of risk potential
Cognitive level: Application

11. A 5-month-old infant is brought to the clinic by his mother, who reports that the infant has nasal congestion, symptoms of a cold, fever, and difficulty breathing. The nurse should first:
1. ask for more history information.
2. perform a respiratory assessment.
3. notify the available physician.
4. take vital signs.

Answer: 2. Any time a relative reports that a child has difficulty breathing, it's imperative for the nurse to do a respiratory assessment immediately. History information and vital signs can be obtained at a later date. After the nurse makes the respiratory assessment, then the physician can be contacted if warranted.

➡ *NCLEX keys*
Client needs category: Safe and effective care environment
Client needs subcategory: Safety and infection control
Cognitive level: Application

12.   A nurse is counseling the mother of a child with attention deficit hyperactivity disorder (ADHD). The mother demonstrates understanding of the teaching when she says:
1.   "When my child comes home from school, the homework is done first."
2.   "I take my child to play in the park as soon as school is over."
3.   "My child loves to sit and watch television after the bus ride home."
4.   "As soon as I arrive home, my child begins to read his favorite book."

Answer: 2. Children with ADHD are impulsive, have high energy levels, and don't follow directions well. An appropriate plan after the child has been in school all day is to allow the child to play to burn up energy; doing so enables the child to concentrate better later.

➡ *NCLEX keys*
Client needs category: Physiological integrity
Client needs subcategory: Physiological adaptation
Cognitive level: Application

13.   An infant is to receive amoxicillin 90 mg three times per day for 10 days to treat otitis media. Amoxicillin suspension is 125 mg/5 ml. How much of the medication should the mother administer at each dosing time? Round your answer to one decimal place.
_____ ml

Answer: 3.6. To calculate the amount to give with each dose, the nurse should use the following formula:
125 mg : 5 ml :: 90 mg : X ml =
(90 mg × 5 ml) ÷ (125 mg × X ml) =
450 ÷ 125 = 3.6

➡ *NCLEX keys*
Client needs category: Physiological integrity
Client needs subcategory: Pharmacological and parenteral therapies
Cognitive level: Application

14.   A school-age child who has hydrocephalus is admitted for a revision of his ventriculoperitoneal shunt. When he returns from surgery, how should the nurse position him?
1.   On his abdomen where he's comfortable
2.   In semi-Fowler's position to prevent aspiration
3.   With the bed flat to prevent a subdural hematoma
4.   On the same side as the shunt repair

Answer: 3. The child should be kept flat to decrease complications that might occur from too rapid a reduction in intracranial fluid. When the fluid is drained too rapidly, a subdural hematoma may result. In children with increased intracranial pressure, the position of choice is with the head of the bed elevated and the child lying on the side opposite the shunt to keep pressure off the shunt valve.

➡ *NCLEX keys*
Client needs category: Physiological integrity
Client needs subcategory: Physiological adaptation
Cognitive level: Application

15.   A 10-month-old infant is admitted to the hospital from the clinic with a probable diagnosis of meningitis. Where should the nurse place the child?
1.   In strict isolation
2.   In respiratory isolation
3.   With other older infants
4.   With another child with meningitis

Answer: 2. The organisms that cause meningitis are transmitted by the spread of droplets. To protect the nursing staff and the family, the infant should be placed in a private room in respiratory isolation until I.V. antibiotics have been administered for 24 hours.

➡ *NCLEX keys*
Client needs category: Safe and effective care environment
Client needs subcategory: Safety and infection control
Cognitive level: Application

16.   Which electrocardiogram (ECG) strip does the nurse expect to see when caring for a child with rheumatic fever?

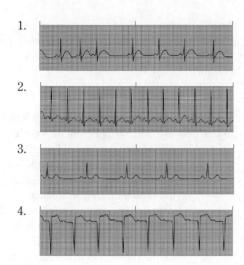

Answer: 4. In children with rheumatic fever, the ECG shows a prolonged PR interval, as seen in strip #4. The first strip shows sinus arrhythmia with a normal (0.12 to 0.2 second) PR interval. The second strip shows sinus tachycardia with a normal PR interval. The third strip illustrates sinus bradycardia, but the PR interval is still within normal limits.

➡ *NCLEX keys*
Client needs category: Physiological integrity
Client needs subcategory: Physiological adaptation
Cognitive level: Analysis

17. A nurse is caring for an infant with bilateral plaster leg casts for congenital clubfoot. Which statement by the parents indicates understanding of the nurse's teaching?
1. "When the casts get dirty, I can wash them with soap and warm water."
2. "I need to frequently check the temperature and color of my child's toes."
3. "I can dry the casts faster with a hair dryer so we can go meet my mother."
4. "When the casts are partly dry, I can coat them with a clear acrylic spray."

Answer: 2. The parents demonstrate understanding when they state that they'll check the temperature and color of the child's toes. Coolness, pale digits, pain, decreased sensation, and absence of pulse may indicate that the cast is too tight, causing neurovascular compromise. Putting water on a plaster cast can soften it and cause it to become misshapen. External heat shouldn't be used to dry the cast because the inside of the cast wouldn't be adequately dried. The cast shouldn't be sprayed with anything that would inhibit the loss of moisture from the plaster.

➡ *NCLEX keys*
Client needs category: Physiological integrity
Client needs subcategory: Reduction of risk potential
Cognitive level: Analysis

18. A nurse is counseling an adolescent who's wearing a Milwaukee brace for scoliosis. The nurse knows that teaching is successful when the adolescent states that the brace must be worn:
1. at night when sleeping.
2. during school hours.
3. 23 hours per day.
4. when eating meals and snacks.

Answer: 3. Routinely, the Milwaukee brace is worn about 23 hours per day. The brace is worn to decrease the thoracic curvature as the adolescent grows. The adolescent can be out of the brace for about 1 hour when showering or exercising.

➡ *NCLEX keys*
Client needs category: Health promotion and maintenance
Client needs subcategory: None
Cognitive level: Application

19. Which instruction should a nurse give the parents of an infant undergoing cleft lip repair?
1. Offer the pacifier as needed.
2. Lay the infant on his abdomen for sleep.
3. Sit the infant up for each feeding.
4. Loosen arm restraints every hour.

Answer: 3. An infant with cleft lip repair is fed in the upright position with a syringe and attached tubing to prevent stress to the suture line from sucking. Pacifiers shouldn't be used during the healing process.

The infant should be put down for sleep on his back or side so that the surgery site isn't traumatized. Arm restraints should be loosened every 2 hours.

➡ *NCLEX keys*
Client needs category: Physiological integrity
Client needs subcategory: Reduction of risk potential
Cognitive level: Application

20. A nurse is assessing an infant with persistent emesis and a provisional diagnosis of pyloric stenosis. For which acid-base imbalance should the nurse assess?
1. Respiratory acidosis
2. Respiratory alkalosis
3. Metabolic acidosis
4. Metabolic alkalosis

Answer: 4. With an excessive loss of potassium, hydrogen, and chloride as a result of persistent emesis, metabolic alkalosis occurs. A compensatory increase in bicarbonate ions is caused by chloride loss. As the result of excessive diarrhea or malnutrition, metabolic acidosis occurs. Respiratory acidosis results from excessive retention of partial pressure of arterial carbon dioxide ($Paco_2$). Respiratory alkalosis results when a loss of $Paco_2$ occurs.

➡ *NCLEX keys*
Client needs category: Physiological integrity
Client needs subcategory: Reduction of risk potential
Cognitive level: Comprehension

21. A nurse is caring for an infant with esophageal atresia and tracheoesophageal fistula. Which statement indicates that the infant's parents understand the diagnosis?
1. "The esophagus ends in a blind pouch so eating can't occur."
2. "There's a connection between the esophagus and the trachea."
3. "The esophagus ends in a blind pouch and there's a tube between the trachea and esophagus."
4. "Stomach acids come back up into the trachea, causing heartburn."

Answer: 3. This statement correctly describes the most common type of esophageal atresia and tracheoesophageal fistula.

➡ *NCLEX keys*
Client needs category: Physiological integrity
Client needs subcategory: Basic care and comfort
Cognitive level: Application

22. A breast-feeding mother of a 6-week-old infant asks the nurse why her infant wasn't diagnosed earlier with congenital hypothyroidism. How should the nurse respond?
1. "Breast-fed infants may not display symptoms until they're weaned."
2. "If you had brought your infant in for a 2-week checkup, you would have been told."
3. "The diagnosis was made earlier but replacement medication won't start yet."
4. "The public health nurse couldn't locate your home."

Answer: 1. Typically, a neonate doesn't exhibit signs of congenital hypothyroidism because of the exogenous source of thyroid hormone supplied by the maternal circulation. It may not be obvious in infants because they have a functional remnant of the thyroid hormone. Breast-fed babies may not manifest symptoms until they're weaned. Telling the mother she missed her 2-week checkup puts the blame on the mother, which isn't necessary. The other options aren't appropriate because the infant was breast-fed — preventing earlier diagnosis.

➡ *NCLEX keys*
Client needs category: Health promotion and maintenance
Client needs subcategory: None
Cognitive level: Application

23. A nurse is teaching a child with diabetes. Which statement by the child indicates that teaching was successful?
1. "Intermediate insulin's action begins 2 to 4 hours after the injection."
2. "Regular insulin should be given early in the morning before breakfast."
3. "Hunger, headache, shakiness, and sweating are all signs of hyperglycemia."
4. "Because exercise increases blood glucose levels, snacks aren't given before exercise."

Answer: 1. Intermediate insulin begins to act within 2 to 4 hours after injection and peaks about 6 to 8 hours after injection. Regular insulin begins to act within 30 minutes and is usually administered right before breakfast. Hunger, headache, shakiness, and sweating are signs of hypoglycemia. Strenuous exercise decreases the blood glucose level, so children engaging in exercise usually need a snack first.

➡ *NCLEX keys*

Client needs category: Physiological integrity
Client needs subcategory: Pharmacological and parenteral therapies
Cognitive level: Application

24. A nurse is teaching the mother of a child with diabetes mellitus. Which statement by the mother shows understanding of why her child needs snacks?
   1.   "Snacks will help my child not want to eat candy with friends."
   2.   "Snacks are given at the time insulin peaks to prevent hypoglycemia."
   3.   "Children can't eat all the calories they need in three meals per day."
   4.   "The insulin shots make my child hungry, so snacks help prevent cheating on the diet."

Answer: 2. The diabetic diet for children includes at least two snacks per day at midafternoon and before bed. Snacks are given at the time insulin peaks to help prevent hypoglycemia. Snacks aren't given to help control the desire for sweets, to ensure sufficient calorie intake, or to prevent the child from cheating on his diet.

➡ *NCLEX keys*

Client needs category: Physiological integrity
Client needs subcategory: Basic care and comfort
Cognitive level: Application

25. An 24-month-old toddler is seen in the clinic for a well checkup. The mother reports that she's in the process of toilet training her child, but the child has many accidents. What should the nurse ask the mother?
   1.   "Does your child understand what's expected?"
   2.   "How many accidents per day does your child have?"
   3.   "Does your child seem to be in pain right before the accident?"
   4.   "What does your child's urine smell like?"

Answer: 4. Asking what the child's urine smells like would yield the most helpful information. Commonly, when a child has a urinary tract infection, the urine has a strong, foul smell. Many 24-month-old children are ready to be toilet trained, and they usually understand what's asked of them. Asking about the number of accidents per day won't provide useful information because the number may vary depending on how much fluid the child drinks. Although the mother may not be able to determine whether the child has pain before an accident, it may be worth asking about after asking about the urine's odor.

➡ *NCLEX keys*

Client needs category: Physiological integrity
Client needs subcategory: Basic care and comfort
Cognitive level: Application

26. A child with a urinary tract infection (UTI) is being treated with an antibiotic for a period of 10 days. Which response by the mother indicates a need for further teaching?
   1.   "My child's urine no longer has an odor, so I stopped his medicine."
   2.   "My child should drink more fluid to help his kidneys function better."
   3.   "My child no longer has a fever, so the medicine must be working."
   4.   "My child can participate in his usual activities as long as he feels up to it."

Answer: 1. The mother requires additional teaching if she states that she stopped giving the antibiotic. An antibiotic should be taken for the entire time it's prescribed. Discontinuing the medication may cause the infection to recur. The other statements indicate understanding of the treatment for a child's UTI.

➡ *NCLEX keys*

Client needs category: Physiological integrity
Client needs subcategory: Pharmacological and parenteral therapies
Cognitive level: Application

27. A child has just returned from surgery for removal of a kidney for Wilms tumor. Which action should the nurse perform first?
1. Offer the child ice chips.
2. Administer pain medication when the child requests it.
3. Take the child's vital signs.
4. Provide games at the child's developmental level.

Answer: 3. The child's vital signs should be taken immediately upon arrival from surgery to determine the baseline and to detect early changes from previous recordings. Following nephrectomy, the child will most likely have a nasogastric tube and won't be allowed ice or fluids by mouth. Pain medication should be administered on a routine schedule to keep the child comfortable. The child should be provided diversions only after sufficient recuperation after surgery.

➡ *NCLEX keys*
Client needs category: Physiological integrity
Client needs subcategory: Basic care and comfort
Cognitive level: Application

28. A mother of a 3-month-old infant calls the clinic and states that her child has a diaper rash. The nurse should advise the mother to:
1. switch to cloth diapers.
2. use baby wipes with each diaper change.
3. leave the diaper open while the infant sleeps.
4. offer extra fluids to the infant until the rash improves.

Answer: 3. Leaving the diaper open while the child sleeps promotes air circulation to the area, improving the condition. There's no need to switch to cloth diapers; in fact, that may make the rash worse. Baby wipes contain alcohol, which may also worsen the condition. Extra fluids won't make the rash better.

➡ *NCLEX keys*
Client needs category: Physiological integrity
Client needs subcategory: Basic care and comfort
Cognitive level: Application

29. A nurse is speaking to the mother of a 5-year-old child who has just burned his arm with hot soup. What advice should the nurse give to the child's mother?
1. Wash the area with soap and water.
2. Spray the area with a pain reliever.
3. Flush the area with tepid water.
4. Bring the child immediately to the clinic.

Answer: 3. When a child has a scald type of burn, it's important to immediately flush the area with tepid water to cool the skin and prevent the burn from progressing. Soap shouldn't be used initially until the area had been flushed well. Spraying the area with pain reliever won't stop the burning process. The child shouldn't be taken to the clinic until the area has been flushed.

➡ *NCLEX keys*
Client needs category: Physiological integrity
Client needs subcategory: Basic care and comfort
Cognitive level: Application

30. A school-age child asks the school nurse how someone gets lice. The nurse should respond that lice are:
1. passed to other children because they don't wash their hands often.
2. spread easily because children share their hats and combs.
3. only spread between children; adults don't have them.
4. hard to spread unless your immune system is depressed.

Answer: 2. Lice are spread easily between children because they share possessions more readily than adults do. Also, children tend to be in closer proximity to each other than adults are.

➡ *NCLEX keys*
Client needs category: Safe and effective care environment
Client needs subcategory: Safety and infection control
Cognitive level: Application

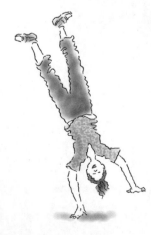

Part VI   Professional issues

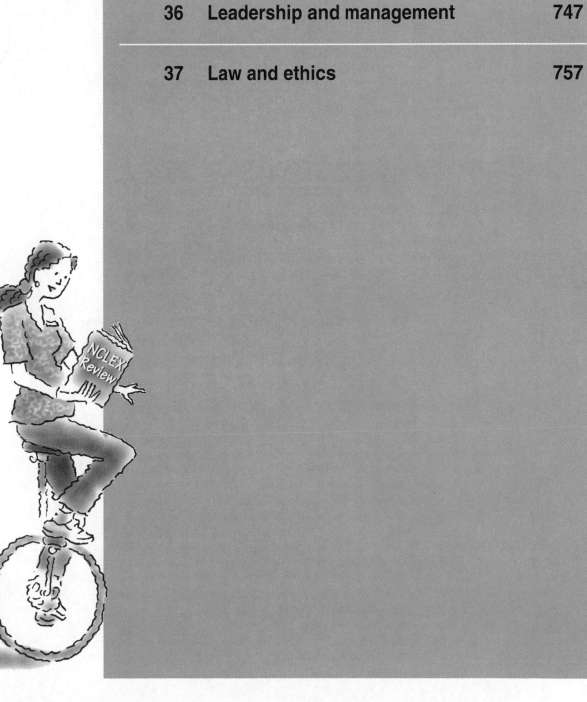

Brush up on key concepts

Management is a process used to make sure a facility's objectives are met. In nursing, management involves coordinating staff to accomplish the facility's objectives in the most efficient, cost-effective manner. You can review the major points of this chapter by consulting the *Cheat sheet* on page 748.

Nurse-manager

A nurse-manager assumes 24-hour accountability for the nursing care delivered in a specific nursing area.

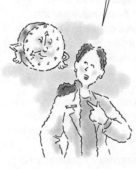

Accountability is an around-the-clock concern for the nurse-manager

Getting the job done
The nurse-manager's responsibilities typically include:
• policy and decision making
• providing adequate staffing for safe, effective client care
• evaluating client care
• providing client-teaching activities
• coordinating nursing services with other client-care services
• supervising and guiding staff members
• evaluating staff performance
• participating in staff recruitment and retention
• providing new staff members with an adequate, individualized orientation
• ensuring that staff members participate in continuing education
• making sure that staff education is appropriate for each member's assigned responsibilities
• planning and implementing budgets

• encouraging staff participation in policy and procedure development and quality monitoring.

MANAGEMENT STYLES
The nurse-manager's job description defines her authority over a specified group of employees and describes her job responsibilities.

What style!
Each manager directs her staff using a different management style. An effective manager commonly uses more than one style. At times, staff should participate in decision making; at other times, staff participation isn't appropriate. The most commonly used management styles include:
• **autocratic** — Decisions are made with little or no staff input. The manager doesn't delegate responsibility. Staff dependence is fostered.
• **laissez-faire** — Little direction, structure, or support is provided by the manager. The manager abdicates responsibility and decision making whenever possible. Staff development isn't facilitated. There's little interest in achieving the goals necessary for adequate client care.
• **democratic** — Staff members are encouraged to participate in the decision-making process whenever possible. Most decisions are made by the group, not the manager. Staff development is encouraged. Responsibilities are carefully delegated to staff to encourage growth and accountability. Positive feedback is given to staff members to encourage professional growth.
• **participative** — Problems are identified by the manager and presented to the staff with several solutions. Staff members are encouraged to provide input but the manager makes the final decision. Negotiation is a

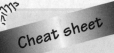

Leadership and management refresher

NURSE-MANAGER
• Assumes 24-hour accountability for the nursing care delivered in a specific nursing area

Management styles
• Autocratic — Decisions are made with little or no staff input. The manager doesn't delegate responsibility. Staff dependence is fostered.
• Laissez-faire — Little direction, structure, or support is provided by the manager. The manager abdicates responsibility and decision making when possible. Staff development isn't facilitated. There's little interest in achieving the goals necessary for adequate client care.
• Democratic — Staff members are encouraged to participate in decision making when possible. Most decisions are made by the group. Staff development is encouraged. Responsibilities are carefully delegated and feedback is given to staff members to encourage professional growth.
• Participative — Problems are identified by the manager and presented to the staff with possible solutions. Staff members are encouraged to provide input but the manager makes the decision. Negotiation is key. The manager encourages staff advancement.

Delegation
• Involves entrusting a task to another staff member
• Helps free the nurse-manager from tasks that can be completed successfully by someone else
• Prepares staff member for career advancement

DISCHARGE PLANNING AND CLIENT TEACHING
• Initiated as soon as possible

Clinical pathways
• Multidisciplinary guidelines for client care
• Documentation tool for nurses and other health care providers
• Provides sequences of multidisciplinary interventions that incorporate teaching, consultation, discharge planning, medications, nutrition, diagnostic testing, activities, treatments, and therapeutic modalities

QUALITY MANAGEMENT
• Continuous quality improvement — Used to continually assess and evaluate the effectiveness of client care
• Benchmarking — Nurse-manager compares best practices from top hospitals with her unit and adapts the unit's practices as needed
• Performance improvement — Establishes a system of formal evaluation of job performance and recommends ways to improve performance and promote professional growth

RESOURCE MANAGEMENT
• Equipment
• Finances and budgets
• Staff

Types of budgets
• Capital — reviewed annually; outlines plan for providing equipment that costs more than $500; nurse-manager determines large, fixed assets or equipment needed within a specified budgetary period (usually 3 to 5 years)
• Operating — day-to-day expenses of a specified nursing area, excluding personnel costs
• Personnel — cost for staffing the unit; based on the number of personnel or full-time equivalents needed

HEALTH CARE DELIVERY SYSTEMS
• Provide payment for health care

Types of health care systems
• Health maintenance organizations (HMOs)— provide comprehensive health services for a designated payment; fixed payment is given to health care provider periodically to cover the costs of health care for each individual enrolled in the HMO
• Preferred provider organizations (PPOs)— negotiate special, reduced rates to attract insurance plan beneficiaries; members' care is paid for if they use a health care provider who's under contract to the PPO
• Managed care organizations — provide beneficiaries with various client care services for an established, agreed-on payment

Managers aren't always leaders

An effective nurse-manager recognizes the valuable role played by a nursing leader. A nursing leader can be any member of the nursing team who encourages her colleagues to achieve the unit goals. Most leaders are excellent role models. They help other staff members develop and improve their nursing skills. They solve problems and work to improve both client care and working conditions at the health care facility.

An effective nurse-manager delegates tasks to staff members. This takes pressure off the manager and helps advance the staff members' careers.

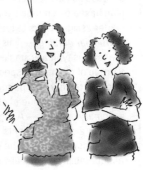

key element of this management style. The manager encourages staff advancement.

Come to an understanding

An effective nurse-manager has a good understanding of each management style. Managers who adopt the autocratic or laissez-faire management style rarely produce effective outcomes. Those who adopt the democratic or participative style are typically successful because these styles foster staff input, goal achievement, and professional growth of staff members. For example, an effective nurse-manager recognizes and fosters the role of the nursing leaders on her staff. (See *Managers aren't always leaders*.)

DELEGATION

One of the most important tasks of the nurse-manager is effective **delegation.** Delegation involves entrusting a task to another staff member. This helps free the nurse-manager from tasks that can be completed successfully by someone else and allows her to focus on other tasks. It also prepares the staff member for career advancement.

The guidelines below can help the nurse-manager with successful delegation. The nurse-manager should:
- recognize that delegation is necessary for effective management
- delegate whenever possible
- delegate tasks only if they're within the scope of practice and skill of the person assigned the tasks
- delegate tasks according to priority (client care must always come first)
- delegate clearly and concisely and include a time frame for completing the task

- provide support and positive feedback when possible.

Although it may be difficult to delegate at first, fostering a working environment that supports autonomy, independence, and professional growth helps with recruitment and retention of staff.

Nursing care delivery systems

Nursing care delivery systems dictate how nursing care is delivered on a nursing unit. Each delivery system has a unique design that must outline:
- who has the responsibility for making client care decisions
- the duration for which client care decisions remain in effect
- work distribution among staff
- procedures for communicating client care.

Special delivery

The nurse-manager should understand the individual delivery systems and choose one that's best for the unit or facility. After a delivery system is chosen, the nurse-manager should evaluate the system regularly to make sure the system meets the needs of the clients. (See *Understanding delivery systems*, page 750.)

To ensure that clients' needs are met, the nurse-manager regularly evaluates nursing care delivery systems.

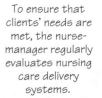

Discharge planning and client teaching

Discharge planning and client teaching go hand in hand; one can't be accomplished without the other.

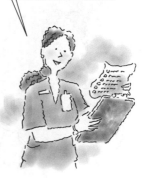

Understanding delivery systems

The members of each nursing unit choose a delivery system that best meets the needs of their clients. The delivery systems listed here are most commonly used today:

• *Team nursing* — A registered nurse leads nursing staff who work together to provide care for a specific number of clients. The team typically consists of registered nurses, licensed practical nurses, and client care attendants. The team leader assesses client needs, plans client care, and revises the care plan based on changes in the client's condition. The team leader assigns tasks to team members as needed.

• *Modular nursing* — This system is similar to team nursing, but the team is typically smaller. A registered nurse is assigned to a group of clients in a specific geographic location. Typically, a registered nurse is paired with a licensed practical nurse to care for a small group of clients.

• *Primary nursing* — A registered nurse plans and organizes care for a group of clients and cares for this group during their entire hospitalization. The registered nurse assumes 24-hour accountability for this group of clients. She delegates care in her absence to other staff members. A registered nurse who cares for the clients in the absence of the primary nurse is called an *associate nurse.* The associate nurse follows the care plan developed by the primary nurse.

• *Total client care nursing* — A registered nurse plans, organizes, and delivers client care for a specific group of clients. If a licensed practical nurse is caring for a group of clients, a registered nurse assesses the clients and plans the care delivered by the licensed practical nurse.

• *Functional nursing* — Each caregiver on a specific nursing unit is given specific tasks that fall into their scope of practice. For example, a registered nurse may administer medications to the entire unit, while a licensed practical nurse performs treatments and the client care attendants provide physical care.

• *Case management* — This form of primary nursing involves a registered nurse who manages the care of an assigned group of clients. This nurse coordinates care with the entire health care team. She helps develop protocols, policies, and procedures and develops a plan to achieve client outcomes.

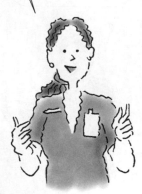

Discharge planning and client teaching are initiated as early in the care process as possible. For clients with scheduled admission dates, teaching begins before hospitalization.

Beginning with admission

The nurse-manager makes sure discharge planning and client teaching are initiated as soon as possible. If the client is admitted to the hospital as an emergency, client teaching should begin as soon as the client's condition stabilizes. For clients with planned admissions, discharge planning should begin before hospitalization. For example, if a client requires a nonemergency surgical procedure, the client should be taught about the procedure and his postoperative care in the physician's office before admission to the hospital. Clients planning outclient treatment should also be taught before admission to the outclient facility.

Follow the clinical pathway

Clinical pathways are multidisciplinary guidelines for client care. A clinical pathway is a documentation tool for nurses as well as other health care providers. It provides the sequences of multidisciplinary interventions that incorporate teaching, consultation, discharge planning, medication, nutrition, diagnostic testing, activities, treatments, and therapeutic modalities.

The goal of a clinical pathway is to achieve realistic expected outcomes for the client and family members. It promotes a professional and collaborative goal for care and practice and assures continuity of care. It should also guarantee appropriate use of resources, which reduces costs and hospital length of stay while also providing the framework for quality management.

Clinical pathways are also used to guide the use of client-teaching tools, such as:

• videos
• audiotapes
• printed materials.

The nurse-manager is responsible for the effectiveness of discharge planning and client teaching. She must collaborate with all members of the interdisciplinary health care team so that all clients attain their maximum state of wellness.

Quality management

Nurse-managers must continuously search for methods to improve the quality of client care. Because change is constant in health care, nurse-managers must think strategically and plan for changes before they arise.

Assess and evaluate

Continuous quality improvement, based on principles from the business world, is a system used to continually assess and evaluate the effectiveness of client care. The nurse-manager uses reports from risk management to assess and evaluate care. Areas that need improvement can be identified by reviewing such incidents as:
- medication errors
- client falls
- treatment errors
- treatment omissions.

Incidents are investigated and a plan is devised to minimize or eliminate the risk of recurrence. Continuous quality improvement calls for constant evaluation of the system for delivering services and the people performing the tasks.

Nothing but the best

Another method for evaluating client care is **benchmarking.** Best practices are taken from the top hospitals and compared with the practices on the manager's unit. The manager then adapts her unit's practices based on how they compare with the best hospitals' practices or benchmarks.

Improving performance and promoting professionalism

Performance improvement, another component of continuous quality improvement, establishes a system of formal evaluation of job performance and recommends ways to improve performance and promote professional growth. Performance evaluations provide recognition, structured feedback, and recommendations for improvement. They also provide an opportunity for both the manager and staff member to clarify performance expectations.

Resource management

Resource management includes the management of:
- equipment
- finances
- staff.

For profit or not

The approach to managing these resources depends on whether the facility is nonprofit or for-profit. Traditionally, health care facilities were nonprofit organizations, making them tax-exempt. Excess revenue was recorded as a positive fund balance, or net worth. This revenue was reinvested in the organization and used to expand or improve services.

Many facilities today are for-profit organizations. The excess revenue generated is divided as a dividend among stockholders or reinvested in the organization. The profit status of the health care facility directs how the financial resources are used.

BUDGET TYPES

Resource management depends on the manager's ability to evaluate the unit's financial performance and prepare the budget accordingly. The **budget** is a plan that directs the use of resources. Nurse-managers must develop three types of budgets:
- capital
- operating
- personnel.

Capital idea

The **capital budget,** which is reviewed annually, outlines a plan for providing equipment needed for the unit that costs more than $500. To prepare the capital budget, the nurse-manager determines what large, fixed assets or pieces of equipment that depreciate are needed within a specified budgetary period (usually 3 to 5 years).

Day-to-day operations

The **operating budget** deals with the day-to-day operating expenses of a specified nursing area excluding personnel costs. Such expenses include medical and nonmedical supplies, certain utilities, small equipment,

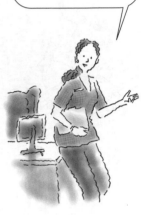

There's always room for improvement when it comes to nursing care. Benchmarking and performance evaluations are two methods used to improve nursing practices.

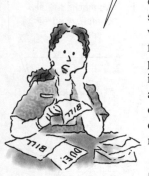

> Resources at any facility include staff, equipment, and finances. Each is a major consideration in budgeting.

and funding for the continuing education and professional development of staff.

Per person

The **personnel budget** identifies the cost for staffing the nursing care unit. The budget is based on the number of personnel or full-time equivalents (FTEs) needed to adequately staff the unit. One FTE is equal to one person working 8 hours per day, 5 days per week, for 52 weeks per year. When calculating the personnel budget, the nurse-manager must include salaries, potential raises, benefits, and anticipated overtime. The nurse-manager compiles her budgets using historical data, client population, staffing needs, equipment needs, and accrediting agency requirements.

Health care delivery systems

Health care delivery systems provide payment for health care. These systems came into existence with the demand for discounted health care services. Health care delivery systems include:

- health maintenance organizations (HMOs)
- preferred provider organizations (PPOs)
- managed care organizations.

Maintenance plan

An **HMO** provides comprehensive health care services to people enrolled in the program for a designated payment. A fixed payment is given to a health care provider periodically to cover the costs of health care for each individual enrolled in the program. This process is known as *capitation*.

Preferred providers

A **PPO** is a health care delivery system that has negotiated a special, reduced rate to attract insurance plan beneficiaries. Members of the PPO have their health care expenses paid for if they use a health care provider who's a provider under contract to the PPO. Members can choose a noncontract provider but must pay additional service fees to cover costs not covered by the PPO.

Cost containment

Managed care organizations provide beneficiaries with various client care services for an established, agreed-on payment. Cost containment measures are in place to monitor and control expenses.

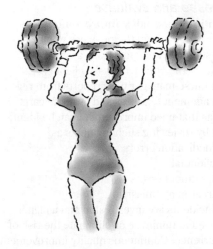

Pump up on practice questions

1. A nurse-manager of an inpatient pediatric unit is at home one evening when she receives a call from a staff nurse informing her of a serious medication error that just occurred on the unit. The nurse-manager was notified because she assumes accountability for what happens on the unit:

1. 5 days per week.
2. 24 hours per day, 7 days per week.
3. 8 hours per day, 7 days per week.
4. 24 hours per day, 5 days per week.

Answer: 2. Nurse-managers are accountable for nursing care on the unit 24 hours per day, 7 days per week.

➡ NCLEX keys
Client needs category: Safe and effective care environment
Client needs subcategory: Management of care
Cognitive level: Application

2. A staff nurse influences the behaviors of her colleagues by guiding and encouraging them. She's an excellent role model but has no formal authority over her peers. This nurse is demonstrating characteristics of which role?
　1. Manager
　2. Autocrat
　3. Leader
　4. Authority
Answer: 3. A leader doesn't always need or have formal power and authority. A leader guides, directs, and enhances the activities of peers and colleagues and is an effective role model. A manager has a formal position of power in an organization and should be an effective leader. An autocrat doesn't seek staff input and doesn't encourage peers or subordinates to grow professionally. Authority is a characteristic of managers and is part of the formal position of power granted to someone as a result of a job description.

➡ NCLEX keys
Client needs category: Safe and effective care environment
Client needs subcategory: Management of care
Cognitive level: Application

3. A nurse-manager is concerned because she received many time-off requests from her staff for the upcoming holiday season. She has come up with several possible solutions to the staffing dilemma and has scheduled a staff meeting to present ideas to the staff. Which management style is this manager demonstrating?
　1. Participative
　2. Democratic
　3. Autocratic
　4. Laissez-faire

Answer: 1. A participative manager identifies problems and presents staff with several possible solutions for discussion. A democratic manager usually allows many decisions to be made by the group. She also solicits the group's ideas about problem solving. An autocratic manager makes decisions without input from staff. A laissez-faire manager provides no direction and abdicates decision making whenever possible.

➡ NCLEX keys
Client needs category: Safe and effective care environment
Client needs subcategory: Management of care
Cognitive level: Application

4. A nurse-manager of a 30-bed surgical unit arrives at work during a snowstorm. She finds that only a licensed practical nurse and two nursing assistants have been able to make the journey to work. Each reporting staff member has skills that can be used to provide care for the clients on the unit. Which nursing care delivery system would be most effective under these circumstances?
　1. Primary nursing
　2. Team nursing
　3. Functional nursing
　4. Case management
Answer: 3. Functional nursing is efficient, requires fewer staff than the other systems, and makes use of the skills of all available staff members. Primary nursing and case management delivery systems require many more registered nurses than are available in this emergency. Team nursing, while requiring fewer registered nurses than primary nursing or case management, doesn't lend itself to the efficient use of skills required in this emergency.

➡ NCLEX keys
Client needs category: Safe and effective care environment
Client needs subcategory: Management of care
Cognitive level: Analysis

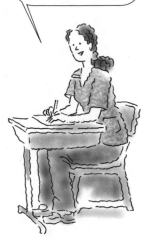

Learn the roles of nursing leaders and nurse-managers. This knowledge will help you pass the exam and will also come in handy when you become a nursing leader or nurse-manager.

5. A registered nurse who works in the preoperative area of the operating room notices that a client is scheduled for a partial mastectomy and axillary lymph node removal the following week. The nurse should make sure that the client is well educated about her surgery by:

1. talking with the nursing staff at the physician's office to find out what the client has been taught and her level of understanding.
2. making sure that the post-anesthesia care unit nurses know what to teach the client before discharge.
3. providing all of the preoperative teaching before surgery.
4. having the post-operative nurses teach the client because she'll be too anxious before surgery.

Answer: 1. The nurse who works in the preoperative area of the operating room should talk to the nurses in the physician's office to find out what the client has been taught. She should then reinforce the teaching and answer any questions the client has. The client will most likely be anxious before her surgery, but the nurse can proceed with teaching. The client will most likely be too sedated to learn about her postoperative care immediately after surgery.

➡ *NCLEX keys*
Client needs category: Safe and effective care environment
Client needs subcategory: Management of care
Cognitive level: Application

6. A nurse-manager of an intensive care unit is interviewing a registered nurse for the team leader position. The nurse appears to be qualified and has excellent references. She states that she's certified in critical care nursing but she misplaced her verification card. Based on her knowledge of her supervisory responsibilities, the nurse-manager should:

1. contact the credentialing center and confirm the nurse's certification.
2. hire the nurse, but tell her that she must provide proof of certification before completing orientation.

3. avoid hiring the nurse because she can't provide proof of certification.
4. trust that the nurse is telling the truth because she has excellent references.

Answer: 1. The nurse-manager must make sure that the nurse is certified as a critical care nurse. She can do this by contacting the credentialing center. In the case of a new hire, the nurse-manager must be sure that the nurse is representing herself truthfully before offering her the position.

➡ *NCLEX keys*
Client needs category: Safe and effective care environment
Client needs subcategory: Management of care
Cognitive level: Application

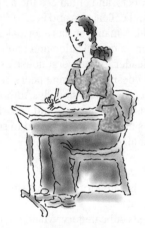

7. A nurse-manager of an outpatient surgery department helps groom her staff for career advancement. Which task can she safely delegate to a staff registered nurse?

1. Ask one of her staff nurses to terminate a client care assistant.
2. Ask two of her staff nurses to schedule staff for the next 2 weeks.
3. Assign 24-hour responsibility to her assistant manager for a period of 2 months.
4. Tell the most experienced staff nurse to select a new nursing care delivery system for use in the department.

Answer: 2. A nurse-manager can only delegate tasks that are within the scope of practice and skill of her subordinates. Scheduling staff falls within this scope. Termination of employees and 24-hour accountability can't be delegated. The selection of a new nursing care delivery system affects the functioning of an entire department and shouldn't be delegated. It should be determined by input from all staff members.

➡ NCLEX keys
Client needs category: Safe and effective care environment
Client needs subcategory: Management of care
Cognitive level: Application

8. A new nurse-manager is trying to determine the best way to implement client teaching in her outpatient surgical center. She decides to gather data from other surgical centers and compare their teaching methods with her center's methods. Which quality improvement process is she using?
1. Benchmarking
2. Risk management
3. Performance improvement
4. Quality management

Answer: 1. Benchmarking is the process of comparing your organization with the effectiveness of organizations formally recognized as some of the best in the business. Risk management is the process of monitoring the organization's adverse occurrences or potential for such occurrences and taking steps to reduce or eliminate these incidents. Performance improvement is the process of evaluating the effectiveness of job performance and taking steps to improve that effectiveness. Quality management is the overall process of evaluating and improving the quality of client services.

➡ NCLEX keys
Client needs category: Safe and effective care environment
Client needs subcategory: Management of care
Cognitive level: Application

9. A nurse-manager of a busy pediatric unit wants to purchase additional computers for client data collection and for online continuing education programs. The total cost is about $1,500. She should include this expense in what portion of her budget?
1. Personnel
2. Operating
3. Capital
4. Managerial

Answer: 3. Equipment that costs more than $500 is typically part of the capital budget. The personnel budget addresses costs related to staffing. The operating budget includes the day-to-day operating expenses of a client care area. Managerial is a general term that doesn't specifically relate to a budget component.

➡ NCLEX keys
Client needs category: Safe and effective care environment
Client needs subcategory: Management of care
Cognitive level: Application

10. A nurse-manager helps clients understand health care delivery systems available to them. One system enables negotiation for a special, reduced rate with specific health care providers. The client then has his care costs provided for by this system. If a client seeks help from such a provider, the provider pays expenses. Which health care delivery system provides this service?
1. Health maintenance organization (HMO)
2. Preferred provider organization (PPO)
3. Managed care
4. Capitation

Answer: 2. A PPO covers medical expenses if its members use the health care services of providers under contract to the organization. An HMO provides comprehensive health care

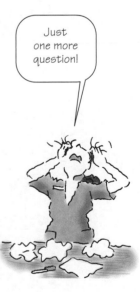

Just one more question!

services to persons enrolled in it for a fixed periodic payment. Managed care organizations provide members with various client-care services for an established, agreed-on payment. Capitation is the fixed rate of payment given to health care providers under contract to an HMO.

➡ *NCLEX keys*

Client needs category: Safe and effective care environment
Client needs subcategory: Management of care
Cognitive level: Knowledge

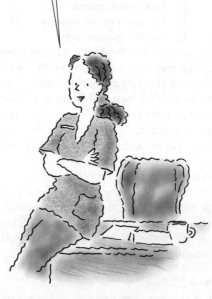

Now that you have your leadership skills down, you can lead us to the next chapter!

37 Law and ethics

Brush up on key concepts

Safe, effective nursing practice requires becoming fully aware of the many legal and ethical issues surrounding professional practice. These issues range from understanding your state's nurse practice act to upholding clients' rights and fulfilling the many legal responsibilities you have as a nurse.

You can review the key points of this chapter at any time, using the *Cheat sheet* on pages 758 and 759.

Nurse practice acts

Each state has a **nurse practice act.** It's designed to protect both the nurse and the public by:
• defining the legal scope of nursing practice
• excluding untrained or unlicensed people from practicing nursing.

Your state's nurse practice act is the most important law affecting your nursing practice. You're expected to care for clients within defined practice limits; if you give care beyond those limits, you become vulnerable to charges of violating your state nurse practice act.

Scope it out
Most nurse practice acts define important concepts, including the scope of nursing practice. In other words, nurse practice acts broadly outline what nurses can and can't do on the job. Make sure that you're familiar with the legally permissible scope of your nursing practice as defined in your state's nurse practice act and that you never exceed its limits. Otherwise, you're inviting legal problems.

Nurse practice acts also outline the conditions and requirements for licensure. To become licensed as a registered nurse, for instance, you must meet certain qualifications such as passing the NCLEX. All states require completion of a basic professional nursing education program. Your state may have additional requirements, including:
• good moral character
• good physical and mental health
• free from criminal conviction
• fluency in English
• free from drug or alcohol addiction.

Nurse practice acts also define requirements for renewing your license, which may include additional education hours as set forth by each state.

Get on board
In every U.S. state and Canadian province, the nurse practice act creates a state or provincial board of nursing. The nurse practice act authorizes this board to administer and enforce rules and regulations about the nursing profession. The board is bound by the provisions of the nurse practice act that created it.

The nurse practice act is the law; the board of nursing can't grant exemptions to it or waive any of its provisions. Only the state or provincial legislature can change the law. In many states and provinces, however, the board of nursing may grant exemptions and waivers to its own rules and regulations.

Moving violations
The nurse practice act also lists violations that can result in disciplinary action against a nurse. Depending on the nature of the violation, a nurse may face state board disciplinary action and liability for her actions.

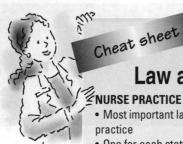

Cheat sheet

Law and ethics refresher

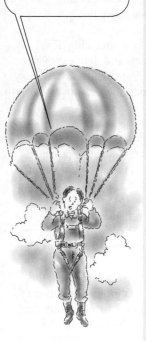

Nurse practice acts define the scope and limits of your professional practice: What you may and may not do on the job.

NURSE PRACTICE ACTS
- Most important law affecting your nursing practice
- One for each state
- Designed to protect nurse and public by defining legal scope of practice and excluding untrained or unlicensed people from practicing nursing
- Outline conditions and requirements for licensure such as passing NCLEX
- Require completion of a basic professional nursing education program; each state may have additional requirements, including good moral character, good physical and mental health, minimum age, fluency in English, absence of drug or alcohol addiction
- Define requirements for renewing a license

INFORMED CONSENT
- Your client's right to be adequately informed about a proposed treatment or procedure
- Responsibility for obtaining informed consent rests with the person who will perform the treatment or procedure (usually the physician).
- The client should be told that he has a right to refuse the treatment or procedure without having other care or support withdrawn and that he can withdraw consent after giving it.

Elements
- Description of the treatment or procedure
- Description of inherent risks and benefits that occur with frequency or regularity (or specific consequences significant to the given client or his designated decision maker)
- Explanation of the potential for death or serious harm (such as brain damage, stroke, paralysis, or disfiguring scars) or for discomforting adverse effects during or after the treatment or procedure
- Explanation and description of alternative treatments or procedures
- Name and qualifications of the person who will perform the treatment or procedure

- Discussion of possible effects of not undergoing the treatment or procedure

Witnessing informed consent
- The client voluntarily consented.
- The client's signature is authentic.
- The client appears to be competent to give consent.

RIGHT TO REFUSE TREATMENT
- Any mentally competent adult may legally refuse treatment if he's fully informed about his medical condition and about the likely consequences of his refusal.
- Some clients may refuse treatment on the grounds of freedom of religion or cultural beliefs.

Grounds for challenging a client's right to refuse treatment
- The client is incompetent.
- Compelling reasons exist to overrule client's wishes such as when the refusal endangers the life of another, when a parent's decision to withhold treatment threatens a child's life, when a client makes statements indicating that he wants to live, and when public interest outweighs the client's right.

Advance directive
- This legal document provides information about the client's wishes for medical decisions in the event that the client becomes incapacitated.
- An advance directive includes a living will and a durable power of attorney for health care.
- The Client Self-Determination Act of 1990 requires facilities to provide clients with information about their rights regarding advance directives, living wills, and durable power of attorney for health care as well as about the facility's policy for implementing them.
- A living will specifies a client's wishes about medical care, including treatment options, in the event that he becomes incompetent or no longer able to express his wishes.

Law and ethics refresher (continued)

RIGHT TO REFUSE TREATMENT (CONTINUED)

- A durable power of attorney for health care designates a person (proxy) to make medical decisions for a client if he becomes incompetent.

HEALTH INSURANCE PORTABILITY AND ACCOUNTABILITY ACT (HIPAA)

- HIPAA was enacted in 2003 to protect privacy and security of medical information.
- Privacy rule protects all oral, written, and electronic health information.
- Protected health information includes individually indentifiable information (such as the client's name, date of birth, Social Security number); health information; demographic information; billing and payment information; information about relatives, household members, and employers; and photos.

MEDICATION ADMINISTRATION

- To guard against malpractice liability, remember the "five rights" formula: right drug, right client, right time, right dosage, right route.
- Nurses have the legal right not to administer drugs they think will harm patients.

NEGLIGENCE AND MALPRACTICE

Negligence

- Failure to exercise the degree of care that a person of ordinary prudence would exercise under the same circumstances

Four criteria for negligence claim

1. A person owed a duty to the person making the claim.
2. The duty was breached.
3. The breach resulted in injury to the person making the claim.
4. Damages were a direct result of the negligence of the health care provider.

Malpractice

- Specific type of negligence
- Violation of professional duty or a failure to meet a standard of care, or failure to use the skills and knowledge of other professionals in similar circumstances

DOCUMENTATION ERRORS

- Complete, accurate, and timely documentation is crucial to the continuity of each client's care.

Functions of well-documented record

- Reflects client care given
- Demonstrates results of treatment
- Helps plan and coordinate care contributed by each professional
- Allows interdisciplinary exchange of information about client
- Provides evidence of nurse's legal responsibilities toward client
- Demonstrates standards, rules, regulations, and laws of nursing practice
- Supplies information for analysis of cost-to-benefit reduction
- Reflects professional and ethical conduct and responsibility
- Furnishes information for continuing education, risk management, diagnosis-related group assignment and reimbursement, continuous quality improvement, case management monitoring, and research

Common documentation errors

- Omissions
- Personal opinions
- Vague entries
- Late entries
- Improper corrections
- Unauthorized entries
- Erroneous or vague abbreviations
- Illegibility and lack of clarity

ABUSE

- Nurse plays a crucial role in recognizing and reporting incidents of suspected abuse.
- Pass the information along to appropriate authorities.
- In many states, failure to report actual or suspected abuse constitutes a crime.

Get it?

Understanding your nurse practice act's general provisions helps you to stay within the legal limits of nursing practice. Interpreting the nurse practice act isn't always easy, however. Nurse practice acts are laws, after all, so they tend to be worded in broad, vague terms, and the wording varies from state to state.

The key point to remember is this: Your state nurse practice act isn't a word-for-word checklist of how you should do your work. Ultimately, you must rely on your own education and knowledge of your facility's policies and procedures.

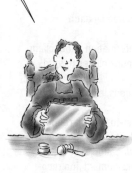

Nurse practice acts are laws; they tend to be worded in broad, vague terms, and the wording varies from state to state.

Declare independence

Most nurse practice acts pose another problem: They state that you have a legal duty to carry out a physician's or a dentist's orders. Yet, as a licensed professional, you also have an ethical and legal duty to use your own judgment when providing client care. When such conflicts arise, don't hesitate to act independently. Follow these guidelines:
• When you think an order is wrong, tell the physician.
• If you're confused about an order, ask the physician to clarify it.
• If the physician fails to correct the error or answer your questions, inform your immediate supervisor or nurse-manager of your doubts. Follow the chain of command established in your facility.

Know your limits

Conflicts of duty can also arise if your state's nurse practice act disagrees with your facility's policies. The nursing service department in each facility develops detailed policies and procedures for staff nurses. These policies and procedures usually specify the allowable scope of nursing practice within the facility. The scope may be narrower than the scope described in your nurse practice act, but it shouldn't be broader.

In other words, your employer can't legally expand the scope of your practice to include tasks prohibited by your nurse practice act. You have a legal obligation to practice within your nurse practice act's limits. Except in a life-threatening emergency, you can't exceed those limits without risking disciplinary action. To protect yourself, compare your facility's policies with your nurse practice act.

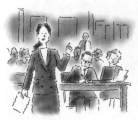

Tell it straight. Reasonable disclosure means the client has a right to know about the risks associated with his diagnosis and treatment.

Change is good

With every new medical discovery or technological innovation, the world of nursing undergoes revision. To align nurse practice acts with current nursing practice, professional nursing organizations and state boards of nursing generally propose revisions to regulations. There's a catch: Nurse practice acts are statutory laws subject to the inevitably slow legislative process, so the law sometimes has trouble keeping pace with medicine.

What does all of this mean for you? To help protect yourself legally, you need to stay current with your state's nurse practice act while you keep up with innovations in health care practice.

Informed consent

Your client has a legal right to be adequately informed about a proposed treatment or procedure. Generally, responsibility for obtaining a client's **informed consent** rests with the person who is to carry out the treatment or procedure (usually the physician). Carrying out a procedure without informed consent can be grounds for charges of assault and battery.

Informed consent involves providing the client (or someone acting on his behalf) with enough information to know:
• what the client is getting into if he decides to undergo the treatment or procedure
• the anticipated consequences if consent is refused or withdrawn.

Nurses may provide clients and their families with information that's within a nurse's scope of practice and knowledge base. However, a nurse can't substitute her knowledge for the physician's input.

Information, please

What should you tell the client? First, he has a right to reasonable disclosure of risks associated with the medical diagnosis and treatment. He also must be given an opportunity to evaluate options, alternatives, and risks before exercising his choice. The basics of informed consent should include:
• description of the treatment or procedure
• description of inherent risks and benefits that occur with frequency or regularity (or specific consequences significant to the given client or his designated decision maker)
• explanation of the potential for death or serious harm (such as brain damage, stroke, paralysis, or disfiguring scars) or for discomforting adverse effects during or after the treatment or procedure
• explanation and description of alternative treatments or procedures

- name and qualifications of the person who is to perform the treatment or procedure
- discussion of the possible effects of not undergoing the treatment or procedure.

The client should also be told that he has a right to refuse the treatment or procedure without having other care or support withdrawn and that he can withdraw consent after giving it.

Can I get a witness?
If you witness a client's signature on a consent form, you attest to three things:
- the client voluntarily consented
- the client's signature is authentic
- the client appears to be competent to give consent.

What they don't know can hurt you
Another potential legal pitfall for nurses is called *negligent nondisclosure*. Let's say, for example, that you believe a client is incompetent to participate in giving consent because of medication or sedation given to him. Perhaps you learn that the practitioner has discussed consent issues with the client when the client was heavily sedated or medicated. Under either of these scenarios, you have an obligation to bring it to the practitioner's attention immediately. If the practitioner isn't available, discuss your concerns with your supervisor.

Always document attempts to reach the practitioner or attending physician in the medical record before allowing the client to proceed with the treatment or procedure. Besides discussing this with the practitioner and your supervisor, you must also assess your client's understanding of the information provided by the practitioner.

When a client is incompetent
A client is deemed mentally incompetent if he can't understand the explanations or can't comprehend the results of his decisions. When a client is incompetent, the practitioner has two alternatives:
- seek consent from the client's next of kin (usually the spouse)
- petition the court to appoint a legal guardian for the client.

Remember, however, that mental illness isn't the same as incompetence. Persons suffering from mental illness have been found competent to give consent because they're alert and, above all, can understand the proposed treatment, risks, benefits, alternatives, and consequences of refusing treatment.

A minor problem
Every state allows an emancipated minor to consent to his own medical care and treatment. Definitions of emancipation vary from state to state, however. Most states allow teenagers to consent to treatment, even though they aren't emancipated, in cases involving pregnancy or sexually transmitted disease.

Right to refuse treatment

The **right to refuse treatment** allows any mentally competent adult to legally refuse treatment if he's fully informed about his medical condition and about the likely consequences of his refusal. As a professional, you must respect that decision.

Most court cases related to the right to refuse treatment have involved clients with a terminal illness (or their families) who want to discontinue life support.

Quality time
More and more, health care providers consider quality end-of-life care as an ethical obligation. But what does end-of-life mean, and how do you measure it? Some researchers point to five "domains," or focal points, that clients view as end-of-life issues. By understanding these domains from the clients' perspectives, nurses can improve the quality of end-of-life care.
- Pain and other symptoms are of concern for many clients.
- Many clients fear "being kept alive" after they can no longer enjoy life; they want to "die with dignity."
- Sense of control is also critical; some clients are adamant about controlling their end-of-life care decisions.

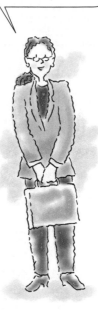

Protect the right of mentally ill clients to informed consent. Remember, under the law, mental illness isn't the same as incompetence.

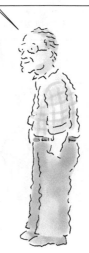

Quality-of-life issues are becoming increasingly important. People like me are demanding to live and die with dignity.

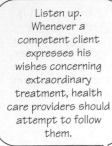

Listen up. Whenever a competent client expresses his wishes concerning extraordinary treatment, health care providers should attempt to follow them.

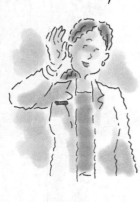

Never ignore a client's request to refuse treatment. Instead, stop preparations for any treatment and notify the physician and your supervisor according to your facility's protocol.

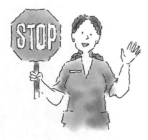

- Many clients tend to seek a psychological outcome rather than a precise treatment decision. For example, some clients feel that their loved ones will be relieved of the burden that difficult end-of-life care decisions entail.
- Many clients express an overwhelming need to communicate with loved ones at this stage of their life. Dying offers important opportunities for growth, intimacy, reconciliation, and closure.

A religious experience

Some clients may refuse treatment on the grounds of freedom of religion or cultural beliefs. Jehovah's Witnesses, for example, oppose blood transfusions, based on their interpretation of a biblical passage that forbids "drinking" blood. Some sect members believe that even a lifesaving transfusion given against their will deprives them of everlasting life. The courts usually uphold their right to refuse treatment because of the constitutionally protected right to religious freedom. However, if the client is a critically ill minor, the court may deny the parents' request to refuse treatment.

Most other religious freedom court cases involve Christian Scientists, who oppose many medical interventions, including medicines.

Planning in advance

Most states have enacted right-to-die laws (also called *natural death laws* or *living will laws*). These laws recognize the client's right to choose death by refusing extraordinary treatment when he has no hope of recovery.

Whenever a competent client expresses his wishes concerning extraordinary treatment, health care providers should attempt to follow them. If the client is incompetent or unconscious, the decision becomes more difficult.

In some cases, the next of kin may express the client's desires for him, but whether this is an honest interpretation of the client's wishes is sometimes uncertain.

Written evidence of the client's wishes, such as an advance directive, provides the best indication of what treatment he would consent to if he could still communicate.

Up to the challenge

There are two grounds for challenging a client's right to refuse treatment: You can claim that the client is incompetent, or you can claim that compelling reasons exist to overrule his wishes.

The courts consider a client incompetent when he lacks the mental ability to make a reasoned decision, such as when he's delirious. The courts also recognize several compelling circumstances that justify overruling a client's refusal of treatment. These include:
- when refusal endangers the life of another
- when a parent's decision to withhold treatment threatens a child's life
- when, despite refusing treatment, the client makes statements indicating that he wants to live
- when the public interest outweighs the client's right.

If your client refuses treatment

Never ignore a client's request to refuse treatment. If your client tells you he's going to refuse treatment or he simply refuses to give consent, follow these guidelines:
- Stop preparations for treatment at once.
- Notify the physician immediately.
- Report your client's decision to your supervisor promptly.

Never delay informing your supervisor, especially if a delay could be life-threatening. Any delay that you're responsible for greatly increases your legal risks.

Advance directive

An **advance directive** is a legal document that provides information about the client's wishes for medical decisions if that client becomes incapacitated. An advance directive includes:
- living will
- durable power of attorney for health care.

General guidelines

The Client Self-Determination Act of 1990 requires facilities to provide clients with written information about their rights regarding advance directives, living wills, and durable power of attorney for health care as well as about the facility's procedure for implementing them. The law also requires the institution to document whether the client has an advance directive.

If your client has an advance directive, take the following steps to safeguard his rights and protect yourself from liability:
• Review your nursing or facility manual for specific directions on what to do. For instance, you may need to inform the client's physician, or you may need to ask your nursing supervisor to inform the facility administration and the legal affairs department.
• With the client's permission, make sure the family knows about the advance directive; if they don't, show them a copy.
• If the client can talk, discuss the will with him, especially if it contains terms that need further definition. As always, objectively document your actions and findings in the client's record.
• If the client drafts an advance directive while under your care, document this in your nurses' notes, describing the circumstances under which the advance directive was drawn up and signed.
• Encourage the client to review the advance directive with his family and physician so that unclear passages can be discussed. Advance directives should also be reviewed periodically to keep pace with changes in technology.

LIVING WILL

A **living will** is a document that specifies a person's wishes about medical care.

I do declare

When a legally competent person draws up a living will, he declares the steps he wants or doesn't want taken when he's incompetent and no longer can express his wishes. Commonly, a living will authorizes the attending physician to withhold or discontinue certain lifesaving procedures under specific circumstances. It may also address treatment options, such as enteral feedings, blood transfusion, antibiotic administration, and dialysis. In some states, however, living wills don't address the issue of discontinuing artificial nutrition and hydration.

Living will laws: The main ingredients

Although living will laws vary from state to state, they generally include such provisions as:
• who may execute a living will
• witness and testator requirements
• immunity from liability for following a living will's directives
• documentation requirements
• instructions on when and how the living will should be executed
• under what circumstances the living will takes effect.

Immunity

Nurses and other health care providers who follow the wishes expressed in a living will authorized by law are generally immune from civil and criminal liability. No matter which state you work in, check your facility's policy and procedures manual, and seek advice from your facility's legal department if needed.

DURABLE POWER OF ATTORNEY FOR HEALTH CARE

A **durable power of attorney for health care** is a document in which the client designates a person (a *proxy*) to make medical decisions for him if he becomes incompetent. This document differs from the usual power of attorney, which requires the client's ongoing consent and deals only with financial issues. Most states have laws authorizing only durable power of attorney for the purpose of initiating or terminating life-sustaining medical treatment.

Health Insurance Portability and Accountability Act

Obtaining highly personal information from a client can be uncomfortable and embarrassing. Reassuring the client that you'll keep all information confidential may help put you both at ease. But stop to think about the legal complexities of this responsibility to maintain the client's right to privacy. What do you do when your client's spouse, other health care professionals, the media, or public health agencies ask

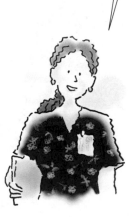

Advance directive laws protect you. Nurses who follow the wishes expressed in an authorized advance directive are generally immune from civil and criminal liability.

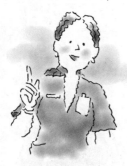

you to disclose confidential information? **The Health Insurance Portability and Accountability Act (HIPAA)** provides the answers.

Some HIPAA action

HIPAA was enacted in 2003 and protects the privacy and security of medical information. Under HIPAA, only those who have a "need to know" are authorized to access client information.

The privacy rule, which is part of HIPAA, consists of national standards that protect all oral, written, and electronic (computer and fax) health information. It allows health care providers to share any information they need to give high-quality health care at the same time that it protects the public by granting clients rights over their health information. All types of heath information are considered confidential, including the client's chart or medical record, conversations about a client's care or treatment, information in the facility's computer system, and billing information. Breeches in confidentiality are subject to fines.

Specific protected health information (PHI) that falls under the privacy rule includes:
• individually identifiable information (such as the client's name, date of birth, Social Security number)
• past, present, and future health information
• demographic information (address, phone number, fax number, or e-mail address)
• billing and payment information
• information about the client's relatives, household members, and employers.

Say "cheese"

Photographs of clients are also considered PHI, so the same protections that apply to written information apply to photos. Permission is needed when the client's name, face, or a unique feature (such as a tattoo) are shown. However, permission isn't required when pictures are taken as part of the client's medical record or when the photo doesn't show enough information to identify the client.

Keeping it confidential

All members of the health care team are responsible for keeping the client's health care records private, including:
• facilities, nursing homes, pharmacies, and clinics
• physicians and dentists
• laboratories and radiology centers
• insurance companies, health maintenance organizations, and most employer group health plans
• certain government programs that pay for health care, such as Medicare and Medicaid.

Strategies and safeguards

To ensure that privacy standards are maintained, health care providers must implement specific strategies to protect their clients' medical information. These strategies include such safeguards as not posting lists of clients' names where the public can see them, not allowing staff to discuss client information in public areas where others can overhear, and disposing of PHI in a proper and confidential manner, usually by shredding it.

Electronic information requires special safeguards to ensure that it's protected, such as assigning computer passwords that allow each employee access only to information necessary to do the employee's job, forbidding employees from sharing or posting passwords, and instructing them to log out of the computer immediately after each use.

When it comes to sharing

In some cases, PHI may be shared — sometimes with prior written permission from the client, sometimes without. Prior written permission is required, for example, when a provider must give information to a client's employer such as in a drug test for employment.

Under other circumstances, PHI can be shared without the client's written permission during the course of:
• treatment — to coordinate care with other health care providers and services, in the case of a medical emergency, or to aid in accurate diagnosis and treatment.
• payment — to bill and collect payment for treatment and services provided.

- health care operations — for quality assessment and improvement, legal issues, auditing, training, and evaluating the performance of health care providers.

The facility may also decide to release information to the client's relatives or significant others if the client can't agree to release information because of illness or injury.

Minor infringements

Minors have the right to privacy, too. In most situations, a parent or legal guardian is authorized to receive and release the minor's PHI. In some circumstances, however, the parent isn't considered the minor's personal representative and therefore doesn't control the minor's PHI. These cases include:
- when there's a reasonable suspicion of parental abuse, neglect, or endangerment
- when state (or other applicable) law stipulates that the minor doesn't require the consent of a parent or other person before he can obtain a particular health care service
- when a court determines someone other than the parent must make treatment decisions for the minor
- when a parent agrees to a confidential relationship between the minor and the physician.

Medication administration

Administering drugs to clients continues to be one of the most important — and, legally, one of the riskiest — tasks you perform.

Getting it right

When administering drugs, one easy way to guard against malpractice liability is to remember the long-standing **"five rights"** formula:
- the right drug
- to the right client
- at the right time
- in the right dosage
- by the right route.

Just say "know"

When you have your nursing license, the law expects you to know about any drug you administer. More specifically, the law expects you to:
- know a drug's safe dosage limits, toxicity, potential adverse effects, and indications and contraindications for use
- refuse to accept an illegible, confusing, or otherwise unclear drug order
- seek clarification of a confusing order from the physician rather than trying to interpret it yourself.

Are there any questions?

If you question a drug order, follow your facility's policies. Usually, you're told to try each of the following actions until you receive a satisfactory answer:
- Look up the answer in a reliable drug reference.
- Ask your charge nurse.
- Ask the facility pharmacist.
- Ask your nursing supervisor or the prescribing physician.
- Ask the chief nursing administrator, if she hasn't already become involved.
- Ask the prescribing physician's supervisor (service chief).
- Get in touch with the facility administration and explain your problem.

An offer you CAN refuse

Nurses have the legal right not to administer drugs they think will harm clients. You may choose to exercise this right when you think:
- the prescribed dosage is too high
- the drug is contraindicated because of possible dangerous interactions with other drugs or with substances such as alcohol
- the client's physical condition contraindicates using the drug.

In limited circumstances, you may also legally refuse to administer a drug on grounds of conscience. Some U.S. states and Canadian provinces have enacted right-of-conscience laws. These laws excuse medical personnel from the requirement to participate in any abortion or sterilization procedure. Under such laws, you may, for example, refuse to give any drug you believe is intended to induce abortion.

Talk about it. All 50 states and the District of Columbia have disclosure laws for child abuse cases. In fact, there may be a criminal penalty for failure to disclose such information.

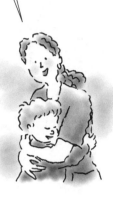

One of the best ways to avoid malpractice is to know the kinds of assignments you're fit to carry out on the job.

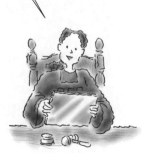

When you refuse to carry out a drug order, make sure that you:
• notify your immediate supervisor so she can make alternate arrangements (assigning a new nurse, clarifying the order)
• notify the prescribing physician (if your supervisor hasn't done so already)
• document that the drug wasn't given and explain why (if your employer requires it).

Protecting yourself

If you make an error in giving a drug, or if your client reacts negatively to a properly administered drug, immediately inform the client's physician and the client or the client's family. Protect yourself by documenting the incident thoroughly. In addition to normal drug-charting information, include information on the client's reaction and any medical or nursing interventions taken.

In the event of error, you should also file a complete incident report. Identify what happened, the names and functions of all personnel involved, and what actions were taken to protect the client after the error was discovered. Follow your facility's procedure for filing a report. The report shouldn't be included in the client's medical record because these reports are used for facility risk management.

Negligence and malpractice

Because nurses are assuming an ever-widening list of client-care responsibilities, it isn't surprising that many nurses are anxious about the possibility of facing a lawsuit some day. Before discussing the specific steps you can take to avoid a lawsuit, here are two terms you need to know more about: negligence and malpractice.

Negligence is usually defined as a failure to exercise the degree of care that a person of ordinary prudence would exercise under the same circumstances. A claim of negligence requires that four criteria be met:
1. A person owed a duty to the person making the claim.
2. The duty was breached.
3. The breach resulted in injury to the person making the claim.

4. Damages were a direct result of the negligence of the health care provider.

Malpractice is a specific type of negligence. It's defined as a violation of professional duty or a failure to meet a standard of care or failure to use the skills and knowledge of other professionals in similar circumstances. You can take steps to avoid tort liability by using caution and common sense and by maintaining heightened awareness of your legal responsibilities. Follow the guidelines below to steer clear of legal pitfalls.

Know your own strengths...and weaknesses

Don't accept responsibilities that you aren't prepared for. If you make an error and then claim you weren't familiar with the unit's procedures, you won't be protected against liability.

You want me to work where?

You may be assigned to work on a specialized unit, which is reasonable as long as you're assigned duties you can perform competently and as long as an experienced nurse on the unit assumes responsibility for the specialized duties. Assigning you to perform total client care on the unit is unsafe if you don't have the skills to plan and deliver that care. Notify your immediate supervisor if you believe an assignment is unsafe.

Delegation 101

Exercise great care as a supervisor when delegating duties because you may be held responsible for subordinates. Inspect all equipment and machinery regularly, and make sure that subordinates use them competently and safely. If someone under your supervision isn't familiar with a piece of equipment, teach how to properly operate it before the subordinate uses it for the first time. Report incompetent health care personnel to superiors through the institutional chain of command.

May I take your order?

Never treat any client without orders from his physician, except in an emergency or per facility protocol. Don't prescribe or dispense medication without authorization. In most cases, only physicians and pharmacists may legally perform these functions.

Don't carry out an order from a physician if you have any doubt about its accuracy or appropriateness. Follow your facility's policy for clarifying ambiguous orders. Document your efforts to clarify the order, and whether the order was carried out.

Watch those medication mix-ups!

Medication errors are the most common and potentially most dangerous of nursing errors. Mistakes in dosage, client identification, or drug selection by nurses have led to vision loss, brain damage, cardiac arrest, and death.

Staying on your client's good side

Trial attorneys have a saying: "If you don't want to be sued, don't be rude." Always remain calm when a client or his family becomes difficult. Clients must be told the truth about errors or adverse outcomes, but this information should be communicated with discretion and sensitivity.

Don't offer opinions

Avoid offering your opinion when a client asks you what you think is the matter with him. If you give your opinion, you could be accused of making a medical diagnosis, which is practicing medicine without a license.

Before you sign on that dotted line...Read!

Never sign your name as a witness without fully understanding what you're signing as well as the legal significance of your signature.

Stick to the FACTs

From a legal standpoint, documented care is as important as the actual care. If a procedure wasn't documented, the courts assume it wasn't performed. Make sure you document all observations, decisions, and actions. The client's chart, when taken into the courtroom, is a nurse's "best evidence" of the care given. The chart should follow the "FACT" rule: be Factual, Accurate, Complete, and Timely.

Assisting in procedures: A word of caution

Don't assist with a surgical procedure unless you're satisfied the client has given proper informed consent. Never force a client to accept treatment he has expressly refused. Don't use equipment that you aren't trained to use or that seems to be functioning improperly.

Use of restraints: Get it in writing

Restraints need to be applied correctly and checked according to the policies and procedures of the facility. Documentation must be exact about the status of the restrained client; the need, number, and kind of restraints used; and the reason for use. An omission or failure to monitor a restrained client may result in a malpractice claim.

An ounce of prevention

Client falls are a very common area of nursing liability. Clients who are elderly, infirm, sedated, or mentally incapacitated are the most likely to fall. The best way to avoid liability is to prevent falls from occurring in the first place. Follow your facility's fall prevention program guidelines, if in place.

Knowing it in advance

Some clients with life-threatening or terminal conditions may choose to exercise their right to a living will or durable power of attorney. Be aware of your state's laws regarding advance directives.

Follow facility policies and procedures

Be familiar with the policies and procedures of the facility where you work. If they're sound and you follow them carefully, they can protect you against a malpractice claim.

Provide a safe environment

When providing care, don't use faulty equipment. Follow your facility's policies and procedures for handling and reporting faulty equipment. Remove the equipment from the client area immediately. Clearly mark the equipment as defective and unusable. Even after repairs are made, don't use the repaired

Being polite has a payoff; it helps protect against liability. Trial attorneys have a saying: "If you don't want to be sued, don't be rude."

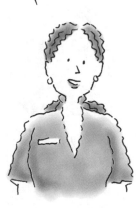

Restraints require restraint. Restraints need to be applied correctly and only when necessary. Monitor clients in restraints according to facility policy to avoid malpractice claims.

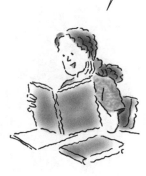

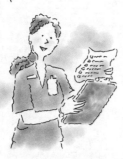

Proper documentation must be detailed and thorough but it's worth the effort. It will protect you and your client.

equipment until technicians demonstrate that the equipment is operating properly. Document the steps you took to handle problems with faulty equipment to show that you followed the facility's policy and procedures.

Documentation errors

Complete, accurate, and timely documentation is crucial to the continuity of each client's care. A well-documented medical record:
- reflects the client care given
- demonstrates the results of treatment
- helps to plan and coordinate the care contributed by each professional
- allows interdisciplinary exchange of information about the client
- provides evidence of the nurse's legal responsibilities toward the client
- demonstrates standards, rules, regulations, and laws of nursing practice
- supplies information for analysis of cost-to-benefit reduction
- reflects professional and ethical conduct and responsibility
- furnishes information for continuing education, risk management, diagnosis-related group assignment and reimbursement, continuous quality improvement, case management monitoring, and research.

Is everything covered?
With a large number of health care professionals involved in each client's care, nursing documentation must be complete, accurate, and timely to foster continuity of care. It should cover:
- initial assessment using the nursing process and applicable nursing diagnoses
- nursing actions, particularly reports to the physician
- ongoing assessment, including the frequency of assessment
- variations from the assessment and plan
- accountability information, including forms signed by the client, location of client valuables, and client education
- notation of care by other disciplines, including physician visits, if practical
- health teaching, including content and response

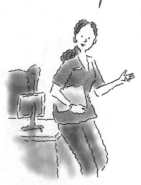

Even seemingly harmless documentation errors can undermine your credibility in court.

- procedures and diagnostic tests
- client response to therapy, particularly to nursing interventions, drugs, and diagnostic tests
- statements made by the client
- client comfort and safety measures.

Avoiding the Big 8
In addition to their potential impact on client care, charting errors or omissions, even if seemingly harmless, undermine your credibility in court. Especially avoid these eight common documentation errors:
1. **Omissions**—Include all significant facts that other nurses need to assess the client. Otherwise, a court may conclude that you failed to perform an action missing from the record or tried to hide evidence.
2. **Personal opinions**—Don't enter personal opinions. Record only factual and objective observations and the client's statements.
3. **Vague entries**—Instead of "Client had a good day," state why: "Client didn't complain of pain."
4. **Late entries**—If a late entry is necessary, identify it as such and sign and date it. Note the date and time you're relating back to.
5. **Improper corrections**—Never erase or obliterate an error. Instead, draw a single line through it, label it "error," and sign and date it.
6. **Unauthorized entries**—Only you should be keeping your records.
7. **Erroneous or vague abbreviations**—Use only standard abbreviations and follow facility policies.
8. **Illegibility and lack of clarity**—Write so that others can read your entry. Use a dictionary if you're unsure of spelling or usage.

Sign language
Sign all notes with your first initial, full last name, and title. Place your signature on the right side of the page as proof that you entered all the information between the previous nurse's signature and your own. If the last entry is unsigned, request that the

nurse who made the entry sign it. Draw lines through empty or remaining spaces to prevent subsequent amendments or additions.

Just what the doctor ordered

Physician's orders fall into three groups: correct as written, ambiguous, and apparently erroneous. If the order is correct as written, initial and check mark each line. Below the physician's signature, sign your name, and indicate the date and time. Ambiguous orders must be clarified with the physician. Document your efforts to clarify the order and whether the order was carried out. If you believe a physician's order is in error, you should refuse to carry it out. Make a record of your refusal together with the reasons and an account of all communication with the physician.

Verbal cues

As a general rule, verbal and telephone orders are acceptable only under acute or emergency circumstances, when the physician can't promptly attend to the client, or according to facility policy. Record the order on the physician's order sheet, note the date and time of the order, and record the order verbatim. On the following line, write "v.v.o." for verified verbal order or "v.t.o." for verified telephone order and record the physician's full name, followed by your signature and the time. To avoid liability, be certain the physician countersigns the order within the time specified by facility policy.

Abuse

As a nurse, you play a crucial role in recognizing and reporting incidents of suspected **abuse.** Abuse can be psychological, physical, sexual, or financial in nature. Abuse victims can be of any age, sex, or socioeconomic group. While caring for clients, you can readily note evidence of apparent abuse. When you do, you must pass the information along to the appropriate authorities. In many states, failure to report actual or suspected abuse constitutes a crime.

Filing a report

Make your report as complete and accurate as possible. Be careful not to let your personal feelings affect the way you make out a report or your decision to file the report.

Abuse cases can raise many difficult emotional issues. Remember, however, that not filing a report can have more serious consequences than filing one that contains an unintentional error. It's better to risk error than to risk breaching the child abuse reporting laws — and, in effect, perpetuating the abuse. Contact your facility's social work department if you have questions about suspected abuse. Always report actual or suspected abuse according to your facility's policies and procedures.

Recognizing the problem

Learn to recognize both the events that trigger abuse and the signs and symptoms that mark the abused and the abuser. Early in your relationship with an abused client, you need to be adept in order to spot the subtle behavioral and interactional clues that signal an abusive situation. Be sure to consider cultural differences so that you don't mistake a client's behavior for a sign of abuse. For example, some cultures don't permit women to make eye contact with men.

Examine the client's relationship with the suspected abuser. For example, abused people tend to be passive and fearful. An abused child usually fails to protest if his parent is asked to leave the examining area. An abused adult, on the other hand, usually wants her abuser to stay with her.

Abused persons may react to facility procedures by crying helplessly and incessantly. They also tend to be wary of physical contact, including physical examinations.

Many facilities have a policy, procedure, or protocol to help nurses and other health care providers make observations that aid the identification of possible abuse victims. Learning these criteria makes spotting victims of abuse a more objective process and prevents cases from going unrecognized.

Managing abuse cases can be a real balancing act. Of course, you need to address the victim's needs, but the abuser needs help, too.

Assessing the abuser

Sometimes the abuser appears overly agitated when dealing with facility personnel; for example, he may get impatient if they don't carry out procedures instantly. At other times, he may exhibit the opposite behavior: a total lack of interest in the client's problems. Alternatively, he may be overly considerate or affectionate while the nursing staff is present.

History lessons

When you take an abuse victim's history, she may be vague about how she was injured and tell different stories to different people. When you ask directly about specific injuries, she may answer evasively or not at all. Sometimes, a victim minimizes or tries to hide her injuries.

Physical clues

Look for characteristic signs of abuse. In most cases of abuse, you find old bruises, scars, or deformities the client can't or won't explain. X-ray examinations may show the presence of many old fractures.

Getting on the SOAP box

Always document your findings objectively; try to keep your emotions out of your charting. One way to do this is to use the *SOAP* technique, which calls for these steps:
• In the subjective (S) part of the note, record information in the client's own words.
• In the objective (O) part, record your personal observations.
• Under assessment (A), record your evaluations and conclusions.
• Under plan (P), list sources of facility and community support available to the client after discharge.

Support for the victim

Many support services have become available for both abusers and their victims. For example, if a female victim is afraid to return to the scene of her abuse, she may find temporary housing in a women's shelter. If no such shelter is available, she may be able to stay with a friend or family member.

Social workers or community liaison workers may also be able to offer suggestions for shelter. Another possibility is a church, synagogue, or mosque, which may have members willing to take the client in. If no shelter can be found, the client may have to stay at the facility for her safety.

Alert the client to state, county, or city agencies that can offer protection. The police department should be called to collect evidence if the client wants to press charges against the abuser. If the client is a child, the law usually requires filing a report with a government family-service agency.

Help for the abuser

You need to evaluate the abuser's ability to handle stress. In some cases, you may be able to refer him to an appropriate local or state agency that can offer help. In most cases, an abuser poses a continued threat to others until he gets help in understanding his behavior and how to change it.

For abusive fathers or mothers, a local chapter of Parents Anonymous (PA) may be helpful. PA, a self-help group made up of former abusers, attempts to help abusing parents by teaching them how to deal with their anger.

Besides helping short-circuit abusive behavior, a self-help group takes abusing parents out of their isolation and introduces them to individuals who can understand their feelings. It also provides help in a crisis, when members may be able to prevent an abusive incident.

Telephone hot lines to crisis intervention services also give abusers someone to talk with in times of stress and crisis and may help prevent abuse. Commonly staffed by volunteers, telephone hot lines provide a link between those who seek help and trained counselors.

These and other kinds of help are also available through family-service agencies and facilities. By becoming familiar with national and local resources, you'll be able to respond quickly and authoritatively when an abuser or his victim needs your help.

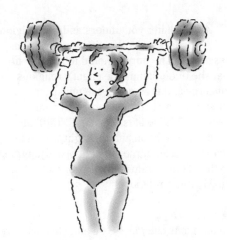

Pump up on practice questions

1. A nurse working at a busy hospital takes steps to challenge an assignment that may not be within the practice limits for nurses in the state where she works. Which law defines the limits of each state's nursing practice?
1. Contract law
2. Nurse Practice Act
3. National Labor Relations Act
4. Food, Drug, and Cosmetic Act

Answer: 2. Each state's Nurse Practice Act is the most important law affecting nursing practice. The law outlines expectations for client care within defined practice limits. Giving care beyond those limits makes the nurse vulnerable to charges of violating the state's nurse practice act. Contract law involves agreements between two or more persons to do some type of remuneration — a "bargained for exchange." National Labor Relations Act allows nurses the right to unionize. Food, Drug, and Cosmetic Act restricts interstate shipment of drugs not approved for human use and outlines the process for testing and approving new drugs.

➡ *NCLEX keys*
Client needs category: Safe and effective care environment
Client needs subcategory: Management of care
Cognitive level: Knowledge

2. A physician orders digoxin (Lanoxin) 4 mg I.V. for a client in rapid atrial fibrillation. How should the nurse proceed?
1. Assess the client's apical heart rate, then administer the dose.
2. Administer 0.4 mg I.V. because the physician most likely meant to write that dosage.
3. Question the physician about the order.
4. Administer the dose, then monitor the client closely.

Answer: 3. As a licensed professional, the nurse has the legal and ethical responsibility to use her own judgment when providing client care. Therefore the nurse should act independently and question the physician's order. The dose ordered is ten times the typical dose. If the nurse administers this dose she could be held accountable for her actions in a court of law.

➡ *NCLEX keys*
Client needs category: Physiological integrity
Client needs subcategory: Pharmacological and parenteral therapies
Cognitive level: Analysis

3. A client undergoing a bronchoscopy needs to sign an informed consent form before the procedure. Which statement by the client indicates that the client understands the teaching?
1. "I can't refuse the procedure after the consent is signed."
2. "I refuse to sign the consent form; another family member can sign for me."
3. "If I refuse to sign the consent form, other treatment will be withdrawn."
4. "Now I know what the alternative treatments and procedures are."

Answer: 4. Informed consent should include an explanation of alternative treatments or procedures. The client should also be told that he has the right to refuse the treatment or procedure without having other care or support withdrawn and that he can withdraw consent after giving it. The client's next of kin can only sign the consent form if the client is deemed incompetent.

Study! Study! Study! Understanding law and ethics is important to you and your clients.

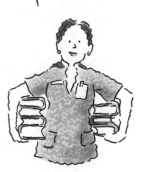

➡ *NCLEX keys*

Client needs category: Safe and effective care environment
Client needs subcategory: Management of care
Cognitive level: Analysis

4. A client is admitted to the hospital with a closed head injury. He's unconscious and requires mechanical ventilation. Which document will most likely be used to make a medical decision for the client?
   1. Durable power of attorney for health care
   2. Power of attorney
   3. Advance directive
   4. Living will

Answer: 1. A durable power of attorney for health care designates a person who is to make medical decisions for the client when he's incompetent to do so. This differs from the power of attorney, which requires the client's ongoing consent and deals only with financial concerns. The durable power of attorney is one component of an advance directive. The living will, also a part of an advance directive, specifies a person's wishes with regard to medical care if he becomes unable to communicate.

➡ *NCLEX keys*

Client needs category: Safe and effective care environment
Client needs subcategory: Management of care
Cognitive level: Application

5. A Jehovah's Witness is admitted to the hospital with upper GI bleeding. The physician orders two units of packed red blood cells administered over 2 hours each. When the nurse tells the client about the order, the client refuses the transfusion. How should the nurse proceed?
   1. Follow the physician's order and administer the transfusion.
   2. Tell the client that she's being ridiculous because she'll die without the transfusion.
   3. Refuse to care for the client because you don't agree with her religious beliefs.

   4. Tell her you understand her religious concerns and notify the physician.

Answer: 4. The nurse should tell the client that she understands the client's religious concerns and then notify the physician. The nurse can't administer the transfusion anyway. This violates the client's right of freedom of religion and the right to refuse treatment. The nurse shouldn't pass judgment on the client or refuse to care for a client based on her religion.

➡ *NCLEX keys*

Client needs category: Safe and effective care environment
Client needs subcategory: Management of care
Cognitive level: Application

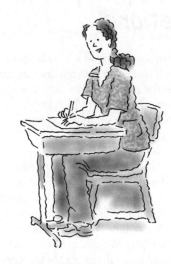

6. A nurse administers a dose of penicillin to a client who suddenly develops hives and difficulty breathing. She notifies the physician and takes emergency measures. What should the nurse include in her documentation?
   1. Document the date, time, and site in which the dose was administered.
   2. In addition to the normal drug charting information, include information about the client's reaction.
   3. In addition to the normal drug charting information, include information about the client's reaction, attempts to notify the physician, and any medical or nursing interventions taken.
   4. Include information about the client's reaction and any nursing interventions taken.

Answer: 3. When a client reacts negatively to a properly administered drug, the nurse should document the normal drug-charting information and also include information about the client's reaction, attempts to notify the physician, and any medical or nursing interventions taken.

➡ *NCLEX keys*

Client needs category: Physiological integrity
Client needs subcategory: Pharmacological and parenteral therapies
Cognitive level: Application

7.   After a medication error is made on her unit, a nurse-manager should expect to receive:
   1.   an incident report.
   2.   an oral report from the nurse.
   3.   a copy of the medication Kardex.
   4.   an order change signed by the physician.

Answer: 1. The nurse should complete an incident report and give it to the nurse-manager, who then gives the report to the risk manager. Incident reports are tools used by management when a client might be harmed. They're used to determine how future problems can be avoided. An oral report doesn't serve as legal documentation. A copy of the medication Kardex isn't sent with the incident report to the risk manager. A physician wouldn't change an order to cover the nurse's mistake.

➡ *NCLEX keys*

Client needs category: Safe and effective care environment
Client needs subcategory: Management of care
Cognitive level: Knowledge

8.   A nurse administers a unit of blood to a client without receiving informed consent. Performing a procedure, such as administering blood products, without receiving informed consent can lead to which charge?
   1.   Assault and battery
   2.   Fraud
   3.   Breach of confidentiality
   4.   Harassment

Answer: 1. Performing a procedure on a client without informed consent can be grounds for charges of assault and battery. Fraud is to cheat someone. Breach of confidentiality refers to conveying information about the client to people who aren't directly involved in his care. Harassment refers to annoying or disturbing an individual.

➡ *NCLEX keys*

Client needs category: Safe and effective care environment
Client needs subcategory: Management of care
Cognitive level: Application

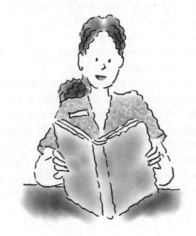

9.   A nurse returns from vacation and finds a new I.V. pump attached to her client's I.V. How should the nurse proceed?
   1.   Read the I.V. pump manual before caring for the client.
   2.   Inform the charge nurse and ask her to provide an educational session about how to use the pump.
   3.   Use the pump because it's somewhat like the old pumps on the unit.
   4.   Refuse to care for the client.

Answer: 2. The nurse should inform the charge nurse that she never used the piece of equipment before and ask the charge nurse to provide an educational session about using the pump. The nurse should review the manual but shouldn't use the pump without an educational session that allows time to practice using the equipment. The nurse should never use a piece of equipment without formal training. A need to use new equipment doesn't automatically justify refusal to care for the client.

➡ *NCLEX keys*
Client needs category: Safe and effective care environment
Client needs subcategory: Management of care
Cognitive level: Application

10. A nurse is caring for a 72-year-old male client who requires insertion of a central venous catheter. Who's responsible for obtaining informed consent?
1. The attending physician
2. The physician who will insert the catheter
3. The charge nurse
4. The nurse assisting with the procedure

Answer: 2. The responsibility for obtaining informed consent typically rests with the person who will perform the treatment or procedure. It isn't the responsibility of the attending physician (unless he's performing the procedure), the charge nurse, or the nurse assisting the physician with the procedure.

➡ *NCLEX keys*
Client needs category: Safe and effective care environment
Client needs subcategory: Management of care
Cognitive level: Application

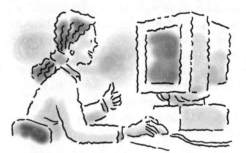

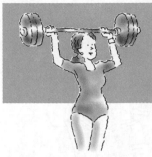

Pump up on more practice questions

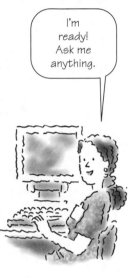

I'm ready! Ask me anything.

1. A client's blood pressure is lower than the specified limits, so the nurse withholds his blood pressure medication. The nurse documents the omission on the medication administration record. Where should she document the reason for withholding the medication if there's no space in the medication administration record?

1. Client care Kardex
2. Progress notes
3. Care plan
4. Nowhere

Answer: 2. If the medication administration record doesn't provide space to document the omission, the nurse should document the reason in the progress notes. The client care Kardex and care plan are used to guide client care; they aren't appropriate forms for documentation. Any time a drug is omitted, the reason for withholding the medication must be documented.

➡ *NCLEX keys*

Client needs category: Safe and effective care environment
Client needs subcategory: Management of care
Cognitive level: Application

2. A client is admitted to your client-care area with a diagnosis of dehydration and pneumonia. After the client is settled in bed, the nurse begins asking questions about his health history. Which action should the nurse avoid when conducting the health history interview?

1. Using general leads to questions
2. Asking open-ended questions
3. Restating information
4. Asking persistent questions

Answer: 4. The nurse should avoid asking persistent questions during the history interview. She should make one or two attempts to get information and then stop. She should respect the client's right to privacy. During the interview the nurse should use general leads, ask open-ended questions, and restate information.

➡ *NCLEX keys*

Client needs category: Safe and effective care environment
Client needs subcategory: Management of care
Cognitive level: Application

3. For a hospitalized client, a physician orders meperidine (Demerol), 75 mg I.M., every 3 hours as needed for pain. However, the client refuses to take injections. Which nursing action is most appropriate?

1. Administering the injection as prescribed
2. Calling the physician to request an oral pain medication
3. Withholding the injection until the client understands its importance
4. Explaining that no other medication can be given until the client receives the injection

Answer: 2. The most appropriate action is to call the physician to request an oral pain medication. By doing so, the nurse is adhering to the client's wishes. Administering an injection without client consent is considered battery and may lead to a lawsuit. Withholding medication without providing an alternative would violate the standards of care. Any attempt to manipulate the client into taking the medication also would violate the standards of care.

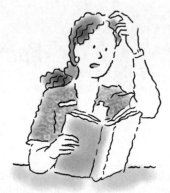

➡ *NCLEX keys*

Client needs category: Safe and effective care environment
Client needs subcategory: Management of care
Cognitive level: Application

4. A nurse is conducting a physical assessment on a 17-year-old female client. The client's mother suspects that the client is sexually active and approaches the nurse, asking to see the chart to confirm her suspicions. How should the nurse address this situation?

1. Inform the mother that she must discuss the matter with the physician.
2. Allow the mother access to the client's chart based on the Family Educational Rights and Privacy Act (FERPA).
3. Discuss the concept of protected health information under the Health Insurance Portability and Accountability Act (HIPAA).
4. Determine if the client is an emancipated minor before releasing the information.

Answer: 3. The Center for Adolescent Health Policy & the Law has stated that it's appropriate for a minor to exercise privacy rights under HIPAA. Therefore, it isn't appropriate for the nurse (or the physician) to discuss the client's information with the client's mother without the client's permission. FERPA protects the confidentiality of minors by defining the term "education records" to include all material containing information related directly to a student and by giving the parents permission to have some control over disclosure of this information. It doesn't apply to health care situations. The client's health information is protected regardless of whether she's emancipated.

➡ *NCLEX keys*

Client needs category: Safe and effective care environment
Client needs subcategory: Management of care
Cognitive level: Analysis

5. While documenting on a client care flow sheet, a nurse notices that she made a mistake. How should the nurse proceed?

1. Use correction fluid and continue to document.
2. Draw a single line through the entry.
3. Cross out the error completely.
4. Erase the error.

Answer: 2. The nurse should draw a single line through the entry and write "error" along with her initials and the date and time above or next to the entry. The nurse should never cover a mistake with correction fluid, completely cross it out, or erase it because this looks as if the nurse is trying to hide something.

➡ *NCLEX keys*

Client needs category: Safe and effective care environment
Client needs subcategory: Management of care
Cognitive level: Application

6. A nurse is conducting a physical assessment on an obese 17-year-old client who has asked for information regarding gastric bypass surgery. Select the statement that best explains informed consent as it applies to this client.

1. The nurse is allowed to provide the client with all information requested regarding the procedure.
2. The nurse should inform the client that he can sign a consent form for the surgical procedure if a parent co-signs with him.

3. The nurse should inform the client that in most states, only the parents can give consent for a minor's medical care.

4. The nurse is allowed to provide the client's legal guardian with all information regarding the procedure.

Answer: 3. A teenage client should be kept informed about medical decisions, but until he's an adult or emancipated, a parent must give consent for the child's care. Providing the client with information on the procedure doesn't address the issue of informed consent. Providing the client's legal guardian with the information wouldn't address the issue of informed consent and would violate the client's right of confidentiality, unless the client has given permission for the nurse to speak with his parents.

➡ NCLEX keys
Client needs category: Safe and effective care environment
Client needs subcategory: Management of care
Cognitive level: Analysis

7. A 42-year-old client admitted with an acute myocardial infarction asks to see his chart. What should the nurse do first?

1. Allow the client to view his chart.
2. Contact the nurse-manager and physician for approval.
3. Ask the client if he has concerns about his care.
4. Tell the client that he isn't permitted to view his chart.

Answer: 3. The client has a legal right to see his chart. However, if he asks to see it, the nurse should first ask him if he has any questions about his care and try to clear up any confusion. The client may be confused about his care. The nurse should check the facility's policy to see whether the chart must be read in the nurse's presence. The nurse should inform the physician and nurse-manager of the client's request.

➡ NCLEX keys
Client needs category: Safe and effective care environment

Client needs subcategory: Management of care
Cognitive level: Application

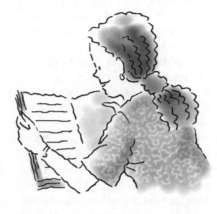

8. A client is to undergo a thoracotomy in the morning. The physician asks the nurse to witness the client's signing of the consent form. What should the nurse do?

1. Make sure the physician thoroughly describes the procedure.
2. Provide emotional support for the client.
3. Make sure the physician explains the risks of undergoing the procedure.
4. Make sure the client is competent, awake, and alert before he signs the consent form.

Answer: 4. Before the nurse witnesses a client's consent, she should make sure that the client is competent, awake, and alert and is aware of what he's doing. Also make sure that the client understands the procedure and the associated risks. Giving the client an explanation doesn't ensure that he understands. The nurse should notify the nurse-manager and the physician if she suspects that the client has doubts about the procedure. Performing a procedure without voluntary consent may be considered battery.

➡ NCLEX keys
Client needs category: Safe and effective care environment
Client needs subcategory: Management of care
Cognitive level: Application

9. A 92-year-old client fell as he attempted to get out of bed on his own. Which information should the nurse include in her documentation of the incident?

1. Describe what she saw and heard and the actions she took when she reached the client.
2. Mention that an incident report was completed.
3. Describe what she thinks occurred.
4. Describe what she was doing when the event occurred.

Answer: 1. The nurse should describe what she saw and heard and the actions she took when she reached the client's bedside as well as the client's account of the incident. She shouldn't document what she thinks occurred. The nurse shouldn't mention that an incident report was completed after charting the event. This destroys the confidential nature of the report and may result in a lawsuit. What the nurse was doing at the time of the incident isn't relevant.

➡ *NCLEX keys*
Client needs category: Safe and effective care environment
Client needs subcategory: Management of care
Cognitive level: Application

10. A client asks to be discharged from the health care facility against medical advice (AMA). What should the nurse do?

1. Prevent the client from leaving.
2. Notify the physician.
3. Have the client sign an AMA form.
4. Call a security guard to help detain the client.

Answer: 2. If a client requests a discharge AMA, the nurse should notify the physician immediately. If the physician can't convince the client to stay, the physician will ask the client to sign an AMA form, which releases the facility from legal responsibility for any medical problems the client may experience after discharge. If the physician isn't available, the nurse should discuss the AMA form with the client and obtain the client's signature. A client who refuses to sign the form shouldn't be detained because this would violate the client's rights. After the client leaves,

the nurse should document the incident thoroughly and notify the physician that the client has left.

➡ *NCLEX keys*
Client needs category: Safe and effective care environment
Client needs subcategory: Management of care
Cognitive level: Application

11. A nursing assistant is assigned to provide morning care to a client. How should the nurse document care given by the assistant?

1. "Morning care provided by B.C., nursing assistant"
2. "Morning care given"
3. There's no need to document morning care.
4. "Morning care given by Betsy Clarke, NA"

Answer: 4. The nurse should document that morning care was given by the nursing assistant, using the nursing assistant's full name and title.

➡ *NCLEX keys*
Client needs category: Safe and effective care environment
Client needs subcategory: Management of care
Cognitive level: Application

12. A nurse administers the wrong I.V. fluid to a client. The hospital's risk manager should receive which information to document the incident?

1. Oral report from the nurse
2. Copy of the client care Kardex
3. Order change written by the physician
4. Incident report

Answer: 4. The risk manager should receive an incident report when a client might be harmed. The incident report is used to determine how future errors can be avoided. An oral report from the nurse doesn't serve as legal documentation. A copy of the client care Kardex isn't sent to the risk manager. A physician shouldn't change an order to cover the nurse's error.

➡ NCLEX keys

Client needs category: Safe and effective care environment

Client needs subcategory: Management of care

Cognitive level: Comprehension

13. When developing a care plan for a client with a do-not-resuscitate order, the nurse should not include which intervention on the care plan?

1. Withdrawing foods and fluids from a competent client under his direction if specified through his living will
2. Administering pain medications as needed and within the prescribed dosage ranges
3. Ensuring access to individuals who can provide spiritual care when requested by a client
4. Administering lethal doses of medications when requested by a competent terminally ill client

Answer: 4. Administration of lethal doses of medications by any health care provider is against the law under any circumstance. Withdrawing foods and fluids is allowed under the law if the client is competent or has a living will that specifies this action. Administering appropriate doses of pain medications as needed and ensuring access to spiritual care, if requested by the client, are appropriate actions by the nurse to ensure competent care.

➡ NCLEX keys

Client needs category: Safe and effective care environment

Client needs subcategory: Management of care

Cognitive level: Analysis

14. A mother brings her 3-year-old child to the emergency department (ED). The mother states that she found blood in her daughter's underwear. The physical examination reveals sexual assault with vaginal penetration. The mother doesn't want the police notified because of the potential publicity. What action should the nurse take?

1. No action is necessary because the mother is the child's legal guardian.
2. Report the findings to the police and have a social worker talk with the mother.
3. Encourage the mother to reconsider her decision.
4. Ask the ED physician to talk to the mother.

Answer: 2. The nurse must report the crime to the authorities regardless of the mother's wishes. Not taking action isn't appropriate. Although the ED physician may talk to the mother and the mother may be encouraged to reconsider her wishes, the crime must be reported and evidence must be collected.

➡ NCLEX keys

Client needs category: Safe and effective care environment

Client needs subcategory: Management of care

Cognitive level: Application

15. A mother brings her child to the emergency department after her husband beat the child. She's afraid to return home. The nurse can refer the mother to several social service agencies. Which agency would be most appropriate?

1. Women's shelter
2. Welfare bureau
3. Children's Protective Services
4. Homeless shelter

Answer: 1. A women's shelter can provide services necessary for both mother and child. The other alternatives may result in separation of the child from the mother and cause further trauma. The welfare bureau is a state agency that provides money, food, or shelter for individuals who need it. It doesn't necessarily deal with children who are victims of abuse. Children's Protective Services will investigate the crime and may want to place the child in a foster home or with other relatives during the investigation. Homeless shelters are voluntary organizations for people in need of shelter and food. They don't necessarily have resources for women and children.

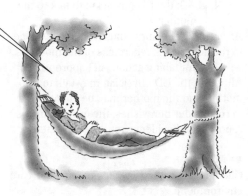

Find a balance between work and rest to maximize your learning experience. Don't forget to take scheduled breaks.

➡ *NCLEX keys*
Client needs category: Safe and effective care environment
Client needs subcategory: Management of care
Cognitive level: Application

16. A registered nurse (RN) is orienting a graduate nurse to the unit. A client is admitted with end-stage leukemia. Which statement made by the graduate nurse should be corrected by the RN?

1. "The client can inform the physician that he doesn't want cardiopulmonary resuscitation if his heart stops beating."
2. "The client could designate another person to make end-of-life decisions when he's no longer able."
3. "The client can write a living will indicating his end-of-life preferences."
4. "The law states that the client must write a new living will each time he's admitted to the hospital."

Answer: 4. The RN needs to inform the graduate that that one living will covers all hospitalizations unless the client decides to make changes. The client typically discusses his wishes with the physician who provides the order for the client care status. A living will explains a person's end-of-life care preferences. A durable power of attorney for health care designates a person to make decisions for the client in the event the client can't make decisions on his own.

➡ *NCLEX keys*
Client needs category: Safe and effective care environment
Client needs subcategory: Management of care
Cognitive level: Analysis

17. A primary nurse is performing an admission assessment on a client admitted with pneumonia. When should the nurse begin discharge planning for this client?

1. When the client's condition is stabilized
2. The day before discharge
3. At the time of admission
4. After the physician writes the discharge order

Answer: 3. Discharge planning should begin as soon as the client is admitted. Beginning the planning as soon as possible gives the staff time to allocate necessary resources the client will require at discharge. Waiting until the client stabilizes, the day before discharge, or after the order is written doesn't allow adequate time for planning.

➡ *NCLEX keys*
Client needs category: Safe and effective care environment
Client needs subcategory: Management of care
Cognitive level: Analysis

18. The nurse-manager is checking a client's chart when she notes that there's no record of an opioid being given to the client even though the nurse on the previous shift signed one out. The client denies receiving anything for pain. Which action should the nurse-manager take first?

1. Notify the pharmacy that the client didn't receive the medication so he doesn't get charged for it.
2. Notify the physician that the client didn't receive the medication.
3. Question the nurse who signed out the opioid to seek clarification about the missing drug.
4. File an incident report.

Answer: 3. The nurse-manager should use a nonthreatening manner to question the nurse who signed out the opioid. If the nurse can't give an adequate explanation, the nurse-manager should follow the facility's procedure to provide help to a staff member who might have a drug-addiction problem. The physician must be notified that the client didn't receive the medication. The pharmacist should be notified of the discrepancies in the opioid count. If policy dictates, the nurse-manager should then file an incident report.

➡ *NCLEX keys*

Client needs category: Safe and effective care environment
Client needs subcategory: Management of care
Cognitive level: Application

19. A charge nurse has been orienting a graduate nurse to the unit. She tells the nurse-manager that she feels the graduate nurse isn't progressing through orientation. Which action by the nurse-manager is most appropriate?
1. Meet with the graduate nurse and formulate a plan to help improve the graduate nurse's performance.
2. Speak with the employee relations director about terminating the graduate nurse.
3. Tell the graduate nurse that if her performance doesn't improve by the deadline she'll be terminated.
4. Encourage the graduate nurse to transfer to a less stressful unit.

Answer: 1. The nurse-manager should meet with the graduate nurse and discuss her perceived weaknesses. Together they should develop a plan to improve the nurse's performance. The other responses don't provide the graduate nurse with the opportunity to improve her performance and they don't provide support to the individual.

➡ *NCLEX keys*

Client needs category: Safe and effective care environment
Client needs subcategory: Management of care
Cognitive level: Application

20. Which client care assignment is most appropriate for a licensed practical nurse (LPN)?
1. An 83-year-old client admitted with heart failure just transferred from the intensive care unit
3. A 35-year-old client admitted 1 day ago with an acute exacerbation of asthma
3. A 44-year-old client with metastatic breast cancer who was prescribed comfort measures
4. A 76-year-old client who underwent an open reduction and internal fixation of her right hip 5 days ago

Answer: 4. The most appropriate assignment for the LPN is the 76-year-old client who underwent an open reduction and internal fixation of the hip 5 days ago. This client is stable and requires physical care; therefore, she's most appropriately cared for by the LPN. The client just transferred from the intensive care unit requires frequent assessment because the client has the potential to become unstable. A 35-year-old client admitted with acute asthma one day ago also requires frequent assessment and should be cared for by a registered nurse. The 44-year-old client being maintained on comfort measures requires frequent assessment and medication titration based on the assessment findings; a registered nurse would most appropriately provide care for this client.

➡ *NCLEX keys*

Client needs category: Safe and effective care environment
Client needs subcategory: Management of care
Cognitive level: Analysis

21. A group of people has identified the lack of documentation when restraints are used. As a result they recommend a change in the facility's documentation form. These people are most likely members of which committee?
1. Quality control
2. Performance improvement
3. The Joint Commission
4. Unit council

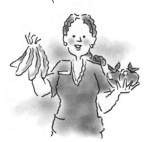

Don't forget: Healthy eating habits help to maintain a healthy mind.

Answer: 2. The performance improvement committee identifies problems who don't meet an established standard and then recommends changes in the facility's policies, procedures, or documentation forms in an effort to improve client care. Quality control is a term used in factory production. The Joint Commission is a private agency that establishes guidelines for the operation of hospitals and other health care facilities. Unit council is a group of individuals who represent the nursing unit and voice concerns of other staff members.

➡ *NCLEX keys*
Client needs category: Safe and effective care environment
Client needs subcategory: Management of care
Cognitive level: Application

22. A nurse failed to administer a medication to a client according to accepted standards. Consequently, the client suffered adverse effects. Failure to provide client care and to follow appropriate standards is called:
1.   breach of duty.
2.   breach of promise.
3.   negligent duty.
4.   tort.
Answer: 1. Breach of duty means that the nurse provided care that didn't meet the accepted standard. When investigating breach of duty, the court asks: How would a reasonable, prudent nurse with comparable training and experience have acted in comparable circumstances?

➡ *NCLEX keys*
Client needs category: Safe and effective care environment
Client needs subcategory: Management of care
Cognitive level: Comprehension

23. A staff nurse goes to the nurse-manager because she feels stressed by her job even though she enjoys the challenge. Which suggestion is best to help the nurse?

1.   "You should consider a position change."
2.   "Take stress management classes."
3.   "Spend more time with your family."
4.   "Try not to take your work home with you."
Answer: 2. Stress management classes teach nurses how to better manage stress in their lives. After identifying factors that contribute to the nurse's stress, alternatives to leaving the nursing job she enjoys may therefore be found. Not spending enough time with her family and taking her work home with her aren't identified as contributing factors in this scenario.

➡ *NCLEX keys*
Client needs subcategory: Safe and effective care environment
Client needs subcategory: Management of care
Cognitive level: Application

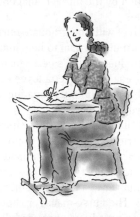

24. A nurse-manager notes that a staff nurse isn't working to full potential. Which strategy by the nurse-manager would best assist the staff nurse?
1.   Assigning the staff nurse several clients with multiple physical problems
2.   Allowing the staff nurse to select her own assignments
3.   Discussing the staff nurse's performance and ways she can improve
4.   Asking the staff nurse to work as an assistant nurse-manager

Answer: 3. The nurse-manager should meet with the staff nurse to discuss her performance and ways she can improve. Assigning the staff nurse several clients with multiple problems would be overwhelming, counterproductive, and unsafe because she has yet to demonstrate the priority-setting and decision-making leadership skills that this client load would require. Letting her select her own assignments could impair the morale of other staff nurses. Having her work as an assistant nurse-manager would be inappropriate until she has demonstrated improved ability and leadership skills.

➡ *NCLEX keys*
Client needs category: Safe and effective care environment
Client needs subcategory: Management of care
Cognitive level: Application

25. Which client should a nurse assess first?
1. A client with a do-not-resuscitate (DNR) order whose blood pressure was 70/34 mm Hg when last measured
2. A client admitted with chest pain 6 hours ago who has had no chest pain since admission to the floor
3. A client just admitted with uncontrolled atrial fibrillation
4. A client who suffered a stroke and requires frequent suctioning

Answer: 3. The nurse should begin by assessing the most acutely ill client; in this case, the newly admitted client with uncontrolled atrial fibrillation. Although the client with a DNR order has low blood pressure, he's most likely terminally ill and doesn't require immediate assessment. The client admitted with chest pain has been without chest pain since admission, so his assessment can be delayed until after the more acute client is assessed. The client who suffered a stroke needs frequent nursing care, but his assessment can be delayed until after the more acute client is assessed.

➡ *NCLEX keys*
Client needs category: Safe and effective care environment
Client needs subcategory: Management of care
Cognitive level: Analysis

26. Which task should a registered nurse (RN) choose to delegate to a nursing assistant? Select all that apply.
1. Assessing a client's pain
2. Taking a client's vital signs
3. Documenting a client's oral intake
4. Performing a blood glucose check
5. Evaluating a client's response to blood pressure medication

Answer: 2, 3, 4. RNs are responsible for all phases of the nursing process, including assessing a client's pain and evaluating a client's response to treatment. An RN may delegate such tasks as taking vital signs, documenting intake and output, and performing blood glucose checks.

➡ *NCLEX keys*
Client needs category: Safe and effective care environment
Client needs subcategory: Management of care
Cognitive level: Analysis

27. A client is being discharged after undergoing abdominal surgery and colostomy formation to treat colon cancer. Which nursing action is most likely to promote continuity of care?
1. Notifying the American Cancer Society of the client's diagnosis
2. Requesting Meals On Wheels to provide adequate nutritional intake
3. Referring the client to a home health nurse for follow-up visits to provide colostomy care
4. Asking an occupational therapist to evaluate the client at home

Answer: 3. Many clients are discharged from acute care settings so quickly that they don't receive complete instructions. Therefore, the first priority is to arrange for colostomy care. The American Cancer Society usually sponsors support groups, which are helpful when the person is ready, but contacting this organization doesn't take precedence over ensuring proper colostomy care. Requesting Meals On Wheels and asking for an occupational therapy evaluation are important but can occur later in rehabilitation.

➡ *NCLEX keys*
Client needs category: Safe and effective care environment
Client needs subcategory: Management of care
Cognitive level: Analysis

28. A client refuses to take his 9 p.m. medication. How should the nurse document this on the medication administration record?
1. Leave the space blank where her initials would typically be written.
2. Circle the time the drug was to be administered.
3. Cross out the time the drug was to be administered.
4. Circle the time the drug was to be administered and record the reason for omission in the progress notes.

Answer: 4. The nurse should circle the time the drug was to be administered and record the reason for omission in the progress notes. Leaving the space blank would be perceived as mistakenly omitting the dose. By crossing out the time the dose was to be administered it may be perceived that the nurse has something to hide and be questioned in a court of law should litigation proceed.

➡ *NCLEX keys*
Client needs category: Safe and effective care environment
Client needs subcategory: Management of care
Cognitive level: Application

29. A nurse-manager notices that a staff nurse isn't providing tracheostomy care to a client according to policy. The nurse's method isn't harmful to the client. How should the nurse-manager proceed?
1. Pull the nurse aside in a private area and tell her that she should review the procedure for tracheostomy care.
2. Do nothing because the nurse's method wasn't harmful to the client.
3. Stop the nurse immediately and tell her she isn't following the facility procedure for tracheostomy care.
4. Wait until the nurse is at the nurses' station with her peers and tell her she should review the procedure

because she wasn't performing tracheostomy care correctly.

Answer: 1. The nurse-manager should pull the nurse aside and tell her that she wasn't performing tracheostomy care according to the established procedure and should review the policy as soon as possible. The nurse-manager shouldn't ignore the nurse's actions because the nurse is performing a procedure that deviates from the accepted policy. Because the nurse is in no way harming the client, the nurse-manager can wait until the nurse finishes and then speak to her in a private location; the nurse-manager shouldn't correct the nurse in front of the client. The nurse-manager shouldn't correct the nurse in front of her peers because this would embarrass the nurse and isn't professional behavior.

➡ *NCLEX keys*
Client needs category: Safe and effective care environment
Client needs subcategory: Management of care
Cognitive level: Analysis

30. Which action can be interpreted as a breach in client confidentiality?
1. A nurse provides the consulting physician with an update of the client's hospital course.
2. An intensive care nurse updates the floor nurse about a client transferred to the intensive care unit 2 days ago.
3. A physician notifies the client's family about the client's diagnosis of epilepsy against the client's wishes.
4. A physician notifies the client's sister because the client has threatened to kill his sister.

Answer: 2. Providing information to a staff nurse who's no longer involved in the client's care can be interpreted as a breach in client confidentiality. Information should be disclosed on a "need to know" basis.

➡ *NCLEX keys*
Client needs category: Safe and effective care environment
Client needs subcategory: Management of care
Cognitive level: Analysis

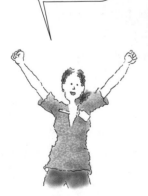

I answered every question correctly! Bring on the exam!

Appendices and index

Physiologic changes in aging

Aging is characterized by the loss of some body cells and reduced metabolism in other cells. These processes cause a decline in body function and changes in body composition. Changes associated with aging occur slowly and gradually, suggesting that, in most cases, they're more obvious with advanced age. For example, skin changes are more obvious in a 95-year-old client than in a 70-year-old client. This chart will help you recognize the gradual changes in body function that normally accompany aging so you can adjust your assessment techniques accordingly.

Area of assessment	Age-related changes
Nutrition	• Protein, vitamin, and mineral requirements usually unchanged • Energy requirements possibly decreased by about 200 calories per day because of diminished activity • Diminished absorption of calcium related to reduced pepsin and hydrochloric acid secretion • Decreased salivary flow and decreased sense of taste (may reduce appetite) • Diminished intestinal motility and peristalsis of the large intestine • Brittle teeth related to thinning of tooth enamel • Decreased biting force • Diminished gag reflex • Limited mobility (may affect frail elder's ability to obtain or prepare food)
Skin	• Facial lines resulting from subcutaneous fat loss, dermal thinning, decreasing collagen and elastin, and up to a 50% decline in cell replacement • Delayed wound healing due to decreased rate of cell replacement • Thinning of skin and decreased skin elasticity (may seem almost transparent) • Brown spots on skin due to localized melanocyte proliferation • Dry mucous membranes and decreased sweat gland output (as the number of active sweat glands declines) • Difficulty regulating body temperature related to decrease in size, number, and function of sweat glands and loss of subcutaneous fat
Hair	• Decreased pigment, causing gray or white hair • Thinning as the number of melanocytes declines • Pubic hair loss resulting from hormonal changes • Facial hair increase in postmenopausal women and decrease in men
Eyes and vision	• Baggy and wrinkled eyelids due to decreased elasticity, with eyes sitting deeper in sockets • Thinner and yellow conjunctivae • Decreased tear production due to loss of fatty tissue in lacrimal apparatus • Corneal flattening and loss of luster • Fading or irregular pigmentation of iris

Area of assessment	Age-related changes
Eyes and vision *(continued)*	• Smaller pupil, requiring three times more light to see clearly; diminished night vision and depth perception • Scleral thickening and rigidity; yellowing due to fat deposits • Vitreous degeneration, revealing opacities and floating debris • Lens enlargement; loss of transparency and elasticity, decreasing accommodation • Impaired color vision due to deterioration of retinal cones • Decreased reabsorption of intraocular fluid, predisposing to glaucoma
Ears and hearing	• Atrophy of the organ of Corti and the auditory nerve (sensory presbycusis) • Inability to distinguish high-pitched consonants • Degenerative structural changes in the entire auditory system
Respiratory system	• Elongated and narrowed nose from continued cartilage growth • Increased anteroposterior chest diameter as a result of altered calcium metabolism and calcification of costal cartilage • Decreased number and size of alveoli • Kyphosis • Respiratory muscle degeneration or atrophy • Declining diffusing capacity • Decreased inspiratory and expiratory muscle strength; diminished vital capacity • Lung tissue degeneration, causing decrease in lungs' elastic recoil capability and increase in residual capacity • Poor ventilation of the basal areas (from closing of some airways), resulting in decreased surface area for gas exchange and reduced partial pressure of oxygen • Oxygen saturation decreased by up to 5% • Drier mucous membranes and decreased ciliary and macrophage activity, heightening risk of pulmonary infection and mucus plugs • Lower tolerance for oxygen debt
Cardiovascular system	• Loss of cardiac contractile strength and efficiency • Progressive decrease in cardiac output with age; up to 35% diminished cardiac output by age 70 • Heart valve thickening, causing incomplete closure (systolic murmur) • Modest increase in left ventricular wall thickness between ages 30 and 80 • Fibrous tissue infiltration of the sinoatrial node and internodal atrial tracts, possibly leading to atrial arrhythmias • Vein dilation and stretching • Gradual decrease in coronary artery blood flow • Increased aortic rigidity, causing increased systolic blood pressure disproportionate to diastolic, resulting in widened pulse pressure

Area of assessment	Age-related changes
Cardiovascular system *(continued)*	• Electrocardiogram changes, such as increased PR interval and shift of QRS axis to the left • Heart rate takes longer to return to normal after exercise • Decreased strength and elasticity of blood vessels, contributing to arterial and venous insufficiency • Decreased ability to respond to physical and emotional stress
GI system	• Atrophy of taste and olfactory receptors • Reduced GI secretions, affecting digestion and absorption • Decreased motility and decreased bowel wall and anal sphincter tone • Liver changes: decreases in weight, regenerative capacity, and blood flow • Decline in hepatic enzymes involved in oxidation and reduction, causing less efficient metabolism of drugs and detoxification of substances
Renal system	• Decline in glomerular filtration rate • Up to 53% decrease in renal blood flow related to reduced cardiac output and atherosclerotic changes • Decrease in size and number of functioning nephrons • Reduction in bladder size, capacity, and muscle tone • Weakening of bladder muscles leading to incomplete emptying • Diminished kidney size • Impaired clearance of drugs • Decreased ability to respond to variations in fluids and electrolytes
Male reproductive system	• Reduced testosterone production, resulting in decreased libido as well as atrophy and softening of testes • Decline in sperm production after age 60 • Prostate gland enlargement, with decreasing secretions • Decreased volume and viscosity of seminal fluid • Slower and weaker physiologic reaction during intercourse, with lengthened refractory period

Female reproductive system	• Declining estrogen and progesterone levels (about age 50) cause:
	  – cessation of ovulation; atrophy, thickening, and decreased size of ovaries
	  – loss of pubic hair and flattening of labia majora
	  – shrinking of vulval tissue, constricted introitus, and loss of tissue elasticity
	  – vaginal atrophy; thin and dry mucous lining; more alkaline pH of vaginal environment
	  – shrinking uterus
	  – cervical atrophy, failure to produce mucus for lubrication, thinner endometrium and myometrium
	  – pendulous breasts; atrophy of glandular, supporting, and fatty tissue
	  – nipple flattening and decreased size
	  – more pronounced inframammary ridges

Area of assessment	Age-related changes
Neurologic system	• Degenerative changes in neurons of central and peripheral nervous system • Decrease in cerebral blood flow • Slower nerve transmission • Gradual decrease in number of brain cells • Hypothalamus less effective at regulating body temperature • Up to 20% neuron loss in cerebral cortex • Slower corneal reflex • Increased pain threshold • Decrease in stage III and IV sleep, causing frequent awakenings; rapid eye movement sleep also decreased
Immune system	• Less vigorous immune system response to stressors • Decline beginning at sexual maturity and continuing with age • Loss of ability to distinguish between self and nonself (autoimmune response) • Loss of ability to recognize and destroy mutant cells, increasing incidence of cancer • Decreased response to antigens • Decreased antibody response, resulting in greater susceptibility to infection • Some active blood-forming marrow replaced by fatty bone marrow, resulting in inability to increase erythrocyte production as readily as before in response to such stimuli as hormones, anoxia, hemorrhage, and hemolysis • Diminished vitamin B_{12} absorption, resulting in reduced erythrocyte mass and decreased hemoglobin level and hematocrit
Musculoskeletal system	• Increased adipose tissue • Diminished lean body mass • Decreased bone mineral density with increased risk of fractures • Decreased height from exaggerated spinal curvature and narrowing intervertebral spaces • Decreased collagen formation and muscle mass; gradual decrease in strength and endurance • Increased viscosity of synovial fluid; more fibrotic synovial membranes
Endocrine system	• Decreased ability to tolerate stress • Blood glucose concentration increases and remains elevated longer than in a younger adult • Diminished levels of estrogen and increasing levels of follicle-stimulating hormone during menopause, causing coronary thrombosis and osteoporosis • Reduced progesterone production • Up to 50% decline in serum aldosterone levels

Selected references

Anatomy & Physiology Made Incredibly Easy, 3rd ed. Philadelphia: Lippincott Williams & Wilkins, 2009.

Assessment Made Incredibly Easy, 4th ed. Philadelphia: Lippincott Williams & Wilkins, 2008.

Baranoski, S., and Ayello, E.A. *Wound Care Essentials: Practice Principles,* 2nd ed. Philadelphia: Lippincott Williams & Wilkins, 2008.

Bickley, L.S., and Szilagyi, P.G. *Bates' Guide to Physical Examination and History Taking,* 10th ed. Philadelphia: Lippincott Williams & Wilkins, 2009.

Bowden, V.R., and Greenberg, C.S. *Pediatric Nursing Procedures,* 2nd ed. Philadelphia: Lippincott Williams & Wilkins, 2008.

Boyd, M.A. *Psychiatric Nursing: Contemporary Practice,* 4th ed. Philadelphia: Lippincott Williams & Wilkins, 2008.

Cardiovascular Care Made Incredibly Easy, 2nd ed. Philadelphia: Lippincott Williams & Wilkins, 2009.

ECG Interpretation Made Incredibly Easy, 5th ed. Philadelphia: Lippincott Williams & Wilkins, 2011.

Fauci, A., et al. *Harrison's Principles of Internal Medicine,* 17th ed. New York: McGraw-Hill, 2009.

Fischbach, F., & Dunning, M.B., eds. *A Manual of Laboratory and Diagnostic Tests,* 8th ed. Philadelphia: Lippincott Williams & Wilkins, 2009.

Hockenberry, M.J., and Wilson, D. *Wong's Nursing Care of Infants and Children,* 8th ed. St. Louis: Mosby–Year Book, Inc., 2007.

Ignatavicius, D.D., and Workman, M.L. *Medical-Surgical Nursing: Patient-Centered Collaborative Care,* 6th ed. Philadelphia: Elsevier, 2010.

Judge, N.L. "Neurovascular Assessment," *Nursing Standard* 21(45):39-44, July 2007.

Karch, A.M. *Focus on Nursing Pharmacology,* 5th ed. Philadelphia: Lippincott Williams & Wilkins, 2010.

Kyle, T. *Essentials of Pediatric Nursing.* Philadelphia: Lippincott Williams & Wilkins, 2008.

Lippincott's Nursing Procedures, 5th ed. Philadelphia: Lippincott Williams & Wilkins, 2008.

Nettina, S.M. *Lippincott Manual of Nursing Practice,* 9th ed. Philadelphia: Lippincott Williams & Wilkins, 2010.

Nursing 2010 Drug Handbook. Philadelphia: Lippincott Williams & Wilkins, 2010.

Pillitteri, A. *Maternal & Child Health Nursing: Care of the Childbearing and Childrearing Family,* 6th ed. Philadelphia: Lippincott Williams & Wilkins, 2010.

Porth, C.M., and Matfin, G. *Pathophysiology: Concepts of Altered Health States,* 8th ed. Philadelphia: Lippincott Williams & Wilkins, 2009.

Professional Guide to Diseases, 9th ed. Philadelphia: Lippincott Williams & Wilkins, 2009.

Smeltzer, S.C., et al. *Brunner & Suddarth's Textbook of Medical-Surgical Nursing,* 12th ed. Philadelphia: Lippincott Williams & Wilkins, 2010.

Taylor, C.R., et al. *Fundamentals of Nursing: The Art and Science of Nursing Care,* 6th ed. Philadelphia: Lippincott Williams & Wilkins, 2008.

Townsend, M.C., and Pedersen, D.D. *Essentials of Psychiatric Mental Health Nursing: Concepts of Care in Evidence-Based Practice.* Philadelphia: F.A. Davis Company, 2008.

Wilson, D., and Hockenberry, M.J. *Wong's Clinical Manual of Pediatric Nursing,* 7th ed. St. Louis: Mosby–Year Book, Inc., 2008.

Index

i refers to an illustration; t refers to a table.

i refers to an illustration; t refers to a table.

i refers to an illustration; t refers to a table.

i refers to an illustration; t refers to a table.

i refers to an illustration; t refers to a table.

i refers to an illustration; t refers to a table.

Notes

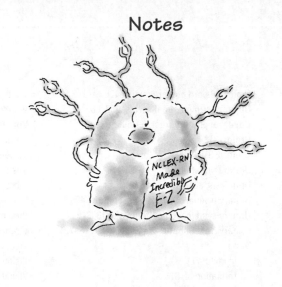

Notes

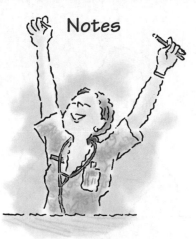

Notes

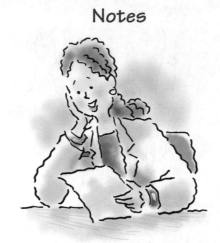

Notes

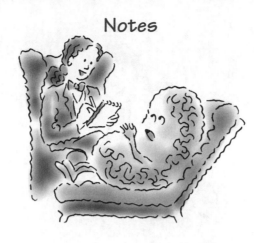

Notes